# Mims'
# Medical Microbiology and Immunology

# Medical Microbiology and Immunology

**Richard V. Goering, BA MSc PhD**
Professor
Department of Medical Microbiology and Immunology
School of Medicine, Creighton University
Omaha, Nebraska, USA

**Hazel M. Dockrell, BA (Mod) PhD**
Professor of Immunology
Faculty of Infectious and Tropical Diseases
London School of Hygiene & Tropical Medicine
London, England, UK

**Mark Zuckerman, MSc FRCPath**
Consultant Virologist and Honorary Reader
South London Specialist Virology Centre
Kings College Hospital NHS Foundation Trust
Department of Infectious Diseases
School of Immunology and Microbial Sciences
King's College London
London, England, UK

**Peter L. Chiodini, OBE BSc MBBS PhD FRCP FRCPath**
Consultant Parasitologist
Hospital for Tropical Diseases, London
Honorary Professor, London School of Hygiene & Tropical Medicine
London, England, UK

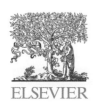

ELSEVIER

EDINBURGH LONDON NEWYORK OXFORD PHILADELPHIA ST LOUIS SYDNEY TORONTO 2025
For additional online content visit Elsevier eBooks+ (eBooks.Health.Elsevier.com)

---

**Notice**

---

ISBN: 978-0-323-93725-2
INTERNATIONAL EDITION: 978-0-443-10747-4

Publisher: Elyse W. O'Grady
Content Development Specialist: Rebecca Gruliow
Project Manager: Gayathri S
Design: Maggie Reid
Illustration Manager: Nijantha Priyadharshini

Printed in India
Last digit is the print number:    9   8   7   6   5   4   3   2   1

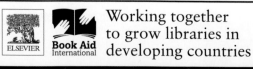

# Foreword to Mims Medical Microbiology, 7th Edition

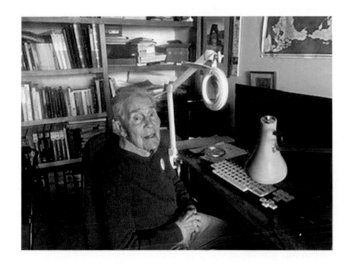

This remains an excellent, well-balanced and useful book. It is more than a mere listing of infectious diseases, and I congratulate the authors.

I'll be a hundred next year and this reminds me that the population as a whole has a bigger proportion of older people now. In this new generation there will be centenarians who will be expecting a heathy old age. If we can find ancient virus sequences in our genome, perhaps we can also help unravel the mysteries of conditions such as Alzheimer disease and macular degeneration.

There will be new infectious diseases and new ideas. I wish you a productive and interesting career.

*Cedric Mims, MD FRCPath*
*Canberra, Australia*
*April 2023*

# Foreword to Mims Medical Microbiology, 6th Edition

When I sat down with immunologist Ivan Roitt to think about writing this book, we agreed that it was to be more than a mere listing of microbial diseases with their diagnosis and treatment. All these infections result from the interplay between microbial cunning in relation to the immunologic and inflammatory defences of the host, and Ivan's contribution meant that the immunology would be relevant and up to date.

During my 60 years as a physician and zoologist in England, America, Africa, and Australia I have been able to study in some detail the mechanism by which microbial parasites enter the body, spread, and cause disease. It was always useful to think of those invaders as parasites, to look at it from their point of view, with the same forces governing the outcome in all cases, whether worms, bacteria, or viruses. It turns out that of all the different living species on earth, nearly half have opted for the parasitic way of life.

While the life of a parasite may sound attractive, with free board and lodging in or on the host, only a few invaders manage to survive those powerful defences. Over millions of years of evolution their ability to avoid or evade the defences has been perfected and should never be underestimated.

Since the first edition of this book we have incorporated several improvements to make learning easier, including case studies, chapter key facts and chapter questions. My hope is that, although what you learn from it will undoubtedly help you with final and board examinations and although over the years many of the details may slip from your memory, you will have retained a useful way of looking at infectious diseases. To put it in military terms, every infection sets in train an armed conflict, with possible disease or death awaiting the loser.

This way of looking at infectious diseases will, I hope, stay with you and prepare you for the astonishing advances and the new treatments that await you during your career — in particular, new diseases from animals or birds, perhaps transmitted by biting insects or bats, as well as possible superstrains of influenza virus from birds that spread effectively in our species and make us ill, and of course new antimicrobial drugs to which resistance is impossible. And we expect an unravelling of the influence on human health of that vast and mysterious collection of resident microbes living in our intestines.

I have always felt a personal as well as a scientific interest in these invaders. They killed both my parents when I was a child long before the development of antibiotics and were responsible for my attacks of measles, mumps, diphtheria, whooping cough, tuberculosis, and, much later, Rift Valley fever in Africa.

*Cedric Mims, MD FRCPath*
*Canberra, Australia*
*October 2016*

# Preface to the seventh edition

*The seventh edition of Mims' Medical Microbiology and Immunology* continues to present the interaction between infectious disease and host response as a give-and-take conflict. Recognition of Cedric Mims's founding contribution and continued interest in this work is seen not only in the title but in his thoughts as expressed in the forewords to both this seventh and the previous edition.

Overall, this edition benefits from significant revision in multiple areas. The introductory chapters continue to present fundamental principles of infectious agents and host defences, including the recognized importance of the human microbiota. Special attention is given to emerging infectious diseases (e.g. SARS-CoV-2, Mpox, *Candida auris*) and the dynamics of persistence and spread in patient populations. Subsequent chapters present major updates in the general principles behind the infectious agent—immune response conflict, followed by a chapter-specific consideration of system-oriented conflict scenarios. Final chapters provide a revised consideration of issues affecting diagnosis and control of the conflict, especially centering on newer molecular (i.e. DNA sequence-based) approaches.

Bibliographic references continue to include current Internet resources. Online access to interactive extras is provided via Elsevier's STUDENT CONSULT website (www.studentconsult.com), including questions and answers, mostly in USMLE format, the Pathogen Parade (infectious agent) index, and the Vaccine Parade index. For the first time ever, a parasitic infection has entered the Vaccine Parade, with the inclusion of a malaria vaccine for use in endemic areas.

In this new edition of *Mims' Medical Microbiology and Immunology* we believe the student will find a logical and unified approach to the subject that is readable, exciting and informative.

*Richard V. Goering, Hazel M. Dockrell,*
*Mark Zuckerman, Peter L. Chiodini*
*2023*

# Contributors and acknowledgments

*Contributors to the 7th edition*

**Alireza Abdolrasouli, PhD FECMM**
Clinical Scientist in Medical Mycology
Department of Infection Sciences
King's College Hospital
London, United Kingdom
*Fungal content*

**Mauricio Arias, MD MSc PhD MRCP FRCPath**
Consultant in Infectious Diseases & Microbiology
Department of Infection Sciences
Kings College Hospital
London, United Kingdom
*Online content*

**Graham Bothamley, PhD MA BM BCh FRCP**
Honorary Professor and Consultant Physician
Homerton University Hospital
Queen Mary University of London
London School of Hygiene & Tropical Medicine
London, United Kingdom
*Contributions to chapters 10, 11, 12, 15, 17, 20*

**Dan Bradshaw, MDres MRCP FRCPath MA BMBCh
DipGUM DFSRH DipHIV**
Consultant Virologist
Virus Reference Department, UK Health Security Agency
Honorary Consultant in Genitourinary Medicine
Imperial College Healthcare NHS Trust
London, United Kingdom
*Online content*

**Carmel Curtis, PhD MRCP FRCPath**
Consultant Microbiologist and Trust
Control Doctor
Clinical Director for Pathology
Department of Infection Sciences
King's College London
London, United Kingdom
*Online content*

**Temi Lampejo, MBBS BSc (Hons) MRCP FRCPath**
Consultant Infectious Diseases Physician and Virologist
King's College Hospital
London, United Kingdom
*Online content*

**Rocío T Martínez Núñez, BSc PhD**
Reader in RNA Biology and Immunity
Department of Infectious Diseases
King's Centre for Lung Health
School of Immunology and Microbial Sciences
Guy's Campus, King's College London
London, United Kingdom
*Online content and Chapter 3*

**Anthony Scott, BM BCh MSc in Epi (LSHTM) DTM&H
FRCP FMedSci**
Professor of Vaccine Epidemiology
Director HPRU in Immunisation
London School of Hygiene & Tropical Medicine
London, United Kingdom
*Chapter 35*

**Ben Zuckerman, MBBS BSc (Hons)**
Specialised Foundation Programme Year 2
Guy's and St Thomas' Hospitals
London, United Kingdom
*Online content and Chapter 26*

*Acknowledgements from prior editions*

**Katharina Kranzer, FRCPath MRCP MBBS MSc PhD**
Professor of Infection Disease Epidemiology
London School of Hygiene & Tropical Medicine
Honorary Consultant in Medical Microbiology
University College London Hospital
London, United Kingdom
*Chapter 33*

**Ivan Roitt, MA DSc (Oxon) FRCPath Hon FRCP (Lond)
FRS**
Emeritus Professor
Centre for Diagnostic and Investigative Oncology
Middlesex University
London, United Kingdom

# A contemporary approach to microbiology

## INTRODUCTION

### Microbes and parasites

**The conventional distinction between microbes and parasites is essentially arbitrary**

Microbiology is sometimes defined as the biology of microscopic organisms, its subject being microbes. Traditionally, clinical microbiology has been concerned with those organisms responsible for the major infectious diseases of humans and whose size makes them invisible to the naked eye. Thus it is not surprising that the organisms included have reflected those causing diseases that have been (or continue to be) of greatest importance in those countries where the scientific and clinical discipline of microbiology developed, notably Europe and the United States. The term *microbes* has usually been applied in a restricted fashion, primarily to viruses and bacteria. Fungi and protozoan parasites have historically been included as more minor contributors, but in general they have been treated as the subjects of other disciplines (mycology and parasitology).

Although there can be no argument that viruses and bacteria are, globally, the most important pathogens, the conventional distinction between these as microbes and the other infectious agents (fungi, protozoa, helminths, arthropod parasites) is essentially arbitrary, not least because the criterion of microscopic visibility cannot be applied rigidly (Fig. Intro.1). Perhaps we should remember that the first microbe to be associated with a specific clinical condition was a parasitic worm—the nematode *Trichinella spiralis*—whose larval stages are just visible to the naked eye (although microscopy is needed for definitive identification). *T. spiralis* was first identified in 1835 and causally related to the disease trichinellosis in the 1860s. Viruses and bacteria comprise just over half of all human pathogen species.

## THE CONTEXT FOR CONTEMPORARY MEDICAL MICROBIOLOGY

Many microbiology texts deal with infectious organisms as agents of disease in isolation, both from other infectious organisms and from the biologic context in which they live and cause disease. It is certainly convenient to consider organisms group by group, to summarize the diseases they cause and to review the forms of available control, but this approach produces a static picture of what is a dynamic relationship between the organism and its host.

The host response is the outcome of the complex interplay between host and parasite. The host response can be discussed in terms of pathologic signs and symptoms and in terms of immune control, but it is better treated as the outcome of the complex interplay between two organisms—host and parasite; without this dimension, a distorted view of infectious disease results. It simply is not true that microbe + host = disease, and clinicians are well aware of this. Understanding why it is that most host–microbe contacts do not result in disease and what changes so that disease does arise is as important as the identification of infectious organisms and a knowledge of the ways in which they can be controlled.

We, therefore, continue to believe that our approach to microbiology, both in terms of the organisms that might usefully be considered within a textbook and in terms of the contexts in which they and the diseases they cause are discussed, provides a more informative and more interesting picture of these dynamic interrelationships. There are many reasons for having reached this conclusion, the most important being the following:

- A comprehensive understanding exists at the molecular level of the biology of infectious agents and of the host–parasite interactions that lead to infection and disease. It is important for students to be aware of this understanding so that they can grasp the connections between infection and disease within both individuals and communities and to use this knowledge in novel and changing clinical situations.
- Clearly the host's response to infection is a coordinated and subtle interplay involving the mechanisms of both innate and acquired resistance, and these mechanisms are expressed regardless of the nature and identity of the pathogen involved. Our present understanding of the ways in which these mechanisms are stimulated and the ways in which they act is very sophisticated. We can see that infection is a conflict between two organisms, with the outcome (resistance or disease) being critically dependent upon molecular interactions. Again, it is essential to understand the basis of this host–pathogen interplay if the processes of disease and disease control are to be interpreted correctly.

**Emerging or reemerging diseases continue to pose new microbiologic problems**

Four other factors have helped to mould our opinion that a broader view of microbiology is needed to provide a firm basis for clinical and scientific practice:

- There is an increasing prevalence of a wide variety of opportunistic infections in patients who are hospitalized or immunosuppressed. Immunosuppressive therapies are now common, as are diseases in which the immune system is compromised—notably, acquired immunodeficiency syndrome (AIDS).
- Newly emerging disease agents continue to be identified, and old diseases previously thought to be under control

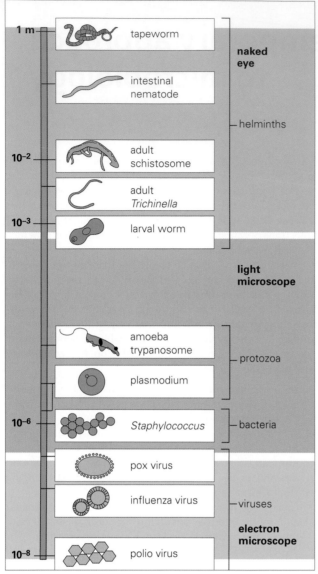

**Fig. Intro.1** Relative sizes of the organisms covered in this book.

good working knowledge of parasitology wherever they are based.

Thus a broader view of microbiology is necessary: one that builds on the approaches of the past but addresses the problems of the present and of the future.

## MICROBIOLOGY PAST, PRESENT AND FUTURE

The demonstration in the 19th century that diseases were caused by infectious agents founded the discipline of microbiology. Although these early discoveries involved tropical parasitic infections and the bacterial infections common in Europe and the United States, microbiologists increasingly focused on the latter, later extending their interests to the newly discovered viral infections. The development of antimicrobial agents and vaccines revolutionized treatment of these diseases and raised hopes for the eventual elimination of many of the diseases that had plagued the human race for centuries. Those in the resource-rich world learned not to fear infectious disease and believed such infections would disappear in their lifetime. To an extent, this was realized; through vaccination, many familiar childhood diseases became uncommon, and those of bacterial origin were more easily controlled by antibiotics. Encouraged by the eradication of smallpox during the 1970s and the success of polio vaccines, the United Nations in 1978 announced programmes to obtain "health for all" by 2000; however, this and other optimistic targets have required reevaluation.

### Infectious diseases are killers in both resource-rich and resource-poor countries

The World Health Organization (WHO) has listed infectious diseases (especially respiratory infections) as second only to heart disease as a global cause of death, although these data were prior to SARS-CoV-2; however, the causes of death vary by region and demographic group. In low- and middle-income countries, infectious diseases are more prevalent than cardiovascular disease, while the reverse is true in high-income countries. The WHO has now listed 12 antibiotic-resistant bacterial pathogens as priorities for the development of new antibiotics, 75% of which are categorized as critical or of high importance; however, infectious diseases frequency and mortality are not evenly distributed worldwide (Fig. Intro.2).

The burden of infectious disease in the resource-poor world is especially concerning. Although sub-Saharan Africa has only ~10% of the world's population, it has the clear majority of human immunodeficiency virus (HIV) infections and AIDS-related deaths and the highest HIV-tuberculosis (TB) coinfection rates. The WHO Africa Region has 95% of the world's malaria cases. TB, HIV/AIDS and dengue are of increasing importance in Southeast Asia and the Pacific, where drug-resistant malaria is also common. Children younger than 5 years are most at risk from infectious diseases. It is obvious that the prevalence and importance of infectious diseases in the resource-poor world are directly linked to poverty.

### Infections continue to emerge or reemerge

On a worldwide basis, infectious diseases continue to emerge in the human population for the first time. Examples include the Middle East respiratory syndrome (MERS) coronavirus,

reemerge as causes of concern. Considering only bacteria, for example, >1500 species are identified as human pathogens.

- The frequency of the major groups of human pathogens can vary depending on several factors, including geographic location, population density and seasonal influence; however, bacterial and viral pathogens are the most common with fungal, protozoa and helminth groups less common but still extremely important.
- Tropical infections now have much greater impact. At least 80 million people travel from resource-rich to resource-poor countries each year, so clinicians in resource-rich settings now see many migrants and tourists who have been exposed to the quite different spectrum of infectious agents found in tropical countries where parasitic infections are much more prevalent. Practicing microbiologists may be called upon to identify and advise on such organisms and therefore require a

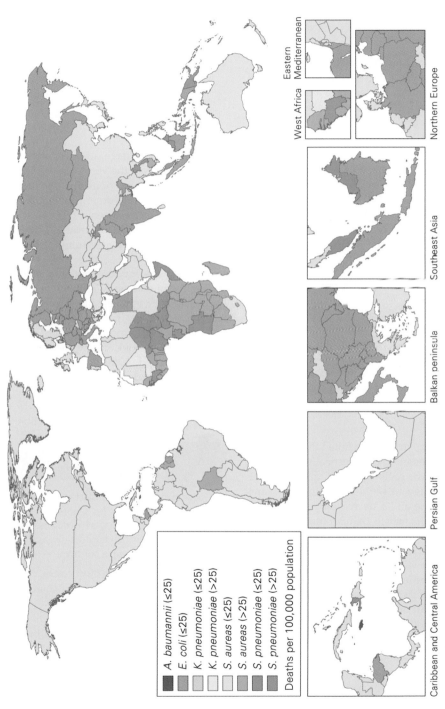

**Fig. Intro.2** Global distribution of age-distributed mortality rates. (Reprinted with permission from Elsevier. GBD 2019 Antimicrobial Resistance Collaborators. Global mortality associated with 33 bacterial pathogens in 2019: a systematic analysis for the Global Burden of Disease Study 2019. *The Lancet.* 2022:400(10369):2221–2248.)

Legend:
- A. baumannii (≤25)
- E. coli (≤25)
- K. pneumoniae (≤25)
- K. pneumoniae (>25)
- S. aureas (≤25)
- S. aureas (>25)
- S. pneumoniae (≤25)
- S. pneumoniae (>25)

Deaths per 100,000 population

Eastern Mediterranean
West Africa
Northern Europe
Southeast Asia
Balkan peninsula
Persian Gulf
Caribbean and Central America

the H7N9 avian influenza virus, Zika virus and, most recently, severe acute respiratory syndrome coronavirus 2 (SARS-CoV-2). Concern regarding the lack of effective antibiotics for treating bacterial infections (see earlier) further underscore the negative global impact of infectious diseases.

### Modern lifestyles and technical developments facilitate transmission of disease

The reasons for the resurgence of infectious diseases are multiple. They include:

- new patterns of travel and trade (especially food commodities), new agricultural practices, altered sexual behaviour, medical interventions and overuse of antibiotics
- the movement of multidrug-resistant bacteria, such as methicillin-resistant *Staphylococcus aureus* and virulent pathogens such as *Clostridioides difficile* from the health care setting into the community (The issue of antimicrobial resistance is compounded in resource-poor countries by inability or unwillingness to complete programmes of treatment and by the use of counterfeit drugs with, at best, partial action. The WHO has now catalogued the existence of >900 counterfeit medical products representing the full spectrum of medical therapies.)
- breakdown of economic, social and political systems especially in the resource-poor world, which has weakened medical services and increased the effects of poverty and malnutrition
- dramatic increase in air travel over the last few decades, which has facilitated the spread of infection and increased the threat of new pandemics. (The Spanish influenza pandemic in 1918 spread along railway and sea links. Modern air travel moves larger numbers of people more rapidly and more extensively and makes it possible for microbes to cross geographic barriers.)

### What of the future?

Predictions based on data from the United Nations and WHO give a choice of scenarios. Optimistically, the aging population, coupled with socioeconomic and medical advances, could be expected to see a fall in the problems posed by infectious disease and a decrease in deaths from these causes. The pessimistic view is that population growth in resource-poor countries (especially in urban populations), the increasing gap between rich and poor countries and continuing changes in lifestyle will result in surges of infectious disease. Even in resource-rich countries, increasing drug resistance and a slowing of developments in new antimicrobials and vaccines will create additional problems in control. Added to these are three additional factors:

- emergence of new human infections, such as a novel strain of influenza virus or a new infection of wildlife origin
- climate change, with increased temperatures and altered rainfall adding to the incidence of vectorborne infection

- threat of bioterrorism, with the possible deliberate spread of viral and bacterial infections to human populations with no acquired immunity or no history of vaccination.

One thing is certain: Whether optimistic or pessimistic scenarios prove true, microbiology will remain a critical medical discipline for the foreseeable future.

## THE APPROACH ADOPTED IN THIS BOOK

The factors outlined in this chapter indicate the need for a text with a dual function:

1. It should provide an inclusive treatment of the organisms responsible for infectious disease.
2. The purely clinical/laboratory approach to microbiology should be replaced with an approach that will stress the biologic context in which clinical/laboratory studies are to be undertaken.

The approach we have adopted in this book is to look at microbiology from the viewpoint of the conflicts inherent in all host–pathogen relationships. We first describe the adversaries: the infectious organisms on the one hand and the innate and adaptive defence mechanisms of the host on the other. The outcome of the conflicts between the two is then amplified and discussed system by system. Rather than taking each organism or each disease manifestation in turn, we look at the major environments available for infectious organisms in the human body such as the respiratory system, the gut, the urinary tract, the blood and the central nervous system. The organisms that invade and establish in each of these are examined in terms of the pathologic responses they provoke. Finally, we look at how the conflicts we have described can be controlled or eliminated at both the level of the individual patient and the level of the community. We hope that such an approach will provide readers with a dynamic view of host–pathogen interactions and allow them to develop a more creative understanding of infection and disease.

### KEY FACTS

- Our approach is to provide a comprehensive account of the organisms that cause infectious disease in humans, from the viruses to the helminths, and to cover the biologic bases of infection, disease, host–pathogen interactions, disease control and epidemiology.

- The diseases caused by microbial pathogens will be placed in the context of the conflict that exists between them and the innate and adaptive defences of their hosts.

- Infections will be described and discussed in terms of the major body systems, treating these as environments in which microbes can establish themselves, flourish and give rise to pathologic changes.

# Contents

*Foreword to the seventh edition by Cedric Mims*   v
*Foreword to the sixth edition by Cedric Mims*   vi
*Preface to the seventh edition*   vii
*Contributors and acknowledgments*   viii
*A contemporary approach to microbiology*   ix
  *Introduction*   ix
  *The context for contemporary medical*
    *microbiology*   ix
  *Microbiology past, present and future*   x
  *The approach adopted in this book*   xii

## SECTION 1 | THE ADVERSARIES – PATHOGENS

**1. Pathogens as parasites**   **2**
  The varieties of pathogens   2
  Living inside or outside cells   3
  Systems of classification   4

**2. The bacteria**   **6**
  Structure   6
  Nutrition   8
  Growth and division   9
  Gene expression   11
  Survival under adverse conditions   14
  Mobile genetic elements   15
  Mutation and gene transfer   20
  The genomics of medically important
    bacteria   23

**3. The viruses**   **27**
  Major groups of viruses   27
  Infection of host cells   28
  Replication   29
  Outcome of viral infection   32

**4. The fungi**   **35**
  Major groups of disease-causing fungi   35

**5. The protozoa**   **40**

**6. The helminths**   **43**
  Life cycles   44
  Helminths and disease   44

**7. The arthropods**   **47**

**8. Prions**   **50**
  A spectrum of neurodegenerative   50
  'Rogue protein' pathogenesis   51
  Development, transmission and diagnosis
    of prion diseases   52
  Prevention and treatment of prion diseases   54

**9. The host–parasite relationship**   **56**
  The microbiota and microbiome   56
  Symbiotic associations   59
  The characteristics of parasitism   60
  The evolution of parasitism   61

## SECTION 2 | THE ADVERSARIES – HOST DEFENCES

**10. The innate defences of the body**   **68**
  Defences against entry into the body   69
  Defences once the microorganism penetrates
    the body   70

**11. Adaptive immune responses bring
    specificity**   **85**
  Lymphoid tissues: primary and
    secondary   85
  Secondary lymphoid organs   88
  Subsets of T cells   88
  Antibody structure and function   91
  Recirculation of T and B cells   92

**12. Cooperation leads to effective immune
    responses**   **97**
  Cooperation means greater efficiency   97
  Opsonization by antibody   97
  Beneficial inflammatory reactions can also be
    enhanced by antibodies   97
  Activation of T cells   98
  B-cell activation   101
  Clonal expansion   102
  Antibody production   102
  Cytokines play an important part in these
    cell–cell interactions   103
  Immunologic memory   103
  Armies must be kept under control   105

## SECTION 3 | THE CONFLICTS

**13. Background to the infectious diseases**   **110**
  Host–parasite relationships   110
  Causes of infectious diseases   114
  The biologic response gradient   116

**14. Entry, exit and transmission**   **117**
  Sites of entry   117
  Exit and transmission   124
  Types of transmission between humans   125
  Transmission from animals   130

**15. Immune defences in action**   **136**
  Complement   137
  Acute phase proteins and pattern
    recognition receptors   137
  Fever   138
  Natural killer cells   138
  Phagocytosis   139
  Cytokines   141
  Antibody-mediated immunity   143
  Cell-mediated immunity   146
  Recovery from infection   149

Contents

16. **Spread and replication** — **152**
Features of surface and systemic infections — 153
Mechanisms of spread through the body — 154
Genetic determinants of spread and replication — 156
Other factors affecting spread and replication — 158

17. **Parasite survival strategies and persistent infections** — **160**
Parasite survival strategies — 161
Concealment of antigens — 162
Antigenic variation — 167
Immunosuppression — 168
Persistent infections — 171

18. **Pathologic consequences of infection** — **176**
Pathology caused directly by microorganisms — 176
Diarrhoea — 180
Pathologic activation of natural immune mechanisms — 180
Pathologic consequences of the immune response — 184
Skin rashes — 188
Viruses and cancer — 189

**SECTION 4 CLINICAL MANIFESTATION AND DIAGNOSIS OF INFECTIONS BY BODY SYSTEM**

19. **Upper respiratory tract infections** — **198**
Rhinitis — 198
Pharyngitis and tonsillitis — 201
Parotitis — 209
Otitis and sinusitis — 210
Acute epiglottitis — 211
Oral cavity infections — 211

20. **Lower respiratory tract infections** — **214**
Laryngitis and tracheitis — 214
Diphtheria — 214
Whooping cough — 216
Acute bronchitis — 217
Acute exacerbations of chronic bronchitis — 217
Bronchiolitis — 218
Respiratory syncytial virus (RSV) infection — 218
Hantavirus pulmonary syndrome (HPS) — 219
Pneumonia — 219
Bacterial pneumonia — 223
Viral pneumonia — 226
Human coronavirus infections — 228
Parainfluenza virus infection — 240
Adenovirus infection — 241
Human metapneumovirus infection — 241
Human bocavirus infection — 241
Influenza virus infection — 241
Measles virus infection — 249
Cytomegalovirus infection — 250
Tuberculosis — 250
Cystic fibrosis — 254
Lung abscess — 254
Fungal infections — 255
Parasitic infections — 256

21. **Urinary tract infections** — **259**
Acquisition and aetiology — 259
Pathogenesis — 260
Clinical features and complications — 261
Laboratory diagnosis — 262
Treatment — 263
Prevention — 264

22. **Sexually transmitted infections** — **266**
STIs and sexual behaviour — 266
Syphilis — 266
Gonorrhoea — 270
Chlamydial infection — 272
Other causes of inguinal lymphadenopathy — 274
Mycoplasmas and nongonococcal urethritis — 275
Other causes of vaginitis and urethritis — 275
Genital herpes — 276
Human papillomavirus infection — 277
Monkeypox, previously a rare viral zoonosis, emerged in 2022 as an STI — 278
Human immunodeficiency virus — 279
Opportunist STIs — 290
Arthropod infestations — 290

23. **Gastrointestinal tract infections** — **291**
Diarrhoeal diseases caused by bacterial or viral infection — 292
Food poisoning: bacterial toxin–associated diarrhoea — 304
Viral causes of diarrhoea — 308
*Helicobacter pylori* and gastric ulcer disease — 312
Parasites and the gastrointestinal tract — 313
Microsporidia — 317
Other intestinal protozoa — 317
Systemic infection initiated in the gastrointestinal tract — 321

24. **Obstetric and perinatal infections** — **337**
Infections occurring in pregnancy — 337
Congenital infections — 338
Infections occurring around the time of birth — 343

25. **Central nervous system infections** — **347**
Invasion of the central nervous system — 347
The body's response to invasion — 348
Meningitis — 349
Encephalitis — 355
Neurologic diseases of possible viral aetiology — 362
Spongiform encephalopathies caused by scrapie-type agents — 362
CNS disease caused by parasites — 362
Brain abscesses — 364
Tetanus and botulism — 364

26. **Infections of the eye** — **367**
Conjunctivitis — 367
Infection of the deeper layers of the eye — 370

27. **Infections of the skin, soft tissue, muscle and associated systems** — **374**
Bacterial infections of skin, soft tissue and muscle — 376
Mycobacterial diseases of the skin — 381
Fungal infections of the skin — 384

Parasitic infections of the skin 389
Mucocutaneous manifestations of viral
  infections 390
Measles virus infection 399
Rubella virus infection 401
Other maculopapular rashes associated
  with viral infections 401
Other infections producing skin lesions 401
Kawasaki disease 401
Viral infections of muscle 402
Postviral fatigue syndrome 402
Parasitic infections of muscle 403
Joint and bone infections 404
Infections of the haemopoietic system 406

**28. Vector-borne infections** **408**
Arbovirus infections 408
Infections caused by rickettsiae 414
Borrelia infections 416
Protozoal infections 418
Helminth infections 425

**29. Multisystem zoonoses** **429**
Viral haemorrhagic fever 429
Arenavirus infections 429
Ebola and Marburg haemorrhagic fevers 432
Q fever 435
Anthrax 435
Plague 436
Yersinia enterocolitica infection 437
Tularaemia 437
Pasteurella multocida infection 438
Leptospirosis 438
Rat-bite fever 439
Brucellosis 440
Helminth infections 441

**30. Fever of unknown origin** **444**
Definitions of fever of unknown origin 444
Causes of FUO 444
Investigation of classic FUO 445
Treatment of FUO 447
FUO in specific patient groups 447
Infective endocarditis 448

**31. Infections in the compromised host** **452**
The compromised host 452
Infections of the host with deficient innate
  immunity due to physical factors 456
Infections associated with secondary
  adaptive immunodeficiency 458
Other important opportunist pathogens 459

**SECTION 5 DIAGNOSIS AND CONTROL**

**32. Diagnosis of infection and assessment
  of host defence mechanisms** **468**
Aims of the clinical microbiology laboratory 468
Specimen processing 469
Cultivation (culture) of microorganisms 470
Identification of microorganisms grown
  in culture 470
Noncultural techniques for the laboratory
  diagnosis of infection 473

Antibody detection methods for the
  diagnosis of infection 481
Assessment of host defence systems 482
Putting it all together: detection, diagnosis
  and epidemiology 484

**33. Epidemiology and control of infectious
  diseases** **485**
What Is Epidemiology? 485
Outcome measurements 485
Types of epidemiologic studies 486
Transmission of infectious disease 490
Vaccine efficacy 493

**34. Attacking the enemy: antimicrobial agents
  and chemotherapy** **495**
Selective toxicity 495
Discovery and design of antimicrobial
  agents 495
Classification of antibacterial agents 497
Resistance to antibacterial agents 497
Classes of antibacterial agents 499
Inhibitors of cell wall synthesis 499
Inhibitors of protein synthesis 506
Inhibitors of nucleic acid synthesis 512
Antimetabolites affecting nucleic acid
  synthesis 514
Other agents that affect DNA 516
Inhibitors of cytoplasmic membrane
  function 516
Urinary tract antiseptics 517
Antituberculosis agents 517
Antibacterial agents in practice 518
Antibiotic assays 520
Antiviral therapy 520
Antifungal agents 532
Antiparasitic agents 534
Control by chemotherapy versus
  vaccination 534
Control versus eradication 538
Use and misuse of antimicrobial
  agents 538

**35. Protecting the host: vaccination** **540**
Vaccination: a 400-year history 540
Aims of vaccination 540
Vaccines can be of different types 541
Vaccines safety 544
Nonspecific beneficial effects of vaccines 546
Vaccines in current use 546
New vaccines in development 554

**36. Specific and nonspecific
  immunotherapy** **559**
Adoptive immunotherapy with T cells 559
Passive immunotherapy with antibodies 560
Nonspecific cellular modulation 563
Correction of host immunodeficiency 564

**37. Infection control** **567**
Common hospital infections 567
Important causes of hospital infection 567
Sources and routes of spread of hospital
  infection 569

Host factors and hospital infection 570
Consequences of hospital infection 571
Prevention of hospital infection 572
Investigating HAI 575
Sterilization and disinfection 579

Index 585

Online only—Pathogen parade
Online only—Vaccine parade
Online only—Multiple choice self-assessment
    questions
Online only—Case studies
Online only—Bibliography—list of useful websites

# SECTION 1

# The Adversaries – Pathogens

| | | |
|---|---|---|
| **1.** | Pathogens as parasites | 2 |
| **2.** | The bacteria | 6 |
| **3.** | The viruses | 27 |
| **4.** | The fungi | 35 |
| **5.** | The protozoa | 40 |
| **6.** | The helminths | 43 |
| **7.** | The arthropods | 47 |
| **8.** | Prions | 50 |
| **9.** | The host–parasite relationship | 56 |

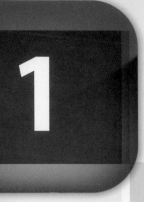

# Pathogens as parasites

## Introduction

The interaction between pathogen and host can be viewed as a parasitic relationship. The pathogenic process involves the establishment, persistence and reproduction of the infecting agent at the expense of the host. How this is accomplished depends on multiple factors, including microbial anatomy, size (macro- vs microparasites) and whether the organisms live inside or outside of host cells. Understanding these issues in the context of a classification system that provides a view of microbe interrelationships provides an important foundation for the study of pathogen–host interaction.

## THE VARIETIES OF PATHOGENS

### Prokaryotes and eukaryotes

A number of important and distinctive biologic characteristics must be taken into account when considering any microorganism in relation to infectious disease. In general, these can be considered in terms of comparative microbial anatomy—the way in which organisms are constructed—and particularly the way in which genetic material and other cellular components are organized.

### All organisms other than viruses and prions are made up of cells

Although viruses have genetic material (DNA or RNA), they are not cellular, and they lack cell membranes, cytoplasm and the machinery for synthesizing macromolecules, depending instead on host cells for this process. Conventional viruses have their genetic material packed inside a protective protein structure termed a *capsid*. The agents (prions), which cause neurodegenerative disorders such as Creutzfeldt-Jakob disease (CJD), variant CJD and kuru in humans and scrapie and bovine spongiform encephalopathy (BSE) in animals lack nucleic acid and consist only of infectious proteinaceous particles.

All other organisms have a cellular organization, being made up of single cells (most microbes) or of many cells. Each cell has genetic material (DNA) and cytoplasm with synthetic machinery and is bounded by a cell membrane.

### Bacteria are prokaryotes; all other organisms are eukaryotes

There are many differences between the two major divisions—prokaryotes and eukaryotes—of cellular organisms (Fig. 1.1). These include the following:

In prokaryotes:

- a distinct nucleus is absent
- DNA is in the form of a single circular chromosome; additional extrachromosomal DNA is carried in plasmids
- transcription and translation can be carried out simultaneously.

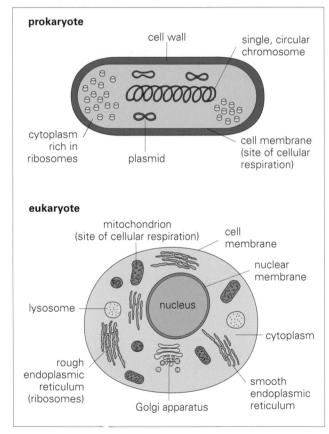

**Fig. 1.1** Prokaryote and eukaryote cells. The major features of cellular organization are shown diagrammatically.

In eukaryotes:

- DNA is carried on several chromosomes within a nucleus.
- the nucleus is bounded by a nuclear membrane
- transcription and translation are carried out separately with transcribed messenger RNA (mRNA) moving out of the nucleus into the cytoplasm for ribosomal translation

- the cytoplasm is rich in membrane-bound organelles (mitochondria, endoplasmic reticulum, Golgi apparatus, lysosomes), which are absent in prokaryotes.

### Gram-negative bacteria have an outer lipopolysaccharide-rich layer

Another important difference between prokaryotes and the majority of eukaryotes is that the cell membrane (plasma membrane) of prokaryotes is covered by a thick protective cell wall. In gram-positive bacteria this wall, made of peptidoglycan, forms the external surface of the cell, whereas in gram-negative bacteria there is an additional outer layer rich in lipopolysaccharides (see Ch. 2). These layers play an important role in protecting the cell against the host immune system and chemotherapeutic agents and in stimulating certain pathologic responses. They also confer antigenicity.

## Microparasites and macroparasites

### Microparasites replicate within the host

There is an important distinction between microparasites and macroparasites that overrides their differences in size. Microparasites (viruses, bacteria, protozoa, fungi) replicate within the host and can, theoretically, multiply to produce a very large number of progeny, thereby causing an overwhelming infection. In contrast, macroparasites (worms, arthropods), even those that are microscopic, do not have this ability: One infectious stage matures into one reproducing stage, and in most cases the resulting progeny leave the host to continue the cycle. The level of infection is, therefore, determined by the number of organisms that enter the body. This distinction between microparasites and macroparasites has important clinical and epidemiologic implications.

The boundary between microparasites and macroparasites is not always clear. The progeny of some macroparasites do remain within the host, and infections can lead to the buildup of overwhelming numbers, particularly in immune-suppressed patients. The roundworms *Trichinella*, *Strongyloides stercoralis* and some filarial nematodes and *Sarcoptes scabiei* (the itch mite) are examples of this type of parasite.

### Organisms that are small enough can live inside cells

Absolute size has other biologically significant implications for the host–pathogen relationship, which cut across the divisions between micro- and macroparasites. Perhaps the most important of these is the relative size of a pathogen and its host's cells. Organisms that are small enough can live inside cells and, by doing so, establish a biologic relationship with the host that is quite different from that of an extracellular organism—one that influences both disease and control.

## LIVING INSIDE OR OUTSIDE CELLS

The basis of all host–pathogen relationships is the exploitation by one organism (the pathogen) of the environment provided by another (the host). The nature and degree of exploitation vary from relationship to relationship, but the pathogen's primary requirement is a supply of metabolic materials from the host, whether provided in the form of nutrients or (as in the case of viruses) in the form of nuclear synthetic machinery. The reliance of viruses upon host synthetic machinery requires an obligatory intracellular habit: Viruses must live within host cells. Some other groups of pathogens (e.g. *Chlamydia*, *Rickettsia*) also live only within cells. In the remaining groups of pathogens, different species have adopted either the intracellular or the extracellular habit or, in a few cases, both. Intracellular microparasites other than viruses take their metabolic requirements directly from the pool of nutrients available in the cell itself, whereas extracellular organisms take theirs from the nutrients present in tissue fluids or, occasionally, by feeding directly on host cells (e.g. *Entamoeba histolytica*, the organism associated with amoebic dysentery). Macroparasites are almost always extracellular (although *Trichinella* is intracellular), and many feed by ingesting and digesting host cells; others can take up nutrients directly from tissue fluids or intestinal contents.

### Pathogens within cells are protected from many of the host's defence mechanisms

As will be discussed in greater detail in Chapter 15, the intracellular pathogens pose problems for the host that are quite different from those posed by extracellular organisms. Pathogens that live within cells are largely protected against many of the host's defence mechanisms while they remain there, particularly against the action of specific antibodies. Control of these infections depends, therefore, on the activities of intracellular killing mechanisms, short-range mediators or cytotoxic agents, although the latter may destroy both the pathogen and the host cell, leading to tissue damage. This problem of targeting activity against the pathogen when it lives within a vulnerable cell also arises when using drugs or antibiotics, as it is difficult to achieve selective action against the pathogen while leaving the host cell intact. Even more problematic is the fact that many intracellular pathogens live inside the very cells responsible for the host's immune and inflammatory mechanisms and, therefore, depress the host's defensive abilities. For example, a variety of viral, bacterial and protozoal pathogens live inside macrophages, and several viruses (including human immunodeficiency virus [HIV]) are specific for lymphocytes.

Intracellular life has many advantages for the pathogen. It provides access to the host's nutrient supply and its genetic machinery and allows escape from host surveillance and antimicrobial defences. However, no organism can be wholly intracellular at all times: If it is to replicate successfully, transmission must occur between the host's cells, and this inevitably involves some exposure to the extracellular environment. As far as the host is concerned, this extracellular phase in the development of the pathogen provides an opportunity to control infection through defence mechanisms such as phagocytosis, antibody and complement. However, transmission between cells can involve destruction of the initially infected cell and so contribute to tissue damage and general host pathology.

### Living outside cells provides opportunities for growth, reproduction and dissemination

Extracellular pathogens can grow and reproduce freely and may move extensively within the tissues of the body. However, they also face constraints on their survival and development. The most important is continuous exposure to components of the host's defence mechanisms, particularly antibody, complement and phagocytic cells.

The characteristics of extracellular organisms lead to pathologic consequences that are quite different from those associated with intracellular species. These are seen most dramatically with the macroparasites, whose sheer physical size, reproductive capacity and mobility can result in extensive destruction of host tissues. Many extracellular pathogens have the ability to spread rapidly through extracellular fluids or to move rapidly over surfaces, resulting in a widespread infection within a relatively short time. The rapid colonization of the entire mucosal surface of the small bowel by *Vibrio cholerae* is a good example. Successful host defence against extracellular parasites requires mechanisms that differ from those used in defence against intracellular parasites. The variety of locations and tissues occupied by extracellular parasites also poses problems for the host in ensuring effective deployment of defence mechanisms. Defence against intestinal parasites requires components of the innate and adaptive immune systems that are quite distinct from those effective against parasites in other sites, and those living in the lumen may be unaffected by responses operating in the mucosa. These problems in mounting effective defence are most acute where large macroparasites are concerned because their size often renders them insusceptible to defence mechanisms that can be used against smaller organisms. For example, worms cannot be phagocytosed; they often have protective external layers, and they can actively move away from areas where the host response is activated.

## SYSTEMS OF CLASSIFICATION

Infectious diseases are caused by organisms belonging to a wide range of different groups: prions, viruses, bacteria, fungi, protozoa, helminths (worms) and arthropods. Each has its own system of classification, making it possible to identify and categorize the organisms concerned. Correct identification is an essential requirement for accurate diagnosis and effective treatment. Identification is achieved by a variety of means, from simple observation to molecular analysis, and classification has been revolutionized by the application of genome sequencing. Many of the major pathogens in all categories have now been sequenced, which has allowed not only more precise identification but also a greater understanding of the interrelationships of members within each taxonomic group.

The approaches used vary between the major groups. For the protozoa, fungi, worms and arthropods, the basic unit of classification is the species, essentially defined as a group of organisms capable of reproducing sexually with one another. Species provide the basis for the binomial system of classification, used for eukaryote and some prokaryote organisms. Species are in turn grouped into a genus (closely related but not interbreeding species). Each organism is identified by two names that indicate the genus and the species, respectively (e.g. *Homo sapiens* and *Escherichia coli*). Related genera are grouped into progressively broader and more inclusive categories.

### Classification of bacteria and viruses

The concept of species is a basic difficulty in classifying prokaryotes and viruses, although the categories of genus and species are routinely used for bacteria. Classification of bacteria has historically used a mixture of easily determined microscopic, macroscopic and biochemical characteristics based on size, shape, colour, staining properties, respiration and reproduction, now also informed by more sophisticated analysis of immunologic and molecular criteria. The former characteristics can be used to divide the organisms into conventional taxonomic groupings, as shown for the gram-positive bacteria in Fig. 1.2 (see also Ch. 2).

### Correct identification of bacteria below the species level is often vital to differentiate pathogenic and nonpathogenic forms

Correct treatment requires correct identification. For some bacteria, important subspecies groups are identified on the basis of their immunologic properties. Cell wall, flagellar and capsule antigens are used in tests with specific antisera to define serogroups and serotypes (e.g. in salmonellae, streptococci, shigellae, *E. coli*). Biochemical characteristics can be used to define other subspecies groupings (biotypes, strains, groups). For example, *Staphylococcus aureus* strains typically release a beta-haemolysin (causing red blood cells

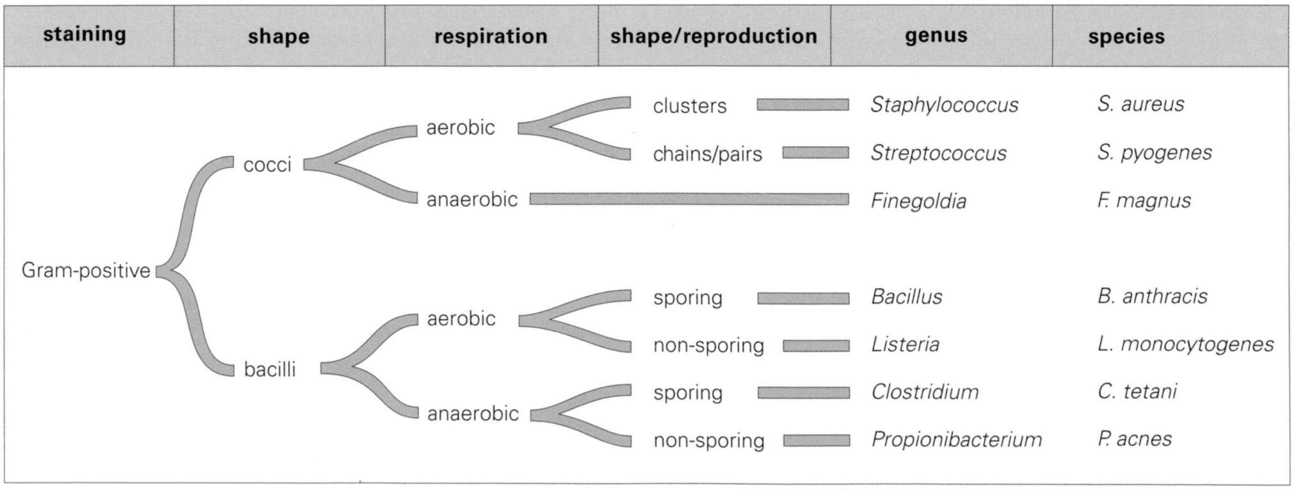

| staining | shape | respiration | shape/reproduction | genus | species |
|---|---|---|---|---|---|
| Gram-positive | cocci | aerobic | clusters | *Staphylococcus* | *S. aureus* |
| | | aerobic | chains/pairs | *Streptococcus* | *S. pyogenes* |
| | | anaerobic | | *Finegoldia* | *F. magnus* |
| | bacilli | aerobic | sporing | *Bacillus* | *B. anthracis* |
| | | aerobic | non-sporing | *Listeria* | *L. monocytogenes* |
| | | anaerobic | sporing | *Clostridium* | *C. tetani* |
| | | anaerobic | non-sporing | *Propionibacterium* | *P. acnes* |

**Fig. 1.2** How the structural and biologic characteristics of bacteria can be used in classification, taking gram-positive bacteria as an example.

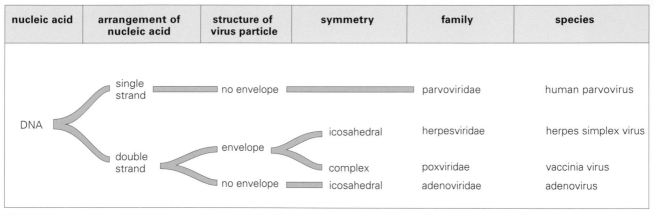

| nucleic acid | arrangement of nucleic acid | structure of virus particle | symmetry | family | species |
|---|---|---|---|---|---|
| DNA | single strand | no envelope | | parvoviridae | human parvovirus |
| | double strand | envelope | icosahedral | herpesviridae | herpes simplex virus |
| | | | complex | poxviridae | vaccinia virus |
| | | no envelope | icosahedral | adenoviridae | adenovirus |

**Fig. 1.3** How the characteristics of viruses can be used in classification, taking DNA viruses as an example.

to lyse). Production of other toxins is also important in differentiating between groups, as in *E. coli*. Antibiotic susceptibility can also be helpful in identification. Matrix-assisted laser desorption ionization time of flight (MALDI TOF) mass spectrometry is increasingly used as a rapid and cost-effective means of identification. Direct genetic approaches are now commonly used in identification and classification such as the use of the polymerase chain reaction (PCR) and probes to detect organism-specific sentinel DNA sequences. These genetic tests are particularly useful for those organisms that grow poorly or not at all in vitro.

### Classification of viruses departs even further from the binomial system

Virus names draw on a wide variety of characteristics (e.g. size, structure, pathology, tissue location, distribution). Groupings are based on characteristics such as the type of nucleic acid present (DNA or RNA), the symmetry of the virus particle (e.g., icosahedral, helical, complex) and the presence or absence of an external envelope, as shown for the DNA viruses in Fig. 1.3 (see also Ch. 3). The equivalents of subspecies categories are also used, including serotypes, strains, variants and isolates and are determined primarily by serologic reactivity of virus material. The influenza virus, for example, can be considered as the equivalent of a genus containing three types (A, B, C) causing infection in people. Identification can be carried out using the stable nucleoprotein antigen, which differs between the three types. The neuraminidase and haemagglutinin antigens are not stable and show variation within types. Characterization of these antigens in an isolate enables the particular variant to be identified, haemagglutinin (H) and neuraminidase (N) variants being designated by numbers (e.g. H5N1, the variant associated with fatal avian influenza; see Ch. 20). A further example is seen in adenoviruses for which the various antigens associated with a component of the capsid can be used to define groups, types and finer subdivisions. The rapid rate of mutation shown by some viruses (e.g., HIV) creates problems for classification. The population present in a virus-infected individual may be genetically quite diverse and may best be described as a quasispecies—representing the average of the broad spectrum of variants present.

### Classification assists diagnosis and the understanding of pathogenicity

Prompt identification of organisms is necessary clinically so that diagnoses can be made and appropriate treatments advised. To understand host–parasite interactions, however, not only should the identity of an organism be known but also as much as possible of its general biology; useful predictions can then be made about the consequences of infection. For these reasons, in subsequent chapters we have included outline classifications of the important pathogens, accompanied by brief accounts of their structure (gross and microscopic), modes of life, molecular biology, biochemistry, replication and reproduction.

## KEY FACTS

- Organisms that cause infectious diseases can be grouped into seven major categories: prions, viruses, bacteria, fungi, protozoa, helminths and arthropods.

- Identification and classification of these organisms are important parts of microbiology and are essential for correct diagnosis, treatment and control.

- Each group has distinctive characteristics (structural and molecular makeup, biochemical and metabolic strategies, reproductive processes) that determine how the organisms interact with their hosts and how they cause disease.

- Many pathogens live within cells where they are protected from many components of the host's protective responses.

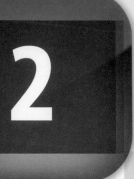

# The bacteria

## Introduction

Although free-living bacteria exist in huge numbers, relatively few species cause disease. The majority of these are well known and well studied; however, new pathogens continue to emerge, and the significance of previously unrecognized infections becomes apparent. Good examples of the latter include Ebola virus disease, Zika fever and severe acute respiratory syndrome coronavirus 2 (SARS-CoV-2); infection with *Legionella*, the cause of Legionnaires' disease, and gastric ulcers, which is associated with *Helicobacter pylori* infection, is a good historical bacterial example.

Bacteria are single-celled prokaryotes, their DNA forming a long circular molecule but not contained within a defined nucleus. Many are motile, using a unique pattern of flagella. The bacterial cell is surrounded by a complex cell wall and often a thick capsule. They reproduce by binary fission, often at very high rates, and show a wide range of metabolic patterns, both aerobic and anaerobic. Classification of bacteria uses both phenotypic and genotypic data. For clinical purposes the phenotypic data are of most practical value and rest on an understanding of bacterial structure and biology (see Fig. 32.2). Detailed summaries of members of the major bacterial groups are given in the Pathogen Parade (see online appendix).

## STRUCTURE

### Bacteria are prokaryotes and have a characteristic cellular organization

The genetic information of bacteria is carried in a long, double-stranded (ds), circular molecule of DNA (dsDNA; Fig. 2.1). By analogy with eukaryotes (see Ch. 1), this can be termed a *chromosome*, but there are no introns; instead, the DNA comprises a continuous coding sequence of genes. The chromosome is not localized within a distinct nucleus; no nuclear membrane is present, and the DNA is tightly coiled into a region known as the *nucleoid*. Genetic information in the cell may also be extrachromosomal, present as small circular self-replicating DNA molecules termed *plasmids*. The cytoplasm contains no organelles other than ribosomes for protein synthesis. Although ribosomal function is the same in both prokaryotic and eukaryotic cells, organelle structure is different. Ribosomes are characterized as 70 S in prokaryotes and 80 S in eukaryotes. (The S unit relates to how a particle behaves when studied under extreme centrifugal force in an ultracentrifuge.) The bacterial 70 S ribosome is specifically targeted by antimicrobials such as the aminoglycosides (see Ch. 34). Many of the metabolic functions performed in eukaryote cells by membrane-bound organelles such as mitochondria are carried out by the prokaryotic cell membrane. In all bacteria except mycoplasmas the cell is surrounded by a complex cell wall. External to this wall may be capsules, flagella and pili. Knowledge of the cell wall and

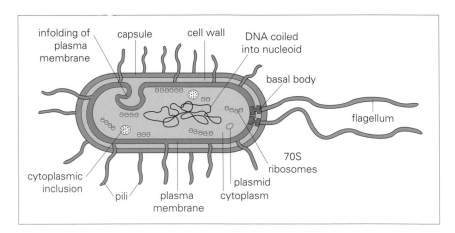

**Fig. 2.1** Diagrammatic structure of a generalized bacterium.

these external structures is important in diagnosis and pathogenicity and for understanding bacterial biology.

### Bacteria are classified according to their cell wall being gram-positive or gram-negative

Gram staining is a basic microbiologic procedure for identification of bacteria (see Ch. 32). The main structural component of the cell wall is peptidoglycan (mucopeptide or murein), a mixed polymer of hexose sugars (*N*-acetylglucosamine and *N*-acetylmuramic acid) and amino acids (Fig. 2.2):

- In gram-positive bacteria the peptidoglycan forms a thick (20–80 nm) layer external to the cell membrane and may contain other macromolecules.
- In gram-negative species the peptidoglycan layer is thin (5–10 nm) and is overlaid by an outer membrane, anchored to lipoprotein molecules in the peptidoglycan layer. The principal molecules of the outer membrane are lipopolysaccharides (LPS) and lipoprotein.

The polysaccharides and charged amino acids in the peptidoglycan layer make it highly polar, providing the bacterium with a thick hydrophilic surface. This property allows gram-positive organisms to resist the activity of bile in the intestine. Conversely, the layer is digested by lysozyme, an enzyme present in body secretions, which, therefore, has bactericidal properties. Synthesis of peptidoglycan is disrupted by beta-lactam and glycopeptide antibiotics (see Ch. 34).

In gram-negative bacteria the outer membrane is also hydrophilic, but the lipid components of the constituent molecules give hydrophobic properties as well. Entry of hydrophilic molecules such as sugars and amino acids is necessary for nutrition and is achieved through special channels or pores formed by proteins called *porins*. The LPS in the membrane confers both antigenic properties (the O antigens from the carbohydrate chains) and toxic properties (the endotoxin from the lipid A component; see Ch. 18).

While staining weakly, gram-positive mycobacteria also possess an outer membrane that contains a variety of complex lipids (mycolic acids). These create a waxy layer that both alters the staining properties of these organisms (the so-called *acid-fast bacteria*) and gives considerable resistance to drying and other environmental factors. Mycobacterial cell wall components also have a pronounced adjuvant activity (i.e. they promote immunologic responsiveness).

External to the cell wall may be an additional capsule of high-molecular-weight polysaccharides (or amino acids in anthrax bacilli) that gives a slimy surface. This provides protection against phagocytosis by host cells and is important in determining virulence. With *Streptococcus pneumoniae* infection, only a few capsulated organisms can cause a fatal infection, but unencapsulated mutants cause no disease.

The cell wall is a major contributor to the ultimate shape of the organism, an important characteristic for bacterial identification. In general, bacterial shapes are categorized as spherical (cocci), rods (bacilli) or helical (spirilla) (Fig. 2.3), although there are variations on these themes.

### Many bacteria possess flagella

Flagella are long helical filaments extending from the cell surface, which enable bacteria to move in their environment. These may be restricted to the poles of the cell, singly (polar) or in tufts (lophotrichous), or distributed over the general surface of the cell (peritrichous). While functionally similar, bacterial flagella are structurally quite different from eukaryote flagella. In addition, the forces that result in movement are generated quite differently, being proton dependent (i.e. driven by movement of hydrogens across the cell membrane) in prokaryotes but adenosine triphosphate (ATP) dependent in eukaryotes. Motility allows positive and negative responses to environmental stimuli such as chemicals (chemotaxis). Flagella are built of protein components (flagellins), which are strongly antigenic. These antigens, the H antigens, are important targets of protective antibody responses.

### Pili are another form of bacterial surface projection

Pili (fimbriae) are more rigid than flagella and function in attachment, either to other bacteria (the sex pili) or to host cells (the common pili). Adherence to host cells involves

**Fig. 2.2** Construction of the cell walls of gram-positive and gram-negative bacteria.

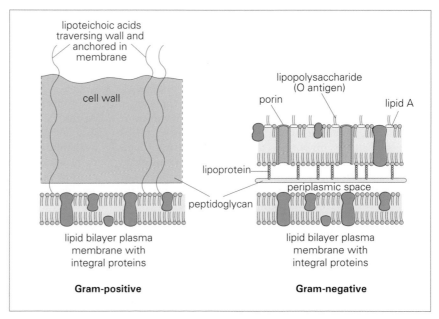

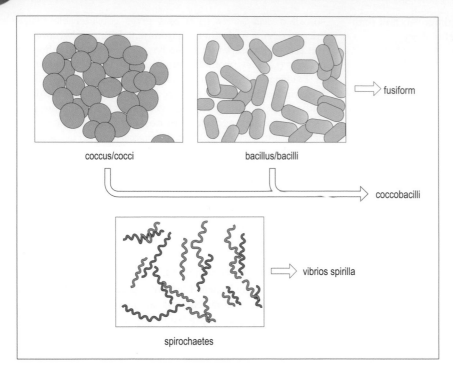

**Fig. 2.3** The three basic shapes of bacterial cells.

coccus/cocci

bacillus/bacilli

fusiform

coccobacilli

vibrios spirilla

spirochaetes

specific interactions between component molecules of the pili (adhesins) and molecules in host cell membranes. For example, the adhesins of *Escherichia coli* interact with fucose/mannose molecules on the surface of intestinal epithelial cells (see Ch. 23). The presence of many pili may help to prevent phagocytosis, reducing host resistance to bacterial infection. Although immunogenic, their antigens can be changed, allowing the bacteria to avoid immune recognition. The mechanism of antigenic variation has been elucidated in organisms such as gonococci and is known to involve recombination of genes coding for constant and variable regions of pili molecules.

## NUTRITION

### Bacteria obtain nutrients mainly by taking up small molecules across the cell wall

Bacteria take up small molecules such as amino acids, oligosaccharides and small peptides across the cell wall. Gram-negative species can also take up and use larger molecules after preliminary digestion in the periplasmic space. Uptake and transport of nutrients into the cytoplasm is achieved by the cell membrane using a variety of transport mechanisms, including facilitated diffusion, which utilizes a carrier to move compounds to equalize their intra- and extracellular concentrations, and active transport in which energy is expended to deliberately increase intracellular concentrations of a substrate. Oxidative metabolism (see later) also takes place at the membrane–cytoplasm interface.

Some species require only minimal nutrients in their environment, having considerable synthetic powers, whereas others have complex nutritional requirements. *E. coli*, for example, can be grown in media providing only glucose and inorganic salts; streptococci, on the other hand, will grow only in complex media providing them with many organic compounds. Nevertheless, all bacteria have similar general nutritional requirements for growth, which are summarized in Table 2.1.

### All pathogenic bacteria are heterotrophic

All bacteria obtain energy by oxidizing preformed organic molecules (carbohydrates, lipids and proteins) from their environment. Metabolism of these molecules yields ATP as an energy source. Metabolism may be aerobic, where the final electron acceptor is oxygen, or anaerobic, where the final acceptor may be an organic or inorganic molecule other than oxygen.

- In aerobic metabolism (i.e. aerobic respiration), complete utilization of an energy source such as glucose produces 38 molecules of ATP.
- Anaerobic metabolism utilizing an inorganic molecule other than oxygen as the final hydrogen acceptor (anaerobic respiration) is incomplete and produces fewer ATP molecules than aerobic respiration.
- Anaerobic metabolism, utilizing an organic final hydrogen acceptor (fermentation), is much less efficient and produces only two molecules of ATP.

Anaerobic metabolism, while less efficient, can thus be used in the absence of oxygen when appropriate substrates are available, as they usually are in the host's body. The requirement for oxygen in respiration may be either obligate or facultative, some organisms being able to switch between aerobic and anaerobic metabolism. Those that use fermentation pathways often use the major product pyruvate in secondary fermentations by which additional energy can be generated. The interrelationship between these different metabolic pathways is illustrated in Fig. 2.4.

The ability of bacteria to grow in the presence of atmospheric oxygen relates to their ability to deal enzymatically with potentially destructive intracellular reactive oxygen species (free radicals, anions containing oxygen, etc.) (Table 2.2).

**Table 2.1** Major nutritional requirements for bacterial growth

| Element | Cell dry weight (%) | Major cellular role |
|---|---|---|
| Carbon | 50 | Molecular building block obtained from organic compounds or $CO_2$ |
| Oxygen | 20 | Molecular building block obtained from organic compounds, $O_2$ or $H_2O$; $O_2$ is an electron acceptor in aerobic respiration |
| Nitrogen | 14 | Component of amino acids, nucleotides, nucleic acids and coenzymes obtained from organic compounds and inorganic sources such as $NH^{4+}$ |
| Hydrogen | 8 | Molecular building block obtained from organic compounds, $H_2O$ or $H_2$; involved in respiration to produce energy |
| Phosphorus | 3 | Found in a variety of cellular components, including nucleotides, nucleic acids, lipopolysaccharide and phospholipids; obtained from inorganic phosphates ($PO_4^{3-}$) |
| Sulphur | 1–2 | Component of several amino acids and coenzymes; obtained from organic compounds and inorganic sources such as sulphates ($SO_4^{2-}$) |
| Potassium | 1–2 | Important inorganic cation, enzyme cofactor, etc. obtained from inorganic sources |

**Table 2.2** Bacterial classification in response to environmental oxygen

| Environmental oxygen | | | |
|---|---|---|---|
| Category | Present | Absent | Oxygen-detoxifying enzymes (e.g. superoxide dismutase, catalase, peroxidase) |
| Obligate aerobe | Growth | No growth | Present |
| Microaerophile | Growth in low oxygen levels | No growth | Some enzymes absent; reduced enzyme concentration |
| Obligate anaerobe | No growth | Growth | Absent |
| Facultative (anaerobe/aerobe) | Growth | Growth | Present |

**Fig. 2.4** Catabolic breakdown of glucose in relationship to final hydrogen acceptor.

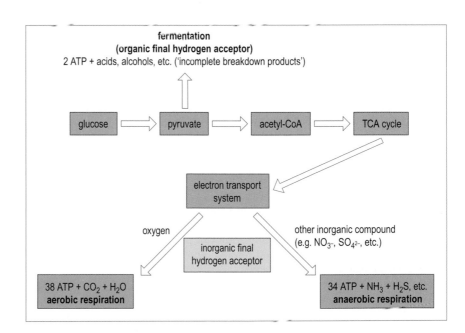

The interaction between these harmful compounds and detoxifying enzymes such as superoxide dismutase, peroxidase and catalase is illustrated in Fig. 2.5 (also see Ch. 10 and Box 10.2).

## GROWTH AND DIVISION

The rate at which bacteria grow and divide depends in large part on the nutritional status of the environment. The growth and division of a single *E. coli* cell into identical daughter cells may occur in as little as 20–30 min in rich laboratory media, whereas the same process is much slower (1–2 h) in a nutritionally depleted environment. Conversely, even in the best environment, other bacteria such as *Mycobacterium tuberculosis* may grow much more slowly, dividing every 24 h. When introduced into a new environment, bacterial growth follows a characteristic pattern depicted in Fig. 2.6. After an initial period of adjustment (lag phase), cell division rapidly occurs, with the population doubling at a constant

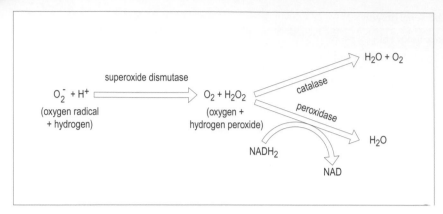

**Fig. 2.5** Interaction between oxygen-detoxifying enzymes.

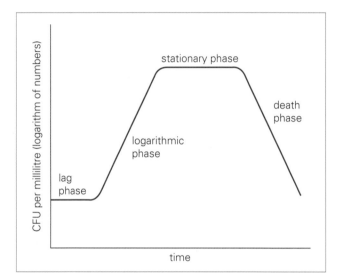

**Fig. 2.6** The bacterial growth curve. CFU, Colony-forming units.

rate (generation time) for a period termed *log* or *exponential phase*. As nutrients are depleted and toxic products accumulate, cell growth slows to a stop (stationary phase) and eventually enters a phase of decline (death).

### A bacterial cell must duplicate its genomic DNA before it can divide

All bacterial genomes are circular, and their replication begins at a single site known as the origin of replication (termed *OriC*). A multienzyme replication complex binds to the origin and initiates unwinding and separation of the two DNA strands, using enzymes called *helicases* and *topoisomerases* (e.g. DNA gyrase). Each of the separated DNA strands serves as a template for DNA polymerase. The polymerization reaction involves incorporation of deoxyribonucleotides, which correctly base pair with the template DNA. Two characteristic replication forks are formed, which proceed in opposite directions around the chromosome. Each of the two copies of the total genetic information (genome) produced during replication comprises one parental strand and one newly synthesized strand of DNA.

Replication of the genome takes approximately 40 min in *E. coli*, so when these bacteria grow and divide every 20–30 min, they need to initiate new rounds of DNA replication before an existing round of replication has finished to provide complete chromosomal copies at an accelerated rate. In such instances, daughter cells inherit DNA that has already initiated its own replication.

### Replication must be accurate

Accurate replication is essential because DNA carries the information that defines the properties and processes of a cell. It is achieved because DNA polymerase is capable of proofreading newly incorporated deoxyribonucleotides and excising those that are incorrect. This reduces the frequency of errors to approximately one mistake (an incorrect base pair) per $10^{10}$ nucleotides copied.

### Cell division is preceded by genome segregation and septum formation

The process of cell division (or septation) involves:

- segregation of the replicated genomes
- formation of a septum in the middle of the cell
- division of the cell to give separate daughter cells.

The septum is formed by an invagination of the cytoplasmic membrane and ingrowth of the peptidoglycan cell wall (and outer membrane in gram-negative bacteria). Septation and DNA replication and genome segregation are not tightly coupled but are sufficiently well coordinated to ensure that the overwhelming majority of daughter cells have the correct complement of genomic DNA.

The mechanics of cell division result in reproducible cellular arrangements when viewed by microscopic examination. For example, cocci dividing in one plane may appear chained (streptococci) or paired (diplococci), while division in multiple planes results in clusters (staphylococci). As with cell shape, these arrangements have served as an important characteristic for bacterial identification.

### Bacterial growth and division are important targets for antimicrobial agents

Antimicrobial agents that target the processes involved in bacterial growth and division include:

- quinolones (ciprofloxacin and levofloxacin), which inhibit the unwinding of DNA by DNA gyrase during DNA replication
- the many inhibitors of peptidoglycan cell wall synthesis (e.g. beta-lactams such as the penicillins, cephalosporins and carbapenems and glycopeptides such as vancomycin).

These are considered in more detail in Chapter 34.

# GENE EXPRESSION

Gene expression describes the processes involved in decoding the genetic information contained within a gene to produce a functional protein or RNA molecule.

## Most genes are transcribed into messenger RNA

The overwhelming majority of genes (e.g. up to 98% in *E. coli*) are transcribed into messenger RNA (mRNA), which is then translated into proteins. Certain genes, however, are transcribed to produce ribosomal RNA species (5 S, 16 S, 23 S), which provide a scaffold for assembling ribosomal subunits; others are transcribed into transfer RNA (tRNA) molecules, which, together with the ribosome, participate in decoding mRNA into functional proteins.

## Transcription

The DNA is copied by a DNA-dependent RNA polymerase to yield an RNA transcript. The polymerization reaction involves incorporation of ribonucleotides, which correctly base pair with the template DNA.

## Transcription is initiated at promoters

Promoters are nucleotide sequences in DNA that can bind the RNA polymerase. The frequency of transcription initiation can be influenced by many factors, for example:

- the exact DNA sequence of the promoter site
- the overall topology (supercoiling) of the DNA
- the presence or absence of regulatory proteins that bind adjacent to and may overlap the promoter site

Consequently, different promoters have widely different rates of transcriptional initiation (of up to 3000-fold). Their activities can be altered by regulatory proteins. Sigma factor (a protein specifically needed to begin RNA synthesis) plays an important role in promoter recognition. The presence of several different sigma factors in bacteria enables sets of genes to be switched on simply by altering the level of expression of a particular sigma factor (e.g. spore formation in gram-positive bacteria).

## Transcription usually terminates at specific termination sites

These termination sites are characterized by a series of uracil residues in the mRNA following an inverted repeat sequence, which can adopt a stem-loop structure that forms as a result of the base pairing of ribonucleotides and interfere with RNA polymerase activity. In addition, certain transcripts terminate following interaction of RNA polymerase with the transcription termination protein rho.

## mRNA transcripts often encode more than one protein in bacteria

The bacterial arrangement seen for single genes (promoter–structural-gene–transcriptional-terminator) is described as monocistronic. However, a single promoter and terminator may flank multiple structural genes, a polycistronic arrangement known as an *operon*. Operon transcription thus results in polycistronic mRNA encoding more than one protein (Fig. 2.7). Operons provide a way of ensuring that protein subunits that make up particular enzyme complexes or are required for a specific biologic process are synthesized

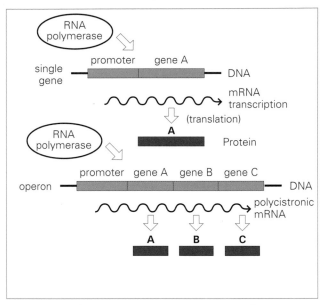

**Fig. 2.7** Bacterial genes are present on DNA as separate discrete units (single genes) or as operons (multigenes), which are transcribed from promoters to give, respectively, monocistronic or polycistronic messenger RNA (mRNA) molecules; mRNA is then translated into protein.

simultaneously and in the correct stoichiometry. For example, the proteins required for the uptake and metabolism of lactose are encoded by the lac operon. Many of the proteins responsible for the pathogenic properties of medically important microorganisms are likewise encoded by operons, for example:

- cholera toxin from *Vibrio cholerae*
- fimbriae (pili) of uropathogenic *E. coli*, which mediate colonization.

## Translation

The exact sequence of amino acids in a protein (polypeptide) is specified by the sequence of nucleotides found in the mRNA transcripts. Decoding this information to produce a protein is achieved by ribosomes and tRNA molecules in a process known as *translation*. Each set of three bases (triplet) in the mRNA sequence corresponds to a codon for a specific amino acid. However, there is redundancy in the triplet code resulting in instances of more than one triplet encoding the same amino acid (i.e. also referred to as *code degeneracy*). Thus a total of 64 codons encode all 20 amino acids as well as start and stop signal codons.

## Translation begins with formation of an initiation complex and terminates at a STOP codon

The initiation complex comprises mRNA, ribosome and an initiator tRNA molecule carrying formylmethionine. Ribosomes bind to specific sequences in mRNA (Shine–Dalgarno sequences) and begin translation at an initiation (START) codon, AUG (i.e. the bases adenosine, uracil, guanine), which hybridizes with a specific complementary sequence (the anticodon loop) of the initiator tRNA molecule. The polypeptide chain elongates as a result of movement of the ribosome along the mRNA molecule and the recruitment of further tRNA molecules (carrying different amino acids), which recognize the subsequent codon triplets. Ribosomes carry out a condensation reaction, which couples the incoming amino acid (carried on the tRNA) to the growing polypeptide chain.

Translation is terminated when the ribosome encounters one of three termination (STOP) codons: UGA, UAA or UAG.

### Transcription and translation are important targets for antimicrobial agents

Such antimicrobial agents include:

- inhibitors of RNA polymerase, such as rifampicin
- a wide array of bacterial protein synthesis inhibitors including macrolides (e.g. erythromycin, aminoglycosides, tetracyclines, chloramphenicol, lincosamides, streptogramins, and oxazolidinones) (see Ch. 34).

## Regulation of gene expression

### Bacteria adapt to their environment by controlling gene expression

Bacteria show a remarkable ability to adapt to changes in their environment. This is predominantly achieved by controlling gene expression, thereby ensuring that proteins are produced only when and if they are required. For example:

- Bacteria may encounter a new source of carbon or nitrogen and consequently switch on new metabolic pathways that enable them to transport and use such compounds.
- When compounds such as amino acids are depleted from a bacterium's environment, the bacterium may be able to switch on the production of enzymes that enable it to synthesize de novo the molecule it requires.

### Expression of many virulence determinants by pathogenic bacteria is highly regulated

This makes sense as it conserves metabolic energy and ensures that virulence determinants are produced only when their particular property is needed. For example, enterobacterial pathogens are often transmitted in contaminated water supplies. The temperature of such water will probably be lower than 25°C and low in nutrients. However, upon entering the human gut there will be a striking change in the bacterium's environment—the temperature will rise to 37°C and there will be an abundant supply of carbon and nitrogen and a low availability of both oxygen and free iron (an essential nutrient). Bacteria adapt to such changes by switching on or off a range of metabolic and virulence-associated genes.

The analysis of virulence gene expression is one of the fastest-growing aspects of the study of microbial pathogenesis. It provides an important insight into how bacteria adapt to the many changes they encounter as they initiate infection and spread into different host tissues.

### The most common way of altering gene expression is to change the amount of mRNA transcription

The level of mRNA transcription can be altered by altering the efficiency of binding of RNA polymerase to promoter sites. Environmental changes such as shifts in growth temperature (from 25°C to 37°C) or the availability of oxygen can change the extent of supercoiling in DNA, thereby altering the overall topology of promoters and the efficiency of transcription initiation. However, most instances of transcriptional regulation are mediated by regulatory proteins, which bind specifically to the DNA adjacent to or overlapping the promoter site, and alter RNA polymerase binding and transcription. The regions of DNA to which regulatory proteins bind are known as *operators* or *operator sites*. Regulatory proteins fall into two distinct classes:

- those that increase the rate of transcription initiation (activators)
- those that inhibit transcription (repressors) (Fig. 2.8).

Genes subject to positive regulation need to bind an activated regulatory protein (apoinducer) to promote transcription initiation. Gene transcription subject to negative regulation is inhibited by the binding of repressor proteins.

### The principles of gene regulation in bacteria can be illustrated by the regulation of genes involved in sugar metabolism

Bacteria use sugars as a carbon source for growth and prefer to use glucose rather than other less well-metabolized sugars. When growing in an environment containing both glucose and lactose, bacteria such as *E. coli* preferentially metabolize glucose and at the same time prevent the expression of the lac operon, the products of which transport and metabolize lactose (Fig. 2.9). This is known as *catabolite repression*. It occurs because the transcriptional initiation of the lac operon is dependent upon a positive regulator: the cyclic adenosine monophosphate (cAMP)–dependent catabolite activator protein (CAP), which is activated only when cAMP is bound. When bacteria grow on glucose the cytoplasmic levels of cAMP are low and so CAP is not activated. CAP is, therefore, unable to bind to its DNA binding site adjacent to the lac promoter and facilitate transcription initiation by RNA polymerase. When the glucose is depleted, the cAMP concentration rises, resulting in the formation of activated cAMP–CAP complexes, which bind the appropriate site on the DNA, increasing RNA polymerase binding and lac operon transcription.

CAP is an example of a global regulatory protein that controls the expression of multiple genes; it controls the expression of over 100 genes in *E. coli*. All genes controlled by the same regulator are considered to constitute a regulon (see Fig. 2.8). In addition to the influence of CAP on the lac operon, the operon is also subject to negative regulation by the lactose repressor protein (LacI; see Fig. 2.9). LacI is encoded by the *lacI* gene, which is located immediately upstream of the lactose operon and transcribed by a separate promoter. In the absence of lactose, LacI binds specifically to the operator region of the lac promoter and blocks transcription. An inducer molecule, allolactose (or its nonmetabolizable homologue, isopropyl-thiogalactoside [IPTG]) is able to bind to LacI, causing an allosteric change in its structure. This releases it from the DNA, thereby alleviating the repression. The lac operon therefore illustrates the fine tuning of gene regulation in bacteria—the operon is switched on only if lactose is available as a carbon source for cell growth but remains unexpressed if glucose, the cell's preferred carbon source, is also present.

### activation – positive gene regulation

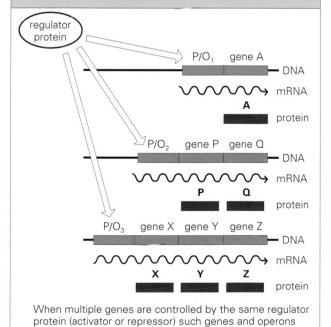

Binding of an activator protein to the operator site (O) causes RNA polymerase to bind to the promoter (P) and initiate messenger RNA (mRNA) transcription

In the absence of the activator protein RNA polymerase fails to bind to the promoter and no mRNA transcription occurs

### repression – negative gene regulation

Binding of a repressor protein to the operator site can inhibit either the binding or activity of RNA polymerase and so block mRNA transcription

In the absence of the repressor protein RNA polymerase can bind to the promoter and initiate mRNA transcription

### regulons – coordinated regulation of multiple genes

When multiple genes are controlled by the same regulator protein (activator or repressor) such genes and operons constitute a regulon

**Fig. 2.8** Expression of genes in bacteria is highly regulated, enabling them to switch genes on or off in response to changes in available nutrients or other changes in their environment. Genes and operons controlled by the same regulator constitute a regulon.

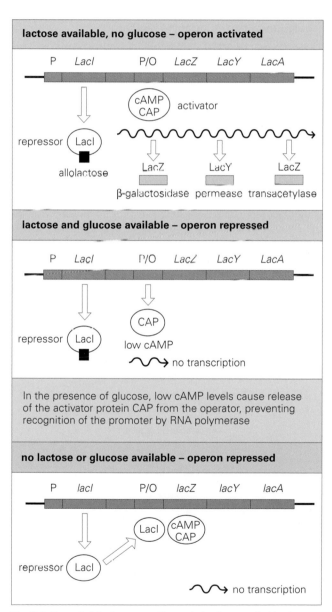

### lactose available, no glucose – operon activated

### lactose and glucose available – operon repressed

In the presence of glucose, low cAMP levels cause release of the activator protein CAP from the operator, preventing recognition of the promoter by RNA polymerase

### no lactose or glucose available – operon repressed

**Fig. 2.9** Control of the lac operon. Transcription is controlled by the lactose repressor protein (LacI, negative regulation) and by the catabolite activator protein (CAP, positive regulation). In the presence of lactose as the sole carbon source for growth, the lac operon is switched on. Bacteria prefer to use glucose rather than lactose, so if glucose is also present, the lac operon is switched off until the glucose has been used.

### Expression of bacterial virulence genes is often controlled by regulatory proteins

An example of such regulation is the production of diphtheria toxin by *Corynebacterium diphtheriae* (see Ch. 20), which is subject to negative regulation if there is free iron in the growth environment. A repressor protein, DtxR, binds iron and undergoes a conformational change that allows it to bind with high affinity to the operator site of the toxin gene and inhibit transcription. When *C. diphtheriae* grow in an environment with a very low concentration of iron (i.e. similar to that of human secretions), DtxR is unable to bind iron, and toxin production occurs.

### Many bacterial virulence genes are subject to positive regulation by two-component regulators

These two-component regulators typically comprise two separate proteins (Fig. 2.10):

- one acting as a sensor to detect environmental changes (such as alterations in temperature)
- the other acting as a DNA-binding protein capable of activating (or repressing in some cases) transcription.

Bacteria may possess multiple two-component regulators recognizing different environmental stimuli. Thus bacteria residing in more complex environments tend to carry increased numbers of two-component regulators.

In *Bordetella pertussis*, the causative agent of whooping cough (see Ch. 20), a two-component regulator (encoded by the Bordatella virulence gene [bvg] locus) controls expression of a large number of virulence genes. The sensor protein BvgS is a cytoplasmic membrane-located histidine kinase that senses environmental signals (temperature, $Mg^{2+}$, nicotinic acid), leading to an alteration in its autophosphorylating activity. In response to positive regulatory signals such as an elevation in temperature, BvgS undergoes autophosphorylation and then phosphorylates, thus activating the DNA-binding protein BvgA. BvgA then binds to the operators of the pertussis toxin operon and other virulence-associated genes and activates their transcription.

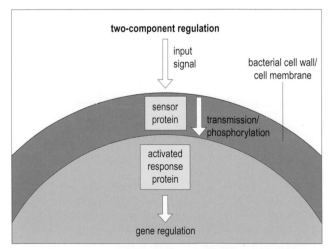

**Fig. 2.10** Two-component regulation is a signal transduction process that allows cellular functions to react in response to a changing environment. An appropriate environmental stimulus results in autophosphorylation of the sensor protein, which, by a phosphotransfer reaction, activates the response protein that affects gene regulation.

In *Staphylococcus aureus*, a variety of virulence genes are influenced by global regulatory systems, the best studied and most important of which is a two-component regulator termed *accessory gene regulator (agr)*. Agr control is complex in that it serves as a positive regulator for exotoxins secreted late in the bacterial life cycle (postexponential phase) but behaves as a negative regulator for virulence factors associated with the cell surface.

The control of virulence gene expression in *V. cholerae* is under the control of ToxR, a cytoplasmic membrane-located protein, which senses environmental changes. ToxR activates both the transcription of the cholera toxin operon and another regulatory protein, ToxT, which, in turn, activates the transcription of other virulence genes such as toxin-coregulated pili, an essential virulence factor required for colonization of the human small intestine.

### In some instances the pathogenic activity of bacteria specifically begins when cell numbers reach a certain threshold

Quorum sensing is the mechanism by which specific gene transcription is activated in response to bacterial concentration. While quorum sensing is known to occur in a wide variety of microorganisms, a classic example is the production of biofilms by *Pseudomonas aeruginosa* in the lungs of patients with cystic fibrosis (CF). The production of these tenacious substances allows *P. aeruginosa* to establish serious long-term infection in patients with CF, which is difficult to treat (see Ch. 20; Fig. 20.25). As illustrated in Fig. 2.11, when quorum-sensing bacteria reach appropriate numbers, the signalling compounds they produce are at sufficient concentration to activate transcription of specific response genes such as those related to biofilm production. Current research is aimed at better understanding the quorum-sensing process in different bacterial pathogens and exploring potential therapeutic approaches (e.g. inhibitory compounds) to interfere with this coordinated mechanism of bacterial virulence.

## SURVIVAL UNDER ADVERSE CONDITIONS

### Some bacteria form endospores

Certain bacteria can form highly resistant spores—endospores—within their cells, and these enable them to survive adverse conditions. They are formed when the cells are unable to grow (e.g. when environmental conditions change or when nutrients are exhausted) but never by actively growing cells. The spore has a complex multilayered coat surrounding a new bacterial cell. There are many differences in composition between endospores and normal cells, notably the presence of dipicolinic acid and a high calcium content, both of which are thought to confer the endospore's extreme resistance to heat and chemicals.

Because of their resistance, spores can remain viable in a dormant state for many years, reconverting rapidly to normal existence when conditions improve. When this occurs, a new bacterial cell grows out from the spore and resumes vegetative life. Endospores are abundant in soils, and those of the *Clostridium* and *Bacillus* are a particular hazard (Fig. 2.12). Tetanus and anthrax caused by these bacteria are both associated with endospore infection of wounds, the bacteria developing from the spores once they are in appropriate conditions.

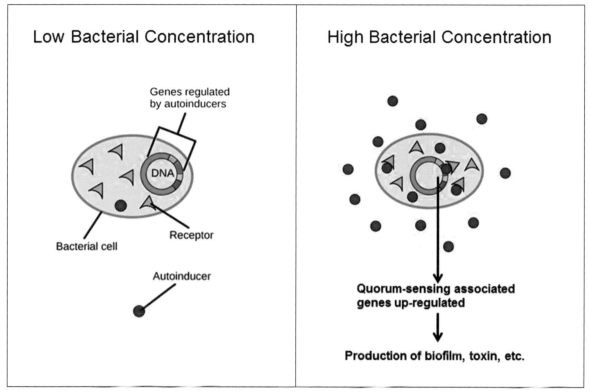

**Fig. 2.11** Quorum sensing bacteria produce autoinducer signalling compounds, which, in sufficient concentration, bind to receptors that activate transcription of specific response genes (for biofilm production, etc.). (Modified from https://www.boundless.com/biology/textbooks/boundless-biology-textbook/cell-communication-9/signaling-in-single-celled-organisms-86/signaling-in-bacteria-391-11617/images/fig-ch09_04_02/.)

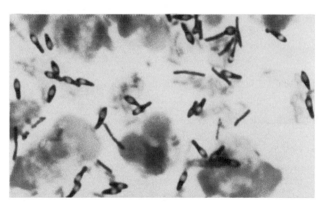

**Fig. 2.12** *Clostridium tetani* with terminal spores.

## MOBILE GENETIC ELEMENTS

The bacterial chromosome represents the primary reservoir of genetic information within the cell; however, a variety of additional genetic elements may also be present, which are capable of independently moving to different locations within a cell or between cells (also termed *horizontal gene transfer*).

### Many bacteria possess small, independently replicating (extrachromosomal) nucleic acid molecules termed *plasmids and bacteriophages*

Plasmids are independent, self-replicating circular units of dsDNA, some of which are relatively large (e.g. 60–120 kb) and others of which are quite small (1.5–15 kb). Plasmid replication is similar to the replication of genomic DNA, although there are differences. Not all plasmids are replicated bidirectionally—some have a single replication fork, and others are replicated like a rolling circle. The number of plasmids per bacterial cell (copy number) varies for different plasmids, ranging from one to thousands of copies per cell. The rate of initiation of plasmid replication determines the plasmid copy number; however, larger plasmids generally tend to have lower copy numbers than smaller plasmids. Some plasmids (broad-host-range plasmids) are able to replicate in many different bacterial species, whereas others have a more restricted host range.

Plasmids contain genes for replication, and, in some cases, for mediating their own transfer between bacteria (*tra* genes). Plasmids may additionally carry a wide variety of additional genes (influencing the overall size of the plasmid), which can confer a variety of advantages to the host bacterial cell (e.g. antibiotic resistance, toxin production).

### Widespread use of antimicrobials has applied a strong selection pressure in favour of bacteria able to resist them

In the majority of cases, resistance to antimicrobials is due to the presence of resistance genes on self-transferrable (conjugative) plasmids (R plasmids; see Ch. 34). These are known to have existed before the era of mass antibiotic treatments, but they have become widespread in many species as a result of selection. R plasmids may carry genes for resistance to multiple antimicrobials. For example, one of the earliest-studied R plasmids, R100, confers resistance to sulphonamides, aminoglycosides, chloramphenicol and tetracycline, and there are many others carrying genes for resistance to an even greater spectrum of antimicrobials. R plasmids can recombine, resulting in individual replicons encoding new combinations of multiple drug resistance.

### Plasmids can carry virulence genes

Plasmids may encode toxins and other proteins that increase the virulence of microorganisms. For example:

- The virulent enterotoxinogenic strains of *E. coli* that cause diarrhoea produce different types of plasmid-encoded enterotoxins that alter the secretion of fluid and electrolytes by the intestinal epithelium (see Ch. 23).
- In *S. aureus*, both an enterotoxin and a number of enzymes involved in bacterial virulence (haemolysin, fibrinolysin) are encoded by plasmid genes.

The production of toxins by bacteria and their pathologic effects are discussed in detail in Chapter 18.

### Plasmids are valuable tools for cloning and manipulating genes

Molecular biologists have generated a wealth of recombinant plasmids to use as vectors for genetic engineering (Fig. 2.13). Plasmids can be used to transfer genes across species barriers so that defined gene products can be studied or synthesized in large quantities in different recipient organisms.

### Bacteriophages are bacterial viruses that can survive outside as well as inside the bacterial cell

Bacteriophages differ from plasmids in that their reproduction usually leads to destruction of the bacterial cell. In general, bacteriophages consist of a protein coat or head (capsid), which surrounds nucleic acid, which may be either DNA or RNA but not both. Some bacteriophages may also possess a tail-like structure, which aids them in attaching to and infecting their bacterial host. As illustrated in Fig. 2.14 for DNA-containing bacteriophages, the virus attaches and injects its DNA into the bacterium, leaving the protective protein coat behind. Virulent bacteriophages instigate a form of molecular mutiny to commandeer cellular nucleic acid and protein to produce new virus DNA and protein. Many new virus particles (virions) are then assembled and released into the environment as the bacterial cell ruptures (lyses), thus allowing the cycle to begin again.

While destruction of the host is always the direct consequence of virulent bacteriophage infection, temperate bacteriophages may exercise a choice. Following infection, they may immediately reproduce in a manner similar to their

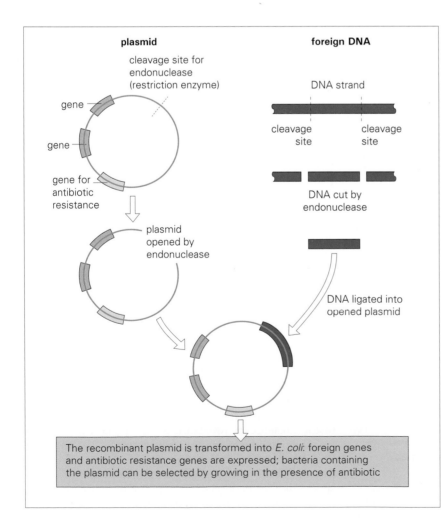

**Fig. 2.13** The use of plasmid vectors to introduce foreign DNA in *E. coli*—a basic step in gene cloning.

**plasmid**

cleavage site for endonuclease (restriction enzyme)

gene

gene

gene for antibiotic resistance

plasmid opened by endonuclease

**foreign DNA**

DNA strand

cleavage site     cleavage site

DNA cut by endonuclease

DNA ligated into opened plasmid

The recombinant plasmid is transformed into *E. coli*: foreign genes and antibiotic resistance genes are expressed; bacteria containing the plasmid can be selected by growing in the presence of antibiotic

**Fig. 2.14** The life cycle of bacteriophages.

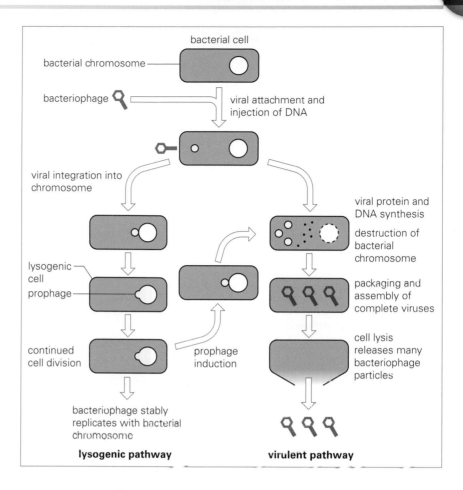

virulent counterparts; however, in some instances they may insert into the bacterial chromosome. This process, termed *lysogeny*, does not kill the cell as the integrated viral DNA (now called a *prophage*) is quiescently carried and replicated within the bacterial chromosome. The lysogenic cell may exhibit new characteristics as a result of expression of genes carried by the prophage (prophage conversion), which in some instances may increase bacterial virulence (e.g. the gene for diphtheria toxin resides on a prophage). Nevertheless, this latent state is eventually destined to end, often in response to some environmental stimulus inactivating the bacteriophage repressor, which normally maintains the lysogenic condition. During this induction process, the viral DNA is excised from the chromosome and proceeds to active replication and assembly, resulting in cell lysis and viral release.

Whether virulent or temperate, bacteriophage infection ultimately results in death of the host cell, which, given current problems with multiple resistance, has sparked a renewed interest in their use as natural antimicrobial agents. A variety of issues related to dosing, delivery, quality control, etc. have impeded the use of bacteriophage therapy in routine clinical practice, however.

## Transposition

Transposable elements are DNA sequences that can jump (transpose) from a site in one DNA molecule to another in a cell. This movement does not rely on host-cell (homologous) recombination pathways, which require extensive similarity between the resident and incoming DNA. Instead, movement involves short target sequences in the recipient DNA molecule where recombination/insertion is directed by the mobile element (site-specific recombination).

Whereas plasmid transfer involves the movement of genetic information between bacterial cells, transposition is the movement of such information between DNA molecules. The most extensively studied transposable elements are those found in *E. coli* and other gram-negative bacteria, although examples are also found in gram-positive bacteria, yeast, plants and other organisms.

### Insertion sequences are the smallest and simplest jumping genes

Insertion sequence elements (ISs) are generally <2 kb in length and only encode functions such as the transposase enzyme, which is required for transposition from one DNA site to another. At the ends of ISs are usually short, inverted repeat sequences (36 nucleotides long in IS*911*), which are also important in the process of locating and inserting into a DNA target (Fig. 2.15A). During the transposition process, a portion of the target sequence is duplicated, resulting in short direct repeat sequences (the same sequence in the same orientation) on each side of the newly inserted IS element. Many aspects of the target selection process remain unclear. While adenine/thymine (A/T)–rich regions of DNA appear to be preferred, some ISs are highly selective, whereas others are generally indiscriminate. Transposition does not rely on enzymatic processes typically used by the cell for homologous recombination (recombination between highly related

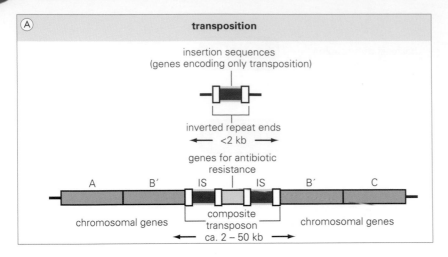

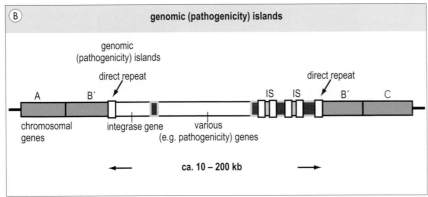

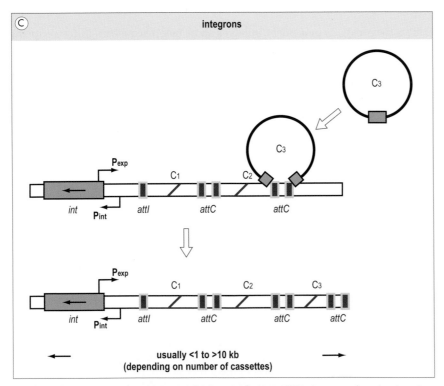

**Fig. 2.15** (A) Transposons (jumping genes) can move from one DNA site to another; they inactivate the recipient gene into which they insert. Transposons often contain genes that confer resistance to antibiotics. (B) Genomic islands are regions of DNA with signature sequences (e.g. direct repeats) indicative of mobility. Their encoded functions increase bacterial fitness (e.g. pathogenicity). (C) Integrons are genetic regions into which independent open reading frames, also termed *gene cassettes*, can integrate and become functional (e.g. under control of the promoter $P_{exp}$). The integration process occurs by site-specific recombination between circular cassettes and their recipient integron, which is directed by an integrase gene (*intI*) with promoter $P_{int}$ and an associated attachment site (*attI*).

DNA molecules) and is thus termed *illegitimate recombination*. The result is a number of ISs in bacterial genomes. For example, some *E. coli* strains carry 19 copies of IS*629* and three copies of IS*677*. Multiple IS copies serve an important function as portable regions of homology throughout a bacterial genome in which homologous recombination may occur between different DNA regions or molecules (e.g. chromosome and plasmid), carrying the same IS sequence. Two IS elements inserting relatively near to each other would allow the entire region to become transposable, further promoting the potential for genetic movement and exchange in bacterial populations.

### Transposons are larger, more complex elements that encode multiple genes

Transposons are >2 kb in size and contain genes in addition to those required for transposition (often encoding resistance to one or more antibiotics) (see Fig. 2.15A). Furthermore, virulence genes, such as those encoding heat-stable enterotoxin from *E. coli*, have been found on transposons.

Transposons can be divided into two classes:

1. composite transposons in which two copies of an identical IS element flank antibiotic-resistance genes (kanamycin resistance in Tn5)
2. simple transposons, such as Tn3 (encoding resistance to beta-lactams).

ISs at the ends of composite transposons may be either in the same or in an inverted orientation (i.e. direct or indirect repeats). Although as part of the composite transposon structure, the terminal IS elements are fully intact and capable of independent transposition.

Simple transposons move only as a single unit, containing genes for transposition and other functions (e.g. antibiotic resistance) with short, inversely oriented sequences (indirect repeats) at each end.

### Mobile genetic elements promote a variety of DNA rearrangements that may have important clinical consequences

The ease with which transposons move into or out of DNA sequences means that transposition can occur:

- from host genomic DNA harbouring a transposon to a plasmid
- from one plasmid to another plasmid
- from a plasmid to genomic DNA.

Transposition onto a broad-host-range self-transferrable (conjugative) plasmid can lead to the rapid dissemination of resistance among different bacteria. The transposition process (whether by ISs or transposons) can be deleterious if insertion occurs within and disrupts a functional gene. However, transpositional mutagenesis has been effectively utilized in the molecular biology laboratory to produce extremely specific mutations without the harmful secondary effects often seen with more generally acting chemical mutagens.

### Other mobile elements also behave as portable cassettes of genetic information

Pathogenicity islands (see Fig. 2.15B) are a special class of mobile genetic elements containing groups of coordinately controlled virulence genes, often with ISs, direct repeat sequences, etc. at their ends. Although originally observed in uropathogenic *E. coli* (encoding haemolysins and pili), pathogenicity islands have now been found in a number of additional bacterial species (*H. pylori*, *V. cholerae*, *Salmonella* spp., *S. aureus* and *Yersinia* spp.). Such regions are not found in nonpathogenic bacteria, may be quite large (up to hundreds of kilobases) and may be unstable (spontaneously lost). Differences in DNA sequence (guanine+cytosine [G+C] content) between such elements and their host genomes and the presence of transposon-like genes support speculation regarding their origin and movement from unrelated bacterial species. The term *genomic island* has been given to DNA sequences similar to pathogenicity islands but not contributing directly to virulence or pathogenicity.

Integrons are mobile genetic elements that are able to use site-specific recombination to acquire new genes in cassette like fashion and express them in a coordinated manner (see Fig. 2.15C). Integrons lack terminal repeat sequences and certain genes characteristic of transposons but, similar to transposable elements, often carry genes associated with antibiotic resistance (see Fig. 34.5).

Another important type of mobile element includes staphylococcal cassette chromosomes (SCCs) such as SCC-*mec*, which not only encodes methicillin resistance but also serves as a recombinational hot spot for the acquisition of other mobile sequences. SCCs influencing virulence and antimicrobial resistance include SCC*capI*, encoding capsular polysaccharide I and SCC$_{476}$ and SCC*mercury*, conferring resistance to fusidic acid and mercury, respectively. The arginine catabolic mobile element (ACME) is a cassette like element potentially contributing to the virulence of the important USA300 community-associated methicillin-resistant *S. aureus* (MRSA) strain originally reported in the United States but now globally disseminated. An example of the interrelationship between the bacterial core genome and additional mobile genetic elements is depicted in Fig. 2.16.

**Fig. 2.16** Linear depiction of the interrelationship between the USA300 methicillin-resistant *Staphylococcus aureus* (MRSA) core genome and key mobile genetic elements SCC*mec*, arginine catabolic mobile element (ACME), two different bacteriophages, two different genomic islands and a pathogenicity island encoding antibiotic resistance and a variety of virulence factors.

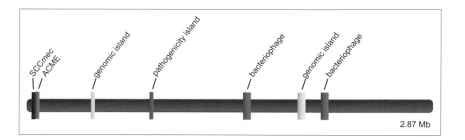

# MUTATION AND GENE TRANSFER

Bacteria are haploid organisms, their chromosomes containing one copy of each gene. Replication of the DNA is a precise process resulting in each daughter cell acquiring an exact copy of the parental genome. Changes in the genome can occur by two processes: mutation and recombination. These processes result in progeny with phenotypic characteristics that may differ from those of the parent. This is of considerable significance in terms of virulence and drug resistance.

## Mutation

### Changes in the nucleotide sequence of DNA can occur spontaneously or under the influence of external agents

While mutations may occur spontaneously as a result of errors in the DNA replication process, a variety of chemicals (mutagens) brings about direct changes in the DNA molecule. A classic example of such an interaction involves compounds known as *nucleotide-base analogues*. These agents mimic normal nucleotides during DNA synthesis but are capable of multiple pairing with a counterpart on the opposite strand. While 5-bromouracil is considered a thymine analogue, for example, it may also behave as a cytosine, thus allowing the potential for a change from T–A to C–G in a replicating DNA duplex. Other agents may cause changes by inserting (intercalating) and distorting the DNA helix or by interacting directly with nucleotide bases to alter them chemically.

Regardless of their cause, changes in DNA may generally be characterized as follows:

- Point mutations—changes in single nucleotides, which alter the triplet code. Such mutations may result in:
  - no change in the amino acid sequence of the protein encoded by the gene because the different codons specify the same amino acid and are therefore silent mutations
  - an amino acid substitution in the translated protein (missense mutation), which may or may not alter its stability or functional properties
  - the formation of a STOP codon, causing premature termination and production of a truncated protein (nonsense mutation).
- More comprehensive changes in the DNA, which involve deletion, replacement, insertion or inversion of several or many bases. The majority of these changes are likely to harm the organism, but some may be beneficial and confer a selective advantage through the production of different proteins.

### Bacterial cells are not defenceless against genetic damage

As the bacterial genome is the most fundamental molecule of identity in the cell, enzymatic machinery is in place to protect it against both spontaneously occurring and induced mutational damage. As illustrated in Fig. 2.17, these DNA repair processes include the following:

- Direct repair, which either reverses or simply removes the damage. This may be regarded as first-line defence. For example, abnormally linked pyrimidine bases in DNA (pyrimidine dimers) resulting from ultraviolet radiation are directly reversed by a light-dependent enzyme through a repair process known as *photoreactivation*.
- Excision repair in which damage in a DNA strand is recognized by an enzymatic housekeeping process and excised, followed by repair polymerization to fill the gap using the intact complementary DNA strand as a template. This is also a primary form of defence, as the goal is to correct damage before it encounters and potentially interferes with the moving DNA replication fork. Some of these housekeeping genes are also part of an inducible system (SOS repair), which is activated by the presence of DNA damage to quickly respond and effect repair.
- Second-line repair, which operates when DNA damage has reached a point where it is more difficult to correct. When normal DNA replication processes are blocked, permissive systems may allow the interfering damage to be inaccurately corrected, allowing errors to occur but improving the probability of cell survival. In other instances in which damage has passed the DNA replication fork, postreplication or recombinational repair processes may cut and paste to construct error-free DNA from multiple copies of the sequence found in parental and daughter strands.

### Bacterial DNA repair has provided a model for understanding similar, more complex processes in humans

DNA repair mechanisms appear to be present in all living organisms as a defence against environmental damage. The study of these processes in bacteria has led to an important understanding of general principles that apply to higher organisms, including issues of cancer and aging in humans. For example, several human disorders are known to be DNA-repair related, including:

- xeroderma pigmentosum, characterized by extreme sensitivity to the sun, with great risk for development of a variety of skin cancers such as basal cell carcinoma, squamous cell carcinoma and melanoma
- Cockayne syndrome, characterized by progressive neurologic degeneration, growth retardation and sun sensitivity not associated with cancer
- trichothiodystrophy, characterized by mental and growth retardation, fragile hair deficient in sulphur and sun sensitivity not associated with cancer.

## Gene transfer and recombination

New genotypes can arise when genetic material is transferred from one bacterium to another. In such instances, the newly transferred DNA is expressed when it:

- inserts into or recombines with the genome of the recipient cell
- is on a plasmid capable of replication in the recipient without recombination.

Recombination can bring about large changes in the genetic material and, as these events usually involve functional genes, they are likely to be expressed phenotypically. DNA can be transferred from a donor cell to a recipient cell by transformation, transduction and conjugation.

**Fig. 2.17** Mechanisms of DNA repair.

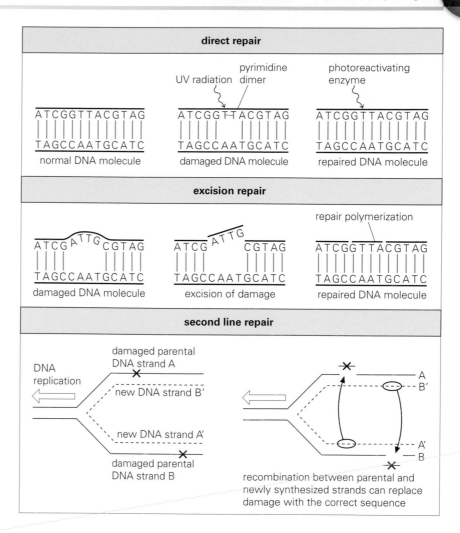

## Transformation

### Some bacteria can be transformed by DNA present in their environment

Certain bacteria such as *S. pneumoniae*, *Bacillus subtilis*, *Haemophilus influenzae* and *Neisseria gonorrhoeae* are naturally competent to take up DNA fragments from related species across their cell walls. Such DNA fragments may result from lysis of organisms, the release of their DNA and its cleavage into smaller fragments, which are then available for uptake by available (competent) recipient cells. Once taken into the cell, chromosomal DNA must recombine with a homologous segment of the recipient's chromosome to be stably maintained and inherited. If the DNA is completely unrelated, the absence of homology prevents recombination and the DNA is degraded. However, plasmid DNA may be transformed into a cell and expressed without recombination. Thus transformation has served as a powerful tool for molecular genetic analysis of bacteria (Fig. 2.18).

Most bacteria are not naturally competent to be transformed by DNA, but competence can be induced artificially by treating cells with certain bivalent cations and then subjecting them to a heat shock at 42°C or by electric shock treatment (electroporation).

Prior to uptake by competent cells, DNA is extracellular, unprotected and thus vulnerable to destruction by environmental extremes (e.g. DNA-degrading enzymes [DNases]). Thus it is the least important mechanism of gene transfer from the standpoint of clinical relevance (e.g. probability of transfer within a patient).

## Transduction

### Transduction involves the transfer of genetic material by infection with a bacteriophage

During the process of virulent bacteriophage replication (or temperate bacteriophage direct replication upon infection, rather than lysogeny), other DNA in the cell (genomic or plasmid) is occasionally erroneously packaged into the virus head, resulting in a transducing particle that can attach to and transfer the DNA it contains into a recipient cell. If chromosomal, the DNA must be incorporated into the recipient genome by homologous recombination to be stably inherited and expressed. As with transformation, plasmid DNA may be transduced and expressed in a recipient without recombination. In either case, this type of gene transfer is known as *generalized transduction* (see Fig. 2.18).

Another form of transduction occurs with temperate bacteriophages since they may integrate at specialized attachment sites in the bacterial genome. As the resulting prophages prepare to enter the lytic cycle, they occasionally incorrectly excise from the site of attachment. This can result

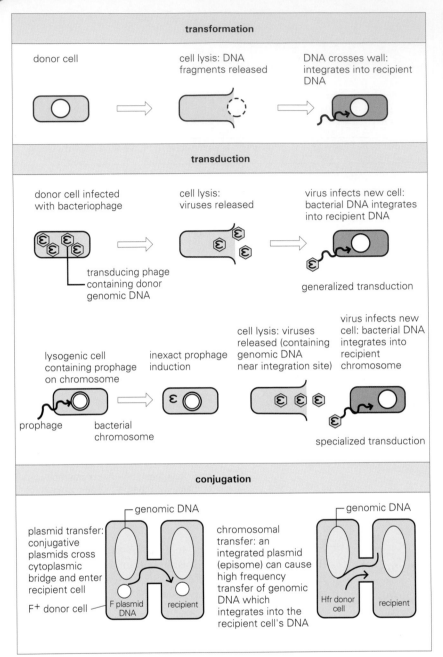

**Fig. 2.18** Different ways in which genes can be transferred between bacteria. With the exception of plasmid transfer, donor DNA integrates into the recipient's genome by a process of either homologous or illegitimate (in the case of transposons) recombination.

in phages containing a piece of bacterial genomic DNA adjacent to the attachment site. Infection of a recipient cell then results in a high frequency of recombinants in which the donor DNA carried by the phage has recombined with the recipient genome in the vicinity of the attachment site. As this specialized transduction is based on specific chromosome–prophage interaction, only genomic DNA (not plasmids) is transferred by this process.

In contrast to transformation, transduced DNA is always protected, thus increasing its probability of successful transfer and potential clinical relevance. Bacteriophages are extremely host-specific parasites, however, and, therefore, they are unable to move any DNA between bacteria of different species.

## Conjugation

### Conjugation is a type of bacterial mating in which DNA is transferred from one bacterium to another

Conjugation is dependent upon the *tra* genes found in conjugative plasmids, which, among other things, encode instructions for the bacterial cell to produce a sex pilus—a tubelike appendage that allows cell-to-cell contact to ensure the protected transfer of a plasmid DNA copy from a donor cell to a recipient (see Fig. 2.18). Because the *tra* genes take up genetic space, conjugative plasmids are generally larger than nonconjugative ones.

Occasionally conjugative plasmids such as the fertility plasmid (F plasmid or F factor) of *E. coli* integrate into the bacterial genome (e.g. facilitated by identical IS elements on both molecules as noted earlier), and such integrated plasmids are called *episomes*. When an integrated F episome attempts conjugative transfer, the duplication-transfer process eventually moves into regions of adjacent genomic DNA, which are carried along from the donor cell into the recipient. Such strains, in contrast to cells containing the unintegrated F plasmid, mediate high-frequency transfer and recombination of genomic DNA (Hfr strains). However, conjugation with Hfr donor cells does not result in complete transfer of the integrated plasmid. Thus the recipient cell does not become Hfr and is incapable of serving as a conjugation donor. The circular nature of the bacterial genome and the relative map positions of different genes were established using interrupted mating of Hfr strains.

When a nonconjugative plasmid is present in the same cell as a conjugative plasmid, they are sometimes transferred together into the recipient cell by the process of mobilization. Conjugative transfer of plasmids with resistance genes has been an important cause of the spread of resistance to commonly used antibiotics within and between many bacterial species since no recombination is required for expression in the recipient. Of all the mechanisms for gene transfer, this rapid and highly efficient movement of genetic information through bacterial populations is clearly of the highest clinical relevance.

## THE GENOMICS OF MEDICALLY IMPORTANT BACTERIA

Bacteria have been historically identified and characterized by phenotypic methods. However, advances in molecular biology have now focused attention on analysis of the bacterial genome as it represents the ultimate source of information regarding bacterial identity, potential for pathogenicity, etc.

### Various targeted approaches to the detection and utilization of genomic sequence information exist

Methods such as the polymerase chain reaction (PCR) and nucleic acid probes have clearly had a pivotal role in providing sequence-based answers to clinical microbiology questions (see Ch. 37).

- *Identification and classification.* The genes encoding ribosomal RNA (16 S, 23 S, 5 S) are typically found together in an operon in which their transcription is coordinated (Fig. 2.19). This rDNA operon is found at least once and often in multiple copies distributed around the chromosome, depending on the bacterial species. (*Borrelia burgdorferi* has one copy; *Clostridioides* [*Clostridium*] *difficile* may have up to 12 copies.) While the rDNA operon contains many conserved sequences (identical in different bacterial species), a portion of the 16 S- and 23 S-encoding regions have been found to be species specific. In between them, an internally transcribed spacer (ITS) region exhibits

sequence variability that may be analysed in PCR products providing utility in differentiating closely related bacterial isolates. Such information may also allow the rapid identification, classification and epidemiology of clinically important microorganisms (see Chs. 32 and 37).

- *Resistance to antimicrobial agents.* Genes specifically mediating antimicrobial resistance are well known (see Ch. 34) and may be detected by a variety of targeted genomic approaches, including PCR and probes.

- *Molecular epidemiology.* While a variety of phenotypic and genotypic methods have been employed to assess interrelationships in clinical isolates (see Ch. 37), epidemiologic analysis has now moved to sequence-based approaches. In contrast to earlier methods, sequence data are highly portable (internet transfer, etc.), less ambiguous (encoded entirely in the characters A, T, G and C that corresponds to the four bases adenine, thymine, guanine and cytosine, respectively) and easily stored in databases.

### Microarrays provide a more global targeted genomic analysis

DNA microarrays are a means for the parallel processing of genomic information. Traditionally molecular biology has operated by analysing one gene in one experiment. Although yielding important information, this approach is time consuming and does not afford ready access to the information (chromosomal organization and multiple-gene interaction) contained within genomic-sequence databases. Microarrays acquire information from multiple queries simultaneously posed to a genomic sequence database (parallel processing). DNA microarrays are based on the principles of nucleic hybridization (A pairs with T; G pairs with C). Although there are a number of variations on the theme, the general format is the arrangement of samples (e.g. gene sequences) in a known matrix on a solid support (nylon, glass, etc.). Using specialized robotics, individual spots may be less than 200 mm in diameter, allowing a single array (often called a *DNA chip*) to contain thousands of spots. Different fluorescently labelled probes of known sequence may then be simultaneously applied followed by monitoring to detect whether complementary binding has occurred.

### DNA microarrays have been especially useful in the identification of mutations and studies on bacterial gene expression

In a number of instances, specific point mutations are clinically important in pathogenic bacteria. Since these changes involve only one nucleotide base, they are often referred to as *single nucleotide polymorphisms (SNPs)*. Resistance to the quinolone class of antibiotics, for example, may result from a single base change within the bacterial *gyrA* gene (see

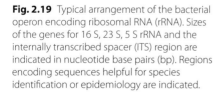

**Fig. 2.19** Typical arrangement of the bacterial operon encoding ribosomal RNA (rRNA). Sizes of the genes for 16 S, 23 S, 5 S rRNA and the internally transcribed spacer (ITS) region are indicated in nucleotide base pairs (bp). Regions encoding sequences helpful for species identification or epidemiology are indicated.

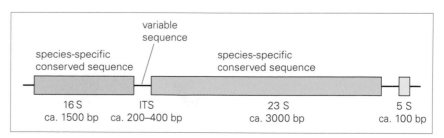

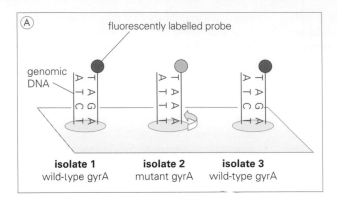

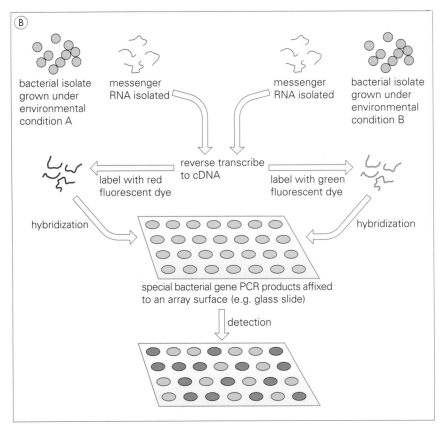

**Fig. 2.20** (A) Microarray detection of mutations and (B) analysis of gene expression. cDNA, complementary DNA synthesized from RNA.

Ch. 34). In the past, such mutations have been detected by PCR amplification of the desired *gyrA* region followed by DNA sequencing and analysis. As illustrated in Fig. 2.20A, DNA microarrays allow *gyrA* amplicons from different bacterial isolates to be applied to the same chip. Two *gyrA* probes (wild type, fluorescently labelled red; mutant, fluorescently labelled green) are applied to the array under conditions so stringent that only 100% homology will result in hybridization. In this way the presence or absence of the specific mutation may be quickly and accurately assessed in a large number of isolates simultaneously.

Studies of gene expression are extremely important to the understanding of numerous bacterial processes, including virulence. For example, analysis might involve a comparison of gene expression (transcription) in an organism under different environmental conditions (see Fig. 2.20B). In such an experiment, genomics can provide data allowing sequences from every known chromosomal gene of the organism to be applied to a unique position on the chip. mRNA (the result

of gene expression) may be isolated from the same bacteria grown under either environmental condition A or B. Using the enzyme reverse transcriptase in a process similar to that naturally employed by retroviruses (see Ch. 3), the mRNA is copied into complementary DNA (termed *cDNA*). Different fluorescent dyes (red or green) are bound to the A or B cDNA, respectively, which is then allowed to hybridize to complementary sequences on the chip. Array spots with red fluorescence will indicate genes expressed in environment A, those appearing green will correspond to genes active in environment B and yellow spots (red + green) will indicate genes active under both conditions.

### Sequence of the entire bacterial chromosome (whole genome sequencing) represents the most global approach to genomic analysis

Targeted sequence-based genomic analysis continues to be of great value in providing results rapidly and comparatively inexpensively. However, the specific nature of these assays is also a limitation since only previously identified genomic regions can be analysed, whereas uncharacterized potentially novel genomic sequences are not detected or investigated. Conversely, whole genome sequencing (WGS) data encompass both characterized and uncharacterized regions of an organism's genome, which may be reanalysed in light of new data to provide information on novel, previously untargeted gene presence and function. Since the first complete bacterial genome sequence was published in 1995, advances in DNA-sequencing techniques have led to a myriad of bacterial pathogens for which the total genomic sequence is known and recorded in the NCBI RefSeq database (https://www.ncbi.nlm.nih.gov/refseq/) (Fig. 2.21). This evolving database represents a powerful resource with enormous application for the understanding and treatment of infectious disease.

### WGS methods continue to evolve in what has been described as generational increments

The scientific literature is somewhat confusing on this issue. The most historically used method for sequencing individual PCR products a few hundred bases in length was developed by Frederick Sanger in 1977. Sanger sequencing is generally considered a first-generation approach. Subsequent next-generation (i.e. next-gen) approaches (more applicable to WGS) have sometimes also been described as second-generation (e.g. parallel sequencing of a group of DNA molecules) or third-generation (sequencing of longer single DNA molecules) approaches.

### Current WGS methods have some common challenges

Current WGS approaches have three basic steps in common (although the specific details differ):

- DNA library preparation
- sequencing
- sequence analysis.

It is important to note that these steps are not fully automated or push-button in nature. Proper preparation of high-quality genomic DNA (i.e. the library) from the organism to be sequenced is critical for a meaningful outcome. The way in which this is accomplished depends on the requirements of the specific DNA-sequencing method. Regardless of the approach, however, the ultimate end product is a computer file containing the sequence data. Thus a computerized approach to sequence analysis is necessary, which can be visualized as having two goals:

- to construct the whole genome as accurately as possible by connecting generated sequences together (assembly)
- genetic analysis of the WGS (i.e. identification of specific genes or gene changes and other genetic signatures of interest).

Depending on the instrumentation, generated sequence lengths (read lengths) may range from several hundred to tens or even hundreds of thousands of base pairs. Since this is less than the total genome size, the sequence reads must be connected to produce the WGS. This is accomplished by computer programs that either identify common overlapping regions in sequence reads (de novo assembly) or connect reads together using a closely related reference genome as a template (reference mapping) (Fig. 2.22A and B, respectively). Ensuring proper quality control (e.g., sequence error rates) is very important but beyond discussion here.

The identification of specific genes, gene changes, and other important genomic information from WGS data is termed *bioinformatics* and involves extensive computer analysis. This is currently the most challenging aspect of WGS data interpretation. There is an intense effort to develop user-friendly software for this purpose, which has currently resulted in an expanding list of free standalone and commercially available software packages dedicated to this purpose. As will be discussed more thoroughly in subsequent chapters (e.g. Ch. 37), bioinformatic analysis has demonstrated that bacterial genomes can be subdivided into core and accessory regions. The core genome represents conserved genes that are found in all members of a bacterial species, while the presence or absence of accessory genomic regions is variable. Taken together, all the core and variable sequences found in members of a bacterial species are termed the *pan-genome*, which is finding increasing use in identifying microorganisms present in specific (e.g. human, environmental) settings (i.e. metagenomics).

### Major groups of bacteria

Detailed summaries of members of the major bacterial groups are given in the Pathogen Parade appendix available online.

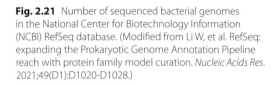

**Fig. 2.21** Number of sequenced bacterial genomes in the National Center for Biotechnology Information (NCBI) RefSeq database. (Modified from Li W, et al. RefSeq: expanding the Prokaryotic Genome Annotation Pipeline reach with protein family model curation. *Nucleic Acids Res*. 2021;49(D1):D1020-D1028.)

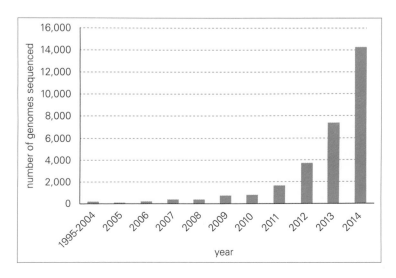

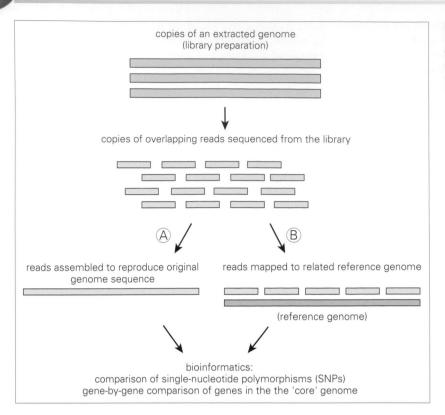

copies of an extracted genome
(library preparation)

copies of overlapping reads sequenced from the library

Ⓐ     Ⓑ

reads assembled to reproduce original
genome sequence

reads mapped to related reference genome

(reference genome)

bioinformatics:
comparison of single-nucleotide polymorphisms (SNPs)
gene-by-gene comparison of genes in the the 'core' genome

**Fig. 2.22** Illustration of the principal steps involved in whole genome sequencing analysis. Overlapping genomic sequences (reads) are ordered and analysed either following (A) de novo sequence assembly or (B) reference mapping to a related genomic template.

## KEY FACTS

- Bacteria are prokaryotes. Their DNA is not contained within a nucleus, and there are relatively few cytoplasmic organelles.

- The cell wall is a key structure in metabolism, virulence and immunity. Its staining characteristics define the two major divisions: the gram-positive and gram-negative bacteria. Flagella may be present and confer motility.

- Bacteria metabolize aerobically and anaerobically and can utilize a range of substrates.

- The bacterial cell walls and their reproductive processes are targets for antimicrobial agents.

- Transcription of bacterial DNA may involve single or multiple genes. The arrangement of promoter and terminal sequences flanking multiple genes forms an operon.

- Bacteria can regulate gene expression to optimize exploitation of their environment.

- Plasmids and bacteriophages are independently replicating extrachromosomal agents. Plasmids may carry genes that affect resistance to antimicrobials or virulence.

- Genetic material can be carried from one bacterium to another in several ways; this can result in the rapid spread of resistance to antimicrobials.

- Genomics is revolutionizing the study of bacterial pathogenicity and the control of associated infections.

## CONFLICTS

Bacteria have many ways of coming out on top in the conflict with the host. A number of them produce highly resistant spores that can survive for long periods in the external world, increasing the chances of infection. Once in the host, there are many ways of evading host responses. For example, some hide within cells, some have external surfaces that prevent host cells from binding to them and others suppress host immunity. Perhaps the most significant advantage bacteria have in their conflict with the host is their ability to sidestep the antibiotics designed to inhibit or eliminate them. Either by mutation, facilitated by their rapid generation/duplication time, or by externally acquired genetic information, they are able to engage in a game of cat and mouse in which repeated introduction of new and improved antimicrobial compounds is met with equally innovative mechanisms of resistance. A classic example of this interaction is seen with the gram-positive bacterium *Staphylococcus aureus*. Although initially susceptible to penicillin, introduced in the 1950s, subsequent development and spread of resistant organisms rendered the antibiotic ineffective. This was countered with the introduction of methicillin in the 1980s, leading to the development of methicillin-resistant *S. aureus* (MRSA), which has now been followed by isolates with resistance to the historically effective antibiotic vancomycin. Unfortunately, a survival-of-the-fittest environment ensures the perpetuation of this conflict, underscoring the importance of the continued development of novel antimicrobial agents.

# The viruses

## Introduction

Viruses differ from all other infectious organisms in their structure and biology, particularly in their reproduction. Although viruses carry conventional genetic information in their DNA or RNA, they lack the synthetic machinery necessary for this information to be processed into new virus material. Viruses are metabolically inert and can replicate only after infecting a host cell and parasitizing the host's ability to transcribe and/or translate genetic information. Viruses infect every form of life. They cause some of the most common and many of the most serious diseases of humans, including cancer. Some insert their genetic material into the human genome, and others can remain latent in different cell types and then reactivate at any time but especially if the body is stressed or the immune system is compromised. Viruses are difficult targets for antiviral agents as it is difficult to target only those cells infected by the virus; however, many can be controlled by vaccines.

## MAJOR GROUPS OF VIRUSES

The classification of viruses into major groups (families) is based on a few simple criteria (see Pathogen Parade available online). These include:

- the type of nucleic acid in the genome
- the number of nucleic acid strands and their polarity
- the mode of replication
- the size, structure and symmetry of the virus particle.

### Viruses share some common structural features

Viruses range from very small (parvovirus, from the Latin *parvus,* meaning "small," at 18–26 nm in diameter) to quite large (vaccinia virus, at 400 nm, is as big as small bacteria). Their genomic organization varies considerably between the different groups, but there are some general characteristics common to all:

- The genetic material, in the form of single-stranded (ss) or double-stranded (ds) or linear or circular RNA or DNA is contained within a coat or capsid made up of a number of individual protein molecules (capsomeres).
- The complete unit of nucleic acid and capsid is called the *nucleocapsid* and often has a distinctive symmetry depending upon the ways in which the individual capsomeres are assembled (Fig. 3.1). Symmetry can be icosahedral, helical or complex.
- In many cases, the entire virus particle (virion) consists only of a nucleocapsid. In others, the virion consists of the nucleocapsid surrounded by an outer envelope or membrane (Fig. 3.2). This is generally a lipid bilayer of host cell origin into which virus proteins are inserted.

### The outer surface of the virus particle is the part that first makes contact with the membrane of the host cell

The structure and properties of the outer surface of the virus particle are therefore of vital importance in understanding the process of infection. In general, naked (envelope-free) viruses

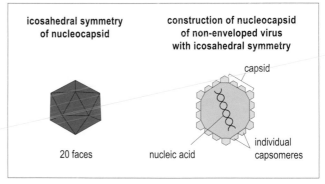

**Fig. 3.1** Symmetry and construction of the viral nucleocapsid.

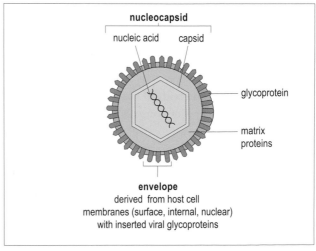

**Fig. 3.2** Assembly of an enveloped virus.

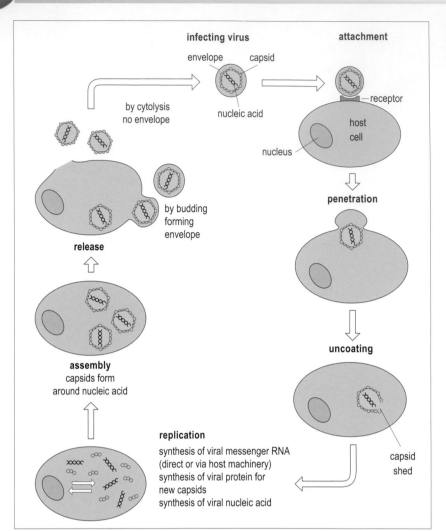

**Fig. 3.3** Stages in the infection of a host's cell and replication of a virus. Several thousand virus particles may be formed from each cell.

are resistant and survive well in the outside world; they may also be acid and bile resistant, allowing infection through the gastrointestinal tract. Enveloped viruses are more susceptible to environmental factors such as drying, gastric acidity and bile. These differences in susceptibility influence the ways in which these viruses can be transmitted and the cells they infect.

## INFECTION OF HOST CELLS

The stages involved in infection of host cells are summarized in Fig. 3.3.

### Virus particles enter the body of the host in many ways

The most common forms of virus transmission (Fig. 3.4; see also Ch. 14) are:

- via inhaled droplets (e.g. rhinovirus, influenza viruses, coronaviruses)
- in food or water (e.g. hepatitis A virus, hepatitis E virus, noroviruses)
- by direct transfer from other infected hosts such as infected body fluids by sexual transmission or blood-borne routes (e.g. human immunodeficiency virus [HIV], hepatitis B virus, Ebola virus)
- from bites of vector arthropods (e.g. yellow fever virus, West Nile virus, Zika virus).

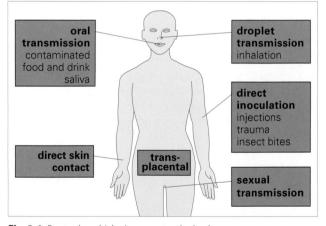

**Fig. 3.4** Routes by which viruses enter the body.

### Viruses show host specificity and usually infect only one or a restricted range of host species. The initial basis of specificity is the ability of the virus particle to attach to the host cell

The process of attachment to, or adsorption by, a host cell depends on general intermolecular forces, then on more specific interactions between the molecules of the

**Table 3.1** Viruses may use more than one receptor to gain entry into the host cell

| Cell membrane receptors for virus attachment | |
|---|---|
| **Virus** | **Receptor molecule** |
| Influenza | Sialic acid receptor on lung epithelial cells and upper respiratory tract |
| Rabies | Acetylcholine receptor Neuronal cell adhesion molecule |
| Human immunodeficiency virus | CD4: primary receptor CCR5 or CXCR4: chemokine receptors |
| Epstein-Barr virus | CD21 (also called CR2) receptor on B cells |
| Human parvovirus B19 | P antigen on erythoid progenitor cells Ku80 antoantigen and α5β1 integrin proposed coreceptors |
| Hepatitis C virus | Scavenger receptor class B, CD81, claudin-1, occluding and very-low-density lipoprotein receptors are host cofactors for viral entry |
| Human rhinoviruses A and B | Intercellular adhesion molecule 1 Low-density lipoprotein receptor |
| Human rhinovirus C | Cadherin-related family member 3—a cell surface protein involved in cell communication |

nucleocapsid in unenveloped viruses or the virus membrane in enveloped viruses, and the molecules of the host cell membrane. In many cases there is a specific interaction with a particular host molecule, which therefore acts as a receptor. This is called *tropism* and is receptor dependent or independent and starts at cell entry. Influenza virus, for example, attaches by its haemagglutinin to a glycoprotein (sialic acid) found on cells of mucous membranes and on red blood cells; other examples are given in Table 3.1. Attachment to the receptor is followed by entry into the host cell.

After fusion of viral and host membranes or uptake into a phagosome, the virus particle is carried into the cytoplasm across the plasma membrane. At this stage, the envelope and/or the capsid is shed and the viral nucleic acid released. The virus is now no longer infective: this eclipse phase persists until new complete virus particles reform after replication. The way in which replication occurs is determined by the nature of the nucleic acid concerned.

## REPLICATION

### Viruses must first synthesize messenger RNA

Viruses contain either DNA or RNA. The nucleic acids are present as single or double strands in a linear (DNA or RNA) or circular (DNA) form. The viral genome may be carried on a single molecule of nucleic acid or on several molecules. With these options, it is not surprising that the process of replication in the host cell is also diverse. In viruses containing DNA, messenger RNA (mRNA) can be

formed using the host's own RNA polymerase to transcribe directly from the viral DNA. The RNA of viruses cannot be transcribed in this way, as host polymerases copy or make RNA from DNA. If RNA-dependent transcription is necessary, the virus must provide its own polymerases. These may be carried in the nucleocapsid or may be synthesized after infection.

### RNA viruses produce mRNA by several different routes

dsRNA viruses contain a negative (–) and a positive (+) sense strand, and the + strand is used directly as mRNA (Fig. 3.5). In ssRNA viruses there are three distinct routes to the formation of mRNA:

1. Where the single strand has the + sense configuration, meaning it has the same base sequence as that required for translation, it can be used directly as mRNA.
2. Where the strand has the negative (–) sense configuration, it must first be transcribed using viral polymerase into a positive sense strand, which can then act as mRNA.
3. Retroviruses follow a completely different route. Their positive sense ssRNA is first made into a negative sense ssDNA, using the viral reverse transcriptase enzyme carried in the nucleocapsid, and dsDNA is then formed, which enters the nucleus and becomes integrated into the host genome. This integrated viral DNA is then transcribed by host polymerase into mRNA.

### Viral mRNA is then translated in the host cytoplasm to produce viral proteins

Once viral mRNA has been formed, it is translated using host ribosomes to synthesize viral proteins (Fig. 3.6). Viral mRNA, which is usually monocistronic, has a single coding region and uses different mechanisms to favour its translation over that of host mRNA from ribosomes so that viral products are synthesized preferentially. In the early phase, the proteins produced are enzymes (regulatory molecules) that will allow subsequent replication of viral nucleic acids; in the later phase, the proteins necessary for capsid formation are produced.

In viruses in which the genome is a single nucleic acid molecule, translation produces a large multifunctional protein, a polyprotein, which is then cleaved enzymatically to produce a number of distinct proteins. In viruses in which the genome is distributed over a number of molecules, several mRNAs are produced, each being translated into separate proteins. After translation, the proteins may be glycosylated, again using host enzymes.

### Viruses must also replicate their nucleic acid

In addition to producing molecules for the formation of new capsids, the virus must replicate its nucleic acid to provide genetic material for packaging into these capsids, resulting in new virions. This process uses viral RNA polymerases.

In positive sense ssRNA viruses such as poliovirus, a polymerase translated from viral mRNA produces negative sense RNA from the positive sense template, which is then transcribed repeatedly into more positive strands. Further cycles of transcription then occur, resulting in the production of very large numbers of positive strands, which are

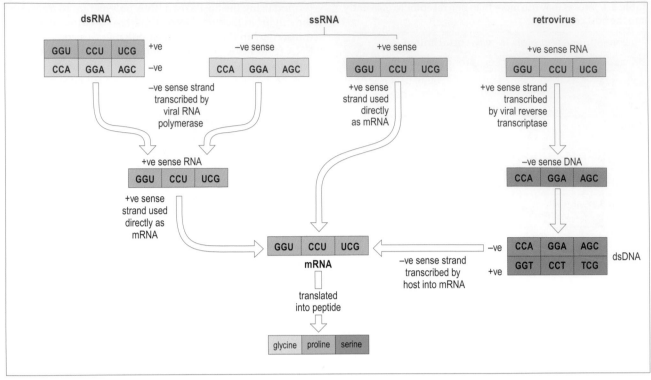

**Fig. 3.5** Ways in which genomic RNA of RNA viruses can be transcribed into messenger RNA (mRNA) before translation into proteins. ds, Double-stranded; ss, single-stranded; +ve, positive sense; −ve, negative sense.

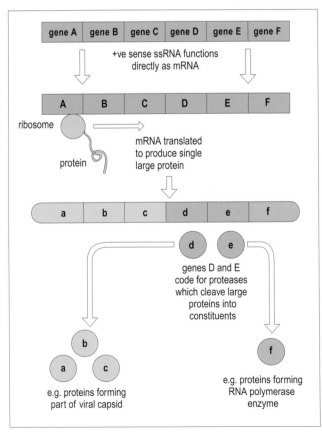

**Fig. 3.6** Translation of viral proteins from messenger RNA (mRNA) and cleavage of viral proteins. +ve, Positive sense; ss, single stranded.

packaged into new particles using structural proteins translated earlier from mRNA (Fig. 3.7).

In negative sense ssRNA viruses, such as rabies virus, transcription by viral polymerase produces positive sense RNA strands for translation into proteins. Some of these proteins are polymerases, which will transcribe the positive sense RNA into new negative sense RNA (see Fig. 3.7) ready to be packaged into new virions. Rabies virus RNA replication occurs in the host cell cytoplasm, but in others, such as measles and influenza virus, RNA replication takes place within the nucleus—large numbers of negative sense RNA molecules being transcribed for packaging into new particles. Nucleic acid replication follows a similar pattern in dsRNA viruses such as rotavirus in that positive sense RNA strands are produced. These then act as templates in a subviral particle for the synthesis of new negative sense strands, which will be packaged with the positive strand as dsRNA in the new virions.

### Replication of viral DNA occurs in the host nucleus—except for poxviruses, where it takes place in the cytoplasm

Viral DNA may become complexed with host histones to produce stable structures. With herpesviruses, mRNA translated in the cytoplasm produces a DNA polymerase that is necessary for the synthesis of new viral DNA; adenoviruses use both viral and host enzymes for this purpose. With retroviruses such as HIV, synthesis of new viral RNA occurs in the nucleus, where the viral DNA that has become integrated into the host genome is transcribed by the host RNA polymerase (see Fig. 3.5). Hepatitis B virus, a partially dsDNA

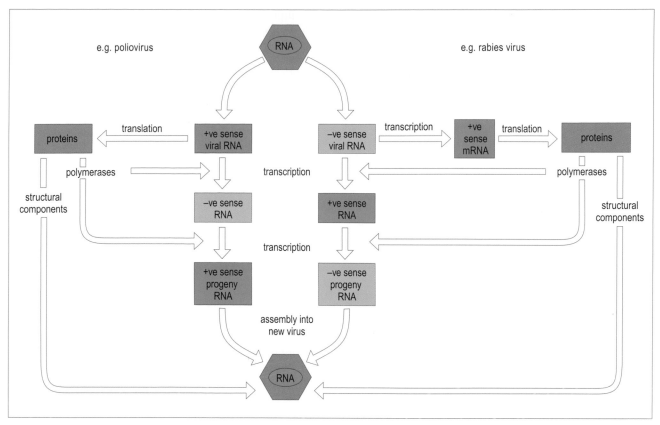

e.g. poliovirus

e.g. rabies virus

**Fig. 3.7** The ways in which genomic RNA of RNA viruses is replicated. +ve, Positive sense; –ve, negative sense; mRNA, messenger RNA.

virus, is unique in using an ssRNA intermediate transcribed from its DNA to synthesize new DNA. Retroviruses and hepatitis B are the only viruses affecting humans that have reverse transcriptase activity (i.e. can copy RNA into DNA).

### The final stage of replication is assembly and release of new virus particles

Assembly of virus particles involves the association of replicated nucleic acid with newly synthesized capsomeres to form a new nucleocapsid. This may take place in the cytoplasm or in the nucleus of the host cell. Enveloped viruses go through a further stage before release. Envelope proteins and glycoproteins, translated from viral mRNA, are inserted into areas of the host cell membrane (usually the plasma membrane). The progeny nucleocapsids associate specifically with the membrane in these areas, via the glycoproteins, and bud through it (Fig. 3.8). The new virus acquires the host cell membrane plus viral molecules as an outer envelope, and viral enzymes, such as the neuraminidase of influenza virus, may assist in this process (see details for influenza virus in Ch. 20). Host enzymes (e.g. cellular proteases) may cleave the initial large envelope proteins, a process that is necessary if the progeny viruses are to be infectious. In herpesviruses, acquisition of a membrane occurs as the nucleocapsids bud from the inner nuclear membrane. Release of enveloped viruses can occur without causing cell death so that infected cells continue to shed virus particles for long periods.

Insertion of viral molecules into the host cell membrane results in the host cell becoming antigenically different. Expression of viral antigens in this way is a major factor in the development of antiviral immune responses.

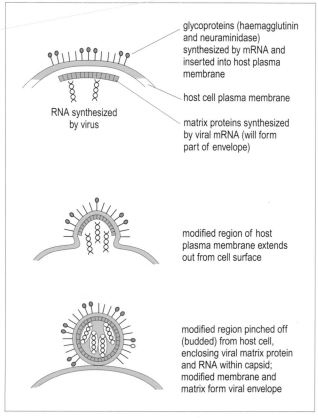

glycoproteins (haemagglutinin and neuraminidase) synthesized by mRNA and inserted into host plasma membrane

host cell plasma membrane

RNA synthesized by virus

matrix proteins synthesized by viral mRNA (will form part of envelope)

modified region of host plasma membrane extends out from cell surface

modified region pinched off (budded) from host cell, enclosing viral matrix protein and RNA within capsid; modified membrane and matrix form viral envelope

**Fig. 3.8** Release of enveloped RNA virus by budding through host cell membrane. Influenza A virus is shown in this example.

## OUTCOME OF VIRAL INFECTION

### Viral infections may cause cell lysis, become chronic or lie latent

In lytic infections the virus goes through a cycle of replication, producing many new virus particles. These are released by cell lysis. This host cell destruction is the typical consequence of infection with polio or influenza viruses. With other infections, such as hepatitis B, the cell may remain alive and continue to release virus particles at a slow rate. These chronic infections are of great epidemiologic importance, as the infected person may act as a symptomless carrier of the virus, providing a continuing source of infection (see Ch. 17). In both lytic and chronic infections, the virus undergoes replication. However, in latent infections, the virus remains quiescent, and the genetic material of the virus may:

- exist in the host cell cytoplasm, such as herpesvirus infections
- be incorporated into the genome, such as retrovirus and hepatitis B virus infections.

Replication does not take place until some signal triggers a release from latency. The stimuli that result in release are not fully understood in all cases. In herpes simplex infection, stress can activate the virus, resulting in an active infection seen as cold sores.

### Some viruses can transform the host cell into a tumour or cancer cell

Lytic, persistent and latent infections involve essentially healthy host cells, although cellular metabolic and regulatory processes can be severely disrupted. Some viruses, however, can transform the host cell, malignant transformation being the change of a differentiated host cell into a tumour or cancer cell (see Ch. 18). Transformed cells show changes in morphology, behaviour and biochemistry. Controlled growth patterns and contact inhibition are lost so that cells continue to divide and form random aggregations. They become invasive and can form tumours. The first human tumour virus was discovered in 1964 when Epstein-Barr virus (EBV) was found by electron microscopic analysis of cells of a tumour called *Burkitt lymphoma* seen in patients of African descent.

However, not all transformed cells give rise to harmful tumours in vivo. Warts, for example, may be benign growths on the skin of the hands or feet caused by one group of papillomaviruses, or genital warts caused by a different group of specific papillomaviruses may lead to cervical cancer.

Cancer-inducing (oncogenic) viruses are found in several different groups, including both DNA and RNA viruses. Of the seven oncogenic viruses affecting humans, which cause 15% of cancers, hepatitis B virus, human papillomaviruses (HPV), Merkel cell virus and human T-cell lymphotropic virus type 1 (HTLV-1) integrate and are therefore part of the host genome. Those that do not integrate are EBV, hepatitis C virus and human herpesvirus type 8 (HHV-8).

Cell proliferation is helped by genes called proto-oncogenes. If these change (e.g. a viral integration event occurs inside a cell cycle regulator gene in the infected cell), the cell can become activated continuously. The changed gene, referred to as an oncogene, causes cell overproliferation and can lead to cancer.

Although the end results of transformation may be similar, the mechanisms involved vary between different viruses. It is a multiple step model, and the end results of cell transformation are similar, but the mechanisms used by these different viruses are diverse and include immune modulation, induced expression of viral and cellular oncogenes and epigenetic changes. High throughput, whole genome sequencing has allowed host–pathogen sequence analysis identifying links between viral integration and changes in gene expression. These techniques demonstrated viral sequences in tumour genomes that, in 2008, resulted in detecting the Merkel cell virus causing Merkel cell carcinoma.

The mechanisms all involve interference with the normal regulation of cell division and response to external growth-promoting and -inhibiting factors. These epigenetic and genetic changes come about after viral nucleic acid is incorporated into the host genome. Finally, cancer is not always the result of some of these infections. Papillomaviruses are present in cervical cancer, but additional cellular events are needed for most of the other viral infections to result in tumours. A classic example is the Rous sarcoma virus, a retrovirus that causes cancer in chickens; 2011 was the 100-year anniversary of Francis Rous demonstrating that this chest tumour could be transmitted by giving tumour extracts that were cell free to chickens related to the same brood. Transformation arises from the introduction into the host genome of a viral oncogene, v-*src*. This codes for an activated and over-expressed protein—tyrosine kinase, an enzyme involved in the phosphorylation of tyrosine residues in target proteins. This leads to some molecular events and changes in phenotype in transformed host cells and subsequent tumorigenesis as a result of the viral infection. A urokinase-type plasminogen activator (PLAU) gene is induced by v-*src* and highly upregulated. PLAU is a protease enzyme that lyses fibrin and breaks down the extracellular matrix, promoting cancer cell adhesion and spread.

More than 20 retroviral oncogenes are now known (Table 3.2). Of the retrovirus family, HTLV-1 is a cancer-causing virus in humans despite neither possessing a viral oncogene nor directly activating a cellular oncogene (see later). In contrast, HIV type 1 and 2 virus infections compromise the host's immune system, resulting in tumours associated with other viruses, including EBV and Kaposi's sarcoma herpesvirus, also known as HHV-8. A larger number of retroviruses cause cancers in animals.

### Tumour formation as a result of viral infection: direct and indirect mechanisms

Viruses associated with cancer may do so by direct means, by expressing viral oncogenes that transform the cell as mentioned earlier. They may also do so indirectly by chronically infecting the cells resulting in inflammation and mutations that result in tumour formation. An example is hepatitis B that activates cell signalling pathways via the HBx oncoprotein.

### Viral oncogenes have probably arisen from incorporation of host oncogenes into the viral genome during viral replication

Oncogenes are designated by short acronyms, preceded by *v* if a viral oncogene is described (e.g. v-*myc*) or by *c* for a

**Table 3.2** Oncogenes, gene products, viruses known to carry them and associated human and animal diseases

| Examples of retroviral oncogenes | | | |
|---|---|---|---|
| **Class of gene product** | **Oncogene** | **Virus** | **Disease** |
| Tyrosine kinases | *fms* | FeLV | Sarcoma |
| | *ros* | ALV | |
| | *src* | ALV | |
| | *yes* | ALV | |
| Serine/threonine kinase | *mos* | MuLV | Sarcoma |
| Examples of human oncogenic viruses | | | |
| | *HBx* | Hepatitis B virus | Hepatocellular carcinoma |
| | *LMP-1, BARF-1* | Epstein-Barr virus | Burkitt lymphoma, B-cell lymphoma, nasopharyngeal carcinoma |
| | *vGPCR* | Human herpesvirus 8 | Kaposi sarcoma, primary effusion lymphoma |
| | *E6, E7* | Human papillomavirus | Cervical, anal, oral cancer |
| | *T antigens* | Merkel cell polyomavirus | Merkel cell carcinoma |
| | *Tax* | Human T-cell leukaemia lymphoma virus | Adult T-cell leukeamia/lymphoma |

ALV/FeLV/MuLV, Avian, feline and murine leukaemia viruses; HBx, hepatitis B x gene; LMP-1, latent membrane protein-1; BARF-1, BamH1-A Reading Frame-1; vGPCR, virus G protein-coupled receptor; E6, E7, early gene; T, tumour; Tax, transcriptional transactivator.

cellular (host) oncogene (e.g. c-*myc*). In HPV infection, recurrent integration of the HPV DNA in upstream regions of c-*myc* causes c-*myc* upregulation, resulting in proliferation and immortalisation of cells. This recurrent integration occurs in other oncogenes that have similar functions, such as *NOTCH1* and *ERBB2*, and tumour suppressor genes. The integration events may cause instability of the genome and resultant changes in gene expression.

Retroviral oncogene sequences can make up as much as 0.03–0.3% of the mammalian genome. Oncogene sequences have been identified in a wide variety of animals, from humans to fruit flies, suggesting that they are conserved because of some valuable function. Which came first, host or viral oncogenes? The fact that host oncogenes contain introns, whereas viral oncogenes do not, and that their chromosomal positions are fixed, implies that they, and not the viral forms, are the original genes.

From what we now know about the gene products of viral oncogenes, we can guess that cellular oncogenes (or proto-oncogenes) probably play an important role in host cell growth regulation. They may code for growth factors themselves, for cell surface receptor molecules that bind specific growth factors, for components of intracellular signalling systems or for gene expression regulatory molecules such as DNA-binding proteins that act as transcription factors.

The Rous sarcoma virus *src* oncogene is incorporated within the viral genome adjacent to the gene coding for viral envelope proteins (Fig. 3.9). Unlike other strongly transforming viruses, the Rous virus has all three genes (*gag, pol, env*) necessary for replication. In the others, termed defective transforming viruses, incorporation of an oncogene results in deletion of genetic material in the regions coding for the *pol* and/or *env* genes, so preventing replication. This becomes possible only with help from genetically complete helper viruses.

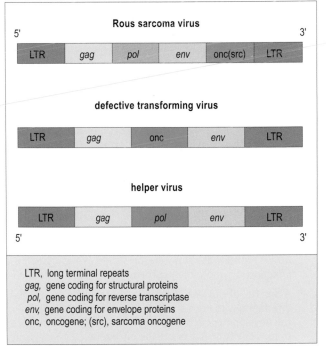

LTR, long terminal repeats
*gag*, gene coding for structural proteins
*pol*, gene coding for reverse transcriptase
*env*, gene coding for envelope proteins
onc, oncogene; (src), sarcoma oncogene

**Fig. 3.9** Rous sarcoma virus can transform the host cell and replicate because it has both the oncogene *src* and a complete genome. Some transforming viruses are defective—they carry the oncogene but lack genes for full replication. Helper viruses can supply these genes.

Oncogenes can be carried from one cell to another within the same host or from one host to another. This can occur through vertical transmission, from mother to baby, through passage of viruses in gametes, across the placenta, or in milk. It can also occur by horizontal transmission, the virus passing in, for example, saliva or urine (see Ch. 14).

Transformation of a cell occurs:

- when viral oncogenes are incorporated into the host genome (as in Rous sarcoma virus)
- when viral DNA is inserted near to a cellular oncogene
- when other mechanisms such as immune signalling, cell metabolism or genetic mutations exist.

Mutations in the oncogene sequence while in the viral genome may occur and single base changes in cellular oncogenes are known to confer the ability to transform normal cells. Viral DNA inserted near a host cell oncogene may alter the expression of that oncogene through disturbance of normal regulatory mechanisms. Altered expression can occur whether the insertion is of a retroviral oncogene or of non-oncogenic viral DNA; it can also occur as a result of exposure to a variety of carcinogens. The products of cellular oncogenes are normally used in series to regulate cellular proliferation in a carefully controlled manner. Viral oncogene products or overexpressed cellular oncogene products short-circuit and overload this complex control system resulting in unregulated cell division.

## KEY FACTS

- Viruses have RNA or DNA but absolutely depend on the host to process their genetic information into new virus particles.

- The outer surface of a virus (capsid or envelope) is essential for host cell contact and entry and determines the capacity to survive in the outside world.

- Viruses can be transmitted in droplets, in food and water, or by intimate contact.

- Replication of viral RNA or DNA is a complex process, making use of host and/or viral enzymes.

- RNA of retroviruses becomes integrated into the host genome.

- New virus particles are released by cell lysis or by budding through the host cell membrane.

- Some viruses, such as herpesviruses, may become latent and require a trigger to resume replication; others replicate at a slow rate, persisting as a source of infection in symptomless carriers.

- A number of viruses transform the host cell by interfering with normal cellular regulation, resulting in the development of a cancer cell. This may be the result of the activity of viral or cellular oncogenes.

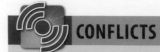

## CONFLICTS

Viruses have developed a cunning strategy as hardy infectious agents as, once they have infected the host cell, they may lie latent or integrate within the host cell DNA and reactivate, potentially transmitting the infection to others. The host may not be too incapacitated, ensuring they can infect those susceptible. In addition, the host needs a full immunosurveillance repertoire to suppress all these viruses waiting to step up to the plate. Once the defences are lowered by stress, immunosuppression or trauma, for example, active viral replication can occur.

Viruses may have a number of options with respect to receptors they can attach to and subsequently infect the host. They may be able to cross species barriers as well and not cause disease in the reservoir host. With respect to transmissibility, their job description includes the ability to exist in blood and other body fluids, to be aerosolized and to be carried by insect vectors. The route of transmission is crucial to maximize their potential for infection. If you, the reader, thought of how you would be a successful virus, you would want to infect as many people as possible, either integrate or lie latent in the host cell and kill neither the cell nor the host so you can continue proliferating. You might also be musing about preferable routes of transmission, so some may say that EBV infection, sealed with a kiss, might be a more desirable option.

To keep the host's immune system on its toes, most of the RNA viruses can subtly change their genetic makeup and drift away from the circulating strain, thus evading the antibody immune response. Alternatively, they may have a number of genotypes with a different susceptibility to antiviral agents, they are not cross-protective, therefore ensuring a multivalent vaccine is required as a preventative measure, and they are associated with a different clinical illness spectrum.

Viruses make full use of the cellular replicative machinery, and, therefore, an antiviral agent has difficulty targeting the virus without affecting the host cell. As a result, most antiviral agents can adversely affect the host. This means that individuals taking certain antiviral agents have to be monitored carefully, as treatment can potentially lead to side effects that include bone marrow suppression, renal toxicity and mitochondrial disorders.

What can the host do to offset all these advantages? Antiviral vaccines have been a major success, behavioural changes can limit the chances of infection and increasingly more precise chemotherapeutic targets are being identified.

# The fungi

## Introduction

**The study of fungi is known as *mycology*, and fungal infections are known as *mycoses***

Fungi are eukaryotes but are quite distinct from plants and animals and occupy their own kingdom. Characteristically they have a thick carbohydrate cell wall containing chitin, glucans, mannans and glycoproteins. They are found either as filamentous fungi (moulds) or as yeasts. Filamentous fungi exist as multinucleate threadlike filaments (hyphae), which may show septation and grow longitudinally and by branching. Yeasts are unicellular, round or oval in appearance and reproduce by budding. Other growth forms such as mushrooms also occur. Fungi are ubiquitous as free-living organisms and are of enormous importance commercially in baking, brewing and pharmaceuticals, producing antibiotics, for example. Some fungi form part of the body's normal flora, and others are common causes of local infections on skin and hair. A number of fungi are associated with significant disease, and many of these are acquired from the external environment. Pathogenic species invade tissues and digest material externally by releasing enzymes; they also take up nutrients directly from host tissues. In recent years invasive fungal disease has assumed much greater prominence in clinical practice as a result of the rise in the number of severely immunocompromised patients.

## MAJOR GROUPS OF DISEASE-CAUSING FUNGI

### Importance of fungi in causing disease

More than 2 million species of fungi are thought to exist and ~150,000 have been described, but only about 300 are identified as pathogens in humans and animals, although the number of pathogenic species is growing. Some of these are cosmopolitan; others are found mainly in tropical regions. Fungi that infect superficially cause relatively minor health problems, but given the large number of cases, they result in considerable morbidity and a significant economic burden on health care systems. Those that invade deeper tissues produce more severe illness and can be life threatening. These systemic forms have become much more serious problems as medical advances have taken place (e.g. immunosuppressive and antibiotic therapies, transplantation, invasive procedures and acquired immunodeficiency syndrome [AIDS]) such that opportunistic infections are now significant components of hospital-acquired infection. Only *Candida* and some dermatophytes are transmitted between humans; the remainder of disease-causing fungal infections are acquired from the environment, including the hospital environment.

### Fungal pathogens can be classified on the basis of their growth forms or the type of infection they cause

Fungi were reclassified down to the level of order in 2007 following advances in fungal molecular taxonomy. Although this has no immediate effect on the practice of clinical microbiology, it will lead to greater understanding of the biology of the kingdom Fungi and the diseases its members may cause.

Examples of branched filamentous forms or yeasts are shown in Figs. 4.1, 4.2, and 4.3. Some show both growth forms in their cycle, with hyphae in the environment and yeasts in humans and are known as dimorphic fungi (e.g. *Histoplasma*). In filamentous forms (e.g. *Trichophyton*), a mass of hyphae forms and is termed a *mycelium*. Asexual reproduction results in the formation of spores (conidia) by which the fungus is dispersed; spores are a common cause of infection after inhalation. In yeasts (e.g. *Cryptococcus*) the characteristic form is the single cell, which reproduces by budding. The bud may remain attached, with further budding and longitudinal growth leading to the formation of chains known as *pseudohyphae*. Thermally dimorphic forms (e.g. *Histoplasma*) form hyphae at environmental temperatures but occur as yeast cells in the body, the switch being temperature induced. Some *Candida* species can produce both yeast and hyphal forms within the body.

The following types of infection (mycoses) are recognized:

- Superficial mycoses in which the fungus grows on body surfaces (skin, hair, nails), external ear canal and eye. Examples are tinea pedis (athlete's foot), otomycosis (fungal ear infection) and fungal keratitis.
- Mucosal infections in which the fungus grows on body mucous membranes (oral, genital) causing oral, oesophageal or genital (vulvovaginal or penile) candidiasis.
- Subcutaneous mycoses in which deeper layers of the skin are involved. Examples are mycetoma (Madura foot), chromoblastomycosis and sporotrichosis. This group of fungal diseases usually develops following transcutaneous trauma. They are also known as *implantation mycoses*.

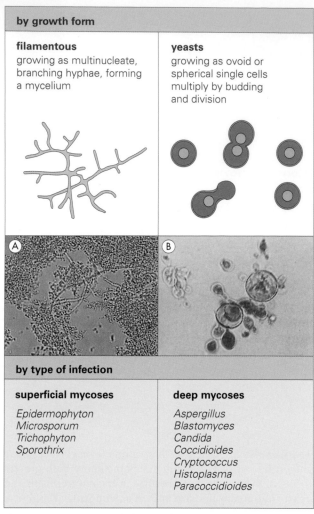

| by growth form | |
| --- | --- |
| **filamentous** <br> growing as multinucleate, branching hyphae, forming a mycelium | **yeasts** <br> growing as ovoid or spherical single cells multiply by budding and division |

| by type of infection | |
| --- | --- |
| **superficial mycoses** | **deep mycoses** |
| *Epidermophyton* <br> *Microsporum* <br> *Trichophyton* <br> *Sporothrix* | *Aspergillus* <br> *Blastomyces* <br> *Candida* <br> *Coccidioides* <br> *Cryptococcus* <br> *Histoplasma* <br> *Paracoccidioides* |

**Fig. 4.1** Two ways to classify fungi that cause disease: by growth form and by type of infection. (A) Hyphae in skin scraping from ringworm lesion. (B) Spherical yeasts of *Histoplasma*. (A, Courtesy D.K. Banerjee; B, courtesy Y. Clayton and G. Midgley.)

- Systemic or deep mycoses with involvement of internal organs. This category includes fungi capable of infecting individuals with normal immunity and the opportunistic fungi that cause disease in patients with compromised immune systems. Examples are invasive aspergillosis, histoplasmosis and systemic candidiasis.

Allergic diseases are often chronic manifestations of hosts' sensitization and immune response to fungi in the respiratory tract. Examples are allergic fungal rhinosinusitis, allergic bronchopulmonary aspergillosis (ABPA) and severe asthma with fungal sensitization.

The superficial mycoses are spread by person-to-person contact (anthropophilic) or animal-to-human contact (zoophilic) (e.g. from cats and dogs) or from soil-to-human contact (geophilic). The subcutaneous mycoses infect humans via the skin (e.g. following skin penetration); the deep mycoses often result from the opportunistic growth of fungi in individuals with impaired immune competence and are primarily acquired via the respiratory tract (see Ch. 31), with intravenous lines being an important portal of entry for *Candida*. Free-living fungi can also cause disease. This occurs indirectly when toxins produced by fungi are present in items used as food (e.g. aflatoxin, a carcinogen produced by *Aspergillus flavus*). In allergic fungal diseases, when spores are inhaled by a human host, an immune response occurs and a hypersensitivity pneumonitis develops (e.g. ABPA).

Many of the fungi that cause disease are normally free living in the environment but can survive in the body if acquired by inhalation or by entry through intravenous cannulas, urinary catheters or wounds. Some fungi are part of the normal flora (e.g. *Candida*) and are innocuous unless the body's defences are compromised (e.g. by underlying malignancy, diabetes mellitus or intravenous drug use). The filamentous forms grow extracellularly, but yeasts can survive and multiply within macrophages and neutrophils. Neutrophils can play a major role in controlling the establishment of invading fungi. Species that are too large for phagocytosis can be killed by extracellular factors released from

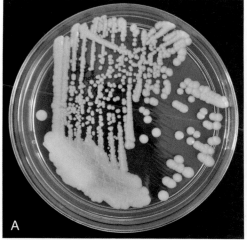

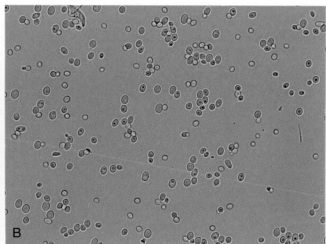

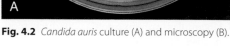

**Fig. 4.2** *Candida auris* culture (A) and microscopy (B).

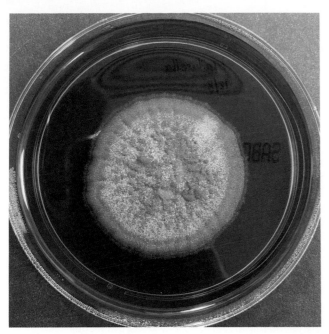

**Fig. 4.3** *Madurella mycetomatis.*

phagocytes as well as by other components of the immune response. Some species, notably *Cryptococcus neoformans*, prevent phagocytic uptake because they are surrounded by a polysaccharide capsule (see Chs. 25 and 31). Until recently, *Pneumocystis jirovecii*, causing an important opportunistic infection in AIDS patients, was classified as a protozoan but it is now regarded as an atypical fungus. It attaches to lung cells (pneumocytes) and can give rise to a fatal pneumonia. The microsporidia, previously thought to be protozoa, now turn out to be closely related to the fungi. The major groups of fungi causing human disease are shown in Table 4.1.

### Control of fungal infection

The echinocandins (e.g. micafungin, anidulafungin, caspofungin) inhibit glucan synthesis in the fungal cell wall. Below the fungal cell wall lies the plasma membrane. Unlike human plasma membranes in which the dominant sterol is cholesterol, the fungal membrane is rich in ergosterol. Compounds that selectively bind to ergosterol can, therefore, be used as effective antifungal agents. These include the polyenes nystatin and amphotericin B. The azoles (e.g. fluconazole, itraconazole, voriconazole) and the allylamines (e.g. terbinafine) inhibit ergosterol synthesis. The pyrimidine analogues (e.g. flucytosine) inhibit nucleic acid synthesis.

**Table 4.1** Summary of fungi that cause important human diseases

| Important fungal diseases | | | | |
|---|---|---|---|---|
| **Type** | **Anatomic location(s)** | **Representative disease** | **Causative organisms** | **Growth form in human body** |
| Superficial | Hair shaft, skin | White piedra<br>Black piedra<br>Pityriasis versicolor<br>Seborrheic dermatitis<br>Tinea nigra | *Trichosporon*<br>*Piedraia hortae*<br>*Malassezia*<br>*Hortaea werneckii* | Y/F |
| Cutaneous | Epidermis, hair, nails | Tinea (ringworm) | *Microsporum, Trichophyton, Epidermophyton, Nannizzia* | F |
| Subcutaneous | Dermis, subcutis | Sporotrichosis<br>Eumycetoma<br>Chromoblastomycosis<br>Lobomycosis | *Sporothrix*<br>Several genera<br>Several genera<br>*Lacazia loboi* | Y[a]<br>F<br>Y/F<br>Yeast-like |
| Systemic | Internal organs | Coccidioidomycosis<br>Histoplasmosis<br>Blastomycosis<br>Paracoccidioidomycosis | *Coccidioides*<br>*Histoplasma*<br>*Blastomyces*<br>*Paracoccidioides* | Form spherules[b]<br>Y<br>Y<br>Y |
| Opportunistic | Internal organs | Cryptococcosis<br>Candidiasis<br>Aspergillosis<br>Mucormycosis<br>Pneumocystis pneumonia<br>Emergomycosis | *Cryptococcus*<br>*Candida*<br>*Aspergillus*<br>Mucorales<br>*Pneumocystis*<br>*Emergomyces* | Y<br>Y[c]<br>F[a]<br>N/A<br>N/A<br>Y[c] |

[a]Growth from the body.
[b]*Coccidioides* has an unusual growth form with yeast-like endospores within a spherule.
[c]Also forms pseudohyphae.
Y, Yeast; F, filamentous; N/A, Y/F forms are not applicable.

## KEY FACTS

- Fungi are distinct from plants and animals, have a thick chitin-containing cell wall and grow as filaments (hyphae) or single-celled yeasts.

- Species causing disease may be acquired from the environment *(Aspergillus)* or occur as part of the normal flora *(Candida)*.

- Infections may be located superficially in cutaneous and subcutaneous sites or in deep tissues.

- Infections are most serious in immunocompromised individuals.

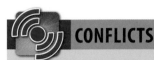

## CONFLICTS

The World Health Organization (WHO) notes evidence indicating that both the incidence and geographic range of fungal diseases are expanding worldwide as a result of global warming and the increase in international travel and trade. In addition, the use of antifungals in agriculture has been linked to rising rates of azole-resistant *Aspergillus fumigatus* infections.

Fungi are versatile; the same species can be both free living in the external environment and cause disease in the human host. Thus there is always a plentiful reservoir of infection. Fungi are physiologically versatile, too, and can grow at a wide range of temperatures. Their asexual reproductive stages (spores or conidia) are small, can be airborne and are easily inhaled. As they have a resistant chitinous cell wall and may produce antiphagocytic factors (polysaccharide capsule), they can be difficult for innate defence systems to deal with. Once past the defences of the respiratory system, many fungi change growth form and invade deeper tissues, often forming a network of elongate hyphae (e.g. in aspergillosis), which are even more difficult to defend against; indeed, immunologic responses may aggravate systemic pathology. The prevalence of infective stages in the environment and the ability of fungi to grow rapidly in the absence of effective defences make fungal infection a major hazard for immunocompromised patients. The balance is further tipped in their favour by the difficulty in diagnosing deep-seated mycoses and by the toxicity to the host of some of the drugs used to treat them. Fortunately, immunologically competent individuals appear to deal well with what must be frequent exposure. However, the potential for disease is always present, and new combatants have joined the conflict.

In 2009 *Candida auris* was isolated in Japan from a patient's external ear canal. Since then, it has been responsible for hospital outbreaks of invasive fungal infections, some of them prolonged, in all five continents involving at least 40 countries. *C. auris* is a formidable opponent because it can be misidentified as a different yeast if biochemical identification methods are used. It colonizes skin for long periods, is usually resistant to fluconazole and is often multidrug resistant. Environmental contamination can take place in health care facilities and result in secondary infections. The US Centers for Disease Control and Prevention considers *C. auris* a public health threat that requires urgent and aggressive action.

There will always be conflicts between host and infecting organisms; given the increasing population of immunocompromised patients, fungi are taking full advantage. First named as recently as 2017, the aptly named genus *Emergomyces* has been responsible for disseminated infection in immunocompromised individuals. Most had advanced human immunodeficiency virus infection; other risk factors were neutropenia, hematologic malignancy, immunosuppressive medication, and solid organ transplants. Particularly dangerous is the fact that emergomycosis can mimic tuberculosis, as well as other fungal infections, notably histoplasmosis and cryptococcosis. Indeed, the histopathologic features of emergomycosis and histoplasmosis are very similar.

Coronavirus disease 2019 (COVID-19)–associated invasive fungal infections are now recognized as important complications in a substantial number of critically ill, hospitalized patients with COVID-19. Three groups of fungal pathogens cause coinfections in COVID-19: *Aspergillus*, Mucorales and *Candida* spp., including *C. auris*. The severe acute respiratory syndrome coronavirus 2 (SARS-CoV-2) infection alters immune and metabolic responses in patients, which, together, produce an inflammatory environment that is highly permissive to fungal infections; however, the underlying mechanisms are complex. Furthermore, immunomodulatory drugs, including corticosteroids and cytokine blockers such as tocilizumab, are used to treat severe COVID-19 infections. These drugs hamper the activation of innate and adaptive antimicrobial responses and, therefore, represent important predisposing factors to secondary fungal infections in this patient population.

In response to these events, in October 2022 WHO published a report that included a priority list of fungal pathogens, cataloguing the 19 fungi that represent the greatest threat to public health (Fig. 4.4). The list aims to drive more research and policy interventions to strengthen the global response to fungal infections and antifungal resistance. This is much needed, as medical mycology has been a relatively neglected branch of microbiology when compared to bacteriology.

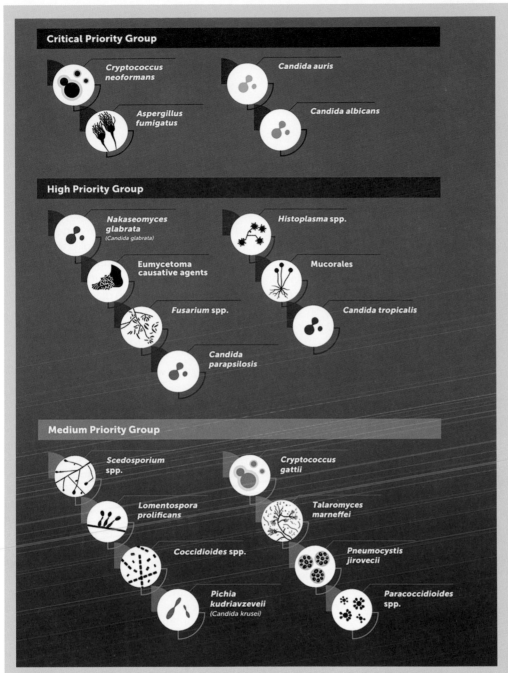

**Fig. 4.4** World Health Organization (WHO) fungal priority pathogens list. (From WHO. *Fungal Priority Pathogens List*. Geneva: Author; 2022.)

# 5

# The protozoa

## Introduction

Twelve diseases in the World Health Organization's (WHO's) list of 20 neglected tropical diseases are caused by parasites, three of them protozoa: Chagas disease, human African trypanosomiasis and leishmaniasis. Protozoa are single-celled animals, ranging in size from 2 to 100 nm. Like human cells, they are eukaryotic, with a discrete nucleus delineated from the cytoplasm by the nuclear membrane. Many protozoal species are free living, but others are important parasites of humans. Some free-living species can infect humans opportunistically. Protozoa continue to multiply in their host until controlled by its immune response or by treatment and thus may cause particularly severe disease in immunocompromised individuals. Protozoal infections are most prevalent in tropical and subtropical regions, but also occur in temperate regions. Protozoa may cause disease directly (e.g. the rupture of red cells in malaria), but more often the pathology is caused by the host's response. Of all the parasitic diseases, malaria presents the most severe global problem and kills ~550,000 people each year, mostly young children.

## Protozoa can infect all the major tissues and organs of the body

Protozoa infect body tissues and organs as:

- intracellular parasites in a wide variety of cells (red cells, macrophages, epithelial cells, brain, muscle)
- extracellular parasites in the blood, intestine or genitourinary system.

The locations of the species of greatest importance are shown in Fig. 5.1. Intracellular species obtain nutrients from the host cell by direct uptake or by ingestion of cytoplasm. Extracellular species feed by direct nutrient uptake or by ingestion of host cells. Parasitic protozoa in the intestine such as *Giardia duodenalis* and *Entamoeba histolytica* generate energy by anaerobic fermentation of glucose and amino acid carbon sources. In contrast, malaria parasites, living in the aerobic environment of the bloodstream, generate energy by glycolysis without subsequent oxidative phosphorylation, an adequate method given the ready availability of glucose in the peripheral blood of humans. Reproduction of protozoa in humans is usually asexual, by binary or multiple division of growing stages (trophozoites). Sexual reproduction is normally absent from the life cycle; however, it is found in the Apicomplexa, a phylum that includes a number of medically important protozoa. Protozoal sexual reproduction occurs in the definitive host. Examples are the insect vector phase of the malaria life cycle and the intestinal epithelial stages of *Toxoplasma* in the cat. *Cryptosporidium* is exceptional in undergoing both asexual and sexual reproduction in humans. Asexual reproduction gives the potential for a rapid increase in number, particularly where host defence mechanisms are impaired. For this reason, some protozoa are most pathogenic in the very young (e.g. *Toxoplasma* in the fetus and in neonates). The human immunodeficiency virus epidemic focused attention on a number of protozoa that give rise to opportunistic infections in immunocompromised individuals. These include the coccidian parasites *Cryptosporidium* and *Cystoisospora*. New parasites continue to emerge (e.g. *Cyclospora cayetanensis*, a foodborne and waterborne cause of diarrhoea that became recognized as a clinical problem in the early 1990s) (Fig. 5.2). *Acanthamoeba*, a free-living amoeba widely distributed in the environment, is becoming increasingly reported as a cause of keratitis, with contact lens wear being the major risk factor.

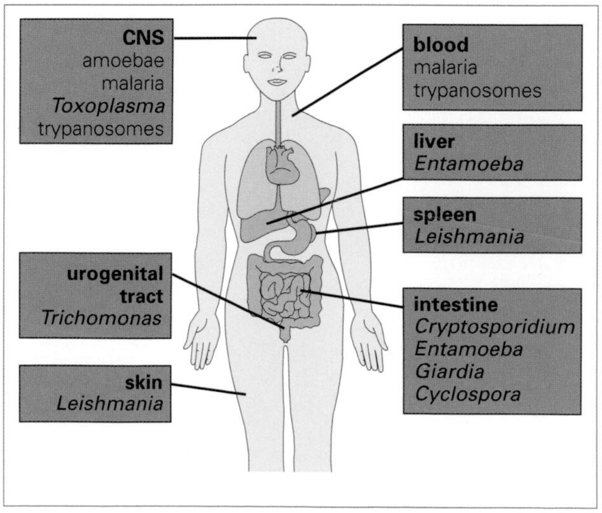

## Protozoa have evolved many sophisticated strategies to avoid host responses

Extracellular species evade immune recognition of their plasma membrane. The interface between host and

**Fig. 5.1** The occurrence of protozoan parasites in the body. CNS, Central nervous system.

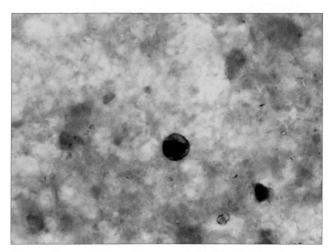

**Fig. 5.2** Oocyst of *Cyclospora cayetanensis*. Modified Ziehl–Neelsen stain. (Courtesy Peter Chiodini.)

extracellular protozoa is the parasite's plasma membrane, and examples of strategies to avoid immune recognition of this surface include the following:

- Trypanosomes undergo repeated antigenic variation of surface antigens.
- Malaria parasites show polymorphisms in dominant surface antigens.
- Amoebae can consume complement at the cell surface.

Intracellular species evade host defence mechanisms. Although intracellular stages are removed from direct contact with antibody, complement and phagocytes, their antigens may be expressed at the surface of the host cell, which can then be a target for cytotoxic effectors. Survival within cells, particularly within macrophages (*Leishmania*, *Toxoplasma*), involves a variety of devices to evade or inactivate the harmful effects of intracellular enzymes or reactive oxygen and nitrogen metabolites. *Toxoplasma* is remarkably effective in that respect, with up to a third of the world's human population estimated to be chronically infected with dormant stages of this organism—no mean feat for a single-celled parasite.

### Protozoa use a variety of routes to infect humans

Many extracellular protozoa are transmitted by ingestion of food or water contaminated with transmission stages such as cysts, but *Trichomonas vaginalis* is transmitted through sexual activity and the trypanosomes by insect vectors. The most important intracellular species—*Plasmodium* and *Leishmania*—are also insect transmitted. *Trypanosoma cruzi*, another insect-transmitted protozoan that has both intracellular and extracellular stages in humans, can additionally be transmitted to the fetus in utero, which is now its main route of acquisition in areas where vectorial transmission has been controlled. *Toxoplasma*, a common and important intracellular protozoan, can be acquired by ingestion or from the mother in utero (Table 5.1).

**Table 5.1** Summary of the location, transmission, and diseases caused by protozoan parasites

| Features of medically important protozoa | | | |
|---|---|---|---|
| **Location** | **Species** | **Mode of transmission** | **Disease** |
| Intestinal tract | *Entamoeba histolytica*<br>*Giardia duodenalis*<br>*Cryptosporidium* spp.<br>*Cystoisospora belli*<br>*Cyctospora cayetanensis* | Ingestion of cysts in food or water | Amoebiasis<br>Giardiasis<br>Cryptosporidiosis<br>Cystoisosporiasis<br>Cyclosporiasis |
| Urogenital tract | *Trichomonas vaginalis* | Sexual | Trichomoniasis |
| Blood and tissue | *Trypanosoma* spp.:<br>*T. cruzi, T. b. gambiense,*<br>*T. b. rhodesiense* | Reduviid bug<br>Tsetse fly | Trypanosomiasis<br>Chagas disease<br>Sleeping sickness |
| | *Leishmania* spp.:<br>*L. donovani* complex<br>*L. tropica, L. major,*<br>*L. Mexicana, L. (Viannia)*<br>*broziliensis* | Sandfly | Visceral leishmaniasis (kala-azar)<br>Cutaneous leishmaniasis<br>Mucosal leishmaniasis |
| | *Plasmodium* spp.:<br>*P. vivax, P. ovale, P. malariae,*<br>*P. falciparum, P. knowlesi* | *Anopheles* mosquito | Malaria |
| | *Toxoplasma gondii* | Ingestion of cysts in raw meat; ingestion of oocysts from cat faeces via environmental contamination | Toxoplasmosis |

## KEY FACTS

- Protozoa are single-celled animals occurring both as free-living organisms and as parasites. Both can cause disease in humans.

- The single most important protozoal disease is malaria, which causes ~550,000 deaths each year.

- Protozoa live both outside and within cells and have complex ways of avoiding the responses of their hosts.

- Most protozoal infections are acquired through ingestion of contaminated water or food or via insect vectors. A few are transmitted from mother to fetus.

## CONFLICTS

Malaria provides a good example of human–protozoan conflict. After a period in the liver, the malaria parasite spends all of its time inside the red cell. It grows, divides and releases new parasites by rupturing the red cell. At this stage, the parasite wins the conflict by hiding away inside the red cell, a nonnucleated cell that cannot respond defensively and does not express major histocompatibility complex class 1 molecules on its surface, helping it to escape from recognition by CD8 T cells. In addition, *Plasmodium falciparum*–infected erythrocytes express antigens on the surface of the red cell, which enables them to adhere to vascular endothelium, a process known as *sequestration* by which they reduce the chance of clearance in the spleen. How can the host protect itself immunologically? It has a number of difficult choices. It can try to destroy the parasite inside the cell by producing toxic mediators, or it can try to destroy the parasite and the cell together by targeting antibodies against antigens from the parasite that appear on the red cell surface, although the parasite presents a moving target as *P. falciparum* is adept at antigenic variation. Both of these are risky strategies. Toxic mediators can affect the host as well as the parasites, particularly if, as in *P. falciparum* malaria, the parasite-infected cells are sequestered inside capillaries in vital organs. Destroying red cells can contribute to anaemia, and the by-products of destruction can be toxic. A significant part of the pathology associated with malaria is, therefore, a cost of the host defending itself—game, set and match to the parasite, although a dead host is of no further use to the parasite. Overall, the human immune response to malaria can achieve a reduction in parasite load, but in most cases it does not result in sterile immunity. Although treatment with antimalarials can be highly effective, if they are given late, the patient may still succumb as a result of complications despite clearance of parasites from the blood. Furthermore, the malaria parasite is adept at developing drug resistance, another example of the moving target.

It is especially difficult to develop vaccines against malaria compared to viruses or bacteria, but at long last humans have a new weapon to deploy in the conflict against malaria. The RTS,S/AS01 malaria vaccine is based on an antigenic subunit of a protein expressed by *P. falciparum* sporozoites, the infective stage of the parasite acquired via an infective mosquito bite. The World Health Organization (WHO) estimates the RTS,S/AS01 vaccine could reduce severe disease in 30% of vaccinated children and recommends its use in regions with moderate to high malaria transmission, with a vaccine schedule starting from 5 months of age. This vaccine alone will not be able to eradicate malaria (by comparison, measles vaccine is ~99% effective), but when used alongside insecticide-treated bed nets, indoor residual insecticide spraying, prompt diagnosis and antimalarial treatment, RTS,S/AS01 represents a significant boost to malaria eradication programmes. Other sporozoite antigen-based malaria vaccines are under development or in clinical trials, and the R21/Matrix-M malaria vaccine has shown promising results in early studies.

Chronic toxoplasmosis represents a stalemate in the conflict between the human host and the parasite. Most infected individuals are well and asymptomatic, but the parasite remains alive albeit dormant in tissue cysts. A dramatic example of the capability of *Toxoplasma* to damage humans is seen with weakening of the host's defences by allogeneic haematopoietic stem cell transplantation (HSCT), the use of which has increased over the last decade, disrupts the stalemate, and tips the balance in favour of *Toxoplasma*. This permits reactivation of tissue cysts in a previously infected individual, with appearance and multiplication of tachyzoites, which can lead to encephalitis, pneumonia and disseminated parasitic infection. Reported mortality of post-HSCT toxoplasmosis is 60% or more, especially with pneumonia or disseminated infection.

# The helminths

## Introduction

The term *helminth* is used for all groups of parasitic worms. Three main groups are important in humans: tapeworms (Cestoda), flukes (Trematoda) and roundworms (Nematoda). The first two belong to the phylum Platyhelminthes, or flatworms; the roundworms are in the separate phylum Nematoda. Platyhelminths have flattened bodies with muscular suckers and/or hooks for attachment to the host. Nematodes (roundworms) have long cylindric bodies and generally lack specialized attachment organs. Helminths are often large organisms with a complex body organization. Although invading larval stages may measure only 100–200 μm, adult worms may be centimetres or even metres long. Infections are commonest in warmer countries, but intestinal species also occur in temperate regions.

### Transmission of helminths occurs in four distinct ways

Transmission routes are summarized in Fig. 6.1. Infection can occur after:

- swallowing infective eggs or larvae via the faecal–oral route
- swallowing infective larvae in the tissues of another host
- active penetration of the skin by larval stages
- the bite of an infected blood-sucking insect vector.

The greater frequency of helminths in tropical climate zones reflects the conditions that favour survival of infective stages and the availability of suitable vectors. The socioeconomic conditions that facilitate faecal–oral spread are present in many parts of the zone, and local practices involved in food preparation and consumption influence helminth prevalence. Elsewhere, infections are commonest in children, in individuals closely associated with domestic animals and in individuals with particular food preferences.

Many helminths live in the intestine, whereas others live in the deeper tissues. Almost all organs of the body can be parasitized. Flukes and nematodes actively feed on host tissues or on the intestinal contents; tapeworms have no digestive system and absorb predigested nutrients via their surface tegument.

The majority of helminths do not replicate within the host, although certain tapeworm larval stages can reproduce asexually in humans. In most, sexual reproduction results in the production of eggs, which are released from the host in faecal material. In others, reproductive stages may accumulate within the host but do not mature. The nematode *Strongyloides* is exceptional in that eggs produced in the intestine can hatch there, releasing larvae that can mature to the infective stage and reinvade the body in the process of autoinfection (Fig. 6.2).

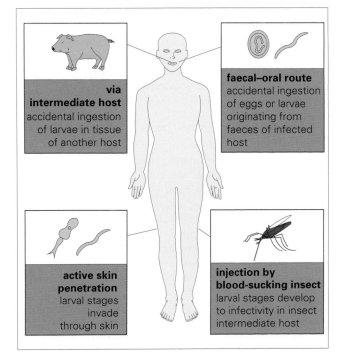

**Fig. 6.1** How helminth parasites enter the body.

**via intermediate host**
accidental ingestion of larvae in tissue of another host

**faecal–oral route**
accidental ingestion of eggs or larvae originating from faeces of infected host

**active skin penetration**
larval stages invade through skin

**injection by blood-sucking insect**
larval stages develop to infectivity in insect intermediate host

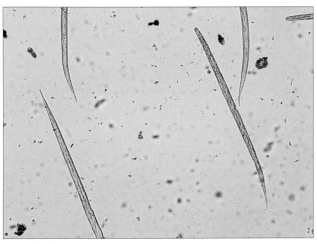

**Fig. 6.2** Filariform larvae, the infective stage of *Strongyloides stercoralis*. (Courtesy Peter Chiodini.)

### The outer surfaces of helminths provide the primary host–parasite interface

In tapeworms and flukes the surface is a complex plasma membrane, and in both there are protective mechanisms to prevent the host from damaging the outer surface. The nematode outer surface is a tough collagenous cuticle, which, although antigenic, is largely resistant to immune attack. However, smaller larval stages may be damaged by host granulocytes and macrophages. Worms release large amounts of soluble antigenic material in their excretions and secretions, and this plays an important role both in immunity and in pathology.

## LIFE CYCLES

### Many helminths have complex life cycles

In direct life cycles, reproductive stages produced by sexually mature adults in one host are released from the body and can develop directly to adult stages after infection of another host via the faecal–oral route (*Ascaris*) or by direct penetration (hookworm). Indirect cycles are those in which reproductive stages must undergo further development in an intermediate host (tapeworms) or vector (filarial worms) before sexual maturity can be achieved in the final host.

### The larvae of flukes and tapeworms must pass through one or more intermediate hosts, but those of nematodes can develop to maturity within a single host

Most flukes are hermaphrodites, except the schistosomes, which have separate sexes. The reproductive organs of tapeworms are replicated along the body (the strobila) in a series of identical segments or proglottids. The terminal gravid proglottids become filled with mature eggs, detach, and pass out in the faeces. The eggs of both flukes and tapeworms develop into larvae that must pass through one or more intermediate hosts and develop into other larval stages before the parasite is again infective to humans. The dwarf tapeworm *Hymenolepis nana*, which is occasionally found in humans, is exceptional as it can go through a complete cycle from egg to adult in the same host.

In nematodes the sexes are separate. Most species liberate fertilized eggs, but some release early-stage larvae directly into the host's body. Development from egg or larva to adult can be direct and occur in a single host, or it may be indirect, requiring development in the body of an intermediate host. Classification of nematodes is complex, and for practical purposes, only two categories of human-specific nematodes are considered here:

- those that mature within the gastrointestinal tract, some of which may migrate through the body during development (e.g. *Ascaris*, hookworms, *Trichinella*, *Strongyloides*, *Trichuris*)
- those that mature in deeper tissues (e.g. the filarial nematodes).

In addition, humans can be infected with the larvae of species that mature in other hosts (e.g. the dog parasites *Toxocara canis* and *Ancylostoma brasiliense*).

## HELMINTHS AND DISEASE

The WHO lists 20 neglected tropical diseases (NTDs), 8 of which are caused by helminths: dracunculiasis, echinococcosis, foodborne trematodiases, lymphatic filariasis, onchocerciasis, schistosomiasis, soil-transmitted helminthiases and taeniasis/cysticercosis. Mainly found in tropical regions, these NTDs are challenging to control, especially those that have complex life cycles, are transmitted by vectors or have animal reservoirs. This is compounded by lack of funding and poor access to health care for those most affected.

### Adult tapeworms are acquired by eating undercooked or raw meat or fish containing larval stages

Tapeworms frequently infect humans, but the adult tapeworms are relatively harmless despite their potential for reaching a large size. Humans can also act as the intermediate hosts for certain species, and the development of larval stages in the body can cause severe disease (Table 6.1).

### The most important flukes are those causing schistosomiasis

Several species of fluke can mature in humans, developing in the intestine, lungs liver and blood vessels. The most important, both in terms of prevalence and pathology, are the blood flukes or schistosomes, the cause of schistosomiasis, also known as *bilharzia*. Three main species—*Schistosoma haematobium*, *S. japonicum* and *S. mansoni*—infect many millions and are responsible for severe disease (Table 6.2). Like all flukes, schistosomes have an indirect life cycle involving stages of larval development in the body of a snail, in this case freshwater aquatic snails. Humans become infected when they come into contact with water-containing infective larvae released from the snails, the larvae penetrating the skin. Other important species are *Clonorchis sinensis*, the oriental liver fluke, and *Paragonimus westermani*, the lung fluke, transmitted by eating raw or undercooked infected freshwater fish or infected freshwater crabs, respectively.

### Certain nematodes are highly specific to humans; others are zoonoses

Several of the many species of nematode that infect humans are highly specific and can mature in no other host. Others have much lower host specificity, being acquired accidentally as zoonoses, with humans acting as either the intermediate or the final host after picking up infection from domestic animals or in food (Table 6.3).

### Survival of helminths in their hosts

Many helminth infections are long lived, the worms surviving in their hosts for many years despite living in parts of the body where there are effective immune defences. How this is achieved has been worked out in several species. Some, such as the schistosomes, disguise themselves from the immune system by binding and incorporating host molecules on their outer surface so they are less easily recognized as foreign invaders—a successful strategy, as some schistosomes have been reported to survive >30 years in the human host. Others actively suppress the host's immune responses by releasing factors that interfere with, or divert, protective responses. For example, the human host shows a degree of immune tolerance to hookworm infection. The worms achieve this by activating regulatory T cells and modulating dendritic cell function. Their ability to do so

**Table 6.1** Summary of the location, transmission and other hosts used by tapeworms that infect humans

| Human tapeworm infections | | | |
|---|---|---|---|
| **Species** | **Acquired from** | **Other hosts** | **Site in humans** |
| **Adult worms** | | | |
| *Taenia saginata* | Larvae in beef | None | Intestine |
| *Taenia solium* | Larvae in pork | None | Intestine |
| *Diphyllobothrium latum* | Larvae in fish | Fish-eating mammals | Intestine |
| *Hymenolepis nana* | Eggs; or larvae in beetles | Rodents | Intestine |
| *Hymenolepis diminuta*[a] | Larvae in insects | Rats, mice | Intestine |
| *Dipylidium caninum*[a] | Larvae in fleas | Dogs, cats | Intestine |
| **Larval worms** | | | |
| *Taenia solium* (cysticercosis) | Eggs in food or water contaminated with human faeces | Pigs | Brain, eyes |
| *Echinococcus granulosus* (cystic echinococcosis; cystic hydatid disease) | Eggs passed by dogs | Sheep | Liver, lungs, brain |
| *Echinococcus multilocularis*[a] (alveolar echinococcosis; alveolar hydatid disease) | Eggs passed by carnivores | Rodents | Liver |
| Pseudophyllidean tapeworms[a] (sparganosis) | Larvae in other hosts | Many vertebrates | Subcutaneous tissues, eyes |
| *Taenia multiceps*[a] | Eggs passed by dogs | Sheep | Brain, eye, subcutaneous tissue |

[a]Rare infections.

**Table 6.2** Summary of the location and transmission of flukes that infect humans

| Human fluke infections | | |
|---|---|---|
| **Species** | **Acquired from** | **Site in humans** |
| *Schistosoma haematobium* *S. japonicum* *S. mansoni* | Penetration of skin by larval stages released from snails | Blood vessels of bladder Blood vessels of intestine Blood vessels of intestine |
| *Clonorchis sinensis* | Ingesting fish infected with larval stages | Liver |
| *Fasciola hepatica* | Ingesting vegetation (e.g. watercress) infected with larval stages | Liver |
| *Paragonimus westermani* | Ingesting freshwater crabs infected with larval stages | Lungs |

is being actively investigated as a potential therapeutic approach to the control of immunologically mediated conditions such as coeliac disease and inflammatory bowel disease. *Trichuris suis* ova, *Trichuris trichiura* ova, larval stages of *Necator americanus* and *Hymenolepis diminuta* have all been used, although results have been variable, and helminth therapy is not widely applied at present. For the future, rather than using the worms themselves, treatments based on helminth-derived immunoregulatory mediators or metabolites, including excretory-secretory products or helminth-induced microbial-derived short chain fatty acids, are likely to be developed.

## KEY FACTS

- Helminths are multicellular (metazoan) worms with distinct tissues and organs that parasitize many parts of the human body, most commonly the gastrointestinal tract.

- Transmission may be direct, through swallowing infective stages or by larvae penetrating the skin, or indirect via intermediate hosts or insect vectors.

- The most serious helminth infection is schistosomiasis, caused by infection with blood flukes. The pathology is primarily due to hypersensitivity reactions to eggs as they pass through tissues.

**Table 6.3** Summary of the location and transmission of nematodes that infect humans

| Human nematode infections | | |
|---|---|---|
| **Species** | **Acquired by** | **Site in humans** |
| **Transmitted person to person** | | |
| *Ascaris lumbricoides* | Ingestion of eggs | Small intestine |
| *Enterobius vermicularis* | Ingestion of eggs | Large intestine |
| Hookworms:<br>    *Ancylostoma duodenale*<br>    *Necator americanus* | <br>Skin penetration by infective larvae<br>Skin penetration by infective larvae | <br>Small intestine<br>Small intestine |
| *Strongyloides stercoralis* | Skin penetration by infective larvae; autoinfection | Small intestine (adults), general tissues (larvae) |
| *Trichuris trichiura* | Ingestion of eggs | Large intestine |
| **Transmitted person to person via arthropod vector** | | |
| *Brugia malayi* | Bite of mosquito-carrying infective larvae | Lymphatics (adults), blood (larvae) |
| *Onchocerca volvulus* | Bite of *Simulium* fly–carrying infective larvae | Skin (larvae, adults), eye (larvae) |
| *Wuchereria bancrofti* | Bite of mosquito–carrying infective larvae | Lymphatics (adults), blood (larvae) |
| *Loa loa* | Bite of deer fly–carrying infective larvae | Subcutaneous tissues (adults), blood (larvae) |
| **Zoonoses transmitted from animals** | | |
| *Angiostrongylus cantonensis* | Ingestion of larvae in snails, crustaceans | Central nervous system (CNS; larvae) |
| *Anisakis simplex* | Ingestion of larvae in fish | Stomach, small intestine (larvae) |
| *Capillaria philippinensis* | Ingestion of larvae in fish | Small intestine (adults, larvae) |
| *Toxocara canis*[a] | Ingestion of eggs passed by dogs | Tissues, eye, CNS (larvae) |
| *Trichinella spiralis*[a] | Ingestion of larvae in pork, or meat of wild mammals | Small intestine (adults), muscles (larvae) |

[a]These species are the commonest in this group.

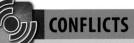

## CONFLICTS

Helminths are typically large parasites, often covered by a protective outer layer so they are difficult for the immune system to deal with—too big for phagocytosis or cytotoxic T cells and unaffected by direct antibody activity. They are often active and mobile and can move away from host defences, damaging host tissues as they do so. Many disguise their outer surfaces or produce immunosuppressive factors. Because they are long lived and able to survive despite immune responses, they can produce chronic disease because of either their activity or misdirected and pathologic host immune responses. Strongyloides is remarkably successful in achieving chronic infection as its life cycle includes an autoinfective process whereby rhabditiform larvae, which are normally passed in the stool to develop further in the soil and become infective filariform larvae, can also transform to that stage while still in the human intestine, thus perpetuating infection in that host for many decades, potentially for life. Reliance on direct infection through faecal–oral contact, or transmission by vectors, makes it difficult to avoid infection when climate and low standards of hygiene combine to tilt the balance in favour of the parasite. Treatment with anthelminthics works against many intestinal worms, but reinfection is almost routine in areas of poor sanitation, necessitating regular retreatment programmes. Those living in the tissues are much more difficult to deal with; for example, echinococcal (hydatid) cysts may require major surgery as well as antiparasitic drugs, and there are still no effective drugs for the treatment of Guinea worm.

# The arthropods

## Introduction

The phylum Arthropoda is the largest in the animal kingdom. It is remarkably diverse and arguably the most successful single group of animals. Arthropods are characterized by having a rigid exoskeleton that contains chitin, a bilaterally symmetrical segmented body and jointed appendages. Examples with which most people will be familiar are crustaceans, centipedes, insects, ticks and mites. The latter three are the most relevant to human disease.

Members of the class Insecta have segmented bodies with a head, thorax, abdomen and three pairs of legs. They usually have wings, but some insects are wingless. Fig. 7.1 shows the structure of an adult mosquito as an example of insect morphology.

Ticks are members of the class Arachnida, which includes spiders. Adult ticks have four pairs of legs; larvae have three pairs.

Mites are also in the class Arachnida. Adults usually have four pairs of legs; larvae have a maximum of three pairs.

Many of these arthropods have adapted to live on humans or use humans as sources of food (blood and tissue fluid). Linked with these feeding habits is the ability of many arthropods to transmit a very wide variety of microbial pathogens. Others, acting as intermediate hosts, may transmit helminth parasites when eaten, and yet other species can inflict dangerous bites and stings.

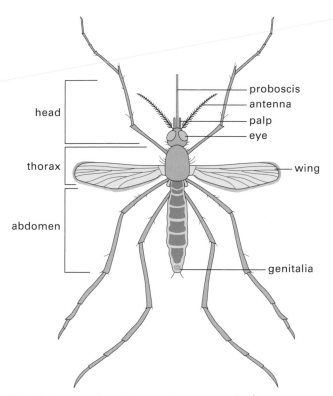

**Fig. 7.1** Structure of an adult mosquito as an example of insect morphology. (Modified from Centers for Disease Control and Prevention. *What Is a Mosquito?* Author; 2020.)

### Many arthropods feed on human blood and tissue fluids

Blood feeders include mosquitoes, midges, biting flies, bugs, fleas and ticks. Some mites also feed in this way — chiggers, the larvae of trombiculid mites, being a familiar example. Contact may be temporary or permanent. Mosquitoes are temporary ectoparasites, feeding for only a few minutes, whereas ticks feed for much longer. The louse *Pediculus humanus* and the crab louse *Phthirus pubis* spend almost all of their lives on humans, feeding on blood and reproducing on the body or in clothing. The scabies mite *Sarcoptes scabiei* (Fig. 7.2) lives permanently on humans, burrowing into the superficial layers of skin to feed and lay eggs. Heavy infections can build up, particularly on individuals with reduced immune responsiveness, causing a severe inflammatory condition (see Ch. 27). In tropical and subtropical regions the larvae (or maggots) of certain flies enter the skin and develop into boil-like lesions under the skin, a condition known as *myiasis*. One remarkable way in which this occurs is exemplified by *Dermatobia hominis,* the human botfly from Central and South America, the adult female of which attaches her eggs to mosquitoes. When the mosquito bites, larvae leave the mosquito and enter human skin at the sites of the mosquito bites.

### Arthropod infestation carries the additional hazard of disease transmission

Arthropods transmit pathogens of all major groups, from viruses to worms, and some (e.g. mosquitoes and ticks)

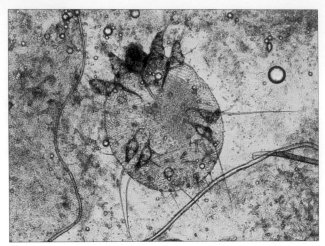

**Fig. 7.2** *Sarcoptes scabiei*, the scabies mite. (Courtesy Peter Chiodini.)

transmit a wide variety of organisms (Table 7.1). The ability to transmit infections acquired from animals to humans poses a constant threat of acquiring zoonoses. Some vectorborne infections, such as yellow fever, have been known for centuries, whereas others, such as the viral encephalitides and Lyme disease, have been recognized more recently (1920s and 1975, respectively). Mosquito-transmitted West Nile virus rapidly became a significant threat in North America after it was first recognized in New York City in 1999, and sporadic cases and outbreaks continue to occur in Europe (see Ch. 28).

### Climate change and arthropod vectors

Arthropods, being poikilothermic organisms, are significantly affected by changes in temperature, which can influence the extent of the geographic area in which they can maintain their populations. Furthermore, within those habitats, the size of their population can be positively or negatively influenced by changes in temperature. Therefore, some geographic areas have become more (and some less) suitable for the survival of arthropod vectors. Changes in rainfall can also have dramatic effects on vectorborne disease (VBD) incidence. However, temperature and rainfall are not the only factors at play, as climate change can induce modifications in land use, water management and the patterns of human activities, all of which affect a local population's exposure to vectorborne pathogens. Thus it is not possible to generalise regarding the impact of climate change on all VBDs, but there are some clear messages of concern, as follows:

The main climatic factors that directly influence VBD ecosystems are temperature and rainfall. A severe example of their effects occurred in Pakistan, commencing in June 2022. The country suffered the worst floods in its history after much heavier monsoon rains, aggravated by heat wave–induced melting of glaciers, all felt to be the result of climate change. As a result, the mosquito population increased significantly, one result of which was a malaria epidemic.

**Table 7.1** Summary of infectious diseases transmitted by arthropods

| Infectious diseases transmitted by arthropods | | |
|---|---|---|
| | **Disease** | **Arthropod vector** |
| **Viruses** | | |
| Arboviruses | Zika virus | Mosquitoes |
| | Dengue fever | Mosquitoes |
| | Yellow fever | Mosquitoes |
| | Encephalitides | Mosquitoes, ticks |
| | Hemorrhagic fevers | Ticks, mosquitoes |
| **Bacteria** | | |
| *Yersinia pestis* | Plague | Fleas |
| *Borrelia recurrentis* | Relapsing fever | Soft ticks |
| *Borrelia burgdorferi* | Lyme disease | Hard ticks |
| *Rickettsias:* | | |
|   *Orientia tsutsugamushi* | Scrub typhus | Larval mites |
|   *R. prowazekii* | Epidemic typhus | Lice (ticks) |
|   *R. mooseri* | Endemic (murine) typhus | Fleas |
|   *R. rickettsii* | Spotted fever | Ticks |
|   *R. akari* | Rickettsial pox | Mites |
| **Protozoa** | | |
| *Trypanosoma cruzi* | American trypanosomiasis (Chagas disease) | Reduviid bugs |
| *T. b. rhodesiense*<br>*T. b. gambiense* | African trypanosomiasis (sleeping sickness) | Tsetse flies |
| *Plasmodium* spp. | Malaria | Mosquitoes |
| *Leishmania* spp. | Leishmaniasis | Sandflies |
| **Worms** | | |
| *Wuchereria* and *Brugia* | Lymphatic filariasis | Mosquitoes |
| *Onchocerca* | Onchocerciasis | *Simulium* flies |
| *Loa loa* | Loiasis (eye worm) | *Chrysops* flies |

With the exception of the zoonotic primate malarias, malaria is an example of a disease with a human host and a single vector, the *Anopheles* mosquito. In contrast, in cases in which an infective organism is maintained in its main reservoir host by an arthropod vector, which can also transmit the pathogen to humans, the result of climate change depends on its effect on both the vector and the reservoir host. For example, Lyme disease has a reservoir maintained by tick transmission in the white-footed mouse *Peromyscus leucopus*, with humans as accidental hosts. In recent years, *Ixodes scapularis,* the vector of Lyme disease in the United States, has extended its range northward. That is concerning in itself, but there has also been expansion of the geographic distribution of the white-footed mouse in the US Midwest and in Canada, associated with shortened winters attributed to climate change. These factors point to a serious risk of an increase in Lyme disease cases taking place in those areas in future years.

Given the remarkable biologic success and adaptability of the arthropods, they are well placed to adapt to and take advantage of climate change in many, although not all, scenarios. Humans face many, challenges in attempting to mitigate their effect on VBD transmission.

## KEY FACTS

- Arthropods of importance in human disease are those that feed on blood or body tissues (insects, ticks, mites) and those that transmit other infections, particularly viruses, bacteria and protozoa.

- Insecticide resistance is a major threat to the success of malaria control and eradication programmes.

## CONFLICTS

Prevention of human infection with insect-transmitted organisms depends very heavily on bite avoidance, as only yellow fever is readily prevented by vaccination. Insect bite avoidance relies on barrier methods (e.g. mosquito nets), insect repellents and insecticides.

Humans pay a price in combatting insects of medical or agricultural importance. For example, the insect nervous system is an important target for some of the major insecticides: The pyrethroid insecticide permethrin, used extensively against mosquitoes, acts on voltage-gated sodium channels in the insect nerve membrane, while organophosphates inhibit anticholinesterase. However, there are important concerns regarding toxicity both in the environment and in humans. For example, the pyrethroids are very toxic to fish and the organophosphates, used extensively in agricultural and environmental pest control in resource-poor settings, are highly toxic to vertebrates. Accidental or deliberate ingestion of organophosphate insecticides is estimated to result in 300,000 deaths a year worldwide.

Furthermore, the insects have fought back and are capable of becoming resistant to insecticides in a variety of ways:

- by changing their metabolism so that their enzyme systems detoxify, destroy or excrete the insecticide more rapidly

- by modifying the site at which the insecticide acts to prevent its binding or interacting there

- by developing barriers to penetration in their outer cuticle, thus slowing absorption of the insecticide into their tissues

- by recognizing the presence of the insecticide and moving away from it when possible.

Ominously, pyrethroid-resistant *Anopheles* mosquitoes can survive up to 1000 times the concentration of insecticide that kills susceptible mosquitoes.

Since 2000, substantial gains have been made in combating malaria using long-lasting insecticidal nets and indoor residual spraying. However, these advances are threatened by the emergence of insecticide resistance. *Anopheles* mosquitoes resistant to at least one class of insecticides have been reported in 90% of malaria-endemic countries, and 32% of them have documented resistance to the pyrethroids, carbamates, organophosphates and organochlorines. Given the presence of multidrug resistance in the malaria parasite *Plasmodium falciparum*, we can be sure that the conflict with this insect-transmitted infection will be long and arduous; and there are many other battles between humans and insects of which insecticide resistance threatens the outcome.

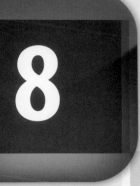

# 8

# Prions

## Introduction

Prions are infectious proteins that acquire alternative conformations and can infect humans, animals and fungi. Prions lack a nucleic acid genome and are highly resistant to all conventional forms of disinfection processes. They are small proteinaceous particles that are modified forms of a normal cellular protein and cause disease by converting normal protein into further abnormal forms.

In humans, prions can cause degenerative changes in the brain: the transmissible spongiform encephalopathies. Creutzfeldt-Jakob disease (CJD) is a fatal human prion disease that has three subtypes: sporadic, inherited and acquired. Kuru is the classic example of acquired CJD, epidemiologic studies confirming human–human transmission due to cannibalistic rituals among the Fore people of Papua New Guinea. In the United Kingdom during the 1990s, individuals developed variant CJD (vCJD) that was associated with eating beef from cows infected with the prion causing bovine spongiform encephalopathy (BSE), known as mad cow disease. In addition, CJD can be acquired exogenously during medical procedures involving contaminated instruments or tissue. Finally, prion-related conditions can arise endogenously by mutation and be inherited.

The prion diseases are part of a spectrum of neurodegenerative disorders in which soluble proteins are modified and accumulate as insoluble beta sheet–rich amyloid fibrils. The other neurogenerative disorders that include different types of dementia are not infectious but are sporadic or inherited, sharing a common pathogenesis. Endogenous sporadic CJD (sCJD) has been known for some time, as well as genetic CJD (or Gerstmann-Sträussler-Scheinker [GSS] disease) and fatal familial insomnia (FFI).

## A SPECTRUM OF NEURODEGENERATIVE DISORDERS—TRANSMISSIBLE SPONGIFORM ENCEPHALOPATHY

Prions lack a nucleic acid genome, are small proteinaceous particles that are modified forms of a normal cellular protein and cause disease by converting normal protein into further abnormal forms. The prion diseases are part of a spectrum of neurodegenerative disorders in which soluble proteins are modified and accumulate as insoluble beta sheet–rich amyloid fibrils. They are infectious proteins that acquire alternative conformations and infect humans, animals and fungi. The biologic function of fungal prions, however, are still unclear and may have detrimental and beneficial effects on the host fungus.

Starting with the acquired subtype of CJD, during the 1990s in the United Kingdom and then in France, individuals developed vCJD, which was associated with eating beef from cows infected with the prion causing BSE, or mad cow disease. The disease modellers reported at the time that this could result in an evolving vCJD epidemic that could involve up to 500,000 people; however, there was insufficient information available to make predictions or calculate risks. In 1990 an infamous episode filmed to reduce the anxiety of the public about eating UK beef involved the agriculture minister and his 4-year-old daughter eating hamburgers. Awful pictures of pyres of burning cattle were in the news

as infected herds were slaughtered to halt the spread of BSE with ~37,000 cows culled in a single year. Subsequently, vCJD was found in humans and was associated with eating BSE-infected beef. vCJD is the most rare form of human prion disease and predominantly presented in people ~30 years of age, with a median survival of 14 months. People often presented with anxiety, withdrawal, and dysphoria before developing cognitive dysfunction, movement disorders and ataxia. Clinically there was a rapid deterioration in muscle and cognitive function that was fatal within months of symptoms developing. Central and limb pain, thought to be thalamic in origin, was also seen early on. Fortunately the incidence of vCJD fell after it peaked at ~29 new diagnoses in 12 countries reporting vCJD figures in 2000 (Fig. 8.1). The huge outbreak of BSE in cattle in the United Kingdom was suppressed, and improvements in food safety had been implemented.

There is also scrapie, a prion that affects sheep and less frequently goats. Apart from the progressively fatal neurologic symptoms, the animals have skin irritation that leads to them rubbing themselves against fences, trees and posts, leading to the name. Finally, there is chronic wasting disease in cervids.

Kuru was thought to have started among the Fore people of Papua New Guinea in the 1920s and fell from the 1950s onwards after they stopped eating the brains of dead people as part of their funeral rituals.

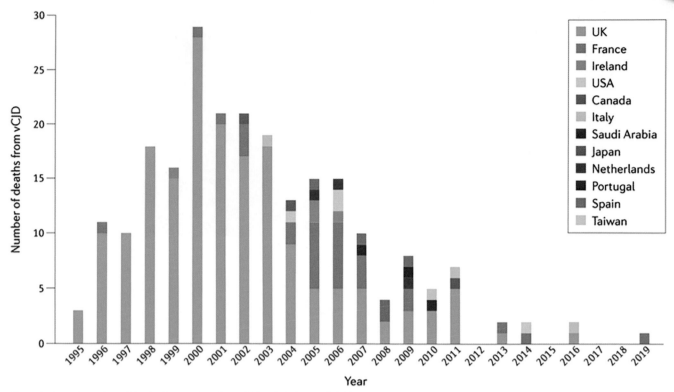

**Fig. 8.1** Annual number of deaths from variant Creutzfeldt-Jakob disease (vCJD) in 12 countries. (From Watson N, et al. The importance of ongoing international surveillance for Creutzfeldt-Jakob disease. *Nature Neuro*. 2021;17:362–379. https://doi.org/10.1038/s41582-021-00488-7; data from the European Creutzveldt-Jakob Disease Surveillance Network [EuroCJD].)

Acquired vCJD is also associated with neurosurgical instruments that had been inadvertently reused after operating on individuals with undiagnosed vCJD. This is because prions are highly resistant to all conventional forms of disinfection processes and bind strongly to metal surfaces. In addition, iatrogenic acquired vCJD had been reported in individuals who received cadaveric pituitary-derived human growth hormone and human dura mater grafts.

Prion-related conditions can arise endogenously by mutation and be inherited, known as sCJD and inherited prion disease (IPD), respectively. Around 85% of people who develop CJD have sCJD, and they are 60–70 years old. The worldwide incidence is 1–2 million. sCJD presents with a fast and progressive dementia, motor dysfunction, visual disturbance, and neuropsychiatric problems and is fatal in a few months. IPD occurs in 10–15% and includes GSS and FFI. They survive for a longer time, and GSS is a progressive ataxia with cognitive and sensory dysfunction. FFI is a progressively worsening sleep disturbance and autonomic system dysfunction.

## ROGUE PROTEIN PATHOGENESIS

### Prions are unique infectious agents

The pathology of the spongiform encephalopathies is characterized by the development of large vacuoles in the central nervous system (CNS). For a long time these diseases were thought to be caused by so-called unconventional slow viruses, but prions were identified, and their characteristics include:

- small size (<100 nm, therefore filterable)
- lack of a nucleic acid genome

- extreme resistance to heat, disinfectants and irradiation (but susceptible to high concentrations of phenol, periodate, sodium hydroxide and sodium hypochlorite)
- slow replication—typically diseases have a long incubation period and usually appear late in life; incubation periods of up to 35 years have been recorded in humans, but vCJD can produce symptoms much more rapidly
- cannot be cultured in vitro
- do not elicit immune or inflammatory responses.

### Prions are host-derived molecules

Studies on scrapie, a fatal transmissible spongiform encephalopathy of sheep and goats, gave some insight into the nature of prions and their role in disease. In the 1960s it had been proposed that proteins could be infectious pathogens and were thought to be involved in scrapie. It was not until 20 years later that Stanley Prusiner demonstrated that the infectious particles purified from hamster brains, having been infected with scrapie, were proteinaceous infectious particles that were called prions. The infectious agent is a host-derived 30–35 kDa glycoprotein (termed prion protein scrapie [PrP$^{Sc}$]) that is associated with the characteristic intracellular fibrils seen in diseased tissue. PrP$^{Sc}$ is derived from a naturally occurring cellular prion protein (PrP$^{C}$), a membrane glycoprotein found most abundantly in the outer membrane of neurones in the central and peripheral nervous systems, but is also found in nonneurologic tissues and organs. PrP$^{C}$ is encoded by the prion protein gene *PRNP* found on chromosome 20 and may have a role in oxidative stress reduction, signal transduction apoptosis and forming

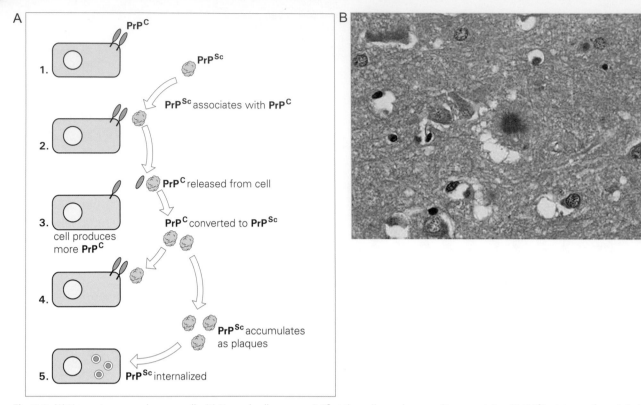

**Fig. 8.2** (A) How prions may damage cells: (1) Normal cells express PrP^C at the cell membrane as linear proteins. (2) PrP^Sc exists as a free globular glycoprotein, which can interact with PrP^C. (3) PrP^C is released from the cell membrane and is converted into PrP^Sc. (4) Cells produce more PrP^C, and the cycle is repeated. (5) PrP^Sc accumulates as plaques and is internalized by cells. (B) Florid plaque. A round amyloid plaque with a dense core is surrounded by multiple small vesicles (haematoxylin and eosin–stained section). (From Mok TH, Mead S. Prion diseases. *Medicine.* 2017;45[11]:fig. 1b.)

and maintaining synapses. This means that it is involved in key physiologic processes in the nervous and immune systems.

Mice with the *PrP^C* gene disrupted are resistant to scrapie, and they show no gross abnormalities. The two proteins have a similar sequence but differ in structure and protease resistance; PrP^Sc is globular and enzyme resistant; PrP^C is linear and enzyme susceptible. The association of PrP^Sc with PrP^C results in conversion of the latter into the abnormal form, the change being largely conformational, from alpha helices to beta-pleated sheets. This conformational change explains why PrP^Sc forms compact protein aggregates that accumulate in the brain. Affected cells produce more PrP^C, and the process is then repeated, the accumulating PrP^Sc aggregating into amyloid fibrils and plaques (Fig. 8.2). PrP^Sc continues to accumulate replacing the normal PrP^C, resulting in neurodegeneration. Replication can lead to very high titres of infectious particles, and up to $10^8$–$10^9$/g of brain tissue have been recorded.

Evidence that the interaction of PrP^Sc with PrP^C causes these events is based on extensive experiments in sheep and mice, the main conclusions being:

- Scrapie infectivity in material copurifies with PrP^Sc.
- Purified PrP^Sc confers greater scrapie activity.
- Mice lacking the *PrP^C* gene do not develop disease when injected with prions.
- Introduction of a *PrP* transgene from a prion donor species (e.g. hamster) into a recipient species (e.g.

mouse) facilitates cross-species transmission, suggesting that homology between the *PrP* genes of donor and recipient is the main molecular determinant of such transmission.

- In vitro, PrP^Sc can convert PrP^C into PrP^Sc, with the transfer of biochemical characteristics.

The development of scrapie in sheep shows strong genetic influences, some breeds being much more resistant than others, and similar genetic effects have been shown in mice. In humans homozygosity for methionine at codon 129 of the prion protein gene is a major determinant of susceptibility to sporadic, iatrogenic and variant CJD. There is also variation in prions, different strains being described. These combinations of host and prion variation result in a spectrum of disease onset and severity. Animal prion diseases (Box 8.1) include scrapie, chronic wasting disease (CWD) and BSE (Fig. 8.3), all of which are sporadic or acquired. CWD affects some North American deer (Fig. 8.4) and Rocky Mountain elk and moose populations. These animals are all hunted and eaten so the concern is that, although CWD has not been transmitted to humans, there is the possibility that this could happen after eating infected meat.

## DEVELOPMENT, TRANSMISSION AND DIAGNOSIS OF PRION DISEASES

There is some evidence that people have a genetic predisposition for sCJD. A naturally occurring polymorphism at codon 129 of the *PrP^C* gene on chromosome 20 codes for the

## Box 8.1     Animal and human prion diseases

| ANIMAL (SPORADIC OR ACQUIRED) | HUMAN |
|---|---|
| Scrapie | Kuru (sporadic and acquired) |
| Chronic wasting disease | CJD (sporadic, inherited, acquired) |
| Bovine spongiform encephalopathy | GSS disease (inherited or sporadic) |
| Transmissible mink encephalopathy | FFI (inherited or sporadic) |
| Feline spongiform encephalopathy | VPSPr (sporadic or familial) |
| Exotic ungulate encephalopathy | |

CJD, Creutzfeldt-Jakob disease; FFI, fatal familial insomnia; GSS, Gerstmann-Sträussler-Scheinker [disease]; VPSPr, variably protease-sensitive prionopathy.

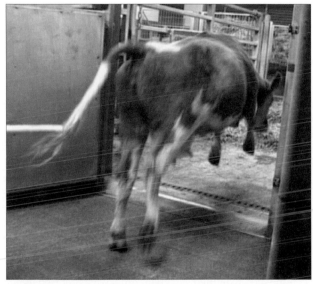

**Fig. 8.3** A cow with bovine spongiform encephalopathy jumping over a minor step. (Copyright © Crown 2003. Courtesy Dr. Timm Konold. Reproduced with permission of the Animal and Plant Health Agency.)

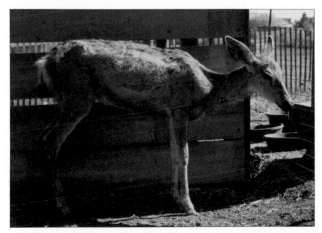

**Fig. 8.4** A deer with chronic wasting disease. (Courtesy Professor Jason Bartz, Department of Medical Microbiology and Immunology, Creighton University School of Medicine, Omaha, NE, USA.)

amino acid methionine or valine. Susceptibility to CJD, as well as the clinical features of the human prion diseases, is strongly influenced by the codon 129 polymorphism. Compared with the unaffected population, people with sCJD are many times more likely to be methionine homozygous (MM genotype) at this locus. Around 40% of people born in Europe have this genotype.

With the exception of prions arising by mutation, transmission and spread of prion disease require exposure to the infective agent. As mentioned previously, having eaten contaminated food, prions survive digestion and are taken up across the intestinal mucosa. They are then carried in lymphoid cells, eventually being transferred into neural tissues and enter the CNS.

### Prions can cross species boundaries

Although prions from one species are more effective in transmitting disease to the same species, transmission can occur between different species (Fig. 8.5). An example of this is the transfer of prions from cattle infected with BSE to humans through consumption of infected meat, which was associated with vCJD. BSE itself arose as a result of transfer to cattle of prions from sheep infected with scrapie, and in 1996 it became clear that human vCJD and BSE were caused by the same prion strain. Unlike CJD itself, vCJD caused disease in younger individuals (age ≥14 years) with a much shorter incubation period. CJD surveillance was started in the United Kingdom in 1990 to identify the number of human infections arising from the UK epidemic of BSE in cattle that was thought to have affected >3 million animals. This estimate was based on the likely number of asymptomatic animals and the clinical diagnosis of BSE made in >180,000 cattle.

vCJD was first reported in the United Kingdom in 1996 by the National CJD Surveillance Unit. Those affected had a clinical and pathologic phenotype distinct from sCJD and were MM genotype at codon 129. vCJD is the only prion disease affecting humans that can be acquired from another species and is caused by BSE. This has also been shown by animal transmission studies in which the infectious agent associated with vCJD was shown to have the same biologic properties as that causing BSE. Epidemiologic studies suggested that the most likely route of transmission was the oral route, the affected individual having eaten beef contaminated with the BSE agent. PrP$^{Sc}$ has been found in the lymphoreticular system, including the tonsils and spleen, as well as neurologic tissues, and the prion may be carried in the blood by lymphocytes.

Overall, by July 2010, 220 people had developed vCJD in 11 countries around the world, 171 of whom were diagnosed in the United Kingdom. Because the incubation period can be very long, it is unclear how many people could have been at risk and asymptomatic. Issues surrounding diagnostic tests included assay sensitivity and specificity, resulting in difficulty in comparing studies. A large study was carried out in the United Kingdom investigating >32,000 anonymized tonsil tissues for disease-related prion protein referred to as PrP$^{CJD}$ from people who underwent an elective tonsillectomy. Of these, 12,753 were from the 1961–1985 birth cohort that included the time most vCJD cases had arisen, and 19,908 were from the 1986–1995 cohort that would potentially have

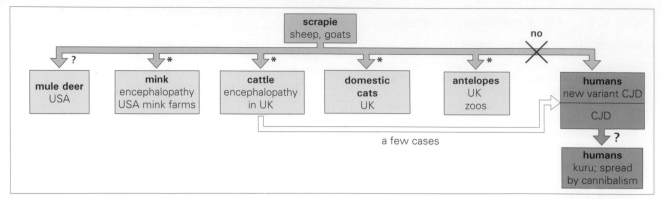

**Fig. 8.5** The spread of scrapie agents between species. Nearly all have been transmitted to laboratory rodents and primates. (* Infections transferred by scrapie-infected sheep materials present in foodstuff. Most of these infectious agents have mutations at amino acid residue 129 of the prion protein, which are thought to cause conversion of the protein into the pathogenic form.) CJD, Creutzfeldt-Jakob disease.

been exposed to BSE-contaminated meat products. PrP$^{CJD}$ was not detected in any samples. By April 2022 the number of deaths in the United Kingdom from confirmed or probable (without neuropathologic confirmation) vCJD totalled 178. That number was much lower than had been predicted by mathematical modellers in the 1990s.

### Prion diseases are difficult to diagnose and treat

Because prions cannot be cultured and there is no immune response, prion disease in its early stages cannot be diagnosed easily. Clinical appearances usually indicate the probable occurrence of prion disease, and tests to confirm vCJD include head magnetic resonance imaging looking for the pulvinar sign (i.e. bilateral hyperintense signals involving the pulvinar thalamic nuclei in the brain), which is a good marker.

In addition, carrying out a lumbar puncture and testing the cerebrospinal fluid (CSF) for 14-3-3 protein, a reliable marker of rapid neuronal destruction, and detecting high levels can be used, although it is more sensitive for sCJD than vCJD. Electroencephalography can also discriminate between sCJD and vCJD.

Tonsillar tissue is a good source of PrP$^{Sc}$ in clinical cases, and these prions can be identified by immunoblotting or immunohistochemistry. Tonsillar and other tissue homogenates can also be tested for the presence of the abnormal prion protein by enzyme immunoassays. These have been used in a number of studies, and the development of diagnostic tests is important not only to make a diagnosis but also from a public health standpoint to prevent infection, as transmission by blood and blood products has been reported. Clinical diagnostic criteria include brain imaging and specific biomarkers in the CSF. Assays such as protein misfolding cyclic amplification based on PrP$^{Sc}$ polymerization were developed, but there were false-positive and -negative results. The amyloid seeding assay, a marker of amyloid formation, was more sensitive but strain dependent. However, the test demonstrating most promise in making the preclinical diagnosis of prion diseases was the brilliantly named real-time quaking-induced conversion assay. The sample is added to recombinant PrP, an amyloid-sensitive fluorescent dye, and a chaotropic agent, and the incubated plate is vigorously shaken (quaked) and fluorescence measured as fibrils form. Femtogram amounts of PrP$^{Sc}$ may be detected.

## PREVENTION AND TREATMENT OF PRION DISEASES

### Prion diseases are incurable

Although there is neither an effective treatment nor vaccine, chemotherapeutic strategies involve stopping the conversion of the normal form of prion protein to the abnormal form PrP$^{Sc}$. Clinical trials of different drugs are difficult due to the disease being rapidly progressive with a diverse range of symptoms that can be challenging to make a rapid diagnosis. Lowering PrP expression has been one of the potential treatments, possibly using antisense oligonucleotides targeting and degrading PrP RNA. Little success has been reported using a number of different agents, including antimalarials and antibiotics (Fig. 8.6) that had been shown to reduce the growth of abnormal prion protein deposits in vitro.

Humanized versions of antibodies that bind to PrP that had activity on prion-infected nerve cells growing in vitro had been prepared for a clinical trial. The hypothesis was that the normal form of PrP required for prions to grow could be removed. Extended survival time was reported when prion-infected mice were treated. As pathogenesis involves recruiting PrP$^C$ into prions, targeting PrP$^C$ is a therapeutic strategy. A study of six patients with CJD given a fully humanised anti-PrP$^C$ monoclonal antibody was reported in 2022, and no clear effect on disease progression and survival time was shown. However, the Medical Research Council Prion Disease Rating Scale scores appeared to stabilize for half the patients when the monoclonal antibody concentration in the CSF had reached the target level.

By understanding the nature of the interactions between PrP$^{Sc}$ and PrP$^C$, ways may be found to regulate the development of disease by reducing or destabilizing the formation of PrP$^{Sc}$. Immunomodulation and mucosal immunization may be potential therapeutic and preventative approaches, especially as the alimentary tract is likely to be the main route of transmission.

### Lessons from kuru

Kuru is a condition that was identified with cannibalistic behaviour in Papua New Guinea. There were >2700 infections between 1957 and 2004, the incubation period of the disease being estimated at >50 years. The fatality rate fell from >200/year in the late 1950s to 6/year in the early 1990s. This reduction followed the prohibition of cannibalistic

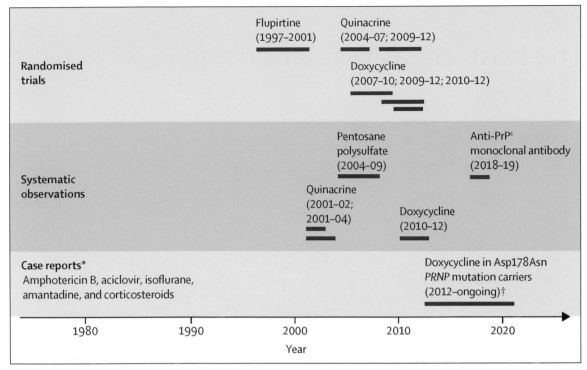

**Fig. 8.6** Progress in trials of potential therapies for Creutzfeldt-Jakob disease. (Reprinted with permission from Elsevier. Zerr I. Investigating new treatments for Creutzfeldt-Jakob disease. *Lancet Neurol.* 2022;21(4):299–300.)

behaviour in the 1950s. A study investigating suspected kuru cases between 1996 and 2004 identified 11 infected individuals. The minimum estimated incubation periods in this group ranged from 34–41 years for women, and the range in males ranged from 39 to at least 56 years. Analysis of the prion protein gene (*PRNP*) showed that most patients with kuru were heterozygous at codon 129.

## KEY FACTS

- Prions are unusual infectious agents causing diseases characterized by changes in the brain (spongiform encephalopathies) and motor disturbances.

- Prions are host-derived glycoproteins and lack a nucleic acid genome. They are extremely resistant to disinfection procedures.

- Transmission of prions is usually by ingestion of contaminated tissues but can occur via medical procedures.

- Diseases in humans caused by prions include kuru, Creutzfeldt-Jakob disease, variant CJD and bovine spongiform encephalopathy.

- The prion diseases are difficult to diagnose, but assays have been developed that could help make a preclinical diagnosis.

## CONFLICTS

Of all the pathogens covered in this book, prions win the human–pathogen conflict. However, one could argue that they may win the battle but lose the war because they kill the host and thus cannot be transmitted further. They are resistant to almost all disinfectant procedures and elicit minimal immune responses. They are never exposed to the outside world and therefore cannot be intercepted. They have no nucleic acids and no metabolic systems, so they cannot be targeted by antimicrobial drugs. Prions can arise by mutation and hijack normal protein-folding control, producing abnormal molecules that are resistant to enzymes. Prions can cross from one species to another and have crossed from animals to humans. Therefore, infection is possible from meat-based food products. The presence of prions in meat is hard to detect; once ingested, prions can travel from the intestine to lymphoid and then to nervous tissues, ultimately causing profound and usually fatal changes in the CNS. Genetic characteristics of potential hosts seem to play an important role in determining the course of disease after exposure. Examples of prion-induced diseases are Creutzfeldt–Jakob disease, variant CJD (linked to mad cow disease) and kuru. These diseases can be diagnosed, but there is currently no effective treatment.

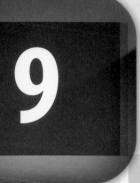

# 9

# The host–parasite relationship

## Introduction

Historically, the study of the host–pathogen (parasite) interrelationship has relied on information gained from the study of specific organisms examined under laboratory conditions. However, advances in molecular biology and DNA sequencing have revealed the existence of microorganisms in the host that cannot be cultured or directly observed. This has led to a quest to understand more completely the full range of microorganisms present in the host, collectively referred to as the *microbiota*, and its genetic content, usually referred to as the *microbiome*. The term *microbiota* is now replacing the phrase *normal flora*, although the latter will still be used on occasion in this book. Analysis of the microbiome is an aspect of what is generally referred to as *metagenomics*: the study of genomic content and diversity in a given environment. Preceding book chapters have focused primarily on organisms that are disease agents. Small numbers may be found in healthy individuals, but their presence in large numbers is usually associated with pathologic changes. The first section of this chapter considers members of the microbiota found in the normal healthy individual, in some cases necessary for normal functioning of the human body but able to cause disease under certain circumstances (e.g. in the newborn or in stressed, traumatized or immunocompromised individuals). Their relationship with the host makes an interesting comparison with that of species that are considered as true parasites or pathogens discussed later in this chapter in the broader context of symbiotic relationships and the evolution of host–parasite relationships.

## THE MICROBIOTA AND MICROBIOME

### Identifying and understanding the microbiota and microbiome

Although the terms *microbiota* and *microbiome* are often used interchangably, the term *microbiota* refers to the living organisms found in a particular environment, such as in the gut where they are referred to as the *gut microbiota*. The term *microbiome* refers to the collection of genomes in an environment but can also include metabolites and structural elements. We will refer to the community of living organisms in an environment as the microbiota and to their genomes as the microbiome.

It has been estimated that humans have $\sim 10^{13}$ cells in the body and $\sim 10^{14}$ bacteria (and 100× more genes) associated with them, the majority in the large bowel. Studies of the microbiota and microbiome rely on advances in high-throughput DNA sequencing and extensive DNA sequence databases. Thus microbial DNA samples can be analysed for (1) the presence of known or new species by comparison with species-specific sequences in a 16S ribosomal gene (see Fig. 2.19) database and (2) potential gene function by comparison of all gene sequences with a database of known genes. Although bacteria are the major contributors to the microbiome, viruses, fungi and protozoa are also regularly found in healthy individuals but are far less frequent. The microbiome content is a consequence of different body areas (e.g. the skin, nose and mouth, intestinal and urogenital tracts) being exposed to or communicating with the external environment.

### The microbiota is acquired rapidly during and shortly after birth and changes continuously throughout life

The organisms present at any given time are influenced by the age, nutrition and environment of the individual. For example, the bowel microbiota of children in developing countries is quite different from that of children in developed countries. In addition, breast-fed infants have lactic acid streptococci and lactobacilli in their gastrointestinal tracts, whereas bottle-fed children show a much greater variety of organisms. Thus the human body can be thought of as a complex of microenvironments with characteristic differences in microbial composition. In this context, organisms present at a given body site of least 95% of individuals are considered to represent a core microbiota, whereas more minor fluctuating organisms represent the variable microbiota.

### The skin is an example of a complex microbiota due to multiple microenvironments

Exposed dry areas are not a good environment for bacteria and, consequently, have relatively few resident organisms on the surface, whereas moister areas (axillae, perineum, between the toes, scalp) support much larger populations. *Staphylococcus epidermidis* is one of the commonest species, making up some 90% of the aerobes and occurring in densities of $10^3–10^4/cm^2$; *Staphylococcus aureus* may be present in the moister regions.

Anaerobic diphtheroids occur below the skin surface in hair follicles and in sweat and sebaceous glands,

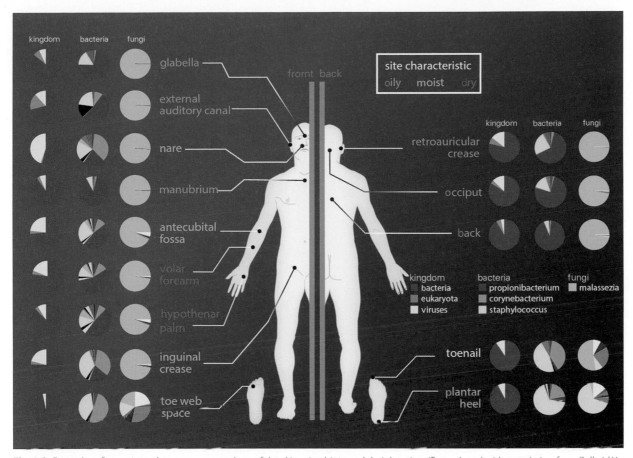

**Fig. 9.1** Examples of organisms that occur as members of the skin microbiota and their location. (Reproduced with permission from Belkaid Y, Segre JA. Dialogue between skin microbiota and immunity. *Science*. 2014;346(6212):954–959. doi:10.1126/science.1260144.)

*Propionibacterium acnes* being a familiar example. Changes in the skin occurring during puberty often lead to increased numbers of this species, which can be associated with acne.

A number of fungi, including *Candida*, occur on the scalp and around the nails. They are infrequent on dry skin but can cause infection in moist skinfolds (intertrigo). An overview of the diversity found in the skin microbiota is shown in Fig. 9.1.

### Both the nose and mouth can be heavily colonized by bacteria

The majority of bacteria here are anaerobes. Common species colonizing these areas include streptococci, staphylococci, diphtheroids and gram-negative cocci. Some of the aerobic bacteria found in healthy individuals are potentially pathogenic (e.g. *S. aureus*, *Streptococcus pneumoniae*, *Streptococcus pyogenes*, *Neisseria meningitidis*); *Candida* is also a potential pathogen.

The mouth contains the widest variety of microenvironments in the body due to both hard and soft surfaces with aerobic and anaerobic niches. The mechanical act of chewing along with the chemical activity of saliva also contributes to oral environmental and microbial diversity. The mucous membranes of the mouth can have the same microbial density as the large intestine, numbers approaching $10^{11}$/g wet weight of tissue.

### Dental caries is one of the most common infectious diseases in developed countries

The prevalence of dental decay is linked to diet as well as to oral hygiene. The surfaces of the teeth and the gingival crevices carry large numbers of anaerobic bacteria. Plaque is a film of bacterial cells anchored in a polysaccharide matrix, which the organisms secrete. When teeth are not cleaned regularly, plaque can accumulate rapidly, and the activities of certain bacteria, notably *Streptococcus mutans* (a member of the oral microbiota), can lead to dental decay (caries) as acid fermented from carbohydrates can attack dental enamel. Dental caries is unique in representing an instance in which a member of the microbiota can cause disease in an immunocompetent host.

### The pharynx and trachea carry their own microbiota

Microorganisms in the pharynx and trachea may include both α- and β-haemolytic streptococci and a number of anaerobes, staphylococci (including *S. aureus*), *Neisseria* and diphtheroids. The respiratory tract is normally quite sterile despite the regular intake of organisms by breathing; however, substantial numbers of clinically normal people may carry the fungus *Pneumocystis jirovecii* (previously known as *Pneumocystis carinii*) in their lungs.

### In the gut, the density of microorganisms increases from the stomach to the large intestine

The stomach normally harbours only transient organisms, its acidic pH providing an effective barrier. However, the gastric mucosa may be colonized by acid-tolerant lactobacilli and streptococci. *Helicobacter pylori*, which can cause gastric ulcers (see Ch. 23), is carried without symptoms by large numbers of people, the bacterium being in mucus and

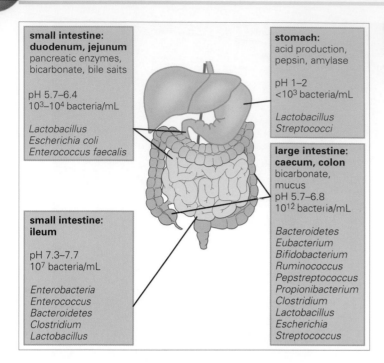

**small intestine: duodenum, jejunum**
pancreatic enzymes, bicarbonate, bile saits

pH 5.7–6.4
$10^3$–$10^4$ bacteria/mL

*Lactobacillus*
*Escherichia coli*
*Enterococcus faecalis*

**stomach:**
acid production, pepsin, amylase

pH 1–2
<$10^3$ bacteria/mL

*Lactobacillus*
*Streptococci*

**small intestine: ileum**

pH 7.3–7.7
$10^7$ bacteria/mL

*Enterobacteria*
*Enterococcus*
*Bacteroidetes*
*Clostridium*
*Lactobacillus*

**large intestine: caecum, colon**
bicarbonate, mucus
pH 5.7–6.8
$10^{12}$ bacteria/mL

*Bacteroidetes*
*Eubacterium*
*Bifidobacterium*
*Ruminococcus*
*Pepstreptococcus*
*Propionibacterium*
*Clostridium*
*Lactobacillus*
*Escherichia*
*Streptococcus*

**Fig. 9.2** Examples of organisms that occur as members of the microbiota of the human gastrointestinal tract and their location. (Adapted from Wisnewsky JA, Doré J, Clement K. The importance of the gut microbiota after bariatric surgery. *Nat Rev Gastroenterol Hepatol.* 2012;9:590–598. doi:10.1038/nrgastro.2012.161.)

neutralizing the local acidic environment. The upper intestine is only lightly colonized ($10^4$ organisms per gram), but populations increase markedly in the ileum, where streptococci, lactobacilli, Enterobacteriaceae and *Bacteroides* may all be present. Bacterial numbers are very high (estimated at $10^{12}$/g) in the large bowel, and many species can be found (Fig. 9.2). The vast majority (95–99%) are anaerobes, *Bacteroides* being especially common and a major component of faecal material; *Escherichia coli* is also carried by most individuals. *Bacteroides* and *E. coli* are among the species capable of causing severe disease when transferred into other sites in the body. Harmless protozoans can also occur in the intestine (e.g. *Entamoeba coli*), and these can be considered as part of the variable microbiota despite being animals.

### The urethra is lightly colonized in both sexes, but the vagina supports an extensive presence of bacteria and fungi

The urethra in both sexes is relatively lightly colonized, although *S. epidermidis*, *Streptococcus faecalis* and diphtheroids may be present. In the vagina the composition of bacterial and fungal microbiota undergoes age-related changes:

- Before puberty, the predominant organisms are staphylococci, streptococci, diphtheroids and *E. coli*.
- Subsequently, lactobacilli predominate, fermenting glycogen for the maintenance of an acid pH, which prevents overgrowth by other vaginal organisms.

A number of fungi occur, including *Candida*, which can overgrow to cause the pathogenic condition thrush if the vaginal pH rises and competing bacteria diminish. The protozoan *Trichomonas vaginalis* may also be present in healthy individuals.

### Advantages and disadvantages of the microbiota

#### Studies of the microbiome have confirmed the benefit of various species to the host

Genetic analysis of the microbiome is needed to identify the many species that may be present in an environment. The contribution of such species to host health is directly shown in instances of dysbiosis, the disruption or disturbance of the microbiota. Broad-spectrum antibiotic therapy can drastically reduce the presence of beneficial microbiota, and the host may then be overrun by introduced pathogens or by overgrowth of organisms normally present in small numbers. After treatment with clindamycin, overgrowth by *Clostridioides difficile*, which survives treatment, can give rise to antibiotic-associated diarrhoea or, more seriously, pseudomembranous colitis.

Ways in which the microbiota inhibits potential pathogens include the following:

- Skin bacteria produce fatty acids, which discourage other species from invading.
- Gut bacteria release a number of factors with antibacterial activity (bacteriocins, colicins) as well as metabolic waste products that help prevent the establishment of other species.
- Vaginal lactobacilli maintain an acid environment, which suppresses growth of other organisms.
- The sheer number of bacteria present in the microbiota of the intestine means that almost all the available ecologic niches become occupied; these species therefore outcompete others for living space.

Gut bacteria also release organic acids, which may have some metabolic value to the host; they also produce B vitamins and vitamin K in amounts that are large enough to be valuable if the diet is deficient. The antigenic stimulation provided by the intestinal flora helps to ensure the normal development of the immune system.

#### Studies of germ-free animals underscore the importance of the microbiota

Germ-free animals tend to live longer presumably because of the complete absence of pathogens, and they develop no caries (see Ch. 19). However, humans acquire microbiota during and immediately after birth, with the accompaniment of intense immunologic activity. Thus the immune system of germ-free animals is less well developed, and they are vulnerable to introduced microbial pathogens, underscoring the important interaction between the microbiota and immune response.

### Problems arise if members of the microbiota spread into previously sterile parts of the body

Examples of this include:

- when the intestine is perforated or the skin is broken
- during extraction of teeth (when *Streptococcus viridans* may enter the bloodstream)
- when organisms from the perianal skin ascend the urethra and cause urinary tract infection.

Members of the microbiota may cause hospital-acquired infection when patients are exposed to treatments that are invasive or that reduce the host's capacity for immune response. Patients suffering burns are also at risk.

As noted earlier, overgrowth by potential pathogens can occur when the composition of the microflora changes (e.g. after antibiotics) or when:

- the local environment changes (e.g. increases in stomach or vaginal pH)
- the immune system becomes ineffective (e.g. acquired immunodeficiency syndrome [AIDS], clinical immunosuppression).

Under these conditions the potential pathogens take advantage of the opportunity to increase their population size or invade tissues, becoming harmful to the host. An account of diseases associated with such opportunistic infections is given in Chapter 31.

## SYMBIOTIC ASSOCIATIONS

All living animals are used as habitats by other organisms; none is exempt from such invasion—bacteria are invaded by viruses (bacteriophages), and protozoans have their own microbiota (e.g. amoebas are natural hosts for *Legionella* *pneumophila* infection). As evolution has produced larger, more complex and better regulated bodies, it has increased the number and variety of habitats for other organisms to colonize. The most complex bodies, those of birds and mammals (including humans), provide the most diverse environments and are the most heavily colonized. Relationships between two species—interspecies associations or symbiosis—are therefore a constant feature of all life.

As the microbiota demonstrates, disease is not the inevitable consequence of interspecies associations between humans and microbes. Many factors influence the outcome of a particular association, and organisms may be pathogenic in one situation but harmless in another. To understand the microbiologic basis of infectious disease, host–microbe associations that can be pathogenic need to be placed firmly in the context of other symbiotic relationships, such as commensalism or mutualism in which the outcome for the host does not normally involve any damage or disadvantage.

### Commensalism, mutualism and parasitism are categories of symbiotic association

All associations in which one species lives in or on the body of another can be grouped under the general term *symbiosis* (literally "living together"). Symbiosis has no overtones of benefit or harm and includes a wide diversity of relationships. Attempts have been made to categorize types of association very specifically, but these have failed because all associations form part of a continuum (Fig. 9.3). Three broad categories of symbiosis—commensalism, mutualism and parasitism—can be identified on the basis of the relative benefit obtained by each partner. None of these categories of association is restricted to any taxonomic group. Indeed, some organisms can be commensal, mutualist or parasitic depending upon the circumstances in which they live (Fig. 9.4).

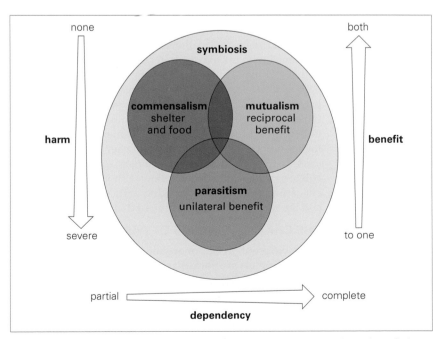

**Fig. 9.3** The relationships among symbiotic associations. Most species are independent of other species or rely on them only temporarily for food (e.g. predators and their prey). Some species form closer associations, termed *symbioses*, and there are three major categories (commensalism, mutualism, parasitism), although each merges with the other and no definition separates one absolutely from the others.

| commensalism – large intestine of humans |
|---|
| *Bacteroides* spp. |
| 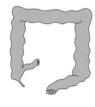 Host provides environment. Bacteria ferment digested food. Present in large numbers ($10^{10}$/g) but usually harmless. May be harmful if tissues damaged (surgery), gut flora changes (antibiotics), or immunity reduced. |

| mutualism – rumen of cattle |
|---|
| *Bacteroides* spp. |
| 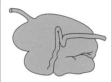 Host provides environment. Bacteria metabolize host food to fatty acids and gases. Host uses fatty acids as energy source. |

| parasitism – large intestine of humans |
|---|
| *Entamoeba histolytica* |
| 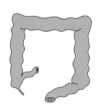 Host provides environment. Protozoa feed on mucosa causing ulcers and dysentery. |

**Fig. 9.4** Examples of commensalism, mutualism and parasitism. These examples show how difficult it is to categorize any organism as entirely harmless, entirely beneficial or entirely harmful.

## Commensalism

### In commensalism, one species of organism lives harmlessly in or on the body of a larger species

At its simplest, a commensal association is one in which one species of organism uses the body of a larger species as its physical environment and may make use of that environment to acquire nutrients.

Like all animals, humans support an extensive commensal microbiota on the skin, in the mouth, and in the alimentary tract. Most of these microbes are bacteria, and their relationship with the host may be highly specialized with specific attachment mechanisms and precise environmental requirements. Normally such microbes are harmless, but they can become harmful if their environmental conditions change in some way (e.g. *Bacteroides*, *E. coli*, *S. aureus*). Conversely, the ability of the intestinal microbiota to prevent colonization by more pathogenic species could also be considered mutualistic, thus the normal definition of commensalism is not very exact because the association can merge into mutualism or parasitism.

## Mutualism

### Mutualistic relationships provide reciprocal benefits for the two organisms involved

Frequently the relationship is obligatory for at least one member and may be for both. Good examples are the bacteria and protozoa living in the stomachs of domestic ruminants, which play an essential role in the digestion and utilization of cellulose, receiving in return both the environment and the nutrition essential for their survival. The dividing line between commensalism and mutualism can be hard to draw. In humans, good health and resistance to colonization by pathogens can depend upon the integrity of the normal commensal enteric bacteria, many of which are highly specialized for life in the human intestine, but there is certainly no strict mutual dependence in this relationship.

## Parasitism

### In parasitism, the symbiotic relationship benefits only the parasite

The terms *parasites* and *parasitism* are sometimes thought to apply only to protozoans and worms, but all pathogens are parasites. Parasitism is a one-sided relationship in which the benefits go only to the parasite, the host providing parasites with their physicochemical environment, their food, respiratory and other metabolic needs and even the signals that regulate their development. Although parasites are thought of as necessarily harmful, this is a view coloured by human and veterinary clinical medicine and by the results of laboratory experimentation. In fact, many parasites establish quite innocuous associations with their natural hosts but may become pathogenic if there are changes in the host's health or if they infect an unnatural host; the rabies virus, for example, coexists harmlessly with many wild mammals but can cause fatal disease in humans. This state of balanced pathogenicity is sometimes explained as the outcome of selective pressures acting upon a relationship over a long period of evolutionary time. It may reflect selection of an increased level of genetically determined resistance in the host population and decreased pathogenicity in the parasite (as has happened with myxomatosis in rabbits, see Fig. 13.2). Alternatively, it may be the evolutionary norm, and unbalanced pathogenicity may simply be the consequence of organisms becoming established in unnatural (i.e. new) hosts. Thus like the other categories of symbiosis, parasitism is impossible to define exclusively except in the context of clear-cut and highly pathogenic organisms. The belief that the ability to cause harm is a necessary characteristic of a parasite is difficult to sustain in any broader view (although it is a convenient assumption for those working with infectious diseases), and the reasons for this are discussed in more detail later.

## THE CHARACTERISTICS OF PARASITISM

### Many different groups of organisms are parasitic, and all animals are parasitized

Parasitism as a way of life has been adopted by many different groups of organisms. Some groups, such as viruses, are exclusively parasitic (see below), but the majority include both parasitic and free-living representatives. Parasites occur in all animals, from the simplest to the most complex, and are an almost inevitable accompaniment of organized animal existence. We can see then that parasitism has been an evolutionary success; as a way of life, it must confer very considerable advantages.

### Parasitism has metabolic, nutritional and reproductive advantages

The most obvious advantage of parasitism is metabolic. The parasite is provided with a variety of metabolic requirements by the host, often at no energy cost to itself, so it can devote a large proportion of its own resources to replication or reproduction. This one-sided metabolic relationship shows a broad spectrum of dependence, both within and between the various groups of parasites. Some parasites are totally dependent upon the host, whereas others are only partly dependent.

### Viruses are completely dependent upon the host for all their metabolic needs

Viruses are at one extreme of the parasite dependency spectrum. They are obligate parasites possessing the genetic information required for production of new viruses but none of the cellular machinery necessary to transcribe or translate this information to assemble new virus particles or to produce the energy for these processes. The host provides not only the basic building blocks for the production of new viruses but also the synthetic machinery and the energy required. Retroviruses go one stage further in dependence, inserting their own genetic information into the host's DNA to parasitize the transcription process. Viruses therefore may represent the ultimate parasitic condition and are qualitatively different from all other parasites in the nature of their relationship with the host (see Ch. 3).

The basis for the fundamental difference between viruses and other parasites is the difference between virus organization and the cellular organization of prokaryotic and eukaryotic parasites. Nonviral parasites have their own genetic and cellular machinery and multienzyme systems for independent metabolic activity and macromolecular synthesis. The degree of reliance on the host for nutritional requirements varies considerably and follows no consistent pattern between the various groups, nor does it follow that smaller parasites tend to be more dependent (e.g. some of the largest parasites, the tapeworms, are wholly reliant upon the host's digestive machinery to provide their nutritional needs). All, of course, receive nutrition from the host, but, whereas some use macromolecular material (proteins, polysaccharides) of host origin and digest it using their own enzyme systems, others rely on the host for the process of digestion as well, being able to take up only low-molecular-weight materials (amino acids, monosaccharides). Nutritional dependence may also include host provision of growth factors that the parasite is unable to synthesize itself. All internal parasites rely upon the host's respiratory and transport systems to provide oxygen, although some respire anaerobically in either a facultative or obligate manner.

### Parasite development can be controlled by the host

The advantage that parasitism confers in reproductive terms makes it vital to coordinate parasite development with the availability of suitable hosts. Indeed, one of the characteristic features of parasites is that their development may be controlled partly or completely by the host, the parasite having lost the ability to initiate or to regulate its own development. At its simplest, host control is limited to providing the cell surface molecules necessary for parasite attachment and internalization. Many parasites, from viruses to protozoa, rely on the recognition of such molecular signals for their entry into host cells, and this process provides the trigger for their replicative or reproductive cycles.

Other parasites, primarily the eukaryotes, require more comprehensive and sophisticated signals, often a complex of signals, to initiate and regulate their entire developmental cycle. The complexity of the signal required for development is one of the factors determining the specificity of the host–parasite relationship. Although the availability of one of the signals entails that parasite development can occur in only one species, host, specificity is high, and although many host species are capable of providing the necessary signals for a parasite, specificity is low.

### Disadvantages of parasitism

The most obvious disadvantage of parasitism arises from the fact that the host controls the development of the parasite. No development is possible without a suitable host, and many parasites will die if no host becomes available. For this reason, several adaptations have evolved to promote prolonged survival in the outside world and so maximize the chances of successful host contact (e.g. virus particles, bacterial spores, protozoan cysts, worm eggs). The prolific replication of parasites is another device to achieve the same end. Nevertheless, where parasites fail to make contact with a host, their powers of survival are ultimately limited. Adaptation to host signals can therefore have a reproductive cost (i.e. the loss of many potential parasites).

## THE EVOLUTION OF PARASITISM

Because so many organisms are parasitic and every group of animals is subject to invasion by parasites, the development of parasitism as a way of life must have occurred at an early stage in evolution and at frequent intervals thereafter. How this occurred is not fully understood, and it may well have been different in different groups of organisms. Some parasites have complex life cycles, too, residing in, for example, two (schistosomiasis) or three (gnathostomiasis) different hosts. In many, parasitism most probably arose as a consequence of accidental contacts between organism and host. Of many such contacts, some would have resulted in prolonged survival, and under favourable nutritional circumstances, prolonged survival would have been associated with enhanced replication, giving the organism a selective advantage within the environment. Many parasites of humans and other mammals may have originated via the route of accidental contact, but it is clear that others have become adapted to these hosts after initially becoming parasitic in other species. For example, parasites of blood-feeding arthropods have ready access to the tissues of the animals on which the arthropods feed. Although the parasite becomes specialized for the nonarthropod host, it may lose the ability to be transmitted by blood feeding. Although the arthropod host is retained in the life cycle, the parasite is faced by competing demands for survival in each host, which probably explains why, for example, arboviruses are restricted to only

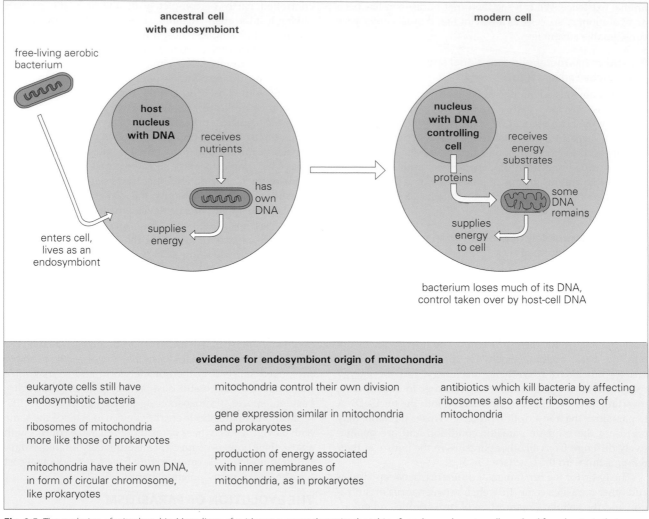

**Fig. 9.5** The evolution of mitochondria. Many lines of evidence suggest that mitochondria of modern eukaryote cells evolved from bacteria that established symbiotic (mutualistic) relationships with ancestral cells.

a few families of RNA viruses and a single DNA virus, African swine fever virus.

### Bacterial parasites evolved through accidental contact

In the case of bacteria, it is easy to see how accidental contact in environments rich in free-living bacteria could lead to successful invasion of external openings such as the mouth and eventual colonization of the gastrointestinal tract. Initially the organisms concerned would have had to be facultative parasites, capable of life both within and outside host organisms (many pathogenic bacteria still have this property [e.g. *Legionella*, *Vibrio*]), but selective pressures would have forced others into obligatory parasitism. Such events are speculative but are supported by the close relationship of enteric bacteria such as *E. coli* with free-living photosynthetic purple bacteria.

### Many bacterial parasites have evolved to live inside host cells

Bacteria that became parasitic by accidental contact would have lived outside host cells at first and would not have had the advantages of being intracellular. The evolution of the intracellular habit required further modifications to allow

survival within host cells but could easily have been initiated by passive phagocytic uptake. Subsequent survival of the pathogen would depend upon the possession of surface or metabolic properties that prevented digestion and destruction by the host cell. The success of intracellular life can be measured not only by the large number of bacteria that have adopted this habit but also by the extent to which some organisms have integrated their biology with that of the host cell. The end point of such integration is perhaps to be seen in the evolution of the eukaryote mitochondrion, which may have evolved from symbiotically associated heterotrophic purple bacteria (Fig. 9.5).

### The pathway of virus evolution is uncertain

Clearly, parasitism by bacteria, which are undoubtedly ancient organisms (they can be traced back 3–5 billion years in the fossil record), depended upon the evolution of higher organisms to act as hosts. Whether the same is true of viruses is open to question and depends upon whether viruses are considered primarily or secondarily simple. If viruses evolved from cellular ancestors by a process of secondary simplification, then parasitism must have evolved long after the evolution of prokaryotes and eukaryotes. If viruses are primitively noncellular, then it is possible that they became parasitic at a very early stage in the evolution of cellular life, at some point when, because of environmental change, independent existence became impossible. A third alternative is that viruses were never anything other than fragments of the nuclear material of other organisms and have in effect always been parasitic. Modern viruses may, in fact, have arisen by all three pathways.

### Eukaryote parasites have evolved through accidental contact

The evolution of parasitism by eukaryotes is likely to have arisen much as it may have done in prokaryotes (i.e. through accidental contact and via blood-feeding arthropods). Examples can be found among protozoan and worm parasites to support this view:

- There are protozoa such as the free-living amoeba *Naegleria,* which can opportunistically invade the human body and cause severe and sometimes fatal disease.
- There are several species of nematode worms that can live either as parasites or as free-living organisms, *Strongyloides stercoralis* being the most important in humans.
- It is likely that trypanosomes (some of which result in sleeping sickness) were primarily adapted as parasites of blood-feeding flies and only secondarily became established as parasites of mammals, although most retain the arthropod in their life cycle.

## Parasite adaptations to overcome host inflammatory and immune responses

We can view the evolution of parasitism and the adaptations necessary for life within another animal as being exactly analogous to the adaptations necessary for life within any other specialized habitat: The environment in which parasites live is merely one of the many to which organisms have become adapted in evolution (comparable with life in soil, fresh water, salt water, decaying material, etc.). However, it is always necessary to remember that in one major respect, parasitism is quite different from any other specialist mode of life. This difference is that the environment in which a parasite lives, the body of the host, is not passive; on the contrary, it is capable of an active response to the presence of the parasite.

The attractiveness of animal bodies as environments for parasites means that hosts are under continual pressures from infection, and these pressures are increased when hosts live:

- close together
- in unsanitary conditions
- in climates that favour the survival of parasite stages in the external world.

### Pressure of infection has been a major influence in host evolution

Pressure of infection has been a major selective influence in evolution, and there is little doubt that it has been largely responsible for the development of the sophisticated inflammatory and immune responses we see in humans and other mammals. In evolutionary terms, all infection has its costs to the host because it diverts valuable resources from the activities of survival and reproduction; thus there has been pressure to develop means of overcoming infection whether or not it causes disease. Of course, this is not the focus of clinical microbiology, which legitimately places emphasis on the costs of infection in terms of frank disease, but it should be remembered because it explains more fully the nature of the continuing battle between host and parasite — the former attempting to contain or destroy, the latter attempting to evade or suppress — and why the emergence of new and the return of old infectious diseases are constant threats.

Parasites are faced with the problems not only of surviving within the environment they experience initially but also of surviving in that environment as it changes in ways that are likely to be harmful to them. The inflammatory and immune responses that follow the establishment of infection are the most important means by which the host can control infections by those organisms able to penetrate its natural barriers and survive within its body. These responses represent formidable obstacles to the continued survival of parasites, forcing them to evolve strategies to cope with harmful changes in their environment. The successful parasite is therefore one that can cope with, or evade, the host's response in one of the ways shown in Table 9.1.

All these adaptations are known to exist within different groups of parasites, and they are well documented in the case of some major human pathogens. Indeed, they are often the very reason why such organisms are major pathogens. Nevertheless, transmission and survival of many parasites depend upon the existence of particularly susceptible host individuals (e.g. children) to provide a continuing reservoir of infective stages.

**Table 9.1** Evasion strategies of parasites

| Evasion strategies | |
|---|---|
| **Strategy** | **Example** |
| Elicit minimal response | Herpes simplex virus: survives in host cells for long periods in a latent stage; no pathology |
| Evade effects of response | Mycobacteria: survive unharmed in granulomas designed to localize and destroy infection |
| Depress host's response | Human immunodeficiency virus: destroys T cells; malaria: depresses immune responsiveness |
| Antigenic change | Viruses, spirochaetes, trypanosomes: all change target antigens so host response is ineffective |
| Rapid replication | Viruses, bacteria, protozoa: produce acute infections before recovery and immunity |
| Survival in weakly responsive individuals | Genetic heterogeneity in host population means some individuals respond weakly or not at all, allowing organism to reproduce freely; examples in all groups |

**Table 9.2** Lifestyle changes and infectious diseases

| Social and behavioural changes and infectious diseases | |
|---|---|
| **The causes** | **The results** |
| Altered environments (e.g. air conditioning) | Water in cooling systems provides growth conditions for *Legionella* |
| Changes in food production and food-handling practices | Intensive husbandry under antibiotic protection leads to drug-resistant bacteria; deep-freezing food, fast-food and inadequately cooked food allow bacteria and toxins to enter body (e.g. *Listeria, Salmonella*) |
| Routine use of antibiotics in medicine | Emergence of antibiotic-resistant bacteria as hazards to hospitalized patients (e.g. methicillin-resistant *Staphylococcus aureus*) |
| Routine use of immunosuppressive therapy | Development of opportunistic infections in patients with reduced resistance (e.g. *Pseudomonas, Candida, Pneumocystis*) |
| Altered sexual habits | Promiscuity increases sexually transmitted diseases (e.g. gonorrhoea, genital herpes, acquired immunodeficiency syndrome) |
| Breakdown of filtration systems, overuse of limited water supplies | Transmission of animal infections leading to diarrhoeal and other infections (e.g. cryptosporidiosis, giardiasis, leptospirosis) |
| Increase in ownership of pets, particularly exotic species | Transmission of animal infections (e.g. *Chlamydia, Salmonella, Toxoplasma, Toxocara*) |
| Increased frequency of journeys to tropical and subtropical countries | Exposure to exotic organisms and vectors (e.g. malaria, viral encephalitis) |

### Changes in parasites create new problems for hosts

From what has already been said, it can be appreciated that there is no such thing as a static host–parasite relationship and that concepts of unchanging pathogenicity or lack of pathogenicity cannot be justified. Each relationship is an arms race: Changes in one member are countered by changes in the other. Quite subtle changes in either can completely change the balance of the relationship (e.g. toward greater or lesser pathogenicity).

A dramatic illustration of this situation was the explosive appearance of individuals with human immunodeficiency virus (HIV) infection in 1981. This group of viruses was originally restricted to nonhuman primates, but changes in the virus permitted extensive infections in humans to the extent that, by 2021, the United Nations Acquired Immunodeficiency Syndrome/World Health Organization (UNAIDS/WHO) estimate of the number of people living with HIV globally was 38.4 million (range 33.9–43.8 million). Similarly, changes in the human coronaviruses allowed human infection from horseshoe bats, causing severe acute respiratory syndrome (SARS), from camels, causing Middle Eastern respiratory syndrome (MERS) and, finally, from SARS-CoV-2, causing the COVID-19 pandemic. There is concern about influenza A viruses that infect a range of animals, including the avian influenza A H5N1 virus, which can spread to humans from infected poultry. Of a different nature, but relevant to the general theme, is the acquisition of drug resistance in bacteria, viruses and protozoa (see Ch. 34). Although the underlying genetic and metabolic changes do not by themselves influence pathogenicity, the expression of such changes in the face of intense and selective chemotherapy certainly does, allowing overwhelming infection to occur with major concerns regarding diminished therapeutic options.

### Host adaptations to overcome changes in parasites

Changes in the host can also alter the balance of a host–parasite relationship. A particularly dramatic example is the intense selection for resistant genotypes in rabbit populations exposed to the myxomatosis virus in the first reported outbreak in the United Kingdom in 1954, which took place concurrently with selection for reduced pathogenicity in the virus itself (see Ch. 13). There are no exactly equivalent examples in humans, but in evolutionary time there have been major selective influences on populations prompting changes to permit survival in the face of life-threatening infections. A good example is the selective pressure exerted by falciparum malaria, which has been responsible for the persistence in human populations of many alleles associated with haemoglobinopathies (e.g. sickle cell haemoglobin). Although these abnormalities are detrimental to varying degrees, they persist because they are (or were) associated with resistance to malarial infection. Studies suggest that malaria may change the frequency of certain human leukocyte antigens in areas where infection is severe.

### Social and behavioural changes can be as important as genetic changes in altering host–parasite relations

Social and behavioural changes can alter host–parasite relations both positively and negatively (Table 9.2). Although many bacterial infections of the intestine have declined in importance with changes in human lifestyle, there are other contemporary microbiologic problems in the resource-rich world whose onset can be traced directly to sociologic, environmental and even medical change. A particularly good example is disease arising from domestication of pets (e.g. toxoplasmosis) because it illustrates that human freedom from some infections arises primarily because of lack of contact with the organisms and not from any innate resistance to the establishment of the infection itself. Diseases arising from contact with infected animals or animal products (zoonotic infections) constitute a constant threat that can be realized by behavioural or environmental changes that alter established patterns of human–animal contact.

## KEY FACTS

- The body is colonized by many organisms (the microbiota), which can be positively beneficial. They live on or within the body without causing disease and play an important role in protecting the host from pathogenic microbes.

- The microbiota is predominantly made up of bacteria but includes viruses, fungi and protozoa.

- Members of the microbiota can be harmful if they enter previously sterile parts of the body. They can also be causes of hospital-acquired infections.

- The usual relationship between the microbiota and the body is an example of beneficial symbiosis; parasitism (in the broad sense, covering all pathogenic microbes) is a harmful symbiosis.

- The biologic context of host–parasite relationships and the dynamics of the conflict between two species in this relationship provide a basis for understanding the causes and control of infectious diseases.

- Changes in medical practice, in human behaviour and (not least) in infectious organisms are broadening the spectrum of organisms responsible for disease.

# The adversaries – host defences

**10.** The innate defences of the body      68

**11.** Adaptive immune responses bring specificity      85

**12.** Cooperation leads to effective immune responses      97

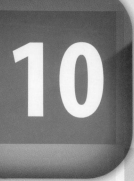

# 10

# The innate defences of the body

## Introduction

The immune system has a challenge. It needs to defend us against pathogens that range in size from the smallest viruses to the large helminth worms. These pathogens may also infect us by different routes, including by aerosol, by ingestion, through the skin, or through sexual contact. In the preceding chapters we have outlined some of the fundamental characteristics of the many types of microparasites and macroparasites (here collectively called *pathogens*) that may infect the body. We will now consider the ways in which the body seeks to defend itself against infection by these organisms, starting with the innate immune responses that are the first line of defence. This chapter will discuss the key cells and molecules involved in innate immunity. These responses can result in inflammation (often necessary but not pleasant), play roles in controlling inflammation and clearing dead cells and regulate all these processes.

### The body has both innate and adaptive immune defences

When an organism infects the body for the first time, the defence systems already in place may well be adequate to prevent replication and spread of the infectious agent, thereby preventing development of disease. These established mechanisms constitute the innate immune system. However, should innate immunity be insufficient to deal with the invasion by the infectious agent, the adaptive immune system then comes into action, although it takes time to reach its maximum efficiency (Fig. 10.1). When it does take effect, it generally eliminates the infecting organism, allowing recovery from disease.

The main feature distinguishing the adaptive response from the innate mechanism is that specific memory of infection is imprinted on the adaptive immune system

so that should there be a subsequent infection by the same agent, a particularly effective response comes into play with remarkable speed. It is worth emphasizing, however, that there is close synergy between the two systems, with the adaptive mechanism greatly improving the efficiency of the innate response and vice versa, and that innate immunity does show some evidence of memory.

The contrasts between these two systems are set out in Table 10.1. On the one hand, the soluble factors such as lysozyme and complement, together with the phagocytic cells, contribute to the innate system, while on the other the T- and B-cell–based mechanisms that produce cytokines and cytotoxicity or antibodies are the main elements of the adaptive immune system. Not only do these lymphocytes provide improved resistance by repeated contact with a given infectious agent, but also the memory with which they become endowed shows very considerable specificity to that infection. For instance, infection with measles virus will induce a memory to that microorganism alone and not to another virus such as rubella.

Both the innate and the adaptive immune systems rely on specialized cells that have particular cell surface receptors and carry out effector functions. Pluripotent hematopoietic stem cells in the bone marrow develop into common myeloid progenitor stem cells or common lymphocyte progenitor stem cells from which the key cells of the innate and the adaptive immune systems develop. These cells will then circulate in the blood and lymph and move into the various lymphoid and other tissues.

The cells of the innate immune system express <100 types of receptors in contrast to the much more extensive repertoire of antigen-specific receptors expressed by T and B cells—there may >$10^{15}$ different antibody specificities expressed by B cells!

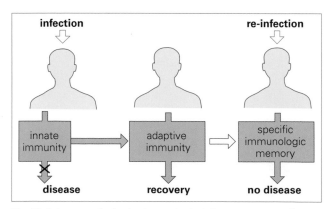

**Fig. 10.1** Innate and adaptive immunity. An infectious organism first encounters the cells and molecules of the innate immune system. If these do not prevent infection, the adaptive immune system is needed with its specific and specialized cells and mediators. Following recovery, specific immunologic memory will prevent reinfection.

**Table 10.1** Comparison of innate and adaptive effector immune systems

| | Innate immune system | Adaptive immune system |
|---|---|---|
| **Major elements** | | |
| Soluble factors | Lysozyme, complement, acute phase proteins (e.g. C-reactive protein), interferons, other cytokines | Antibody Cytokines |
| Cells | Phagocytes Innate lymphoid cells, including natural killer cells | T cells B cells |
| Receptors | <100 invariant receptors (includes pathogen recognition receptors, complement receptors, etc.) | T-cell receptors (repertoire $\sim10^8$, with $10^{61}$ possible Variable (V), Diversity (D) and Joining (J) combinations) B cell receptors (antibody repertoire $10^{15}$–$10^{18}$) (both clonally expressed with extensive variation) |
| **Response to microbial infection** | | |
| First contact | + | + |
| Second contact | ++ | + + ++ |
| | Broad specificity; no specific memory | Antigen specificity; specific memory |
| | Resistance not improved by repeated contact | Resistance improved by repeated contact |

Innate immunity used to be referred to as natural and adaptive as acquired. The two systems are bridged by innate lymphoid cells, and innate immunity is needed for an effective adaptive immune response. Humoral immunity due to soluble factors uses antibody (made by B cells) to provide specific protection, whereas cellular immunity relies on antigen-specific T cells. If the same organism persists or is encountered a second time, a more effective specific adaptive response to its antigens is induced. Although this immunologic memory largely relies on memory B cells and memory T cells, some cells of the innate immune system can show a form of memory, although this lacks the antigen specificity shown by T and B cells.

## DEFENCES AGAINST ENTRY INTO THE BODY

### A variety of biochemical and physical barriers operate at the body surfaces

Before an infectious agent can penetrate the body, it must overcome biochemical and physical barriers that operate at the body surfaces. One of the most important of these is the skin, which is normally impermeable to the majority of infectious agents. Many bacteria fail to survive for long on the skin because of the direct inhibitory effects of lactic acid and fatty acids present in sweat and sebaceous secretions and the lower pH to which they give rise (Fig. 10.2). However, should there be skin loss as can occur in burns or damage through trauma, for example, infection becomes a major problem.

The membranes lining the inner surfaces of the body secrete mucus, which acts as a protective layer outside the epithelium, inhibiting the adherence of bacteria to the epithelial cells, thereby preventing them from gaining access to the body. Microbial and other foreign particles trapped within this adhesive mucus may be removed by mechanical means such as ciliary action, coughing and sneezing. The flushing actions of tears, saliva and urine are other mechanical strategies that help to protect the epithelial surfaces. In addition, many of the secreted body fluids contain microbicidal factors (e.g. the acid in gastric juice, spermine and zinc in semen, lactoperoxidase in milk, lysozyme in tears, nasal secretions and saliva).

Harmless commensal organisms that are part of our microbiota (see Ch. 9) also protect us through microbial antagonism. These commensal organisms suppress the growth of many potentially pathogenic bacteria and fungi at superficial sites, firstly by virtue of their physical advantage of previous occupancy, especially on epithelial surfaces, secondly by competing for essential nutrients, and

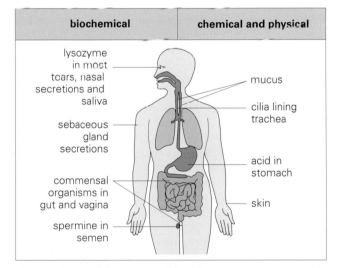

**Fig. 10.2** Exterior defences. Most of the infectious agents encountered by an individual are prevented from entering the body by a variety of biochemical and physical barriers. The body tolerates a huge number of commensal and harmless organisms, now collectively called the *microbiota*; these organisms may prevent pathogens from invading through competition and have a major impact on immune function.

thirdly by producing inhibitory substances such as acid or colicins. The latter are a class of bactericidins that have a number of modes of action, including binding to the negatively charged surface of susceptible bacteria and forming a voltage-dependent channel in the membrane, which kills by destroying the cell's energy potential.

Keratinocytes in the skin can sense pathogens and secrete antimicrobial peptides and cytokines, while deeper into the skin a range of other cell types such as dendritic cells, innate lymphoid cells (ILCs), mast cells and T lymphocytes contribute to host defence.

## DEFENCES ONCE THE MICROORGANISM PENETRATES THE BODY

Despite the general effectiveness of the various barriers, microorganisms can often successfully penetrate the body. When this occurs, two main defensive strategies come into play, based on:

- the destructive effect of soluble antimicrobial factors, such as defensins and cathelicidin
- the mechanism of phagocytosis, involving engulfment and killing of microorganisms by specialized cells, the professional phagocytes.

There are two types of antimicrobial molecules secreted by epithelial cells as well as by phagocytic cells. The **defensins**, which are small cationic peptides, are directly toxic to not only bacteria but also to fungi and encapsulated viruses; some are made by epithelial cells in mucosa and Paneth cells in the gut, and others are made by neutrophils and cytotoxic T cells. Cathelicidin is another useful molecule with antibacterial effects (see Ch. 15).

### Phagocytes

The innate immune system has an efficient way of removing and killing pathogens or particles larger than 0.5–1 µM: phagocytosis. Phagocytes engulf the pathogens and, if we are lucky, kill them. The phagocytes consist of two major cell families first defined by zoologist Elie Metchnikoff (Box 10.1; Fig. 10.3):

- the larger macrophages; some are resident in tissues, but most develop from monocytes circulating in the blood and are summoned to the site of an active infection
- the smaller neutrophils, which are generally referred to as *neutrophils* or *polymorphs* (polymorphonuclear neutrophils [PMNs]) because they have a segmented multilobed nucleus and their cytoplasmic granules do not stain with haematoxylin and eosin (Fig. 10.4).

As a very crude generalization, the PMNs provide the major phagocytic defence against pyogenic (pus-forming) bacteria, whereas the macrophages are best at combating organisms capable of living within the cells of the host. Neutrophils are closely related to eosinophils and basophils but are more phagocytic. They are also effective against fungi.

Monocytes develop from myeloid precursor cells in the bone marrow and then circulate in the blood. Most monocytes in the blood are termed *classical monocytes* and express the CD14 marker; a small subset that express both the CD14 and CD16 markers patrol the endothelial surfaces.

Dendritic cells can also phagocytose microorganisms but less efficiently; immature dendritic cells are more phagocytic than mature dendritic cells. Dendritic cells come in two main types, myeloid (mDC) and plasmacytoid (pDC) dendritic cells (Table 10.2). The mDCs can be subdivided into Langerhans cells in the skin, dermal or interstitial dendritic cells and monocyte-derived dendritic cells. Dendritic cells play a major role as antigen-presenting cells, and the process of antigen presentation will be discussed later in Chapter 12.

### Macrophages are widespread throughout the tissues

Monocytes can settle in tissues where they develop into macrophages. The majority of tissue-resident macrophages originate during embryogenesis and enter the tissue where they differentiate into a macrophage that has properties

### Box 10.1   Lessons in Microbiology

**Elie Metchnikoff—father of phagocytosis**

Metchnikoff (1845–1916) was a Russian zoologist who became fascinated by how cells deal with bacteria. He observed that if he introduced a rose thorn into a transparent starfish larva, the thorn became surrounded by motile cells. He then went on to investigate mammalian leukocytes, showing that they could engulf microorganisms, which he termed *phagocytosis*. He defined two types of phagocytes: the smaller microphage (now called a *neutrophil*) and the larger macrophage. We now know that phagocytosis is further enhanced when the humoral components antibody and complement are present.

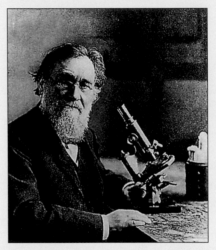

**Fig. 10.3**  Elie Metchnikoff, the father of phagocytosis. (Courtesy the Wellcome Institute Library, London.)

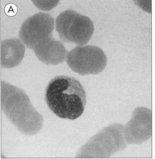 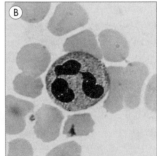

**Fig. 10.4**  Phagocytic cells. (A) Blood monocyte and (B) polymorphonuclear neutrophil, both derived from bone marrow stem cells. (Courtesy P.M. Lydyard.)

particular to the site they have entered (Fig. 10.5). They are concentrated in the lung (alveolar macrophages), liver (Kupffer cells), lining of lymph node medullary sinuses and splenic venous sinusoids where they are well placed to filter out foreign material. Other examples are the brain microglia, kidney mesangial cells, synovial A cells and osteoclasts in bone. These tissue macrophages are long-lived cells that depend upon mitochondria for their metabolic energy and show elements of rough-surfaced endoplasmic reticulum

**Table 10.2** Dendritic cells come in two main types: myeloid and plasmacytoid

| | Myeloid dendritic cells | Plasmacytoid dendritic cells |
|---|---|---|
| Origin | Common myeloid precursor cells | Common lymphoid precursor cells |
| Tissue location | Epidermis, mucosa, lymphoid tissues | T-cell areas of lymphoid tissues |
| Myeloid markers (e.g. CD14) | Yes | No |
| Main cytokines produced | IL-8, IL-12 | Type I interferons |

IL, Interleukin.

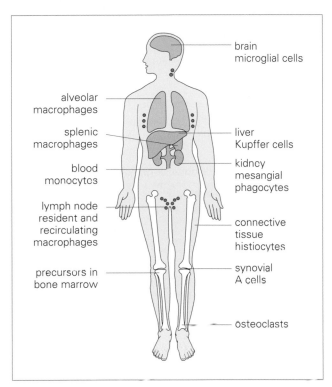

**Fig. 10.5** The mononuclear phagocyte system. Most tissue macrophages are derived very early in life and differentiate in the organs to which they have homed.

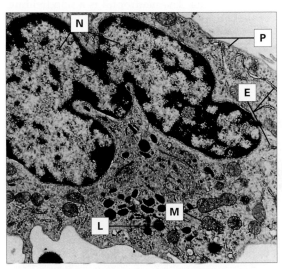

**Fig. 10.6** Monocyte (× 8000), with horseshoe nucleus (N). Phagocytic and pinocytic vesicles (P), lysosomal granules (L), mitochondria (M) and isolated profiles of rough-surfaced endoplasmic reticulum (E) are evident. (Courtesy B. Nichols; Copyright © Rockefeller University Press.)

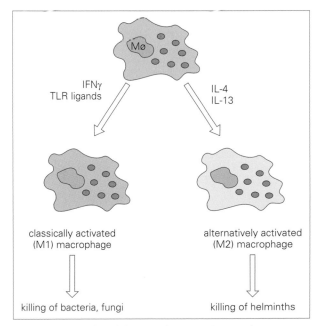

**Fig. 10.7** Classically and alternatively activated macrophages. Macrophages can be activated in two ways to form activated macrophages that can kill different types of pathogens. Interferon gamma (IFNγ) derived from natural killer cells, ILC1 cells or Th1 T cells and Toll-like receptor (TLR) ligands will induce classically activated (M1) macrophages; IL-4 and IL-13 from Th2 T cells will induce alternatively activated (M2) macrophages. Alternatively activated macrophages also play a role in tissue repair. IL, Interleukin; Th, T helper.

required to produce the formidable array of different secretory proteins that these cells generate.

Throughout life, bone marrow promonocytes develop into circulating blood monocytes (Fig. 10.6; also see Fig. 10.4) and finally become mature macrophages, which are enriched in tissues in states of disease and inflammation. Collectively these cells are termed the *mononuclear phagocyte system* (see Fig. 10.5).

Macrophages live much longer than neutrophils or monocytes but have other interesting properties. If the cytokine interferon gamma (IFNγ) is around, they can become activated, becoming more efficient at killing intracellular pathogens. This is an example in which innate cell function is enhanced by adaptive immunity, as some T cells as well as the innate natural killer (NK) cells make IFNγ. These IFNγ-activated macrophages are called *classically activated*, or *M1 macrophages*. Other cytokines such as interleukin (IL)–4 and IL-13 drive the development of *alternatively activated*, or *M2 macrophages* (Fig. 10.7). These two macrophage subsets play particular roles in our defence against intracellular infections and helminth infections.

## Neutrophils possess a variety of enzyme-containing granules

The neutrophil is the dominant white cell in the bloodstream and, like the macrophage, shares a common haemopoietic stem cell precursor with the other cell types found in the blood. It has no mitochondria but uses its abundant cytoplasmic glycogen stores for its energy requirements; therefore, glycolysis enables these cells to function under anaerobic conditions such as those in an inflammatory focus. The neutrophil is a nondividing, short-lived cell with a segmented nucleus; the cytoplasm

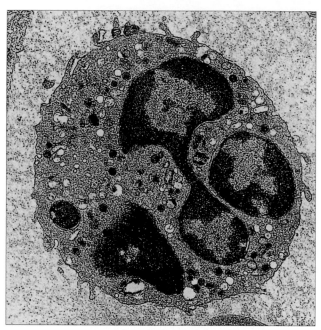

**Fig. 10.8** The neutrophil. The multilobed nucleus and primary azurophilic, secondary specific and tertiary lysosomal granules are well displayed. There is an overlap in the contents between some of the granules. Typical conventional lysosomes with acid hydrolase are also seen. (Courtesy D. McLaren.)

is characterized by an array of granules (Fig. 10.8; Table 10.3). Neutrophils can produce IL-8 as well as other chemokines and cytokines. They provide a major defence against extracellular and acute bacterial infections such as with staphylococci or streptococci, but they also play a role in chronic infections—in tuberculosis, a very chronic intracellular bacterial infection, neutrophils in the lungs may contain phagocytosed mycobacteria.

Some of the key differences between neutrophils and macrophages are shown in Table 10.4.

## Phagocytosis and killing

We will now return to the major function of phagocytes, phagocytosis, and how phagocytosis results in killing of the ingested organism.

### How do phagocytes sense infection?

Before the professional phagocyte can phagocytose a microorganism, it must first attach to the phagocyte surface.

**Table 10.3** Neutrophil cytoplasmic granules

| Primary azurophilic granules | Secondary specific granules | Tertiary granules |
|---|---|---|
| Lysozyme | Lysozyme | Lysozyme |
| Myeloperoxidase | Cytochrome $b_{558}$ | Cytochrome $b_{558}$ |
| Elastase | Gelatinase (matrix metalloproteinase (MMP9) | Gelatinase (MMP9) |
| Cathepsins | Lactoferrin | |
| Acid hydrolases | Collagenase matrix metalloproteinase (MMP8) | |
| Defensins | | |
| Bactericidal permeability increasing protein | | |

**Table 10.4** The major phagocytic cells—PMNs and macrophages—differ in a number of important respects

| Cell | Neutrophil | Macrophage |
|---|---|---|
| Site of production | Bone marrow | Bone marrow or tissues |
| Duration in blood | 7–10 h | 20–40 h (monocyte) |
| Average life span | 4 days | Months–years |
| Numbers in blood | $(2.5–7.5) \times 10^9/L$ | $(0.2–0.8) \times 10^9/L$ |
| Numbers in tissues | (Transient) | $100 \times$ blood |
| Principal killing mechanisms | Oxidative, nonoxidative | Oxidative, nitric oxide, cytokines |
| Activated by | TNF, IFNγ, GM-CSF, microbial products | TNF, IFNγ, GM-CSF, microbial products (e.g. LPS) |
| Important deficiencies | CGD Myeloperoxidase Chemotactic Chediak-Higashi | Lipid storage diseases |
| Major secretory products | Lysozyme | Over 80, including lysozyme, cytokines (TNFα, IL-1), complement factors |

CGD, Chronic granulomatous disease; GM-CSF, granulocyte-macrophage colony-stimulating factor; IFN, interferon; IFNγ, interferon gamma; IL, interleukin; LPS, lipopolysaccharide; PMN, polymorphonuclear neutrophil; TNF, tumour necrosis factor; TNFα, tumour necrosis factor alpha.

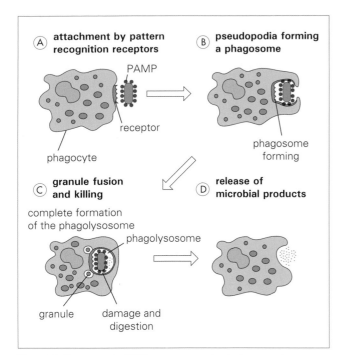

**Fig. 10.9** Phagocytosis. (A) Phagocytes attach to microorganisms (*blue icon*, not shown to scale) via their cell surface receptors, which recognize pathogen-associated molecular patterns (PAMPs) such as lipopolysaccharide. (B) If the membrane now becomes activated by the attached infectious agent, the pathogen is taken into a phagosome by pseudopodia, which extend around it. (C) Once inside the cell, the various granules fuse with the phagosome to form a phagolysosome. (D) The infectious agent is then killed by a battery of microbicidal degradation mechanisms, and the microbial products are released.

Pattern recognition receptors (PRRs) on the phagocyte surface bind repeating pathogen-associated molecular patterns (PAMPs) (Fig. 10.9).

The Toll-like receptors (TLRs) are a major family of PRRs. The TLRs are so-called because of their similarity to the Toll receptor in the fruit fly *Drosophila*, which, in the adult fly, triggers an intracellular cascade generating the expression of antimicrobial peptides in response to microbial infection. A series of cell surface TLRs acting as sensors for extracellular infections have been identified (Fig. 10.10), which are activated by microbial elements such as peptidoglycan, lipoproteins, mycobacterial lipoarabinomannan, yeast zymosan and flagellin.

Other PRRs displayed by phagocyte on the cell surface include the cell-bound C-type (calcium-dependent) lectins, of which the macrophage mannose receptor is an example, and scavenger receptors, which recognize a variety of anionic polymers and acetylated low-density proteins. Some TLRs (TLR 3, 7, 9) are also found in the endosomal environment where they recognize PAMPs such as the unmethylated guanosine–cytosine sequences of bacterial DNA and double-stranded RNA from RNA viruses (see Fig. 10.10). There are also cytoplasmic PRRs such as NOD-like and RIG-like receptors that can recognize pathogens. The NOD-like receptors recognize diaminopimelic acid from gram-negative bacteria (NOD-1) and bacterial muramyl dipeptide (NOD-2), and once engaged, induce nuclear factor (NF)–κB activation. Bacterial flagellin is also recognized by NOD-like receptors. Cytoplasmic receptors also sense viruses—retinoic acid-inducible gene-1 (RIG-1) receptors sense viral RNA and signal via interferon-regulated factors to induce IFNs.

Infections usually result in damaged and dying cells that need to be removed and that are recognized because they express damage-associated molecular patterns (also called *alarmins*) such as abnormal host DNA (as well as pathogen-derived DNA). An example of a sensor for double-stranded DNA is STING, which stands for *st*imulator of *in*terferon *g*enes. Damaged cells are also recognized by TLRs, C-type lectin receptors, other molecules such as heat shock proteins and inflammasomes (see later).

#### The phagocyte is activated through PAMP recognition

Signals are sent through the phagocyte's receptors to initiate the ingestion phase by activating an actin–myosin contractile system that sends arms of cytoplasm around the organism until it is completely enclosed within a vacuole (phagosome) (Fig. 10.11; see also Fig. 10.9). Shortly afterward, the cytoplasmic granules fuse with the phagosome and discharge their contents around the captive microorganism.

#### Opsonization increases phagocytosis

Pathogens can be opsonized or coated by the binding of plasma proteins from the complement system. Opsonization increases the efficiency of uptake of the particle or pathogen. This process becomes even more efficient if specific antibodies are around and can bind to receptors for the constant Fc end of the antibody molecule on the macrophage surface. The phagocytes have receptors for the C3a and C5a complement components (see later). These complement components are examples of molecules that recognize PAMPs. Other phagocytic receptors include dectin-1, the mannose receptor and scavenger receptors. As well as internalizing the pathogen, other G protein–coupled receptors on phagocytes sense bacteria and trigger killing mechanisms such as production of reactive oxygen species.

#### The internalized pathogen is the target for a fearsome array of killing mechanisms

As phagocytosis is initiated, the attached microbes also signal through one of the PRRs to engineer an appropriate defensive response to the different types of infection through a number of NF-κB–mediated responses. This activation of a unique plasma membrane–reduced nicotinamide adenine dinucleotide phosphate (NADPH) oxidase reduces oxygen to a series of powerful microbicidal agents, namely superoxide anion, hydrogen peroxide, singlet oxygen and hydroxyl radicals (Fig. 10.12). Subsequently the peroxide, in association with myeloperoxidase, generates a potent halogenating system from halide ions, which is capable of killing both bacteria and viruses.

As superoxide anion is formed, the enzyme superoxide dismutase acts to convert it to molecular oxygen and hydrogen peroxide but, in the process, consumes hydrogen ions. Therefore, initially there is a small increase in pH, which facilitates the antibacterial function of the families of cationic proteins derived from the phagocytic granules (Box 10.2). These molecules damage microbial membranes by the proteolytic action of cathepsin G and by direct adherence to the microbial surface. The defensins have an amphipathic structure, which allows them to interact with and disrupt

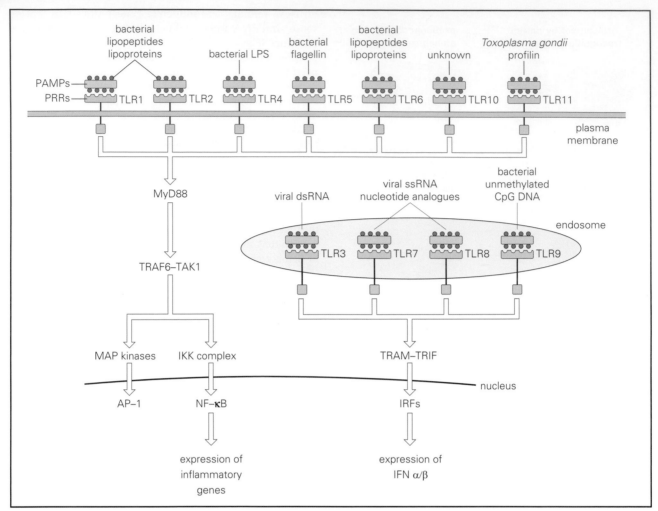

**Fig. 10.10** Recognition of pathogen-associated molecular patterns (PAMPs) by a subset of pattern recognition receptors (PRRs) termed Toll-like receptors (TLRs). TLRs reside within plasma membrane or endosomal membrane compartments, as shown. All TLRs have multiple *N*-terminal leucine-rich repeats forming a horseshoe-shaped structure that acts as the PAMP-binding domain. Upon engagement of the TLR ectodomain with an appropriate PAMP (some examples are shown), signals are sent that ultimately activate the activation protein 1 (AP-1), nuclear factor-κB (NF-κB) and/or interferon-regulated factor (IRF) transcription factors, as shown. NF-κB and IRF transcription factors then direct the expression of numerous antimicrobial gene products such as cytokines and chemokines, as well as proteins that are involved in altering the activation state of the cell. There are also cytosolic PRRs that can sense bacterial peptidoglycan (NOD-like receptors), viral RNA (RIG-like receptors) and cytosolic DNA sensors. MyD88 is a signalling adaptor that is part of the supramolecular organizing centre; TRAF6 is a ubiquitin ligase; TAK1 phosphorylates the mitogen-activated protein (MAP) kinases; the IKK complex contains I kappa kinases; TRAM is a signalling adaptor molecule; TRIF is TIR domain containing adaptor inducing IFNβ. TLR10 ligands may include HIV-gp41.

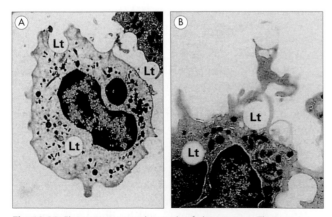

**Fig. 10.11** Electron micrographic study of phagocytosis. These two micrographs show human phagocytes engulfing latex particles (Lt). (A) × 3000; (B) × 4500. (Courtesy C.H.W. Horne.)

the structure and function of microbial membranes. These antibiotic peptides reach extraordinarily high concentrations within the phagosome and act as disinfectants against a wide spectrum of bacteria, fungi and enveloped viruses. Other important factors are:

- lactoferrin, which complexes iron to deprive bacteria of essential growth elements
- lysozyme, which splits the proteoglycan cell wall of bacterianitric oxide, which, together with its derivative, the peroxynitrite radical, can also be directly microbicidal (Fig. 10.13).

The pH now falls so that the dead or dying microorganisms are extensively degraded by acid hydrolytic enzymes that are derived from lysosomes that have fused with the phagosome to produce a phagolysosome, and the degradation products are released to the exterior. These digestive enzymes need an acidic pH to function effectively.

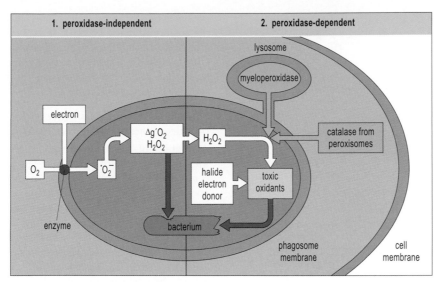

**Fig. 10.12** Oxygen-dependent microbicidal activity during the respiratory burst. The enzyme nicotinamide adenine dinucleotide phosphate (NADPH) oxidase in the phagosome membrane reduces oxygen by the addition of electrons to form superoxide anion ($^{\cdot}OH_2^-$). This can then give rise to hydroxyl radicals ($^{\cdot}OH$), singlet oxygen ($\Delta g'O_2$) and hydrogen peroxide ($H_2O_2$), all of which are potentially toxic. If lysosome fusion occurs, myeloperoxidase or, in some cases, catalase from peroxisomes acts on peroxides in the presence of halides to generate toxic oxidants such as hypohalite. (Modified from Male D, Peebles RS, Male, V. *Immunology*, ed 9, Mosby Elsevier; 2021.)

## Box 10.2 ◻ Oxygen-independent antimicrobial mechanisms

| MOLECULE | FUNCTION |
|---|---|
| Cathepsin G | Damage to microbial membranes |
| Elastase | Damage to microbial membranes |
| Defensins (low molecular weight) | Damage to microbial membranes |
| Cationic proteins (high molecular weight) | Damage to microbial membranes |
| Bactericidal permeability increasing protein | Damage to microbial membranes |
| Lactoferrin | Complex with iron |
| Lysozyme | Splits peptidoglycan in bacterial cell wall |
| Acid hydrolases | Degrade dead pathogens |

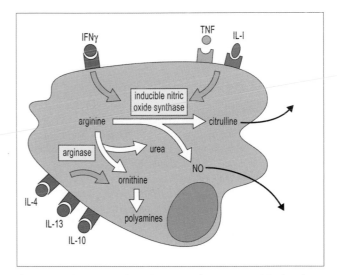

**Fig. 10.13** The nitric oxide pathway. Interferon gamma (IFNγ) and other inflammatory cytokines cause production of inducible nitric oxide synthase (i-NOS, also known as *NOS2*). i-NOS combines oxygen with guanidino nitrogen of L-arginine to give nitric oxide (NO•), which is toxic for bacteria and tumour cells. Toxicity may be increased by interactions with products of the oxygen reduction pathway, leading to the formation of peroxynitrites. Cell activation by Th2-type cytokines promotes breakdown of arginine to ornithine and urea. Polyamines are products of ornithine, which promote collagen synthesis and cell proliferation. (Modified from Male D, Peebles RS, Male V. *Immunology*, ed 9, Mosby Elsevier; 2021.)

NF-κB activation can also lead to the release of proinflammatory mediators. These include the antiviral IFNs, the small protein cytokines (IL-1β, IL-6, IL-12) and tumour necrosis factor alpha (TNFα, a proinflammatory cytokine produced by macrophages and other cell types), which activate other cells through binding to specific receptors, and chemokines such as IL-8, which represent a subset of chemoattractant cytokines.

### Phagocytes are mobilized and targeted onto the microorganism by chemotaxis

Phagocytosis cannot occur unless the bacterium first attaches to the surface of the phagocyte, and clearly this cannot happen unless both have become physically close to each other. There is therefore a need for a mechanism that mobilizes phagocytes from afar and targets them onto the bacterium. Many bacteria produce chemical substances such as formyl methionyl peptides, which directionally attract leukocytes in a process called *chemotaxis*. However, this is a relatively weak signalling system, and evolution has provided the body with a far more effective magnet that uses a complex series of proteins collectively termed *complement*.

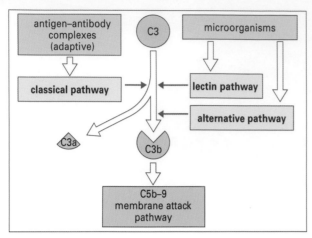

**Fig. 10.14** The complement pathways. There are three complement pathways, which, although initiated in different ways, all generate a C3 covertase, which converts C3 to C3b, the central event of the complement system. C3b in turn activates the terminal lytic membrane attack pathway. The first stage in the classical pathway is the binding of antigen to antibody. The alternative pathway does not require antibody and is initiated by the covalent binding of C3b to hydroxyl and amine groups on the surface of various microorganisms. The lectin pathway is also triggered by microorganisms in the absence of antibody, with sugar residues on the pathogen surface providing the binding sites. The alternative and lectin pathways provide antibody-independent innate immunity, whereas the classical pathway represents a more recently evolved link to the adaptive immune system. (Modified from Male D, Peebles RS, Male V. *Immunology*, ed 9, Mosby Elsevier; 2021.)

## Activation of the complement system

Complement resembles blood clotting, fibrinolysis and kinin formation in being a major triggered enzyme cascade system. Such systems are characterized by their ability to produce a rapid, highly amplified response to a trigger stimulus mediated by a cascade phenomenon in which the product of one reaction is the enzymic catalyst of the next. There are three ways in which complement can be activated: through the classical pathway in which C1q binds to antibody-antigen complexes (but even here there are innate initiators such as C-reactive protein [CRP] or natural antibody), through the recognition of lectins such as mannan-binding lectin and ficolins by PAMPs, and through what is rather misleadingly called the *alternative complement pathway* in which complement is directly activated by bacteria (Fig. 10.14; Table 10.5). All three pathways lead to inflammation and cell lysis.

The most abundant and most central component in the complement cascade is C3 (complement components are designated by the letter C followed by a number), and the cleavage of this molecule is at the heart of all complement-mediated phenomena. In normal plasma, C3 undergoes spontaneous activation at a very slow rate to generate the split product C3b. This can complex with another complement component, factor B, which is then acted upon by a normal plasma enzyme, factor D, to produce the C3-splitting enzyme $\overline{C3bBb}$. This C3 convertase can then split new molecules of C3 to give C3a (a small fragment) and further C3b. This represents a positive feedback circuit with potential for runaway amplification; however, the overall process is restricted to a slow turnover rate by powerful regulatory mechanisms that break down the unstable soluble-phase C3 convertase into inactive cleavage products (Fig. 10.15). In the presence of certain molecules, such as the carbohydrates on the surface of many bacteria, the C3 convertase can become attached and stabilized against breakdown. Under these circumstances, there is active generation of new C3 convertase molecules, and what is known as the *alternative complement pathway* is activated (Fig. 10.16).

### Complement synergizes with phagocytic cells to produce an acute inflammatory response

Activation of the alternative complement pathway with the consequent splitting of very large numbers of C3 molecules has important consequences for the orchestration of an integrated antimicrobial defence strategy (see Fig. 10.16). Large numbers of C3b molecules produced in the immediate vicinity of the microbial membrane bind covalently to that surface and act as opsonins (molecules that make the particle they coat more susceptible to engulfment by phagocytic cells; see later). This C3b, together with the C3 convertase, acts on the next component in the sequence, C5, to produce a small fragment, C5a, which, together with C3a, has a direct effect on mast cells to cause their degranulation (Fig. 10.17). This results in the release not only of mediators of vascular permeability but also of factors chemotactic for neutrophils (Table 10.6). The circulating equivalent of the tissue mast cell, the basophil, is also shown in Fig. 10.17.

The vascular permeability mediators increase the permeability of capillaries by modifying the intercellular forces between the endothelial cells of the vessel wall. This allows the leakage or exudation of fluid and plasma components, including more complement, to the site of the infection. These mediators (see Table 10.6) also upregulate molecules such as intercellular adhesion molecule-1 and E-selectin, which bind to specific complementary molecules on the neutrophils and encourage them to stick in stages to the walls of the capillaries, a process termed *margination*.

The chemotactic factors, on the other hand, provide a chemical gradient that attracts marginated neutrophils from their intravascular location through the walls of the blood vessels to the site of the C3b-coated bacteria that initiated the whole activation process. Neutrophils have a receptor for C3b on their surface, and, as a result, the opsonized bacteria adhere very firmly to the surface of these newly arrived cells.

The processes of capillary dilation (erythema), exudation of plasma proteins and of fluid (oedema) due to hydrostatic and osmotic pressure changes, and the accumulation of neutrophils are features of the acute inflammatory response and result in a highly effective way of focusing phagocytic cells onto complement-coated microbial targets.

The macrophage can also be stimulated by certain bacterial toxins, such as the lipopolysaccharides by the action of C5a and by the phagocytosis of C3b-coated bacteria to secrete other potent mediators of acute inflammation independently of the mast cell–directed pathway (Fig. 10.18).

### C9 molecules form the membrane attack complex, which is involved in cell lysis

We have already introduced the idea that, following the activation of C3, the next component to be cleaved is C5; the larger C5b fragment that results becomes membrane bound. This subsequently binds components C6, C7 and C8, which form a complex capable of inducing a critical

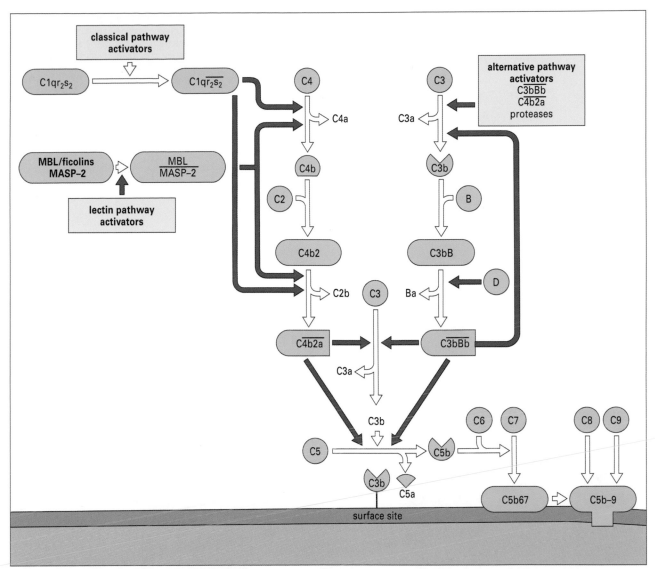

**Fig. 10.15** Outline of complement activation. The proteins of the classical and alternative pathways are assigned numbers (e.g. C1, C2). Many of these are zymogens (i.e. proenzymes that require proteolytic cleavage to become active). The cleavage products of complement proteins are distinguished from parent molecules by suffix letters (e.g. C3a, C3b). The proteins of the alternative pathway are called *factors* and are identified by single letters (e.g. factor B, which may be abbreviated to FB or just B). Components are shown in green, conversion steps as white arrows, and activation/cleavage steps as red arrows. The classical pathway is activated by the cleavage of C1r and C1s following association of C1qr2s2 with classical pathway activators, including immune complexes. Activated C1s cleaves C4 and C2 to form the classical pathway C3 convertase C4b2a. Cleavage of C4 and C2 can also be effected via mannose-binding lectin (MBL) associated serine proteinase-2 (MASP-2) of the lectin pathway, which is associated with MBL or ficolin. The alternative pathway is activated by the cleavage of C3 to C3b, which associates with factor B and is cleaved by factor D to generate the alternative pathway C3 convertase C4b2a. The initial activation of C3 happens to some extent spontaneously, but this step can also be mediated by classical or alternative pathway C3 convertases or a number of other serum or microbial proteases. Note that C3b generated in the alternative pathway can bind more factor B and generate a positive feedback loop to amplify activation on the surface. Note also that the activation pathways are functionally and structurally analogous, and the diagram emphasizes these similarities. For example, C3 and C4 are homologous, as are C2 and factor B, and MASP-2 is homologous to C1r and C1s. Either the classical or alternative pathway C3 convertases may associate with C3b bound on a cell surface to form C5 convertases, C4b2a3b or C3bBbC3b, which split C5. The larger fragment C5b associates with C6 and C7, which can then bind to plasma membranes. The complex of C5b67 assembles C8 and multiple molecules of C9 to form a membrane attack complex (MAC), C5b–9. (Modified from Male D, Peebles RS, Male V. *Immunology*, ed 9, Mosby Elsevier; 2021.)

**Table 10.5** Complement pathways

|  | **Classical pathway** | **Lectin pathway** | **Alternative pathway** |
|---|---|---|---|
| Triggered by | Ag-Ab immune complexes | Mannose binding lectin, collectin-11, ficolins | Microbial polysaccharides, properdin |
| Initial event | C1q binding to generate C1qr2s2 to cleave C4 | MBL or Ficolin binding to MASP-2 to cleave C4 | Generation of C3bBb and C4b2c |
| Metal ion dependency | $Ca^{2+}$ | $Ca^{2+}$ | $Mg^{2+}$ |
| End result | Cleavage of C3 | Cleavage of C3 | Cleavage of C3 |

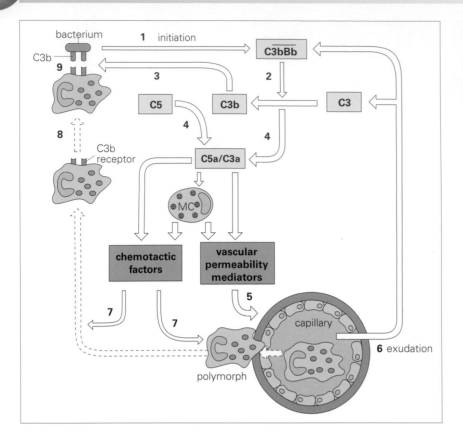

**Fig. 10.16** The defensive strategy of the acute inflammatory reaction initiated by bacterial activation of the alternative complement pathway. Activation of the C3bBb C3 convertase by the bacterium (1) leads to the generation of C3b (2) (which binds to the bacterium [3]), C3a and C5a (4), which recruit mast cell (MC) mediators. These in turn cause capillary dilation (5), exudation of plasma proteins (6), and chemotactic attraction (7) and adherence of neutrophils to the C3b-coated bacterium (8). Note that C5a itself is also chemotactic. The neutrophils are then activated for phagocytosis and the final kill (9).

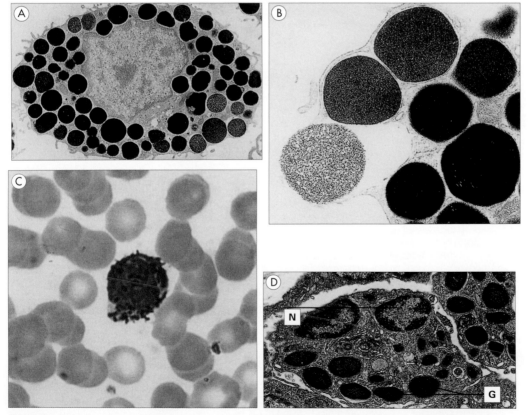

**Fig. 10.17** Electron micrographs of mast cells and basophils. These show (A) a resting rat peritoneal mast cell with its electron-dense granules (× 6000) and (B) a granule in the process of exocytosis (× 30,000). The morphology of a circulating human basophil is shown in (C), which shows a typical basophil with its deep violet-blue granules in a blood film stained with Wright's stain (× 1500) and in (D), an electron micrograph image of the ultrastructure of a basophil in guinea pig skin showing the nuclei (N) and characteristic randomly distributed granules (G) (× 6000). (A and B, Courtesy T.S.C. Orr; C and D, courtesy D. McLaren.)

**Table 10.6** The major inflammatory mediators that control blood supply and vascular permeability or modulate cell movement

| Inflammatory mediators | | |
|---|---|---|
| **Mediator** | **Main source** | **Actions** |
| Histamine | Mast cells, basophils | Increased vascular permeability, smooth muscle contraction, chemokinesis |
| 5-Hydroxytryptamine (5HT – serotonin) | Platelets, mast cells (rodent) | Increased vascular permeability, smooth muscle contraction |
| Platelet activating factor (PAF) | Basophils, neutrophils, macrophages | Mediator release from platelets, increased vascular permeability, smooth muscle contraction, neutrophil activation |
| Interleukin-8 (IL-8, CXCL8) | Mast cells, endothelium, monocytes and lymphocytes | Neutrophil and monocyte localization |
| C3a | Complement C3 | Mast cell degranulation, smooth muscle contraction |
| C5a | Complement C5 | Mast cell degranulation, neutrophil and macrophage chemotaxis, neutrophil activation, smooth muscle contraction, increased capillary permeability |
| Bradykinin | Kinin system (kininogen) | Vasodilation, smooth muscle contraction, increased capillary permeability, pain |
| Fibrinopeptides and fibrin breakdown products | Clotting system | Increased vascular permeability, neutrophil and macrophage chemotaxis |
| Prostaglandin $E_2$ (PGE$_2$) | Cyclo-oxygenase pathway, mast cells | Vasodilation, potentiates increased vascular permeability produced by histamine and bradykinin |
| Leukotriene $B_4$ (LTB$_4$) | Lipoxygenase pathway, mast cells | Neutrophil chemotaxis, synergizes with PGE$_2$ in increasing vascular permeability |
| Leukotriene $D_4$ (LTD$_4$) | Lipoxygenase pathway | Smooth muscle contraction, increasing vascular permeability |

Other mediators are generated from the coagulation process. Chemotaxis refers to directed migration of granulocytes up the concentration gradient of the mediator, whereas chemokinesis describes randomly increased motility of these cells.
From Male D, Brostoff J, Roth DB, et al. *Immunology*, ed 7, Mosby Elsevier; 2006.

**Fig. 10.18** A role for the macrophage (*Mø*) in the initiation of acute inflammation. Stimulation induces macrophage secretion of mediators. Blood neutrophils stick to the adhesion molecules on the endothelial cell and use them to provide traction as they force their way between the cells, through the basement membrane (with the help of secreted elastase) and up the chemotactic gradient. During this process they become progressively activated by neutrophil-activating peptide 2 (NAP-2). ELAM-1, Endothelial cell leukocyte adhesion molecule 1; ICAM-1, intercellular adhesion molecule 1; IL-1, interleukin-1; IL-8, interleukin-8; LTB$_4$, leukotriene B$_4$; NAP-1, neutrophil-activating peptide 1; PGE$_2$, prostaglandin E$_2$; PMN, polymorphonuclear neutrophil; TNFα, tumour necrosis factor alpha.

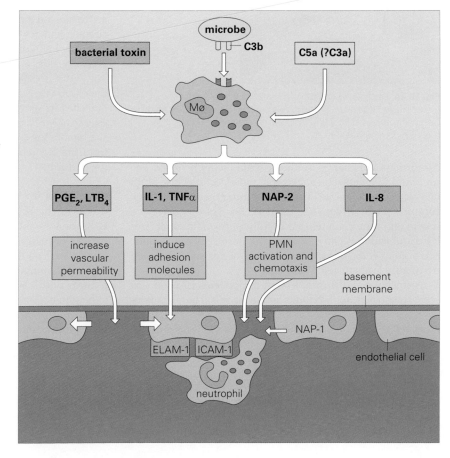

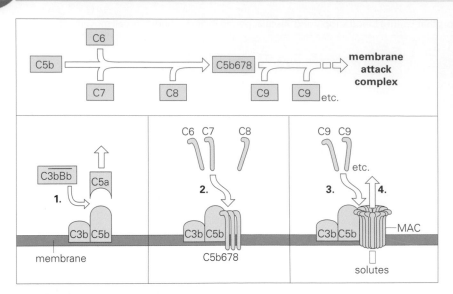

**Fig. 10.19** Assembly of the C5b-9 membrane attack complex (MAC). (1) Recruitment of a further C3b into the C3bBb enzymic complex generates a C5 convertase, which cleaves C5a from C5 and leaves the remaining C5b attached to the membrane. (2) Once C5b is membrane bound, C6 and C7 attach themselves to form the stable complex C5b67, which interacts with C8 to yield C5b678. (3) This unit has some effect in disrupting the membrane but primarily causes the polymerization of C9 to form tubules traversing the membrane. The resulting tubule is referred to as a MAC. (4) Disruption of the membrane by this structure permits the free exchange of solutes, which are primarily responsible for cell lysis.

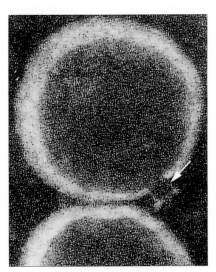

**Fig. 10.20** Electron micrograph of the membrane attack complex. The funnel-shaped lesion (*arrow*) is due to a human C5b–9 complex that has been reincorporated into lecithin liposomal membranes (× 234 000). (Courtesy J. Tranum-Jensen and S. Bhakdi.)

conformational change in the terminal component C9. The unfolded C9 molecules become inserted into the lipid bilayer and polymerize to form an annular membrane attack complex (MAC) (Figs. 10.19 and 10.20). This behaves as a transmembrane channel that is fully permeable to electrolytes and water; because of the high internal colloid osmotic pressure of cells, there is a net influx of sodium ($Na^+$) that frequently leads to cell lysis.

As mentioned, the complement components C3a and C5a were chemotactic for basophils and mast cells. These granulocytes also have specialized granules as illustrated in Fig. 10.17. Mast cell degranulation results in release of histamine and heparin as well as certain cytokines such as IL-8, and the type 2 cytokines IL-4 and IL-13.

### Eosinophils act against large parasites

It takes little imagination to realize that the professional phagocytes (neutrophils and monocytes/macrophages) are far too small to be capable of physically engulfing larger

parasites such as helminths. An alternative strategy, such as killing by an extracellular surface attack of the type discussed earlier, would seem to be a more appropriate form of defence. Eosinophils, the final type of granulocyte that plays a role in innate immunity, appear to have evolved to fulfil this role. These polymorphonuclear relatives of the neutrophil have distinctive cytoplasmic granules, which stain strongly with acidic dyes (Fig. 10.21) and have a characteristic ultrastructural appearance. The core of the granule contains a major basic protein (MBP), while the matrix contains an eosinophilic cationic protein, a peroxidase and a perforin-like molecule. Eosinophils have surface receptors for C3b and, when activated, generate copious amounts of active oxygen metabolites. Eosinophils make up 2–5% of circulating leukocytes in healthy individuals.

Many helminths can activate the alternative complement pathway but, although resistant to C9 attack, their coating with C3b allows adherence to the eosinophils through their C3b surface receptors. Once activated, the eosinophil launches its extracellular ammunition, which includes the release of MBPs and the cationic protein to damage the parasite membrane, with a possibility of a further chemical burn from the oxygen metabolites and leaky pore formation by the perforins.

### Inflammation—a double-edged sword

Complement activation can induce inflammation, which is needed to mobilise cells, increase vascular permeability and hopefully help invading pathogens to be removed and killed. Too much inflammation is, however, not a good thing. Inflammation has four classical features: rubor or redness with vasodilation via nitric oxide, calor (heat due to heightened metabolism and use of glycolysis), dolor (pH, stretch receptors etc.), and tumour (swelling due to vascular permeability and oedema, with cell infiltrates).

### Inflammasomes

Within the cytoplasm of phagocytes, special complexes of cytoplasmic proteins called *inflammasomes* recruit and activate critical enzymes such as caspases. The enzyme caspase 1 cleaves a precursor molecule to produce the cytokines IL-1α and Il-1β, which act synergistically with TNFα. Different types

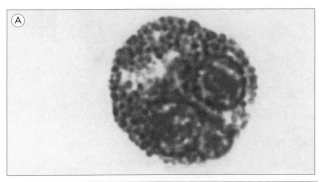

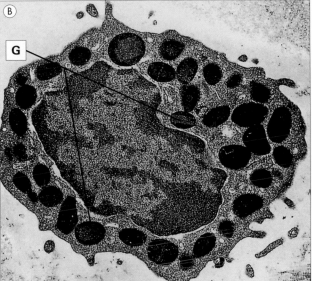

**Fig. 10.21** The eosinophil granulocyte is capable of extracellular killing of parasites (e.g. worms) by releasing its granule contents. (A) Morphology of the eosinophil. This blood smear enriched for granulocytes shows an eosinophil with its multilobed nucleus and heavily stained cytoplasmic granules. Leishman's stain (× 1800). (B) Electron micrograph showing the ultrastructure of a guinea pig eosinophil. The mature eosinophil contains granules (G) with central crystalloids (× 8000). (A, Courtesy P. Lydyard; B, courtesy D. McLaren.)

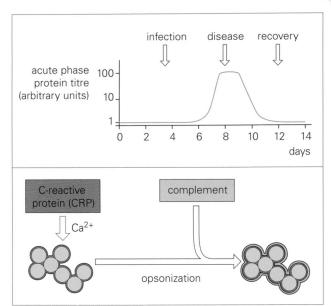

**Fig. 10.22** Acute phase proteins, here exemplified by C-reactive protein (CRP), are serum proteins that increase rapidly in concentration (sometimes up to 100-fold) following inflammation induced by infection (*graph*). They are important in innate immunity to infection. CRP recognizes and binds in a calcium ($Ca^{2+}$)-dependent fashion to molecular groups found on a wide variety of bacteria and fungi. In particular, it uses its pattern recognition to bind the phosphocholine moiety of pneumococci. The CRP acts as an opsonin and activates complement with all the associated sequelae. Another acute phase protein, mannose-binding protein reacts with not only mannose but also several other sugars, enabling it to bind to a wide variety of gram-negative and gram-positive bacteria, yeasts, viruses and parasites, subsequently activating the complement system and phagocytic cells. The structurally related ficolins typically recognize pathogen-associated molecular patterns containing *N*-acetylglucosamine and can activate the lectin complement pathway.

of inflammasomes are activated by different bacterial components; for example, the NLRP3 inflammasome recognizes the PAMPs discussed earlier, bacterial flagellin activates the NLRP4 inflammasome and the AIM2 inflammasome senses cytoplasmic viral DNA. Once activated, a form of proinflammatory cell death called *pyropoptosis* occurs in which the cell swells up in size, lyses and releases its cytoplasmic contents. Special proteins from the gasdermin family are needed to induce this form of cell death, which can release bacteria from macrophages that can then be phagocytosed and killed by neutrophils. Of course, the inflammasomes themselves then have to be regulated through a series of regulator proteins.

## Acute phase proteins

Certain proteins in the plasma, collectively termed *acute phase proteins*, increase in concentration in response to early alarm mediators such as the cytokines IL-1, IL-6 and TNF that are released as a result of infection or tissue injury. Many acute phase reactants such as mannose-binding lectin and CRP increase dramatically during inflammation (Fig. 10.22). Like the professional phagocytes, both use PRRs to bind to molecular patterns on the pathogen (PAMPs)

to generate defensive effector functions. Other acute phase reactants show more moderate rises, usually less than five-fold (Table 10.7). This response involves a considerable energy and resource cost for the host, and these proteins have a wide range of roles that include homeostatic roles as well as pathogen defence. Acute phase proteins such as CRP can be used clinically as a marker of inflammation.

## Other extracellular antimicrobial factors

There are many microbicidal agents that operate at short range within phagocytic cells but also appear in various body fluids in sufficient concentration to have direct inhibitory effects on infectious agents. For example, lysozyme is present in fluids such as tears and saliva in amounts capable of acting against the proteoglycan wall of susceptible bacteria. Other proteins such as collectins bind to carbohydrates on microbial surfaces (see Ch. 15). Whether agents that normally act over a short range, such as reactive oxygen metabolites or TNF, can reach concentrations in the body fluids that are adequate to allow them to act at a distance from the cell producing them is less certain.

### Interferons are a family of broad-spectrum antiviral molecules

IFNs are widespread throughout the animal kingdom and are discussed further in Chapter 15. They were first recognized by the phenomenon of viral interference in which a

**Table 10.7** Acute phase proteins produced in response to infection in the human

| Acute phase reactant | Function |
|---|---|
| **Dramatic increases in concentration** | |
| C-reactive protein | Fixes complement, opsonizes |
| Mannose-binding lectin | Fixes complement, opsonizes |
| Secretory phospholipase A2 | Kills gram-positive bacteria |
| Serum amyloid A protein | Unknown |
| **Moderate increases in concentration** | |
| α₁ Proteinase inhibitors | Inhibit bacterial proteases |
| α₁ Antichymotrypsin | Inhibits bacterial proteases |
| α₁ Acid glycoprotein | Unknown but binds many drugs/lipophilic compounds |
| C3, C9, factor B | Increase complement function |
| Ceruloplasmin | O₂ scavenger |
| Fibrinogen | Coagulation |
| Angiotensin | Blood pressure |
| Haptoglobin | Binds haemoglobin |
| Fibronectin | Cell attachment |

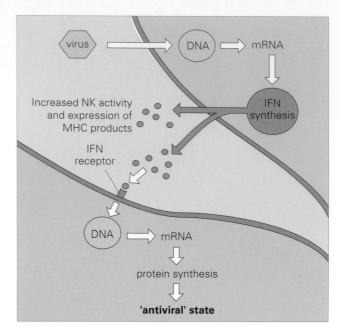

**Fig. 10.23** The action of interferon (IFN). A virus infecting a cell induces the production of the type I interferons IFNα/β. These are released and bind to IFN receptors on other cells. The IFNs induce the production of antiviral proteins, which are activated if virus enters the second cell, and increased synthesis of surface MHC molecules, which enhance susceptibility to cytotoxic T cells (see Ch. 11). MHC, Major histocompatibility complex; NK, natural killer.

cell infected with one virus is found to be resistant to super-infection by a second unrelated virus. Leukocytes produce many different alpha interferons (IFNα), whereas fibroblasts and probably all cell types synthesize IFNβ; these are collectively called *type 1 interferons* (another type of interferon [IFNγ] is made by NK cells and other ILCs as discussed later, as well as by the Th1 subset of T cells [see Fig. 11.10]). When cells are infected by a virus, they synthesize and secrete IFNα and IFNβ, which bind to specific receptors on nearby uninfected cells. The bound IFN exerts its antiviral effect by facilitating the synthesis of two new enzymes that interfere with the machinery used by the virus for its own replication. The mechanism of action of IFN is discussed more fully in Chapter 15; the net result is to set up a cordon of infection-resistant cells around the site of virus infection, so restraining its spread (Fig. 10.23). IFN is highly effective in vivo, as supported by experiments in which mice injected with an antiserum to murine IFN were found to be killed by several hundred times less virus than was needed to kill the controls. It should be emphasized, however, that type 1 IFN seems to play a significant role in recovery from, rather than prevention of, viral infections.

### NK cells recognize virally infected cells, allowing them to be killed

Viruses need to infect host cells to utilize the host cell's machinery to replicate. Clearly it is in the interests of the host to try to kill such infected cells before the virus has had a chance to reproduce. NK cells are cytotoxic cells that appear to have evolved to carry out just such a task. These are large granular lymphocytes (Fig. 10.24) that recognize virus-infected or stressed cells, allowing them to be differentiated from normal cells; this clever discrimination is mediated by activating receptors on the NK cells such as NKG2D, which

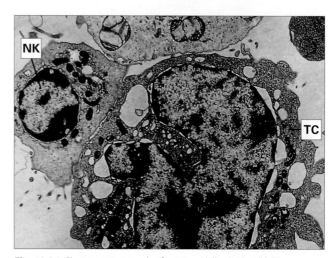

**Fig. 10.24** Electron micrograph of a natural killer (NK) cell killing a tumour cell (TC). NK cells bind to and kill IgG antibody-coated and noncoated tumour cells. It is essential for the membranes of the two cells to be in contact for the NK cell to deliver the kiss of death (× 4500). (Courtesy P. Lydyard.)

recognize ligands on the infected cell that are related to major histocompatibility complex (MHC) class I molecules, and inhibitory receptors that bind to MHC class I molecules on normal cells, generating signals that counteract those from the activating receptors. Activation of the NK cell results in the extracellular release of its granule contents into the space between the target and effector cells. These contents include perforin molecules, which resemble C9 in many respects, especially in their ability to insert into the membrane of the target cell and polymerize to form annular transmembrane pores, like the MAC. This permits the entry of another

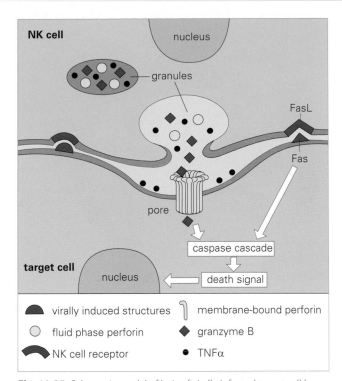

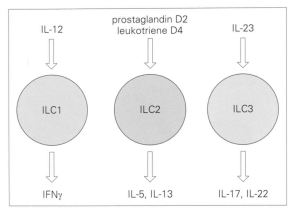

**Fig. 10.26** Innate lymphoid cells. There are three main groups of innate lymphoid cells (ILC1, 2, and 3) that respond to different signals of inflammation or tissue damage and that produce particular cytokines, including those illustrated. Natural killer cells are similar to ILC1s. IFNγ, Interferon gamma; IL, interleukin.

**Fig. 10.25** Schematic model of lysis of virally infected target cell by a natural killer (NK) cell. If the NK cell receptors bind to the surface of the virally infected cell, and if signals from activation receptors exceed those from the inhibitory receptors that recognize normal major histocompatibility complex (MHC) class I molecules, there is exocytosis of granules and release of cytolytic mediators into the intercellular cleft. A calcium-dependent conformational change in the perforin enables it to insert and polymerize within the membrane of the target cell to form a transmembrane pore, which allows entry of granzyme B into the target cell, where it causes programmed cell death (apoptosis). A backup cytolytic system using engagement of the Fas receptor with its ligand (FasL) can also trigger apoptosis, as can binding of granule-derived tumour necrosis factor (TNF) to its receptor. Unlike the pattern recognition receptor–mediated activation of phagocytes by intracellular components—so-called danger-associated molecular patterns (DAMPs)—released on *necrotic* cell death typically caused by tissue trauma, burns and other nonphysiologic stimuli, cells undergoing *apoptotic* death do not activate the immune system because they express surface molecules such as phosphatidyl serine, which mark them out for phagocytic removal before they release their intracellular DAMPs.

granule protein, granzyme B, which leads to death of the target cell by apoptosis (programmed cell death), a process mediated by a cascade of proteolytic enzymes termed *caspases*, which terminates with effector caspases that process the cell for clearance, including the ultimate fragmentation of DNA by a Ca-dependent endonuclease (Fig. 10.25).

Subsidiary mechanisms that can activate the caspase pathway include engagement of Fas (CD95) on the target cell by Fas ligand (CD178, a member of the TNF superfamily) and binding of TNF released from the NK granules to surface receptors. TNF was first recognized as a product of activated macrophages known to be capable of killing certain other cells, particularly some tumour cells.

### Innate lymphoid cells

The NK cells discussed earlier are one of a larger group of innate lymphocytes (Fig. 10.26). As we will see in Chapter 11, in many ways ILCs duplicate functions of the subsets of T cells; however, like NK cells, they lack the specific antigen receptors expressed by T cells and do not have PRRs. Instead, they respond to tissue damage in terms of cytokines, alarmins and inflammatory mediators secreted by myeloid or epithelial cells. ILCs are derived from bone marrow precursors and, different from the circulating NK cells, are resident in the tissues, including skin, lung and intestine. There are three main groups of ILCs: group 1 ILCs make IFNγ (type 1 response), group 2 ILCs make IL-5 and IL-13 (type 2 response) and group 3 ILCs make IL-17 and IL-22 (initiator and regulatory roles), although, as we will see later for T cells, there can be some plasticity in which exposure to particular cytokines will alter the cytokines produced by ILCs.

### Mobilising the cells and mediators of innate immunity

All these defensive cells and effector molecules have to reach the site of infection to be useful (Fig. 10.27). This is achieved by increasing capillary permeability using the complement component C5a and other inflammatory mediators (Table 10.6) and by the production of chemotactic factors. For example, the cytokine IL-6 plays a major role in provoking a proinflammatory response.

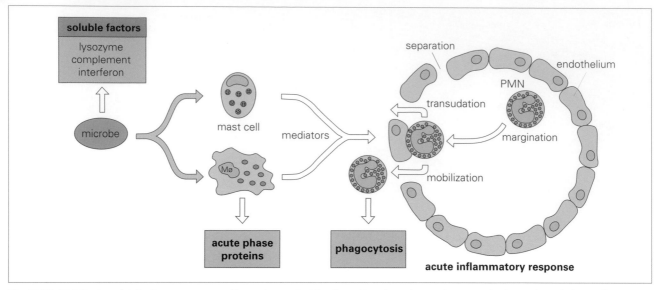

**Fig. 10.27** Mobilization of defensive components of innate immunity. Microbes, either through complement activation or through direct effects on macrophages (Mø), release mediators that increase capillary permeability to allow transudation of plasma bactericidal molecules and to chemotactically attract plasma neutrophils from the bloodstream to the infection site. PMN, Polymorphonuclear neutrophil.

## KEY FACTS

- The innate system of immune defence consists of formidable barriers to prevent pathogens entering the body's tissues followed by a second line of defence by phagocytes and circulating soluble factors. Colonization of the body by normally nonpathogenic (opportunistic) microorganisms occurs whenever there is a hereditary or acquired deficiency in any of these functions.

- Pathogens are recognized in extracellular, cell surface and intracellular compartments, and a protective response is set in motion.

- The main phagocytic cells are polymorphonuclear neutrophils and macrophages. The pathogens are then killed by a variety of mechanisms: reactive oxygen species, acidic pH and enzymes such as lysozyme.

- Complement acts as a first response to infection in an amplifying cascade to ensure a rapid response. Complement can be activated through different pathways, called the *classical, alternate* and *lectin pathways*, centred around the C3a and C5a components. Complement components induce inflammation, improve phagocytosis through opsonization and can cause direct lysis of bacteria or cells by punching holes in their membranes.

- The degranulation of C3b-bound eosinophils can damage larger parasites and might stop large parasites from establishing a foothold in potential hosts.

- Inflammation can be initiated by tissue macrophages and induced by bacterial toxins C5a or C3b-coated bacteria to release TNF, $LTB_4$, $PGE_2$, the neutrophil chemotactic factor IL-8 and a neutrophil-activating peptide.

- Acute phase proteins in the blood, such as CRP, support the inflammatory response.

- Type 1 IFNs can block viral replication.

- Virally infected cells can be killed by NK cells following increased recognition by activation receptors that overcomes inhibitory signals from normal MHC class I recognition. NK cells is one of the group 1 ILCs that are activated by IL-12. ILCs lack the ability to sense pathogens directly but respond to tissue damage and inflammation.

- Phagocyosis is the mechanism used to dispose of most microbes, and the mobilization and activation of these cells by orchestrated responses such as the acute inflammatory response is a key feature of innate immunity. However, not every organism is susceptible to phagocytosis or even to killing by complement or lysozyme, which explains why the additional specificity of the adaptive immune response is needed; this is explored in Chapter 11.

# Adaptive immune responses bring specificity

## Introduction

### How can the immune system recognize an extensive repertoire of foreign antigens in an efficient way?

To protect us against pathogens—those that we have never been exposed to as well as those we have met before—the immune system needs to be permanently on stand-by but in an effective and efficient way. There are many instances in which the cells and molecules of innate immunity are insufficient to cope effectively with these infections, and a greater degree of specificity is needed. Cells that defend us against different types of infections and that have specialized functions are required. This is where the antigen-specific T and B lymphocytes come to our defence.

However, the immune system faces the same challenge as many armies—how to defend the body when it is unknown what the next threat will be or where an attack will be launched. Will it need specialized marines, pilots or ground troops and where should they be based? It has solved this dilemma by having cells recirculate through the body and by sending out signals to attract its troops to the site of attack. Once it has the troops it needs, they also need to work together, as discussed in Chapter 12.

## LYMPHOID TISSUES: PRIMARY AND SECONDARY

The cells that provide the immune system with its exquisite antigen specificity are lymphocytes (Fig. 11.1). When not activated, T and B lymphocytes, now usually called *T* and *B cells*, have a small rim of cytoplasm and are often referred to as *resting*. Once activated, they become larger and more granular and are called *lymphoblasts*. Although resting T and B cells look similar, luckily they (and many other cell types) can be distinguished by the surface antigens they express, often referred to as *markers*. Most of these have been given cluster of differentiation (CD) numbers, a designation to allow antibodies that recognize different epitopes on the same molecule to be grouped together (Table 11.1). Cell subsets also express key transcription factors, discussed later for T cells and innate lymphoid cells (ILCs), and such genetic markers are increasingly used (see Fig. 11.10).

The tissues of the immune system divide into those where the lymphocytes develop—the primary lymphoid organs—and the secondary lymphoid organs where immune responses are initiated and where the mature cells wait while on stand-by (Fig. 11.2).

Like the cells of the innate immune system, B cells develop in the bone marrow (chickens have a specialized organ for this called the *bursa of Fabricius*). Each mature B cell expresses antibody of one specificity on its surface, formed by splicing different variable and constant region genes together, and the first stages of these gene rearrangements take place in the bone marrow. B cells that recognize self-antigens are deleted at this stage as these cells would only cause autoimmunity. The bone marrow also contains the precursors of T cells. The presence of these and many other precursor stem cells in the bone

marrow explains why bone marrow transplants work so well to replace damaged cells. The bone marrow is critical for both production and replacement of the cells of the immune system.

Immature T cells have a specialized organ in which they develop, called the *thymus*. The thymus carries out two important roles: giving positive survival signals to immature cells to keep them alive but also carrying out negative selection to remove cells that might cause damage by recognizing our own cells (or self). T-cell maturation is therefore a more complicated process than the production of a useful repertoire of antigen recognition receptors in B cells.

Once the cells needed for innate and acquired immunity are mature, they circulate via the blood and lymph, which also allows them to enter the specialized secondary lymphoid organs such as spleen, lymph nodes and lymphoid tissues associated with the gut (gut-associated lymphoid tissue [GALT]) and the mucosa (mucosa-associated lymphoid tissue [MALT]). When needed, the cells of the immune system can reach anywhere in the body, particularly if there is inflammation.

### The thymus is a highly specialized organ producing mature T cells

T cells, like B cells, natural killer (NK) cells and ILCs develop from a common lymphoid progenitor cell in the bone marrow. In the thymus, T cells develop from immature pre-T cells or thymbocytes into mature T cells (Fig. 11.3). In the outer cortex the immature thymocytes first receive maturation signals, including interleukin 7 (IL-7) produced by cortical epithelial cells. They already express the main T-cell marker antigen CD3 but now also start to express both CD4

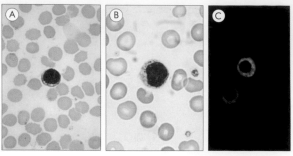

**Fig. 11.1** Lymphocytes and plasma cells. (A) Small B and T lymphocytes have a round nucleus and a high nuclear:cytoplasmic ratio. (B) A large granular lymphocyte with a lower nuclear:cytoplasmic ratio, an indented nucleus and azurophilic cytoplasmic granules. Fewer than 5% of T helper cells and 30–50% of cytotoxic T cells, γδ T cells and natural killer cells have this morphology. (C) Antibody formed when B cells differentiate into plasma cells, here stained with fluoresceinated anti-human IgM (green) and rhodaminated anti-human IgG (red) showing extensive intracytoplasmic staining. Note that plasma cells produce only one class of antibody as the distinct staining reveals. (A and B, stained with Giemsa, courtesy A. Stevens and J. Lowe; C, modified from Zucker-Franklin A, et al. *Atlas of Blood Cells: Function and Pathology*, ed 2, vol. 11, EE Ermes; Lea and Febiger; 1988.)

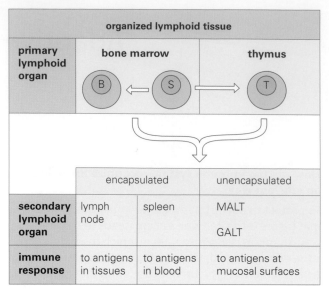

**Fig. 11.2** Organized lymphoid tissue. Haemopoietic stem cells (S) arising in the bone marrow differentiate into common lymphoid progenitor cells and then into immunocompetent B and T cells in the primary lymphoid organs. The T and B cells colonize the secondary lymphoid tissues where immune responses are organized. GALT, Gut-associated lymphoid tissue; MALT, mucosa-associated lymphoid tissue.

**Table 11.1** Useful CD markers that can be used to identify different cell types

| CD molecule | Cell expression | Function |
|---|---|---|
| CD3 (δ, γ, ε-chains) | All T cells | Signal transduction from T-cell antigen receptor |
| CD4 | CD4 T cells | Binds to MHC II |
| CD8 (α-, β-chains) | CD8 T cells | Binds to MHC I |
| CD14 | Monocytes/macrophages, dendritic cells, neutrophils | Binds LPS–LPS binding protein complex |
| CD16α (FcRIIIA) | NK cells, macrophages | Fc receptor for IgG, phagocytosis, antibody-dependent cellular cytotoxicity (ADCC) |
| CD19 | B cells | B-cell activation |
| CD20 | B cells | B-cell activation? |
| CD25 (α-chain) | Activated T and B cells; Tregs | Binds IL-2 |
| CD45 | Splice variants CD45RA on naive T cells, CD45RO on antigen-experienced/memory T cells (also on B cells) | Splice variant of common leukocyte antigen |
| CD69 | Activated T cells, B cells, NK cells | Early activation marker |
| CD158 (killer Ig-like receptor, KIR) | NK cells, T-cell subset | Activation/inhibition of NK cells (interaction with MHC I) |
| CD159a (NKG2D) | NK cells | Activation/inhibition of NK cells (interaction with MHC I) |
| CD206 (mannose receptor) | Monocytes/macrophages | Phagocytosis of microorganisms |

ADCC, antibody-dependent cellular cytotoxicity; CD, cluster of differentiation (antibodies that recognize the same chain or molecule); Ig, immunoglobulin; IL, interleukin; LPS, lipopolysaccharide; MHC, major histocompatibility class; NK, natural killer; Treg, regulatory T cell.

and CD8, two surface markers that will later identify the CD4 and CD8 T-cell subsets. If the thymus is absent, as in the congenital DiGeorge syndrome in humans or in nude (athymic) mice, no mature T cells develop. The thymus decreases in size as we age, but it is still capable of producing some new T cells in adults.

The next step involves complicated genetic rearrangements similar to those that occur in B cells as they differentiate (see later). The repertoire or number of potential shapes or antigens that need to be recognized by T cells is very large, but the T-cell receptor (TCR) repertoire is generated in a very efficient way, by combining and splicing different

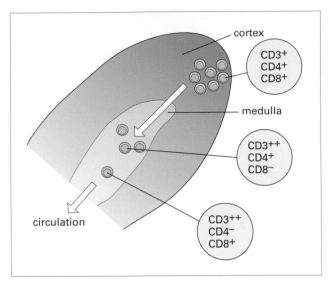

**Fig. 11.3** Structure and function of the thymus. The bilobed thymus is subdivided into lobules by fibrous trabeculae. The most immature thymocytes are found in the outer cortex, where gene rearrangement to form the T-cell receptor occurs. Following positive and negative selection once in the medulla the T cells start to express only CD4 or CD8 before entering the circulation via blood vessels. CD, Cluster of differentiation.

gene segments together, just as for the antibody molecule described later. The alpha (α) chain contains variable (V) and joining (J) gene segments that are combined with a constant or C region (Fig. 11.4). The second beta (β) chain combines V, diversity (D) and J gene segments as well as its own C regions. Further diversity results from reading the D segments of the β-chain in all three reading frames and from adding N and P nucleotides to the V–D and D–J junctions of the α-chain and the V–J junctions of the β-chain. A subset of T cells expresses a γδ–TCR rather than an αβ–TCR, but if the α-chain is expressed, this results in the deletion of the Vδ region, committing the cell to express an αβ-TCR. Again, as in the antibody molecules, the most variable regions are in the complementarity-determining region hypervariable loops on the α- and β-chains. But the TCR does have important differences from immunoglobulin—it is not secreted, it does not change its C regions and there is no somatic mutation to further increase the repertoire of antigens that can be recognized. Another critical difference between the TCR and antibody is that the TCR only recognizes antigen presented by a major histocompatibility complex (MHC) molecule as we will discuss further in Chapter 12, while antibody binds to or recognizes free antigen.

Two further selection processes take place in the thymus. First, only those T cells whose TCR can recognize self-MHC molecules presenting self-peptides are given a survival signal by thymic cortical epithelial cells in a process that is called *positive selection*. Any T cells unable to recognize antigens presented by the individual's MHC molecules would be useless and only occupy valuable space, so they are better deleted. A final step of maturation in the thymus involves negative selection through which any T cell whose TCR binds too strongly to the self-MHC molecules is deleted by apoptosis (programmed cell death) as these cells could be dangerous, inducing autoimmunity with an immune

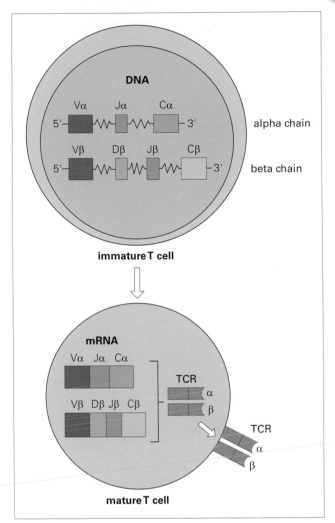

**Fig. 11.4** T-cell receptor (TCR) rearrangement. Rearrangement of the gene segments for the α- and β-chains (or γ- and δ-chains) of the TCR is similar to that for the immunoglobulin heavy and light chains. Spliced transcribed RNA codes for the individual α- and β-chains that are expressed on the T-cell surface with specificity for a peptide presented in the peptide-binding groove of major histocompatibility complex molecules. The combination of V, J and C gene segments for the α-chain and of V, D, J and C gene segments for the β-chain provides even greater total diversity in antigen recognition than for the immunoglobulin molecule.

response against the body or self. This process involves medullary thymic epithelial cells. From the combinations of gene segments and chains, there is a T-cell repertoire even larger than that of the starting B-cell repertoire; however, this repertoire ($10^{61}$ possible combinations but after positive and negative selections probably $10^8$ different TCRs) does not expand further in the periphery owing to mutation, as is the case for antibodies. All the T cells expressing a particular TCR are called a *clonotype*.

During these selection processes the T cells express the signature T-cell antigen CD3 and are positive for both the CD4 and CD8 antigens. In the medulla the T cells then become either CD4 or CD8 positive and start expressing more of the CD3 antigen. To become a CD4 T cell or a CD8 T cell, the CD8 gene is silenced in a CD4 T cell, and vice versa, which requires epigenetic modifications.

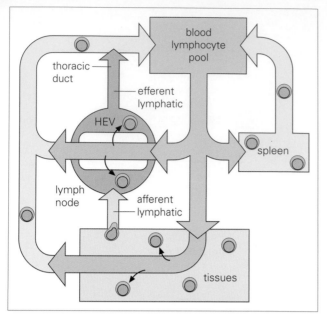

**Fig. 11.5** Recirculation of T and B cells. The lymphocytes move through the circulation and enter the lymph nodes via the specialized endothelial cells of the postcapillary venules (HEV). They leave through the efferent lymphatic vessels and pass through other lymph nodes, finally entering the thoracic duct, which empties into the circulation at the left subclavian vein (in humans). Lymphocytes enter the white pulp areas of the spleen in the marginal zones; they pass into the sinusoids of the red pulp and leave via the splenic vein. (Modified from Roitt IM, Brostoff J, Male D. *Immunology*, ed 6, Elsevier Science; 2002.)

(Epigenetic modifications involve changes to the promotor and enhancer regions of genes, including the methylation of cytosines, and modification of the histone tails of nucleosomes.) The T cells that enter the circulation are mature CD3 T cells expressing a functional TCR and CD4 or CD8. However, in immunology speak, they are still naive T cells as they have not yet been activated by the signals they receive when they recognize antigen presented by self-MHC. The thymus medulla also contains structures called *Hassall corpuscles*, formed of epithelial cells and what are probably dead T cells.

Once ready, the naive T cells join the naive B cells (and innate immune cells) in the blood. They can then enter the secondary lymphoid organs (spleen, lymph nodes, MALT, GALT) and recirculate around the body through the lymphatic vessels and the blood (Fig. 11.5). They can also enter other tissues. And most importantly, they can go to sites of infection and inflammation when they are needed.

### Maturation of B cells

B cells mature in the fetal liver before birth and subsequently in the bone marrow. First one and then the second chain of the B-cell antigen receptor, the antibody molecule, are expressed. As for T cells, B cells only mature if they express a functional antigen receptor, and they die by clonal deletion if they are strongly self-reactive to avoid generation of autoantibodies, although the B cell can try to modify a self-reactive antigen receptor through further gene rearrangement in a process called gene editing in which the B cell undergoes another round of V-J recombination in its light chain. Once a mature B cell is produced, it

will enter the circulation and can move into the secondary lymphoid organs.

## SECONDARY LYMPHOID ORGANS

Lymphoid organs like the lymph nodes and spleen are compartmentalized into T- and B-cell areas containing mature T and B cells. In the lymph node, B cells are found in B-cell follicles surrounded by T-cell zones in which T cells respond to antigens brought there by dendritic cells (Fig. 11.6). B and T cells both enter through the high endothelial venules but are then directed to their respective B- and T-cell zones by particular chemokines. T cells express CCR7, which binds to CXCL19 and CXCL21 expressed by stromal cells in the T-cell regions. B cells are attracted to the B-cell follicles where the CXCR5 on their surface binds to CXCL13 on the surface of follicular dendritic cells. The B-cell primary follicles develop into germinal centres where B cells are activated and proliferate following antigen stimulation; once they become mature plasma cells that secrete large quantities of antibody, they move into the medulla. In the spleen B cells are again found in follicles, in this case in the white pulp, surrounded by T cells in an area called the *periarteriolar lymphoid sheath*.

The MALT also contains foci of lymphocytes in Peyer's patches, where lymphocytes can respond to antigens from the environment and particularly to the heavy bacterial load in the intestine by producing immunoglobulin A (IgA) antibodies for mucosal secretions. IgA antibodies will opsonize bacteria for phagocytosis rather than activating complement. Immune responses in the gut are damped down so the beneficial commensal bacteria in the gut can survive. The lymphocytes that form the MALT recirculate between these mucosal tissues using specialized homing receptors (Fig. 11.7). There are further fat-associated lymphoid clusters in the pleural, pericardial and peritoneal cavities.

## SUBSETS OF T CELLS

Just as there are subsets of ILCs, subsets of T cells also develop specialized functions.

T cells can be subdivided by function (e.g. as helper, cytotoxic and regulatory T cells) and by production of particular cytokines or cytotoxic mediators. CD4 T cells are generally referred to as *T-helper (Th) cells* and CD8 T cells as *T-cytotoxic cells*, although both CD4 and CD8 T cells can have a variety of functions. The initial division of CD4 helper T cells into Th1 and Th2 T cells, making the defining cytokines interferon gamma (IFNγ) and IL-4, respectively, has been expanded to include Th17 T cells making IL-17, Th9 T cells found in skin and mucosal surfaces making IL-9, which activates mast cells, and regulatory T cells (Treg) making the immunosuppressive cytokines transforming growth factor-β (TGFβ) and IL-10. Another T-cell subset, follicular helper T cells (Tfh) provide specialized help to B cells. Tfh help germinal centres to develop in the secondary lymphoid organs and secrete IL-21 and IL-4 (Fig. 11.8). Further activation markers such as CD69 and CD25 identify activated T cells, and finally more markers can distinguish naive T cells (CD45RA) from antigen-stimulated effector cells or memory cells (CD45RO) that will provide better and faster protection if we meet the same infection again. Within the cell there are signalling cascades and transcription factors associated with these functions. As more sophisticated ways

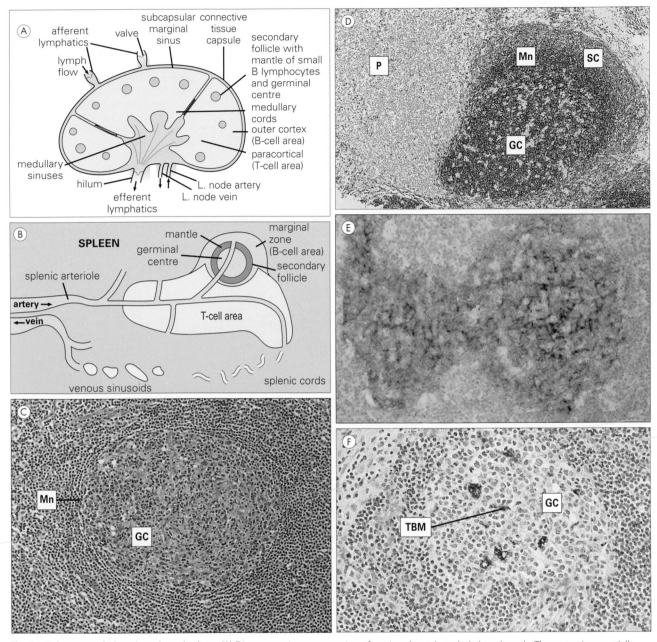

**Fig. 11.6** Structure of a lymph node and spleen. (A) Diagrammatic representation of section through a whole lymph node. The cortex is essentially a B-cell region where differentiation within the germinal centres of secondary follicles to antibody-forming plasma cells and memory cells occurs. (B) Diagrammatic representation of spleen showing B- and T-cell areas. (C) Structure of a secondary follicle. A large germinal centre (GC) is surrounded by the mantle zone (Mn). (D) Distribution of B cells in lymph node cortex. Immunochemical staining of B cells for surface immunoglobulin shows that they are concentrated largely in the secondary follicle, GC, Mn and between the capsule and the follicle—the subcapsular zone (SC). A few B cells are seen in the paracortex (P), which contains mainly T cells. (E) Follicular dendritic cells in a secondary lymphoid follicle. This lymph node follicle is stained with enzyme-labelled monoclonal antibody to demonstrate follicular dendritic cells. (F) GC macrophages. Immunostaining for cathepsin D shows several macrophages localized in the GC of a secondary follicle. These macrophages, which phagocytose apoptotic B cells, are called tingible body macrophages (TBM). (A and B, Courtesy A. Stevens and J. Lowe; C–F, from Male D, Brostoff J, Roth DB, et al. *Immunology*, ed 7, Mosby Elsevier; 2006.)

of analysing individual T cells have been developed, it has become clear that the immune system does not always keep T cells in these clearly defined subsets, there may be subsets within these subsets and T cells can show the ability to change from one subset to another, a phenomenon known as plasticity. This is presumably another way in which the immune system can generate more T cells of the type it needs to defend the body against a particular infection, as and when they are needed.

Like CD4 T cells, CD8 T cells can make cytokines, such as IFNγ and IL-4, but are also good at killing virus-infected target cells. The CD8 T cell recognizes viral peptides derived from cytoplasmic viruses that presented by MHC class I molecules on the host cell surface. Once activated, the T cell can punch holes in the infected target cell membrane using molecules such as perforin and granulysin with structural similarities to the C9 terminal complement component. NK cells can also kill target cells using

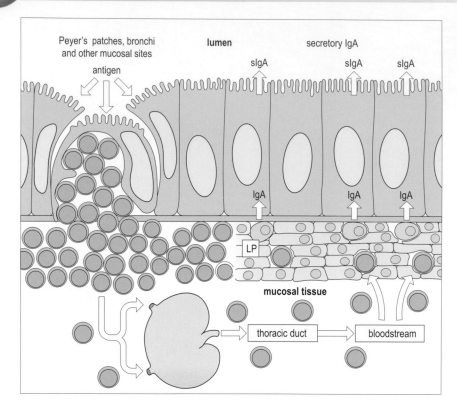

**Fig. 11.7** Mucosa-associated lymphoid tissue (MALT). Lymphoid cells, which are stimulated by antigen in Peyer's patches (or the bronchi or another mucosal site), migrate via the regional lymph nodes and thoracic duct into the bloodstream and thence to the lamina propria (LP) of the gut or other mucosal surfaces, which might be close to or distant from the site of priming. Thus lymphocytes stimulated at one mucosal surface may become distributed selectively throughout the MALT system. This is mediated through specific adhesion molecules on the lymphocytes and the mucosal high-walled endothelium of the postcapillary venules. (Modified from Roitt IM, Brostoff J, Male D. *Immunology*, ed 6, Elsevier Science; 2002.)

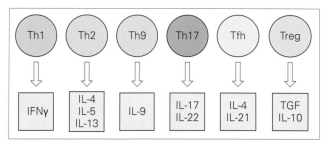

**Fig. 11.8** CD4 T-cell subsets. CD4 helper T cells can develop into a number of CD4 T-cell subsets in response to stimulation with particular cytokines; using particular transcription factors and gene regulators, these T cells then produce particular cytokines that carry out distinct functions. Th1 and Th2 cells are now often called *type 1 and 2* as the same patterns of cytokines can also be produced by CD8 T cells. Note that the frequencies of the different T cell subsets differ—Th1 and Th2 are the most numerous and Th9 is found in the smallest numbers—and that within each cell type there may be further subsets. IFN, Interferon; IL, interleukin; TGF, transforming growth factor; Th, T-helper cell; Tfh, follicular helper T cells; Treg, regulatory T cell.

perforin. Other ways cytotoxic T cells can kill is by using granzyme, a molecule that is delivered into the target cells but that can kill some pathogens directly, and by inducing apoptosis (programmed cell death) through Fas–FasL (CD95-CD178) interactions (Fig. 11.9).

### Why do we need so many types of T cell?

Firstly, the immune system has to defend us from a range of pathogens: bacteria, viruses and parasites. This requires specialized immune cells, but within the complexity of all these

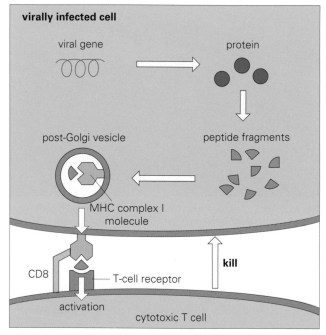

**Fig. 11.9** Cytotoxic T lymphocytes are activated when their specific cell surface receptors recognize an infected cell by binding to a surface MHC class I molecule that is associated with a peptide fragment derived from a degraded intracellular viral protein. The cytotoxic cells then kill the virally infected cells using cytolytic granules containing perforin and granzyme released into the contact zone between the T cell and the target cell or by inducing apoptosis, programmed cell death, in the infected cell. Cytotoxic CD8 cells can be serial killers, killing a number of virally infected cells. CD, Cluster of differentiation; MHC, major histocompatibility complex.

**Fig. 11.10** Parallels between the main CD4 T-cell subsets and innate lymphoid cell *(ILC)* subsets. ILC1, ILC2 and ILC3 cells use the same transcription factors and produce similar cytokines to the CD4 Th1, Th2 and Th17 subsets. Thus both ILC1 and Th1 cells provide protection against intracellular pathogens, ILC2 and Th2 help with defence against helminths and ILC3 and Th17 help with protection against fungi. Natural killer cells can be grouped with ILC1; they also make IFNγ but do not depend on the transcription factor T-bet. The ILC subsets develop from a common lymphocyte precursor (CLP) in the bone marrow; the CD4 subsets develop from naive CD4 T cells. CD, Cluster of differentiation; GATA, GATA transcription factor; IFN, interferon; IL, interleukin; ROR, RAR-related orphan receptor; Th, T helper cell.

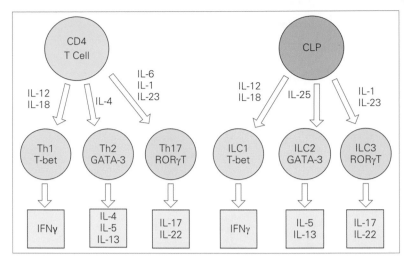

subsets, there is also redundancy in which evolution has resulted in not only type 2 or Th2 CD4 T cells but also type 2 CD8 T cells, and there are parallels in cytokine production between the Th1 and Th2 subsets and ILC types ILC1 and ILC2 (Fig. 11.10). These parallels illustrate why it is better to refer to type 1 (proinflammatory, making IFNγ), type 2 (anti-inflammatory, making IL-4) and type 3 (regulatory, making TGFβ and IL-10) cytokine responses. All T cells, B cells, NK cells and ILCs develop from common lymphocyte progenitor cells in the bone marrow.

## ANTIBODY STRUCTURE AND FUNCTION

The antibody molecule is the B cell's antigen recognition molecule. The term *antigen* was given to the parts of foreign microorganisms that were *anti*body *gen*erating. Antibodies are expressed on the surface of the B cells where they can bind to parts of an antigen directly, but they can also be secreted by the B cell as soluble antibodies.

All antibodies have the same four-chain structure, with two longer heavy chains and two shorter light chains (Fig. 11.11). Their specificity is determined by the sequences of three hypervariable regions on both the heavy chain and the light chain that together form the fragment antigen binding (Fab) region. These hypervariable regions are also called *complementarity-determining regions*, as their sequence is complementary to the antigen. The molecule has a flexible hinge joint where the Fab region joins the constant, or Fc region. How strongly the single antigen-binding site binds to the antibody defines the antibody affinity.

Just as for the TCR, the chains of the antibody molecule are put together by splicing variable, diversity, joining and constant region gene segments together (Fig. 11.12). The heavy chains are formed from splicing V, D, J and C region genes together, while the light chains have V, J and C genes. All of this requires recombination signal sequences, a number of enzymes and epigenetic changes to the chromatin. This generates a huge repertoire of antibodies, enabling the immune system to have antibodies that are able to recognize the many pathogenic threats we may face.

The antigen-binding sites at the end of the two arms of the antibody molecule recognize three-dimensional shapes or antigens. These can be formed by the three-dimensional shape of a molecule or a linear sequence of amino acids.

Antibodies can also recognize sugars, lipids and nucleic acids as antigens—it is the shape that determines how well they bind to, or recognize, an antigen. The strength of the binding of the bivalent basic IgG antibody molecule (or the four-valent secretory IgA or the 10 binding sites of the pentavalent IgM antibody molecule) defines the overall strength of binding or avidity. High affinity and avidity binding is important to prevent the antibody from dissociating from its antigen, as this binding is not irreversible. During an immune response the affinity of the antibodies made can increase, owing to somatic mutation in the Fab (variable) region and selection of higher affinity antibodies. The repertoire of naive B cells is estimated to be $\sim 1 \times 10^7$. With somatic mutation there could theoretically be $10^{15}$–$10^{18}$ different antibodies in the mature antibody repertoire, but there is just not enough space (or probably need) in the body for all of these.

### Antibodies come in different classes and subclasses with different structures and functions

B cells initially make IgD, with two heavy and two light chains, which is expressed on the surface of naive B cells. The clever thing is that this basic antibody molecule can retain its antigen specificity but change its other properties encoded in the sequence of the Fc region. This **class switching** involves switching the constant or C regions of the heavy and light chains but fusing them to the same antigen-binding sequences that give the antibody its antigen specificity. Alternative splicing combines the same Fab regions from the IgD molecule with the Fc region for IgM, which forms a pentameric IgM antibody that is particularly good at agglutinating bacteria and binding complement, and then with the Fc region for IgG. The IgG molecule itself comes in different subclasses with different functions (IgG1, IgG2, IgG3, IgG4 in humans). The bivalent secretory IgA molecules protect mucosal surfaces, and IgE antibodies help defend us against helminth parasites as well as unwanted allergies (Table 11.2). The antibody molecules themselves are part of an immunoglobulin superfamily of molecules that includes not only the antibodies, the TCR and MHC molecules but also a number of other molecules found in the plasma membranes of the cell that have similar domain structures.

The process of stimulating B cells to proliferate, so that useful B-cell clones expand, with further increases in the

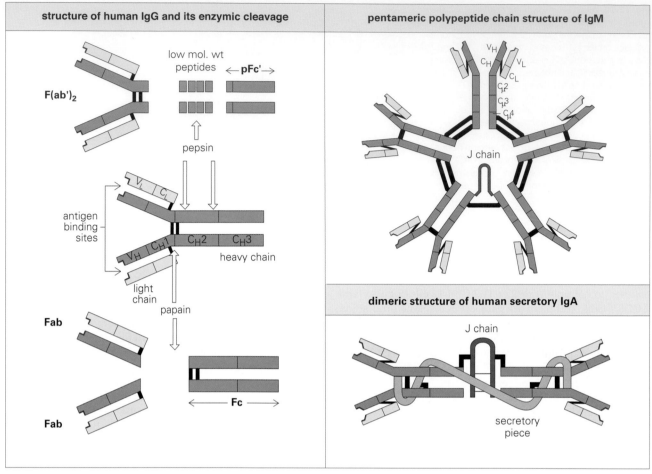

**Fig. 11.11** The structure of immunoglobulins. The basic structure of immunoglobulins is a unit consisting of two identical light polypeptide chains and two identical heavy polypeptide chains linked together by disulphide bonds *(black bars)*. Each chain is made up of individual globular domains. Different antibodies have different $V_L$ and $V_H$ domains, the highly variable regions of the light and heavy chains, respectively. This hypervariability is confined to three loops on the $V_L$ and three on the $V_H$ domains. These make up the antigen-binding site *(highlighted in red)*. In contrast, the remaining domains ($C_L$, $C_H1$, etc.) are relatively constant in amino acid structure. Cleavage of human immunoglobulin G (IgG) by pepsin induces a divalent antigen-binding fragment, $F(ab')_2$ and a pFc' fragment composed of two terminal $C_H3$ domains. Papain produces two univalent antigen-binding fragments, Fab, and an Fc portion containing the $C_H2$ and $C_H3$ heavy chain domains. Polymerization of the basic immunoglobulin units to form IgM and IgA is catalysed by the joining *(J)* chain. The portion of the transporter (which transfers IgA across the mucosal cell to the lumen) that remains attached to the IgA is termed the *secretory piece*.

affinity of the antibodies they make due to somatic hyper-mutation, and class switching and differentiation of B cells into plasma cells, takes place in the germinal centres of the lymph nodes and spleen. Some memory B cells are also exported to provide better protection against future attacks by the same pathogen, as discussed in Chapter 12.

### Subsets of B cells

There are also subsets of B cells (Table 11.3). The main B-cell subset responsible for producing the most effective antibod-ies and that undergoes both class switching and somatic mutation of the antibodies they make are the follicular B cells, but these require help from T cells, which will be dis-cussed further in Chapter 12. These B cells can develop into plasma cells and memory B cells (see Fig. 12.10). Marginal zone B cells can respond to antigens without help from T cells but produce only short-lived plasma cells; similar B-1 cells are found in mucosal tissues. These B cells derive from

precursors in the liver rather than the bone marrow. Some B cells are initially activated in extrafollicular locations, but these cells only generate short-lived plasma cells.

## RECIRCULATION OF T AND B CELLS

Naive T and B cells can move from the thymus and the bone marrow into the secondary lymphoid organs where they are activated, whereas activated effector T and B cells can migrate into tissues and to sites of inflammation and tissue injury. Migration requires adhesion to endothelial cells in the postcapillary venules. Adhesion needs selectins, adhe-sion molecules that bind carbohydrates with relatively low affinity, and integrins, a larger family of 30 adhesion mol-ecules that mediate tighter binding. There are also members of the immunoglobulin superfamily (as they have an immu-noglobulin-like chain) that mediate binding, such as inter-cellular adhesion molecule 1 (ICAM-1) or leukocyte func-tion—associated antigen 3 (LFA-3) that can act as ligands for

**Fig. 11.12** Differentiation events leading to the expression of unique sIgM monomers on the surface of an immunocompetent B lymphocyte. There are 45 germline $V_H$ genes encoding the major portion of the variable region, with 23 minigene segments encoding the D segment and 6 for the J region. As the cell differentiates, $V_H$, D and J gene segments on one chromosome randomly fuse to generate lymphocytes with a very wide range of individual heavy chain variable domains. There are separate loci for the genes encoding the kappa and lambda light chains. Variable region light chain domains are formed by random $V_L$ to J recombination—there are 35 and 30 kappa and lambda V genes with 5 and 4 J regions for each. Finally, the variable and constant region genes, respectively, recombine to encode a single antibody molecule expressed on the mature B-cell surface as an sIgM antigen receptor. When activated for antibody production, the transmembrane segment of IgM, which normally holds the molecule on the surface, is spliced out at the RNA stage and the soluble form of the IgM is secreted. Subsequently, heavy chain constant region gene switching can occur to generate the various immunoglobulin classes (IgG, IgA, etc.). Leader sequences have been omitted for simplicity.

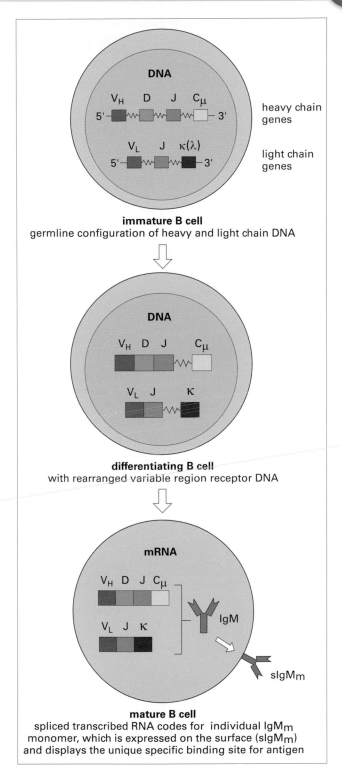

**immature B cell**
germline configuration of heavy and light chain DNA

**differentiating B cell**
with rearranged variable region receptor DNA

**mature B cell**
spliced transcribed RNA codes for individual $IgM_m$ monomer, which is expressed on the surface ($sIgM_m$) and displays the unique specific binding site for antigen

integrins (Fig. 11.13). Naive T and B cells use L-selectin and the integrin LFA-1 to reach the secondary lymphoid organs (naive T cells also use LFA-4). To enter sites of inflammation and infection, effector and memory T cells use LFA-1, very late antigen 4 (VLA-4) and the integrin $\alpha_4\beta_7$, while the tissue-homing central memory T cells also use L-selectin to enter tissues. The ligand for LFA-1 is ICAM-1, which is expressed on cytokine-activated endothelial cells. VLA-4 binds to vascular cell adhesion molecule 1 (Table 11.4). Some T cells remain in tissues once there, as tissue-resident T cells (e.g. memory T cells for Epstein-Barr virus are retained in the tonsils by local production of the cytokine IL-15 that down-regulates the sphingosine-1-phosphate molecule they need to exit the tonsil).

Chemokines (Table 11.5) also play a key role in attracting T and B cells to the right place. There are as many as

**Table 11.2** Biologic properties of major immunoglobulin (Ig) classes in the human

| Designation | IgG | IgA[a] | IgM | IgD | IgE |
|---|---|---|---|---|---|
| Major characteristics | Most abundant internal Ig | Protects external surfaces | Very efficient against bacteria | Mainly lymphocyte receptor | Initiates inflammation; raised in parasitic infections; causes allergy symptoms |
| Valency[b] | 1 | 1 (monomer)/2 (dimer with secretory piece) | 5 | 1 | 1 |
| Half-life[c] | ++ | + | + | + | + |
| Antigen binding | + + | + + | + + | + + | + + |
| Complement fixation (classical)[d] | + + | − | + + + | + | − |
| Cross placenta[c] | + + | − | − | − | − |
| Fix to homologous mast cells and basophils | − | − | − | − | + + |
| Binding to macrophages and neutrophils for opsonisation | (IgG1, IgG3 best) | + | − | − | + |

[a]Dimer in external secretion carries secretory piece; IgA dimer and IgM contain J-chains.
[b]Valency or number of four-chain molecules, each with two antigen-binding sites.
[c]Half-life ranges from 2–5 days (+) to 3–4 weeks (++) and is dependent on the ability to bind the neonatal Fc receptor FcRn; IgG3 is more short-lived than IgG1, 2 or 4. Ability to cross the placenta also depends on size and ability to bind FcRn.
[d]IgG1 and IgG3 are best at complement fixation; IgG2 fixes complement weakly and IgG4 not at all.

**Table 11.3** B-cell subsets

| Subset | Follicular B cells[a] | Marginal zone B cells | B-1 B cells |
|---|---|---|---|
| Location | Lymphoid tissues, blood | Lymphoid tissues, blood (man) | Mucosal tissues, peritoneal cavity, pleural cavity |
| Markers | CD19, CD23, MHCII, Fc receptors | IgM, CD27 | IgM, CD20, CD27, CD43 |
| Function | Produce high-affinity T-dependent mainly IgG antibodies to protein antigens; generate B-cell memory | T-independent[b] IgM low-affinity antibodies to polysaccharides | T-independent IgM low-affinity antibodies to polysaccharides |

An additional subpopulation of suppressor B cells has been proposed.
[a]Follicular B cells form the majority of B cells.
[b]Most but not all marginal zone B cells make T-independent antibodies. Note that B cells can also present antigens to T cells.

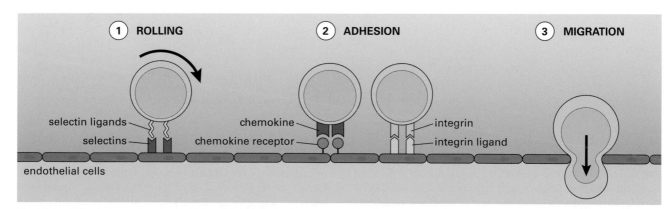

**Fig. 11.13** Cell recruitment into tissues. This occurs in sequential stages. First, (1) cytokines such as tumour necrosis factor and interleukin 1 induce the expression of selectins on endothelial cells, enabling cells expressing selectin ligands to start to roll along the endothelial surface, then (2) chemokines on the endothelial surface bind to chemokine receptors on the cells, leading to stronger more stable integrin binding, which halts the movement of the cell, and finally (3) the cell can transmigrate out of the blood vessel into the tissues.

**Table 11.4** Important adhesion molecules

| Family | Molecule | Distribution | Ligand | Cell types bound |
|---|---|---|---|---|
| Selectins | L-selectin (CD62L) | Neutrophils, monocytes, naive and central memory T cells, naive B cells | Sialyl Lewis X or PNAd, Gly-CAM1, CD34, MAdCAM1 | Endothelium |
| | E-selectin (CD62E) | Activated endothelium (activated by TNF, IL-1) | Sialyl Lewis X (e.g. CLA-1) | Neutrophils, monocytes, effector and memory T cells |
| | P-selectin (CD62P) | Activated endothelium (activated by thrombin or histamine) | Sialyl Lewis X on glycoproteins, PSGL-1 | Neutrophils, monocytes, effector and memory T cells |
| Integrins | LFA-1 (CD11a, CD18) | Neutrophils, monocytes, naive and central memory T cells, naive B cells | ICAM-1, ICAM-2 (upregulated by cytokines) | Endothelium[a] |
| | Mac-1 (CD11b, CD18) | Neutrophils, monocytes, dendritic cells | ICAM-1 (CD54), ICAM-2 (CD102) | Endothelium[a] |
| | VLA-4 (CD49a, CD29) | Monocytes, T cells (naive, effector, memory) | VCAM-1 (CD106) | Endothelium[a] |
| | $\alpha_4\beta_1$ (CD49d, CD29) | Monocytes, macrophages, lymphocytes | VCAM-1 (CD106) | Gut endothelium |
| | $\alpha_4\beta_7$ (LPAM-1) | Lymphocytes | MAdCAM-1 | Endothelium |
| Immunoglobulin superfamily | ICAM-1 (CD54) | Dendritic cells, lymphocytes, activated blood vessels | Integrins LFA-1, Mac-1 | Neutrophils, monocytes, naive T and B cells |
| | LFA 3 (CD58) | Antigen-presenting cells, lymphocytes | CD2 | Neutrophils, monocytes, naive T and B cells |

[a]Upregulated when activated by cytokines.
CLA-1, Cutaneous lymphocyte antigen 1; ICAM, intercellular adhesion molecule; LFA-1, leukocyte function-associated antigen 1; MAC-1, macrophage integrin-1; MAdCAM-1, mucosal addressin adhesin molecule-1; PNAd, peripheral node addressin; VCAM, vascular cell adhesion molecule; VLA-4, very late antigen 4.

**Table 11.5** Some important chemokines

| Chemokines | Receptor | Distribution | Function in recruitment |
|---|---|---|---|
| CCL19, CCL21 | CCR7 | Dendritic cells, naive T cells | Migration to paracortical areas in lymphoid tissues |
| CXCL13 | CXCR5 | B cells, Tfh cells | Migration to B-cell follicles in lymphoid tissues |
| CXCL9, CXCL10 (IP-10) | CXCR3 | Activated T cells | Migration to sites of inflammation |
| CXCL1, CXCL2, CXCL8 (IL-8) | CXCR1, CXCR2 | Neutrophils | Migration to sites of inflammation and infection |
| CCL2 (MCP-1), CCL3 (MIP-1α) | CCR2; CCR1, CCR5 | Leukocytes, monocytes/macrophages | Migration to sites of infection |
| CCL4 (MIP-1β) | CCR5[a] | Dendritic, monocyte, T cell, NK cells | Migration to sites of inflammation and infection |
| CCL5 (RANTES) | CCR1, CCR3, CCR5 | Leukocytes | Mixed leukocyte recruitment |
| CC11 (Eotaxin) | CCR3 | Eosinophils, basophils, Th2 T cells | Migration to sites of inflammation |

[a]Also acts as HIV coreceptor.
IP-10, Interferon-γ induced protein-10; MCP-1, monocyte chemotactic protein 1; MIP-1α/β, macrophage inflammatory protein-α/β.

50 chemokines playing roles in cell migration, activation and chemotaxis grouped into those with a CXC structure (α-chemokines) or CC structure (β-chemokines) depending on whether there is an extra amino acid (X) in between two cysteines; fractalkine helps recruit T cells, NK cells and monocytes and has a CX3CL1 structure, whereas the small lymphotactins have a XCL1 structure and help with T cell and NK cell recruitment.

Naive T cells are directed to the T-cell areas of lymphoid organs by the chemokines CCL19 and CCL21, which bind to CCR7 on the naive T-cell surface. B cells are attracted into the white pulp in the spleen and into germinal centres by the chemokine CXCL13, which binds to CXCR5 on the B-cell surface. Mature plasma cells move out of the lymphoid organs and enter particular tissues based on the antibody they produce (e.g. IgA-producing plasma cells move to mucosal sites as they express the integrin $\alpha_4\beta_7$, and the chemokine receptors CCR9 and CCR10 that bind to Mad-CAM-1, CCL25 and CCL28 on mucosal epithelial cells). Naive T and B cells will be retained in lymphoid tissue while they become activated.

As well as this increased adhesion and attraction to lymphoid tissues of naive T and B cells, the activated T and B cells are also attracted to sites of inflammation and infection by chemotaxis in response to signals alerting the body that there are invaders about or that tissue damage is occurring as for the cells of the innate immune system (see Table 11.5). Crossing the endothelium also causes some activation of phagocytes, making them more phagocytic and increasing the production of mediators.

## KEY FACTS

- The lymphoid system has primary lymphoid organs such as the thymus and bone marrow, where the T and B cells develop and secondary lymphoid organs such as the lymph nodes and spleen, where the mature T and B cells are activated to carry out their functions.

- The cells of the immune system recirculate through the body in the blood and lymph and are attracted to sites of infection by mechanisms that sense pathogens and markers of inflammation.

- The cells of the adaptive immune system, the T cells and B cells, are antigen specific—each T or B cell has multiple copies of a single receptor on its surface that recognizes antigen. These antigen receptors are made by splicing a number of gene segments together, allowing a large repertoire of antigens to be recognized.

- T cells only recognize antigens presented in the groove of an MHC molecule by an antigen-presenting cell, whereas the antibody that forms the antigen recognition molecule on a B cell can recognize and bind to free antigen or to whole pathogens.

- There are subsets of both T and B cells that carry out specialized functions; some of these functions are similar to those seen in the cells of the innate immune system.

- T and B cells, as well as phagocytic cells, get to sites of inflammation and infection by binding to endothelial cells using selectins and integrins and migrating into the tissues; cells are also attracted by chemokines.

- Once the body has its armies of antigen-specific T and B cells as well as the cells of the innate system, it is ready to defend us against a range of pathogens in an efficient and effective way.

# Cooperation leads to effective immune responses

## Introduction

Once the immune system has a full arsenal of innate and antigen-specific adaptive immune responses at its disposal, it needs to exploit these effectively in defending the body against pathogens. To deliver a protective immune response, the various players must work together. Opsonization with antibodies and complement increases the efficiency of phagocytosis of microbes. Antigens are presented to T cells by professional antigen-presenting cells (APCs). More than one signal is needed to activate T cells, and although B-cell activation is simpler, it also usually requires T-cell help and cascades of intracellular events. Activated effector T cells can act directly through cell–cell contact to kill an infected cell but also produce soluble cytokines as messengers that act on other cells. Once the immune response has successfully dealt with an invader, it needs to be shut down. This chapter will discuss the many ways in which the cells of the innate and adaptive immune systems and their products interact to provide effective immunity against infections.

## COOPERATION MEANS GREATER EFFICIENCY AND SPECIFICITY

Antibodies on their own can serve useful functions, such as blocking the activity of toxins, but combining antibodies with the phagocytes of the innate immune system delivers more effective phagocytosis through opsonization. Additional activation of the complement system will further enhance removal of pathogens and result in beneficial inflammation and lysis of infected cells.

T cells recognize processed antigen presented by APCs, unlike the B cells that can recognize free antigen or antigens on the surface of a pathogen. Nevertheless, to deliver effective antibody responses, T cells need to provide help to B cells through a specialized subset of T follicular helper cells. Subsets of CD4 Th cells also provide help to cytotoxic CD8 T cells and can activate macrophages, making them more effective at killing intracellular organisms. Many of these interactions involve cell–cell contact and signalling, but others are mediated by cytokines delivered into the cell–cell contact zone or immunologic synapse.

As both T and B cells have antigen-specific receptors, they can be increased in number as required through clonal expansion. Although the rapid expansion of large numbers of antigen-specific T and B cells is beneficial, once the infection has been dealt with, an excess of these cells would only occupy valuable space and so the numbers are reduced by apoptosis. In case we are threatened by the same pathogen again, the immune system maintains highly specialized elite troops on standby—these antigen-specific memory T and B cells are ready to be deployed and are already trained to kill or to secrete antibodies or cytokines. Finally, all these troops must be kept from getting out of control, so regulatory T cells and mechanisms of immune suppression are needed.

## OPSONIZATION BY ANTIBODY ENHANCES PHAGOCYTOSIS AND LEADS TO COMPLEMENT ACTIVATION

Although antibodies can, by themselves, carry out useful functions such as blocking toxins from binding to their receptors, they work best when cooperating with phagocytes. Opsonization of a microbe when antigen-specific antibodies bind to its surface antigens will make it easier for the phagocyte to phagocytose the microbe. The Fc portion of the antibody molecule can bind to Fc receptors expressed on the phagocyte (Fig. 12.1). As noted in Chapter 11, some antibody classes and subclasses are good at activating the complement cascade, and additional opsonization with C3b, which then binds to the C3b receptor, further enhances phagocytosis (Fig. 12.2). Antibody-coated bacteria can also bind complement leading to lysis. The combined presence of complement and antibodies has a dramatic effect on survival of extracellular bacteria (Fig. 12.3). This illustrates how the innate and adaptive immune systems work together to deal with the removal of microbes.

## BENEFICIAL INFLAMMATORY REACTIONS CAN ALSO BE ENHANCED BY ANTIBODIES

As well as increasing the rate of removal of pathogens, antibodies and complement enhance inflammation, with release of cytokines from macrophages. Activation of complement, as well as certain proinflammatory cytokines and mediators such as chemokines, increases vascular permeability, thus enabling greater numbers of circulating monocytes as well as other leukocytes to access the site of an infection. Other cytokines will attract and activate neutrophils. Adhesion molecules will then enhance binding to the vascular endothelium.

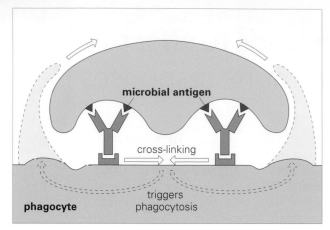

**Fig. 12.1** The binding of a microbe to a phagocyte by more than one antibody cross-links the antibody (Fc) receptors on the phagocyte surface and triggers phagocytosis of the microorganism, which is engulfed by the extending cytoplasmic projections.

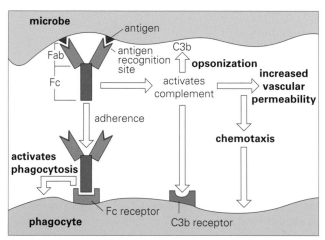

**Fig. 12.2** The antibody adaptor molecule. Antibodies (antiforeign bodies) are produced by host lymphocytes on contact with invading microbes, which act as antigens (i.e. generate antibodies). Each antibody (see Fig. 11.11) has a recognition site (Fab) enabling it to bind antigen and a backbone structure (Fc) capable of some secondary biologic action such as activating complement and phagocytosis. Thus in the present case, antibody bound to the microbe activates complement and initiates an acute inflammatory reaction. The C3b generated fixes to the microbe and, together with the antibody molecules, facilitates adherence to Fc and C3b receptors on the phagocyte and thence microbial ingestion.

Mast cells express receptors for immunoglobulin E (IgE) antibodies. Cross-linking of these receptors will result in signalling and mast cell degranulation also leading to increased polymorph chemotaxis and vascular permeability (Fig. 12.4).

## ACTIVATION OF T CELLS INVOLVES ANTIGEN-PRESENTING CELLS AND ADDITIONAL COSTIMULATORY SIGNALS

Once a T cell is mature, it enters the circulation, expressing a T-cell receptor (TCR) on its surface. This receptor is designed to recognize antigen, or rather short linear peptides, presented in the groove of a major histocompatibility

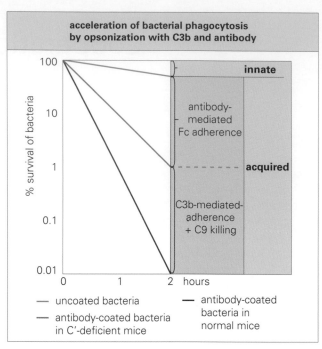

**Fig. 12.3** The slow rate of phagocytosis of uncoated bacteria (innate immunity) is increased many times by acquired immunity through coating with antibody and then C3b (opsonization). Killing may also take place through the C5–9 terminal complement components. This is a hypothetic but realistic situation; the natural proliferation of the bacteria has been ignored.

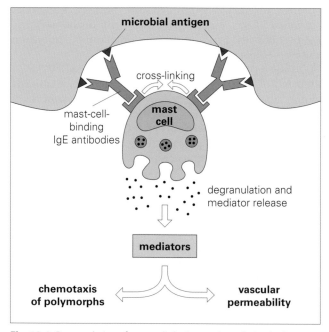

**Fig. 12.4** Degranulation of mast cells by interaction of microbial antigen with specific antibodies of the immunoglobulin E (IgE) class, which bind to special receptors on the mast cell surface. The cross-linking of receptors caused by this interaction leads to the release of mediators, which induce an increase in vascular permeability and attract neutrophils (i.e. they provoke an acute inflammatory reaction at the site of the microbial antigen).

**Fig. 12.5** Migration and maturation of interdigitating dendritic cells (IDCs). The precursors of the IDCs are derived from bone marrow stem cells. They travel via the blood to nonlymphoid tissues. These immature IDCs (e.g. Langerhans cells in skin) are specialized for antigen uptake. Subsequently, they travel via the afferent lymphatics to take up residence within secondary lymphoid tissues, where they express high levels of major histocompatibility complex (MHC) class II and costimulatory molecules such as B7. Both the DCs and the naive T cells express the chemokine receptor CCR7 and so colocalize in the lymphoid tissues. DCs are highly specialized for the activation and differentiation of naïve T cells, which are effected through three signals: (1) T-cell receptor (TCR) binding to MHC/peptide complex, (2) B7–CD28 costimulation and (3) cytokine release. (Modified from Roitt IM, Delves PJ. *Roitt's Essential Immunology*, ed 10, Blackwell Science; 2001.)

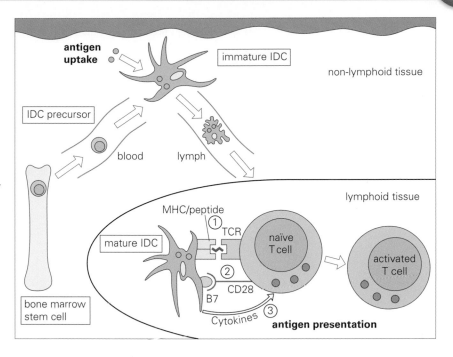

complex (MHC) molecule. The peptides are presented to the T cells by highly efficient professional APCs called *dendritic cells* (DCs; Fig. 12.5) within the T-cell areas of the secondary lymphoid organs. The DCs found in lymphoid organs express greater numbers of the MHC molecules on their surface compared with those found resident in tissues. The DCs also need to be good at providing costimulatory signals (see later). Macrophages and even B cells can also present antigens to T cells, but, although macrophages are better at phagocytosis than DCs, both macrophages and B cells have lower expression of MHC and costimulatory molecules than do the DCs in lymphoid tissues, although following activation, this can be increased.

CD4 T cells recognize and respond to peptides presented by MHC class II molecules that are derived from the degradation of proteins from phagocytosed organisms; the CD8 T cells recognize peptides derived from antigens in the cytoplasm that are presented by MHC class I molecules. The peptide-binding cleft or groove of the MHC class I molecule is closed at the ends and so binds only short peptides of 8–9 amino acids in length (Fig. 12.6), whereas the MHC class II molecules have clefts that are open at the ends so the peptides can be up to 30 amino acids long. These MHC molecules are highly heterogeneous, so some people will respond well to particular peptides and others weakly or not at all (leaving what is called a *hole* in their antigen-recognition repertoire). But before there can be an immune response, the peptides have to be loaded into the grooves of the MHC molecules (Fig. 12.7).

To be presented in the groove of the MHC class I molecule, antigens must first get into the cytoplasm of the cell. There they are degraded by a special organelle called a proteasome. Next a transporter—imaginatively called transporter associated with antigen processing—is needed to get the peptides to where the MHC class I molecules are located within the lumen of the endoplasmic reticulum. MHC I molecules with empty grooves are selected by a molecule

called tapasin, and once the peptide has bound into the MHC I groove the molecule is ready to begin its journey to the cell surface through the Golgi region and via exocytic vesicles. As the MHC class I molecule has a groove with closed ends, only peptides of eight to nine amino acids will fit comfortably.

Organisms that are phagocytosed or antigens that are endocytosed (taken up into membrane-bound endosomes) are degraded following fusion with lysosomes containing hydrolytic enzymes. The MHC class II molecules are found in a special type of endosome that also contains other key molecules needed to help transfer foreign peptides into the MHC class II groove. First, the invariant chain that has been occupying the groove must be removed through initial degradation to form a shorter CLIP peptide and then exchanged for the foreign peptide by a peptide exchanger molecule called *HLA-DM*. Fusion of the two types of endosome, those containing the foreign peptides and those with the MHC molecules, results in suitable foreign peptides occupying the MHC class II groove. The ends of the MHC class II groove are open so any peptide that hangs out from the ends can be trimmed to a final length of 13–30 amino acids. The MHC class II molecule is then cycled out to be expressed on the surface of the cell. Simple really!

The MHC antigens or human leukocyte antigens are highly variable, so different individuals can respond to or recognize different peptide antigens. MHC tetramer reagents can be made containing four copies of a particular labelled MHC class I molecule binding a specific antigen and used to stain antigen-specific CD8 T cells, which will only bind T cells whose TCR recognizes the same peptide presented by the same MHC molecule. It is now also possible to make ferritin-containing complexes with 12 MHC-peptide complexes, which are more sensitive reagents for staining antigen-specific T cells. Tetramers with MHC class II antigens are more complex to make as there are two variable MHC chains.

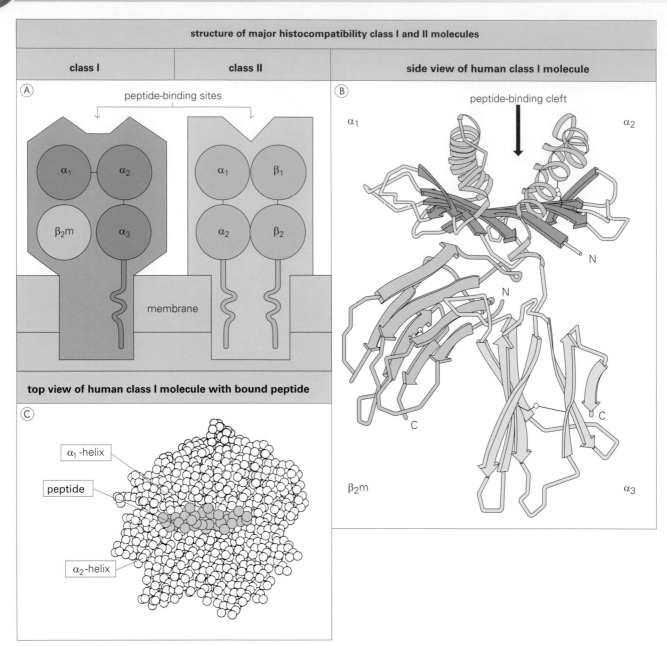

| structure of major histocompatibility class I and II molecules | | |
|---|---|---|
| **class I** | **class II** | **side view of human class I molecule** |

(A) peptide-binding sites

(B) peptide-binding cleft

top view of human class I molecule with bound peptide

(C)

α₁ -helix

peptide

α₂ -helix

**Fig. 12.6** Class I and II major histocompatibility complex (MHC) molecules. (A) Diagram showing domains and transmembrane segments; the α-helices and β-pleated sheets are viewed end-on. (B) Side view of human class I molecule (HLA-A2) based on X-ray crystallographic structure showing the cleft and the typical immunoglobulin folding of the α₃ and β₂-microglobulin (β₂m) domains (four antiparallel β-strands on one face and three on the other). The strands making the β-pleated sheet are shown as thick grey arrows in the amino to carboxyl direction, and α-helices are represented as helical ribbons. The inside-facing surfaces of the two helices and the upper surface of the β-pleated sheet form a cleft that binds the peptide. (C) Top view of a peptide bound tightly within the MHC class I cleft, in this case peptide 309–317 from HIV-1 reverse transcriptase bound to HLA-A2. This is the view seen by the combining site of the T-cell receptor described later. (B, Modified from Bjorkman PI, Saper MA, Samraoui B, et al. The foreign antigen binding site and T cell recognition regions of class I histocompatibility antigens. *Nature.* 1987;329:512; C, modified from Vignali DAA, Strominger JL. Co-receptor function and the characteristics of MHC-bound peptides: a common link? *The Immunologist.* 1994;2:93–99.)

### T cells need additional signals for activation

If a CD4 or CD8 T cell recognizes the peptide MHC complex on the surface of an APC, often referred to as its *cognate antigen*, this provides the first signal for T-cell activation. However, a second signal is also required, delivered by the binding of a molecule called *CD28* on the T cell to the B7 molecule on the APC; without this second signal, tolerance rather than activation occurs. If both the antigen-recognition

and second signals are sent, then T-cell activation results, helped by T-cell expression of CD40 interacting with CD40L on the APCs and leading to additional cytokine release from the DC. T-cell activation involves a cascade of intracellular enzymes. The TCR itself does not have a cytoplasmic tail capable of delivering such signals—instead signalling occurs through the associated gamma (γ), delta (δ), epsilon (ε) and zeta (ζ) chains of the CD3 molecule. This signalling

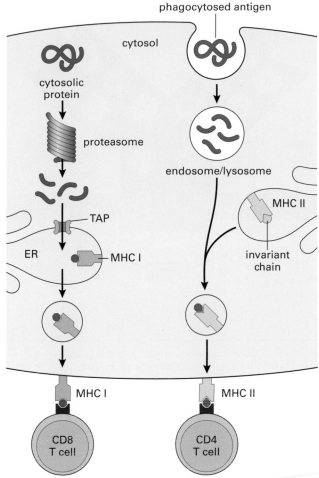

**Fig. 12.7** Pathways of antigen presentation by major histocompatibility complex (MHC) class I and II molecules. Antigens in the cytosol of the cells (e.g. viral antigens) get degraded in proteasomes and transported into the endoplasmic reticulum (ER) with the help of the transporter associated with antigen processing (TAP) before being loaded onto the MHC I molecules and recycled out onto the cell membrane for presentation of their peptides to CD8 T cells. Phagocytosed or endocytosed antigens are degraded after fusion with lysosomes and replace the invariant chain that stabilizes the MHC II molecules until they have bound peptide. Once on the cell surface, the MHC II–peptide complex will activate antigen-specific CD4 T cells.

involves the phosphorylation of protein kinases, and for TCR signalling through the CD3 chains, there are immunoreceptor tyrosine-based activation motifs (ITAMs) available for tyrosine phosphorylation. ITAMs consist of two copies of the sequence (tyrosine—any amino acid—any amino acid—leucine). Sometimes the kinase enzymes associate with the intracellular portion of a coreceptor such as the CD4 α-chain or the CD8 α- and β-chains (Fig. 12.8).

The molecular interactions between the T cell and the APC take place within a contact zone known as the *immunologic synapse*, where lipid rafts help bring the molecules on the two cells together. The central zone of the synapse that contains the TCR and associated coreceptors is called the *central supramolecular activation cluster (SMAC)*, which is surrounded by a peripheral area that contains adhesins. Cytokines are also secreted directly into this synapse.

The immunoglobulin molecule on the surface of a B cell is also unable to signal directly and is associated with two invariant chains, Igα and Igβ, that contain ITAMs. For natural killer cells that lack both CD3 and immunoglobulin on their surface, signalling occurs through their own ITAM-containing DAP12 protein.

### Complex intracellular signalling cascades follow the phosphorylation of ITAMs

T cells use a particular kinase Lck to phosphorylate the ITAMs of the TCR complex. Next the tyrosine kinase ZAP-70 binds to the phosphorylated ITAMs leading to phosphorylation of the adaptor protein linker for activation of T cells (LAT). The following steps are even more complex, involving assembly of enzyme scaffold proteins, adaptor molecules and a host of enzymes, but the end result is the production of transcription factors such as nuclear factor of activated T cells (NFAT) and nuclear factor kappa B (NFKB), and changes in metabolism, $Ca^{2+}$, adhesion properties and cytoskeletal reorganization, leading to cell activation and ultimately cell division.

### T cells with a γδ TCR and other invariant T cells recognize nonprotein antigens

A smaller family of T cells has a TCR with γ- and δ-chains rather than the usual αβ-TCR. These γδ-T cells recognize nonprotein antigens, including phosphorylated molecules and lipids, presented by CD1 molecules that lack the diversity seen in the classical MHC I molecules. Other invariant T cells called *mucosal-associated invariant (MAIT)* T cells are found in the mucosa and that recognize vitamin D metabolites from bacteria and fungi presented by MR1, another invariant MHC-like molecule.

### Superantigens and mitogens stimulate many T cells

Some superantigens can stimulate any TCR expressing particular families of Vβ genes directly, independently of their antigen specificity, activating up to 20% of all T cells. Staphylococcal enterotoxin B can do this, leading to extensive T-cell activation and a cytokine storm due to the excessive cytokine release that results; this is both a way of avoiding a focused specific immune response (see Ch. 17) and inducing immunopathology (see Ch. 18). Both T and B cells can also be stimulated nonspecifically by mitogens (e.g. the red kidney bean–derived phytohaemagglutinin or concanavalin A for T cells and pokeweed mitogen for B cells). These mitogens can be useful tools for immunologists but are best avoided in real life, which is why it is important to boil uncooked red kidney beans well!

## B-CELL ACTIVATION

The antibody expressed on the surface of a B cell acts as its antigen receptor binding either linear sequences or three-dimensional shapes on the antigen. Antigens reach lymphoid follicles via afferent lymphatics or the subcapsular sinuses and are presented to follicular B cells by follicular DCs or macrophages, but they are not processed by APCs. B-cell activation signals from the ITAM motifs on the associated Igα and Igβ chains are amplified if C3d binds to CR2 receptors on the B cells, and further signals may come from pathogen-associated molecular patterns on the microbe inducing TLR signalling (see Fig. 12.8).

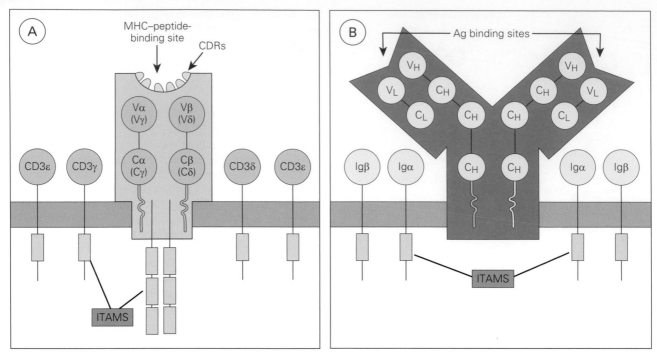

**Fig. 12.8** Activation of T and B cells. (A) The T-cell receptor on αβ-T cells consists of an α- and β-chain each composed of a variable (V) and a constant (C) domain resembling the immunoglobulin Fab antigen-binding fragment in structure. The highly variable (complementarity-determining) regions (CDRs) on the variable domains contact the major histocompatibility complex (MHC)–peptide antigen complex. This produces a signal that is transduced by the invariant CD3 complex composed of γ-, δ-, ε- and ζ- or η-chains through their cytoplasmic immune receptor tyrosine-based activation motifs (ITAMs), which contact protein tyrosine kinases. γδ-T cells (see later) have receptors composed of γ- and δ-chains as indicated in the figure. (B) Antibody acts as the B-cell receptor, but as this does not have intracellular signalling domains, the activation signals are transduced through the Igα and Igβ chains. B cells are activated more strongly if C3d binds to the CR2 receptor. CD, Cluster of differentiation; Ig, immunoglobulin.

Additional signals are provided by T cells (see later) and type 2 cytokines.

## CLONAL EXPANSION

Each T and B cell expresses its own antigen receptor, either a TCR or an Ig molecule. Clonal expansion enables a large increase in the numbers of antigen-specific T or B cells. A lymphocyte expressing a receptor for a particular antigen or part of that antigen (the epitope) is activated as described earlier, leading to a clone of cells with the same receptor (and the same function) (Fig. 12.9). Although some bystander proliferation of nonantigen-specific cells occurs through the release of cytokines such as IL-2 that act as growth factors, clonal expansion is a very effective way of producing more of the cells you need on demand.

The principle of clonal expansion can be used to generate a clone of T cells expressing the same TCR. The T-cell clone must be stimulated by antigen presentation of the epitope it recognizes, as well as growth factors such as IL-2 and IL-7, but can be maintained in tissue culture without being immortalized by fusion with a tumour cell or transformed by infection with a tumour virus. However, these days it is more common to investigate the properties of individual T cells using single cell RNA sequencing.

## ANTIBODY PRODUCTION INVOLVES A SERIES OF STEPS WITHIN THE GERMINAL CENTRE

To make an effective antibody response is a complicated process! First, the antigen-specific B cells needs to be activated and needs to proliferate. However, whereas all the daughter clones of a particular T cell will express exactly the same TCR, somatic mutation in the immunoglobulin genes leads to antibodies of greater affinity, as well as switching of the class and subclass of antibody made by the B cell (Fig. 12.10). An enzyme called *activation-induced cytidine deaminase* drives the development of somatic mutations in the immunoglobulin V region genes of germinal centre B cells and initiates isotype switching.

### T-cell help for antibody production

Within germinal centres in the secondary lymphoid organs, T-cell help is needed for effective B-cell development and to help the affinity maturation of the antibodies produced (Fig. 12.11). The specialized T cells providing this help in the lymph nodes and spleen are called *follicular helper T cells (Tfh)*. The Tfh respond to IL-6 and chemokines such as CXCL13 and move into the germinal centre; IL-6 activates the STAT 3 transcription factor and then the Tfh lineage-defining transcription factor Bcl-6. Contact between the Tfh and the B cell at the junction of the T- and B-cell areas in lymphoid tissues involves costimulatory molecules such as CD28 as well as through the TCR/MHC, but B-cell help is also mediated by IL-4 and IL-21 secreted by the Tfh. IL-21 is particularly important in promoting the proliferation of B cells and their differentiation into plasma cells that produce large quantities of antibody. Tfh in germinal centres are critical for the development of high-affinity B cells; one study found that antiviral IgG antibodies decreased by 98% if Tfh were not present.

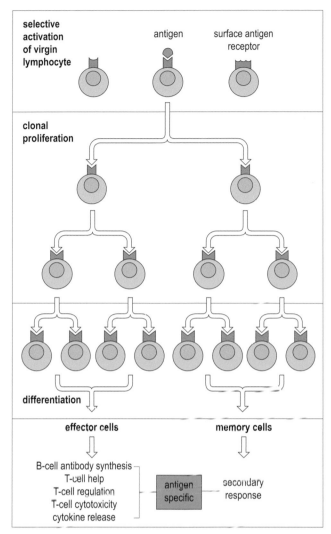

**Fig. 12.9** Generation of a large population of effector and memory cells by clonal proliferation after primary contact of B or T cell with antigen. A fraction of the progeny of the original antigen-reactive lymphocytes becomes nondividing long-lived memory cells, whereas the others become the effector cells of humoral or cell-mediated immunity. Memory cells provide a large pool of antigen-specific cells that are activated more easily than naive T or B cells.

Tfh cells seem to be very permissive for viral production in early human immunodeficiency virus (HIV) infection; they are reduced in number as infection progresses, but they are maintained in those individuals (called elite controllers) who control their HIV infection without progression.

#### Sometimes B cells can make antibodies without T-cell help

Some antigens, called *T-independent antigens*, can stimulate B cells to make antibodies directly, without help from T cells. Just as T cells expressing TCRs with different specificities can be activated by superantigens, B cells expressing different immunoglobulins can also be activated by polyclonal activators called *thymus-independent* or *TI-1 antigens*, such as lipopolysaccharide or bacterial DNA, that activate the B cell via Toll-like receptors—in effect acting as B-cell mitogens (Fig. 12.12). These thymus-independent antigens do not induce affinity maturation or B-cell memory responses.

A second type of T-cell independent antigen has repeating determinants such as those found on the polysaccharide capsules of some bacteria. These are presented to marginal zone B cells by marginal zone macrophages in the spleen or to B cells by macrophages in the subcapsular sinus of lymph nodes. The repeating determinants cross-link the immunoglobulins on the B cell, leading to B-cell activation. But again, the antibody response is not optimal as mainly IgM antibody is produced, although it is useful to be able to generate rapid antibodies to *Streptococcus pneumoniae* polysaccharide, for example, with complement activation by the IgM Fc region.

#### Monoclonal antibody technology exploits clonal expansion and transformation to produce large quantities of monoclonal antibodies

B cells are harder to maintain in culture than T cells, but fusing an individual B cell to a myeloma cell will result in a clone of transformed B cells, producing antibody of one specificity called *monoclonal antibodies* (Fig. 12.13, Box 12.1). Monoclonal antibodies are now widely used in medicine (e.g. to block cytokines such as tumour necrosis factor alpha [TNFα; see Fig. 15.9] for diagnosis [see Ch. 32] or in immunotherapy [see Ch. 36]). The monoclonal antibody can be humanized through inserting the critical antigen recognition CDR regions into the basic structure of a human antibody, preventing it from being recognized as foreign.

### CYTOKINES PLAY AN IMPORTANT PART IN THESE CELL–CELL INTERACTIONS

As seen already, to make an effective T-cell or antibody response requires cooperation between cells of different types. In addition to direct cell–cell contact, which triggers signalling cascades, cytokines are secreted into the contact zone or immunologic synapse between the cells. Cytokines that are secreted by one cell can also act as a molecular messenger on the cell itself in an autocrine manner, but most often they act on another cell in a paracrine reaction. The APC delivers cytokines such as IL-12 to the CD4 T cell; the T cell itself secretes growth factors such as IL-2 and cytokines that will help B-cell production of antibodies as well as drive the development of M1 or M2 macrophages. (Some of these many interactions are listed in Table 12.1.) A large number of cytokines are now known, and some have redundant functions; many can be grouped into families by their functions (e.g. inducing type 2 cytokine responses or their structure with homologies in their cytokine-binding domains and their intracellular signalling domains). In general, cytokines act between adjacent cells; when they are found in large quantities in the circulation, it is usually bad news. Some infections can trigger a massive release of cytokines in a cytokine storm, which causes a lot of pathology; this was thought to be responsible for the multitude of deaths caused by the Spanish H1N1 influenza outbreak in 1918 and can be triggered by superantigens such as staphylococcal enterotoxin B.

### IMMUNOLOGIC MEMORY ENABLES A SECOND INFECTION WITH THE SAME MICROBE TO BE DEALT WITH MORE EFFECTIVELY

Once the body has dealt with an infection, the adaptive immune system keeps some of the antigen-specific cells it has generated on standby as memory T and B cells. When a

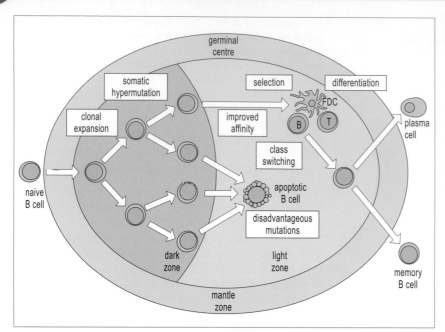

**Fig. 12.10** Structure and function of the germinal centre in B-cell development. One or a few B cells in the dark zone proliferate actively. This proliferation leads to clonal expansion and is accompanied by somatic hypermutation of the immunoglobulin V region genes. B cells with the same specificity but various affinities are, therefore, generated. In the light zone, B cells with disadvantageous mutations or with low affinity undergo apoptosis and are phagocytosed by macrophages (see Fig. 11.6F). Cells with appropriate affinity encounter the antigen on the surface of the follicular dendritic cells (FDCs) and, with the help of CD4 T cells, undergo class switching, leaving the follicle as memory B-cell or plasma cell precursors. (From Male D, Brostoff J, Roth DB, et al. *Immunology*, ed 7, Mosby Elsevier; 2006.)

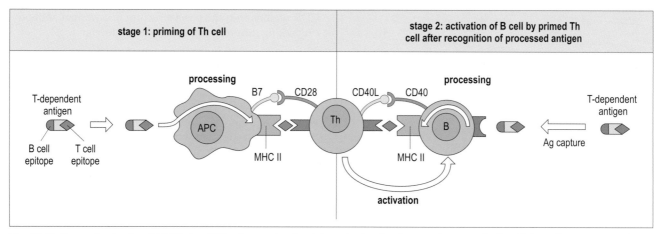

**Fig. 12.11** The mechanism by which T-helper (Th) cells are primed and then stimulate B cells to synthesize antibody to T-dependent antigens with the help of the cognate costimulatory pairs B7/CD28 and CD40L/CD40. See text for a detailed description of the sequence of events. Ag, Antigen; APC, antigen-presenting cell; CD40L, CD40 ligand; MHC, major histocompatibility complex.

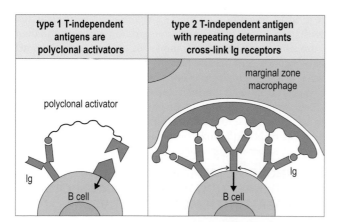

**Fig. 12.12** B-cell activation by T-independent antigens. Some antigens can directly activate the B cells, others with repeating structures cross-link specific antibodies on the B-cell surface. Ig, Immunoglobulin.

naive T cell has recognized and been activated by its specific antigen presented by the right MHC molecule, it changes both its ability to secrete cytokines (or make cytotoxic mediators) and some of its surface antigens or markers. There are different subsets of memory T cells that express particular markers and that are found in particular locations (Table 12.2). Central memory T cells can recirculate through the peripheral lymphoid tissues as they express the chemokine receptor CCR7. Effector memory T cells are better at migrating to sites of inflammation. Other tissue-resident T memory cells are mainly located in epithelia. CD4 T cells need to provide help to CD8 T cells to generate a good CD8 memory T-cell response. Meanwhile, memory B cells are mainly located in the spleen and lymph nodes. Human memory B cells express CD27, one member of the TNF receptor family of receptors. As noted, T-independent antigens do not induce B-cell memory.

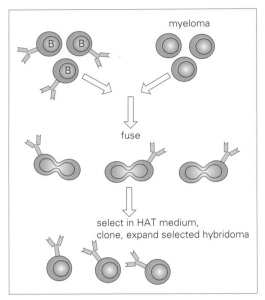

**Fig. 12.13** Production of monoclonal antibodies. Mouse spleen cells from immunized mice are fused to myeloma cells using polyethylene glycol. As the myeloma cells lack the enzyme hypoxanthine–guanine phosphoribosyltransferase, culture in medium containing hypoxanthine aminopterin thymidine (HAT) allows only fused hybridoma cells to survive, and these cells can then be cloned by limiting dilution. Those hybridomas making the antibody you want can then be selected. Newer techniques use genetic engineering to clone the DNA from selected antibody variable light chain (VL) and variable heavy chain (VH) regions.

---

## Box 12.1    Monoclonal Antibodies

Georges Kohler and Cesar Milstein first published how to make monoclonal antibodies in 1975. A single B cell (from an animal immunized with the antigen of interest) is fused to a myeloma cell, giving an immortalized cell making antibody of a single specificity. This technology has revolutionized both immunology and medicine, and Kohler and Milstein shared the Nobel Prize for Physiology or Medicine in 1984, along with Niels Jerne "for theories concerning the specificity in development and control of the immune system and the discovery of the principle for production of monoclonal antibodies." Monoclonal antibodies are used to identify cell surface and intracellular molecules using flow cytometry. They are the basis of many diagnostic assays for infection and are used therapeutically.

---

Memory cells are easier to activate than naive cells and are present at higher frequencies than antigen-specific naive cells so will generate a faster and more effective antigen-specific immune response when they are restimulated. For antibody responses, secondary or memory responses will consist mainly of IgG and IgA antibodies that will be of higher affinities than those produced in the primary response. Immunologic memory can last for long periods — when the isolated Faroe Islands had a measles epidemic in 1846, those who had measles in the previous epidemic in 1781 were still immune! Although, in some cases, reexposure to the same antigens may boost memory responses, memory cells can be maintained without antigen, presumably through cytokine

stimulation. Memory T cells express a molecule called *Bcl-2* that promotes cell survival and a receptor for IL-7 that seems important for the maintenance of memory T cells. Memory CD8 T cells also depend on IL-15 for their survival and seem to have larger clones but of fewer different antigen specificities than memory CD4 T cells; they also need CD4 T-cell help for their development and long-term maintenance. Different virus infections result in the expansion of different types of memory cells (see Fig. 15.15).

Although memory T cells or their descendants may be long-lived, too much antigen stimulation can result in the memory T cells losing function and becoming old or senescent, at which point they start to reexpress the naive T-cell marker CD45RA.

## ARMIES MUST BE KEPT UNDER CONTROL

An immune response will naturally wane once an infection has been dealt with and its antigens removed, thus stopping the stimulation of antigen-specific cells. The now-unwanted antigen-specific cells that are not retained as memory cells die due to a lack of cytokines such as IL-2 and IL-7 that promote cell division, but these cytokines also increase the expression of molecules like Bcl-2 that are antiapoptotic, and so without them the cell is more likely to undergo death by apoptosis. Apoptosis, or programmed cell death, can be induced by either of two pathways: an intrinsic pathway associated with the expression of Bim or an extrinsic pathway of apoptosis that is activated through Fas (CD95), a molecule that has an intracellular death domain and is a member of the TNF receptor superfamily. The body does not have enough space to keep cells that are currently not needed, so apoptosis is a useful way to rid them. Cytotoxic T cells express FasL on their surface and use induction of apoptosis as one way in which they kill infected target cells.

To control and downregulate excessive immune responses that might cause immunopathology, the body also uses a number of other mechanisms, including blocking costimulatory signals needed for cell activation and inhibitory cytokines, some of which are secreted by specialized regulatory T cells (Fig. 12.14). Regulatory T cells (Treg) secrete cytokines that inhibit cytokine secretion and T-cell function, such as IL-10 (originally called *cytokine synthesis inhibitory factor*) and transforming growth factor beta (TGFβ). Tregs can develop in the thymus where they are associated with tolerance to self-antigens, while Tregs that develop in lymphoid tissues are responsible for the downregulation of immune responses induced by infection. Tregs express the transcription factor FoxP3 and high levels of CD25, the α-chain of the IL-2 receptor, but low levels of the IL-7 receptor. The *FoxP3* gene is demethylated, and this epigenetic modification results in greater FoxP3 transcription; TGFβ also stimulates FoxP3 expression. There are also regulatory B cells.

To prevent the immune system from making immune responses to the body's own cells and thus inducing autoimmunity, other processes can be used. A state of anergy or tolerance (self-tolerance) can be induced (Fig. 12.15). For example, T cells can become unresponsive or anergic to an antigen if they receive the first TCR-MHC activating signal without costimulation. This may be a useful way of ensuring that T cells recognizing self-tissue antigens not found in the thymus (and so not able to direct the removal of such

**Table 12.1** Cytokines that play major roles in cell–cell cooperation and induction of adaptive immune responses

| Factor | Receptor family | Source | Actions |
|---|---|---|---|
| IL-1 α/β | IL-1 | Macrophages | Induce inflammation |
| IL-2 | Type I | T cells | T-cell proliferation |
| IL-3 | Type I | T cells | Pluripotent growth |
| IL-4 | Type I | T cells | B-cell proliferation and IgE selection, Th1 suppression |
| IL-5 | Type I | T cells | B-cell growth, IgA and eosinophil differentiation |
| IL-6 | Type I | Macrophages, T cells | B-cell differentiation, induce acute phase proteins |
| IL-7 | Type I | T cells | B- and T-cell proliferation |
| IL-9 | Type I | T cells | Activates mast cells, after induction with TGFβ and IL-4 |
| IL-10 | Type II | T cells | Inhibition of Th1 cytokine production |
| IL-12 | Type I | Monocytes, Mφ | Induction of Th1 cells |
| IL-13 | Type I | T cells | Inhibits mononuclear phagocyte inflammation: proliferation and differentiation of B cells |
| IL-15 | Type I | Dendritic cells | Maintenance of CD8 T-memory cells |
| IL-17 | IL-17 | CD4 T cells | Proinflammatory; stimulates production of cytokines, including TNFα, IL-1β, IL-6, IL-8, G-CSF |
| IL-18 | IL-1 | Macrophages | Induces IFNγ production by T cells; enhances NK cytotoxicity |
| IL-21 | Type I | Th cells | NK differentiation; B activation; T-cell costimulation induces acute phase reactants |
| IL-22 | Type II | T cells | Inhibits IL-4 production by Th2; induces production of antimicrobial proteins by epithelial cells |
| IL-23 | Type I | Dendritic cells | Induces proliferation and IFNγ production by Th1; induces proliferation of memory cells |
| IL-26 | Type II | Th17 T cells | Lysis of membranes of gram-negative bacteria |
| IL-33 | IL-1 | Epithelial cells, endothelial cells | Induces secretion of type 2 cytokines (IL-4, IL-13) in T cells, ILCs |
| IFNγ | Type II | T cells, NK cells | Antiviral, activation of macrophages, inhibition of Th 2 cells, MHC class I and II induction |
| TGFβ | TGFβ | T cells/macrophages | Inhibits activation of NK and T cells, macrophages; inhibits proliferation of B and T cells, promotes wound healing |

The cytokines can be grouped by which receptor family they belong to.
BM, Bone marrow; G-CSF, granulocyte colony-stimulating factor; GM-CSF, granulocyte-macrophage colony-stimulating factor; IFN, interferon; IL, interleukin; ILC, innate lymphoid cell; M-CSF, macrophage colony-stimulating factor; NK, natural killer cell; PMN, polymorphonuclear neutrophil; TGFβ, transforming growth factor beta.

**Table 12.2** Human memory CD4 T-cell subsets

|  | Naive T cells | Effector T cells | Effector memory T cells | Central memory T cells | Tissue-resident memory T cells |
|---|---|---|---|---|---|
| Tissue location | Blood, lymphoid tissues | Blood, lymphoid tissues | Peripheral tissues, mucosal tissues | Lymphoid tissues | Peripheral tissues |
| CD45 isotype | RA | RO | RO | RO | RO |
| CCR7 | ++ | + | − | + | ± |
| CD62L (L-selectin) | ++ | + | ± | + | ± |
| Proliferative ability | ± | +++ | ± | ++ | + |
| Cytokines produced | IL-2 | IFNγ, IL-4/5/13, IL-17 | IFNγ, IL-4/5/13, IL-17 | IL-2 | IFNγ |
| BCL-2 (antiapoptotic) | − | − | + | + | + |

Tissue resident memory T cells also express CD69 and CD103 (αE integrin). There are also similar types of memory CD8 T cells. All memory cells depend on IL-7 for survival, and CD8 memory cells also require IL-15. BCL-2, B-cell lymphoma 2; CCR7, C-C chemokine receptor 7; CD, cluster of differentiation; IFN, interferon; IL, interleukin.

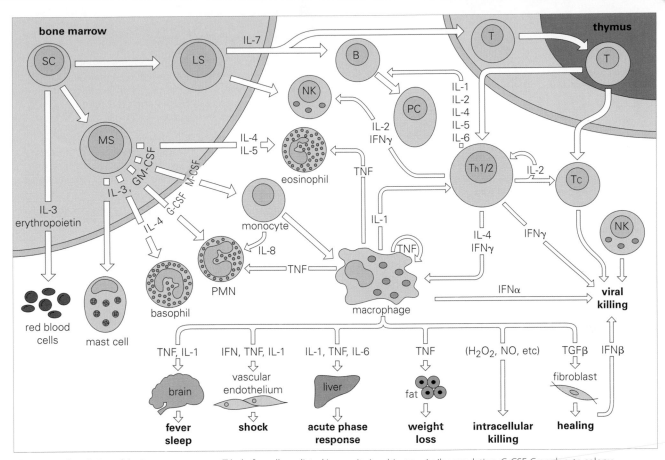

**Fig. 12.14** Regulation of the immune response. T help for cell-mediated immunity is subject to similar regulation. G-CSF, Granulocyte colony-stimulating factor; GM-CSF, granulocyte-macrophage colony-stimulating factor; $H_2O_2$, hydrogen peroxide; LS, lymphoid stem cell; M-CSF, macrophage colony-stimulating factor; MS, myeloid stem cell; NK, natural killer cell; NO, nitric oxide; PC, plasma cell; PMN, polymorphonuclear lymphocyte; SC, stem cell; Tc, cytotoxic T cell; TGFβ, transforming growth factor beta; Th, T-helper cell; TNF, tumour necrosis factor. (Modified from Playfair JHL. *Immunology at a Glance*, Blackwell Science; 2001.)

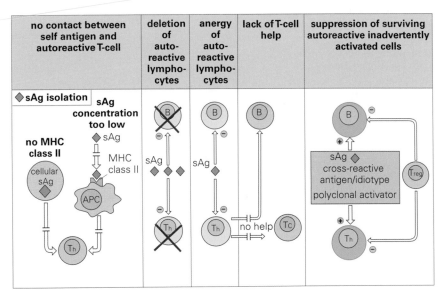

**Fig. 12.15** Mechanisms of peripheral self-tolerance. Self antigens (sAg) will not stimulate autoreactive T-helper (Th) cells if they are anatomically isolated, if there is too low a concentration of processed peptide–major histocompatibility complex class II (MHC II) molecules, or if there is no MHC II on the cell. Both B and T cells can be deleted by clonal deletion via apoptosis or made anergic (unresponsive) by contact with self-antigen without a costimulatory signal or via an inhibitory receptor, by lack of T cell help or be suppressed by regulatory T cells or cytokines. Th cells are the most readily tolerized population, and surviving autoreactive B cells and cytotoxic T (Tc) cells cannot function without T-cell help. Cells that are dead, unresponsive or suppressed are shown in grey. APC, Antigen-presenting cell. (Modified from Delves PJ, et al. *Roitt's Essential Immunology*, ed 11, Blackwell Science; 2006.)

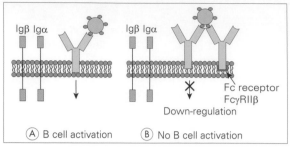

**Fig. 12.16** B-cell downregulation through antibody feedback. Normally B cells are activated when antigen is recognized by antibody expressed on the surface of the B cell leading to signalling through the B-cell receptor immunoglobulin (Ig)α- and Igβ-chains, with the subsequent involvement of SRC kinases, scaffold proteins and tyrosine phosphorylation leading to activation of phosphatidyl inositol triphosphate (PIP3) kinase (A). If antigen binds to both the B-cell surface receptor and to antibody bound to the FcγRIIβ receptor, this inhibitory Fc receptor blocks signalling and B-cell activation by activating the Fc receptor-associated SHIP phosphatase that converts PIP3 to phosphatidyl biphosphate (PIP2) (B).

T cells before their export from the thymus) do not induce autoimmunity. T-cell tolerance can also be induced by inhibitory molecules such as CTLA-4 binding to B7-1 on the APC. CTLA-4 has a much higher affinity for B7 than CD28, so it will bind strongly but does not give a costimulatory signal. Another inhibitory receptor molecule PD-1 is similar to CD28 and expressed on activated T cells, binding to PD-L1 and PD-L2. PD-1 signals through its cytoplasmic tail, leading to activation of a phosphatase enzyme SHP2 and counteracting the positive activating signals sent by MHC-TCR engagement and costimulation. Expression of PD-1 is upregulated on T cells during chronic infections. B cells can also be made anergic (unresponsive) if they have weak binding to a self-antigen, can be deleted through apoptosis, or suppressed in the same ways as T cells. B cells have one additional way of downregulating antibody production (antibody feedback), when antibody binds to the FcRγRIIA receptor, which has an immunoreceptor tyrosine-based inhibition motif in its cytoplasmic domain leading to removal of PIP3 and blocking further antibody production (Fig. 12.16). Finally, there is an interesting phenomenon called *oral tolerance* that must have developed to prevent immune reactions to food antigens and the gut microbiome.

## KEY POINTS

- To make an effective, specific immune response, cooperation between the cells of the innate and adaptive immune systems is needed, including multiple steps such as antigen presentation to T cells, T- and B-cell activation and cytokine secretion.

- Activation of T and B cells involves more than just antigen recognition, including specialized costimulatory as well as cytokine signals, that results in activation of intracellular signalling cascades, metabolic changes and ultimately cell division.

- Cell division will produce clones of daughter T cells of the same antigen specificity; B cells further fine-tune their antigen specificity during an immune response due to somatic mutation, leading to antibodies of greater affinity.

- After the infection has been controlled, the number of antigen-specific T and B cells declines due to cell death, but some remain as memory cells, enabling a faster and more efficient response to reinfection with the same organism.

- The effector cells are also kept from getting out of control and causing tissue damage by regulatory cells such as Tregs and suppressive cytokines such as IL-10 and TGFβ.

# The Conflicts

| 13. | Background to the infectious diseases | 110 |
| 14. | Entry, exit and transmission | 117 |
| 15. | Immune defences in action | 136 |
| 16. | Spread and replication | 152 |
| 17. | Parasite survival strategies and persistent infections | 160 |
| 18. | Pathologic consequences of infection | 176 |

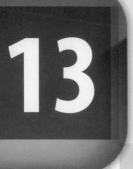

# 13

# Background to the infectious diseases

## Introduction

Vertebrates have been continuously exposed to microbial infections throughout their hundreds of millions of years of evolution. Disease or death was the penalty for inadequate defences. Therefore they have developed:

- highly efficient methods for recognizing foreign invaders
- effective inflammatory and immune responses to restrain the growth and spread of foreign invaders and to eliminate them from the body.

The fundamental bases of these defences have been described in Chapters 10–12. If these defences were completely effective, microbial infections would be scarce and terminated rapidly, as microorganisms would not be allowed to persist in the body for long periods.

### Microbes rapidly evolve characteristics that enable them to overcome the host's defences

Microorganisms faced with the antimicrobial defences of the host species have evolved and developed a variety of characteristics that enable them to bypass or overcome these defences and carry out their obligatory steps for survival (Table 13.1). Unfortunately, microorganisms evolve with extraordinary speed in comparison with their hosts. This is partly because they multiply much more rapidly, the generation time of an average bacterium being ≤1 h, compared with about 20 years for the human host. Rapid evolutionary change is also favoured in bacteria that can hand over genes (carried on plasmids) directly to other bacteria, including unrelated bacteria. Antibiotic resistance genes, for instance, can then be transferred rapidly between species. This rapid rate of evolution ensures that pathogens are always many steps ahead of the host's antimicrobial defences. Indeed, if there are possible ways

around the established defences, microorganisms are likely to have discovered and taken advantage of them. Infectious microorganisms therefore owe their success to this ability to adapt and evolve, exploiting weak points in the host's defences as outlined in Table 13.2 and Figs. 13.1 and 13.2. The host, in turn, has had to respond to such strategies by slowly improving defences, adding extra features, having multiple defence mechanisms with overlap and a good deal of duplication.

## HOST–PARASITE RELATIONSHIPS

### The speed with which host adaptive responses can be mobilized is crucial

Every infection is a race between the capacity of the microorganism to multiply, spread and cause disease and the ability of the host to control and finally terminate the infection (see Fig. 13.1). For instance, a 24-h delay before an important host response comes into operation

**Table 13.1** Successful infectious microorganisms must take certain obligatory steps

| Obligatory steps for infectious microorganisms | | |
|---|---|---|
| **Step** | **Requirement** | **Outcome** |
| Attachment ± entry into body | Evade natural protective and cleansing mechanisms | Entry (infection) |
| Local or general spread in the body | Evade immediate local defences | Spread |
| Multiplication | Increase numbers (although many will die in the host or en route to new hosts) | Multiplication |
| Evasion of host defences | Evade immune and other defences long enough for the full multiplication cycle in the host to be completed | Avoid killing by host defences |
| Shedding from body (exit) | Leave body at a site and on a scale that ensures spread to fresh hosts | Transmission |
| Cause damage in host | Not strictly necessary but often occurs[a] | Pathology, disease |

[a]The last step, cause damage in host, is not strictly necessary, but a certain amount of damage may be essential for shedding. The outpouring of infectious fluids in the common cold or diarrhoea, for instance, or the trickle from vesicular or pustular lesions is required for transmission to fresh hosts.

**Table 13.2** Some examples of host defences and microbial evasion strategies

**Host's defences and the microbe's answer**

| Defence | Microbial answer | Mechanism | Example |
|---|---|---|---|
| Mechanical and other barriers | Bind firmly to epithelial surface | Surface molecule on microbe attaches to receptor molecule on host epithelial cell | Influenza, rhinovirus, Chlamydia, gonococci |
| | Interfere with ciliary activity | Produce ciliotoxic/ciliostatic molecule | Bordetella pertussis, pneumococci, Pseudomonas |
| Host cell membranes as barrier to pathogen | Traverse host cell membrane | Fusion protein in viral envelope | Influenza, HIV |
| | Enter cell by active penetration | Microbial enzymes mediate cell penetration | Trypanosoma cruzi, Toxoplasma gondii |
| Phagocytic and immediate host defences | Microbe ingested and killed by phagocyte | Inhibit phagocytosis | Pneumococci, Treponema pallidum, Haemophilus influenzae |
| | | Microbial outer wall or capsule impedes phagocytosis | |
| | Inhibit phagosome–lysosome fusion | Sulphatides of Mycobacterium tuberculosis inhibit fusion | M. tuberculosis |
| | Interfere with signal transduction in macrophage | Induction of SOCS proteins | Toxoplasma gondii |
| | Resist killing and multiply in phagocyte | Exit from phagosome into cytoplasm (Listeria) | Brucella spp., Listeria monocytogenes, measles, dengue viruses |
| Host molecules (lactoferrin, transferrin etc.) restrict availability of free iron needed by microbe | Microbe competes with host for iron | Microbe possesses avidly iron-binding siderophores | Pathogenic Neisseria, Escherichia coli, Pseudomonas |
| Complement activated with antimicrobial effects | Inactivate complement components | Production of an elastase | Pseudomonas aeruginosa |
| | Interfere with complement-mediated phagocytosis | C3b receptor on microbe competes with that on phagocyte and complement access blocked | Candida albicans, T. gondii, M protein of Streptococcus pyogenes |
| Infected host produces interferons to inhibit virus replication | Induce a poor interferon response | Core antigen of hepatitis B suppresses IFNβ production | Hepatitis B, rotaviruses |
| | Insensitive to interferons | Prevent activation of interferon-induced enzymes | Adenovirus |

Continued

**Table 13.2** Some examples of host defences and microbial evasion strategies —cont'd

**Host's defences and the microbe's answer**

| Defence | Microbial answer | Mechanism | Example |
|---|---|---|---|
| Immune defences | | | |
| Infected host produces antibody | Destroy antibody | Bacterium produces IgA protease | Gonococci, *H. influenzae*, streptococci, *Neisseria meningitidis* |
| | Display Fc receptor on microbial surface | Antibody bound to microbe in upside-down position | Staphylococci (protein A), trypanosomes, certain streptococci, herpes simplex virus, cytomegalovirus |
| Infected host produces antimicrobial cell-mediated immune response | Invade T cells, and interfere with their function or kill them | Virus envelope molecule binds to CD4 on helper T-cell surface | HIV |
| | Induce regulatory T cells | Suppress beneficial immunity | *Bordetella pertussis*, *M. tuberculosis*, *Helicobacter pylori*, HIV |
| Antimicrobial immune response recognizes infected cells and destroys them | Microbe in cells fails to display microbial antigens on cell surface | Viral antigens not synthesized | Herpes simplex virus latent in sensory neurons |
| | | Virus inhibits transport of MHC class I molecules to cell surface, thus avoiding recognition by CD8 T cell | Cytomegalovirus, adenovirus |
| Effective immune response produced | Vary microbial antigens in individual host or during spread in host community | Switch on different surface antigens | *Trypanosoma brucei*, *Borrelia recurrentis* |
| | | Mutation, genetic recombination | Influenza virus, streptococci, gonococci |

Although inflammation is not listed as a host defence in its own right, many of these defences depend on local inflammation. Inflammation (see Ch. 10) means an increased blood supply and the delivery of antibodies, complement, immune cells, and phagocytes to the site of infection. In the days before antibiotics, people applied hot poultices to staphylococcal boils and abscesses to increase the amount of inflammation and hasten recovery. Microbes that interfere with the action of complement or with chemotaxis (staphylococci, streptococci, *P. aeruginosa*, herpes simplex viruses) will thereby tend to reduce inflammation.
HIV, Human immunodeficiency virus; IFNβ, interferon beta; MHC, major histocompatibility complex; SOCS, suppressor of cytokine signalling.

**Fig. 13.1** Every infection is a race. Delays in mobilizing host adaptive defences can lead to disease or death.

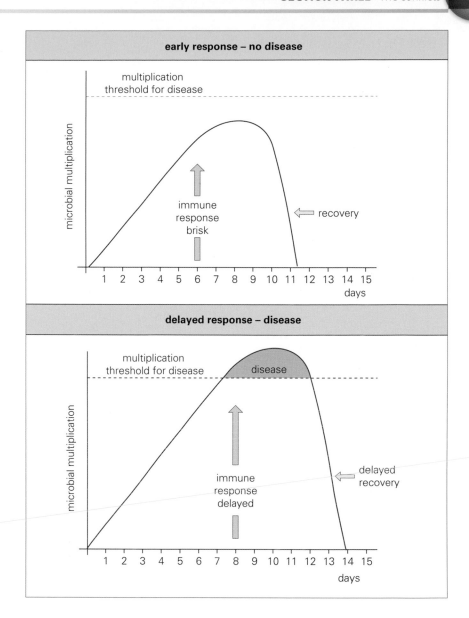

can give a decisive advantage to a rapidly growing micro-organism. From the host's point of view, it may allow enough damage to cause disease. More importantly, from the pathogen's point of view, it may give the microbe the opportunity to be shed from the body in larger amounts or for an extra 1–2 days. A pathogen that achieves this will be rapidly selected for in evolution.

### Adaptation by both host and parasite leads to a more stable balanced relationship

The picture of conflict between host and parasite, usually and appropriately described in military terms, is central to an understanding of the biology of infectious disease. As with military conflicts, adaptation on both sides (Box 13.1) tends to lessen the damage and incidence of death in the host population, leading to a more stable and balanced relationship. The successful parasite gets what it can from the host without causing too much damage; in general, the more ancient the relationship, the less the damage. Many microbial parasites, not only the normal flora (see Ch. 9) but also meningococci and pneumococci and others, live

for the most part in peaceful coexistence with their human host.

Some microorganisms remain at body surfaces, perhaps spreading locally but failing to invade deeper tissues. These include the common cold viruses, wart viruses, mycoplasmas and skin fungi. Often the disease is mild, but severe illness can occur when powerful toxins are produced and act either locally (cholera) or at distant sites (diphtheria).

Infecting microorganisms can gain entry to a healthy host and cause disease in three ways (Fig. 13.3):

- microorganisms with specific mechanisms for attaching to, or penetrating, the body surfaces (most viruses and certain bacteria)
- microorganisms introduced by biting arthropods (e.g. malaria, plague, typhus, yellow fever)
- microorganisms introduced into otherwise normal healthy hosts via skin wounds or animal bites (clostridia, rabies, *Pasteurella multocida*).

Microorganisms are also able to infect a normal healthy host when surface or systemic defences are impaired

## Box 13.1 ■ Lessons in Microbiology

### Myxomatosis

Myxomatosis provides a well-studied classic example of the evolution of an infectious disease unleashed on a highly susceptible population. This viral disease, which is spread mechanically by mosquitoes, normally infects South American rabbits *(Sylvilagus brasiliensis)*, but they remain perfectly well, developing only a virus-rich skin swelling at the site of the mosquito bite. The same virus in the European rabbit *(Oryctolagus cuniculus)* causes a rapidly fatal disease.

Myxomavirus was successfully introduced into Australia in 1950 as an attempt to control the rapidly increasing rabbit population. Initially, >99% of infected rabbits died (see Fig. 13.2), but then two fundamental changes occurred:

1. New, less lethal strains of virus appeared and replaced the original strain. This occurred because rabbits infected

with these strains survived for longer and their virus was therefore more likely to be transmitted.

2. The rabbit population changed its character, as those that were genetically more susceptible to the infection were eliminated. In other words, the virus positively selected the more resistant host, and the less lethal virus strain proved to be a more successful parasite. If the rabbit population had been eliminated, the virus would also have died out, but the host–parasite relationship quite rapidly settled down to reach a state of better balanced pathogenicity, and by the 1970s, only about half the rabbits died from infection. Australian rabbits have since faced a new threat: a calicivirus introduced from Europe, which spreads by contact and causes a lethal haemorrhagic disease.

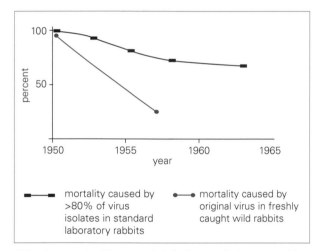

**Fig. 13.2** Evolution of a pathogen within a host species. Myxomatosis is the best-studied example of the appearance of a highly lethal pathogen in a host population that gradually settles down to a state of more balanced pathogenicity. *Vibrio cholerae* has progressed in this direction.

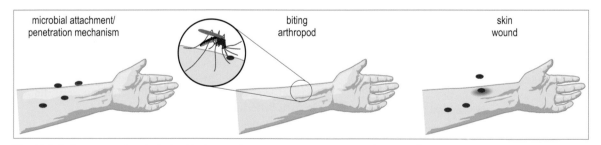

**Fig. 13.3** Pathogens can invade the healthy host in three main ways. Invasion may also occur if the host is immunosuppressed.

(see Ch. 31), as occurs with burns, insertion of foreign bodies (cannulas and catheters), urinary tract infections in men (stones, enlarged prostate; see Ch. 21), bacterial pneumonia following initial viral damage (postinfluenza) or depressed immune responses (immunosuppressive drugs or diseases such as acquired immunodeficiency syndrome).

## CAUSES OF INFECTIOUS DISEASES

### Many microbes commonly cause infection

Humans are host to many different microorganisms. In addition to the scores of microbes that form the normal flora or microbiota, there are many that quite commonly cause infection, some of them remaining in the body for many years afterward. Against this rich background of parasitic activity, how do we prove that a certain microorganism is the culprit in any given disease? In some instances (anthrax, cholera, tetanus, malaria) the causative microorganism is identified and incriminated at an early stage; in others it is not so easy.

### Koch's postulates to identify the microbial causes of specific diseases

In 1890 Robert Koch (Box 13.2) set out as postulates the following criteria he felt to be necessary for a microorganism to be accepted as the cause of a given disease:

- The microbe must be present in every case of the disease.
- The microbe must be isolated from the diseased host and grown in pure culture.
- The disease must be reproduced when a pure culture of the organism is introduced into a nondiseased-susceptible host.
- The microbe must be recoverable from an experimentally infected host.

In the early days of microbiology, Koch's postulates brought a welcome clarity. The germ theory of disease causation had only recently been set out following Koch's classic studies on anthrax (1876) and tuberculosis (1882), and methods for isolating microbes in pure culture and identifying them were only just being developed. However, modifications were needed to include certain bacterial diseases and the new world of viral diseases. The microbe could not always be grown in the laboratory (*Treponema pallidum*, wart viruses, *Mycobacterium leprae*), and for certain microbes (hepatitis B, Epstein-Barr virus [EBV]) there were (initially) no susceptible animal species. Therefore the criteria have been modified on several occasions to accommodate these problems, including the need for sequence-based identification of the infectious organisms, the challenges of viruses and the complexities of microbial interactions.

### Conclusions about causation are now reached using enlightened common sense

Nowadays, with our vastly increased technology and understanding of infection, those early attempts to make lists and apply rigid criteria may seem old-fashioned. Perhaps we can now reach conclusions about causation using common sense. For instance, we recognize that diseases sometimes do not appear until many years after a specific infection (subacute sclerosing panencephalitis; see Ch. 25, Creutzfeldt-Jakob disease; see Ch. 8). Molecular genetic techniques may now identify previously uncultivable causative organisms. The polymerase chain reaction was used to amplify and sequence small amounts of mRNA from the bowel of patients with Whipple's disease, a rare multisystem disorder. A unique 16S mRNA was identified belonging to the previously uncharacterized, uncultivable bacterium *Tropheryma whipplei*. Nevertheless, grey areas remain, especially in diseases of possible or probable microbial aetiology in which the pathogen does not act alone. Cofactors

---

## Box 13.2 ■ Lessons in Microbiology

### Robert Koch (1843–1910)

In 1876, while in general practice in Berlin, Robert Koch (Fig. 13.4) isolated the anthrax bacillus and became the first to show a specific organism as the cause of a disease. In 1882 he discovered *Mycobacterium tuberculosis* as the cause of tuberculosis. He then went on to lead an expedition to Egypt and India in 1883 and discovered the cause of cholera: *Vibrio cholerae*.

Koch was the founder of the germ theory of disease, which maintained that certain diseases were caused by a single species of microbe. In 1890 he set out his postulates as ground rules. New techniques were necessary to meet the exacting requirements of the postulates, and Koch became the first to grow bacteria in colonies, initially on potato slices, and later, with his pupil Julius Petri (who gave his name to Petri dishes), on solid gelatin media.

Koch himself could not reproduce cholera in animals, however, and not all microbes could be cultivated. His original rules therefore had to be modified. Nevertheless, he brought order and clarity to medicine; previously diseases were attributed to miasmas (malaria is derived from *mal aria*, "bad air") or mists, to punishments from the gods or devils or to unfortunate conjunctions of the stars and planets. However, there was resistance to his ideas. A distinguished Munich physician, Max Von Petternkofer, believed that he had disproved the new theory when he drank a pure culture of *V. cholerae* and suffered no more than mild diarrhoea!

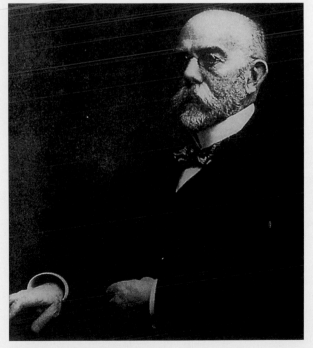

**Fig. 13.4** Robert Koch (1843–1910).

**Table 13.3** The likelihood of developing clinical disease varies with the infection and often depends upon age

| Frequency of clinically apparent disease | |
|---|---|
| **Infection** | **Approximate percent with clinically apparent disease** |
| *Pneumocystis jirovecii*[a] | 0 |
| Epstein-Barr virus (child age 1–5 yr) | 1 (30–75% in young adults) |
| Poliomyelitis (child) | 24[b] |
| Malaria (child age 1–5 yr) | 25 (2% in adults) |
| Rubella | 50 |
| Influenza (young adult) | 60 |
| Whooping cough Typhoid Anthrax | }>90 |
| Gonorrhoea (adult male) Measles | }99 |
| Rabies | }100 |

[a]Formerly *P. carinii.*
[b]1% develop paralytic poliomyelitis.

or genetic and immunologic factors in the host may play a vital part. Examples include:

- the cancers associated with viruses (hepatitis B, genital wart viruses, EBV)
- diseases of possible microbial origin in which a number of different pathogens may be involved (postviral fatigue syndrome, exacerbations of multiple sclerosis)
- diseases that might be infectious but occur in only a very small proportion of genetically predisposed individuals (rheumatoid arthritis, juvenile diabetes mellitus).

## THE BIOLOGIC RESPONSE GRADIENT

### It is uncommon for a pathogen to cause exactly the same disease in all infected individuals

A physician must be able to make a diagnosis when only some of the possible signs and symptoms are present. The exact clinical picture depends on many variables such as infecting dose and route, age, sex, presence of other pathogens, nutritional status and genetic background. Infections such as measles or cholera give a fairly consistent disease picture, but others such as syphilis cause such a wide spectrum of pathology that Sir William Osler (1849–1919) stated, "He who knows syphilis knows medicine."

There is great variation not only in the nature but also in the severity of clinical disease. Many infections are asymptomatic in >90% of individuals, the clinically characterized illness applying to only an occasional unfortunate host (Table 13.3). This illness can be mild or severe. Asymptomatically infected individuals are important because, although they develop immunity and resistance to

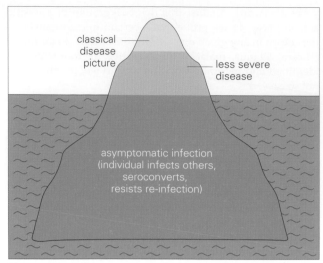

**Fig. 13.5** The iceberg concept of infectious disease.

reinfection, they are not identified, move normally in the community and can infect others. Clearly there is little point in isolating a clinically infected patient when there is a high frequency of asymptomatically infected and infectious individuals in the community. This phenomenon can be represented as an iceberg (Fig. 13.5). In addition, individuals can be infectious before they develop symptoms.

## KEY FACTS

- Faced with host defences (see Chs. 10–12), the pathogens (see Chs. 1–7) have developed mechanisms to bypass them, and, in turn, the host defences have had to be modified, although slowly, in response.

- There is a conflict between the pathogen and host, and every infectious disease is the result of this ancient battle. Details of the host–pathogen conflict are given in Chapters 13–18, an outline of diagnostic methods in Chapter 32 and a central account of infectious diseases according to the body systems involved in Chapters 19–31.

- Speed matters. Every infection is a race between (1) microbial replication and spread and (2) the mobilization of host responses.

- Some organisms can invade a healthy host but others gain entry with help – injected via insect bite or gaining entry through wounds.

- Molecular techniques have helped identify the cause of a disease.

- Pathogens do not necessarily produce the same disease in all infected individuals. A biologic response gradient causes a spectrum that can range from an asymptomatic to a lethal infection.

# Entry, exit and transmission

## Introduction

### Microorganisms must attach to, or penetrate, the host's body surfaces.

The mammalian host can be considered as a series of body surfaces. To establish themselves on or in the host, microorganisms must either attach to or penetrate one of these body surfaces. The outer surface, covered by skin or fur, protects and isolates the body from the outside world, forming a dry, horny, relatively impermeable outer layer. Elsewhere, however, there has to be more intimate contact and exchange with the outside world. Therefore, in the alimentary, respiratory and urogenital tracts where food is absorbed, gases exchanged and urine and sexual products released, respectively, the lining consists of one or more layers of living cells. In the eye, the skin is replaced by a transparent layer of living cells: the conjunctiva. Well-developed cleansing and defence mechanisms are present at all these body surfaces, and entry of microorganisms always has to occur in the face of these natural mechanisms. Successful microorganisms, therefore, possess efficient mechanisms for attaching to, and often traversing these body surfaces. Transmission depends on the interaction with both the host interaction and the external environment. Nonenveloped viruses are quite robust and are infectious during the various conditions that they meet (e.g. enteroviruses in the gastrointestinal tract are quite acid resistant and stable over a wide pH range). Clearly the longer a microorganism can survive outside a host, the greater the chance of transmission. The crucial variable factors are the environment and its heat, pH and moisture.

## Receptor molecules

There are often specific molecules on pathogens that bind to receptor molecules on host cells, either at the body surface (viruses, bacteria) or in tissues (viruses). These receptor molecules, of which there may be more than one, are not present for the benefit of the virus or other infectious agent; they have specific functions in the life of the cell. Very occasionally, the receptor molecule is present only in certain cells, which are then uniquely susceptible to infection. Examples include the main receptor and coreceptors for human immunodeficiency virus (HIV); namely, the cluster of differentiation antigen 4 (CD4) and the coreceptors CC chemokine receptor 5 (CCR5) and/or CXC chemokine receptor 4 (CXCR4). The B-cell CR2/CD21 receptor binds the Epstein-Barr virus envelope protein gp350, and alpha-dystroglycan (DG) of Schwann cells is a receptor that *Mycobacterium leprae* binds to and allows invasion into peripheral nerve cells and development of leprosy. DG is a versatile cell surface molecule and can be used by arenaviruses such as Lassa fever virus. In these cases, the presence of the receptor molecule determines microbial tropism and accounts for the distinctive pattern of infection. Receptors are therefore critical determinants of cell susceptibility, not only at the body surface but in all tissues. After binding to the susceptible cell, the microorganism can multiply at the surface (mycoplasma, *Bordetella pertussis*) or enter the cell and infect it (viruses, chlamydia; see Ch. 16).

## Exit from the body

Microorganisms must also exit from the body if they are to be transmitted to another host. They are either shed in large numbers in secretions and excretions or are available in the blood for uptake (e.g. by blood-sucking arthropods or needles).

## SITES OF ENTRY

### Skin

#### Microorganisms gaining entry via the skin may cause a skin infection or infection elsewhere

Microorganisms that infect or enter the body via the skin are listed in Table 14.1. On the skin, microorganisms other than residents of the normal flora (see Ch. 9) are soon inactivated, especially by fatty acids (skin pH is ~5.5), and probably by substances secreted by sebaceous and other glands, and certain peptides formed locally by keratinocytes protect against invasion by group A streptococci. Materials produced by the normal flora of the skin also protect against infection. Skin bacteria may enter hair follicles or sebaceous glands to cause styes and boils or teat canals to cause staphylococcal mastitis.

Several types of fungi such as the dermatophytes (i.e. tinea corporis [ringworm] and tinea pedis [athlete's foot]) infect the nonliving keratinous structures, including the stratum corneum, hair and nails, produced by the skin.

**Table 14.1** Microorganisms that infect via the skin

| Microorganism | Disease | Comments |
|---|---|---|
| Arthropod-borne viruses | Fever and various organ systems can be affected such as: West Nile encephalitis Japanese encephalitis Yellow fever Zika virus-related microcephaly Congo–Crimean haemorrhagic fever | 150 distinct viruses, transmitted by bite of infected arthropod |
| Rabies virus | Rabies | Bite or scratch from infected terrestrial mammal, licking broken skin, contact with bat saliva |
| Human papillomaviruses | Warts | Infection restricted to epidermis |
| Staphylococci | Boils | Commonest skin invaders |
| *Rickettsia* | Typhus, spotted fevers | Infestation with infected arthropod |
| *Leptospira* | Leptospirosis | Contact with water containing infected animal urine |
| Streptococci | Impetigo, erysipelas | Concurrent pharyngeal infection in one-third of cases |
| *Bacillus anthracis* | Cutaneous anthrax | Systemic disease following local lesion at inoculation site |
| *Treponema pallidum* and *T. pertenue* | Syphilis, yaws | Warm, moist skin susceptible |
| *Yersinia pestis*, *Plasmodia* | Plague, malaria | Bite from infected rodent flea or mosquito |
| *Trichophyton* spp. and other fungi | Ringworm, athlete's foot | Infection restricted to skin, nails, hair |
| *Ancylostoma duodenale Necator americanus* *Ancylostoma ceylanicum* | Intestinal hookworm disease | Silent entry of larvae through skin (i.e. bare feet) *A. duodenale* and *N. americanus* worldwide and *A. ceylanicum* in some regions mostly eosinophilic enteritis |
| Filarial nematodes | Filariasis | Bite from infected mosquito, midge, blood-sucking fly |
| *Schistosoma* spp. | Schistosomiasis | Larvae (cercariae) from infected snail penetrate skin during wading or bathing |

Some remain restricted to the skin (papillomaviruses, ringworm); others enter the body after infecting the skin (syphilis) or after mechanical transfer across the skin (arthropod-borne infections, schistosomiasis).

Infection is established as long as the parasites' rate of downward growth into the keratin exceeds the rate of shedding of the keratinous product. When the latter is very slow, as in the case of nails, the infection is more likely to become chronic.

Wounds, abrasions, or burns are more common sites of infection. Even a small break in the skin can be a portal of entry if microorganisms such as streptococci, water-borne leptospira or blood-borne hepatitis B virus are present at the site. A few pathogens such as leptospira or the larvae of *Ancylostoma* and *Schistosoma* can traverse the unbroken skin by their own activity.

### Biting arthropods

Biting arthropods such as mosquitoes, ticks, fleas, and sandflies (see Ch. 28) penetrate the skin during feeding and can thus introduce infectious agents or parasites into the body. The arthropod transmits the infection and is an essential part of the life cycle of the microorganism. Sometimes the transmission is mechanical, the microorganism contaminating the mouth parts without multiplying in the arthropod. In most cases, however, the infectious agent multiplies in the arthropod and, as a result of millions of years of adaptation, causes little or no damage to that host. After an incubation period, it appears in the saliva or faeces and is transmitted during a blood feed. The mosquito, for instance, injects saliva directly into host tissues as an anticoagulant, whereas the human body louse defecates as it feeds, and *Rickettsia*

*rickettsii*, which is present in the faeces, is introduced into the bite wound when the host scratches the affected area.

### The conjunctiva

The conjunctiva can be regarded as a specialized area of skin. It is kept clean by the continuous flushing action of tears, aided every few seconds by the window cleaner action of the eyelids. Therefore the microorganisms such as chlamydia and gonococci that can infect the normal conjunctiva of a baby having been delivered through a bacterially infected birth canal must have efficient attachment mechanisms (see Ch. 26). Interference with local defences due to decreased lacrimal gland secretion or conjunctival or eyelid damage allows even nonspecialist microorganisms to establish themselves. Contaminated birth canals, fingers, flies or towels carry infectious material to the conjunctiva, examples including herpes simplex virus infections leading to keratoconjunctivitis or chlamydial infection resulting in trachoma. Antimicrobial substances in tears, including lysozyme, an enzyme and certain peptides, have a role in defence.

### Respiratory tract
**Some microorganisms can overcome the respiratory tract's cleansing mechanisms**

Air normally contains suspended particles, including smoke, dust and microorganisms. Efficient cleansing mechanisms deal with these constantly inhaled particles. With

~500–1000 microorganisms/m³ inside buildings, and a ventilation rate of 6 L/min at rest, as many as 10,000 microorganisms/day are introduced into the lungs. In the upper or lower respiratory tract, inhaled microorganisms, like other particles, will be trapped in mucus, carried to the back of the throat by ciliary action, and swallowed. Those that invade the normal healthy respiratory tract have developed specific mechanisms to avoid this fate. Ventilation of buildings has been highlighted especially during the COVID-19 pandemic.

### Interfering with cleansing mechanisms

The ideal strategy is to attach firmly to the surfaces of cells forming the mucociliary sheet. Specific molecules on the organism, often called *adhesins*, bind to receptor molecules on the susceptible cell (Fig. 14.1). Examples of such respiratory infections are given in Table 14.2.

Inhibiting ciliary activity is another way of interfering with cleansing mechanisms. This helps invading microorganisms establish themselves in the respiratory tract. *B. pertussis*, for instance, not only attaches to respiratory epithelial cells but also interferes with ciliary activity; other bacteria (Table 14.3) produce various ciliostatic substances of generally unknown nature.

### Avoiding destruction by alveolar macrophages

Inhaled microorganisms reaching the alveoli encounter alveolar macrophages, which remove foreign particles and keep the air spaces clean. Most microorganisms are destroyed by these macrophages, but one or two pathogens have learnt either to avoid phagocytosis or to avoid destruction after phagocytosis. Tubercle bacilli, for instance, survive in the macrophages, and respiratory tuberculosis is thought to be initiated in this way. Inhalation of as few as 5–10 bacilli is enough. The vital role of macrophages in antimicrobial defences is dealt with more thoroughly in Chapter 15. Alveolar macrophages are damaged following inhalation of toxic asbestos particles and certain dusts, and this leads to increased susceptibility to respiratory tuberculosis.

## Gastrointestinal tract

### Some microorganisms can survive the intestine's defences of acid, mucus and enzymes

Apart from the general flow of intestinal contents, there are no particular cleansing mechanisms in the intestinal tract. Diarrhoea and vomiting could be considered to be extreme

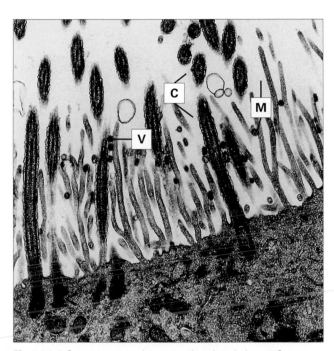

**Fig. 14.1** Influenza virus attachment to ciliated epithelium. Influenza virus particles (V) attached to cilia (C) and microvilli (M). Electron micrograph of thin section from organ culture of guinea pig trachea 1 h after addition of the virus. (Courtesy R.E. Dourmashkin.)

**Table 14.2** Microbial attachment in the respiratory tract

| Microorganisms | Disease | Microbial adhesion | Receptor on host cell |
|---|---|---|---|
| Influenza A virus | Influenza | Haemagglutinin | Sialyloligosaccharides |
| Rhinovirus | Common cold | Capsid protein | ICAM-1 (CD54) |
| Coxsackieviruses | Common cold; hand, foot, and mouth disease (vesicles); rashes; aseptic meningitis | Capsid protein | Coxsackievirus and adenovirus receptor (CAR)—multifunctional cellular protein |
| Parainfluenza virus type 1, respiratory syncytial virus | Respiratory illness | Envelope protein | Insulin-like growth factor-1 receptor (IGFR-1) triggers the activation of protein kinase C zeta that recruits nucleolin from the nucleus to the plasma membrane. Nucleolin is an entry coreceptor. |
| *Mycoplasma pneumoniae* | Atypical pneumonia | Mediated by the terminal organelle, a membrane-bound extension of the mycoplasma-infected cell | Sialylated glycoproteins |
| *Haemophilus influenza, Streptococcus pneumonia* | Respiratory disease | Surface molecule | B-glucan receptor Platelet-activating factor (PAF) |
| Measles virus | Measles | Haemagglutinin | CD46 |

CD46, Cluster of differentiation 46 is a membrane cofactor protein involved in complement regulation; ICAM-1, intercellular adhesion molecule-1; integrins, family of adhesion receptors (e.g. laminin receptor) expressed on many cell types.

**Table 14.3** Interference with ciliary activity in respiratory infections

| Cause | Mechanisms | Importance |
|---|---|---|
| Infecting bacteria interfere with ciliary activity (*Bordetella pertussis, Haemophilus influenzae, Pseudomonas aeruginosa, Mycoplasma pneumoniae*) | Production of ciliostatic substances (tracheal cytotoxin from *B. pertussis*, at least two substances from *H. influenzae*, at least seven from *P. aeruginosa*) | + + |
| Viral infection | Ciliated cell dysfunction or destruction by influenza, measles | + + + |
| Atmospheric pollution (automobiles, cigarette smoking) | Acutely impaired mucociliary function | ? + |
| Inhalation of unhumidified air (indwelling tracheal tubes, general anaesthesia) | Acutely impaired mucociliary function | + |
| Chronic bronchitis, cystic fibrosis | Chronically impaired mucociliary function | + + + |

Although pathogens can actively interfere with ciliary activity (first item), a more general impairment of mucociliary function also acts as a predisposing cause of respiratory infection.

**Table 14.4** Microbial attachment in the intestinal tract

| Microorganism | Disease | Attachment site | Mechanism |
|---|---|---|---|
| Poliovirus | Poliomyelitis | Intestinal epithelium | Viral capsid protein attaches to a specific receptor, called Pvr (polio virus receptor) or CD155, a cellular glycoprotein |
| Rotavirus | Diarrhoea | Intestinal epithelium | Viral outer capsid protein VP4 attaches to host cell glycans and then interacts with several coreceptors during postattachment steps |
| *Vibrio cholera* | Cholera | Intestinal epithelium | Multivalent adhesion molecule (MAM) 7 is an outer membrane protein mediating host cell attachment |
| *Escherichia coli* (EPEC and EHEC) | Diarrhoea | Intestinal epithelium | Bacteria inject translocated intimin receptor (Tir), an effector, that inserts into host cell plasma membrane acting as a receptor for the bacterial surface protein called intimin |
| *Salmonella typhi* | Enteric fever | Ileal epithelium | Bacterial adhesins bind to host cell receptors |
| *Shigella* spp. | Dysentery | Colonic epithelium | Shigella surface protein, IscA, acts as an adhesin and interacts with host cells after activating a type III secretion system, triggering its uptake into epithelial cells |
| *Giardia lamblia* | Diarrhoea | Duodenal and jejunal epithelium | Protozoa bind to mannose-6-phosphate on host cell; also have mechanical sucker—the ventral disc |
| *Entamoeba histolytica* | Dysentery | Colonic epithelium | Lectin on surface of amoeba binds host cell |
| *Ancylostoma duodenale* | Hookworm | Intestinal epithelium | Buccal capsule |

examples. Under normal circumstances, multiplication of resident bacteria is counterbalanced by their continuous passage to the exterior with the rest of the intestinal contents. Ingestion of a small number of nonpathogenic bacteria, followed by growth in the lumen of the alimentary canal, produces only relatively small numbers within 12–18 h, which is the normal intestinal transit time.

Infecting bacteria must attach themselves to the intestinal epithelium (Table 14.4) if they are to establish themselves and multiply in large numbers. They will then avoid being carried straight down the alimentary canal to be excreted with the rest of the intestinal contents. The concentration of microorganisms in faeces depends on the balance between the production and removal of bacteria in the intestine. *Vibrio cholerae* (Figs. 14.2 and 14.3) and rotaviruses both establish specific binding to receptors on the surface of intestinal epithelial cells. For *V. cholerae*, establishment in surface mucus may be sufficient for infection and pathogenicity. The fact that certain pathogens infect mainly the large bowel (*Shigella* spp.) or small intestine (most salmonellae, rotaviruses) indicates the presence of

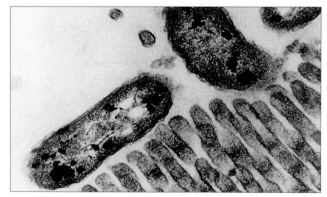

**Fig. 14.2** Attachment of *Vibrio cholerae* to brush border of rabbit villus. Thin section electron micrograph (×10,000). (Courtesy E.T. Nelson.)

specific receptor molecules on mucosal cells in these sections of the alimentary canal.

Infection sometimes involves more than mere adhesion to the luminal surface of intestinal epithelial cells. *Shigella flexneri*, for example, can only enter these cells from the basal

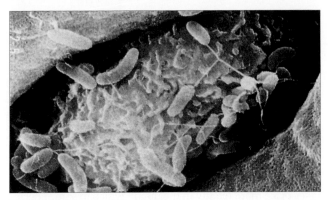

**Fig. 14.3** Adherence of *Vibrio cholerae* to M cells in human ileal mucosa. (Courtesy T. Yamamoto.)

surface. Initial entry occurs after uptake by M cells, highly specialized within the epithelium and initiate mucosal immune responses by taking the bacteria to the lymphoid tissue and the bacteria then invade local macrophages. This gives rise to an inflammatory response with an influx of polymorphs, which, in turn, causes some disruption of the epithelial barrier. Bacteria can now enter on a larger scale from the intestinal lumen and invade epithelial cells from below. The bacteria enhance their entry by exploiting the host's inflammatory response.

### Crude mechanical devices for attachment

Crude mechanical devices are used for the attachment and entry of certain parasitic protozoans and worms. *Giardia lamblia*, for example, has specific molecules for adhesion to the microvilli of epithelial cells but also has its own microvillar-sucking disk. Hookworms attach to the intestinal mucosa by means of a large mouth capsule containing hooked teeth or cutting plates. Other worms (e.g. *Ascaris*)

maintain their position by bracing themselves against peristalsis, while tapeworms adhere closely to the mucus covering the intestinal wall, the anterior hooks and sucker playing a relatively minor role for the largest worms. A number of worms actively penetrate into the mucosa as adults (*Trichinella*, *Trichuris*) or traverse the gut wall to enter deeper tissues (e.g. the embryos of *Trichinella* released from the female worm and the larvae of *Echinococcus* hatched from ingested eggs).

### Mechanisms to counteract mucus, acids, enzymes, and bile

*Successful intestinal pathogens must counteract or resist mucus, acids, enzymes and bile.* Mucus protects epithelial cells, perhaps acting as a mechanical barrier to infection. It may contain molecules that bind to microbial adhesins, therefore blocking attachment to host cells. It also contains pathogen-specific secretory IgA antibodies, which protect the immune individual against infection. Motile microorganisms (*V. cholerae*, salmonellae, certain strains of *Escherichia coli*) can propel themselves through the mucous layer and are therefore more likely to reach epithelial cells to make specific attachments; *V. cholerae* also produces a mucinase, which probably helps its passage through the mucus. Nonmotile microorganisms, in contrast, rely on random and passive transport in the mucous layer.

As might be expected, microorganisms that infect by the intestinal route are often capable of surviving in the presence of acid, proteolytic enzymes and bile. This also applies to microorganisms that shed from the body by this route (Table 14.5).

All organisms infecting by the intestinal route must run the gauntlet of acid in the stomach. *Helicobacter pylori* has evolved a specific defence (Box 14.1). The fact that tubercle bacilli resist acid conditions favours the establishment of

**Table 14.5** Microbial properties that aid success in the gastrointestinal tract

| Property | Examples | Consequence |
|---|---|---|
| Specific attachment to intestinal epithelium | Poliovirus, rotavirus, *Vibrio cholerae* | Microorganism avoids expulsion with other gut contents and can establish infection |
| Motility | *V. cholerae*, certain *Escherichia coli* strains | Bacteria travel through mucus and are more likely to reach susceptible cell |
| Production of mucinase | *V. cholerae* | May assist transit through mucus |
| Acid resistance | *Mycobacterium tuberculosis* | Encourages intestinal tuberculosis (acid-labile microorganisms depend on protection in food bolus or in diluting fluid) and increased susceptibility in individuals with achlorhydria |
| | *Helicobacter pylori* | Establish residence in stomach |
| | Enteroviruses (poliovirus, coxsackieviruses, echoviruses), hepatitis A virus | Infection and shedding from gastrointestinal tract |
| Bile resistance | *Salmonella*, *Shigella*, enteroviruses | Intestinal pathogens |
| | *Enterococcus faecalis*, *E. coli*, *Proteus*, *Pseudomonas* | Establish residence |
| Resistance to proteolytic enzymes | Reoviruses in mice | Permits oral infection |
| Anaerobic growth | *Bacteroides fragilis* | Most common resident bacteria in anaerobic environment of colon |

## Box 14.1 ▪ Lessons in Microbiology

### How to survive stomach acid: the neutralization strategy of *Helicobacter pylori*

This bacterium was discovered in 1983 and was shown to be a human pathogen when two courageous doctors, Warren and Marshall in Perth, Western Australia, drank a potion containing the bacteria and developed gastritis. The infection spreads from person to person by the gastro–oral or faecal–oral route, and 150 years ago nearly all humans were infected as children. Today, in countries with improved hygiene, this is put off until later in life, until at the age of 50 more than half of the population has been infected. The clinical outcome includes peptic ulcer, gastric cancer, and gastric mucosa-associated lymphoid tissue (MALT) lymphoma; host, bacterial, and environmental factors are thought to be involved. Genetic susceptibility is implicated in both acquiring and clearing *H. pylori* (HP) infection. After being eaten, the bacteria have a number of strategies resulting in adaptation to the host gastric mucosa having attached by special adhesins to the stomach wall. These include host mimicry leading to evasion of the host response and genetic variation. Most pathogens (e.g. *Vibrio cholerae*) are soon killed at the low pH encountered in the stomach. *H. pylori*, however, protects itself by releasing large amounts of urease, which acts on local urea to form a tiny cloud of ammonia round the invader. The attached bacteria induce apoptosis in gastric epithelial cells, as well as inflammation, dyspepsia and occasionally a duodenal or gastric ulcer, so that treatment of these ulcers is by antibiotics rather than merely antacids. Some 90% of duodenal ulcers are due to HP infection, and the rest are due to aspirin or nonsteroidal antiinflammatory drugs. The bacteria do not invade tissues; they stay in the stomach for years, causing asymptomatic chronic gastritis. Up to 3% of infected individuals develop chronic active gastritis and progress to intestinal metaplasia, which can lead to stomach cancer. *H. pylori* was the third bacterium for which the entire genome was sequenced; several gene products have been characterized, and key developments include understanding the genetic variation of genes encoding the outer membrane proteins and host adaptation.

intestinal tuberculosis, but most bacteria are acid sensitive and prefer slightly alkaline conditions. For instance, volunteers who drank different doses of *V. cholerae* contained in 60 mL saline showed a 10,000-fold increase in susceptibility to cholera when 2 g of sodium bicarbonate was given with the bacteria. The minimum disease-producing dose was $10^8$ bacteria without bicarbonate and $10^4$ bacteria with bicarbonate. Similar experiments have been carried out in volunteers with *Salmonella typhi*, and the minimum infectious dose of 1000–10,000 bacteria was again significantly reduced by the ingestion of sodium bicarbonate. Infective stages of protozoa and worms resist stomach acid because they are protected within cysts or eggs. Unenveloped viruses are also at an advantage as they resist hot, acidic and dry environments.

When the infecting microorganism penetrates the intestinal epithelium (*Shigella*, *S. typhi*, hepatitis A, other enteroviruses) the final pathogenicity depends on:

- subsequent multiplication and spread
- toxin production
- cell damage
- inflammatory and immune responses.

### Microbial exotoxin, endotoxin and protein absorption

Microbial exotoxins, endotoxins and proteins can be absorbed from the intestine on a small scale. Diarrhoea generally promotes the uptake of protein, and absorption of protein also takes place more readily in the infant, which in some species needs to absorb antibodies from milk. In addition to large molecules, particles the size of viruses can be taken up from the intestinal lumen. This occurs in certain sites such as those where Peyer patches occur. Peyer patches are isolated collections of lymphoid tissue lying immediately below the intestinal epithelium, which in this region is highly specialized, consisting of so-called M cells (see Fig. 14.3). M cells take up particles and foreign proteins and deliver them to underlying immune cells with which they are intimately associated by cytoplasmic processes.

## Urogenital tract

### Microorganisms gaining entry via the urogenital tract can spread easily from one part of the tract to another

The urogenital tract is a continuum, so microorganisms can spread easily from one part to another, and the distinction between vaginitis and urethritis, or between urethritis and cystitis, is not always easy or necessary (see Chs. 21 and 22).

### Vaginal defences

The vagina has no cleansing mechanisms, and repeated introductions of a contaminated, sometimes pathogen-bearing foreign object (the penis) makes the vagina particularly vulnerable to infection, forming the basis for sexually transmitted diseases (see Ch. 22). Nature has responded by providing additional defences. During reproductive life, the vaginal epithelium contains glycogen owing to the action of circulating estrogens, and certain lactobacilli colonize the vagina, metabolizing the glycogen to produce lactic acid. As a result, the normal vaginal pH is ~5, which inhibits colonization by all except the lactobacilli and certain other streptococci and diphtheroids. Normal vaginal secretions contain up to $10^8$/mL of these commensal bacteria. If other microorganisms are to colonize and invade, they must either have specific mechanisms for attaching to vaginal or cervical mucosa or take advantage of minute local injuries during sexual intercourse (genital warts, syphilis) or impaired defences (presence of tampons, estrogen imbalance). These are the microorganisms responsible for sexually transmitted diseases.

### Urethral and bladder defences

The regular flushing action of urine is a major urethral defence, and urine in the bladder is normally sterile.

The bladder is more than an inert receptacle, and in its wall there are intrinsic, but poorly understood, defence mechanisms. These include a protective layer of mucus and the ability to generate inflammatory responses and produce secretory antibodies and immune cells.

### Mechanism of urinary tract invasion

The urinary tract is nearly always invaded from the exterior via the urethra, and an invading microorganism must first and foremost avoid being washed out during urination. Specialized attachment mechanisms have therefore been developed by successful invaders (e.g. gonococci) (Fig. 14.4). A defined peptide on the bacterial pili binds to a syndecan-like proteoglycan on the urethral cell, and the cell is then induced to engulf the bacterium. This is referred to as parasite-directed endocytosis and occurs with chlamydia.

The foreskin is a handicap in genitourinary infections because sexually transmitted pathogens often remain in the moist area beneath it after detumescence, giving them increased opportunity to invade. All sexually transmitted infections (STIs) are more common in uncircumcised males.

Intestinal bacteria (mainly *E. coli*) are common invaders of the urinary tract, causing cystitis. The genitourinary anatomy is a major determinant of infection (Fig. 14.5). Spread to the bladder is no easy task in the male, where the flaccid urethra is 20 cm long. Therefore urinary infections are rare in males unless organisms are introduced by catheters or when the flushing activity of urine is impaired (see Ch. 21). The foreskin causes trouble, again, in urinary tract infection by faecal bacteria. These infections are more common in uncircumcised infants because the prepuce may harbour faecal bacteria on its inner surface.

Things are different in females. Not only is the urethra much shorter (5 cm), but it is also very close to the anus (see Fig. 14.5), which is a constant source of intestinal bacteria. Urinary infections are about 14 times more common in women, and at least 20% of women have a symptomatic urinary tract infection at some time during their life. The invading bacteria often begin their invasion by colonizing the mucosa around the urethra and probably have special attachment mechanisms to cells in this area. Bacterial invasion is favoured by the mechanical deformation of the urethra and surrounding region that occurs during sexual intercourse, which can lead to urethritis and cystitis. Bacteriuria is about 10 times more common in sexually active than inactive women.

### Oropharynx

#### Microorganisms can invade the oropharynx when mucosal resistance is reduced

Commensal microorganisms in the oropharynx are described in Chapter 19.

#### Oropharyngeal defences

The flushing action of saliva provides a natural cleansing mechanism (about 1 L/day is produced, needing 400 swallows), aided by masticatory and other movements of the tongue, cheek and lips. On the other hand, material borne backwards from the nasopharynx is firmly wiped against the pharynx by the tongue during swallowing, and pathogens therefore have an opportunity to enter the body at this site. Additional defences include secretory IgA antibodies, antimicrobial substances such as lysozyme, the normal flora, and the antimicrobial activities of leukocytes present on mucosal surfaces and in saliva.

#### Mechanisms of oropharyngeal invasion

Attaching to mucosal or tooth surfaces is obligatory for both invading and resident microorganisms. For instance, different types of streptococci make specific attachments via lipoteichoic acid molecules on their pili to the buccal epithelium and tongue (resident *Streptococcus salivarius*), to teeth (resident *S. mutans*), or to pharyngeal epithelium (invading *S. pyogenes*).

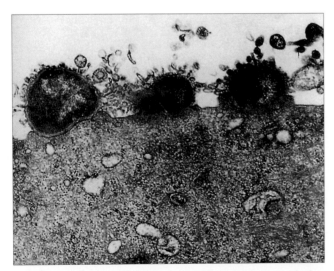

**Fig. 14.4** Adherence of gonococci to the surface of a human urethral epithelial cell. (Courtesy P.J. Watt.)

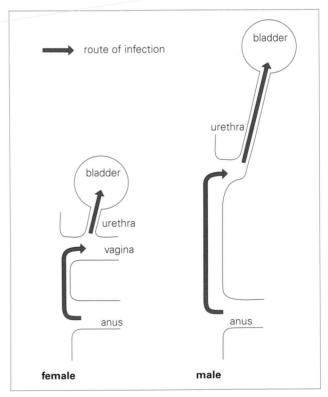

**Fig. 14.5** The female urogenital tract is particularly vulnerable to infection with faecal bacteria mainly because the urethra is shorter and nearer to the anus.

Factors that reduce mucosal resistance allow commensal and other bacteria to invade, as in the cases of gum infections caused by vitamin C deficiency or of *Candida* invasion (thrush) promoted by changed resident flora after broad-spectrum antibiotics. When salivary flow is decreased for 3–4 h, as between meals, there is a four-fold increase in the number of bacteria in saliva. In dehydrated patients, salivary flow is greatly reduced, and the mouth soon becomes overgrown with bacteria. As at all body surfaces there is a shifting boundary between good behaviour by residents and tissue invasion according to changes in host defences.

## EXIT AND TRANSMISSION

### Microorganisms have a variety of mechanisms to ensure exit from the host and transmission

Successful pathogens must leave the body and then be transmitted to fresh hosts. Highly pathogenic microbes (e.g. Ebola virus, *Legionella pneumophila*) will have little impact on host populations if their transmission from person to person is uncommon or ineffective. Nearly all pathogens are shed from body surfaces, this being the route of exit to the outside world. Some, however, are extracted from inside the body by vectors (e.g. the blood-sucking arthropods that transmit yellow fever, malaria, and filarial worms). Table 14.6 lists the types of infection and their role in the transmission of the pathogen and provides a summary of the host defences and the ways in which they are evaded. Transfer from one host to another forms the basis for the epidemiology of infectious disease (see Ch. 33).

Transmission depends upon three factors:

- the number of microorganisms shed
- the microorganism's stability in the environment
- the number of microorganisms required to infect a fresh host (the efficiency of the infection).

### Number of microorganisms shed

Obviously the more virus particles, bacteria, protozoa, and eggs that are shed, the greater is the chance of reaching a fresh host. There are, however, many hazards. Most of the shed microorganisms die, and only an occasional one survives to perpetuate the species.

### Stability in the environment

Microorganisms that resist drying spread more rapidly in the environment than those that are sensitive to drying (Table 14.7). Microorganisms also remain infectious for longer periods in the external environment when they are resistant to thermal inactivation. Certain microorganisms have developed special forms (e.g. clostridial spores, amoebic cysts) that enable them to resist drying, heat inactivation and chemical insults, and this testifies to the importance of stability in the environment. If still alive, microorganisms are more thermostable when they have dried. Drying directly

**Table 14.6** Types of infection and their role in transmission

| Type of infection | Host defences | Evasion mechanism of pathogen | Examples | Value of evasion mechanism in transmission |
|---|---|---|---|---|
| Respiratory tract | Mucociliary clearance | Adhere to epithelial cells, interfere with ciliary action | Influenza viruses Pertussis | Essential |
| | Alveolar macrophage | Replicate in alveolar macrophage | *Legionella* Tuberculosis | Essential |
| Intestinal tract | Mucus, peristalsis | Adhere to epithelial cells | Rotavirus *Salmonella* | Essential |
| | Acid, bile | Resist acid, bile | Poliovirus | Essential |
| Reproductive tract | Flushing action of urine and genital secretions, mucosal defences | Adhere to urethral and vaginal epithelial cells | Gonococcus *Chlamydia* | Essential |
| Urinary tract | Flushing action of urine | Adhere to urethral and epithelial cells | *Escherichia coli* | No value |
| | | Reach urine from tubular epithelium | Polyomavirus | Valuable |
| Central nervous system (CNS) | Enclosed in bony box of skull and vertebral column | Reach CNS via nerves or blood vessels that enter skull or vertebral column | Bacterial meningitis Viral encephalitis | No value |
| Skin mucosa | Layers of constantly shed cells (mucosa) | Invade skin and mucosa from below | Varicella Measles | Essential |
| | Dead keratinized cell layers (skin) | Infect basal epidermal layer | Papillomaviruses | Essential |
| | | Infect via minor abrasions | Staphylococci Streptococci | Essential |
| | | Penetrate intact skin | Schistosomiasis Ancyclostomiasis | Essential |
| Vascular system | Skin | Infection of host by biting vector, replication in blood cells or in vascular endothelial cells | Malaria Yellow fever | Essential |

For each type of host defence, the successful pathogen has an answer, which may or may not be important for transmission.

**Table 14.7** Microbial resistance to drying as a factor in transmission

| Stability on drying | Examples | Consequence |
|---|---|---|
| Stable | Tubercle bacilli<br>Staphylococci | } Spread more readily in air (dust, dried droplets) |
| | Clostridial spores<br>Antrax spores<br>*Histoplasma* spores | } Spread readily from soil |
| Unstable | *Neisseria meningitidis*<br>Streptococci<br>*Bordettella pertussis*<br>Influenza virus<br>Measles virus | } Require close (respiratory) contact |
| | Gonococci<br>HIV<br>*Treponema pallidum* | } Require close (sexual) contact |
| | *Vibrio cholerae*<br>Leptospira | } Spread via water, food |
| | Yellow fever virus<br>Malaria<br>Trypanosomes | } Spread via vectors (i.e. remain in a host) |
| | Larvae/eggs of worms | Need moist soil (except pinworms) |

Pathogens that are already dehydrated, such as spores, are also more resistant to thermal inactivation. Spores can survive for years in soil. HIV, Human immunodeficiency virus.

from the frozen state (freeze drying) can make them very resistant to environmental temperatures. The fact that spores and cysts are dehydrated accounts for much of their stability. Microorganisms that are sensitive to drying depend for their spread on close contact, vectors, or contamination of food and water for spread.

## Number of microorganisms required to infect a fresh host

The efficiency of the infection varies greatly between microorganisms and helps explain many aspects of transmission. For instance, volunteers ingesting 10 *Shigella dysenteriae* bacteria (from other humans) will become infected, whereas as many as $10^6$ *Salmonella* spp. (from animals) are needed to cause food poisoning. The route of infection also matters. A single tissue culture infectious dose of a human rhinovirus instilled into the nasal cavity causes a common cold and, although this dose contains many virus particles, about 200 such doses are needed when applied to the pharynx. As few as 10 gonococci can establish an infection in the urethra, but many thousand times this number are needed to infect the mucosa of the oropharynx or rectum.

## Other factors affecting transmission

Genetic factors in microorganisms also influence transmission. Some strains of a given microorganism are, therefore, more readily transmitted than others, although the exact mechanism is often unclear. Transmission can vary independently of the ability to do damage and cause disease (pathogenicity or virulence).

Activities of the infected host may increase the efficiency of shedding and transmission. Coughing and sneezing are reflex activities that benefit the host by clearing foreign material from the upper and lower respiratory tract, but they also benefit the microorganism. Strains of microorganism that are more able to increase fluid secretions or irritate respiratory epithelium will induce more coughing and sneezing than those less able and will be transmitted more effectively. Similar arguments can be applied to the equivalent intestinal activity: diarrhoea. Although diarrhoea eliminates the infection more rapidly (prevention of diarrhoea often prolongs intestinal infection), from the pathogen's point of view it is a highly effective way of contaminating the environment and spreading to fresh hosts.

## TYPES OF TRANSMISSION BETWEEN HUMANS

Microorganisms can be transmitted to humans by humans, vertebrates, and biting arthropods. Transmission is most effective when it takes place directly from human to human. The most common worldwide infections are spread by the respiratory, faecal–oral, or sexual route. A separate set of infections is acquired from animals, either directly from vertebrates (the zoonoses) or indirectly from biting arthropods. Infections acquired from other species are either not transmitted or transmit very poorly from human to human. Types of transmission are illustrated in Fig. 14.6.

### Transmission from the respiratory tract

#### Respiratory infections spread rapidly when people are crowded together indoors

This is a subject that has come under close scrutiny given the COVID-19 pandemic (see Ch. 20). An increase in nasal secretions with sneezing and coughing promotes effective shedding from the nasal cavity. In a sneeze (Fig. 14.7) up to 20,000 droplets are produced, and during a common cold, for instance, many of them will contain virus particles.

A smaller number of microorganisms (hundreds) are expelled from the mouth, throat, larynx, and lungs during coughing (whooping cough, tuberculosis). Talking is a less important source of airborne particles but does produce them, especially when the consonants *f, p, t,* and *s* are used. It

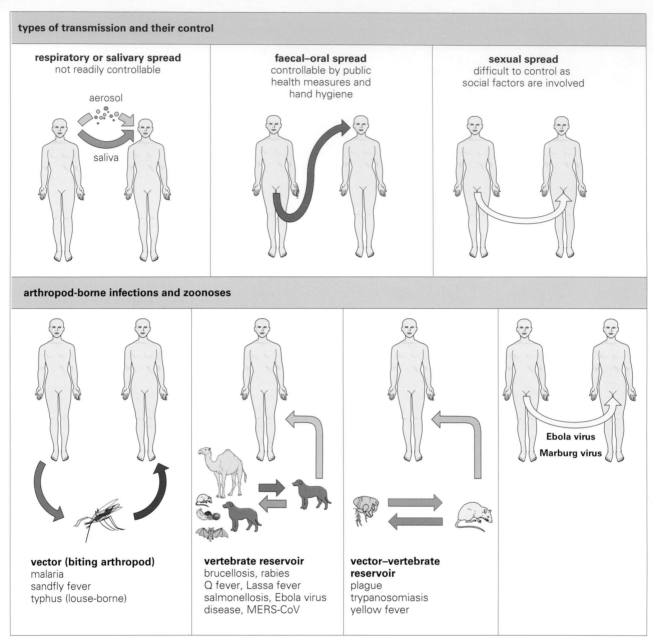

**types of transmission and their control**

| respiratory or salivary spread | faecal–oral spread | sexual spread |
| --- | --- | --- |
| not readily controllable | controllable by public health measures and hand hygiene | difficult to control as social factors are involved |

aerosol

saliva

**arthropod-borne infections and zoonoses**

**vector (biting arthropod)**
malaria
sandfly fever
typhus (louse-borne)

**vertebrate reservoir**
brucellosis, rabies
Q fever, Lassa fever
salmonellosis, Ebola virus
disease, MERS-CoV

**vector–vertebrate reservoir**
plague
trypanosomiasis
yellow fever

Ebola virus

Marburg virus

**Fig. 14.6** Types of transmission and their control. Arthropod-borne infections and zoonoses can be controlled by controlling vectors or by controlling animal infection; there is virtually no person-to-person transmission of these infections, except for pneumonic plague and Ebola virus infection (see Ch. 29).

is surely no accident that many of the most abusive words in the English language begin with these letters, so that a spray of droplets (possibly infectious) is delivered with the abuse!

The size of inhaled droplets determines their initial localization. The largest droplets fall to the ground after travelling ~4 m, and the rest settle according to size. Those 10 μm or so in diameter can be trapped on the nasal mucosa. The smallest (1–4 μm diameter) are kept suspended for an indefinite period by normal air movements, and particles of this size are likely to pass the turbinate baffles in the nose and reach the lower respiratory tract.

When people are crowded together indoors, respiratory infections spread rapidly (e.g. the common cold in schools and offices and meningococcal infections in military recruits). This is perhaps why respiratory infections are common in winter. The air in ill-ventilated rooms is also more humid, favouring survival of suspended microorganisms such as streptococci and enveloped viruses. Air conditioning is another factor, as the dry air leads to impaired mucociliary activity. Respiratory spread is, in one sense, unique. Material from one person's respiratory tract can be taken up almost immediately into the respiratory tract of other individuals. This is in striking contrast to the material expelled from the gastrointestinal tract, and it helps explain why respiratory infections spread so rapidly when people are indoors.

Handkerchiefs, hands and other objects can carry respiratory virus infection from one individual to another, although coughs and sneezes provide a more dramatic

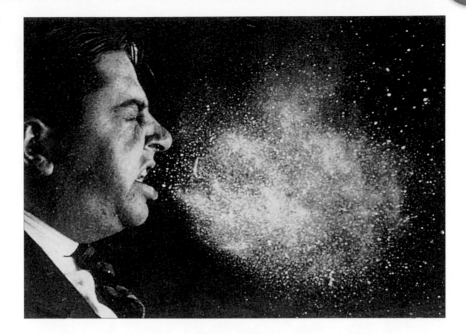

**Fig. 14.7** Droplet dispersal following a violent sneeze. Most of the 20,000 particles seen are coming from the mouth. (Reprinted with permission from American Association for the Advancement of Science. Moulton FR, ed. *Aerobiology*. Publication of the American Association for the Advancement of Science, No. 17, Washington; 1942.)

route. Transmission from the infected conjunctiva is referred to in Chapter 26.

The presence of receptors (see Table 14.2) and local temperature as well as initial localization can determine which part of the respiratory tract is infected. For instance, it can be assumed that rhinoviruses arrive in the lower respiratory tract on a large scale, but they fail to grow there because, like leprosy bacilli, they prefer the cooler temperature of the nasal mucosa.

## Transmission from the gastrointestinal tract

### Intestinal infection spreads easily if public health and hygiene are poor

The spread of an intestinal infection is assured if public health and hygiene are poor, the pathogen appears in the faeces in sufficient numbers, and there are susceptible individuals in the vicinity. Diarrhoea gives it an additional advantage, and the key role of diarrhoea in transmission has been referred to earlier. During most of human history there has been a large-scale recycling of faecal material back into the mouth, and this continues in resource-poor countries. The attractiveness of the faecal–oral route for microorganisms and parasites is reflected in the great variety that are transmitted in this way.

Intestinal infections have been to some extent controlled in resource-rich countries. The great public health reforms of the 19th century led to the introduction of adequate sewage disposal and a supply of purified water. For instance, in England 200 years ago, there were no flushing toilets and no sewage disposal, and much of the drinking water was contaminated. Cholera and typhoid spread easily, and in London, the Thames became an open sewer. Today, as in other cities, a complex underground disposal system separates sewage from drinking water. Intestinal infections are still transmitted in resource-rich countries, but via food and fingers rather than by water and flies. Therefore although each year in the UK there are dozens of cases of typhoid acquired on visits to resource-poor countries, the infection is not transmitted to others.

The microorganisms that appear in faeces usually multiply in the lumen or wall of the intestinal tract, but there are a few that are shed into bile. For instance, hepatitis A enters bile after replicating in liver cells.

## Transmission from the urogenital tract

### Urogenital tract infections are often sexually transmitted

Urinary tract infections are common, but most are not spread via urine. Urine can contaminate food, drink and living space. Examples of some infections that are spread by urine are listed in Table 14.8.

### Sexually transmitted infections

Microorganisms shed from the urogenital tract are often transmitted as a result of mucosal contact with susceptible individuals, typically as a result of sexual activity. If there is a discharge, organisms are carried over the epithelial surfaces, and transmission is more likely. Some of the most successful sexually transmitted microorganisms (gonococci, chlamydia) therefore induce a discharge. Other microorganisms are transmitted effectively from mucosal sores (ulcers; e.g. *Treponema pallidum*, herpes simplex virus, and monkeypox [mpox] virus). Mpox was added to the list of STIs in 2022 after increasing infections were found in men who have sex with men as the main group affected (Fig. 14.8). The human papillomaviruses are transmitted from genital warts or from foci of infection in the cervix where the epithelium, although apparently normal, is dysplastic and contains infected cells (see Ch. 22).

The transmission of STIs is determined by social and sexual activity. Changes in the size of the human population and way of life have had a dramatic effect on the epidemiology of STIs. More opportunities to have sexual encounters have arisen owing to increasing population density, increased movement of people, social media and the internet and the knowledge that STIs are treatable and pregnancy is avoidable. In addition, the contraceptive pill

**Table 14.8** Human infections transmitted via urine

| Infection | Details | Value in transmission |
|---|---|---|
| Schistosomiasis | Parasite eggs excreted in bladder | +++ |
| Typhoid | Bacterial persistence in bladder scarred by schistosomiasis | + |
| Polyomavirus infection | Commonly excreted in urine | ? |
| Cytomegalovirus infection | Commonly excreted in infected children | ? |
| Leptospirosis | Infected rats and dogs excrete bacteria in urine | ++ |
| Lassa fever (and South American haemorrhagic fevers) | Persistently infected rodent excretes virus in urine | +++ |

Schistosomiasis is the major infection transmitted in this way, the eggs undergoing development in snails before reinfecting humans. Viruses are shed in the urine after infecting tubular epithelial cells in the kidney.

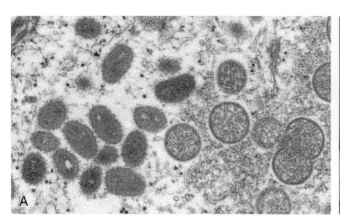
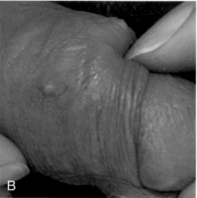

**Fig. 14.8** (A) Electron microscopy of monkeypox virus. (B) Monkeypox genital lesion. (A, From Luigi P, et al. Monkeypox: a novel pitfall in clinical dermatology. *Trav Med Infect Dis*. 2022;50: fig.1D; B, from Huang T-S, et al. The first imported case of monkeypox in Taiwan. *J Formosan Med Assoc*. 2023;122(1):73–77, fig.1.)

reduced the use of mechanical barriers to conception. Condoms have been shown to reliably retain and reduce the transmission potential of herpes simplex virus, HIV, chlamydia and gonococci in simulated sexual intercourse tests of the syringe and plunger type (see Ch. 22).

STIs are, however, transmitted with far less speed and efficiency than respiratory or intestinal infections. Frequent sexual activity is not enough without involving multiple partners because those in a stable partnership can do no more than infect each other. Changes in sexual practices have led to a dramatic rise in the incidence of STIs.

As almost all mucosal surfaces of the body can be involved in sexual activity, microorganisms have had increasing opportunity to infect new body sites. The meningococcus, a nasopharyngeal resident, has therefore sometimes been recovered from the cervix, the male urethra and the anal canal, while gonococci and chlamydia can infect the throat and anal canal. It is no surprise that genito–oro–anal contacts have sometimes allowed intestinal infections such as *Salmonella*, *Giardia*, hepatitis A virus, *Shigella* and pathogenic amoebae to spread directly between individuals despite good sanitation and sewage disposal. Mpox also emerged as a worldwide STI in 2022 with human-to-human transmission being more evident in comparison with previous outbreaks in Central and West Africa.

### Semen as a source of infection

It might be expected that semen is involved in the transmission of infection, and this is the case in viral infections of animals such as blue tongue and foot and mouth disease. In humans, cytomegalovirus that is shed from the oropharynx is also often present in large quantities in semen, and the fact that it is also recoverable from the cervix suggests that it is sexually transmitted. Hepatitis B virus and HIV are also present in semen and are STIs, but Ebola virus has been found in seminal fluid for up to a median period of 204 days, with around 20% persistence at 1 year in older age groups with more severe infections. Zika virus, a mosquito-borne flavivirus emerged in 2015, spread to >86 countries and was associated with adverse birth outcomes. Zika viral RNA could be detected in semen, but the viral load fell within 3 months after illness onset, but was positive in one man for 281 days.

### Perinatal transmission

The female genital tract can also be a source of infection for the newborn child (see Ch. 24). During passage down an infected birth canal, microorganisms can be wiped onto the conjunctiva of the infant or inhaled, leading to a variety of conditions such as conjunctivitis, pneumonia and bacterial meningitis.

### Transmission from the oropharynx

#### Oropharyngeal infections are often spread in saliva

Saliva is often the vehicle of transmission. Microorganisms such as streptococci and tubercle bacilli reach saliva during upper and lower respiratory tract infections, while certain viruses infect the salivary glands and are transmitted in this way. Paramyxovirus, herpes simplex virus,

**Table 14.9** Human infections transmitted via saliva

| Microorganism | Comments |
|---|---|
| Herpes simplex virus | Infection generally during childhood |
| Cytomegalovirus Epstein-Barr virus | Adolescent/adult infection is common |
| Rabies virus | Shed in saliva of infected dogs, wolves, jackals, bats |
| Pasteurella multocida | Bacteria in upper respiratory tract of dogs, cats appear in saliva and are transmitted via bites, scratches |
| Streptobacillus moniliformis | Present in rat saliva and infects humans (rat bite fever) |

**Table 14.10** Human infections transmitted via the skin

| Microorganism | Disease | Comments |
|---|---|---|
| Staphylococci | Boils, carbuncles, neonatal skin sepsis | Pathogenicity varies, skin lesions or nose picking are common sources of infection |
| Treponema pallidum | Syphilis | Mucosal surfaces more infectious than skin |
| Treponema pertenue | Yaws | Regular transmission from skin lesions |
| Streptococcus pyogenes | Impetigo | Vesicular (epidermal) lesions crusting over, common in children in hot, humid climates |
| Staphylococcus aureus | Impetigo | Less common; bullous lesions, especially in newborn |
| Dermatophytes | Skin ringworm | Different species infect skin, hair, nails |
| Herpes simplex virus | Herpes simplex, cold sore | Up to $10^6$ infectious units/mL of vesicle fluid |
| Varicella-zoster virus | Varicella, zoster | Vesicular skin lesions occur but transmission is usually respiratory[a] |
| Coxsackievirus A16 | Hand, foot and mouth disease | Vesicular skin lesions, but transmission faecal and respiratory |
| Papillomaviruses | Warts | Many types[b] |
| Leishmania tropica | Cutaneous leishmaniasis | Skin sores are infectious |
| Sarcoptes scabei | Scabies | Eggs from burrow transmitted by hand (also sexually) |

[a]Except in zoster in which a localized skin eruption occurs.
[b]Generally direct contact, but plantar warts are commonly spread following walking barefoot on contaminated floors such as swimming pool surrounds.

cytomegalovirus and human herpes virus type 6 are shed into saliva. In young children, fingers and other objects are regularly contaminated by saliva, and each of these infections is acquired by this route. Epstein-Barr virus is also shed into saliva but is transmitted less effectively perhaps because it is present only in cells or in small amounts. In resource-rich countries, people often escape infection during childhood and become infected as adolescents or adults during the extensive salivary exchanges (mean 4.2 mL/h) that accompany oral encounters of the deep and meaningful kind. Saliva from animals is the source of a few infections, and these are included in Table 14.9.

## Transmission from the skin

### Skin can spread infection by shedding or direct contact

Dermatophytes (fungi such as those that cause ringworm) are shed from skin and from hair and nails, the exact source depending on the type of fungus (see Ch. 27). Skin is also an important source of certain other bacteria and viruses, as outlined in Table 14.10.

### Shedding to the environment

The normal individual sheds desquamated skin scales into the environment at a rate of about $5 \times 10^8$/day, the rate depending on physical activities such as exercise, dressing and undressing. The fine white dust that collects on indoor surfaces, especially in hospital wards, consists largely of skin scales. Staphylococci are present, and different individuals show great variation in staphylococcal shedding, but the reasons are unknown.

Transmission by direct contact or by contaminated fingers is much more common than following release into the environment, and microorganisms transmitted in this way include potentially pathogenic staphylococci and human papillomaviruses.

## Transmission in milk

Milk is produced by a skin gland. Microorganisms are rarely shed into human milk, and examples include HIV, cytomegalovirus and human T-cell lymphotropic virus 1 (HTLV-1), but milk from cows, goats and sheep can be important sources of infection (Table 14.11). Bacteria can be introduced into milk after collection.

## Transmission from blood

### Blood can spread infection via arthropods or needles

Blood is often the vehicle of transmission. Microorganisms and parasites spread by blood-sucking arthropods (see later) are effectively shed into the blood. Infectious agents present in blood, including hepatitis B and C viruses and HIV, and are also transmissible either in unscreened transfused blood or when blood-contaminated needles are used for injections

**Table 14.11** Human infections transmitted via milk

| Microorganism | Type of milk | Importance in transmission |
|---|---|---|
| Cytomegalovirus | Human | + (postnatal) |
| Human immunodeficiency virus | Human | + |
| Human T-cell lymphotropic virus 1 | Human | + |
| *Brucella* | Cow, goat, sheep | + + |
| *Mycobacterium bovis* | Cow | + + |
| Coxiella burnetii (Q fever) | Cow | + |
| *Campylobacter jejuni* | Cow | + + |
| *Salmonella* spp.<br>*Listeria monocytogenes*<br>*Staphylococcus* spp.<br>*Streptococcus pyogenes*<br>*Yersinia enterocolitica* | Cow | + |

Human milk is rarely a significant source of infection. All pathogens listed are destroyed by pasteurization.

or intravenous drug misuse. Intravenous drug misuse is a well-known factor in the spread of these infections. Unfortunately, in parts of the resource-poor world, disposable syringes tend to be used more than once, without being properly sterilized in between. The prolonged outbreak of hepatitis C virus genotype 4 infection in Egypt was thought to have originated from the time when parenteral antischistosomal treatment with injectable antimony was given in mass campaigns, involving reused syringes, from the 1950s to the 1980s. To prevent this, the World Health Organization encouraged the use of syringes in which, for instance, the plunger cannot be withdrawn once it has been pushed in.

Blood is also the source of infection in transplacental transmission, which generally involves initial infection of the placenta (see Ch. 24).

### Vertical and horizontal transmission

#### Vertical transmission takes place between parents and their offspring

When transmission occurs directly from parents to offspring via, for example, sperm, ovum, placenta (Table 14.12), milk or blood, it is referred to as vertical. This is because it can be represented as a vertical flow down a page (Fig. 14.9), just

**Table 14.12** Human infections transmitted via the placenta

| Transplacental transmission of infection | |
|---|---|
| **Microorganism** | **Effect** |
| Rubella virus, cytomegalovirus | Placental lesion, abortion, stillbirth, organ malformation |
| HIV | HIV infection in babies and infants and AIDS if undiagnosed |
| Hepatitis B virus | Hepatitis B infection, but most occur peri- or postnatally |
| *Treponema pallidum* | Stillbirth, congenital syphilis with malformation |
| *Listeria monocytogenes* | Meningoencephalitis |
| *Toxoplasma gondii* | Stillbirth, CNS disease |

AIDS, Acquired immunodeficiency syndrome; CNS, central nervous system; HIV, human immunodeficiency virus.

like a family pedigree. Other infections, in contrast, are said to be horizontally transmitted, with an individual infecting other individuals by contact, respiratory or faecal–oral spread. Vertically transmitted infections can be subdivided as shown in Table 14.13. There are many retrovirus sequences present in the normal human genome known as endogenous retroviruses. These DNA sequences are too incomplete to produce infectious virus particles, but they can be regarded as amazingly successful parasites. In addition, some of them may confer benefit, for example, by coding for proteins that help coordinate early stages of fetal development. They survive within the human species, watched over, conserved and replicated as part of our genetic constitution.

## TRANSMISSION FROM ANIMALS

### Humans and animals share a common susceptibility to certain pathogens

Humans live in daily contact, directly or indirectly, with a wide variety of other animal species, both vertebrate and invertebrate, sharing not only a common environment but also a common susceptibility to certain pathogens. The degree to which animal contacts transmit infection depends upon the type of environment and nature of the contact. The former can be urban, rural, tropical, temperate, hygienic or unsanitary. The latter may be close contact made with vertebrate animals used for food or as pets and with invertebrate animals adapted to live or feed on the human body. Less intimate contact is made with many other species, which nevertheless may transmit pathogens equally well. For convenience, animal-transmitted infections can be divided into two categories:

- those involving arthropod and other invertebrate vectors
- those transmitted directly from vertebrates (zoonoses).

More detailed accounts of these infections are given in Chapters 28 and 29.

### Invertebrate vectors

#### Insects, ticks and mites (bloodsuckers) are the most important vectors spreading infection

By far the most important vectors of disease belong to these three groups of arthropods: insects, ticks and mites. Many species are capable of transmitting infection, and a wide

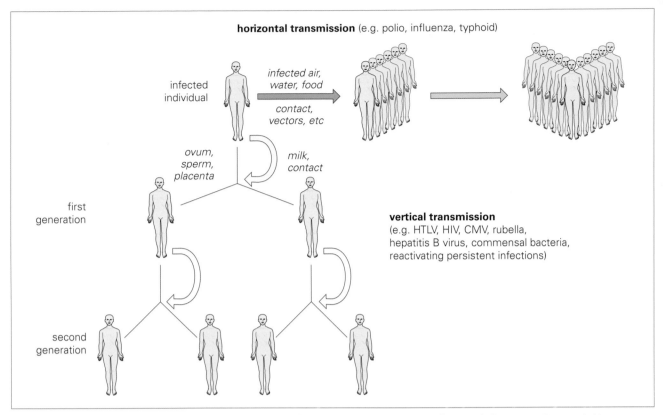

**Fig. 14.9** Vertical and horizontal transmission by infection. Most infections are transmitted horizontally, as might be expected in crowded human populations. Vertical transmission becomes more important in small isolated communities. CMV, Cytomegalovirus; HIV, human immunodeficiency virus; HTLV, human T-cell lymphotropic virus.

**Table 14.13** Types of vertical transmission

| Type | Route | Examples |
|------|-------|----------|
| Prenatal | In utero | Rubella, cytomegalovirus, syphilis, toxoplasmosis, hepatitis B, HIV |
| Perinatal | Infected birth canal | Gonococcal/chlamydial conjunctivitis, herpes simplex |
| Postnatal | Milk<br>Direct contact with blood at delivery | Cytomegalovirus, HIV, HTLV-1<br>Hepatitis B virus, HIV, HTLV-1 |
| Germline | Viral DNA sequences in human genome | Endogenous retroviruses make up to 8% of the human genome, and their role is still unclear |

HIV, Human immunodeficiency virus; HTLV, human T-cell lymphotropic virus.

range of organisms is transmitted (Table 14.14). In the past, insects have been responsible for some of the most devastating epidemic diseases (e.g. fleas and plague, lice and typhus). Even today, one of the world's most important infectious diseases—malaria—is transmitted by the *Anopheles* mosquito. The distribution and epidemiology of these infections are determined by the climatic conditions that allow the vectors to breed and the organism to complete its development in their bodies. Some diseases are therefore purely tropical and subtropical, including malaria, sleeping sickness and yellow fever; others are much more widespread such as plague and typhus. However, with climate change and increased travel, some viral infections are being seen in previously unaffected regions (e.g. West Nile virus and chikungunya infections reported in Italy; Zika virus infections in the Americas, Africa, and other regions of the world).

### Passive carriage

Insects may carry pathogens passively on their mouth parts, on their bodies, or within their intestines. Transfer onto food or onto the host occurs directly as a result of the insect feeding, regurgitating or defecating. Many important diseases such as trachoma can be transmitted in this way by common species such as houseflies and cockroaches.

Blood-feeding species have mouth parts adapted for penetrating skin to reach blood vessels or to create small pools of blood (Fig. 14.10). The ability to feed in this way provides access to organisms in the skin or blood. The mouth parts can act as a contaminated hypodermic needle, carrying infection between individuals.

### Biologic transmission

This is much more common, the blood-sucking vector acting as a necessary host for the multiplication and development

**Table 14.14** Arthropod-borne pathogens

| Arthropod-borne pathogens | | | |
|---|---|---|---|
| **Arthropods** | | **Pathogens** | **Diseases** |

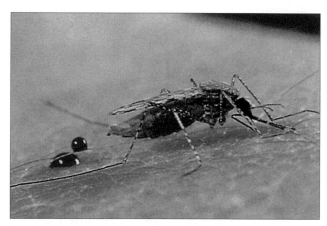

| Pathogens | Diseases |
|---|---|
| Flaviviruses | Yellow fever<br>Dengue<br>Zika microcephaly<br>West Nile<br>Japanese encephalitis |
| Bunyaviruses | Haemorrhagic fevers |
| Yersinia | Plague, tularemia |
| Rickettsias | Q fever, spotted fevers, typhus, nickettsial pox |
| Spirochaetes | Relapsing fever, Lyme disease |
| Trypanosomes | Sleeping sickness, Chagas disease |
| Leishmania | Leishmaniasis |
| Plasmodium | Malaria |
| Nematodes | Lymphatic filariases, loiasis, onchocerciasis |

*Arthropods (left diagram): Insects — Houseflies, Sandflies, Mosquitoes, Blackflies, Lice, Fleas, Hemiptera bugs, Midges, Tabanids; Acarids — Ticks, Mites. Pathogens (right of diagram): Viruses, Bacteria, Protozoa, Helminths.*

**Fig. 14.10** Female *Anopheles* mosquito feeding. (Courtesy C.J. Webb.)

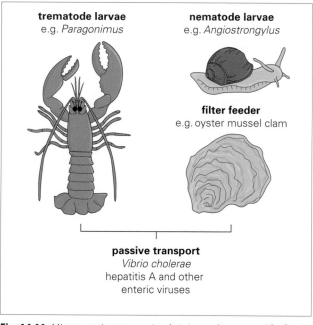

**trematode larvae**
e.g. *Paragonimus*

**nematode larvae**
e.g. *Angiostrongylus*

**filter feeder**
e.g. oyster mussel clam

**passive transport**
*Vibrio cholerae*
hepatitis A and other
enteric viruses

**Fig. 14.11** Microorganisms transmitted via invertebrates used for food. Filter-feeding molluscs living in estuaries near sewage outlets are a common source of infection.

of the pathogen. Almost all of the important infections (listed in Table 14.14) are transmitted in this way. The pathogen is reintroduced into the human host, after a period of time, at the next blood meal. Transmission can be by direct injection, usually in the vector's saliva (malaria, yellow fever), or by contamination from faeces or regurgitated blood deposited at the time of feeding (typhus, plague).

### Other invertebrate vectors spread infection either passively or by acting as an intermediate host

Many invertebrates used for food convey pathogens (Fig. 14.11). Perhaps the most familiar are the shellfish (molluscs and crustaceans) associated with food poisoning, acute gastroenteritis, and hepatitis. These filter feeders accumulate viruses and bacteria in their bodies, taking them in from contaminated waste, then transferring them passively. In other cases, the relationship between the pathogen and the invertebrate is much closer. Many parasites, especially worms, must undergo part of their development in the invertebrate before being able to infect a human. Humans are infected when they eat the invertebrate (intermediate) host. Dietary habits are therefore important in infection, an extreme example being kuru. Other unusual links include lassa fever from eating the African soft-furred rat *Mastomys natalensis*, a delicacy in some areas of the world, and hepatitis E virus infection from eating undercooked pork sausages, venison, wild boar meat or shellfish.

**Table 14.15** Zoonoses: human infections transmitted directly from vertebrates (birds and mammals)

| Pathogens | Vertebrate vector | Diseases |
|---|---|---|
| **Viruses** | | |
| Arenaviruses | Mammals | Lassa fever, lymphocytic choriomeningitis, Bolivian haemorrhagic fever |
| Poxviruses | Mammals | Cowpox, orf |
| Hepatitis E virus | Pigs | Hepatitis E |
| Rhabdoviruses | Mammals | Rabies |
| SARS coronavirus[a] | Monkeys, Himalayan palm civets, raccoon dogs, cats, dogs, rodents | SARS (severe acute respiratory syndrome) |
| MERS coronavirus[a] | Camels | MERS (Middle East respiratory syndrome) |
| Avian influenza viruses[a] | Chickens | Influenza A H5N1 and other strains |
| **Bacteria** | | |
| *Bacillus anthracis* | Mammals | Anthrax |
| *Brucella* | Mammals | Brucella |
| *Chlamydia* | Birds | Psittacosis |
| *Leptospira* | Mammals | Leptospirosis (Weil's disease) |
| *Listeria* | Mammals | Listeriosis |
| *Salmonella* | Birds, mammals | Salmonellosis |
| *Mycobacterium tuberculosis* | Mammals | Tuberculosis |
| **Fungi** | | |
| *Cryptococcus* | Birds | Meningitis |
| *Dermatophytes* | Mammals | Ringworm |
| **Protozoa** | | |
| *Cryptosporidium* | Mammals | Cryptosporidiosis |
| *Giardia* | Mammals | Giardiasis |
| *Toxoplasma* | Mammals | Toxoplasmosis |
| **Helminths** | | |
| *Ancylostoma* | Mammals | Hookworm disease |
| *Echinococcus* | Mammals | Hydatid disease |
| *Taenia* | Mammals | Tapeworms |
| *Toxocara* | Mammals | Toxocariasis (visceral larval migrans) |
| *Trichinella* | Mammals | Trichinellosis |

[a]Poor transmission from person to person, but they may at any time change and develop the capacity for efficient transmission.

Aquatic molluscs (snails) are necessary intermediate hosts for schistosomes—the blood flukes. They become infected by larval stages, which hatch from eggs passed into water in the urine or faeces of infected people. After a period of development and multiplication, large numbers of infective stages (cercariae) escape from the snails. These can rapidly penetrate through human skin, initiating the infection that will result in adult flukes occupying visceral blood vessels (see Ch. 28).

## Transmission from vertebrates

### Many pathogens are transmitted directly to humans from vertebrate animals

Strictly, the term zoonoses can apply to any infection transmitted to humans from infected animals, whether this is directly by contact or eating or indirectly via an invertebrate vector. Here, however, zoonoses are used to describe infections of vertebrate animals that can be transmitted directly. Many pathogens are transmitted in this way (Table 14.15) by a variety of different routes, including contact, inhalation, bites, scratches, contamination of food or water and ingestion as food.

The epidemiology of zoonoses depends upon the frequency and the nature of contact between the vertebrate and the human hosts. Some are localized geographically, being dependent, for example, on local food preferences. Where these involve eating uncooked animal products such as fish or amphibia, a variety of parasites, especially tapeworms and nematodes, can be acquired. Others are associated with occupation (e.g. if this involves contact with raw animal products): butchers, in the case of toxoplasmosis and Q fever, or

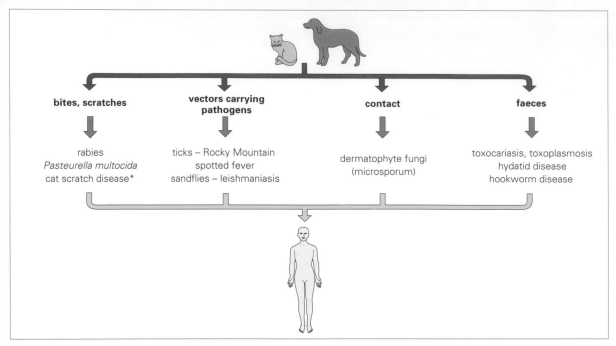

**Fig. 14.12** Man's best friends? Zoonoses transmitted from dogs and cats. *A benign infection with skin lesions and lymphadenopathy shown to be due to a bacterium *Bartonella henselae*.

frequent contact with domestic stock as can happen with farm workers in the case of brucellosis and dermatophyte fungi. In urban areas, zoonoses are most likely to be acquired by eating or drinking infected animal products or by contact with dogs, cats and other domestic pets. Hepatitis E virus infections were regarded as a sporadic cause of hepatitis in Europe until studies reported in 2015 that blood transfusion recipients developed the infection having received blood from asymptomatic hepatitis E viraemic donors. Eating undercooked pork sausages, as well as other more exotic meat products, was associated with transmission, and it was reported as a zoonotic infection of pigs (see Ch. 23).

**Domestic pets or pests?**

Dogs and cats are the most common domestic pets, and both are reservoirs of infection for their owners (Fig. 14.12). The pathogens concerned are spread by contact, bites and scratches, by vectors, and by contamination with faecal material. Major infections transmitted in these ways include toxocariasis from dogs and toxoplasmosis from cats. Both are almost universal in their distribution.

Humans may acquire hydatid disease from tapeworm eggs passed in dog faeces where dogs are used for herding domestic animals and have access to infected carcasses. In rural areas of many countries this has been, or remains, an important infection.

Many species of birds are kept as pets, and some can pass on serious infections to those in contact with them. Contact is usually through inhalation of infected particulate material. Perhaps the most important of these is psittacosis caused by *Chlamydophila* (formerly *Chlamydia*) *psittaci*, which despite the common name parrot fever can be acquired from many avian species.

The recent trend in resource-rich countries toward keeping unusual or exotic pets, especially reptiles, exotic birds, and mammals, raises new risks of zoonotic infection. Many reptiles, for example, pass human-infective *Salmonella* spp. in their droppings. Exotic birds and mammals can carry a range of viruses that could be transmitted under the correct conditions such as mpox (Box 14.2). Diagnosis of infections under these circumstances can be difficult if the physician does not know of the existence of such pets.

---

**Box 14.2 ■ Lessons in Microbiology**

**Viral zoonosis involving exotic animals outside their normal environment**

Human monkeypox (mpox) virus infection was named in 1970, having first been isolated in Denmark in 1958 after outbreaks of a rash illness in captive cynomolgus monkeys. The first human mpox infections detected outside Africa were reported in the United States in 2003. Most individual infections had been seen in Central and West Africa and small outbreaks in the Democratic Republic of Congo.

Mpox virus is a double-stranded DNA virus in the family *Poxviridae* and genus *orthopoxvirus* that includes smallpox and cowpox. It is a zoonosis, and, although the animal reservoir is not clear, some rodents in Central and West African tropical rainforests, including Gambian pouched rats (Fig. 14.13), have been implicated, with infected monkeys as intermediate hosts. Clearly humans and other animals are susceptible, with the 2022 global outbreak of human mpox demonstrating how infections can go viral.

**Fig. 14.13** Gambian pouched rat. (From Bentz EJ, Ophir AG. Chromosome scale genome assembly of the African giant pouched rat (*Cricetomys ansorgei*) and evolutionary analysis reveals evidence of olfactory specialization. *Genomics* 2022;114[6], fig.1.)

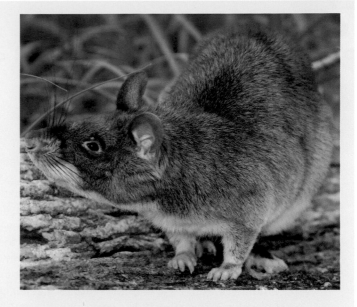

On May 24, 2003, a 3-year-old girl (Patient 1) with cellulitis and fever after a bite from Prairie Dog 1 on May 13 was reported to the Wisconsin Division of Public Health. The prairie dog had developed eye discharge, papular skin lesions, and lymphadenopathy on May 13 having been bought 2 days earlier. It died on May 20, and only bacterial contamination was detected in an enlarged submandibular lymph node. No similar illnesses were reported until June 2 when public health was notified about a Wisconsin meat inspector and distributor of exotic animals (Distributor 2, Patient 4). He had been bitten and scratched by a prairie dog on May 18, and a nodular skin lesion developed at the scratch site on May 23. Fever, rigors, sweats and lymphadenopathy began on May 26, and he was admitted to hospital. On June 3 the teams found out he had sold two prairie dogs to the index patient's family. Public health case finding and animal activities were initiated. At the same time a poxvirus had been detected by electron microscopy in a skin lesion from Patient 2 (the mother of Patient 1), who became ill on May 26. This was shown to be an orthopoxvirus. By June 7 there were 11 patients with confirmed or suspected mpox linked to prairie rats housed with Gambian pouched rats imported from Ghana to Texas. An ill Gambian giant rat had been part of the group and transmitted the virus to prairie dogs housed in the same exotic-animal facility. Altogether, by July 30 there were 72 confirmed or suspected infected individuals. The clinical course was self-limited. Control measures included home isolation, quarantine of infected and exposed mammals, and surveillance of all whom had been exposed to ill patients or prairie dogs. Nobody received vaccinia immunoglobulin or smallpox immunisation that could confer protection.

## KEY FACTS

- To establish infection in the host, pathogens must attach to, or pass across, body surfaces.

- Many pathogens have developed chemical or mechanical mechanisms to attach themselves to the surface of the respiratory, urogenital, or alimentary tracts. In the skin they generally depend on entry via small wounds or arthropod bites.

- Pathogens must exit from the body after replication to be transmitted to fresh hosts. This also takes place across body surfaces.

- Efficient shedding of pathogens from the skin or respiratory, urogenital or alimentary tracts and delivery into the blood or dermal tissues for uptake during arthropod feeding are vital stages in their life cycles.

- Many human infections come from animals, either directly (zoonoses) or indirectly (via blood-sucking arthropods), and the incidence of these infections depends on exposure to infected animals or arthropods.

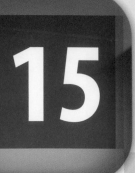

# 15 Immune defences in action

## Introduction

The immune system has a number of defence strategies at its disposal with which to attack and neutralize the threats from invading pathogens. As discussed in Chapters 10–12, these include both innate and adaptive cells and soluble cytokine mediators. Although they lack the dramatic specificity and memory of adaptive (i.e. T- and B-cell–based) immune mechanisms, the innate defences are vital to survival, particularly in invertebrates in which they are the only defence against infection.

In addition to these nonspecific mechanisms, the immune system enables the specific recognition of antigens by T and B cells as part of adaptive immunity. Broadly speaking, antibodies are particularly important in combating infection by extracellular microbes, particularly pyogenic bacteria, while T-cell immunity is required to control intracellular infections with bacteria, viruses, fungi or protozoa (Fig. 15.1). Their value is illustrated by the generally disastrous results of defects in T and/or B cells or their products, discussed in more detail in Chapter 31. This chapter gives examples of how these different types of immunity contribute to and collaborate in the body's defences against pathogens.

### Antimicrobial peptides protect the skin against invading bacteria

A number of proteins that are expressed at epithelial surfaces and by neutrophils, (polymorphonuclear neutrophils, or PMNs) can have a direct antibacterial effect. These include beta defensins, dermicidins and cathelicidins. Defensins form 30–50% of neutrophil granules and disrupt the lipid membranes of bacteria. Dermicidin is made by sweat glands and is secreted into sweat; it is active against *Escherichia coli*, *Staphylococcus aureus* and *Candida albicans*. Cathelicidin has potent antimicrobial effects against most gram-positive and gram-negative bacteria. The precursor cathelicidin protein is cleaved into two peptides, one of which, LL37, is not only toxic to microorganisms but also binds lipopolysaccharide (LPS). Cathelicidin is active against methicillin-resistant *S. aureus*, showing it has a therapeutic potential. Mice, for which PMNs and keratinocytes are unable to make cathelicidin, become susceptible to infection with group A *Streptococcus*. Cathelicidin also plays a role in immunity to *Mycobacterium tuberculosis* through its action on vitamin D.

Another interesting innate defence mechanism is the formation of neutrophil extracellular traps (NETs). NETs are formed from decondensed unwound DNA, with neutrophil granule proteins and myeloperoxidase, and can bind both gram-positive and gram-negative bacteria, although they may not always be killed (Fig. 15.2). NETs can damage fungal hyphae that are too large to be phagocytosed; the key molecule here seems to be calprotectin, which is released from the NETs. Of course, the bacteria can fight back, in this case, through secreting DNAases or by having capsules to prevent entrapment. NETs can also cause tissue damage and promote cancer metastases, so DNAse treatment is being investigated as a treatment to break down NETs.

Lysozyme is one of the most abundant antimicrobial proteins in the lung. Genetically engineered transgenic mice with a lot more lysozyme activity than control mice in their bronchoalveolar lavage were much better at killing group B streptococci and *Pseudomonas aeruginosa* (Fig. 15.3).

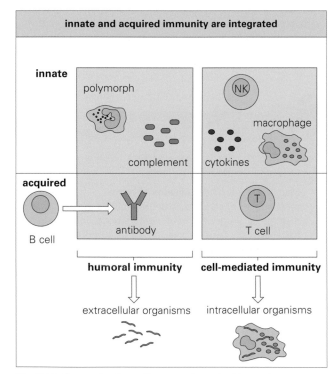

**Fig. 15.1** The mechanisms of innate and acquired immunity are integrated to provide the basis for humoral and cell-mediated immunity. Deficiencies of humoral immunity predispose to infection with extracellular organisms, and deficiencies of T-cell–mediated responses are associated primarily with intracellular infections.

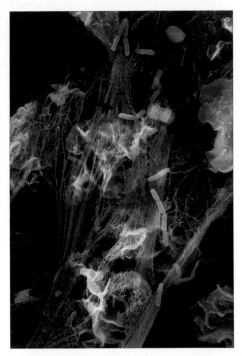

**Fig. 15.2** Neutrophil extracellular traps can trap bacteria. These chromatin-containing complexes can trap bacteria such as *Shigella* (illustrated). (Courtesy Dr. Volker Brinkmann, Max Planck Institute for Infection Biology, Berlin.)

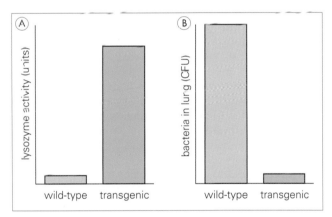

**Fig. 15.3** Transgenic mice making greater amounts of lysozyme are more resistant to infection with *Pseudomonas aeruginosa*. (A) The transgenic mice have eighteen fold more lysozyme activity than the wild-type control mice. (B) The transgenic mice showed much greater killing of *P. aeruginosa* in the lungs following intratracheal infection than did the wild-type mice. CFU, Colony-forming unit. (Modified from Akinbi HT, et al. Bacterial killing is enhanced by expression of lysozyme in the lungs of transgenic mice. *J Immunol*. 2000;165:5760–5766.)

## COMPLEMENT

### The alternative pathway and lectin-binding pathways of complement activation are part of the early defence system

The basic biology of the complement system and its role in inducing the inflammatory response and promoting chemotaxis, phagocytosis and vascular permeability are described in Chapter 10. Complement can also directly damage microorganisms as part of the early response to infection. Lack of the central complement component C3 leads to infection with a wide range of pyogenic bacteria. Patients deficient in later complement components C5, C6, C7, C8 or C9 are unable to eliminate *Neisseria* (*gonococci* and *meningococci*), with an increased risk of developing septicaemia or becoming a carrier. This suggests that these bacteria require the extracellular lytic pathway for elimination.

All three pathways can be activated by the innate system, but activation through the classical pathway is the only one for which antibodies improve the response. It should be recognized that the complement classical pathway activation is most efficiently activated by immunoglobulin M (IgM).

## ACUTE PHASE PROTEINS AND PATTERN RECOGNITION RECEPTORS

### C-reactive protein is an antibacterial agent produced by liver cells in response to cytokines

Among the acute phase proteins produced during inflammatory reactions, C-reactive protein (CRP) is particularly interesting in being an antibacterial agent, although most of this activity has so far been shown against *Streptococcus pneumoniae*. CRP is a pentameric beta globulin, somewhat resembling a miniature version of IgM (molecular weight 130,000 compared with 900,000 for IgM), and a member of the pentraxin family. It reacts with phosphorylcholine in the wall of some streptococci and subsequently activates both complement and phagocytosis. CRP is produced by liver cells in response to cytokines, particularly interleukin 6 (IL-6; see Fig. 10.22), IL-1 and tumour necrosis factor (TNF), and levels can rise as much as 1000-fold in 24 h—a much more rapid response than that of antibody production. Therefore CRP levels are often used to monitor inflammation (e.g. in rheumatic diseases). Serum amyloid P (SAP) is another short pentraxin that binds to phosphatidylethanolamine on bacterial membranes, whereas the long chain pentraxin, PTX3, along with CRP and SAP, activates the classical complement pathway by binding C1q. SAP and PTX3 enhance the phagocytosis of *Aspergillus fumigatus*, while PTX3 modulates the inflammatory response to *Klebsiella pneumoniae*. The other acute phase proteins are also produced in increased amounts early in infection and have not only antimicrobial activity but also can act as opsonins or antiproteases, be involved in the fibrinolytic or anticoagulant pathways or play an immunomodulatory role. For example, many of the complement components are acute phase proteins. Those with a role in protection against infection are also termed *pattern recognition receptors*, such as mannose-binding lectin (MBL). The acute phase protein splA$_2$ (a member of the secretory phospholipase A$_2$ family) is important in protection against gram-positive bacteria in serum. Some acute phase proteins such as LPS-binding protein may reduce pathology by binding toxic bacterial products such as LPS.

### Collectins and ficolins

Collectins are proteins with three or six subunits, each containing a calcium-dependent lectin head and a collagen-like tail, that bind to carbohydrate molecules expressed on bacterial and viral surfaces. This results in cell recruitment, activation of the alternative complement cascade and macrophage activation. Two collectins, the surfactant proteins A and D, are able to inhibit bacterial growth and opsonize bacteria directly, leading to phagocytosis and activation of complement. Surfactant protein A has been shown to play a role in the innate defence of the lung against infection with group B streptococci. Mice deficient in surfactant protein A are much more susceptible to infection, developing greater pulmonary infiltration and dissemination of bacteria to the spleen, compared with those able to produce the collectin. Polymorphisms in the surfactant A and D genes have also been linked to susceptibility to respiratory syncytial virus, as these surfactants act as opsonins for the virus.

MBL is another collectin found in serum. Binding of MBL to carbohydrates containing mannose or fucose on microorganisms leads to complement activation through the MBL pathway. Bacteria opsonized by MBL bind to the C1q receptor on macrophages, leading to phagocytosis. Many individuals have low serum concentrations of MBL due to mutations in the *MBL* gene or its promoter. A study of children with malignancies showed that MBL deficiency increased the duration of infections. Lung surfactant proteins A and D and MBL bind to the surface spikes or S protein of the severe acute respiratory syndrome (SARS) virus (see Ch. 20), and so people with low MBL genotypes may be at increased risk of SARS infection. Lung surfactants also bind to the S protein on SARS coronavirus 2 (SARS-CoV-2).

Ficolins are plasma proteins with a similar structure to collectins that bind *N*-acetylglucosamine and lipotechoic acid from the cell walls of gram-positive bacteria. Ficolins 1, 2 and 3 and MBL bind to the surface of *Leishmania braziliensis* promastigotes.

## Macrophages can recognize bacteria as foreign using Toll-like receptors

Toll-like receptors (TLRs) on macrophages and other cells bind conserved microbial molecules such as LPS (endotoxin), bacterial DNA, double-stranded RNA or bacterial flagellin pathogen-associated molecular patterns (see Ch. 10) leading to the release of proinflammatory cytokines and increased expression of major histocompatibility complex (MHC) molecules and costimulatory molecules, thus enhancing antigen presentation and usually leading to the activation of T-helper 1 (Th1) cells. The single nucleotide polymorphism Asp299Gly within the *TLR4* gene (TLR4 binds endotoxin) is more common in children who die from severe meningococcal disease compared with survivors.

Microbes in the cytosol of a cell can also be recognized as foreign using another family of pattern recognition receptors called *nucleotide-binding and oligomerization leucine-rich repeat receptors (NLRs)*. Some NLRs can sense bacterial or viral DNA, leading to activation of inflammasomes, which are complexes of proteins, and ultimately leading to the secretion of IL-1β and other proinflammatory cytokines. One way in which SARS-CoV-2 induces hyperinflammation is through its N protein activating the NLR3 inflammasome. NLRs can also induce a process called *autophagy* in which normal cytoplasmic contents are degraded after fusion with autolysosomes.

## FEVER

A raised temperature almost invariably accompanies infection (see Ch. 30). In many cases, the cause can be traced to the release of cytokines such as IL-1 or IL-6, which play important roles in both immunity and pathology (see Ch. 10).

## It is probably unwise to generalize about the benefit or otherwise of fever

Several microorganisms have been shown to be susceptible to high temperature. This was the basis for the fever therapy of syphilis by deliberate infection with blood-stage malaria for which Julius Wagner-Jaurgg won the Nobel Prize for Medicine in 1927, and the malaria parasite itself may also be damaged by high temperatures, although it is obviously not eliminated. In general, however, one would predict that successful parasites would be adapted to survive episodes of fever; indeed the stress or heat-shock proteins produced by both mammalian and microbial cells in response to stress of many kinds, including heat, are thought to be part of their protective strategy. On the other hand, several host immune mechanisms might also be expected to be more active at slightly higher temperatures as all enzyme reaction rates increase with a temperature rise; examples are complement activation, membrane function, lymphocyte proliferation and the synthesis of proteins such as antibody and cytokines.

## NATURAL KILLER CELLS

### Natural killer cells are a rapid but nonspecific means of controlling viral and other intracellular infections

Natural killer (NK) cells provide an early source of cytokines and chemokines during infection until there is time for the activation and expansion of antigen-specific T cells. NK cells can provide an important source of interferon gamma (IFNγ) during the first few days of infection. NK cell cytokine production can be secreted by cytokines such as IL-12 and IL-18, which are secreted by macrophages in response to LPS or other microbial components. As well as IFNγ, NK cells can make TNFα and, under some conditions, the downregulatory cytokine IL-10. Some tissues such as the gut need their own special populations of innate lymphoid cells (ILC3 cells), which make large amounts of the cytokine IL-22 to help defend the gut against certain intestinal pathogens.

NK cells can also act as cytotoxic effector cells, lysing host cells infected with viruses and some bacteria as they make both cytotoxic granules and perforin. They recognize their targets by means of a series of activating and inhibitory receptors that are not antigen specific. The main NK-cell–activating receptors are called *killer cell Ig-like receptors (KIRs)*; others are carbohydrate-binding C-type lectins such as NKG2D, which bind the MHC-like MIC-A and MIC-B molecules that are expressed on virus-infected cells and tumour cells. The inhibitory receptors recognize the complex of MHC class I and self-peptide; if both this inhibitory receptor and another NK-cell–activating receptor are engaged, the NK cell will not be activated, and a healthy cell will not be killed. However, if there is insufficient MHC class I on the cell surface, the inhibitory receptor is not engaged, and the NK cell is activated to kill the target cell. This is an effective strategy, as some viruses inhibit MHC class I expression on the cells they infect. NK cells are therefore a more rapid but less specific means of controlling viral and other intracellular infections. The importance of NK cells is highlighted by the ability of mice lacking both T and B cells (severe combined immunodeficiency) to control some virus infections, and

**Table 15.1** Natural killer cells play an important role in controlling infections

| Infections where natural killer cells have been shown to help control infection | |
| --- | --- |
| **Human** | **Mouse** |
| Human cytomegalovirus (human herpesvirus 5) | Mouse cytomegalovirus |
| Vesicular stomatitis virus | Herpes simplex virus |
| Herpes simplex virus | Vaccinia virus |
| Human papillomavirus | Influenza virus |
| Human immunodeficiency virus | *Toxoplasma gondii* |
| Epstein-Barr virus (EBV) | EBV in human reconstituted mice |
| | Malaria |
| | *Trypanosoma cruzi* |

humans with NK-cell defects are susceptible to certain viruses (Table 15.1). NK cells can also lyse red cells containing malaria parasites (Fig. 15.4).

NK cells and the other ILCs form a bridge between the innate and adaptive immune responses, and their function may be enhanced by components of adaptive immunity. NK cells can show some immunologic memory, which may result from epigenetic modifications, so perhaps their full abilities are not yet appreciated!

## NKT cells and γδT cells

Two further small populations of cells may play a role in infection by responding to nonprotein antigens from pathogens. A small group of cells express both NK-cell and T-cell markers and are so-called *NKT cells*; they can also recognize lipid antigens presented by CD1 molecules that are similar to MHC class I molecules but less polymorphic. The γδT cells are classical T cells that express a T-cell receptor (TCR) with γ and δ chains rather than an αβ TCR; they respond to microbial lipids and small phosphorylated antigens also presented by MHC class I–like molecules that have limited polymorphism. γδT cells are often found at epithelial surfaces and make up approximately 10% of the intraepithelial lymphocytes in the human gut.

## PHAGOCYTOSIS

### Phagocytes engulf, kill and digest would-be parasites

Perhaps the greatest danger to the would-be parasite is to be recognized by a phagocytic cell, engulfed, killed and digested (Fig. 15.5). A description of the various stages of phagocytosis is given in Chapter 10. Phagocytes (principally macrophages) are normally found in tissues where invading microorganisms are more likely to be encountered. In addition, phagocytes present in the blood (principally the neutrophils, or PMNs) can be rapidly recruited into the tissues when and where required. Only approximately 1% of the normal adult bone marrow reserve of $3 \times 10^{12}$ PMNs is present in the blood at any one time, representing a turnover of approximately $10^{11}$ PMNs per day. Most macrophages remain within the tissues, and well under 1% of our phagocytes are present in the blood as monocytes. PMNs are short lived, but macrophages can live for many years (see later).

### Intracellular killing by phagocytes

#### Phagocytes kill organisms using either an oxidative or a nonoxidative mechanism

The mechanisms by which phagocytes kill the organisms they ingest are traditionally divided into oxidative and nonoxidative, depending upon whether the cell consumes oxygen in the process. Respiration in PMNs is nonmitochondrial and anaerobic, and the burst of oxygen consumption, the so-called *respiratory burst* (see Fig. 10.12) that accompanies phagocytosis represents the generation of microbicidal reactive oxygen intermediates (ROIs).

#### Oxidative killing involves the use of ROIs

The importance of ROIs in bacterial killing was revealed by the discovery that PMNs from patients with chronic granulomatous disease (CGD) did not consume oxygen after phagocytosing staphylococci. Patients with CGD have one of three kinds of genetic defect in a PMN membrane enzyme system involving nicotinamide adenine dinucleotide phosphate oxidase (PHOX; see Ch. 31). The normal activity of this system is the progressive reduction of atmospheric oxygen to water with the production of ROIs such as the superoxide ion, hydrogen peroxide and free hydroxyl radicals, all of which can be extremely toxic to microorganisms (Table 15.2).

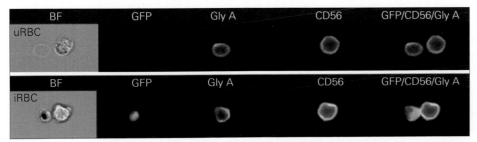

**Fig. 15.4** Natural killer (NK) cells can bind to and kill malaria-infected erythrocytes. The upper panels show uninfected human red blood cells (uRBCs), and the bottom ones show red cells infected with *Plasmodium falciparum* (iRBC). The transgenic malaria parasites are labelled with green fluorescent protein (GFP), the red cell membrane with blue phycoerythrin-labelled glycophorin A (Gly A), and the NK cell membrane with yellow phycoerythrin–cyanine 7 tandem protein. The NK cells expressing the NK cell marker CD56 bind only to the malaria-infected erythrocytes, as shown in the merged images. BF, Bright field; CD56, cluster of differentiation 56. (Courtesy Samuel Sherratt, London School of Hygiene & Tropical Medicine.)

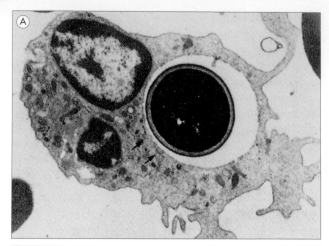

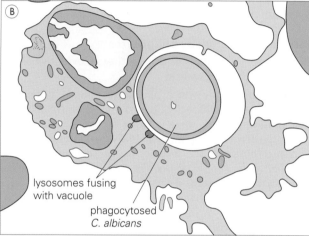

lysosomes fusing
with vacuole

phagocytosed
*C. albicans*

**Fig. 15.5** (A) Electron micrograph and (B) diagrammatic representation of neutrophil containing phagocytosed *Candida albicans* (× 7000). (Courtesy H. Valdimarsson.)

**Table 15.2** Some organisms killed by reactive oxygen and nitrogen species

| Bacteria | Fungi | Protozoa |
|---|---|---|
| *Staphylococcus aureus* | *Candida albicans* | *Plasmodium* |
| *Escherichia coli* | *Aspergillus* | *Leishmania* (nitric oxide) |
| *Serratia marcescens* | | |

Patients with CGD are unable to kill staphylococci and certain other bacteria and fungi, which consequently cause deep chronic abscesses. They can, however, deal with catalase-negative bacteria such as pneumococci because these produce, not destroy, their own hydrogen peroxide in sufficient amounts to interact with the cell myeloperoxidase, producing the highly toxic hypochlorous acid. The defective PMNs from patients with CGD can be readily identified in vitro by their failure to reduce the yellow dye nitroblue tetrazolium to a blue compound (the NBT test; see Ch. 32).

### Antimicrobial effects of ROIs

ROIs can damage cell membranes (lipid peroxidation), DNA and proteins (including vital enzymes), but in some cases it may be the altered pH that accompanies the generation of ROIs that does the damage. Killing of some bacteria and fungi (e.g. *E. coli*, *Candida*) occurs only at an acid pH, while killing of others (e.g. staphylococci) occurs at an alkaline pH. There may also be a need for protease activity (e.g. cathepsins, elastase), with enzyme solubilization occurring as a result of the influx of $H^+$ and $K^+$ into the phagocytic vesicle.

### Cytotoxic lipids prolong the activity of ROIs

As already mentioned, one of the targets of the toxic ROIs is lipid in cell membranes. ROIs are normally extremely short lived (fractions of a second), but their toxicity can be greatly prolonged by interaction with serum lipoproteins to form lipid peroxides. Lipid peroxides are stable for hours and can pass on the oxidative damage to cell membranes, both of the parasite (e.g. malaria-infected red cell) and of the host (e.g. vascular endothelium). The cytotoxic activity of normal human serum to some blood trypanosomes has been traced to the high-density lipoproteins.

## Nonoxidative killing

### Nonoxidative killing involves the use of the phagocyte's cytotoxic granules

Oxygen is not always available for killing microorganisms; indeed, some bacteria grow best in anaerobic conditions (e.g. the Clostridia of gas gangrene), and oxygen would in any case be in short supply in a deep tissue abscess or a tuberculosis (TB) granuloma. Phagocytic cells, therefore, also contain other cytotoxic molecules. The best studied are the proteins in the various PMN granules (Table 15.3) that act on the contents of the phagosome as the granules fuse with it. Note that the transient fall in pH accompanying the respiratory burst enhances the activity of the cationic microbicidal proteins and defensins. Neutrophil serine proteinases have homology to the cytotoxic granzymes released by cytotoxic T cells.

Another phagocytic cell, the eosinophil, is particularly rich in cytotoxic granules (see Table 15.3). The highly cationic (i.e. basic) contents of these granules give them their characteristic acidophilic staining pattern. Five distinct eosinophil cationic proteins are known and seem to be particularly toxic to parasitic worms, at least in vitro. Because of the enormous difference in size between parasitic worms and eosinophils, this type of damage is limited to the outer surfaces of the parasite. The eosinophilia typical of worm infections is presumably an attempt to cope with these large and almost indestructible parasites. Both the production and level of activity of eosinophils is regulated by T cells and macrophages and mediated by cytokines such as IL-5 and TNFα.

Monocytes and macrophages also contain cytotoxic granules. Unlike PMNs, macrophages contain little or no myeloperoxidase but secrete large amounts of lysozyme. Lysozyme is an antibacterial molecule that attacks peptidoglycan in the cell wall of bacteria, which is particularly effective against gram-positive bacteria where it has easier access to the peptidoglycan. Macrophages are extremely sensitive to activation by bacterial products (e.g. LPS) and T-cell cytokines (e.g. IFNγ). Activated macrophages have a greatly enhanced ability to kill both intracellular and extracellular targets.

## Nitric oxide

A major secreted product of the activated macrophage is nitric oxide (NO), one of the reactive nitrogen intermediates

**Table 15.3** Contents of polymorphonuclear leukocyte and eosinophil granules

| Polymorphonuclear neutrophils (PMNs) and eosinophil granule contents | | |
|---|---|---|
| **PMN** | | **Eosinophil** |
| *Primary (azurophil)* | *Specific (heterophil)* | *Cationic* |
| Myeloperoxidase | Lysozyme | Peroxidase |
| Acid hydrolases | Lactoferrin | Cationic proteins |
| Cathepsins G, B, D | Alkaline phosphatase | ECP |
| Defensins | NADPH oxidase | MBP |
| BPI | Collagenase | Neurotoxin |
| Cationic proteins | Histaminase | Lysophospholipase |
| Lysozyme | | |

BPI, Bactericidal permeability increasing protein; ECP, eosinophil cationic protein; MBP, major basic protein; NADPH, nicotinamide adenine dinucleotide phosphate.

(RNIs) generated during the conversion of arginine to citrulline by arginase (see Fig. 10.13). NO is strongly cytotoxic to a variety of cell types, and RNIs are generated in large amounts during infections (e.g. leishmaniasis, malaria).

## CYTOKINES

### Cytokines contribute to both infection control and infection pathology

Early studies with supernatants from cultures of lymphocytes and macrophages revealed a family of non-antigen–specific molecules with diverse activities, which were involved in cell-to-cell communication. These are now collectively known as *cytokines*. Cytokines play many crucial roles in protection against infectious diseases. The way in which these molecules acquired their sometimes rather misleading names and the bewildering overlap of function between molecules of quite different structure are described in detail in Chapter 12.

Cytokines are of importance in infectious disease for two contrasting reasons:

• They can contribute to the control of infection.
• They can contribute to the development of pathology.

The latter harmful aspect, of which TNFα in septic shock is a good example, is discussed in Chapter 18. The beneficial effects can be direct or more often indirect via the induction of some other antimicrobial process.

### Interferons

The best-established antimicrobial cytokines are the interferons (Table 15.4). The name is derived from the demonstration in 1957 that virus-infected cells secreted a molecule

**Table 15.4** Human interferons

| | Type I IFNα | Type I IFNβ | Type II IFNγ | Type III IFNλ |
|---|---|---|---|---|
| Alternative name | Leukocyte IFN | Fibroblast IFN | Immune IFN | |
| Principal source | All cells | All cells | Th1 T cells NK cells, ILC1 | Epithelial cells, dendritic cells |
| Inducing agent | Viral infection (DNA, ± ssRNA) | Viral infection (DNA, ± ssRNA) | Antigen or mitogen (Th1 T cells) | Viral infections (DNA, ± ssRNA or dsRNA) |
| Number of species | 22[a] | 1 | 1 | 4[b] |
| Chromosomal location of gene(s) | 9 | 9 | 12 | 19 |
| Antiviral activity | +++ | +++ | + | ++ |
| **Immunoregulatory activity** | | | | |
| Macrophage activation | Polarization to M1 macrophages | − | +++ | − |
| T-cell function | + (enhances activation) | + (enhances activation | + | + (proliferation, Th1/Th17 cytokines) |
| MHC I upregulation | + | + | + | − |
| MHC II upregulation | − | − | + | − |

± ssRNA, Negative or positive sense single-stranded ribonucleic acid (RNA); dsRNA, double-stranded RNA; IFN, interferon; MHC, major histocompatibility complex; NK, natural killer; ILC, innate lymphoid cell; M1, classically activated macrophage; Th, T helper.
[a]Each species coded by a different gene; in addition to IFNα and IFNβ, there are three other type I interferons: IFN-ω, IFN-ε, and IFN-κ.
[b]European/Asian ancestry individuals mostly lack the gene for IFNλ-4.

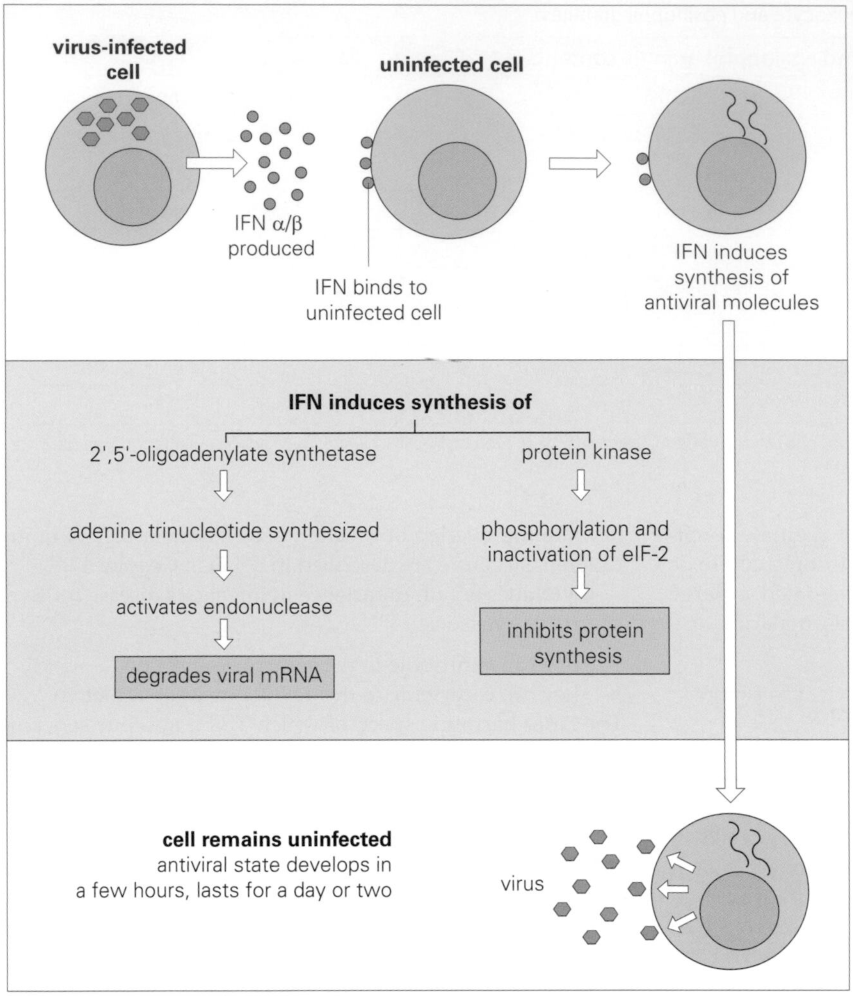

**Fig. 15.6** The molecular basis of type I interferon (IFN) α/β action. eIF-2, Eukaryotic initiation factor 2.

that interfered with viral replication in bystander cells. IFNs of all three types (I IFNαβ, II IFNγ, III IFNλ) interact with specific receptors on most cells, following which they induce an antiviral state via the generation of at least two types of enzymes: a protein kinase and a 2',5'-oligoadenylate synthetase. Both enzymes result in the inhibition of viral RNA translation and therefore of protein synthesis (Fig. 15.6).

## IFNα and IFNβ constitute a major part of the early response to viruses

IFNα and IFNβ (type I IFNs) are produced rapidly within 24 h of infection and constitute a major part of the early response to viruses.

Type I IFNs can also inhibit virus assembly at a later stage (e.g. retroviruses), while many of their other effects contribute to the antiviral state (e.g. by the enhancement of cellular MHC expression and the activation of NK cells and macrophages) (Fig. 15.7). Unlike cytotoxic T cells, type I IFNs normally inhibit viruses without damaging the host cell. In animal experiments, treatment with antibodies to IFNα greatly increases susceptibility to viral infection; treatment with IFNα has proved useful for some human virus infections, notably chronic hepatitis B (see Ch. 23). Cleverly, it seems that once viral DNA has been sensed in the cytoplasm of the infected cell, by cyclic guanosine

monophosphate–adenosine monophosphate synthase, the heterodinucleotide cyclic GMP–AMP (called *cGAMP*) can not only trigger a protein that stimulates interferon expression (STING), but also the cGAMP can be packaged into newly produced viruses, which means the virus itself carries stimulators of antiviral interferons into the next cell it infects!

Although best known for their antiviral activity, type I IFNs have recently been shown to be induced by, and active against, infections with a wide range of organisms, including rickettsia, mycobacteria and several protozoa. A study of gene expression in patients with TB identified activation of many genes induced by type I IFNs as well as by type II IFNγ.

IFNγ (type II immune IFN) is mainly a T-cell product and is therefore produced later, although an early IFNγ response may be mounted by NK cells and type 1 ILCs. The role of IFNγ is discussed further under T cells (see later). Some intracellular organisms (e.g. *Leishmania*) can counteract the effect of IFNγ on MHC expression, thereby facilitating their own survival.

Type III IFNs (most information is known about IFNλ) also play a role in immunity to viruses. The *NSP1* gene in rotavirus induces proteosomal degradation of IFN-inducing factors, thus stopping the production of IFNs. A mutation in the *NSP1* gene restores IFN production (Fig. 15.8). Both type I and type III IFNs are produced, and IFNλ may be

**Fig. 15.7** The multiple activities of interferons (IFNs) in viral immunity. CD, Cluster of differentiation; IL, interleukin; MHC, major histocompatibility complex; NK, natural killer.

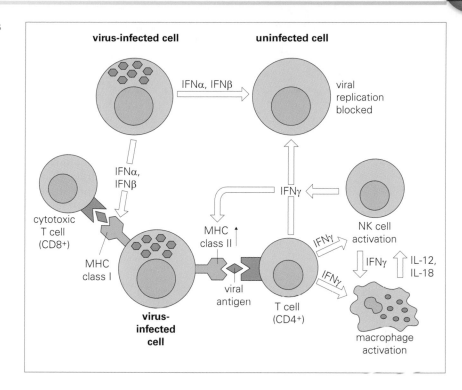

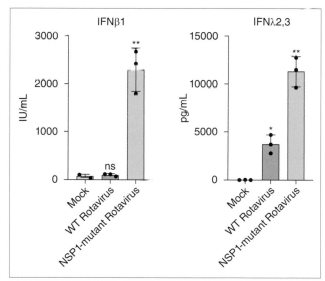

**Fig. 15.8** A mutation in the rotavirus *NSP1* gene restores induction of both type I and type III interferons. Interferon production in a cell line infected with wild-type (WT) rotavirus or rotavirus with a mutation in nonstructural protein 1 (NSP1) showed how the WT rotavirus uses NSP to prevent production of type I IFNβ1 and type III IFNs λ2,3. ns, Not significant; *, P < .01; **, P < .0001 compared to mock-infected control cells. (Modified from Doldan P, Dai J, Metz-Zumaran C, et al. Type III and not type I interferons efficiently prevent the spread of rotavirus in human intestinal epithelial cells. *J Virol*. 2022;96(17):e0070622.)

particularly important in blocking viral replication in intestinal epithelial cells.

### Other cytokines

#### TNF production can be good or bad

A striking example of a potentially useful role for TNF in infection is illustrated by what happened when a humanized antibody against TNF was used to treat patients with

rheumatoid arthritis and Crohn disease. A number of treated patients developed TB soon after starting therapy (Fig. 15.9); others developed *Listeria*, *Pneumocystis* or *Aspergillus* infections. Patients should now be tested for latent TB before starting treatment with a TNF-blocking antibody. However, TNF is also thought to contribute to the pathology of TB and that of malaria (see Ch. 18). The requirement to have not too little and not too much of a mediator that would induce damaging pathology, rather than an amount that is just right, is sometimes referred to as the *Goldilocks principle*. Paradoxically, TNF concentration is raised in human immunodeficiency virus (HIV) infection and has been found to enhance the replication of HIV in T cells, a positive feedback with worrying potential. The role of T-cell–derived cytokines such as IFNγ in immunity to infection is discussed later.

### ANTIBODY-MEDIATED IMMUNITY

The key property of the antibody molecule is to bind specifically to antigens on the foreign microbe. In many cases this is followed by secondary binding to other cells or molecules of the immune system (e.g. phagocytes, complement). These are discussed later, but first some general features that influence the effectiveness of the antibody response should be mentioned.

#### Speed, amount and duration

Because of the cell interactions involved and the need for proliferation of a small number of specific precursor lymphocytes, a primary antibody response can be dangerously slow in reaching protective levels. The classic example before penicillin became available was lobar pneumonia in which the race between bacterial multiplication and antibody production was neck-and-neck for about 1 week, at which point one side or the other dramatically won. Nowadays, of course, vaccines and antibiotics have intervened to improve the patient's chances. Experiments with specially

143

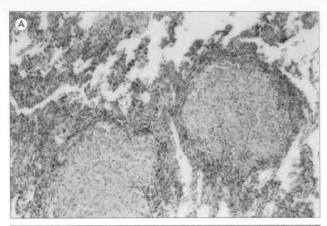

**Fig. 15.9** Photomicrographs of lung specimens from patients with tuberculosis (A) who did not (× 100) or (B) who did (× 100) receive infliximab, a humanized antibody to TNFα. In the patient without infliximab treatment, there are well-formed granulomas; in the patient with anti-TNF treatment, there is minimal granuloma formation but much fibrosis and inflammation. (From Keane J, et al. Tuberculosis associated with infliximab, a tumor necrosis factor alpha-neutralizing agent. *N Engl J Med*. 2001;345:1098–1104.)

bred lines of mice suggest that the speed and size of an antibody response is under the control of a large number of genes, and the same is undoubtedly true in humans. To help provide cover while specific antibodies are produced, there are some preexisting natural antibodies that are usually low-affinity and cross-reactive IgM antibodies.

The rate of replication of the microorganism must also be considered. Replication rates, as indicated by doubling times (see Ch. 16), vary from <1 h (most viruses, many bacteria) to days or even weeks (mycobacteria, *Treponema pallidum*). Microorganisms tend to grow more slowly in vivo than in vitro, which shows that the host environment is generally hostile. When the incubation period is only a few days (e.g. rhinovirus, rotavirus, cholera), the antibody response is too slow to affect the initial outcome, and rapidly produced cytokines such as IFNs are more important.

Usually the antibody response continues as long as antigen is present, although some downregulation may occur in very prolonged responses, presumably in an effort to limit immunopathology (see Ch. 18). The lifelong immunity that follows many virus infections may often be due to regular boosting by viruses in the community, but sometimes (e.g. yellow fever) there is no obvious boost, yet antibodies persist for decades. Such persistence of immunologic memory may

be due to the nonspecific stimulation of memory B and T cells by cytokines during responses to other antigens, a process called *bystander activation*.

## Affinity

It seems self-evident that a higher antigen-binding affinity would make antibody more useful, and passive protection experiments have confirmed this. Affinity is determined by both the germline antibody gene pool and somatic mutation in individual B lymphocytes and appears to be under genetic control, which is separate from that controlling the total amount of antibody made. A tendency toward a low antibody affinity to the tetanus toxoid vaccine has been found in some subjects, particularly those with predominantly IgG4 responses, and there is strong evidence from mouse experiments that failure to develop high-affinity antibody responses can predispose to immune complex disease.

## Antibody classes and subclasses (isotypes)

The different Fc portions of the antibody molecule are responsible for most of the differences in antibody function (see Ch. 11). Switching from one to another while preserving the same Fab portion allows the immune system to try out different effector mechanisms against the microbial invader. This flexibility is not total. For example, T-independent antigens such as some polysaccharides induce mainly IgM antibodies, T cells being required for the switch to IgE and helpful for IgG switching. IgG antibodies to polysaccharides tend to be mainly IgG2, whereas IgG antibodies to protein are mainly IgG1. The poor development of IgG2 in children younger than age ~2 years explains their lack of response to bacteria with polysaccharide capsules (e.g. *S. pneumoniae*, *Haemophilus influenzae*). Antibodies to viruses are predominantly IgG1 and IgG3, and those to helminths are IgG4 and IgE. Antigens encountered via the digestive tract induce mainly IgA, which is processed during its passage through epithelial cells to sIgA, the only type of antibody that can function in this protease-rich intestinal environment; the gut microbiota may induce T-independent IgA class switching through interactions with intestinal epithelial cells.

## Blocking and neutralizing effects of antibody

Simple binding of antibody molecules to a microbial surface is often enough to protect the host. It may physically interfere with the receptor interaction necessary for microbial entry (e.g. of a virus into a cell) or with the binding of a toxin to its host receptor. This is the basis of many life-saving vaccines against viruses or bacterial toxins. Such vaccines need to generate high-affinity antibodies, and T-cell help will be needed.

Blocking of attachment and entry can be effective against all organisms that use specific attachment sites, whether viral, bacterial or protozoal (see Ch. 14). An important exception is those organisms that parasitize the macrophage, such as the virus of dengue fever; here the presence of a low concentration of IgG antibody can enhance infection by promoting attachment to Fc receptors (see Ch. 18).

A more subtle blocking effect of antibody is interference with essential surface components of the parasite, particularly if these are enzymes or transport molecules. The successful pathogen takes steps to protect such components whenever possible, as described in Chapter 17.

## Immobilization and agglutination

Immunoglobulin antibodies, particularly the large pentameric IgM, are the same order of size as some of the smaller viruses and larger than the thickness of a bacterial flagellum (Fig. 15.10), so the simple physical attachment of antibody can considerably restrict the activities of motile organisms. In addition, the multivalent design of the antibody molecules enables it to link together two or more organisms, as can readily be demonstrated in the bacterial agglutination tests (Fig. 15.11). The protective value of agglutination in vivo is hard to assess; once clumped, most organisms are probably rapidly phagocytosed, but clumps of still-motile trypanosomes can be seen in the blood of infected animals with enough serum antibodies. Agglutination reactions in vitro can be useful in diagnosis (see Ch. 32).

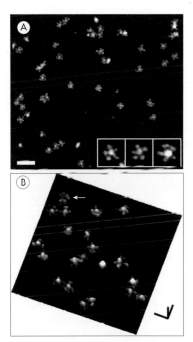

**Fig. 15.10** (A, B) The immunoglobulin M (IgM) molecule. The free form of IgM adopts a starlike configuration (*arrow*), as shown in the image obtained with low temperature atomic force microscopy. (From Czajkowsky DM. The human IgM pentamer is a mushroom-shaped molecule with a flexural bias. *PNAS*. 2009;106:14960–14965.)

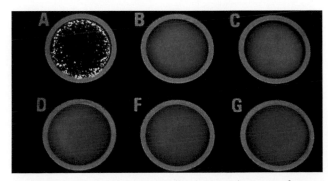

**Fig. 15.11** Bacterial agglutination. Well A shows agglutination of group A streptococci with latex particles coated with anti-group A antibodies. (Courtesy D.K. Banerjee.)

## Lysis

Lysis of bacteria in the presence of complement provides another convenient assay for the presence of antibody (IgG and IgA). However, lysis probably plays a major protective role in only a restricted range of infections, notably those caused by *Neisseria* and some viruses (see Ch. 17).

## Opsonization

Whether by the direct binding of the immunoglobulin CH2 and CH3 regions to Fc receptors or via the activation of complement to allow C3b to bind to its receptor, opsonization represents the most important overall function of the antibody molecule. Telling evidence for this is the general similarity in the effects on the patient of defects in antibody, complement (up to and including C3) and phagocytic cells (see Ch. 31). It is estimated that the rate of phagocytosis is enhanced by up to 1000-fold by antibody and complement acting together (Fig. 15.12). Lobar pneumonia due to *S. pneumoniae* again provides a good example: IgG antibody against the capsule allows neutrophils to phagocytose the organisms, converting a lung virtually solid with fluid, fibrin and phagocytic cells into the normal breathing apparatus. Note that the later complement components C5–C9 are not required, so that deficiencies of these do not predispose to bacterial infection in general (see Ch. 31). Of course, the effectiveness of opsonization depends on the phagocytic cell being capable of finishing off the ingested organism. This is not the case, however, with organisms that inhibit or avoid the normal intracellular killing processes of which mycobacteria are a typical example (see Ch. 17).

### Antibody-dependent cellular cytotoxicity

In the case of larger organisms (worms being the most obvious example), phagocytosis is clearly not a possibility. However, several types of cells, having made contact with the parasite through antibody and Fc receptors in the same way as phagocytes do, can inflict damage extracellularly through antibody-dependent cellular cytotoxicity. These include most conventional phagocytes, eosinophils and degranulation of NK cells via CD16 Fc gamma-receptor III binding.

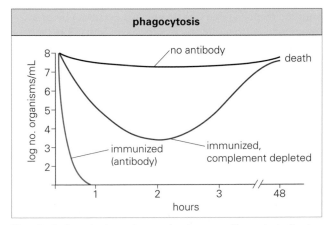

**Fig. 15.12** Opsonization enhances the clearance of bacteria. Antibody and complement together accelerate the clearance of pneumococci from the blood of mice (*blue line*), depletion of complement allows some opsonization if antibody is present but fails to control the infection (*red line*).

**Table 15.5** Antibody and cell-mediated immunity (CMI) in resistance to systemic infections

| Type of resistance | Antibody | CMI |
|---|---|---|
| Recovery from primary infection | Yellow fever, polioviruses, coxsackieviruses<br>Streptococci, staphylococci<br>*Neisseria meningitidis*<br>*Haemophilus influenzae*<br>*Candida* spp.<br>*Giardia duodenalis*<br>Malaria[a] | Poxviruses (e.g. ectromelia [mice], vaccinia [humans])<br>Herpes-type viruses: herpes simplex, varicella-zoster, cytomegalovirus<br>LCM virus (mice)<br>Tuberculosis<br>Leprosy<br>Systemic fungal infections<br>Chronic mucocutaneous candidiasis[b] |
| Resistance to reinfection | Nearly all viruses, including measles, most bacteria | Tuberculosis<br>Leprosy |
| Resistance to reactivation of latent infection | | Varicella-zoster, cytomegalovirus, herpes simplex, tuberculosis, *Pneumocystis jiroveci*[c] |

Either antibody or CMI is known to be the major factor in these examples. But in many other infections there is no information, and sometimes both types of immunity are important. It is likely that CMI is also involved in resistance to activation of latent tuberculosis infection.
CMI, Cell-mediated immunity; LCM, Lymphocytic choriomeningitis.
[a]Protection is incomplete and short lived.
[b]Both Th1 and Th17 cells may be involved.
[c]Formerly *P. carinii*.

Indeed, the precise way in which antibody protects against infection is, in the majority of cases, still unknown. For example, the enormous production of IgA in the intestine, which may amount to half of all antibodies produced in the body, suggests the vital importance of mucosal protection, yet deficiency of IgA is relatively common and not particularly serious.

Table 15.5 gives some examples of common infections normally controlled by antibody. Once again, it must be emphasized that the presence of antibody by no means denotes a protective role. It may be directed against irrelevant or noncritical microbial antigens, or the infection may be of a type that is not primarily controlled by antibody, as with many intracellular infections (e.g. TB, typhoid, herpesvirus). The best indication of the value of antibody comes from antibody-deficiency syndromes (see Ch. 31).

## CELL-MEDIATED IMMUNITY

T cells form the second main component of the adaptive immune response (see Chs. 11 and 12). Some act by producing cytokines that induce macrophage activation or help antibody production, and others act by their direct cytotoxic action on infected target cells. In both cases the T cell needs to see the combination of specific peptide and MHC molecule that is recognized by its TCR. Some examples in which T-cell–mediated immunity is important in resistance to systemic infections are given in Table 15.5.

### T-cell immunity correlates with control of bacterial growth in leprosy

In leprosy there is a spectrum of disease ranging from the paucibacillary tuberculoid form to the multibacillary lepromatous disease. *Mycobacterium leprae*–specific T-cell immunity, as measured by lymphocyte proliferation, secretion of Th1 cytokines such as IFNγ or delayed-type hypersensitivity skin testing, is found in patients with tuberculoid leprosy but is absent in patients with lepromatous leprosy (see Ch. 27). The value of T-cell stimulation

leading to macrophage activation and bacterial killing is clearly illustrated by experiments in which lepromatous leprosy patients' skin lesions were injected with IFNγ. This resulted in an influx of T cells and macrophages into the skin lesions and a reduction in the number of bacteria. Another good example of the protective role of IFNγ and Th1 immunity is seen in animal models of *Leishmania* infection: some mouse strains such as C57BL/6 are resistant to disease, controlling the infection and making a good Th1 cytokine response, whereas other susceptible strains such as BALB/c cannot control parasite growth and fail to make IFNγ (Table 15.6).

### Further evidence for the protective effects of IFNγ

The protective effects of making IFNγ, which then binds to its specific receptor on macrophages and induces macrophage activation and the production of antimicrobial molecules, are illustrated very clearly by the consequences of a failure in IFNγ synthesis or of binding to its receptor. Mice, in which the gene for IFNγ has been inactivated (knocked out), become very susceptible to intracellular infections. Rare individuals with mutations in the genes for the IFNγ receptor have been identified. Such individuals

**Table 15.6** Cytokine production in the spleens of mice infected with *Leishmania major*

| Protective influence of IFNγ in *Leishmania* infection | | | |
|---|---|---|---|
| Mouse strain | Phenotype | IFNγ (Th1) | IL-4 (Th2) |
| C57BL/6 | Resistant | + | - |
| BALB/c | Susceptible | - | + |

The resistant phenotype (C57BL/6 mice) was associated with the production of the T helper 1 (Th1) cytokine interferon gamma (IFNγ), whereas the susceptible phenotype was associated with the production of the Th2 cytokine interleukin 4 (IL-4). (From Heinzel FP, et al. Reciprocal expression of interferon gamma or interleukin 4 during the resolution or progression of murine leishmaniasis. *J Exp Med*. 1989;169:59.)

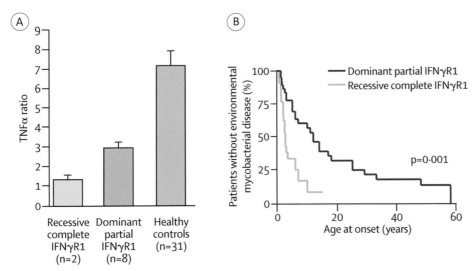

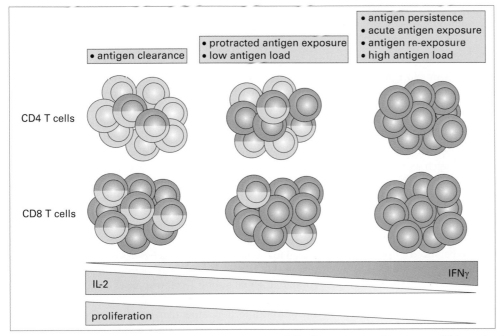

**Fig. 15.13** Genetic mutations in the interferon gamma (IFNγ) receptor 1 cause susceptibility to mycobacterial disease. Individuals with recessive complete or dominant partial IFNγR1 mutations were tested for the ability of peripheral blood mononuclear cells to secrete TNFα in response to IFNγ and LPS, compared to cells from healthy controls (A), or for time from birth to onset of first episode of environmental mycobacterial disease shown in a Kaplan-Meier curve (B). (Reprinted with permission from Elsevier. Dorman SE, et al. Clinical features of dominant and recessive interferon γ receptor 1 deficiencies. *Lancet*. 2004;364:2113–2121.)

cannot respond to IFNγ and are susceptible to infections with mycobacteria (Fig. 15.13) or to disseminated infections following bacille Calmette-Guérin (BCG) vaccination.

Some bacteria evade these protective Th1 responses by inducing antigen-specific regulatory T cells that produce transforming growth factor beta (TGFβ) or IL-10 that down-regulate IFNγ production.

### Cytokine signatures

T cells can make a variety of cytokines, but it may be most useful if particular combinations of cytokines are made by the same cell. For example, polyfunctional T cells that make IFNγ, TNFα and IL-2 make greater quantities of IFNγ than those T cells that make only IFNγ and are associated with control of the size of *Leishmania* lesions in the mouse.

**Fig. 15.14** Cytokine signatures. The balance between virus-specific T cells secreting interferon gamma (IFNγ, *purple cells*) and T cells secreting interleukin 2 (IL-2, *yellow cells*) that proliferate better varies with the antigen load and the type of viral infection. Acute infections such influenza have a high antigen load; following clearance of virus the antigen load falls and IL-2–producing cells predominate particularly in the CD4 T-cell population; in a chronic controlled infection such as Epstein-Barr virus (EBV), chronic cytomegalovirus (CMV) or human immunodeficiency virus type 1 (HIV-1) in long-term nonprogressors there is production of both IL-2 and IFNγ-secreting T cells as well as polyfunctional cells that make both cytokines; in chronic infection with high antigen load such as progressive HIV-1 infection, IFNγ-producing cells with a limited ability to proliferate predominate. CD, Cluster of differentiation. (Modified from Pantaleo G, Harari A. Functional signatures in antiviral T-cell immunity for monitoring virus-associated diseases. *Nat Rev Immunol*. 2006;6:417–423.)

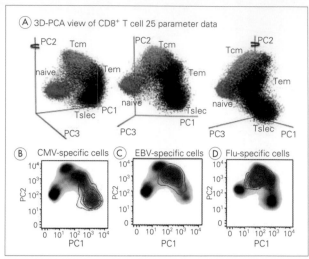

(A) 3D-PCA view of CD8⁺ T cell 25 parameter data

(B) CMV-specific cells  (C) EBV-specific cells  (D) Flu-specific cells

**Fig. 15.15** Different viral infections have different types of memory CD8 T cells. (A) Cytometry by time-of-flight uses specific heavy-metal–labelled antibody to label cells, followed by mass spectrometry to identify the binding of specific antibodies by individual T cells. Human peripheral blood T cells were analysed for expression of 25 parameters that included T-cell markers, memory T-cell markers, activation and functional markers. (B–D) Virus-specific T cells are identified using tetramers with cytomegalovirus (CMV), Epstein-Barr virus (EBV) and influenza peptides. The 25 parameters are then grouped by principal component analysis (PCA). The three-dimensional (3D) visualization of the PCA in (A) shows that human naive CD8 T cells develop into Tcm and Tem cells; Tslec cells, a smaller group of short-lived effector cells, are shown in red. The plots in B–D show tetramer-positive cells specific for CMV, EBV or influenza, respectively, in red. The phenotypes of the memory CD8 T cells differ in the three viral infections: CMV infection shows Tem with more short-lived effector cells, EBV infection shows most Tem and the more acute influenza infection has more Tcm. Tcm, Central memory T cells; Tem, effector memory T cells; Tslec, short-lived effector T cells. (Modified from Newell EW, Sigal N, Bendall SC, et al. Cytometry by time-of-flight shows combinatorial cytokine expression and virus-specific cell niches within a continuum of CD8⁺ T cell phenotypes. *Immunity.* 2012;36:142–152.)

During viral infections, the pattern or biosignature of cytokines produced by T cells may vary with clearance of infection or antigen load during a chronic infection (Fig. 15.14). For example, primary infection with HIV or cytomegalovirus (CMV) induces mainly IFNγ-producing T cells; in influenza, IL-2–producing cells predominate after viral clearance; chronic viral infection such as EBV or HIV in nonprogressors seems to lead to a mixed IFNγ and IL-2 signature, but with progressive HIV infection and a higher antigen load, this signature shifts to dominant IFNγ production. The balance between effector T cells and resting memory T cells will also change from acute to chronic disease with HIV. Healthy people have balanced populations of naive, effector and memory T cells in both the CD4 and CD8 compartments; in acute HIV the effector CD8 T cells expand, but with chronic infection the naive and memory CD4 T cells are lost. The phenotype of the memory cells will also differ in different types of infection (Fig. 15.15). New techniques such as cytometry by time-of-flight, which uses larger panels of antibodies tagged with metals to surface and intracellular markers than was possible in fluorescence-based flow cytometry, or spectral flow cytometry and other single cell analyses, are revealing even more subsets of memory cells.

## Th17 T cells

The division of CD4 T cells into Th1 and Th2 T cells aided our understanding of immunity to many infections. However, another CD4 subset making IL-17 and Th17, induced by the cytokines IL-23 and IL-1β, contributes to antimicrobial immunity. There are six IL-17 family members, IL17A–IL17F, but IL-17A is usually called *IL-17*. The focus has been on CD4 T cells making IL-17, but it can also be made by CD8 T cells, ILCs, NK cells, γδT cells and even mast cells. Th17 cells are induced by IL-23, a member of the IL-12 family, and make IL-22, which helps maintain epithelial barriers. Th17 cells play a role in immunity against a number of bacterial infections, including *K. pneumoniae, S. pneumoniae, E. coli, S. aureus, Listeria monocytogenes* and *C. albicans*. Patients with psoriasis treated with a monoclonal antibody to IL-17A/F developed more oral candidiasis. One way in which IL-17 works is by inducing neutrophil recruitment and production of antimicrobial peptides. Some patients with chronic mucocutaneous candidiasis have signalling defects leading to problems with production of Th17 cells and increased susceptibility to *Candida*. IL-17 in combination with IFNγ can also induce activation of macrophages and neutrophils, increasing bacterial killing, while IL-17 and IL-22 may help killing of Leishmania parasites through induction of nitric oxide. Another role for Th17 cells is to secrete IL-26, a cytokine that forms pores in the membranes of gram-negative bacteria leading to lysis of *E. coli, P. aeruginosa* and *K. pneumoniae*. IL-17 along with IL-22 may also help restrict tissue damage during episodes of inflammation. Whether IL-17 plays an important role in viral infections is still not clear, and there is a lot more to learn about the IL-17 family. It is also worth noting that IL-17 can induce pathology as a result of inflammation, and monoclonal antibodies to IL-17 are therefore being used to treat a number of autoimmune diseases.

## T-cell responses can be exploited in diagnostic tests for tuberculosis

There are two types of tests that measure T-cell responses to *M. tuberculosis*: the tuberculin skin test and the newer IFNγ release assays (IGRAs). The tuberculin skin test (Mantoux test) is a delayed-type hypersensitivity skin test in which induration induced by the intradermal injection of purified protein derivative from *M. tuberculosis* is measured 2–3 days later. However, the Mantoux skin test is positive in those with either latent infection or active TB disease. Worse, many of the antigens in the purified protein derivative preparation of *M. tuberculosis* used as the antigen in this test are cross-reactive with those in other mycobacteria, including BCG and nontuberculous environmental mycobacteria. This means that BCG-vaccinated subjects and those not exposed to *M. tuberculosis* itself may have a positive Mantoux skin test, so a higher cutoff is used to exclude those with such cross-reactivity. Those with a large skin test response are at increased risk of developing TB, showing that strong T-cell responses can be induced during disease progression and that a strongly positive skin test can indicate infection rather than immunity. Skin tests can also be used to screen for T-cell anergy (e.g. by using candidin), as most individuals will have been exposed to *Candida*.

More specific IGRAs that measure IFNγ release in response to peptides from antigens present in *M. tuberculosis* and not found in BCG or most environmental mycobacteria are now available (see Ch. 20). However, again, these tests will be positive in those with latent TB infection or with active TB disease.

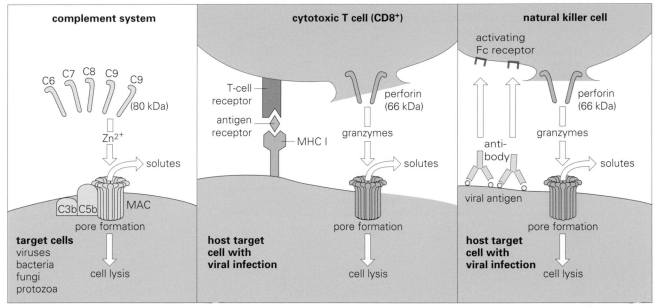

**Fig. 15.16** Comparison of the lytic mechanisms of cytotoxic cells and the complement system. The FcγRIII receptor (CD16) on the natural killer cell binds immunoglobulin IgG1 and IgG3 antibodies; other activating receptors are NKG2C and NKG2D. CD, Cluster of differentiation; MAC, membrane attack complex; MHC, major histocompatibility complex; $Zn^{2+}$, zinc ion.

### Cytotoxic T cells kill by inducing leaks in the target cell

The well-known cytotoxic T lymphocyte (CTL) is unusual in that both antigen-specific recognition and killing of the target are carried out by the same cell. The recognition step involving a peptide from an antigen that becomes associated with a class I MHC molecule is discussed in Chapter 12; it displays the high degree of specificity characteristic of all adaptive responses. Antigenic stimulation is necessary to induce the formation of cytotoxic granules, which are not present in naive CD8 T cells. The granule contents are delivered into the contact zone between the cytotoxic T cell and its target cell, and nearby cells are spared. A useful marker called CD107 of lysosomal-associated membrane protein-1 is left on the surface of the cytotoxic T cell once a T cell has released its granules.

The killing mechanism, however, is relatively nonspecific. It involves the induction of leaks or pores in the target cell membrane by the insertion of perforin, a 66 kDa molecule that, when polymerized, is structurally and functionally similar to the terminal complement component C9 (80 kDa; Fig. 15.16). Granzymes are found as proenzymes in acidic granules where they bind to serglycin; once cleaved by cathepsin, they enter the target cell and induce apoptosis. A recent study has shown that, once inside a target cell infected with bacteria or protozoa such as *Listeria* or *Toxoplasma*, granulysin, which is a third component of human lytic granules, enables granzymes to kill the bacteria and parasites in a process similar to apoptosis. Target cell death can also be caused by apoptosis, a suicide programme built into all cells that is induced by Fas/FasL interactions, granzymes and TNFα. Leakage of cell contents may also contribute to cell death.

These mechanisms are thought to operate principally against virus-infected cells (such as EBV, hepatitis, HIV, influenza, CMV), but they can also kill cells infected with other intracellular pathogens, including *Listeria* or *Toxoplasma*.

Most cytotoxic T cells are CD8 positive, recognizing MHC class I–restricted peptide epitopes, but cytotoxicity can also be mediated by CD4 T cells and by γδT cells. It may seem unexpected that CD8 T cells are activated in some intracellular bacterial infections such as TB in which the mycobacteria should be within phagosomes, but microbial antigens or even the bacteria may escape into the cytoplasm of the host cell, allowing the antigens to be picked up and presented by MHC I molecules. CD8 activation may also result from a process called cross-priming in which bacterial antigens taken up by a dendritic cell are processed for MHC class I presentation as well as MHC class II presentation. In some cases, apoptotic blebs released by apoptotic, infected macrophages may be taken up by dendritic cells. Unfortunately the lysis of an infected target cell may not always kill the intracellular pathogen, but its release from its hideaway could lead to subsequent killing by a more highly activated macrophage (Fig. 15.17).

Another interesting recent finding is that not all CD8 T cells can act as effector cytotoxic T cells. More human CD8 T cells express granzyme A than the preformed effector molecule perforin. In HIV infection, two-thirds of the CD8 T cells express granzymes, but only one-third express perforin. This may explain why virus-infected cells escape killing by antigen-specific CD8 T cells in HIV infection. Finally, some CD4 T cells can express cytotoxic markers and kill infected target cells, too.

The cytotoxic molecules used by cytotoxic T cells are shown in Table 15.7. These cytotoxic cells are also important in dealing with tumour cells.

### RECOVERY FROM INFECTION

The everyday concept of an infectious disease is one in which the patient is ill for a period of days to months and then recovers. In many cases they are subsequently immune to the disease. In such circumstances, one can be fairly certain that adaptive (lymphocyte-based) mechanisms have been at work because (1) the existence of disease symptoms implies that natural defence mechanisms, which act rapidly, did not succeed in eliminating the parasite; (2) a period of days or weeks

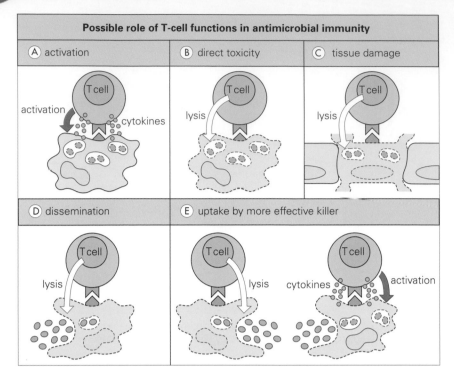

**Possible role of T-cell functions in antimicrobial immunity**

(A) activation

(B) direct toxicity

(C) tissue damage

(D) dissemination

(E) uptake by more effective killer

**Fig. 15.17** Possible roles for T cells in immunity to intracellular pathogens. (A) The T cell activates intracellular killing mechanisms by secretion of cytokines such as IFNγ (e.g. in a macrophage). (B) The T cell directly kills cell and parasite. (C) The T cell destroys vital tissue in the process of killing the parasite. (D) By lysing cells the T cell allows still-living parasites to disseminate. (E) Parasites released in this way may be phagocytosed by a host cell that is better at intracellular killing. (Modified from Kaufmann SH. In vitro analysis of the cellular mechanisms involved in immunity to tuberculosis. *Rev Infect Dis*. 1989;11[2]:S448–S454.)

**Table 15.7** Some important cytotoxic molecules in cytotoxic T-cell and natural killer cell granules that operate against infectious organisms

| Cytotoxic molecules | Properties | Effect |
|---|---|---|
| Perforin | Monomer; forms pore once polymerized | Pore allows entry of granzymes into cell |
| Granzymes[a] | Proenzymes cleaved by cathepsin | Induce apoptosis |
| Granulysin (human cells only) | Alters membrane permeability | Delivers granzymes to intracellular bacteria and protozoa |

[a]Human granzyme B can also play a beneficial role in wound healing.

is typical of the time that adaptive immune mechanisms take to reach maximal levels; and (3) subsequent immunity is a sign of the immunologic memory exclusive to T and B cells, which possess the ability to specifically recognize antigens, to proliferate into clones and to survive as memory cells. Thus the older individuals are, the better they are adapted to the environment, until old age begins to weaken the immune system itself.

In the early stages of an infection, however, adaptive immunity may need some assistance. Since the lymphocytes are programmed to recognize the shapes of antigenic epitopes, they cannot distinguish virulent from harmless parasites and must rely on recognizing danger signals; nor can they know which type of immune response will be most effective. Often one mechanism is responsible for recovery and another for resistance to reinfection (e.g. cytotoxic cells and IFN in recovery from measles, antibody in prevention of a second attack). In many infections there is still controversy as to which of the numerous responses that can be detected are useful, harmful or neutral. The reason for an individual's failure to recover (or suffer) from an infection can also be hard to pinpoint. If the infection is one from which most people recover (e.g. measles) or from which they do not suffer at all (e.g. *Pneumocystis*), then an immunodeficiency should be considered (see Ch. 31). Infections that are rapidly fatal in normal individuals (e.g. Lassa fever) are frequently those to which the human immune system

has not been exposed, as they are normally maintained in animals and only accidentally infect humans (see Zoonoses, Ch. 29). If the infection normally runs a prolonged course without either being eliminated or killing the host, however, the parasite can be considered successful, and this success will be due to one or more survival strategies. These are the subject of Chapter 17.

### Nutrition may have more subtle effects on immunity to infection

Even if an immunodeficiency state is not present, other factors may affect how a person copes with an infection. For example, during starvation or malnutrition, concentrations of the hormone leptin (which is produced by adipocytes and among other functions induces PMN activation) fall. Mice that fasted for 2 days had higher numbers of *S. pneumoniae* in their lungs than did normally fed animals, but if the fasted animals were given leptin, the number of PMNs in the lungs increased and the bacterial counts fell (Fig. 15.18). Leptin-deficient mice are highly susceptible to bacterial infections such as *Klebsiella* and *Listeria*. However, being obese is not good either—it is worth noting that obese people seem to be more susceptible to many more types of infections than those of a normal weight.

Other factors that affect how well the immune system works include stress, the microbiota, exercise, seasonality and genetics.

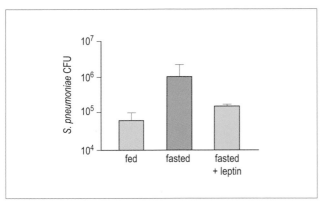

**Fig. 15.18** Leptin can restore host defence against *Streptococcus pneumoniae* in fasted mice. Colony-forming units (CFU) of bacteria in the lung were measured after normal feeding (*orange column*), in animals fasted for 48 h (*purple column*) or fasted but given leptin (*blue column*), 24 h after infection with *S. pneumoniae*. (Modified from Mancuso P, et al. Leptin corrects host defense defects after acute starvation in murine pneumococcal pneumonia. *Am J Respir Crit Care Med*. 2006;173:212–218.)

## KEY FACTS

- Protection against infectious organisms that penetrate the outer barriers of the skin and mucous membranes is mediated by a variety of early defence mechanisms, which constitute innate immunity.

- These early defence mechanisms occur more rapidly but are less specific than the adaptive mechanisms based on antigen-specific lymphocyte (T- and B-cell) responses.

- Important early defence mechanisms include the acute phase response, the complement system, IFNs, phagocytic cells, NK cells and other innate lymphoid cells. Together these act as a first line of defence during the initial hours or days of infection.

- Adaptive immunity mediated by antibody and T cells is responsible for recovery from infection in many cases, although these mechanisms take days to weeks to reach peak efficiency.

- Sometimes, as in the common viral infections, cell-mediated immunity is responsible for recovery from infection and antibody for the maintenance of immunity.

- Failure to recover from infection may be due to some deficiency of host immunity or to successful evasion strategies used by the microorganism.

# 16 Spread and replication

## Introduction

### An infection may be a surface infection or a systemic infection

Many successful microorganisms multiply in epithelial cells at the site of entry on the body surface but fail to spread to deeper structures or through the body. Local spread takes place readily on a fluid-covered mucosal surface, often aided by ciliary action, and large-scale movements of fluid spread the infection to more distant areas on the surface. This is obvious in the gastrointestinal tract. In the upper respiratory tract, high winds (coughing, sneezing) can splatter infectious agents onto new areas of mucosa or into the openings of sinuses or the middle ear, while the gentler downward trickle of mucus during sleep may seed an infectious agent into the lower respiratory tract. As a result, large areas of the body surface can be involved within a few days, with shedding to the exterior. There is not enough time for a primary immune response to be generated, and therefore nonadaptive responses—interferon, natural killer cells—are more important in controlling the infection. These surface infections therefore show a hit-and-run pattern.

In contrast, other microorganisms spread systemically through the body via lymph or blood. They often undergo a complex or stepwise invasion of various tissues before reaching the final site of replication and shedding to the exterior (e.g. measles, typhoid). Surface and systemic infections and their consequences are compared in Fig. 16.1.

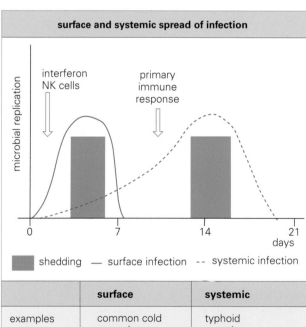

**Fig. 16.1** Surface and systemic infections. IFN, Interferon; NK, natural killer.

| | surface | systemic |
|---|---|---|
| examples | common cold gonorrhoea bacillary dysentery | typhoid measles |
| incubation period | <1 week | >1 week |
| recovery mechanism | non-adaptive* (IFN, NK) | adaptive (immune response) |

*if there is pre-existing immunity (memory), a secondary immune response comes into operation within 1–2 days

## FEATURES OF SURFACE AND SYSTEMIC INFECTIONS

### A variety of factors determine whether an infection is a surface or a systemic infection

What prevents surface infections from spreading more deeply? Why do the pathogens that cause systemic infections leave the relatively safe haven of the body surface to spread through the body, where they will bear the full onslaught of host defences? These are important questions. For instance, what are the factors that persuade meningococci residing harmlessly on the nasal mucosa to invade deeper tissues, reach the blood and meninges and cause meningitis? The answer is not known.

Temperature is one factor that can restrict pathogens to body surfaces. Rhinovirus infections, for instance, are restricted to the upper respiratory tract because they are temperature sensitive, replicating efficiently at 33°C but not at the temperatures encountered in the lower respiratory tract (37°C). *Mycobacterium leprae* is also temperature sensitive, which accounts for its replication being more or less limited to nasal mucosa, skin and superficial nerves.

The site of budding is a factor that can restrict viruses to body surfaces. Influenza and parainfluenza viruses invade surface epithelial cells of the lung, but they are liberated by budding from the free (external) surface of the epithelial cell, not from the basal layer from where they could spread to deeper tissues (Fig. 16.2).

Many microorganisms are obliged to spread systemically because they fail to spread and multiply at the site of initial infection, the body surface. In the case of measles or typhoid, there is, for unknown reasons, next to no replication at the site of initial respiratory or intestinal infection. Only after spreading through the body systemically are large numbers of microorganisms delivered back to the same surfaces where they multiply and are shed to the exterior. Other microorganisms need to spread systemically because they have committed themselves to infection by one route, while major replication and shedding occurs at a different site. The pathogen must reach the replication site, and there is then no need for extensive replication at the site of initial infection.

For instance, mumps and hepatitis A viruses infect via the respiratory and alimentary routes, respectively, but must spread through the body to invade and multiply in salivary glands (mumps) and liver (hepatitis A).

### In systemic infections, there is a stepwise invasion of different tissues of the body

This stepwise invasion is demonstrated by measles (Fig. 16.3) and typhoid (Fig. 16.4) infections. Although the final sites of multiplication may be essential for pathogen shedding and transmission (e.g. measles), they are sometimes completely unnecessary from this point of view (e.g. meningococcal

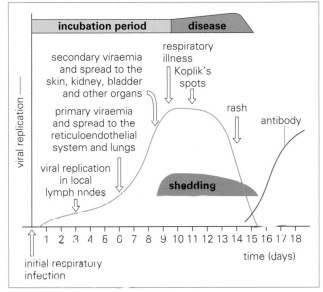

**Fig. 16.3** The pathogenesis of measles. Virus invades body surfaces from the blood, traversing blood vessels to reach surface epithelium first in the respiratory tract where there are only one to two layers of epithelial cells, then in mucosae (Koplik spots) and finally in the skin (rash).

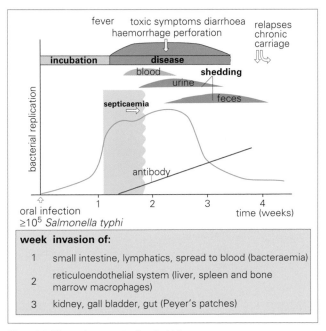

**Fig. 16.4** The pathogenesis of typhoid fever.

| week | invasion of: |
|------|--------------|
| 1 | small intestine, lymphatics, spread to blood (bacteraemia) |
| 2 | reticuloendothelial system (liver, spleen and bone marrow macrophages) |
| 3 | kidney, gall bladder, gut (Peyer's patches) |

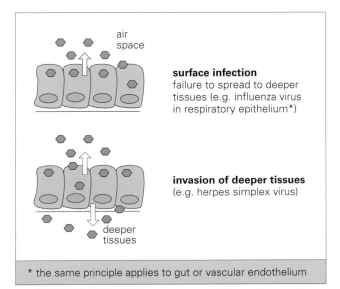

surface infection
failure to spread to deeper tissues (e.g. influenza virus in respiratory epithelium*)

invasion of deeper tissues
(e.g. herpes simplex virus)

* the same principle applies to gut or vascular endothelium

**Fig. 16.2** Topography of virus release from epithelial surfaces can determine the pattern of infection.

**Table 16.1** Replication rates of different microorganisms

| Microorganisms | Situation | Mean doubling time |
|---|---|---|
| Most viruses | In cell[a] | <1 h |
| Many bacteria (e.g. *Escherichia coli*, staphylococci) | In vitro | 20–30 min |
| *Salmonella typhimurium* | In vitro<br>In vivo | 30 min<br>5–12 h |
| *Mycobacterium tuberculosis* | In vitro<br>In vivo | 24 h<br>Many days |
| *Mycobacterium leprae*[b] | In vivo | 2 wk |
| *Treponema pallidum*[b] | In vivo | 30 h |
| *Plasmodium falciparum* | In vitro/in vivo (erythrocyte or hepatic cell) | 8 h |

[a]But some viruses show greatly delayed replication or delayed spread from cell to cell.
[b]But cannot be cultivated in vitro.

meningitis, paralytic poliomyelitis). These pathogens are not shed to the exterior after multiplying in the meninges or spinal cord.

For the pathogen, systemic spread is fraught with obstacles, and a major encounter with immune and other defences is inevitable. Microorganisms have, therefore, been forced to develop strategies for bypassing or countering these defences (see Ch. 17).

### Rapid replication is essential for surface infections

The rate of replication of the infecting microorganism is of central importance, and doubling times vary from 20 minutes to several days (Table 16.1). Hit-and-run (surface) infections need to replicate rapidly, whereas a microorganism that divides every few days (e.g. *Mycobacterium tuberculosis*) is likely to cause a slowly evolving disease with a long incubation period. Microorganisms nearly always multiply faster in vitro than they do in the intact host, as might be expected if host defences are performing a useful function. In the host, microorganisms are phagocytosed and killed, and the supply of nutrients may be limited. The net increase in numbers is slower than in laboratory cultures in which pathogens are not only free from attack by host defences, but also every effort has been made to supply them with optimal nutrients, susceptible cells and so on.

## MECHANISMS OF SPREAD THROUGH THE BODY

### Spread to lymph and blood

#### Invading pathogens encounter a variety of defences on entering the body

After traversing the epithelium and its basement membrane at the body surface, invading pathogens face the following defences:

- Tissue fluids containing antimicrobial substances (antibody, complement).
- Local macrophages (histiocytes). Subcutaneous and submucosal macrophages are a threat to microbial survival.
- The physical barrier of local tissue structure. Local tissues consist of various cells in a hydrated gel matrix; although viruses can spread by stepwise invasion of cells, invasion is more difficult for bacteria, and those that spread effectively sometimes possess special spreading factors (e.g. streptococcal hyaluronidase).
- The lymphatic system. The rich network of the lymphatic system soon conveys microorganisms to the battery of phagocytic and immunologic defences awaiting them in the local lymph node (Fig. 16.5). Macrophages, strategically placed in the marginal and other lymph sinuses, constitute an efficient filtering system for lymph.

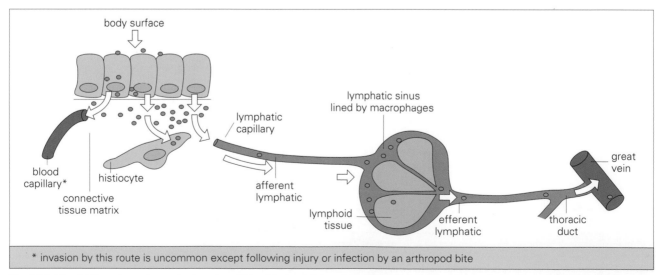

**Fig. 16.5** Microbial invasion and spread to lymph and blood. Pathogens (or other particles) beneath surface epithelium readily enter local lymphatics.

The infection may be halted at any stage, but, by multiplying locally or in lymph nodes and by evading phagocytosis, the microorganism can ultimately reach the bloodstream. Therefore a minor injury to the skin followed by a red streak (inflamed lymphatic) and a tender, swollen local lymph node are classic signs of streptococcal invasion. Most bacteria cause a great deal of inflammation when they invade in this way. In the early stages, lymph flow increases, but eventually, if there is enough inflammation and tissue damage in the node itself, the flow of the lymph may cease. In contrast, viruses and other intracellular microorganisms often invade lymph and blood silently and asymptomatically during the incubation period; this is facilitated when they infect monocytes or lymphocytes without initially damaging them.

## Spread from blood

### The fate of microorganisms in the blood depends upon whether they are free or associated with circulating cells

Viruses or small numbers of bacteria can enter the blood without causing a general body disturbance. For instance, transient bacteraemias are fairly common in normal individuals and may occur after defecation or brushing teeth, but the bacteria are usually filtered out and destroyed in macrophages lining the liver and spleen sinusoids. Under certain circumstances, the same bacteria have a chance to localize in less well-defended sites such as congenitally abnormal heart valves in the case of viridans streptococci, causing infective endocarditis, or in the ends of growing bones in the case of *Staphylococcus aureus* osteomyelitis.

If microorganisms are free in the blood, they are exposed to body defences such as antibodies and phagocytes. However, if they are associated with circulating cells, these cells can protect them from host defences and carry them around the body. For example, many viruses (e.g. Epstein-Barr virus, rubella) and intracellular bacteria (*Listeria*, *Brucella*) are present in lymphocytes or monocytes, and, if not damaged or destroyed, these carrying cells protect and transport them. Malaria infects erythrocytes.

On entering the blood, microorganisms are exposed to macrophages of the reticuloendothelial system. Here, in the sinusoids where blood flows slowly, they are often phagocytosed and destroyed. But certain microorganisms survive and multiply in these cells (*Salmonella typhi*, *Leishmania donovani*, yellow fever virus). The microorganism may then:

- spread to adjacent hepatic cells in the liver (hepatitis viruses) or splenic lymphoid tissues (measles virus)
- reinvade the blood (*S. typhi*, hepatitis viruses).

### Each circulating microorganism invades characteristic target organs and tissues

If uptake by reticuloendothelial macrophages is not complete within a short time or if large numbers of microorganisms are present in the blood, there is an opportunity for localization elsewhere in the vascular system. Why each circulating microorganism invades characteristic target organs and tissues (Table 16.2) is not completely understood, but may be due to:

- specific receptors for the microorganism leading to localization on the vascular endothelium of certain target organs

**Table 16.2** Circulating microorganisms that invade organs via small blood vessels

| Pathogen | Disease | Principal organs invaded[a] |
|---|---|---|
| **Viruses** | | |
| Hepatitis B virus | Hepatitis B | Liver |
| Rubella virus | Congenital rubella | Placenta (fetus) |
| Varicella-zoster virus | Chickenpox | Skin, respiratory tract |
| Polio virus | Poliomyelitis | Brain, spinal cord |
| Mumps virus | Mumps | Parotid, testes, ovaries, central nervous system, pancreas |
| Zika virus | Microcephaly | Brain |
| **Bacteria** | | |
| *Rickettsia rickettsii* | Rocky Mountain spotted fever | Skin |
| *Treponema pallidum* | Secondary syphilis | Skin, mucosae |
| *Neisseria meningitidis* | Meningitis | Meninges |
| **Protozoa** | | |
| *Trypanosoma cruzi* | Chagas disease | Heart, skeletal muscle |
| *Plasmodium* spp. | Malaria | Liver |
| **Fungi** | | |
| *Talaromyces marneffei* | Talaromycosis | Skin |
| *Cryptococcus neoformans* | Cryptococcosis | Brain |
| **Helminths** | | |
| *Schistosoma* spp. (larvae) | Schistosomiasis | Veins of bladder, bowel |
| *Ascaris lumbricoides* (larvae) | Ascariasis | Lung |
| *Ancylostoma duodenale* (larvae) | Hookworm | Lung |

[a]In liver and sinusoids; elsewhere, in capillaries and venules.

- subsequent colonization and replication
- accumulation of circulating pathogens in sites where there is local inflammation because of the slower flow and sticky endothelium in inflamed vessels.

After localization and organ invasion, the replicating pathogen is shed from the body if the organ has a surface with access to the outside world. It may also be shed back into the bloodstream, either directly or via the lymphatic system.

## Spread via nerves

### Certain viruses spread via peripheral nerves from peripheral parts of the body to the central nervous system and vice versa

Tetanus toxin reaches the central nervous system (CNS) by this route. Rabies, herpes simplex virus and varicella-zoster virus travel in axons, and, although the rate is slow, being accounted for by axonal flow (up to 10 mm/h), this movement is important in the pathogenesis of these infections. Rabies not only reaches the CNS largely by peripheral nerves but also takes the same route from the CNS when it invades the salivary glands. Few, if any, host defences are in a position to control this type of viral spread once nerves are invaded.

An uncommon route of spread to the CNS is via olfactory nerves with axons terminating on olfactory mucosa. For instance, certain free-living amoebae (e.g. *Naegleria* spp.) found in sludge at the bottom of freshwater pools may take this route and cause meningoencephalitis in swimmers. Viruses and bacteria in the nasopharynx (e.g. meningococci, poliovirus) generally spread to the CNS via the blood.

## Spread via cerebrospinal fluid

### Once microorganisms have crossed the blood–cerebrospinal barrier, they spread rapidly in the cerebrospinal fluid spaces

Such microorganisms can then invade neural tissues (e.g. echoviruses, mumps virus) as well as multiply locally (*Neisseria meningitidis*, *Haemophilus influenzae*, *Streptococcus pneumoniae*) and possibly infect ependymal and meningeal cells.

## Spread via other routes

### Rapid spread from one visceral organ to another can take place via the pleural or peritoneal cavity

Both the pleural and peritoneal cavities are lined by macrophages, as if in expectation of such invasion, and the peritoneal cavity contains an antimicrobial armoury consisting of the omentum (the abdominal policeman) and many lymphocytes, macrophages and mast cells. Injury or disease in an abdominal organ provides a source of infection for peritonitis as do chest wounds or lung infections for pleurisy.

## GENETIC DETERMINANTS OF SPREAD AND REPLICATION

### The pathogenicity of a microorganism is determined by the interplay of a variety of factors

These factors are referred to in Chapters 13 and 17. A distinction is sometimes made between pathogenicity and virulence. Virulence implies a quantitative measure of pathogenicity. For instance, it can be expressed as the number of organisms necessary to cause death in 50% of individuals (i.e. lethal dose 50, or LD50). Nearly all pathogenicity factors are controlled by host and microbial genes. It has long been known that there are host genetic influences on susceptibility to infectious disease and that mutations in microorganisms affect their pathogenicity. A number of these genetic factors have been revealed by the application of molecular genetics techniques, and, as a result, it is increasingly possible to identify the specific gene products involved. Progress has also been made, although with greater difficulty, in understanding the mode of action of these gene products.

### Genetic determinants in the host

#### The ability of a microorganism to infect and cause disease in a given host is influenced by the genetic constitution of the host

At a relatively gross level, some human pathogens either do not infect other species or infect only closely related primates (e.g. measles, trachoma, typhoid, hepatitis B, warts), whereas others infect a very wide range of hosts (e.g. rabies, anthrax). Also, within a given host species, there are genetic determinants of susceptibility. The best examples are found in animals, but there are examples for human disease (see later).

One example at the molecular level is the sickle cell gene and susceptibility to malaria. Malaria merozoites (see Ch. 28) parasitize red blood cells and metabolize haemoglobin, freeing haem and using globin as a source of amino acids. The sickle cell gene causes a substitution of the amino acid valine for glutamic acid at one point in the b-polypeptide chain of the haemoglobin molecule. The new haemoglobin (haemoglobin S) becomes insoluble when reduced and precipitates inside the red cell envelope, distorting the cell into the shape of a sickle. In homozygous individuals there are two of these genes, and the individual has the disease sickle cell anaemia because the red cells are so fragile that they sickle under normal circumstances. But in the heterozygote (sickle cell trait), the gene is less harmful and provides resistance to severe forms of *Plasmodium falciparum* malaria, which ensures its selection in endemic malarial regions. The gene would be eliminated from populations after 10 to 20 generations unless it conferred some advantage. Restriction endonuclease analyses of the gene in Indian and West African populations revealed it arose independently in these malarious countries. Homozygotes, however, show increasing susceptibility to other infections, particularly *S. pneumoniae*, as a result of splenic dysfunction following repeated splenic infarcts.

Other examples are individuals who are nonsecretors of ABO blood groups due to homozygosity for a fucosyltransferase 2 variant that is critical for AB antigen synthesis and are completely resistant to norovirus infections that cause diarrhoea. Almost total resistance to human immunodeficiency virus 1 infection and new variant Creutzfeldt-Jakob disease is seen in individuals homozygous for a 32-base pair deletion in the *CCR5* chemokine receptor gene and those homozygous for valine at codon 129 of the prion protein gene, respectively.

The P blood group antigens are attachment sites for bacteria. Uropathogenic *Escherichia coli* binds the Pk antigen, and people with the P1k phenotype are at high risk of urinary tract infections and pyelonephritis. In addition, the *P. vivax* malarial parasite binds to Duffy-positive red blood cells, and people who are Duffy negative are relatively resistant to infection. Those with the p phenotype cannot develop parvovirus B19 infection as the

## Box 16.1 ■ Lessons in Microbiology

### Genetically determined susceptibility to infection

There are several classic examples of susceptibility to infectious disease determined by unidentified but presumably genetic factors in the human host.

### The Lubeck disaster due to vaccination with virulent tubercle bacilli

In Lubeck, Germany, between December 1929 and April 1930, three oral doses of living tubercle bacilli, instead of attenuated (vaccine) bacilli, were inadvertently given to 251 infants <10 days old. There were 72 deaths, 135 developed clinical tuberculosis but recovered and were alive and well 12 years later, while 44 became tuberculin positive but remained well. Each received the same inoculum, and it seems likely that the differences in outcome were largely due to genetic factors in the host. This disaster was a setback for early bacille Calmette–Guérin (BCG) enthusiasts. Dr. George Deycke, in whose laboratory the contaminated batch of BCG had been produced (but never tested for virulence before use), was tried, found guilty of manslaughter and injury by negligence and sent to prison, together with the director of the Lubeck Health Office.

### Identical twins are affected similarly by respiratory tuberculosis

A study of tuberculosis in twins when at least one twin had the disease showed that, for identical twins, the other twin was affected in 87% of cases. With nonidentical twins, the equivalent figure was only 26%. In addition, the identical twins had a similar type of clinical disease.

### A military misfortune due to contamination of yellow fever vaccine with hepatitis B virus

In 1942, >45,000 US military personnel were vaccinated against yellow fever but were inadvertently injected at the same time with hepatitis B virus present as a contaminant in the human serum used to stabilize the vaccine. There were 914 clinical cases of hepatitis, of which 580 were mild, 301 moderate, and 33 severe. Even with a given batch of vaccine, the incubation period varied in the range of 10–20 weeks. Serologic tests were not then available, so the number of subclinical infections is unknown. In this case both physiologic and genetic influences on susceptibility may have played a part.

**Table 16.3** Examples of attenuation of pathogens following repeated passage in vitro

| Pathogen | Passage | Attenuated (live) product |
| --- | --- | --- |
| *Mycobacterium bovis* | 10 years of repeated passage in glycerin–bile–potato medium | Bacille Calmette–Guérin (BCG) vaccine |
| Rubella virus | 27 passages in human diploid cells | Rubella vaccine (Wistar RA 27/3) |

receptor for B19 is the P antigen or globoside on the red blood cell. Thus heterogeneity in blood group antigens could have developed to protect humans against a variety of pathogens.

### Susceptibility often operates at the level of the immune response

A poor immune response to a given infection can lead to increased susceptibility to disease, whereas an immune response that is too vigorous may lead to immunopathologic disease (see Ch. 18). Of particular importance are the major histocompatibility complex (MHC) genes on chromosome 6, coding for MHC class II (human leucocyte antigen [HLA] DP, DQ, DR) antigens and controlling specific immune responses. For example, susceptibility to leprosy is strongly influenced by MHC class II genes. People with the HLA DR3 antigen are more susceptible to tuberculoid leprosy, whereas those with HLA DQ1 are more susceptible to lepromatous leprosy.

Studies of identical twins (Box 16.1) provide evidence that genetic determinants affect susceptibility to tuberculosis. The present-day European population shows considerable resistance to this disease. During the great epidemics of pulmonary tuberculosis in Europe in the 17th through 19th centuries, genetically susceptible individuals were weeded out. In 1850 mortality rates in Boston, New York, London, Paris and Berlin were over 500/100,000, but with improvements in living conditions, these fell to 180/100,000 by 1900, and they have fallen even more since then. However, previously unexposed populations, especially in Africa and the Pacific Islands, show much greater susceptibility to respiratory tuberculosis. In the Plains Indians living in the Qu'Appelle Valley reservation in Saskatchewan, Canada, in 1886 tuberculosis spread through the body to infect glands, bones, joints and meninges, giving a death rate of 9000/100,000.

### Genetic determinants in the pathogen

#### Virulence is often coded for by more than one microbial gene

Virulence is determined by numerous factors such as adhesion, penetration into cells, antiphagocytic activity, production of toxins and interaction with the immune system. Consequently, different genes and gene products are involved in different ways and at different stages in pathogenesis.

Under natural circumstances, microorganisms are constantly undergoing genetic change (i.e. mutations). The single-stranded RNA viruses in particular show very high mutation rates. Mutations affecting surface antigens undergo rapid selection in the host under immune pressure (antibody, cell-mediated immunity), as in the case of the rapidly evolving M proteins of streptococci and the capsid proteins of picornaviruses. In addition, genetic changes in bacteria are often due to acquisition or loss of genetic elements such as integrins, pathogenicity islands, transposons and plasmids (see Chs 3 and 34).

Changes in the virulence of a microorganism take place during artificial culture in the laboratory. For instance, in the classic procedure for obtaining a live vaccine, a microorganism is repeatedly grown (passaged) in vitro, and this generally leads to reduced pathogenicity in the host. The new strain is then referred to as *attenuated* (Table 16.3).

Our understanding of the genetic basis for microbial pathogenicity has advanced, owing to genetic manipulation techniques such as cloning, site-specific mutagenesis and clustered regularly interspaced short palindromic repeats (CRISPR)–Cas9. For instance, by introducing or deleting/inactivating genome segments, the virulence genes can be identified. CRISPR-Cas9 is an editing technique borrowed from bacteria. In 1987 it was found that *E. coli* had a system that could cut out parts of viral DNA when attacked and store it to ensure they could recognize it and had a defence for it if needed in the future. The technique allows editing of parts of the genome by deleting, adding or altering the DNA sequence. The Cas9 enzyme cuts the two strands of DNA at a specific place in the genome so that bits of DNA can then be added or removed. This is done by a predesigned small piece of RNA sequence (~20 bases long) nested in a longer piece of RNA that acts as a scaffold that binds to DNA. The small piece of RNA, known as a guide RNA, directs the Cas9 enzyme to the part of the genome of interest where it is cut, damaging the DNA. The cellular RNA repair machinery takes over, thus the change is introduced.

Major advances in genomics, including high-throughput rapid DNA sequencing and bioinformatics, have made major contributions to our understanding of virulence genes and conditions affecting their expression. This has allowed sequencing of the entire genome for many infectious agents (bacteria and viruses). This information has facilitated the assignment of virulence functions to specific loci and greatly improved our understanding of the way microorganisms sense and respond to the host environment.

## OTHER FACTORS AFFECTING SPREAD AND REPLICATION

Various other factors have an influence on susceptibility to infectious disease (Table 16.4). In most cases it is not known whether this involves differences in microbial spread and

**Table 16.4** Host factors influencing susceptibility to infectious diseases

| Factor | Example | Alteration in susceptibility | Mechanism |
|---|---|---|---|
| Host genetics | Human immunodeficiency virus (HIV) | Delayed progression to acquired immunodeficiency syndrome (AIDS)<br>Protection against HIV | Human leucocyte antigen (HLA)-A, -B, -C heterozygosity<br>C-C Chemokine receptor (CCR) *Δ32* mutation coreceptor heterozygosity<br>CCR5 *Δ32* mutation coreceptor homozygosity |
| | Tuberculosis (TB) | Increased susceptibility | Variants in major histocompatibility complex (MHC) class II region |
| | Leprosy | Increased susceptibility | Human leukocyte antigen – DR isotype (HLA-DR) region |
| | Malaria | Protection against malaria | Haemoglobinopathies: sickle cell anaemia, thalassaemia, glucose-6-phosphate dehydrogenase deficiency |
| | Hepatitis C | Resolution of infection | Polymorphisms in the gene encoding interferon (IFNλ3) interleukin (previously *IL28B*) |
| | Parvovirus B19 | Protection against parvovirus infection | Individuals with the p phenotype (red blood cell P antigen is the cell receptor for parvovirus B19) |
| Pregnancy | Hepatitis E virus | Maternal mortality 10–30% in third trimester | ?Increased metabolic burden for liver in pregnancy/immune response |
| | Zika virus | Congenital Zika syndrome, especially fetal microcephaly | Zika virus antigen found in cytoplasm of degenerating and necrotic neurons and glial cells |
| | Urinary infections | Pyelonephritis more common | Reduced peristalsis in ureter |
| Malnutrition | Measles | More severe; more lethal | Vitamin A deficiency; depressed CMI |
| Age | Respiratory syncytial virus | More severe; more lethal in infant | Small diameter of airways |
| | Mumps, chickenpox, Epstein-Barr virus infection | More severe in adult | ?Increased immunopathology |
| Atmospheric pollution | Raised sulphur dioxide levels | Excess acute respiratory disease | ?Interference with mucociliary defences |
| | Silicosis | Increased susceptibility to tuberculosis | ?Damage to lung macrophages |
| Foreign bodies | Necrotic bone fragments | Chronic osteomyelitis more common | Antimicrobial defences less effective in necrotic tissue |
| | Necrotic tissues | Increased susceptibility to *Clostridium perfringens* | Anaerobic necrotic tissues favour bacterial growth |

**Table 16.4** Host factors influencing susceptibility to infectious diseases—cont'd

| Factor | Example | Alteration in susceptibility | Mechanism |
|--------|---------|------------------------------|-----------|
| Stress, hormones | Decreased glucocorticoid production: Addison disease | Increased susceptibility to infection | ?Hypersensitivity to inflammatory/immune responses |
| | Increased glucocorticoid production: steroid therapy | Increased susceptibility to infection | Reduction in protective immune/inflammatory responses |

CMI, Cell-mediated immunity.

replication or differences in host immune and inflammatory responses. Infections in hosts with immunologic and other defects are described in Chapter 31.

### The brain can influence immune responses

When stress (a loosely used word) is associated with malnutrition or crowding, it may be difficult to disentangle the separate influences of these various factors on susceptibility to infection as in the case of tuberculosis. The brain can, however, influence immune responses, acting via the hypothalamus, pituitary and adrenal cortex. It has long been known that glucocorticoids, which have powerful actions on immune cells, are needed for resistance to infection and trauma. A shortage of glucocorticoids, as in Addison disease, or an excess, as with steroid therapy, results in increased susceptibility to infection (see Table 16.4). In addition, the brain and the endocrine and immune systems often use the same molecular messengers: cytokines, peptide hormones and neurotransmitters. Neural cells, for instance, have receptors for interferons and for interleukins IL-1, IL-2, IL-3 and IL-6, and thymic lymphocytes can produce prolactin and growth hormone. Immune–neuroendocrine crosstalk now has molecular respectability and provides an acceptable basis for the influence of the brain on immunity and infectious disease.

## KEY FACTS

- Infections restricted to the body surfaces (e.g. common cold, *Shigella* dysentery) have shorter incubation periods than do systemic infections (e.g. measles, typhoid), and adaptive (immune) host responses tend to be less important.

- Pathogens with a slow growth rate (e.g. *M. tuberculosis*) tend to cause diseases that evolve slowly.

- Spread through the body takes place primarily via lymph and blood. The fate of circulating pathogens depends on whether they are free or present in circulating blood cells.

- Uptake by reticuloendothelial cells in liver and spleen focuses infection into these organs, but specific localization in the vascular bed of other organs (e.g. mumps virus

in salivary glands, meningococci in meninges) is not understood.

- Viruses can spread in either direction along nerve axons, and this is important in the pathogenesis of recurrent herpes simplex virus infection, varicella zoster and rabies.

- Pathogenicity and virulence are strongly influenced by genetic factors in the host (e.g. tuberculosis in identical twins) and by genetic factors in the pathogen (e.g. sickle cell trait in *P. falciparum* malaria).

- Our understanding of virulence has been greatly enhanced by advances in molecular biology, which have allowed sequence analysis of entire microbial genomes and a clearer view of microbial response to the host environment.

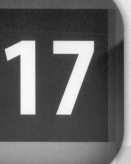

# Parasite survival strategies and persistent infections

## Introduction

### The most common pathogens have developed answers to host defences

So far, we have concentrated on the battery of mechanisms available to the host, both innate and adaptive, to keep out and destroy pathogens. Powerful as these are, they are obviously not 100% effective; otherwise healthy people would never have infections. In fact, most of the common infectious organisms described in this book have developed answers to host defences that enable them to survive as human parasites. They successfully infect humans and are of concern to the physician precisely because they have developed strategies for evading or actively interfering with host defences. This may take the form of several skirmishes before there is a decisive battle outcome, with the pathogen looking for a suitable environment where it might avoid the host immune response.

## Strategies to evade innate nonadaptive defences such as the phagocyte

These are many and include the following:

- *Avoiding being killed by phagocytes.* Successful parasites have evolved numerous ingenious antiphagocytic devices (Fig. 17.1). These range from avoiding being phagocytosed, not being killed if phagocytosed and killing or inhibiting the phagocyte itself. Some bacteria such as *Mycobacterium tuberculosis* inhibit phagosome-lysosome fusion; others such as *Listeria* break out of the phagolysosome by punching holes in the membranes and escaping into the cytoplasm. If a microorganism can survive within the phagocyte, this poses a very serious challenge to the host.
- *Interfering with ciliary action* (see Table 14.3).
- *Interfering with neutrophil extracellular traps (NETs).* Bacteria such as *Staphylococcus aureus* try to avoid being trapped by NETs (Fig. 15.2) by secreting DNAses; *Leishmania* promastigotes produce 3'-nucleotidase/nuclease to help their escape from NETs. However, sometimes organisms want to increase NET formation; *M. avium intracellulare* strains induce NET formation and interleukin 8 (IL-8) production, leading to attraction of more neutrophils and inflammation and leading to the progression of lung infection.
- *Production of biofilms.* Staphylococci produce biofilms to help their survival.
- *Interfering with the activation of complement.* Microorganisms can acquire or mimic complement regulators, actively inhibit complement components or enzymatically destroy complement components. A variety of pathogens can bind complement regulators, including *Escherichia coli*, streptococci and *Candida albicans*. The smallpox and vaccinia viruses produce proteins that mimic host complement regulators. *S. aureus*, streptococci, herpes simplex virus (HSV), *Schistosoma* and *Trypanosoma* express complement inhibitors. The parasite *T. cruzi* expresses five complement regulatory proteins on its surface. *Pseudomonas* bacteria produce an elastase that inactivates the C3b and C5a components of complement; other

proteases that destroy complement components are produced by *Pseudomonas*, *Serratia marcescans* and *Schistosoma mansoni*. *S. aureus* has a surface immunoglobulin binding protein and an extracellular fibrinogen binding protein that generate plasmin to degrade C3 and C3b. Another strategy is to physically block complement lysis — the insertion of the C567 complex is prevented by the long side chains of the cell wall polysaccharides of smooth strains of *Salmonellae* and by the capsules of staphylococci, which do not activate complement, and the cell wall of gram-positive bacteria prevents lysis by the complement membrane attack complex (Fig. 17.2). However, some pathogens take the opposite approach, choosing to enter host cells by exploiting opsonization with complement components: Human immunodeficiency virus (HIV)–1 and *M. tuberculosis* exploit the CR3 receptor in this way.

- *Producing iron-binding molecules.* Nearly all bacteria need iron, but the host's iron-binding proteins such as transferrin limit the availability of this element. Accordingly, certain bacteria (e.g. *Neisseria*) produce their own powerful iron-binding proteins to circumvent the shortage.
- *Blocking type I interferons.* Host cells respond to double-stranded DNA (dsDNA) and double-stranded RNA (dsRNA) from infecting pathogens (including all viruses) by forming interferons alpha (IFNα) and beta (IFNβ); dsDNA in the cytoplasm is detected through the STING cytosolic DNA sensing pathway and dsRNA through cytoplasmic RIG-like receptors. These are produced rapidly, within 24 h after infection, and are part of the innate immune response (see Ch. 10). Certain viruses are either poor inducers of interferons (hepatitis B) or produce molecules that block the action of interferons in cells (hepatitis B, HIV, adenoviruses, Epstein-Barr virus [EBV], rotavirus, vaccinia virus).

### Many pathogens target the TLR signalling pathway

Signalling through the macrophage Toll-like receptors (TLRs; see Ch. 10) is essential for activation of many antimicrobial defences. The TLRs provide a series of cell surface and intracellular receptors with which the cell can sense

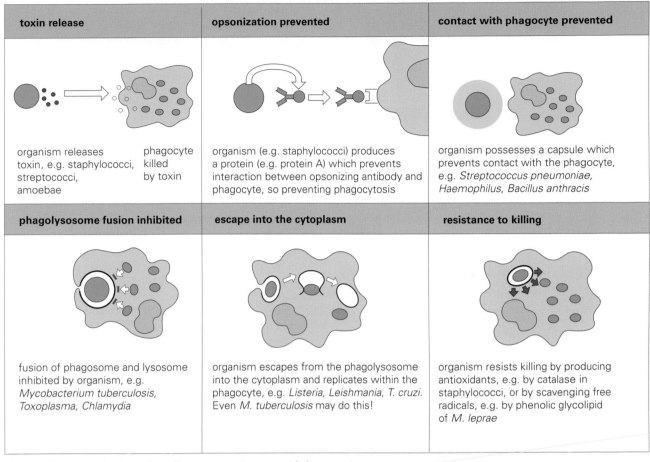

| toxin release | opsonization prevented | contact with phagocyte prevented |
|---|---|---|
| organism releases toxin, e.g. staphylococci, streptococci, amoebae    phagocyte killed by toxin | organism (e.g. staphylococci) produces a protein (e.g. protein A) which prevents interaction between opsonizing antibody and phagocyte, so preventing phagocytosis | organism possesses a capsule which prevents contact with the phagocyte, e.g. *Streptococcus pneumoniae*, *Haemophilus*, *Bacillus anthracis* |
| **phagolysosome fusion inhibited** | **escape into the cytoplasm** | **resistance to killing** |
| fusion of phagosome and lysosome inhibited by organism, e.g. *Mycobacterium tuberculosis*, *Toxoplasma*, *Chlamydia* | organism escapes from the phagolysosome into the cytoplasm and replicates within the phagocyte, e.g. *Listeria*, *Leishmania*, *T. cruzi*. Even *M. tuberculosis* may do this! | organism resists killing by producing antioxidants, e.g. by catalase in staphylococci, or by scavenging free radicals, e.g. by phenolic glycolipid of *M. leprae* |

**Fig. 17.1** Various mechanisms adopted by microorganisms to avoid phagocytosis.

infectious organisms. These receptors are clearly very important to host defence, as there are now >70 examples of bacteria and viruses interfering with signalling through the TLRs (Table 17.1). Following TLR binding, a complex series of intracellular events take place, with the TLR cytoplasmic tail interacting with adaptor molecules, recruiting serine threonine kinases, ubiquitin ligases, production of a polyubiquitin scaffold, further phosphorylation events in protein complexes and the eventual activation and translocation to the nucleus of transcription factors such as nuclear factor kappa B. Most of these steps can be targeted by bacteria or viruses.

Adaptor proteins allow larger signalling complexes to be made that elicit a response from the cell to the environment. For example, hepatitis C virus can cleave the adaptor molecule TRIF that interacts with TLR3 and 4, blocking signalling.

### Strategies to evade adaptive defences

#### Strategies to evade adaptive defences are more sophisticated than those for evading innate defences

The strategies that pathogens use to evade or interfere with adaptive (immune) defences are more sophisticated than those for evading innate defences because antigen-specific lymphocytes have cell receptors that can recognize virtually any shape (B cells) or amino acid sequence (T cells), provided it is not identical to self. For example:

- The polysaccharide capsules of bacteria and the fungus *Cryptococcus neoformans* prevent nonimmune contact between phagocytes and the bacterial cell wall but are quickly recognized as foreign by B-cell surface receptors (immunoglobulin), leading to the formation of antibody with consequent opsonization and phagocytosis of the organism.
- Many microorganisms such as bacteria and fungi can resist intracellular destruction by macrophages, but if their peptides are presented in association with major histocompatibility complex (MHC) molecules on the macrophage surface, their presence is detected by T cells. This enables T-helper (Th) cells to produce macrophage-activating cytokines like interferon gamma (IFNγ) and cytotoxic T (Tc) cells to kill the infected cell.

In both these examples, the T and B cells are behaving like a highly specialized and sharply observant secret police force that is more effective than the cells of the innate immune system.

### PARASITE SURVIVAL STRATEGIES

Parasite survival strategies can take as many forms as there are parasites, but they can be usefully classified by the immune component that is evaded and the means selected to do this. They enable the pathogen to undergo what are often quite lengthy periods of growth and spread during the incubation period before being shed and transmitted to the next host, as occurs in hepatitis B and tuberculosis. Shedding of the pathogen for just a few extra days after clinical recovery also gives more extensive transmission in the community, and this is a worthwhile result for the pathogen. A person who has recovered from norovirus or rotavirus may remain infectious for up to 2 weeks after recovery from the clinical symptoms.

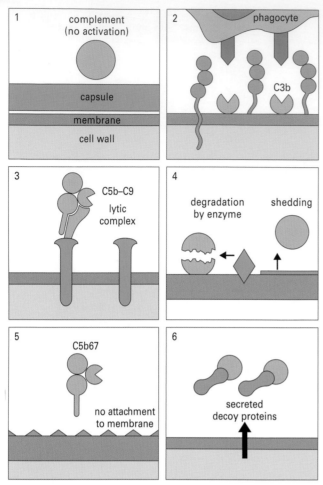

**Fig. 17.2** Bacteria avoid complement-mediated damage by a variety of strategies. (1) An outer capsule or coat prevents complement activation. (2) An outer surface can be configured so that complement receptors on phagocytes cannot obtain access to fixed C3b. (3) Surface structures can be expressed that divert attachment of the lytic membrane attack complex from the cell membrane. (4) Membrane-bound enzyme can degrade fixed complement or cause it to be shed. (5) Complement inhibitors can be captured onto the surface. (6) Direct inhibition of the C3 and C5 convertases blocks complement activation. (Panels 1–4 from Male D, Brostoff J, Roth DB, et al. *Immunology*, Mosby Elsevier; 2021.)

## Viruses are particularly good at hindering immune defences

Viruses are able to impede immune defences for a number of reasons:

- Their invasion of tissues and cells is often silent. Unlike most bacteria, they do not form toxins, and, as long as they do not cause extensive cell destruction, there is no sign of illness until the onset of immune and inflammatory responses, sometimes several weeks after infection, as occurs in hepatitis B virus (HBV) and EBV infections.
- Viruses such as rubella virus, wart viruses, HBV and EBV can infect cells for long periods without adverse effects on cell viability.

## Some pathogens are able to persist in the host for even longer

Certain pathogens can remain (persist) in the host for many years or, often, for life. From the pathogen's point of view, persistence is worthwhile only if shedding occurs during the persistence (Box 17.1).

Virus latency is a type of persistence and is based on an intimate molecular relationship with the infected cell. The viral genome continues to be present in the host without continuously producing antigens or infectious material until the virus reactivates (becomes patent).

## Strategies for evading host defences include causing a rapid hit-and-run infection

One evasion strategy for microorganisms is to cause a rapid hit-and-run infection. The pathogen invades, multiplies and is shed within a few days, before adaptive immune defences have had time to come into action. Infections of the body surfaces (rhinoviruses, rotaviruses) come into this category. Otherwise, the principal strategies employed by parasites to elude the lymphocyte adaptive responses are concealment of antigens, antigenic variation and immunosuppression.

## CONCEALMENT OF ANTIGENS

A spy in a foreign country can conceal their presence from the police by hiding, by never venturing out of doors, or

**Table 17.1** Many pathogens interfere with the Toll-like receptor (TLR) signalling pathways

| Step targeted | Pathogen | Result |
|---|---|---|
| TLR expression | *Filaria* | ↓NF-κB activation |
| TLR binding | *Staphylococcus aureus* | SSL3 and SSL4 proteins bind TLR2 ectodomain; production of biofilms also reduces TLR2 and TLR9 signalling |
| Supramolecular organizing centre | *Escherichia coli* | Blocks TIR–TIR interactions |
| TRAF6 and TAK1 protein ubiquitination and activation | Epstein-Barr virus | Deubiquinates TRAF6 |
| Mitogen-activated protein kinases | Ebola virus | Blocks p38 phosphorylation |
| IKK complex | Vaccinia virus | Binds IKKβ |
| Transcription factors | *Shigella flexneri* | Inhibits nuclear translocation of NF-κB |

The complex signalling pathways that follow TLR binding are targeted by a range of pathogens. TLRs interact first with intracellular sorting adaptor proteins that recruit signalling adaptor proteins with formation of a supramolecular organizing centre where multiprotein complexes coordinate responses to microbes and cytokines. These activate an E3 ubiquitin ligase and further proteins activate mitogen-activated protein kinases. The I kappa kinase (IKK) complex enables ubiquinization that promotes further activation and signalling, which ultimately leads to activation of transcription factors that translocate to the nucleus (see Fig. 10.10). SSL, Staphylococcal superantigen-like; TIR, Toll/IL-1 receptor/resistance (TIR domains on TLRs and adaptor proteins; TAK, transforming growth factor beta (TGFβ)–activated kinase; TRAF, tumour necrosis factor (TNF) receptor–associated family.

For more details, see Rosadini CV, Kagan JG. Early innate immune responses to bacterial LPS. *Curr Opin Immunol.* 2015;32:61–70.

## Box 17.1 ■ Lessons in Microbiology

### Trail of illness from a slippery cook

In 1901 Mary Mallon, from Long Island, New York, took a job as cook with a family in New York City. Soon afterward, the family washerwoman and a visitor to the house became ill with enteric fever (typhoid). Mary moved to another job and a few weeks later all seven family members plus two of the servants came down with enteric fever. Similar infections followed her movements as a cook, and in 1906 the authorities tried to dissuade her from such work. She was indignant at the suggestion that she was carrying a dangerous germ, knowing that she was healthy, and failed to keep promises to have regular checks and give up work. She was suspicious of officials and aggressive, on one occasion advancing toward the questioner brandishing a carving knife. She was later arrested and put in an isolation hospital. After appealing to the US Supreme Court, she was released in 1910 promising not to work as a cook. Then in 1914 typhoid epidemics broke out in a hospital and in a sanatorium where she had worked as a cook. She was traced, living under a false name, and in the interests of public safety she was detained permanently on North Brother Island, where she died in 1938. In her cooking career she had been responsible for about 200 cases of typhoid in eight different families and had started seven epidemics of the disease. Her favourite recipe, an iced peaches dessert, may have been a good source of infection.

Mary had recovered fully from an attack of typhoid earlier in life, but she had gallstones; this enabled the bacteria to persist in her gallbladder for many years, appearing intermittently in the faeces. About 5% of cases become carriers in either the gallbladder or the urinary bladder, and they play a central role as foci of infection. Nowadays, Mary would have to have acquired her original infection in a region such as the Indian subcontinent, where typhoid is endemic. Each year there are ~21 million typhoid cases worldwide, 300 of which are confirmed cases in the United States, most being travellers to the Indian subcontinent (see also Ch. 23).

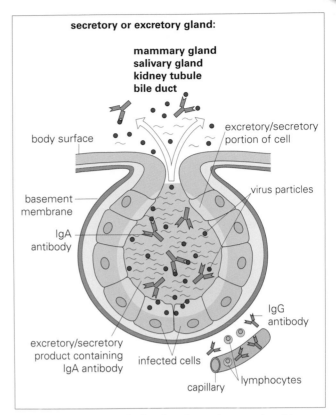

**Fig. 17.3** Viral infection of cell surfaces facing the external world. Infection of the surface epithelium of, for instance, a secretory or excretory gland allows direct shedding of the virus to the exterior, as well as avoidance of host immune defences. Ig, Immunoglobulin.

by adopting the disguise of a local. Parasites have the same options. Places to hide include the interior of host cells (although the MHC molecules act as informers for this compartment, picking up and transporting microbial peptides to the cell surface where they will be recognized) and particular sites in the body where lymphocytes do not normally circulate (privileged sites, the equivalent of no-go areas or safe houses).

### Remaining inside cells without their antigens being displayed on the surface prevents recognition

If a pathogen can remain inside cells without allowing its antigens to be displayed on the cell surface, it will remain unrecognized (incognito) as far as immune defences are concerned. Even if specific antibody and T-cell responses have been induced, the pathogen inside such a cell is unaffected. Persistent latent viruses such as HSV in sensory neurones behave in this way. During reactivation, antigenic boosting of immune defences is, however, inevitable.

Other strategies are possible. Several viruses (HIV in macrophages, coronaviruses) display their proteins secretly on the walls of intracellular vacuoles instead of at the cell surface and bud into these vacuoles. Adenoviruses have taken more

active steps to avoid antigen display. One of the adenoviral proteins (E19) combines with class I MHC molecules and prevents their passage to the cell surface so that infected cells are not recognized by Tc cells.

### Colonizing privileged sites keeps the pathogen out of reach of circulating lymphocytes

The vast numbers of pathogens that colonize the skin and the intestinal lumen, together with those that are shed directly into external secretions, are effectively out of reach of circulating lymphocytes. They are exposed to secretory antibodies, which, although able to bind to the microbe (e.g. influenza virus) and render it less infectious, are generally unable to kill the pathogen or control its replication in or on the epithelial surface (Figs. 17.3 and 17.4). A local inflammatory response, however, can enhance host defences.

Within the body it is more difficult to avoid lymphocytes and antibodies, but certain sites are safer than others. These include the central nervous system, joints, testes and placenta. Here, lymphocyte circulation is less intense, there may be fewer dendritic cells to present foreign antigens and access of antibodies and complement is more restricted. Soluble factors such as TGFβ or cell-bound inhibitors such as CD200, PD-1 and FasL also help to induce tolerance rather than a protective immune response in these shielded sites; however, as soon as inflammatory responses are induced, then lymphocytes, monocytes and antibodies are rapidly delivered and the site loses its privilege.

Additional privileged sites can be created by the infectious organism itself. A good example is the cystic echinococcal

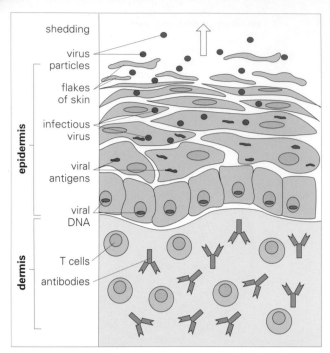

**Fig. 17.4** Wart virus replication in epidermis—a privileged site? Cell differentiation such as keratinization controls virus replication, and, as a result, virus matures when it is physically removed from immune defences.

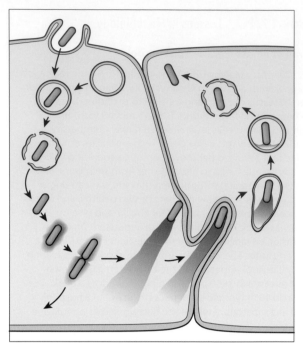

**Fig. 17.6** *Listeria* can move directly from cell to cell. Moving directly from one cell into another enables the bacteria to evade any harmful antibodies they might otherwise be exposed to. (Modified from Portnoy DA. Yogi Berra, Forrest Gump, and the discovery of Listeria actin comet tails. *Mol Biol Cell*. 2012;23(7):1141–1145.)

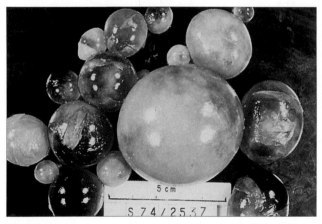

**Fig. 17.5** Cystic echinococcal (cystic hydatid) cysts. Multiple, fluid-filled cysts in a surgical specimen. The lung is a common site. Growing within a cyst is a survival strategy for *Echinococcus granulosus*. (Courtesy J.A. Innes.)

(cystic hydatid) cyst that develops in the liver, lung or brain around larval stages (protoscoleces) of the tapeworm *Echinococcus granulosus* (Fig. 17.5), inside which they can survive even though the blood of the host contains protective antibody. The TB granuloma (see Ch. 20) was thought to wall off the infection, but this is probably only true once the granuloma has calcified, as before then it seems both cells and antigens at least may leave.

Perhaps the most highly privileged site of all is host DNA, and this is occupied by the retroviruses. Retroviral RNA is transcribed by the enzyme reverse transcriptase into DNA as a necessary part of the replicative cycle, and this then becomes integrated into the DNA of the host cell (see Ch. 22). Once integrated, and as long as there is no cell damage and viral products are not expressed on the cell surface where they can be recognized by immune defences, the virus enjoys total anonymity. This is what makes complete removal of virus from a patient infected with HIV such a daunting task. The intragenomic site becomes even more privileged if the egg or sperm is infected. The viral genome will then be present in all embryonic cells and transferred from one generation to another as if it were the host's own DNA. Luckily, this does not happen with HIV or with human T-cell lymphotropic virus 1 and 2. However, the endogenous retroviruses of humans present in profusion as DNA sequences in our genome but not expressed as antigens come into this category. They are part of our inheritance. This surely represents the ultimate step in parasitism at the borderline between infection and heredity.

### Cell–cell spread is another effective way of avoiding exposure to harmful extracellular molecules

*Listeria* exploits its listeriolysin molecule to punch a hole in the phagosome membrane and escape into the cytoplasm of the cell. It can also move from cell to cell with minimal exposure to the exterior. It acts on actin regulatory factors, inducing the production of actin-rich protrusions, which can essentially inject the *Listeria* bacteria directly into the next cell without the immune system getting a chance to attack it (Fig. 17.6).

### Mimicry sounds like a useful strategy but does not prevent the host from making an antimicrobial response

If the pathogen can in some way avoid inducing an immune response, this can be regarded as a concealment of its antigens. One method is by mimicking host antigens, as such self antigens are not recognized as foreign. Some parasite-derived molecules resemble those of the host (Table 17.2). In the case of viral proteins, mimicry based on amino acid sequence homology (sharing of 8–10 consecutive amino acids) is seen to be common when sequence comparisons are made between viral

**Table 17.2** Some examples of mimicry or uptake of host antigens by parasites

| Pathogen's strategy | Parasite | Corresponding host antigen |
|---|---|---|
| Mimicry | Streptococci (M protein and N-acetyl-beta-D-glucosamine) | Cardiac myosin |
| | Mycobacterium tuberculosis | 65 kDa heat shock protein |
| | Treponema | Cardiolipin[a] |
| | Plasmodium falciparum | Vitronectin, thrombospondin[b] |
| | Trypanosoma cruzi | Heart myosin, nerve |
| Antigen uptake | Neisseria meningitidis, Trypanosoma cruzi trypomastigotes | Complement factor H |
| | Cytomegalovirus | $\beta_2$-Microglobulin |
| | Schistosoma | Glycolipids, HLA I, HLA II |
| | Ascaris | Blood group A, B antigens |

HLA, Human leukocyte antigen (major histocompatibility antigen).
[a]Basis for the original Wasserman-antibody test for syphilis developed in 1906.
[b]The homologous malaria protein thrombospondin-related anonymous protein shares an 18 amino acid sequence with the circumsporozoite protein that mediates binding to hepatocytes.

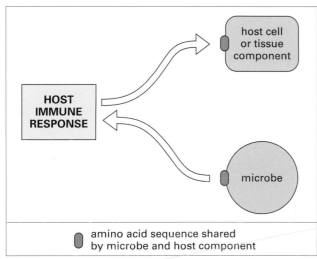

**Fig. 17.7** Molecular mimicry. Molecular mimicry by the pathogen can induce host cell damage. For example, rheumatic heart disease following streptococcal infection is caused by antibodies reacting with meromyosin (a component of myosin), the cross-reacting determinant.

and host proteins. Perhaps the most celebrated example is the cross-reaction between group A beta-haemolytic streptococci and human myocardium. This cross-reaction underlies the development of rheumatic heart disease following repeated streptococcal infection because of antibody made against the cross-reacting determinant meromyosin (Fig. 17.7). The fact that the host makes such autoantibodies shows that, in this case, mimicry does not prevent an antimicrobial host response.

### Pathogens can conceal themselves by taking up host molecules to cover their surface

This is illustrated in Table 17.2. A superb example of this is the blood fluke *Schistosoma*, as the schistosomulae acquire a surface coat of host blood group glycolipids and MHC antigens from the plasma. Such a parasite must indeed be virtually invisible to a T or B cell. For unknown reasons, this strategy is essentially restricted to helminths. Schistosomulae also take up decay, accelerating factor from human red cells, which blocks C3 activation and so complement-mediated lysis, while *T. cruzi* trypomastigotes bind factor H with the same effect.

The uptake of immunoglobulin molecules by a pathogen seems to be a more widespread phenomenon. A number of

viruses and bacteria produce immunoglobulin-binding proteins, which are displayed on their surface and bind immunoglobulin molecules of all specificities in an immunologically useless upside-down position (Fig. 17.8). This prevents the access of specific antibodies or T cells to the pathogen or the infected cell. *Mycoplasma* produce a unique immunoglobulin-binding protein that was recognized only in 2014; a better-known bacterial protein that binds immunoglobulins is staphylococcal protein A, a cell wall protein excreted from virulent staphylococci that inhibits the phagocytosis of antibody-coated bacteria. Certain herpesviruses (HSV, varicella-zoster virus [VZV], cytomegalovirus [CMV]) code for molecules that act as Fc receptors for IgG, and streptococci produce an Fc receptor for IgA.

### Immune modulation

Modulation of the host immune response by the pathogen can prevent this response from being an effective one. An alternative strategy for the pathogen is to avoid inducing an immune response or to induce a poor and ineffective response. Possible methods include:

- infection during early embryonic life
- the production of large quantities of the microbial antigen or of antigen–antibody complexes
- upsetting the balance between cell and antibody-mediated immune responses—or between Th cell 1 and 2 responses
- reducing the numbers or function of T or B cells by inducing apoptosis or leading to T-cell exhaustion as in sepsis
- inducing regulatory T cells (Tregs) or molecules that downregulate protective immunity.

Some vectors also help with immune evasion (e.g. ticks that cause Lyme disease secrete evasins that block chemokines, and the sandflies that transmit *Leishmania* have salivary proteins that increase immunomodulatory IL-10 production).

### Infection during early embryonic life

Before full development of the immune system, a time when antigens present are regarded as self, infection could possibly result in immune tolerance. However, in intrauterine infection with CMV, rubella virus and syphilis, the fetus does eventually produce IgM antibody, which is detectable in umbilical cord blood, but cell-mediated responses are more seriously impaired. Children with congenital CMV or rubella fail to develop lymphoproliferative responses to

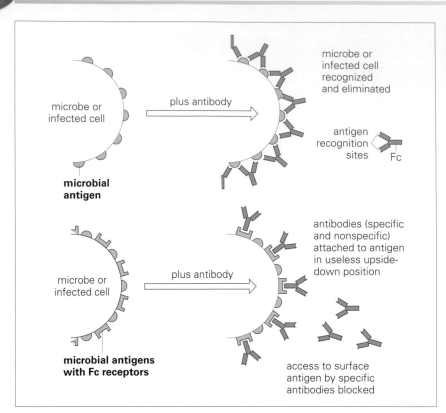

microbe or infected cell

plus antibody

microbe or infected cell recognized and eliminated

**microbial antigen**

antigen recognition sites

Fc

microbe or infected cell

plus antibody

antibodies (specific and nonspecific) attached to antigen in useless upside-down position

**microbial antigens with Fc receptors**

access to surface antigen by specific antibodies blocked

**Fig. 17.8** Evasion through production of Fc receptors. The production of Fc receptors is of some benefit to pathogens (e.g. staphylococci, streptococci, herpes simplex virus, varicella-zoster virus and cytomegalovirus).

CMV or rubella antigens and consequently take years to clear the virus from the body (see Ch. 24). In some cases, infection in the neonatal period is more likely to result in tolerance than infection in later life. Therefore neonatal infection with HBV frequently results in permanent carriage of the virus.

## Production of large quantities of microbial antigen or antigen–antibody complexes

Large quantities of microbial antigen or antigen–antibody complexes circulating in the body can cause immune tolerance to that antigen. Anergy, as evidenced by normal antibody but depressed cell-mediated immune responses to the invading pathogen, is seen in disseminated coccidioidomycosis and cryptococcosis as well as in visceral and diffuse cutaneous leishmaniasis, in each case associated with large amounts of microbial antigen in the circulation.

## Upsetting the balance between type 1 and type 2 cytokine responses

Resistance to infection often depends upon a suitable balance between Th1 and Th2 responses (see Ch. 11). Good defence against tuberculosis and herpesviruses needs cell-mediated immunity, whereas antibody is required to protect us against polioviruses or *Streptococcus pneumoniae*. In active tuberculosis, T cells making IL-4 can be detected with a reduction in the beneficial Th1 cytokine response. By inducing an ineffective type of Th2 response rather than effective Th1 activation, a pathogen can promote its own survival.

An altered Th1:Th2 balance can also drive macrophages to be classically activated or alternatively activated. Saliva from the *Leishmania* sandfly vector can reduce Th1 and increase Th2 cytokine production and IL-10, thus reducing macrophage activation by inducing alternatively activated macrophages. In helminth infections, as well as allergy, Th2 cytokines such as IL-4 and IL-13 induce alternatively activated macrophages

**Table 17.3** Infections in which regulatory T cells are induced

| | |
|---|---|
| *Bordetella pertussis* | Inhibit Th1 immunity |
| *Mycobacterium tuberculosis* | Inhibit Th1 immunity |
| *Helicobacter pylori* | Control peptic ulcer disease |
| Hepatitis B virus | Associated with viral load in serum |
| Hepatitis C virus | Suppress cytotoxic T-cell responses but also pathology |
| Herpes simplex virus | Reduce extent of inflammation |
| *Plasmodium falciparum* | Associated with higher parasitaemia |

Th, T-helper cell.

(classically activated macrophages are those activated by IFNγ). The Th2 cytokines play a role in helminth expulsion from the gut, with direct effects on epithelial cells and goblet cells, including mucous production and enhanced gut mobility through smooth muscle contraction and fluid secretion.

## Regulatory T cells

Some bacteria evade protective Th1 responses by inducing antigen-specific Tregs (originally called suppressor T cells). Tregs can be found in healthy individuals but can also be induced by exposure to antigen in the presence of transforming growth factor beta (TGFβ) and IL-10. *Bordetella pertussis* infection induces Tregs specific for its filamentous haemagglutinin and pertactin. These Tregs produce TGFβ and IL-10 and thus suppress Th1 immunity to two vital bacterial components that help the bacteria attach to host cells. Tregs are induced by many other bacteria, including *M. tuberculosis* in which lung granulomas contain Tregs and increased expression of TGFβ with reduced T-cell activation and production of beneficial IFNγ, during malaria infection and by some helminth antigens (Table 17.3).

**Fig. 17.9** Antigenic variation as a microbial strategy. The change in antigens may take place in the originally infected individual, enabling the pathogen to undergo renewed growth (e.g. in the variant surface genes in trypanosomiasis, relapsing fever [see Ch. 28]) or it may take place as the pathogen passes through the host population, enabling it to reinfect a given individual (e.g. influenza).

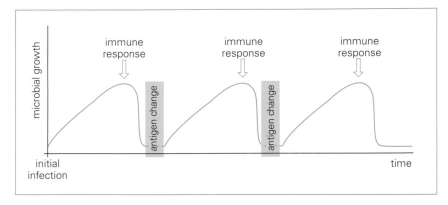

## ANTIGENIC VARIATION

Reverting to the metaphor of a spy in foreign territory, there is another way to confuse the enemy: by repeated changes in appearance. The African trypanosome, the causative organism of sleeping sickness, does this, and so do a wide range of other protozoa, viruses and bacteria. Antigenic variation can occur during:

- the course of infection in a given individual
- spread of the pathogen through the host community (Fig. 17.9).

As a strategy for evading host immune responses, antigenic variation depends upon variation occurring in antigens for which recognition is involved in protection. Antigenic variation is common as the pathogen passes through the host community. It tends to be more important in longer-lived hosts, such as humans in whom microbial survival is favoured by multiple reinfections during the lifetime of an individual. It is more common in infections limited to respiratory or intestinal epithelium for which the incubation period is <1 week and the pathogen can infect, multiply and be shed from the body before a significant secondary immune response is generated. During systemic infections (e.g. measles, mumps, typhoid) the incubation period is longer, and secondary responses have more opportunity to be mobilized and control an infection by an antigenic variant. Accordingly, antigenic variation is not an important feature of these systemic infections.

At the molecular level, there are three main mechanisms for antigenic variation: mutation, recombination and gene switching.

### The best-known example of mutation is the influenza virus

As the influenza virus spreads through the community, there are repeated mutations in the genes coding for haemagglutinin and neuraminidase (see Ch. 20), causing small antigenic changes that are sufficient to reduce the effectiveness of B- and T-cell memory built up in response to earlier infections. This is called *antigenic drift*. Human rhinoviruses and enteroviruses also evolve rapidly and show a similar antigenic drift. Antigenic drift could account for the wealth of antigenic types of staphylococci, streptococci and pneumococci. During earlier poliovirus epidemics, mutations occurred at the rate of about two base substitutions per week, some of them involving the main antigenic sites on the virus. HIV (see Ch. 22) undergoes antigenic drift, but in this case it occurs during infection of a given individual, which is why this infection is difficult for the immune system to control. Mutations affecting the epitopes recognized by Tc cells are the source of escape mutants.

### The classic example of antigenic variation using gene recombination involves influenza A virus

More extensive and sudden alterations in antigens can take place by the exchange of genetic material between two different pathogens. The classic example is genetic shift in influenza A virus (Fig. 17.10; also see Ch. 20). When human and avian virus strains recombine, a completely new strain of influenza A virus suddenly emerges, expressing a haemagglutinin or neuraminidase of avian origin. This new virus, not previously experienced by the present population, gives rise to an influenza pandemic. The 2009-2010 swine flu epidemic, which originated in Mexico, was caused by a H1N1 virus—segments of its genome were identified in flu isolates almost 20 years earlier, but gene reassortment led to the new pandemic strain (see Fig. 17.10). Surprisingly, it now seems that the 1918 Spanish flu pandemic may not have been caused by antigenic shift but instead by an avian flu that became able to infect humans.

### Mutations in the Severe acute respiratory syndrome coronavirus 2 (SARS-CoV-2) virus led to variants of concern

As discussed in Chapter 33, during the coronavirus disease 2019 (COVID-19) pandemic, mutations in the viral genome led to variants of concern that proved to be more infectious than the original virus. The greater the quantity of virus in circulation and the higher the number of infected individuals, the more likely the chance of mutations that will either reduce the efficacy of protective antibodies and vaccination or modify the infection.

### Gene switching was first demonstrated in African trypanosomes

Gene switching represents the most dramatic form of antigenic variation and was first demonstrated in the African trypanosomes, *Trypanosoma brucei gambiense* and *T. b. rhodesiense* (see Ch. 28). These organisms carry genes for ~1000 quite distinct surface molecules known as *variant surface glycoproteins (VSGs)*, which cover almost the entire surface and are immunodominant. The trypanosome can switch from using one gene to another, much as a B cell does with the immunoglobulin heavy chain–constant genes. This explains why a sequence of antigenically unrelated infections occurs at approximately weekly intervals, although *T. brucei* expresses several VSGs in each wave of parasitaemia. This enables the trypanosome to persist while the immune system is constantly trying to catch up with it. The main stimulus for each gene switch is possibly the antibody response itself, as there are plenty of antibodies to VSG in the blood, but the exact mechanism is not clear. About 10% of the trypanosome genome consists of surface coat genes, but this is a worthwhile investment for the parasite.

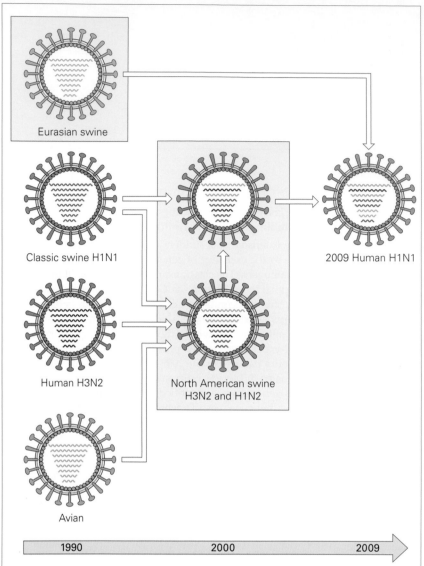

**Fig. 17.10** Antigenic shift in influenza. The major surface antigens of influenza virus are haemagglutinin and neuraminidase. Haemagglutinin is involved in attachment to cells, and antibodies to haemagglutinin are protective. Antibodies to neuraminidase are much less effective. The influenza virus can change its antigenic properties slightly (antigenic drift) or radically (antigenic shift). Pandemics can arise when there is antigenic shift with reassortment of genes. The diagram shows the origins of the 2009 pandemic influenza A (H1N1). The official influenza antigen nomenclature is based on the type of haemagglutinin (H1, H2, etc.) and neuraminidase (N1, N2, etc.) expressed on the surface of the virion. Note that, although new strains replace old strains, the internal antigens remain largely unchanged. (Modified from Trifonov V, Khiabanian H, Rabadan R. Geographic dependence, surveillance and origins of the 2009 influenza A (H1N1) virus. *N Engl J Med*. 2009;361:115–119.)

Image labels: Eurasian swine; Classic swine H1N1; Human H3N2; Avian; North American swine H3N2 and H1N2; 2009 Human H1N1; 1990; 2000; 2009

## Gene conversion can result in the relapsing infections

Gene conversion is thought to be responsible for the relapsing persistent course of certain other infections, including that by *Borrelia*. *B. burgdorferi* moves genes from 15 silent cassettes into the surface-bound lipoprotein gene, *vlsE*, in a process called *segmental gene conversion*, which results in diversity in six central regions of the *vlsE* gene. Gonococci also show great antigenic variation as they circulate through the host community, including through genetic recombination in their pilin genes. Here, there is recombination with a sequence from one of the many silent copies of *pilS* being transferred to the *pilE* gene using a gene conversion system involving a number of DNA repair genes including *RecA* and *RecF*.

## Stage-specific antigens provide another useful strategy to evade immunity

Some parasites have more complicated life cycles than bacteria or viruses and need to display stage-specific molecules that are restricted to each part of the life cycle. So, while the immune system is busy trying to recognize and respond to malaria antigens expressed on the invading sporozoites in the liver, parasites in the blood stage of infection express different antigens on the surface of infected red cells and merozoites. The sexual forms of the parasite that will continue the life cycle once back in the mosquito express further novel gametocyte antigens. Some of these stage-specific antigens such as the circumsporozoite protein are being targeted as malaria vaccines (see Ch. 35), although protection against the liver stage must be complete to prevent blood-stage infection. Other parasites with stage-specific antigens are the schistosomes and the filarias.

## IMMUNOSUPPRESSION

### Many virus infections cause a general temporary immunosuppression

A large variety of microorganisms cause immunosuppression in the infected host. The mechanism is not fully understood, but it often involves invasion of the immune system by the pathogen—in other words, "to evade, invade." The host shows a depressed immune response to antigens of the infecting pathogen (antigen-specific suppression) or, more commonly, to both antigens of the infecting pathogen and unrelated antigens. HIV is one of the most spectacular but by no means the only pathogen that interferes with the immune system in this way (Table 17.4). HIV causes death of CD4 T cells, resulting in a disastrous loss of T-cell function.

**Table 17.4** Depressed immune responses in microbial infections

| Parasite | Feature of immunosuppression | Mechanism |
|---|---|---|
| **Viruses** | | |
| HIV | ↓Ab ↓CMI, long lasting | ↓CD4[a] T cells; immunosuppression by gp41; reduced antigen presentation by infected APC |
| Epstein-Barr virus | ↓CMI, temporary | Includes polyclonal activation of infected B cells[a] |
| Measles | ↓CMI, temporary[b] | Differentiation blocked in infected T and B cells[c] |
| Varicella-zoster virus, mumps | ↓CMI, temporary | Infection of T cells |
| **Bacteria** | | |
| *Mycobacterium leprae* (lepromatous leprosy) | ↓CMI | Polyclonal activation of B cells, production of IL-4 and IL-10 |
| **Protozoa and helminths** | | |
| *Trypanosoma* | ↓Ab ↓CMI | Regulatory T cells, production of IL-10, ↓T-cell proliferation |
| *Plasmodium* | ↓Ab ↓CMI | Regulatory T cells, ↓antigen presentation |
| *Toxoplasma* | ↓CMI | ↓CD4 T cells, IFNγ, IL-1β, apoptosis, ROS |
| *Leishmania* | ↓CMI | Production of IL-10 and TGFβ |
| Filarias[d] | ↓CMI | ↓CD4 T cell proliferation, ↓Th1 and upregulation Th2 |

Ab, Antibody; APC, antigen-presenting cell; CMI, cell-mediated immunity, HIV, human immunodeficiency virus; IFN, interferon; IL, interleukin; ROS, reactive oxygen species.
[a]For HIV, the depressed responses are seen later, after initial neutralizing antibody and cytotoxic cell responses. There are many possible mechanisms involved in HIV immunosuppression, but decreased numbers of CD4 T cells is probably the most important.
[b]The *BCRF-1* gene of the virus codes for an IL-10–like molecule that enhances antibody rather than protective CMI responses.
[c]Patients with a positive tuberculin skin test become temporarily negative during measles infection. Measles also stops macrophages producing IL-12, a molecule needed for the Th1-type (protective) immune response.
[d]The ES-62 filarial antigen can inhibit the proliferation of CD4 T cells and B2 B cells.

To induce antigen-specific immunosuppression would bring most benefit to the invading pathogen, but a general immunosuppression, as long as it is temporary, may give the pathogen enough time to grow, spread and be shed before being eliminated. This is what happens in many virus infections. A lasting general immunosuppression would be detrimental to the pathogen because susceptibility to other infections would cause unnecessary damage to the host species. From this point of view, HIV certainly overstepped the mark.

### Different pathogens have different immunosuppressive effects

Immunosuppression by pathogens often involves actual infection of immune cells:

- T cells (HIV, measles)
- B cells (EBV)
- macrophages (HIV, CMV, *Leishmania*)
- dendritic cells (HIV).

This may result in impaired cell function (e.g. blocking of cell division or of release of IL-2 [or other cytokines]) or in cell death.

Additional immunosuppressive actions taken by pathogens include the release of immunosuppressive molecules. For instance, the gp41 polypeptide formed by HIV acts as an immunologic anaesthetic, temporarily blocking T-cell function. Other pathogens (poxviruses, herpesviruses, *T. cruzi*) release molecules that interfere with the action of complement or with immunologically important cytokines such as IL-2, IFNs (see earlier) or tumour necrosis factor.

### Certain pathogen toxins are immunomodulators

A particularly dramatic form of immune interference is practised by the staphylococci. Many strains liberate exotoxins (staphylococcal enterotoxins, epidermolytic toxin and toxic shock syndrome toxin [TSST-1]) that are responsible for disease. At first sight, producing these toxins seems to be of no advantage to the staphylococci, but it is now recognized that they have extremely powerful immunomodulatory actions—they are the most potent T-cell mitogens known and act at picomolar concentrations. They function as superantigens and, after binding to MHC class II molecules on antigen-presenting cells, act as polyclonal activators of T cells bearing particular families of genes in their T-cell receptors (Fig. 17.11). A large proportion (2–20%) of all T cells then respond by dividing and releasing cytokines; only 0.001–0.01% are capable of doing this in response to a regular antigen. Although most of us make antibodies to TSST-1, about 1 in 5 do not and so are more susceptible to developing TSS. Staphylococcal enterotoxin-B can be used by immunologists to nonspecifically activate T cells in vitro. Similar molecules are produced by certain streptococci and mycoplasmas.

Possible mechanisms by which the staphylococcal toxins may interfere with immune defences include:

- excessive local liberation of cytokines by activated cells in a cytokine storm
- killing of T cells or other immune cells with pore-forming toxins
- diversion of T cells of all specificities into immunologically unproductive activity by polyclonal activation.

The fungus *C. albicans* produces a secreted toxin called *candidalysin*, which is necessary for mucosal invasion by fungal hyphae. The toxin causes epithelial cell damage but also triggers a danger signal alert to the immune system that this normally surface-colonizing yeast has become invasive.

Less dramatic polyclonal activation is seen in many other infections. Pathogens may cause polyclonal activation of B cells as well as T cells (e.g. in EBV and HIV infections), and this can be interpreted as an immunodiversion by the infecting

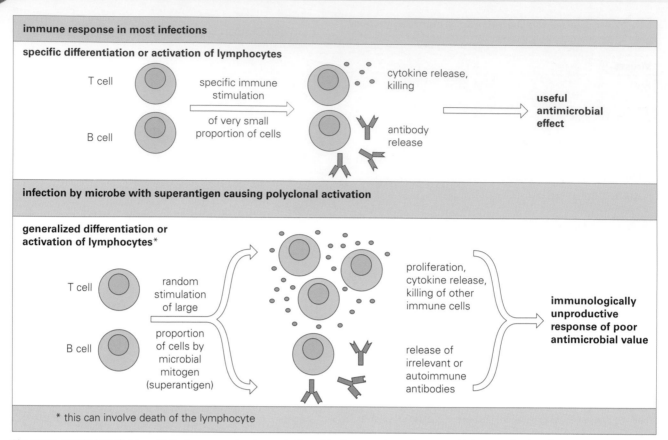

**Fig. 17.11** Microbial interference with the immune system by production of T-cell superantigens. Some microbial toxins will induce the proliferation of families of T cells resulting in activation of a much larger number of cells than is seen with antigens. This leads to excessive release of cytokines and severe illness.

pathogen or in the case of EBV as production of a supply of B cells in which the virus can grow. One consequence is that a range of irrelevant, sometimes autoimmune, antibodies are formed (e.g. heterophile antibodies in EBV infection). Finally, some persistent infections just wear out the immune system, resulting in T-cell exhaustion or immune senescence in which the T cells become less good at proliferating and lose the ability to make IL-2. CMV does this, as does HIV.

### Successful pathogens often interfere with signalling between immune cells, with cytotoxic T-cell recognition or with host apoptotic responses

Many pathogens interfere with host molecules such as cytokines, chemokines, MHC, and apoptotic and complement receptors, all of which are essential components of host defence. Many DNA viruses code for fake molecules or fake cell receptors for the host molecules, and this disrupts the antimicrobial response. HSV produces a molecule, glycoprotein C, that functions as a receptor for C3b. It is present on the virus particle and on the infected cell and interferes with complement activation, protecting both the virus and the infected cell from destruction by antibody and complement.

EBV produces a homologue of IL-10, a cytokine initially called *cytokine synthesis inhibitory factor*. *M. tuberculosis* binds to the DC-SIGN receptor on macrophages, and this induces IL-10 production by the infected macrophages, which again favours the infecting pathogen. Furthermore, *M. tuberculosis* and other intracellular organisms (*Leishmania major*, *Histoplasma capsulatum*) inhibit IL-12 production by the infected macrophages. Th1 T cells are therefore not activated by IL-12 to form IFNγ, and the immune response is again diverted from the protective Th1

response. Another way to block production of beneficial IFNγ is exploited by *Toxoplasma gondii*, which stops the STAT1 transcription factor from dissociating from DNA.

Adenoviruses and herpesviruses prevent Tc cells from killing infected cells by reducing MHC class I expression and thus antigen expression on the target cell.

A strategy useful for one pathogen is not necessarily good for others. For example, a local cell infected with a virus can commit suicide by undergoing apoptosis, a useful defence if it takes place before virus replication is complete. So certain viruses (HSV, EBV, HIV) code for proteins that interfere with apoptosis, permitting long-term infection of the cell. Other viruses, however, such as measles, induce apoptosis, as do certain bacteria (*Shigella flexneri*, *Salmonella*) after encountering macrophages, enabling them to escape destruction while the parasite *T. gondii* blocks apoptosis. It may be useful to induce apoptosis in one cell but not in another. Thus HIV inhibits apoptosis in the infected immune cell but induces apoptosis in neighbouring uninfected cells.

### Some pathogens interfere with the local expression of the immune response in tissues

Some pathogens do not interfere with the development of an immune response but, instead, actively interfere with its expression in tissues; for instance *Neisseria gonorrhoeae*, *S. pneumoniae* and many strains of *Haemophilus influenzae* liberate a protease that cleaves human IgA antibody. These bacteria are residents or invaders of mucosal surfaces on which IgA antibodies operate, and the ability to produce such an enzyme seems unlikely to be mere coincidence.

## PERSISTENT INFECTIONS

### Persistent infections represent a failure of host defences

One way of looking at persistent infections (Table 17.5) is to regard them as failures of host defences that should control microbial growth and spread and eliminate the pathogen from the body. The pathogen may persist in:

- a defiant infectious form, as with hepatitis B in the blood or the schistosome in the blood vessels of the alimentary tract or bladder

**Table 17.5** Examples of persistent infections in humans

| Microorganism | Site of persistence | Infectiousness of persistent microorganism | Consequence | Shedding of microorganism to exterior |
|---|---|---|---|---|
| **Viruses** | | | | |
| Herpes simplex virus | Dorsal root ganglia | + | Reactivation, cold sore | + |
| | Salivary glands | + | Not known | + |
| Varicella-zoster virus | Dorsal root ganglia | + | Reactivation, zoster | + |
| Cytomegalovirus | Lymphoid tissue | + | Reactivation ± disease | + |
| Epstein-Barr virus | Lymphoid tissue | + | Lymphoid tumour | − |
| | Epithelium | − | Nasopharyngeal carcinoma | − |
| | Salivary glands | + | Not known | + |
| Hepatitis B and C viruses | Liver (virus shed into blood) | + | Chronic hepatitis: liver cancer | + |
| Adenoviruses | Lymphoid tissue | + | Not known | + |
| Polyomaviruses BK and JC (humans) | Kidney | − | Reactivation (immunosuppression) | + |
| HTLV-1 and 2 | Lymphoid and other tissues | + | HTLV-1 T-cell leukaemia, neurologic disease HTLV-2 neurologic disease | − |
| Paramyxovirus | Brain | ± | Subacute sclerosing panencephalitis | − |
| HIV | Lymphocytes, macrophages | + | Chronic infection | + |
| ***Chlamydia*** | | | | |
| *Chlamydia trachomatis* | Conjunctiva | + | Chronic disease and blindness | + |
| ***Rickettsia*** | | | | |
| *Rickettsia prowazekii* | Lymph node | ? | Activation | + |
| **Bacteria** | | | | |
| *Salmonella typhi* | Gallbladder, urinary tract | + | Intermittent shedding in urine, faeces | + |
| *Mycobacterium tuberculosis* | Lung-macrophages | | Constant interaction with local tissues until inflammation that induces tissue destruction occurs (immunocompetent adults) or replication is unrestricted (immunosuppression, old age) | + |
| *Treponema pallidum* | Disseminated | ± | Chronic disease | − |
| **Parasites** | | | | |
| *Plasmodium vivax* and *P. ovale* | Liver | Only for red cells | Activation, clinical malaria | + Via subsequent erythrocytic cycle then a mosquito vector |
| *Toxoplasma gondii* | Lymphoid tissue, muscle, brain | ± | Activation, neurologic disease | − |
| *Trypanosoma cruzi* | Blood, macrophages | + | Chronic disease | + Via reduviid bug vector |
| *Schistosoma mansoni* | Gut | + | Chronic disease | Eggs |
| Filarias | Lymphatics, lymph nodes, subcutaneous tissue | + | Chronic disease | + Via insect vector |

Shedding to the exterior takes place either directly (e.g. via skin lesions, saliva, urine) or indirectly (e.g. via the blood [hepatitis B] or an insect vector [malaria]). Sometimes a persistent oprgansim is viable and would be infectious if eaten by its definative host.

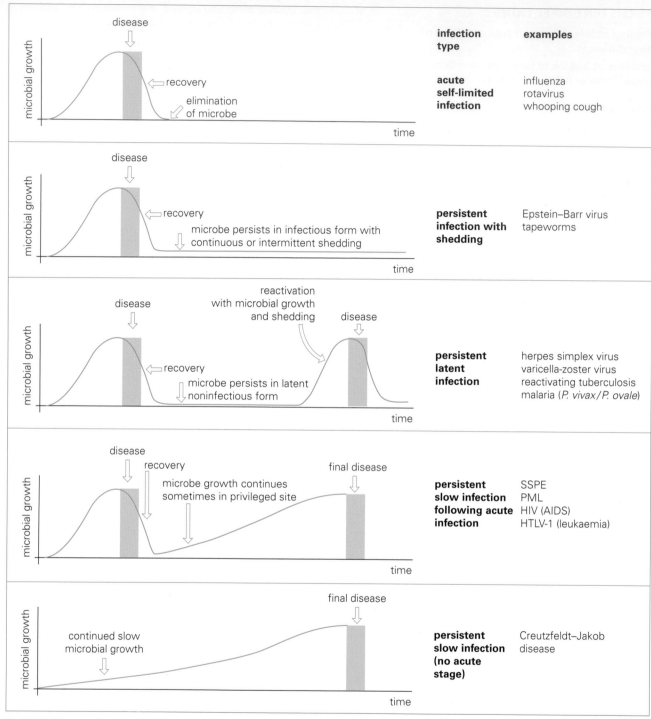

**Fig 17.12** Patterns of acute and persistent infections. For some pathogens (e.g. cytomegalovirus), the distinction between persistence in infectious form and true latency is not clear. AIDS, Acquired immunodeficiency syndrome; HIV, human immunodeficiency virus; HTLV-1, human T-cell leukaemia virus 1; PML, progressive multifocal leukoencephalopathy; SSPE, subacute sclerosing panencephalitis.

- a form with low or partial infectivity (e.g. adenoviruses in the tonsils and adenoids)
- a metabolically altered state, such as in latent *M. tuberculosis* in which the slowing of metabolism is a response to bacterial stress in the phagolysosome and latency may be more of an incubation period
- a completely noninfectious form.

Latent virus infections are classic examples of this type of persistence. For example, HSV DNA persists in sensory neurons, in the dorsal root ganglia. During latency, a single latency-associated transcript is highly expressed in the neurons, in contrast to the ≥80 proteins produced in the lytic cycle in epithelial cells. This latency-associated transcript plays a role in silencing the HSV lytic genes. The viral genome is not integrated with host DNA, and, instead of being linear, it is circular and exists in free episomal form. It now seems that epigenetics (through which DNA transcription can be regulated) plays a major role in controlling viral latency. This impacts on the frequency of reactivation and in maintenance of the latent reservoir of virus.

## Latent infections can become patent

Latent infections are so-called because they can become patent. This is where they become of great medical interest, and the legacy of latent herpesvirus infections in humans is described in Chapter 27. Different patterns of persistent infections are illustrated in Fig. 17.12. Persistent infections are important for four main reasons:

1. They can be reactivated many years later and represent a reservoir of infection within the individual and community.
2. They are sometimes associated with chronic disease, as in the case of chronic hepatitis B infections, subacute sclerosing panencephalitis following measles and acquired immunodeficiency syndrome (AIDS).
3. They are sometimes associated with cancers, such as hepatocellular carcinoma with HBV, Burkitt lymphoma and nasopharyngeal carcinoma with EBV.
4. From the microbial viewpoint, they enable the infectious agent to persist in the host community (Box 17.2).

## Reactivation of latent infections

### Reactivation is clinically important in immunosuppressed individuals

Reactivation occurs in immunocompromised patients and is of major clinical importance in those immunosuppressed as a result of chronic infection and disease, such as HIV and AIDS, tumours (including leukaemias and lymphomas) or in those immunosuppressed following transplantation. Reactivation also occurs during naturally occurring periods of immunocompromise, the most important of these being pregnancy and old age. From the pathogen's point of view, latency is an adaptation that allows reactivation with renewed growth and shedding of the infectious agent during these naturally occurring periods.

Features of reactivation in herpesvirus infections are described in Chapters 22 and 27.

New imaging techniques have shown that latency in tuberculosis is a more active state than was previously recognized, with some granulomas in the lung showing metabolic activity while others are more silent. There is interest in identifying gene expression signatures that would predict

---

### Box 17.2 ■ Lessons in Microbiology

#### Persistence is of survival value for the pathogen

Persistence without any further shedding, as occurs in subacute sclerosing panencephalitis and progressive multifocal leukoencephalopathy (see Ch. 25), is of no survival value, but there are obvious advantages if the pathogen is also shed either continuously or intermittently. This is especially true when the host species consists of small isolated groups of individuals (Fig. 17.13). Measles, for instance, is not normally a persistent infection. It infects only humans, does not survive for long outside the body and has nowhere else to go (i.e. there is no animal reservoir). Without a continued supply of fresh susceptible humans, the virus could not maintain itself and would become extinct. At all times there must be an individual acutely infected with measles. From studies of island communities it is clear that a minimum of ~500,000 humans is needed to maintain measles without reintroduction from outside. In Palaeolithic times, when humans lived in small, isolated groups, measles could not have existed in its present form.

In contrast, persistent and latent infections are admirably adapted for survival under these circumstances. Varicella-zoster virus (VZV) can maintain itself in a community of <1000 individuals. Children get chickenpox, the virus persists in latent form in sensory neurones, and later in life the virus reactivates to cause shingles. By this time a new generation of susceptible individuals has appeared, and the shingles vesicles provide a fresh source of virus.

Serologic studies show that the viral infections prevalent in small, completely isolated Indian communities in the Amazon basin are persistent or latent (e.g. due to adenoviruses, polyomaviruses, papillomaviruses, herpesviruses) rather than nonpersistent (e.g. due to influenza, measles, poliovirus). The same principles apply to nonviral infections. Those present in small communities are either persistent (e.g. typhoid, respiratory tuberculosis) or have an animal reservoir for maintenance of the pathogen.

---

those individuals progressing from latent to active tuberculosis so that they could be treated before they infect others.

#### It is useful to distinguish two stages in viral reactivation

The first event in reactivation (Fig. 17.14), the resumption of viral activity in the latently infected cell, involves transcription of immediate-early genes. In the case of HSV this can be triggered by sensory stimuli arriving in the neuron from skin areas responding to sunlight, by trauma such as dental procedures, by other infections or by hormonal influences.

The second event involves the spread and replication of the reactivated virus. HSV must travel down the sensory axon to the skin or mucosal surface, infect and spread in subepithelial tissues and then in the epithelium, finally forming a virus-rich vesicle (>1 million infectious units per millilitre of vesicle fluid). All this takes at least 3–4 days. This second stage is less mysterious than the first and can be controlled by the immune system. Therefore cold sores may be associated with poor lymphocyte responses to HSV antigens and zoster with declining cell-mediated responses to VZV antigens in older people.

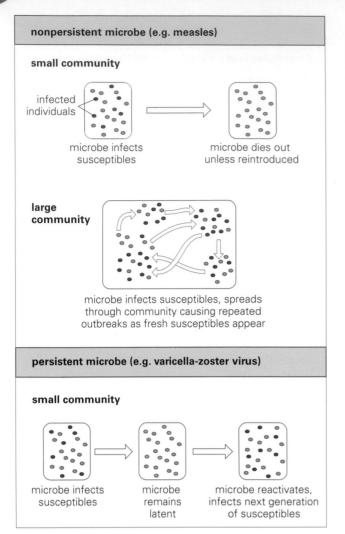

**nonpersistent microbe (e.g. measles)**

**small community**

infected individuals

microbe infects susceptibles

microbe dies out unless reintroduced

**large community**

microbe infects susceptibles, spreads through community causing repeated outbreaks as fresh susceptibles appear

**persistent microbe (e.g. varicella-zoster virus)**

**small community**

microbe infects susceptibles

microbe remains latent

microbe reactivates, infects next generation of susceptibles

**Fig. 17.13** Persistence is a microbial survival strategy.

The first stage probably occurs more frequently because immune defences often arrest the process during the second stage before final production of the lesion. As many as 10–20% of HSV reactivation episodes are thought to be non-lesional with burning, tingling and itching at the site but no signs of a cold sore. Also, zoster may involve no more than the sensory prodrome associated with virus reactivation and replication in sensory neurones; skin lesions are prevented by host defences.

Reactivation of EBV and CMV with appearance of the virus in saliva or blood is generally asymptomatic. In immunologically deficient individuals, however, reactivation may progress to cause clinical disease: either hepatitis and pneumonitis in the case of CMV or post-transplant lymphoma and the rarer hairy tongue leukoplakia due to EBV (see Ch. 31).

## Pathogens are clever and often use a number of these evasion strategies

The most successful pathogens have evolved multiple ways by which to interfere with what would otherwise be damaging immune responses. The many ways used by *S. aureus* is one example of this (Table 17.6) and shows how hard such pathogens have to work to evade the immune response. Similarly, CMV exploits many mechanisms, including interfering with dendritic cell maturation, and so with antigen presentation, antibody-mediated immunity, cytokine function and apoptosis. CMV infection may mostly be silent but is quietly pushing otherwise useful T cells toward exhaustion and senescence. The only good thing is that, through understanding these evasion mechanisms, we have learned more about how the immune system works.

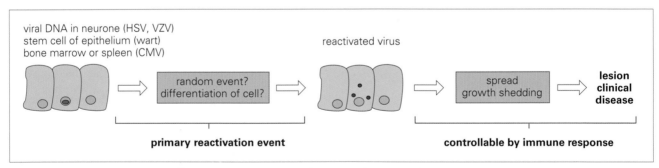

viral DNA in neurone (HSV, VZV)
stem cell of epithelium (wart)
bone marrow or spleen (CMV)

reactivated virus

random event? differentiation of cell?

spread growth shedding

**lesion clinical disease**

**primary reactivation event**

**controllable by immune response**

**Fig. 17.14** Two stages in reactivation of latent viruses. CMV, Cytomegalovirus; HSV, herpes simplex virus; VZV, varicella-zoster virus.

**Table 17.6** Examples of the many evasion mechanisms used by *Staphylococcus aureus*

| Molecule | Mechanism | Effect on immune response |
|---|---|---|
| Staphylococcal protein A | Binds immunoglobulin Fc and Fab | Blocks phagocytosis; B-cell apoptosis |
| Staphylococcal complement inhibitor family | Bind classical and alternative pathway C3 convertases[a] | Block complement activation |
| Extracellular fibrinogen-binding protein | Inhibits C3b-mediated opsonization | Block phagocytosis |
| Extracellular complement-binding protein | Inhibits C3b-mediated opsonization | Block phagocytotosis |
| Complement 4 binding protein | Inhibits C3b-mediated opsonization | Block phagocytosis |
| Staphylococcal superantigen-like protein 7 | Binds to C5 and IgA | Blocks C5 convertase |
| Chemotaxis inhibitory protein | Blocks recruitment of neutrophils and leukocytes | Reduced phagocytosis and inflammation |
| Staphylokinase | Binds to neutrophil α-defensins | Blocks bactericidal activity |
| α-Toxin | Pore forming | Lyse epidermal, stromal and immune cells |
| Bicomponent leukotoxins (i.e. PVL) | Pore forming | Lyse epidermal, stromal and immune cells |
| Phenol-soluble modulins | Pore forming | Lyse epidermal, stromal and immune cells |
| Toxic shock syndrome toxin-1 | Nonspecific activation of T cells | Nonprotective activation and exhaustion of T cells |
| Staphylococcal enterotoxins (SEA, SEB, SEC, SE-1X) | Nonspecific activation of T cells | Nonprotective activation and exhaustion of T cells |

PVL, Panton-Valentine leucocidin toxin made by some types of *S. aureus*.
[a]C4b2b and C3bBb.
Modified from Miller LS, Fowler VG, Shukla SK, et al. Development of a vaccine against Staphylococcus aureus invasive infections: evidence based on human immunity, genetics and bacterial evasion mechanisms. *FEMS Microbiol Rev.* 2020;44(1):123–153.

## KEY FACTS

- Many successful parasites have adopted strategies for evading immune responses. These enable them to stay in the body long enough to complete their business of infection and shedding to fresh hosts. Some parasites persist indefinitely in the body.

- Mechanisms of immune evasion include:

  - concealing parasite antigens from the host (staying inside host cells, infecting privileged sites)

  - changing parasite antigens, either in the infected individual (e.g. trypanosomiasis) or during spread through the host population (e.g. influenza)

  - direct action on immune cells (e.g. HIV on CD4 T cells) or on immune signalling systems (e.g. production of fake cytokine molecules)

  - local interference with immune defences (complement activation, production of IgA proteases, Fc receptors).

- During some persistent infections, the pathogen may continue to multiply and be able to infect others (e.g. HIV, hepatitis B).

- In other persistent infections, the pathogen enters into a latent state and, later in life, reactivates with renewed multiplication and the ability to infect others (e.g. herpesviruses, *M. tuberculosis*).

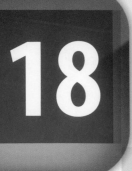

# 18

# Pathologic consequences of infection

## Introduction

Infections can cause a range of unwanted symptoms, sometimes caused by the microbe itself and sometimes by the immune response to infection. Inflammation is beneficial but also unpleasant. A range of other hypersensitivity responses can be damaging to the host. Some viruses can cause cancer. We will now review these unwanted results of infections and how the immune system responds.

### Symptoms of infections are produced by the microorganisms or by the host's immune responses

Symptoms that appear rapidly after the acquisition of an infection are usually due to the direct action of molecules secreted by the invading microbe. A virus in a cell may cause metabolic shutdown or lyse the cell. Bacteria, however, provoke most of their acute effects by releasing toxins but may also cause distress by inducing inflammation. The inflammatory response is of course an important component of host protection, vascular permeability being vital for the rapid mobilization of cells such as neutrophils, and serum components such as complement and antibody. Inflammation is therefore intrinsically a healthy sign, and it is interesting that some virulent bacteria (e.g. staphylococci) try to inhibit the inflammatory response.

### Pathologic changes are often secondary to the activation of immunologic mechanisms that are normally thought of as protective

These may involve the innate or the adaptive immune system or, more usually, both (Fig. 18.1). Tissue damage resulting from adaptive immune responses is usually referred to as immunopathology and is quite common in infectious diseases, particularly those that are chronic and persistent. The immunologic basis of these mechanisms of tissue damage is described in Chapter 15. The killing of viral-infected cells by cytotoxic T cells will obviously lead to the death of the infected cells as well as the invader.

Certain viruses can cause permanent malignant changes in cells as a result of direct, indirect and a mixture of both types of mechanisms. Seven viruses that infect humans cause up to 15% of human cancers around the world. These include human T-cell lymphotropic virus type 1 (HTLV-1; lymphomas, leukaemias), Epstein-Barr virus (EBV; nasopharyngeal carcinoma and Burkitt's lymphoma [BL]), human papillomaviruses (HPV; cervical cancer), hepatitis B (HBV) and C virus (HCV) infections (liver cancer), human immunodeficiency virus (HIV; immunosuppression leads to the development of cancers such as Kaposi's sarcoma (KS) and primary effusion lymphoma associated with human herpesvirus type 8 [HHV-8] and EBV lymphoma) and the rare Merkel cell polyomavirus (Merkel cell carcinoma of the skin). Cofactors may be involved. Immunisation programmes for HBV and HPV infections have reduced the incidence of liver and cervical cancer, respectively.

## PATHOLOGY CAUSED DIRECTLY BY MICROORGANISMS

### Direct effects may result from cell rupture, organ blockage or pressure effects

Organisms that multiply in cells and subsequently spread usually do so by rupturing the cell. Many viruses and some intracellular bacteria and protozoa behave in this way (Table 18.1), but many others do not. For example, viruses or bacteria may remain latent (e.g. herpes simplex virus [HSV] and varicella-zoster virus in nerve ganglia, and *Mycobacterium tuberculosis* in macrophages), and many viruses can bud from a cell without disrupting it. The type of cell infected may also have an influence on survival of the organism. Thus although HIV causes lysis of CD4 T cells, macrophages are more resistant to both infection and lysis. Other direct effects include:

- blockage of major hollow viscera by helminths
- blockage of lung alveoli by dense growth (e.g. of *Pneumocystis*)
- mechanical effects of large cysts (e.g. *Echinococcus*).

### Bacteria may produce enzymes to promote their survival or spread

A number of bacteria release enzymes that break down the tissues or the intercellular substances of the host, allowing the infection to spread freely. Among these enzymes are hyaluronidase, collagenase, DNase and streptokinase. Some staphylococci release a coagulase that deposits a protective layer of fibrin onto and around the cells, thus localizing them.

### Exotoxins are a common cause of serious tissue damage, especially in bacterial infection

The pathogen may actively secrete exotoxins (Table 18.2) that cause direct damage to cells (Fig. 18.2). In some cases, these are clearly part of its strategy for entry, spread or defence against the host, but sometimes they seem to be of little or no benefit to the pathogen.

Most exotoxins are proteins and are often coded not by the bacterial DNA but in plasmids (e.g. *Escherichia coli*) or

**Fig. 18.1** Pathologic effects of infection: a general scheme. Infectious parasitic organisms can cause disease directly (*top*) or indirectly via overactivation of various immune mechanisms, either innate (*middle*) or adaptive (*bottom*). IFN, Interferon; IgE, immunoglobulin E; IL, interleukin; Mφ, macrophage; PMN, polymorphonuclear neutrophil; TNF, tumour necrosis factor.

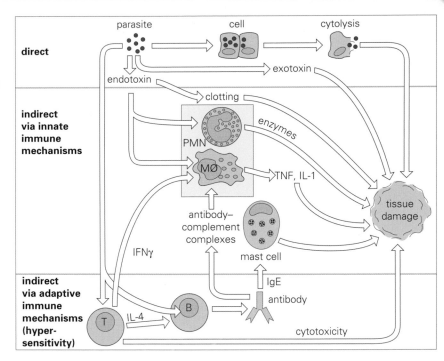

**Table 18.1** Examples of organisms that directly damage tissue

| Organism | Cell or tissue damaged | Mechanism |
|---|---|---|
| **Viruses** | | |
| Poliovirus | Neurones | |
| Rhinovirus | Lower respiratory tract epithelium | |
| Human immunodeficiency virus | CD4 T cells, macrophages | Cytopathic |
| Coxsackievirus | Pancreatic beta cells, cardiac cells | |
| Rotavirus | Enterocytes | |
| **Bacteria** | | |
| *Streptococcus mutans* | Teeth | Acid production |
| **Fungi** | | |
| *Histoplasma* | Macrophages | Damaged macrophage releases cytokines |
| **Protozoa** | | |
| *Plasmodium* | Erythrocytes | Damaged erythrocyte removed |
| **Helminths** | | |
| *Ascaris* | Intestinal occlusion | Mechanical |
| | Biliary occlusion | Mechanical, inflammation |
| *Echinococcus* | Hydatid cyst | Pressure effects |

Many organisms directly damage or destroy the tissues they infect. This is especially common with cytopathic viruses.

phages (e.g. botulism, diphtheria, scarlet fever). In some cases, they consist of two or more subunits, one of which is required for binding and entry to the cell while the other switches on or inhibits some cellular function.

Powerful toxins are generally secreted from extracellular pathogens. Microbes that multiply in cells cannot afford to cause serious damage at too early a stage, and such toxins therefore tend to be less prominent in intracellular infections due to *Mycobacteria*, *Chlamydia* or *Mycoplasma*.

For example, leprosy patients with lepromatous disease can live with huge bacterial loads for many years. Although many toxins can kill host cells, lower concentrations may be important by causing dysfunction in immune or phagocytic cells. For example, concentrations of streptolysin well below the cell-killing level will inhibit leukocyte chemotaxis, and the staphylococcal enterotoxins and exfoliative toxins also have immunomodulatory activity at exceedingly low (nanogram to picogram) levels.

**Table 18.2** Some important exotoxins in disease

| Organism | Exotoxin | Tissue damaged | Action | Disease |
|---|---|---|---|---|
| **Bacteria** | | | | |
| Clostridium tetani | Tetanus toxin | Neurones | Spastic paralysis | Tetanus |
| Clostridium botulinum | Neurotoxin | Nerve–muscle junction | Flaccid paralysis | Botulism |
| Corynebacterium diphtheriae | Diphtheria toxin | Throat, heart, peripheral nerve | Inhibits protein synthesis | Diphtheria |
| Shigella dysenteriae | Enterotoxin | Intestinal mucosa | Destroys mucosal cells | Dysentery |
| Escherichia coli | Enterotoxin | Intestinal epithelium | Fluid loss from intestinal cell | Gastroenteritis |
| Vibrio cholerae | Enterotoxin | Intestinal epithelium | Fluid loss from intestinal cell | Cholera |
| Staphylococcus aureus | α-haemolysin | Red and white cells (via cytokines) | Haemolysis | Abscesses |
| | Enterotoxins[a] | Intestinal cells | Induces vomiting, diarrhoea | Food poisoning |
| | TSST1 | T cells | Release of cytotoxins | Toxic shock syndrome |
| Streptococcus pyogenes | Streptolysin O and S | Red and white cells | Haemolysis | Haemolysis, pyogenic lesions |
| | Erythrogenic | Skin capillaries | Skin rash | Scarlet fever |
| Bacillus anthracis | Cytotoxin | Lung | Pulmonary oedema | Anthrax |
| Bordetella pertussis | Pertussis toxin | Trachea | Kills epithelium | Whooping cough |
| Listeria monocytogenes | Haemolysin | Leukocytes, monocytes | Cell lysis | Listeriosis |
| **Fungi** | | | | |
| Aspergillus fumigatus | Aflatoxin | Liver | Carcinogenic | ? Liver damage/cancer[b] |
| **Protozoa** | | | | |
| Entamoeba histolytica | Enterotoxin | Colonic epithelium | Cell lysis | Amoebic dysentery |

Many bacteria and a few other organisms damage host tissues by secreting exotoxins, some examples of which are shown here. Some bacterial exotoxins are among the most powerful toxins known. Vaccination, by inducing antibody, is often very effective in protection.

[a] S. aureus has five enterotoxins: SEA, SEB, SEC, SED and SEE. Staphylococcal enterotoxins and toxic shock syndrome toxin (TSST-I) are superantigens that activate T cells expressing particular Vβ genes in their T-cell receptors.

[b] In turkeys and pigs from A. fumigatus–contaminated ground nuts, but not so far in humans.

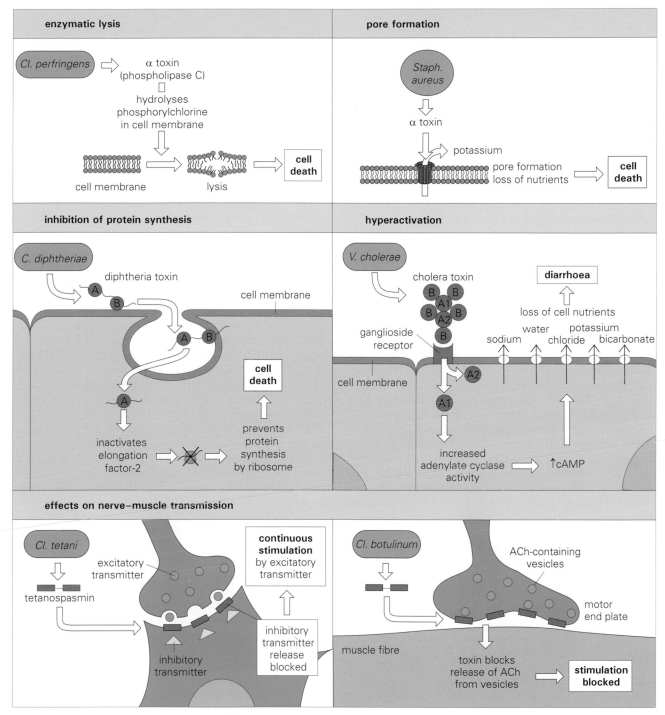

**Fig. 18.2** The mode of action of some exotoxins. Bacterial toxins act in a variety of ways. Often the toxin is a two-chain molecule, one chain being concerned with entry into cells while the other has inhibitory activity against some vital function. ACh, Acetylcholine; cAMP, cyclic adenosine monophosphate; C, *Corynebacterium*; Cl, *Clostridium*; Staph, *Staphylococcus*; V, *Vibrio*.

## Toxins may damage or destroy cells and are then known as haemolysins

Cell membranes can be damaged enzymatically by lecithinases or phospholipases, or by insertion of pore-forming molecules, which destroy the integrity of the cell. The collective term for such toxins is haemolysins, although many cells other than red blood cells can be affected. Both staphylococci and streptococci produce pore-forming toxins; pseudomonads release enzymatic haemolysins. The staphylococcal alpha haemolysin is secreted as a soluble monomer but binds to a membrane protein to form a heptamer, making a beta-barrel pore in the membrane.

## Toxins may enter cells and actively alter some of the metabolic machinery

Characteristically, these toxin molecules have two subunits. The A subunit is the active component, while the B subunit is a binding component needed to interact with receptors on the cell membrane. When binding occurs, the A subunit, or the whole toxin–receptor complex, is taken into the cell by endocytosis, and the A subunit becomes activated. Two well-studied toxins of this type are those of diphtheria (see Ch. 20) and cholera (Ch. 23).

## Diphtheria toxin blocks protein synthesis

Diphtheria toxin is synthesized as a single polypeptide and binds by the B subunit to target cells (see Fig. 18.2). The polypeptide is partially cleaved, and then the entire toxin–receptor complex is internalized. The A subunit then splits off and passes into the cytosol, where it inactivates the transfer of amino acids from transfer RNA to the polypeptide chain during translation of mRNA by ribosomes. It does this by catalysing attachment of adenosine diphosphate (ADP) ribose to the elongation protein (ADP ribosylation), effectively blocking protein synthesis.

## Cholera toxin results in massive loss of water from intestinal epithelial cells

Cholera toxin is released as a complex of five B subunits surrounding the A subunit. The latter is cleaved into two fragments: A1 and A2, held by disulphide bonds. The B subunits bind to ganglioside receptors on intestinal epithelial cells, leading to internalization of the A subunits, which then separate from one another (see Fig. 18.2). The A1 portion then ADP-ribosylates one of the regulatory molecules involved in the production of cyclic adenosine monophosphate (cAMP). As a result, the regulatory molecule is unable to turn off cAMP production. The increased levels of cAMP in the cell change the sodium/chloride flux across the cell membrane, resulting in a massive outflow of water and electrolytes from the cell and causing the profuse diarrhoea of cholera. The exotoxins of *E. coli* and salmonella have similar actions, as does pertussis toxin.

## Tetanus and botulinum toxins are among the most potent affecting nerve impulses

These toxins are extremely potent and active at low doses. Tetanus and botulinum toxins have the characteristic A + B structure, the B subunit binding to ganglioside receptors on nerve cells. The internalized A subunit of tetanus is carried by axonal transport from the point of production to the central nervous system, where it interferes with synaptic transmission in inhibitory neurones by blocking neurotransmitter release. This allows the excitatory transmitter to continuously stimulate the motor neurones, causing spastic paralysis. Botulinum toxin enters the body via the intestine, escaping digestion and crossing the gut wall. The toxin affects peripheral nerve endings at the neuromuscular junction, blocking presynaptic release of acetylcholine. This prevents muscle contraction, causing flaccid paralysis.

## Inactivation of toxins without altering antigenicity results in successful vaccines

Toxins can often be inactivated (e.g. by formaldehyde) without altering their antigenicity, and the resulting toxoids are among the most successful of all vaccines (see Ch. 35), the classic examples being diphtheria and tetanus toxoids. Toxins are generally more highly conserved

in their structure than the surface antigens of the organism secreting them. This allows for more effective cross-immunity and explains, for example, why scarlet fever (caused by streptococcal erythrotoxin) usually occurs only once, whereas streptococcal infections recur almost indefinitely.

## Toxins as magic bullets

An interesting offshoot of the two-subunit structure of toxins is that, by changing the specificity of the part responsible for attachment, the specificity of the toxin for a particular cell type can be changed. An example is the plant toxin ricin—the A subunit can be attached to a monoclonal antibody to make it a specific poison for tumour cells that can be targeted to the cell cytoplasm with a signal peptide, inducing apoptosis.

# DIARRHOEA

## Diarrhoea is an almost invariable result of intestinal infections

Diarrhoea is one of the major causes of death in children worldwide, with rotavirus as the main culprit (see Ch. 23). In industrialized regions, bacterial pathogens such as *Campylobacter* and nontyphoidal *Salmonella* are increasingly important, and *Clostridium difficile* and norovirus infections are a problem in hospitals, particularly in the elderly. Another culprit is the enterotoxigenic strains of *E. coli*, which can produce a heat-stable toxin (ST) and a heat-labile toxin (LT-I); diarrhoea can be caused by *E. coli* strains that produce one or both toxins.

Diarrhoea can be considered as a means for the host to rid itself rapidly of the infectious organism and for the infection to spread to other hosts. Diarrhoea is a feature of a wide range of organisms. While toxins are often the cause (e.g. cholera, shigella), microbial invasion and damage to epithelial cells may also be important. The pathophysiology, with changes in electron transport or loss of enterocytes, has been elucidated in some cases. Many of the organisms causing diarrhoea can be picked up from food, but the term food poisoning is usually reserved for those cases where toxins are already present in the food rather than being generated during the growth of organisms in the intestine (Fig. 18.3). As would be expected, food poisoning causes symptoms earlier (i.e. hours after exposure rather than days) (Table 18.3). Some viruses, especially norovirus infections, sometimes referred to as causing winter vomiting disease, cause outbreaks of diarrhoea and vomiting particularly in closed groups or communities such as in hospitals or on cruise ships. Since the COVID-19 pandemic in 2020–2022, norovirus outbreaks have increased in the United Kingdom and in winter 2023 were most common in care homes and nurseries. In a single week in February 2023, 54 outbreaks were reported in England.

# PATHOLOGIC ACTIVATION OF NATURAL IMMUNE MECHANISMS

## Overactivity can damage host tissues

The very potent innate immune mechanisms discussed in Chapter 15 have inbuilt safety as far as specificity is concerned. They have had to evolve in the constant presence of the host's self antigens, to which they do not therefore

**Fig. 18.3** Outbreak of bloody diarrhoea caused by enterohaemorrhagic *Escherichia coli* (EHEC) 0157 in South Wales, in 2005. The verotoxin produced by EHEC causes diarrhoea and is similar to the *Shigella* toxin. The first cases had all eaten school dinners containing cooked meats from a single supplier. Of the total 157 reported cases, 65% were in school-aged children. Thirty-one people were admitted to hospital, and one child died. NPHS, National Public Health Service. (Modified from: The Public Inquiry into the September 2005 Outbreak of *E. coli* 0157 in South Wales. Chairman H. Pennington, March 2009. http://mrsaactionuk.net/pdfs/reportecoli.pdf.)

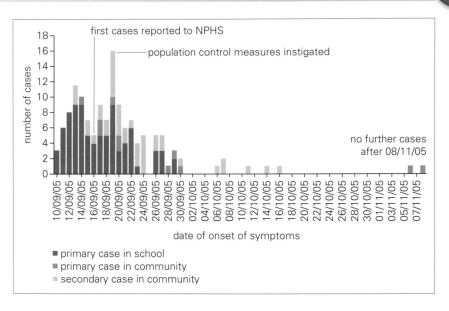

**Table 18.3** Infectious causes of diarrhoea

|  | Onset | Source |
|---|---|---|
| **Food poisoning (due to preformed toxin in food)** | | |
| *Staphylococcus aureus* | 1–6 h | Cream, meat, poultry |
| *Clostridium perfringens* | 8–20 h | Reheated meat |
| *Clostridium botulinum* | 12–36 h | Canned food |
| *Bacillus cereus* | 1–20 h | Reheated foods |
| **Intestinal infections** | | |
| Rotavirus | 2–5 days | Faecal–oral |
| Norovirus | 1–2 days | Faecal–oral |
| *Salmonella* | 1–2 days | Eggs, food |
| *Clostridium difficile* | 1–2 days | Faecal–oral |
| *Shigella* | 1–4 days | Faecal–oral |
| *Campylobacter* | 1–4 days | Poultry, domestic animals |
| *Vibrio cholerae* | 2 days | Faecal–oral |
| *Escherichia coli* | 1–4 days | Food |
| *Yersinia enterocolitica* | Days–weeks | Pets (e.g. dogs) |
| *Giardia duodenalis* <br> *Entamoeba histolytica* | 1–2 weeks <br> Days–weeks | } Contaminated water |
| *Cryptosporidium* <br> *Cystoisospora belli* | } Days–weeks | } Faecal–oral opportunistic (e.g. in AIDS) |

Worldwide, infectious diarrhoea is the major cause of infant mortality.

respond. However, they are not so well controlled quantitatively, and there are many cases when overactivity damages not only an invading parasite but also innocent host tissues. The expression of natural immunity often causes a certain amount of inflammation—and this can be severe, with tissue damage. Complement, neutrophils and tumour necrosis factor (TNF) play important roles.

Microbial endotoxin activates the immune system and induces cytokines, causing a bewildering variety of biologic effects (Fig. 18.4). At the clinical level it can be responsible for septic shock.

### Endotoxins are typically lipopolysaccharides

Endotoxins of bacteria and other microorganisms have a deceptively similar name to exotoxins but are profoundly different in their significance. Unlike exotoxins, these are integral parts of the microbial cell wall and are normally released only when the cell dies. Endotoxins are particularly

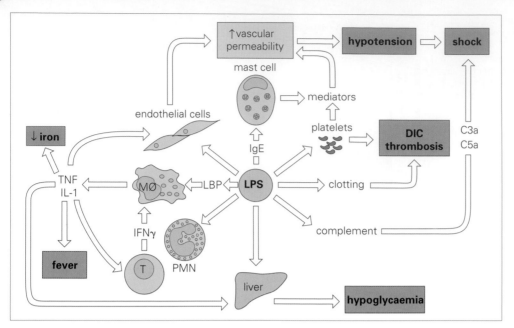

**Fig. 18.4** The many activities of bacterial endotoxin. Lipopolysaccharide (LPS) activates almost every immune mechanism as well as the clotting pathway and, as a result, LPS is one of the most powerful immune stimuli known. DIC, Disseminated intravascular coagulation; IFN, interferon; IL, interleukin; LBP, LPS binding protein; Mφ, macrophage; PMN, polymorphonuclear neutrophil; TNF, tumour necrosis factor.

characteristic of gram-negative bacteria. A typical lipopoly-saccharide (LPS) endotoxin is composed of:

- a conserved lipid portion (lipid A) inserted into the cell wall, responsible for much of the toxic activity
- a conserved core polysaccharide
- the highly variable *O*-polysaccharide, responsible for the serologic diversity, which is a feature of organisms such as salmonellae and shigellae.

LPSs stimulate an extraordinary range of host responses—or perhaps one should say a wide range of responses have evolved to respond to LPSs. These include LPS-binding protein (the LPS–LPS binding protein complex then binds to CD14 on macrophages and dendritic cells) and TLR4 (see Ch. 10). In the words of Lewis Thomas, "When we sense lipopolysaccharide, we are likely to turn on every defence at our disposal" (see Fig. 18.4). Evidently, the body needs to be aware of invading gram-negative bacteria at the earliest possible stage.

Clinically, the most important effects of LPS are fever and vascular collapse (shock). As mentioned in Chapter 15, fever may benefit host or parasite, or both, and is currently considered to be mainly due to the action of two cytokines, inter-leukin 1 (IL-1) and TNF, on the hypothalamus. Both these cytokines are produced by macrophages in response to LPS (and to analogous molecules from other organisms; see later) (Box 18.1).

### Endotoxin shock is usually associated with systemic spread of organisms

The commonest example of endotoxin (or septic) shock is septicaemia with gram-negative bacteria such as *E. coli* or *Neisseria meningitidis*. However, many other organisms also release molecules that stimulate TNF and/or IL-1 production (Table 18.4) and therefore function in part like LPS, although they are primarily unrelated in structure. In the toxic shock syndrome of young women with staphylococcal infections

of the genital tract, toxic shock syndrome toxin is the media-tor; it acts as a superantigen, activating a large proportion (up to one in five) of all T cells (see Ch. 17) that express par-ticular Vβ genes in their T-cell receptors. Activating an enor-mous number of T cells produces enough cytokine to cause the toxic effect.

Septic shock, however, is a complex phenomenon, and other bacterial components such as peptidoglycans may play a part. Disseminated intravascular coagulation (DIC), hypo-glycaemia and cardiovascular failure are features of septic shock. In streptococcal infections, the culprits are pyrogenic (erythrogenic) exotoxins released by the bacteria.

The involvement of cytokines in the pathogenesis of shock is by no means a purely academic concern because it suggests the possibility of treatment by antagonists of these cytokines (e.g. by monoclonal antibodies or inhibi-tors) rather than by antibodies to the toxins themselves, which are of enormous antigenic diversity. However, so far monoclonal antibodies to endotoxin have not proved to be effective.

### The cytokine most closely linked to disease is TNF

Raised concentrations of TNF in the serum have been shown to correlate with severity in patients with meningococ-cal septicaemia and with *Plasmodium falciparum* malaria. However, animal experiments indicate that, in such cases, TNF probably synergizes with other cytokines such as IL-1 and interferon gamma (IFNγ), to produce its full effects. In meningococcal disease, TNF concentrations in blood and cerebrospinal fluid can change independently, the former being raised in septicaemia and the latter in meningitis; it therefore appears that the production and/or effects of TNF can be restricted to a particular body compartment.

In some cases, it may be worth suppressing inflammation with steroids (e.g. a randomized trial in which dexametha-sone was given to patients with acute bacterial meningitis

## Box 18.1 Lessons in Microbiology

### Is it a cold—or is it flu?

The common cold is usually caused by a rhinovirus or a coronavirus. Real influenza, caused by the influenza virus, usually has a more sudden onset, and the combination of fever and a cough has a predictive value of ~80%. But what causes the symptoms of sore throat, sneezing, nasal discharge and nasal congestion?

Sore throat symptoms are thought to be caused by prostaglandins and bradykinin acting on sensory nerve endings in the airway. Sneezing is triggered by inflammatory mediators in the nose and nasopharynx acting on the trigeminal nerves. The plasma-rich exudate that forms part of the nasal discharge can change from clear to yellow/green during an upper respiratory infection. The colour reflects the recruitment of leukocytes into the airway lumen. If large numbers of leukocytes are present, the green protein myeloperoxidase found in the azurophil granules of neutrophils gives the discharge a green colour. Nasal congestion occurs later in infection, when inflammatory mediators such as bradykinin cause the large veins in the nasal epithelium to dilate. Common cold viruses do not cause such damage to the airway epithelium, and infection may not create a cough—but influenza usually causes serious damage to the respiratory epithelium. Fever is mainly caused by IL-1 and IL-6. It also seems that cytokines are responsible for muscle aches and pains by causing the breakdown of muscle proteins. Of course, TNF was originally called cachexin because of its ability to cause muscle wasting or cachexia.

Sometimes in past flu epidemics, such as the Spanish flu in 1918, people died very quickly, within a few days of infection, which seems too fast for secondary infections to be responsible. Reconstructed viruses with the same haemagglutinin and neuraminidase seem to cause severe inflammation, and it is possible that excessive cytokine release, in a cytokine storm, caused the pathology.

**Table 18.4** Important endotoxins and functionally related molecules that induce TNF

| Organisms | Toxin |
|---|---|
| **Bacteria** | |
| ***Gram-negative*** | |
| *Salmonella*<br>*Shigella*<br>*Escherichia coli*<br>*Neisseria meningitidis* | LPS |
| ***Gram-positive*** | |
| *Staphylococcus aureus* | TSST1 |
| *Mycobacteria* | Lipoarabinomannan |
| *Bordetella pertussis* | Endotoxin |
| **Fungi** | |
| Yeasts | Zymosan |
| **Protozoa** | |
| *Plasmodium* | Phospholipids (exoantigens) |

Most endotoxins are lipopolysaccharides (LPS) and exert their main effects by stimulating cytokine release. LPS can also induce the secretion of other cytokines such as interleukin 1. TSST1, Toxic shock syndrome toxin.

showed that corticosteroid reduced mortality). Antibodies can be used to block inflammatory mediators: anti-TNF monoclonal antibodies are now used to treat rheumatoid arthritis. The immune system itself also tries to control inflammation during sepsis by producing antiinflammatory mediators such as IL-10 and TGFβ.

There may also be strain differences in the ability of bacteria to induce inflammation; *Haemophilus influenzae* strains isolated from patients with chronic obstructive pulmonary disease exacerbations induce more inflammation than do colonizing strains not associated with the worsening of symptoms (Fig. 18.5).

### Complement is involved in several tissue-damaging reactions

The activation of complement is a vital part of immunity to many bacteria, viruses and protozoa (see Chs. 10 and 15). Complement can, however, be involved in tissue-damaging reactions such as immune complex disease, which also involves antibody and usually neutrophils (polymorphonuclear leukocytes [PMNs]). Complement also plays an important role in the acute inflammatory response by generating the chemotactic factors C3a and C5a (see Ch. 10). Animal experiments suggest that C5a contributes to cardiac problems during sepsis, as it binds to C5a receptors on cardiomyocytes (cardiomyocytes are also damaged by LPS itself and by inflammatory cytokines such as IL-1, TNF and IL-6).

Direct activation of complement by LPS may contribute to the shock induced by toxic amounts of this endotoxin, in which the levels of complement components (e.g. C3) drop profoundly; this response appears to involve both the classical and the alternative complement pathways, which are activated by the lipid and polysaccharide components, respectively. C3a and C5a are produced in large amounts, and there is frequently a severe decrease in the number of PMNs because of aggregation of these cells, adherence to vessel walls and their activation to release toxic molecules, both oxidative and nonoxidative. When this occurs in the pulmonary capillaries, severe pulmonary oedema may result—the acute respiratory distress syndrome (ARDS).

### Disseminated intravascular coagulation is a rare but serious feature of bacterial septicaemia

DIC can be a feature of bacterial (e.g. meningococcal) septicaemia but is also seen in some virus infections such as Ebola fever (Ch. 29). The relative contributions of immune complexes, platelets and direct activation of the clotting pathway via the effect of LPS on Hageman factor remain controversial. For example, the haemorrhagic phenomena of yellow

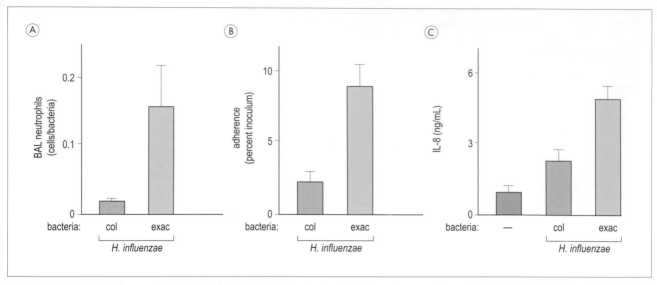

**Fig. 18.5** *Haemophilus influenzae* strains isolated from patients with chronic obstructive pulmonary disease (COPD) induce more inflammation than colonizing strains not associated with worsening of symptoms. *H. influenzae* strains from patients with COPD exacerbations (exac) induce greater numbers of neutrophils (A), more adherence to airway epithelial cells (B) and more IL-8 (C) than do isolates associated with colonization (col). BAL, Bronchoalveolar lavage; IL-8, interleukin 8. (Modified from: Chin CL, et al. *Haemophilus influenzae* from patients with chronic obstructive pulmonary disease exacerbation induce more inflammation than colonizers. *Am J Respir Crit Care Med*. 2005;172:85–91.)

fever are probably secondary to coagulation defects due to the extensive liver damage, whereas in dengue (haemor-rhagic) fever it has been suggested that there is immune complex deposition in blood vessels. However, in all these haemorrhagic syndromes the role of cytokines such as TNF also needs to be considered.

## PATHOLOGIC CONSEQUENCES OF THE IMMUNE RESPONSE

### Overreaction of the immune system is known as hypersensitivity

Adaptive immune responses are vital to defence against infection, as witnessed by the increased susceptibility to infectious disease of immunodeficient patients (see Ch. 31). The antimicrobial effects of T- and B-cell responses act mainly by focusing or enhancing nonspecific effector mechanisms (see Ch. 11). This may also enhance the pathologic effects outlined earlier. The tissue-damaging effects of hypersensitivity are referred to as immunopathologic. Coombs and Gell in 1958 classified hypersensitivity into four types based on the immunologic mechanism underlying the tissue-damaging reaction.

### Each of the four main types of hypersensitivity can be of microbial or nonmicrobial origin

Hypersensitivity of microbial origin includes some of the most serious of these responses (Table 18.5). Organisms of many sorts can be involved, but one common feature is that the infection is prolonged, with continuous or repeated antigenic stimulation.

### Type I hypersensitivity

These reactions are often called immediate, as they can occur within minutes, when the allergen triggers the degranulation of mast cells precoated with specific IgE antibodies.

### Allergic reactions are a feature of helminth infections

The most dramatic allergic (type I) reaction is that following the rupture of an *Echinococcus granulosus* (cystic hydatid) cyst. Slow leakage of worm antigens ensures that the patient's mast cells are sensitized with specific IgE, and the massive flood of antigens on rupture may cause acute fatal anaphylaxis, with vascular collapse and pulmonary oedema. Even the small amount of antigen used in the now supersed Casoni intradermal skin test can have this effect, although this is rare.

Another helminth associated with high levels of IgE is *Ascaris*, but here the pathologic consequences are mainly respiratory, with eosinophilic infiltrates and asthmatic episodes corresponding to passage of the parasite through the lung. The itchy rashes characteristic of helminth infections when their larvae die in the skin are probably also of this type, an example being swimmer's itch due to cercariae released from snails infected with human, animal or avian schistosomes.

Why allergic reactions are such a feature of helminth infections is not clear, but they may be due to some feature of the antigens; in addition, it has been suggested that IgE plays a role in protection against helminths. One would hope so, as in all other respects this class of antibody appears to be nothing but a nuisance.

Some insect venoms cause severe and life-threatening systemic reactions called anaphylaxis. One-third of beekeepers are sensitized to bee venom and have venom-specific IgE; the main honeybee allergen is Api m 1. Some insect allergens are enzymes such as hyaluronidases or dipeptidylpeptidases that are cross-reactive between species such as bees and wasps. Hypersensitivity can be demonstrated through skin prick or basophil activation tests. Venom immunotherapy can induce tolerance through desensitization, reducing the risk of a future systemic reaction by 90%.

Allergic diseases are more common than they used to be, and it has been proposed that this may be because most of us now grow up in an environment that is too clean. The hygiene

**Table 18.5** Hypersensitivity of microbial origin

| Coombs and Gell classification | Principal mechanism | Examples |
|---|---|---|
| Type I (allergic/anaphylactic) | IgE, mast cells, Th2 cytokines | Helminths<br>*Ascaris*<br>*Echinococcus granulosus* (ruptured cyst)<br>? Viral skin rash<br>? Upper respiratory tract<br>Viral infections |
| Type II (cytotoxic) | IgM and IgG to surface antigens<br>Complement<br>Cytotoxic cells | Virus-infected cells<br>Malaria-infected erythrocytes<br>Autoantibodies in:<br>    *Mycoplasma*<br>    Streptococci<br>    *Trypanosoma cruzi* |
| Type III (immune complex mediated) | Immune complexes with IgM or IgG<br>Complement<br>PMN | In tissues:<br>    Allergic alveolitis<br>    Actinomycosis<br>In blood vessels:<br>    Glomerulonephritis<br>    Malaria<br>    Streptococci<br>    Hepatitis B<br>    Syphilis |
| Type IV (cell mediated) | T cells (Th1, Th17, CTL)<br>Cytokines<br>Macrophages (and other nonspecific cells) | Granuloma<br>Tuberculosis<br>Leprosy (tuberculoid)<br>Schistosomiasis (eggs)<br>*Histoplasma*<br>Mononuclear infiltration ± cell damage in many virus infections with CD4 and CD8 T-cell–derived cytokines and macrophages playing roles<br>Viral rashes |
| Autoimmunity | Cross-reaction with host | Streptococcal myocarditis |
| | Polyclonal B-cell activation | Human African trypanosomiasis |

All four classic types of hypersensitivity can be induced by infectious organisms, types II and III being the most commonly encountered. Note that some mechanisms mediating hypersensitivity also take part in protective immunity. PMN, Polymorphonuclear neutrophil.

hypothesis proposes that, if we are exposed to a range of bacterial and viral infections in infancy, this may prevent the development of more harmful allergies by promoting a bias toward Th1 cytokine production. Certainly people living in Africa seem to have had more exposure to antigenic stimulation, age for age, than those living in Europe, with more memory T cells and fewer naive T cells, although this may also be due to earlier infections with viruses such as cytomegalovirus. Slightly surprisingly, it seems that infections with helminths, which induce copious Th2 responses, also protect against development of atopy possibly because they outcompete the allergen-specific IgE on mast cells. Other factors such as innate immunity and regulatory T cells that act to reduce harmful immune responses causing immunopathology may be involved.

## Type II hypersensitivity

### Type II reactions are mediated by antibodies to the infectious organism or autoantibodies

Strictly speaking, type II reactions are mediated by antibody (usually IgG but also IgM) leading to cytotoxicity, either extracellular or intracellular (e.g. after phagocytosis). Antibody binds to the cell and, if complement is activated, the cell is lysed. An important distinction can be made between antibodies to the (foreign) infectious organism and autoantibodies; the former kill host cells because they display foreign antigens, whereas the latter bind to unaltered host antigens, and both types of response occur in infectious disease (see Table 18.5).

### In blood-stage malaria, malarial antigens attach themselves to host cells

Antibody binding and then complement-mediated lysis of red cells leads to autoimmune haemolytic anaemia. It has been shown that the haemolytic anaemia of blood-stage malaria is due not to autoantibody, as previously thought, but to antibodies to parasite-derived antigens that have been picked up by red cells. In some cases, it may be the antigen–antibody complex that binds to the cell. A similar reaction (blackwater fever) can occur following treatment of malaria (usually *P. falciparum*, very occasionally *P. vivax* or *P. malariae*) with amino-alcohol drugs such as quinine or mefloquine.

**Antimyocardial antibody of group A β-haemolytic streptococcal infection is the classic autoantibody triggered by infection**

This reaction is due to the presence of the same cross-reacting carbohydrate antigen on the bacterium and the myocardium, causing rheumatic heart disease with damage to the cardiac valve. However, as more protein sequences are obtained and compared, numerous other similar examples have come to light, and it is possible that cross-reaction between microbial and human antigens may underlie a number of diseases of currently unknown origin. Whether this mimicry of host antigens has any survival value to the microbe is discussed in Chapter 17.

## Type III hypersensitivity

### Immune complexes cause disease when they become lodged in tissues or blood vessels

Immune complexes cause pathology if they are made in excess, if they are not removed properly from the circulation and if they deposit in blood vessels leading to vasculitis, in joints giving arthritis or in tissues such as the kidney resulting in glomerulonephritis.

The formation of immune complexes can lead to phagocytosis and removal of antigen but also to complement activation. Complications occur when the complexes escape removal by the phagocytes of the reticuloendothelial system and become lodged in the tissues or blood vessels, attracting complement and neutrophils. Release of lysosomal enzymes then results in local damage, which is particularly serious in small blood vessels, especially in the renal glomeruli. Immune complex disease is a major cause of both acute and chronic

glomerulonephritis, and the majority of cases are probably the result of infection. There is also an important group in which autoantigen–autoantibody complexes are responsible (e.g. DNA–anti-DNA in systemic lupus erythematosus [SLE]), but even these may ultimately be the consequence of viral infection or reactivation—there is an association between EBV infection and SLE, particularly in younger patients.

Like most other immunopathologic conditions, immune complex deposition is usually a feature of chronic infection (e.g. malaria). However, a persistent antigenic stimulus is not the only prerequisite, indicated by the fact that the most serious form of malarial nephropathy is found in *P. malariae* (quartan) malaria, which progresses despite successful treatment of the infection, whereas the nephropathy of *P. falciparum* (malignant tertian) malaria typically recovers after the infection has been cured. Predisposing factors may include a poor antibody response (in terms of amount or affinity), a particular tendency of the antigen itself to bind to vascular endothelium, or inhibition of the normal function of phagocytes or complement in removing circulating complexes.

Acute glomerulonephritis occurs as a rare but serious complication of streptococcal infection (see Ch. 19) and is at least partly due to localization in glomeruli of immune complexes containing streptococcal antigens (Fig. 18.6). Neutrophil infiltration and alterations in the basement membrane cause leakage of albumin, even red cells, into the urine. The glomerulonephritis appears a few weeks after the infection has been terminated. When complexes are deposited over a long period (malarial nephropathy), the mesangial cell intrusions and fusion of foot processes cause a more irreversible impairment of glomerular function (chronic glomerulonephritis).

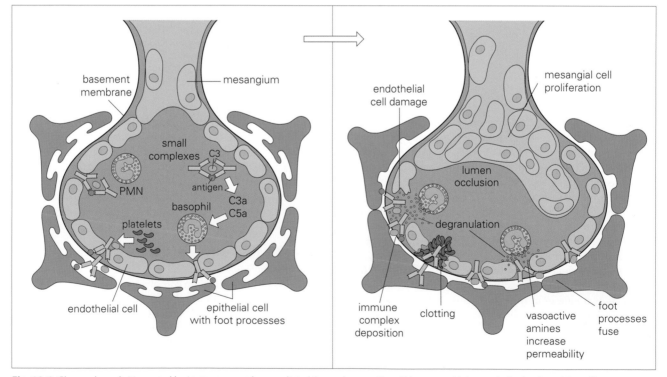

**Fig. 18.6** Glomerulonephritis caused by immune complex–mediated tissue damage. Type III hypersensitivity results in the deposition of immune complexes in the blood vessel walls, particularly at sites of high pressure, filtration or turbulence such as the kidney. Large complexes deposit on the glomerular basement membrane, whereas small ones pass through the basement membrane and then deposit on the epithelial side of the glomerulus. PMN, Polymorphonuclear neutrophil.

## Occupational diseases associated with inhalation of fungi are the classic examples of immune complex deposition in the tissues

Immune complex deposition in the tissues, made famous by the work of Arthus on antigens injected into the skin of animals with preexisting antibody (mainly IgG), manifests as a combination of thrombosis in small blood vessels and necrosis in the tissues due to PMN degranulation (Fig. 18.7). The best-studied examples are the occupational diseases associated with inhalation of fungi (e.g. farmer's lung, pigeon-fancier's disease, maple bark stripper's disease) in which chronic inflammation of the lung can lead to a state of destruction and fibrosis known as extrinsic allergic alveolitis, an unfortunate name as classic (IgE-mediated) allergy does not seem to be involved.

## Another well-known example of immune complex disease was serum sickness

Serum sickness follows repeated injections of foreign protein, leading to circulating immune complexes, which deposit in the kidneys (see Fig. 18.6), skin and joints. This was common in the preantibiotic days of passive serotherapy with horse serum for diphtheria (see Ch. 36). To prevent a similar reaction to monoclonal antibodies used as immunotherapy, antibodies are now genetically engineered so that as much of the molecule as possible is humanized, and some are now fully human.

## Type IV hypersensitivity

### Cell-mediated immune responses invariably cause some tissue destruction that may be permanent

Despite the examples of antibody-mediated tissue damage discussed earlier, the antibody response generally achieves its purpose in eliminating invading organisms without any trace of damage to the host. Cell-mediated (type IV) hypersensitivity responses with the activation of both T cells and macrophages invariably cause some tissue destruction, which may be reparable if not too prolonged, but over time cytokines such as TGFβ and IL-13 can act on myofibroblasts leading to fibrosis and even calcification (Table 18.6).

**Fig. 18.7** The Arthus reaction. Microbial antigens that enter the tissues (e.g. fungal particles in the lung) encounter antibodies and form immune complexes. These activate complement and initiate chemotaxis of polymorphonuclear neutrophils (*PMNs*), and degranulation of these and tissue mast cells. The resulting inflammatory response is further potentiated by damage induced by PMN-derived lysosomal enzymes.

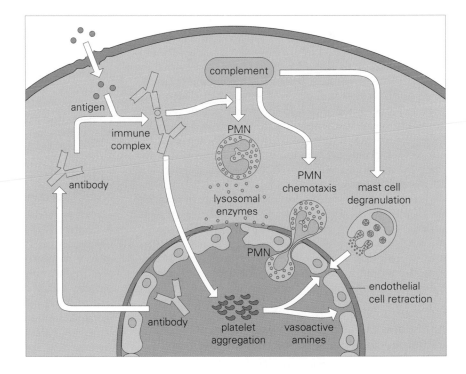

**Table 18.6** Cell-mediated immunity in protection and disease

| Cell-mediated responses | | | |
|---|---|---|---|
| **Immune cells or molecules** | **Protective effect against** | **Pathologic effect** | **Skin test** |
| Cytotoxic T cells (CD8) | Virus infections<br>*Theileria* (Mycobacteria)[a] | Local tissue loss | |
| Basophils, T cells | ? | Inflammation | 24 h (Jones-Mote reaction) |
| T cells (CD4)<br>Macrophages<br>Cytokines<br>Giant cells<br>Epithelioid cells<br>Eosinophils | Intracellular organisms<br>Viruses<br>Bacteria<br>Fungi<br>Protozoa<br>Worms | Mononuclear cell infiltration<br>Granuloma<br>Fibrosis<br>Calcification | } Delayed/tuberculin type (>2 days) |

[a]A role for CD8 T cells in protection against *M. tuberculosis* has been proposed.

## From the medical viewpoint, granuloma formation is the most important type IV hypersensitivity response

The cell-mediated response to microbial antigen is responsible for granuloma formation and plays a major role in diseases such as tuberculosis, tuberculoid leprosy, lymphogranuloma inguinale and *Toxocara* infection. Some granulomas tend to undergo necrosis (e.g. caseation in tuberculosis) whereas others do not (e.g. leprosy, sarcoidosis), which may be explained in terms of the different pattern of cytokines involved. TNF, often in association with some microbial products, is especially likely to cause necrosis through its effects on vascular endothelium. In tuberculosis the granuloma has an outer ring of lymphocytes, while myeloid cells are found in the core, including the multinucleated giant cells typical of such granulomas. However, there are also unexpected findings: the lymphocyte cuff contains not just CD4 and CD8 T cells but B cells, while the centre contains monocytes and neutrophils as well as macrophages, with expression of downregulatory molecules such as IDO-1 and PD-L1, as well as TGFβ.

### The clinical features of schistosomiasis are produced by cell-mediated immunity

The price paid for protective cell-mediated immunity is particularly well illustrated by the helminth disease schistosomiasis. *Schistosoma mansoni* (the blood fluke) lays eggs in the mesenteric venous system, some of which become lodged in small portal vessels in the liver. Strong cell-mediated reactions to secreted enzymes lead to granulomatous reactions around each egg, resulting in egg destruction and sparing of liver parenchyma from the toxic effects of the egg enzymes. However, the coalescent granulomas ultimately cause portal fibrosis, with portal hypertension, oesophageal varices and haematemesis (see Ch. 23).

The rather unexpected effect of malnutrition in reducing the incidence and severity of certain diseases (e.g. typhus, malaria) may be attributable to a reduction in immunopathology, though in the majority of diseases (e.g. measles, meningococcal infection, tuberculosis) the reverse is true. Indeed, poor nutrition may be a major factor predisposing to the greater severity of many common infections in tropical countries.

### Antibodies can also cause enhancement of pathology, as in dengue infection

Most cases of dengue haemorrhagic fever occur in people who get a second infection with the dengue virus. Neutralizing antibodies bind to an epitope on the envelope dimer. The problem is that there are four dengue serotypes that can differ by as much as 30% in the amino acid sequence of their envelope proteins. After infection with a second serotype, the concentration and avidity of the antibodies that have been generated to the first serotype will not be sufficient to prevent the new infection but will enhance virus uptake as antibody binding to the virus leads to greater internalization through Fc binding (Fig. 18.8). The viral load falls as the fever falls, but this is when the most severe symptoms and pathology appear, including leakage of plasma from capillaries, haemorrhage and shock, at least partly due to excessive inflammatory cytokine release in a cytokine storm. Antibody-dependent enhancement of infection has been

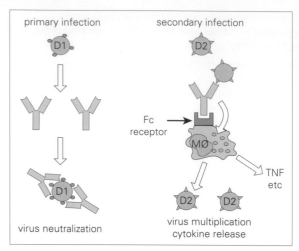

**Fig. 18.8** Antibody-dependent enhancement in dengue (D) infection. A primary infection with one of the four dengue serotypes generates protective neutralizing antibodies to the E protein. A subsequent infection with a different serotype can lead to severe pathology with vascular leakage as a result of virus multiplication and cytokine release. It is thought that cross-reactive antibodies from the first infection are insufficient in quantity or avidity to neutralize the second serotype but do enable the virus to enter monocytes/macrophages through Fc receptor binding. Mφ, Macrophage; TNF, tumour necrosis factor.

reported in one study of Nicaraguan children with previous Zika virus infection in which it enhanced the future risk of dengue virus 2 disease and dengue virus 2 and 3 severity, in humans, due to cross-reactivity between the envelope proteins of these two Flaviviruses. This has been a cause for concern in the development of dengue and Zika virus vaccines.

## SKIN RASHES

### A variety of skin rashes have an immunologic origin

The ways in which infections can affect the skin are detailed in Chapter 27, but some rashes are considered to be immunologically mediated. For example, the characteristic skin rash of measles is absent in children with T-cell deficiency (e.g. thymic aplasia or DiGeorge syndrome), who instead develop a fatal systemic infection indicating that the skin lesions are T-cell mediated and are associated with cell-mediated immunity. In contrast, if children with T-cell deficiency are vaccinated with live vaccinia virus, they develop an inexorable spreading skin lesion, which is clearly a direct and not an immunopathologic effect.

Table 18.7 lists the more common skin conditions of immunologic origin in which an infectious organism is thought to be involved.

### The SARS-CoV-2 coronavirus causes lung immunopathology

For some individuals at least, infection with SARS-CoV-2 led to a severe infection requiring hospitalization that was sometimes fatal. The pneumonia induced showed tissue damage caused by the virus, followed by local and then systemic inflammation. Excessive production of proinflammatory cytokines, including IL-1, IL-6, IL-17 and TNFα, caused a cytokine storm and ARDS with lung damage. The inflammatory response involved emergency myelopoiesis and vascular damage. The systemic inflammation was associated

**Table 18.7** Skin rashes and their immunologic basis

| Organism | Disease | Character | Pathogenic basis |
|---|---|---|---|
| **Viruses** | | | |
| Measles | Measles | Maculopapular rash | } T cells, immune complexes, allergy |
| Rubella | German measles | Maculopapular rash | ? Immune mediated |
| Enterovirus | Hand, foot, mouth | Vesicular Erythematous | Viral cytopathic Viral ? immune mediated |
| Varicella-zoster | Chickenpox/zoster | Vesicular rash | Viral cytopathic |
| Human immunodeficiency virus | Acquired immunodeficiency syndrome | Maculopapular | Lymphocytic infiltrate |
| Epstein-Barr virus | Glandular fever | Erythematous rash Transient erythematous rash | Idiosyncratic antibody development to ampicillin Viral ? immune mediated |
| Parvovirus B19 | Erythema infectiosum | Erythematous rash | Immune complexes |
| **Bacteria** | | | |
| *Streptococcus pyogenes* | Scarlet fever | Erythematous rash | Erythrogenic toxin |
| *Treponema pallidum* *T. pertenue* | Syphilis Yaws | } Disseminated infectious rash in secondary stage | Immune complexes |
| *Salmonella typhi* | Typhoid, enteric fever | Sparse rose spots | Immune complexes |
| *Neisseria meningitidis* | Meningitis, spotted fever | Petechial or maculopapular lesions | Immune complexes |
| *Mycobacterium leprae* | Tuberculoid leprosy | Hypopigmented skin lesions | T cells, macrophages |
| *Rickettsia prowazeki* and others | Typhus | Maculopapular or haemorrhagic rash | Thrombosis |
| **Fungi** | | | |
| Dermatophytes | Dermatophytid or allergic rash | | Immune complexes ? |
| *Blastomyces dermatitidis* | Blastomycosis | Papule or pustule developing into granuloma | Hypersensitivity to fungal antigens, T cells |
| **Protozoa** | | | |
| *Leishmania tropica* | Cutaneous leishmaniasis | Papules ulcerating to form crusted infectious sores | T cells, macrophages |

Many skin rashes represent immunologic reactions occurring in the skin. It is suspected that several skin diseases of unknown origin are in fact caused by viruses, either directly or indirectly.

with reductions in T cells, natural killer cells and dendritic cells in the blood; patients with stronger CD4 and CD8 T-cell responses tended to have milder disease. Some of the patients with more severe disease had antibodies to IFNα and IFNω, leading to reduced viral clearance, depressed type 1 and increased type 2 T-cell cytokine responses and more plasmablasts.

## VIRUSES AND CANCER

A variety of RNA and DNA viruses can cause permanent malignant changes within cells (Table 18.8). An account of proviruses and oncogenes (genes causing malignancy) is included in Chapter 3. Various human cancers have been shown to be associated with such oncogenic viruses (Table 18.9). Around 16% of all human cancers are associated with seven virus infections and causing ~1 million deaths annually. Some of these include cancers associated with HIV infection. Three types of cancer, namely KS, non-Hodgkin lymphoma (NHL) and cervical cancer, are part of the classification of an acquired immunodeficiency syndrome

(AIDS) defining diagnosis, consistent with advanced HIV infection. The resulting immunosuppression and loss of immune control over HHV-8 (KS-associated herpesvirus), EBV-associated diffuse large B-cell and central nervous system NHL and HPV-associated cervical cancer leads to these cancers developing. There are latent and lytic components to the life cycles of these viruses. Few genes are expressed in latent infections, allowing the virus to reside in specific sites with the potential for reactivation but enabling infected cells to undergo future malignant change. The virus can disseminate in the lytic stage by release from infected cells. Some of the genes expressed can also promote tumour development. This part of the viral replicative cycle may therefore be of more importance in virus-associated malignancy. HIV-infected individuals are also at higher risk of developing HPV-associated anal cancer and HBV-associated liver cancer. As always, cancer prevention is the aim, and two vaccines against HPV and HBV are available and effective, with other vaccines being developed (see Ch. 35).

**Table 18.8** Malignant transformation

| Changes | Details |
|---|---|
| Morphology | Loss of shape; rounding |
| | Decreased adhesion to surface |
| Growth, contact | Loss of contact inhibition of growth and movement |
| | Increased ability to grow from a single cell |
| | Increased ability to grow in suspension |
| | Capacity for continued growth (immortalization) |
| Cellular properties | DNA synthesis induced |
| | Chromosomal changes |
| | Appearance of new antigens (viral or cellular in origin) |
| Biochemical properties | Loss of fibronectin |
| | Reduced cAMP |

These changes occur when tumour viruses cause transformation of cultured cells. Many of these changes are obviously relevant for tumour production in vivo. cAMP, Cyclic adenosine monophosphate.

### Human T-cell lymphotropic virus type 1 is associated with adult T-cell leukaemia/lymphoma

HTLV-1 and HTLV-2 are retroviruses that have no oncogenes (see Ch. 3). An aggressive haematologic malignancy called adult T-cell leukaemia/lymphoma (ATLL) is reported in ~5% of HTLV-1 infections. HTLV-1 proviral DNA is detectable in the cellular DNA of individuals with ATLL.

Although reported around the world, HTLV-1 infection is endemic in South Japan, the Caribbean islands, West and Central Africa and parts of South America. Less is known about the geographic distribution of HTLV-2, which was first isolated from an individual with atypical hairy T-cell leukaemia but has no association with malignancy. This virus can be found in certain Amerindian tribes and is associated with neurologic and other chronic inflammatory conditions. Transmission is by breastfeeding and sexual intercourse, cellular blood products (blood donation) and rarely by organ transplantation.

The carcinogenic nature of HTLV-1 is not due to activation of a cellular oncogene but the result of a multistage process with a number of somatic mutations accumulating over time. These oncogenic driver events are key to tumour progression. It is now thought that the mitotic replicative error over time since infection in infancy is the main mechanism of oncogenesis. The two key HTLV-1 regulatory genes, *tax* and *HBZ*, were thought to be oncogenes, but their products may contribute to oncogenesis by causing genetic instability, promoting cell proliferation and helping maintain the malignant ATLL clone.

These infections are described in more detail in Chapter 27.

### EBV is associated with nasopharyngeal carcinoma and some lymphomas

EBV is associated with the development of nasopharyngeal carcinoma (NPC; see Ch. 19), which is common in South China and other parts of Asia (8–30 cases/100,000 people/year, but higher in men than women), less common in parts of North and South Africa and rare elsewhere in the world. The reason for this restricted geographic and specific ethnic group distribution is unknown. There are different types of NPC, and EBV is strongly associated with nonkeratinizing squamous cell as well as undifferentiated carcinoma. There is no convincing evidence for specific carcinogenic EBV strains, but these effects could be due to local cocarcinogens such as nitrosamines in salted fish. EBV DNA can be demonstrated in the cancer cells, but the precise mechanism for carcinogenesis is unknown; cellular oncogenes have not been implicated. There is a complex interplay between EBV,

**Table 18.9** Viruses and human cancer

| Viruses | Cancer | Strength of association | Viral genome in cancer cells | Cofactor |
|---|---|---|---|---|
| Epstein-Barr virus | Burkitt's lymphoma | ++ | + | Malaria |
| | Nasopharyngeal carcinoma | ++ | + | Nitrosamines |
| | Hodgkin disease | + | + | – |
| Human papillomavirus | Cervical cancer | ++ | + | – |
| | Oropharyngeal cancer | ++ | + | – |
| | Skin cancer | + | + | Genetic predisposition ? UV light |
| HHV-8 (KSHV) | Kaposi sarcoma | ++ | + | HIV immunosuppression |
| Hepatitis B virus | Liver cancer | ++ | + | ? Aflatoxin |
| Hepatitis C virus | Liver cancer | ++ | – | – |
| HTLV-1 | T-cell leukaemia | ++ | + | – |

Many viruses transform cells in culture, but only a few are important in human cancer. The associations are strongly supported by studies of naturally occurring or experimentally induced cancers in animals. HHV-8, Human herpesvirus 8; HIV, human immunodeficiency virus; HTLV-1, human T-cell lymphotropic virus 1; KSHV, Kaposi sarcoma–associated herpes virus; UV, ultraviolet.

host genetics and environmental factors, including tobacco smoking, dietary components and occupational exposure.

With respect to NPC pathogenesis, the clonal origin of EBV infection suggests childhood infection may lead to early initiation of NPC. The EBV latent proteins affect the tumour microenvironment by driving a rapid clonal expansion of EBV-infected cells. This results in a number of genetic and epigenetic events and NPC progression. The EBV lytic phase produces infectious virions that spread EBV infection to other cells inducing genetic instability in infected premalignant cells. There is dysregulation of genes involved in DNA repair, cell cycle checkpoint and anti-oncogenesis. EBV also affects the innate immune response by disrupting chemokine and cytokine signalling pathways.

People at high risk of developing NPC have high IgA titres to EBV capsid antigen a year or more before clinical symptoms appear. This helps detect early stage NPC and can be used to monitor the response to treatment and prognosis.

There have been advances in management of NPC, with chemotherapy and radiotherapy and a number of immunotherapeutic approaches.

### EBV is associated with Burkitt's lymphoma

Burkitt's lymphoma (BL), a tumour of immature B cells, occurs in parts of East Africa, such as Uganda, and in Papua New Guinea in 6–14-year-old children, especially boys.

BL was the first human cancer to be associated with EBV and shown to have a chromosomal translocation activating an oncogene (MYC protooncogene), a gene that can transform a cell into a cancer cell. The World Health Organization classification of three clinical variants of BL is:

- endemic (eBL), which is found mostly in Africa and is associated with malaria endemicity and EBV infection. However, epidemiologic studies have shown that other factors and/or possible genetic predisposition may also play a part to cause eBL
- sporadic (sBL), which is seen outside Africa and is rarely associated with EBV infection. Driver genes are those that contribute to tumour progression and are present in sBL
- immunodeficiency related.

EBV DNA is present in the tumour cells, but most of the many copies of the EBV genes are not integrated into the host cell DNA. The tumour is probably caused by the action of EBV on B cells, causing them to proliferate and making activation of cellular oncogenes more likely. The cellular oncogene c-*myc* is translocated from chromosome 8 to the immunoglobulin heavy chain locus on chromosome 14, where it is expressed. As a result, the B cell may be prevented from entering the resting stage. There is also downregulation of adhesion and human leukocyte antigen (HLA) molecules, so that the EBV-containing cells, which are normally subject to immune control, develop into tumour cells. The BL cells also show other chromosomal abnormalities, but their role in tumorigenesis is unclear.

The fact that EBV is a common worldwide infection, whereas BL, like NPC, is restricted geographically, points once again to the involvement of local cofactors, perhaps chemical or infectious cocarcinogens. Malaria is a recognized cofactor in BL, and *P. falciparum* can repeatedly infect African children causing chronic antigenic stimulation and consequent proliferation of latently EBV-infected B memory cells, inducing polyclonal B-cell expansion and lytic cycle EBV reactivation. Expansion of latently infected B cells increases the chance of a c-*myc* translocation, seen in all BL. Another hypothesis is that malaria coinfection impairs EBV-specific T-cell responses with loss of viral immune surveillance and control.

### EBV is also associated with Hodgkin's lymphoma and lymphomas in immunosuppressed individuals, including post-transplant lymphoproliferative disease

EBV has been shown to be associated with classical Hodgkin's lymphoma, as seen in childhood and older adulthood. There is increasing evidence for EBV infection to have a role in specific lymphoma subtypes, including diffuse large B-cell lymphomas and angioimmunoblastic T-cell lymphomas.

Post-transplant lymphoproliferative disorder (PTLD) is associated with immunosuppressive drugs given after solid organ or haematopoietic allogeneic stem cell transplantation. Most are B-cell lymphomas, and one-third develop in the first 12 months post-transplantation (early PTLD), half of which are EBV driven. A 5-year incidence study reported PTLD development in 0.6–9% in adult and 2–16% in paediatric transplant recipients.

Higher risk of PTLD involves donor (D) to recipient (R) EBV VCA IgG serology mismatches (D positive/R negative or D negative/R positive). EBV viraemia monitoring post-transplant is important. The lowest risk of PTLD is in kidney transplant recipients, compared to heart and lung transplant recipients, due to more intensive use of immunosuppression. The large number of EBV-infected donor lymphocytes within specific organs may be another factor. The age of the transplant recipient is a factor, too, with greatest risk at the youngest and older ages. HLA mismatch and specific HLA types in recipients are associated with higher risk, but some donor haplotypes are protective.

As cytotoxic T cells police EBV infection, when host immunosuppression reduces T-cell surveillance then uncontrolled lymphoproliferation can result. Reducing immunosuppression in EBV-driven PTLD may, however, result in graft rejection. Alternative treatment is usually required involving targeted monoclonal antibodies, namely rituximab, which acts on the B-cell CD20 receptor used for EBV entry and in cytotoxic chemotherapy regimes.

EBV-associated primary cerebral lymphoma may occur in HIV-infected individuals. The role of HIV is mostly indirect and is related to immunosuppression or B-cell activation. About 30% of AIDS-related lymphomas are BL. Counterintuitively, since the advent of combined antiretroviral therapy (cART) there has been an increased risk for developing Hodgkin's lymphoma, which may be partly due to the increase in the age of the population living with HIV due to cART (a downside effect of immune reconstitution). This is because Hodgkin's lymphoma is associated with EBV infection, and immune reconstitution increases the stimulation of B cells in which EBV exists episomally.

### Certain HPV infections are associated with cervical cancer

Papillomavirus infections are ubiquitous, transmitted by direct contact and associated with a number of epithelial hyperproliferative diseases. There are five genera, one of which, the alphapapillomavirus genus, includes the high-risk HPV types involved in anogenital and some head and neck cancers. Two others, the beta- and gammapapillomavirus genera, are the skin HPV types found widely on the skin surface. The viral life cycle is intertwined with the host keratinocyte cells' differentiation cycles. After small epithelial abrasions in skin or mucosal surfaces, these cells in the basal skin layer are exposed to HPV, and the viral DNA becomes episomal and replicates with the host DNA using host synthetic machinery.

There are clear associations between the development of cervical cancer and infection with some of the ~200 subtypes of HPV (see Chs. 3, 22 and 27). It has been suggested that the vaginal microbiota (VM), the microbial flora in that site, could play both a protective and a destructive role in HPV persistence. Using high-throughput gene sequencing, higher microbial diversity was detected in the VM of HPV-positive compared with HPV-negative women. It is possible that the composition of the VM could influence the host's innate immune response, susceptibility to infection and development of cervical disease.

Most HPV infections resolve within 24 months, but those that do not account for >80% of cervical cancers, the remainder being penile, vulval, rectal and oropharyngeal cancers, which are also associated with HPV. The HPV high-risk types include 16 and 18; low-risk types include 6 and 11. The latter cause cervical lesions but have a lower risk of progression to malignancy. HPV vaccine programmes were started in 2009 (see Ch. 35).

In most primary and metastatic cancer cells, the HPV genomes are present in integrated form within the host genome, and certain viral oncoprotein genes referred to as E6 and E7 are transcribed and translated. Integration occurs at different chromosomal locations, and the E6 and E7 open-reading frames seem to be involved in transformation of epithelial cells and in maintenance of the transformed state, probably by binding to and inactivating tumour-suppressing cellular proteins concerned with regulation of the cell cycle. E6 is involved in upregulating telomerase activity, maintaining telomere integrity during cell division and mediating degradation of p53, a tumour-suppressor protein; E7 binds and inactivates the retinoblastoma proteins (pRb). Both these activities are critical in HPV-induced oncogenesis and result in genome instability, accumulation of oncogene mutations, uncontrolled cell growth and eventually cancer. The viral E6 and E7 proteins drive cell proliferation in the nasal and parabasal cell layers at sites such as the cervix, where neoplastic changes can occur. There are functional differences in E6 and E7 that may explain the presence of high-risk and low-risk HPV types. For example, the low-risk E7 proteins differ from the high-risk ones in the way they associate with the pRb, while the high-risk E7 protein binds to and degrades other proteins that control cell cycle entry and reentry in basal and upper epithelial cell layers. Cervical cancer is an uncommon sequel to infection with the low-risk types of HPV, and cocarcinogens such as cigarette smoke and HSV have been implicated.

### HPV infection is also associated with squamous cell carcinoma of the skin

Betapapillomaviruses have been associated with the development of nonmelanoma skin cancer, together with ultraviolet (UV) radiation. They may help initiate skin carcinogenesis in what is termed a hit-and-run action by exacerbating the accumulation of UV radiation–induced DNA breaks and somatic mutations. Unlike in cervical cancer, where the E6 and E7 oncoproteins alter the host immune response to establish persistent infection and promote cellular transformation, E6 and E7 expression of skin HPV types is not needed to maintain the skin cancer phenotype.

People with the rare autosomal recessive disease epidermodysplasia verruciformis (EV) are infected with up to 20 different but less common types of HPV, and 30–60% of EV patients between 20 and 40 years of age develop multiple squamous cell carcinomas (SCCs) of the skin. Of these tumours, 90% contain HPV-5, -8, -14 and -20 DNA. These HPV types may act as cocarcinogens with UV light or immunosuppression in the development of nonmelanoma skin cancers, the most common form of skin tumours in populations with fair skin.

HPVs may also play a role in the genesis of 90% of the skin cancers that appear in immunosuppressed organ transplant recipients, and cutaneous warts are common in these patients. In addition, there are reports that skin cancers in healthy individuals may be associated with HPV infection.

Head and neck SCC are caused mostly by exposure to tobacco and alcohol. It was thought that oropharyngeal SCC (OPSCC) would fall as public health programmes were increasingly successful in reducing smoking rates. However, the incidence of OPSCC plateaued and then increased, associated with HPV-16. HPV-positive OPSCC was associated with exposure to high-risk HPV and was found to have wild-type p53 and high levels of p16, a marker of HPV DNA integration into nuclear DNA. In the United States, 5% annual increases in the rate of OPSCC diagnosis have been reported particularly in males with multiple sexual partners and/or orogenital partners. Increases in incidence of OPSCC have also been seen in Europe and Australia.

### HBV and HCV are major causes of liver cancer (hepatocellular carcinoma)

In 2020, ~900,000 people worldwide were diagnosed with liver cancer, of whom ~800,000 people died. Reports estimate that ~56% are related to HBV and 20% to HCV. Bearing in mind liver cancer is the sixth most diagnosed cancer, these are treatable infections, and HBV can be prevented by immunisation.

The results, in sequential order, of chronic active hepatitis (CAH) include hepatocyte necrosis, chronic inflammation, cytokine production, fibrosis and cirrhosis. Therefore CAH is a major driver for the development of hepatocellular carcinoma (HCC).

Individuals with active hepatitis B infections are 20-fold more likely to develop HCC than are uninfected individuals. The oncogenic process depends on a number of predisposing factors that are both viral and host derived (Fig. 18.9). HCC is the outcome of chronic necroinflammatory liver disease associated with higher levels of HBV replication as well as the host immune response. Moreover, some HBV mutant strains and specific genotypes may be associated with HCC development. Integrated HBV sequences found in HCC tumour cells may activate cellular oncogenes that encode proteins linked with controlling cell signalling, proliferation and viability, such as the *myc* family. Chronic inflammation, associated with increased liver cell proliferation, induces

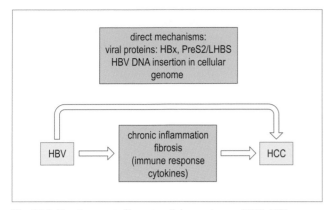

**Fig. 18.9** Development of hepatocellular carcinoma (HCC). HBV, Hepatitis B virus; HBx, hepatitis B virus x protein; PreS2-LHBS, PreS2 mutant large surface antigen.

several rearrangements of the integrated HBV genome that can generate chromosomal instability. The relationship between HBV DNA integration and either activation or inactivation of specific genes in the pathogenesis of HCC is complex. Specific HBV proteins such as the intriguingly named HBx, as well as the L envelope protein (HBsAg can enhance the IL-6-STAT3 pathway involved in tumour growth and development), have important roles in cellular transformation. HBx protein has a key role in HBV replication and HCC progression by:

- integrating into the hepatocyte genome and affecting genomic stability
- inducing epigenetic modifications (i.e. DNA methylation, histone acetylation)
- inducing oxidative stress by interacting with mitochondria and other proteins
- regulating protooncogene activation and tumour suppressor gene inactivation
- transactivating cellular promoters and enhancers and regulating inflammatory proliferation-related signalling pathways such as NF-κB and Jak1/STAT
- binding to p53 in cell cytoplasm, inhibiting p53-dependent apoptosis and DNA repair
- upregulating vascular endothelial growth factor and angiogenic factor ang2 promoting angiogenesis.

The hepatitis B virus S gene codes for hepatitis B surface antigen in three segments, namely PreS1, PreS2 and S. The PreS2 mutant large surface antigen (PreS2-LHBS) is an oncoprotein that induces liver cirrhosis and liver cancer.

Finally, HBV and HCV coinfection may act in concert with chronic alcohol consumption in liver carcinogenesis.

HCC is more common in certain parts of the world, such as Africa and Southeast Asia, and this may be due to the presence of cocarcinogens (e.g. aflatoxin). However, the closely related hepadnavirus of woodchucks (Box 18.2) causes the same tumour in these animals in the apparent absence of cocarcinogens.

The mechanism by which HCV causes HCC is indirect, as HCV sequences are not integrated into tumour cells. It is thought that the persistent hepatocyte damage and inflammation in HCV carriers, together with the effects of cytokines on the development of fibrosis and hepatocyte proliferation, results in HCC. HCV has a direct action via specific viral proteins interacting with host cell factors modulating pathways

---

### Box 18.2 ■ Lessons in Microbiology

#### The many faces of hepatitis B

Classic epidemiologic studies on hepatitis B virus in Taiwan showed two things. First, 90% of those infected in infancy developed chronic HBV infections, as did 23% of those infected at 1–3 years, but only 3% of those infected as university students. Second, among 3454 individuals with chronic HBV infection, there were 184 cases of hepatocellular carcinoma, whereas there were only 10 cases among 19,253 of those with past HBV infection. Some 80% of all liver cancers are due to hepatitis B.

Worldwide there are ~350 million individuals with chronic HBV infection; therefore with liver cancer causing up to 2 million deaths each year, hepatitis B virus is second only to tobacco as a human carcinogen.

Very similar viruses infect woodchucks, ground squirrels and Pekin ducks. In northwest United States, 30% of woodchucks have a chronic HBV infection, and most develop liver cancer in later life. In this host, the virus infects not only liver cells but also lymphoid cells in the spleen, peripheral blood and thymus, and pancreatic acinar cells and bile duct epithelium.

Transmission by individuals with chronic HBV infection has been reported in different healthcare settings, but hepatitis B immunisation and advances in antiviral therapy are reducing these incidents.

---

such as cell signalling and proliferation and apoptosis that result in malignant transformation of liver cells.

HCV core, NS3, NS5A and NS5B proteins can:

- promote cell proliferation
- regulate cytokines, oxidative stress, apoptosis
- cause liver disease progression.

HCV NS5A and NS3 can also bind to P53 and downregulate the expression of cell cycle regulation genes. HCV core protein can induce oxidative DNA damage and inhibit apoptosis.

Once cirrhosis is established, the annual incidence of HCC is 1–7% per year. In addition, HCV is associated with mixed cryoglobulinaemia, a lymphoproliferative disorder that can develop into B-cell non-Hodgkin's lymphoma.

### Several DNA viruses can transform cells in which they are unable to replicate

Extensive studies have been carried out concluding that despite high oncogenicity in vitro and in laboratory animals, these viruses do not seem to be important in human cancer. For instance:

- Human adenoviruses transform cells in culture and cause sarcomas experimentally in hamsters. About 10% of the adenovirus genome integrates, and the T antigen is expressed. However, adenoviruses are not associated with human cancer.
- Polyomavirus (from the Latin *poly*, "many" and *oma*, "tumours"), a mouse papovavirus, and simian vacuolating virus 40 (SV40), a monkey papovavirus, both cause tumours in experimentally inoculated hamsters. The viral DNA is integrated into the DNA of tumour cells, and T antigens are expressed. Are these viruses, or their human equivalents (BK and JC viruses), linked with human cancers? An incident occurred ~30 years ago

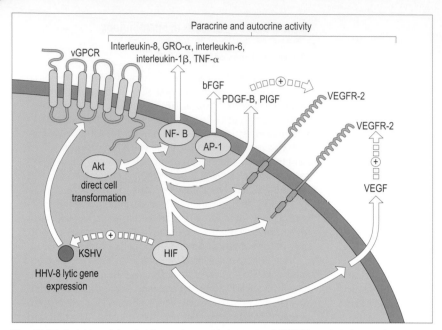

**Fig. 18.10** Activities of the viral G protein–coupled receptor (vGPCR) protein in human herpesvirus 8 (HHV-8). The constitutively active vGPCR of HHV-8 may promote the development of Kaposi sarcoma by means of a variety of mechanisms. Signalling by vGPCR activates Akt, an activated protein kinase that directly induces cell transformation. The vGPCR also results in the production of a variety of other factors, including the nuclear factor (NF)-κB-dependent factors interleukin (IL)-8, growth-related protein alpha (GRO-α), IL-6, IL-1β, tumour necrosis factor alpha (TNFα), AP-1-dependent basic fibroblast growth factor (bFGF), platelet-derived growth factor B (PDGF-B) and placental growth factor (PlGF). Some but not all studies have found that vGPCR induces secretion of vascular endothelial growth factor (VEGF), and there is evidence that this secretion may be mediated by hypoxia-inducible factor (HIF). Also, vGPCR upregulates the expression of the VEGF receptors 1 and 2 (VEGFR-1 and VEGFR-2, respectively). PlGF, VEGF and other factors can act in an autocrine or paracrine fashion to promote Kaposi's sarcoma. KSHV, Kaposi's sarcoma–associated herpes virus. (Modified from: Yarchoan R. Key role for a viral lytic gene in Kaposi's sarcoma. *N Engl J Med*. 2006;355:1383–1385, with permission.)

when thousands of children were accidentally inoculated with SV40 virus present in certain batches of poliovirus vaccine. The formalin inactivation procedure had failed to kill the SV40 virus present in the monkey kidney cells in which the polio vaccine had been grown. There was, however, no consequent increase in tumour incidence in the SV40-infected individuals. Nevertheless, evidence is accumulating that JC, BK and SV40 viruses are associated with certain cancers of the brain, with certain lymphomas and with other tumours, although a causative role has not been established.

### Kaposi's sarcoma is caused by HHV-8 infection

Kaposi's sarcoma (KS) is a multicentric tumour that involves massive proliferation of endothelial cells (see Ch. 27). It was described in 1872 by Moritz Kaposi, a Hungarian dermatologist, and HHV-8 DNA was identified in 1994 from a lesion in an individual with AIDS-associated KS. HHV-8, referred to originally as the KS-associated herpesvirus, is transmitted both by sexual intercourse and by saliva (but also by blood and organ donors) and is present in the tumours.

Other malignancies associated with HHV-8 include primary effusion lymphoma and multicentric Castleman's disease.

KS was originally a rare skin tumour seen in the Mediterranean but also sub-Saharan African population. After 1981 and the advent of the AIDS pandemic, KS was seen more frequently.

HHV-8 latently infects most tumour cells in lymphomas and KS. As a result, they are resistant to antiviral drugs targeting herpesviruses in the lytic cycle of replication. One of the HHV-8 lytic genes encodes the viral G protein–coupled receptor (vGPCR), a constitutively active cellular chemokine receptor. vGPCR signalling can result in cell proliferation, the production of angiogenic factors and, in an animal model, KS-like lesions (Fig. 18.10). Moreover, there are indirect mechanisms involved in oncogenesis relating to altered T-cell responses and HHV-8 immunoregulation.

HHV-8 has developed strategies to evade innate and specific immunity, affect cell signalling, induce proliferation and prevent apoptosis of infected cells, thus promoting oncogenesis and angiogenesis.

The incidence of KS fell sharply in individuals infected with HIV after the advent of cART. However, in 2018 it was reported that KS was the global-leading cancer among HIV-infected individuals with AIDS. KS treatment is aimed at immune reconstitution by giving cART. Localized treatment is usually avoided, and systemic treatment involves chemotherapy using liposomal anthracycline agents.

### Bacteria associated with cancer

The association between *Helicobacter pylori* and stomach and duodenal cancer, including gastric mucosa-associated lymphoid tissue lymphoma, is discussed in Chapter 23. It is thought that a number of inflammatory reactions are triggered as a result of *H. pylori* colonizing the stomach mucosa leading to chronic atrophic gastritis. This sets off a cascade of mucosal changes resulting in intestinal metaplasia, dysplasia and carcinoma. The question is whether there are other environmental or genetic cofactors involved in oncogenesis. The tumour is associated with chronic inflammation secondary to *H. pylori* colonization, but it is thought that the bacterium alone is not sufficient for cancer to develop.

## KEY FACTS

Tissue damage or disease can be caused by infectious organisms in a number of ways.

- Infectious organisms may destroy cells directly (e.g. cytopathic viruses), release toxins that destroy cells or their cellular function (e.g. staphylococcal or tetanus toxins), overstimulate normal defence systems (e.g. LPS) or stimulate excessive or prolonged adaptive responses.

- Such effects of infectious organisms on defence systems may be antibody or T-cell mediated and are collectively known as hypersensitivity reactions or immunopathology.

- Some viruses have been shown to be involved in the initiation of tumours, with the viral genome being found in the cancer cells. The restricted geographic distribution of some of these tumours may be due to the local presence of cocarcinogens.

# Clinical Manifestation and Diagnosis of Infections by Body System

| | | |
|---|---|---|
| 19. | Upper respiratory tract infections | 198 |
| 20. | Lower respiratory tract infections | 214 |
| 21. | Urinary tract infections | 259 |
| 22. | Sexually transmitted infections | 266 |
| 23. | Gastrointestinal tract infections | 291 |
| 24. | Obstetric and perinatal infections | 337 |
| 25. | Central nervous system infections | 347 |
| 26. | Infections of the eye | 367 |
| 27. | Infections of the skin, soft tissue, muscle and associated systems | 374 |
| 28. | Vector-borne infections | 408 |
| 29. | Multisystem zoonoses | 429 |
| 30. | Fever of unknown origin | 444 |
| 31. | Infections in the compromised host | 452 |

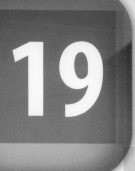

# Upper respiratory tract infections

## Introduction

The air we inhale contains millions of suspended particles, including microorganisms, most of which are harmless. However, the air may contain large numbers of pathogenic microorganisms if someone is near an individual with a respiratory tract infection. Efficient cleansing mechanisms (see Chs. 10 and 14) are therefore vital components of the body's defence against infection of both the upper and lower respiratory tract. Infection takes place against the background of these natural defence mechanisms, and it is then appropriate to ask why the defences have failed. For the upper respiratory tract, the flushing action of saliva is important in the oropharynx, and the mucociliary system in the nasopharynx traps invaders. As on other surfaces of the body (see Ch. 9), a variety of microorganisms live harmoniously in the upper respiratory tract and oropharynx (Table 19.1); they colonize the nose, mouth, throat and teeth and are well adapted to life in these sites. Normally they are well-behaved guests, not invading tissues and not causing disease; however, as in other parts of the body, resident microorganisms can cause trouble when host resistance is weakened. In addition, a host of invaders cause upper respiratory tract symptoms that may progress to the lower respiratory tract, depending on the pathogen.

### The upper and lower respiratory tracts form a continuum for infectious agents

We distinguish between upper and lower respiratory tract infections, but the respiratory tract from the nose to the alveoli is a continuum as far as infectious agents are concerned (Fig. 19.1). There may, however, be a preferred focus of infection (e.g. the nasopharynx for coronaviruses and rhinoviruses); but parainfluenza viruses, for instance, can infect the nasopharynx to give rise to a cold, as well as the larynx and trachea resulting in laryngotracheitis (croup) and occasionally the bronchi and bronchioles resulting in bronchitis, bronchiolitis, or pneumonia.

### Generalizations can be made about upper and lower respiratory tract infections

1. Although many microorganisms are restricted to the surface epithelium, some spread to other parts of the body before returning to the respiratory tract, oropharynx and salivary glands (Table 19.2).
2. Two groups of pathogens can be distinguished: professional and secondary invaders (Table 19.3).
3. Professional invaders are those that successfully infect the normally healthy respiratory tract. They generally possess specific properties that enable them to evade local host defences such as the attachment mechanisms of respiratory viruses (Table 19.4). Secondary invaders cause disease only when host defences are already impaired (see Table 19.3).
4. The symptoms of an upper respiratory tract infection include fever, rhinitis and pharyngitis or sore throat. It

is not just respiratory pathogens that cause these symptoms; cytomegalovirus (CMV) and Epstein-Barr virus (EBV) infections are included in this chapter but are associated only with the fever and pharyngitis components. They are both part of a glandular fever differential diagnosis.

## RHINITIS

### Molecular diagnostic tests have demonstrated a much wider range of viruses that cause colds compared with older techniques

Viruses are the most common invaders of the nasopharynx, and a great variety of types (see Table 19.4) are responsible for the symptoms referred to as the common cold. They induce a flow of virus-rich fluid, called *rhinorrhea*, from the nasopharynx, and when the sneezing reflex is triggered, then large numbers of virus particles are discharged into the air. Transmission is therefore by aerosol and by virus-contaminated hands (see Ch. 14). Most of these viruses possess surface molecules that bind them firmly to host cells or to cilia or microvilli protruding from these cells. As a result they are not washed away in secretions and are able to initiate infection in the normally healthy individual. Virus progeny from the first-infected cell then spread to neighbouring cells and via surface secretions to new sites on the mucosal surface. After a few days, damage to epithelial cells and the secretion of fluid containing inflammatory mediators such as bradykinin lead to common cold–type symptoms (Fig. 19.2).

**Table 19.1** The normal flora of the respiratory tract

| Type of resident[a] | Microorganism |
|---|---|
| Common residents (>50% normally) | Oral streptococci<br>*Neisseria* spp.<br>*Moraxella*<br>Corynebacteria<br>*Bacteroides*<br>Anaerobic cocci (*Veillonella*)<br>Fusiform bacteria[b]<br>*Candida albicans*[b]<br>*Streptococcus mutans*<br>*Haemophilus influenzae* |
| Occasional residents (<10% normally) | *Streptococcus pyogenes*<br>*Streptococcus pneumoniae*<br>*Neisseria meningitidis* |
| Uncommon residents (<1% normally) | *Corynebacterium diphtheriae*<br>*Klebsiella pneumoniae*<br>*Pseudomonas*<br>*Escherichia coli*[c]<br>*Candida albicans*[c] |
| Residents in latent state in tissues[d]:<br>Lung<br>Lymph nodes<br>Sensory neurone/dorsal root ganglia | *Pneumocystis jirovecii*,<br>*Mycobacterium tuberculosis*<br>Cytomegalovirus, Epstein-Barr virus<br>Herpes simplex virus, Varicella-zoster virus |

[a]All except tissue residents are present in the oronasopharynx or on teeth.
[b]Present in mouth; also *Entamoeba gingivalis*, *Trichomonas tenax*, micrococci, *Actinomyces* spp.
[c]Especially after antibiotic treatment.
[d]All except *M. tuberculosis* are present in most humans.

**Table 19.2** Pathogens that gain entry via the upper respiratory tract

| Type | Examples |
|---|---|
| Restricted to surface | Rhinoviruses<br>Influenza<br>*Streptococci* (in throat)<br>*Chlamydia* (conjunctivitis)<br>Diphtheria<br>Pertussis<br>*Candida albicans* (thrush) |
| Spread through body | Measles, mumps, rubella<br>EBV, CMV<br>*Chlamydophila psittaci*[a]<br>Q fever<br>*Cryptococcosis* |

After entry via the respiratory tract, pathogens either stay on the surface epithelium or spread through the body. CMV, Cytomegalovirus; EBV, Epstein-Barr virus.
[a]Formerly *Chlamydia psittaci*.

## Viral coinfections are being detected using more sensitive tests

In view of the large variety of viruses and because common colds are generally mild and self-limiting with no systemic spread in healthy individuals, determination of the aetiology is helpful from both a management and an epidemiologic perspective. In particular, molecular diagnostic tests of higher sensitivity and specificity detect a wider range of viruses, and coinfections have been seen where before only one pathogen was identified. This has had an impact on diagnosis, especially when the lower respiratory tract is involved, as for instance with influenza viruses or in children with respiratory syncytial virus (RSV) infection.

The revolution in laboratory diagnosis meant that older methods of cell culture looking for a viral cytopathic effect or adding red cells to detect haemagglutinating viruses, as well as immunofluorescence detecting viral antigens in exfoliated cells in samples such as nasopharyngeal aspirates or throat swabs (see Fig. 19.5), have been superseded in many parts of the world by molecular diagnostic tests. The severe acute respiratory syndrome coronavirus 2 (SARS-CoV-2) pandemic resulting in coronavirus disease 2019 (COVID-19) accelerated the widespread use of real-time multiplex polymerase chain reaction (PCR), which may be performed in laboratories or as point-of-care tests.

Collecting an acute and convalescent serum sample and looking for a rise in virus-specific antibodies can confirm the diagnosis retrospectively, but now, together with virus isolation in cell culture and immunofluorescence, these tests are mostly found in reference laboratory settings rather than in routine diagnostic services.

Due to the increased sensitivity in detecting respiratory viruses by PCR, together with automated sample extraction and detection methods, many laboratories use molecular methods for making a diagnosis using combined nose and throat swab samples. These swabs can be used instead of collecting nasopharyngeal aspirates that are more invasive and lead to aerosol production—an infection control issue.

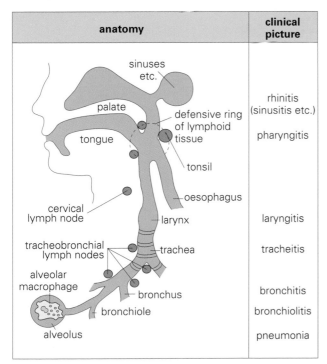

| anatomy | clinical picture |
|---|---|
| sinuses etc. | rhinitis (sinusitis etc.) |
| palate | |
| defensive ring of lymphoid tissue | pharyngitis |
| tongue | |
| tonsil | |
| oesophagus | |
| cervical lymph node | |
| larynx | laryngitis |
| tracheobronchial lymph nodes | |
| trachea | tracheitis |
| alveolar macrophage | |
| bronchus | bronchitis |
| bronchiole | bronchiolitis |
| alveolus | pneumonia |

**Fig. 19.1** The respiratory tract as a continuum.

**Table 19.3** The two types of respiratory invader—professional or secondary

| Type | Requirement | Examples |
|---|---|---|
| Professional invaders (infect healthy respiratory tract) | Adhesion to normal mucosa (in spite of mucociliary system) | Respiratory viruses (influenza, coronaviruses, rhinoviruses)<br>*Streptococcus pyogenes* (throat)<br>*Streptococcus pneumoniae*<br>*Chlamydia* (psittacosis, chlamydial conjunctivitis and pneumonia, trachoma) |
| | Ability to interfere with cilia | *Bordetella pertussis*<br>*Mycoplasma pneumoniae*<br>*S. pneumoniae* (pneumolysin) |
| | Ability to resist destruction in alveolar macrophage | *Legionella*<br>*Mycobacterium tuberculosis* |
| | Ability to damage local (mucosal, submucosal) tissues | *Corynebacterium diphtheriae* (toxin)<br>*S. pneumoniae* (pneumolysin) |
| Secondary invaders (infect when host defences impaired) | Initial infection and damage by respiratory virus (e.g. influenza virus) | *Staphylococcus aureus*<br>*S. pneumoniae*, pneumonia-complicating influenza |
| | Local defences impaired (e.g. cystic fibrosis) | *S. aureus*<br>*Pseudomonas* |
| | Chronic bronchitis, local foreign body or tumour | *Haemophilus influenzae*<br>*S. pneumoniae* |
| | Depressed immune responses (e.g. acquired immunodeficiency syndrome, neoplastic disease) | *Pneumocystis jirovecii*<br>Cytomegalovirus<br>*M. tuberculosis* |
| | Depressed resistance (e.g. elderly, alcoholism, renal or hepatic disease) | *S. pneumonia*<br>*S. aureus*<br>*H. influenzae* |

**Table 19.4** Respiratory viruses and their mechanisms of attachment

| Virus | Types involved | Attachment mechanisms | Disease |
|---|---|---|---|
| Human coronaviruses (HCoV) | SARS-CoV and SARS-CoV-2<br>MERS-CoV<br>HCoV-229E<br>HCoV-OC43<br>HCoV-NL63<br>HCoV-HKU1 | Spike glycoprotein is involved in binding to sialic acids at surface of host cells.<br>The receptor for the highly pathogenic HCoV:<br>SARS-CoV and SARS-CoV-2 is angiotensin-converting enzyme 2.<br>The receptor for MERS-CoV is dipeptidyl peptidase 4. | Severe acute respiratory syndrome (SARS)<br>COVID-19<br>Middle East respiratory syndrome (MERS)<br>Common cold |
| Influenza virus | A, B, C | Haemagglutinin binds to *N*-acetylneuraminic acid (sialic acid)–containing glycoprotein on cell surface | May also invade lower respiratory tract |
| Enteroviruses, including coxsackie virus A (24 types), echoviruses (34 types), enteroviruses (116 serotypes) | Many | Capsid protein binds to ICAM-1 type molecule on cell[b] | Common cold; also oropharyngeal vesicles (herpangina) and hand, foot and mouth disease (A16, EV71) |
| Rhinoviruses (>100 types)[a] | All | Capsid protein binds to ICAM-1 type molecule on cell[b] | Common cold but can be severe in immunocompromised patients |
| Parainfluenza virus (4 types) | 1, 2, 3, 4 | Viral envelope protein binds to glycoside on cell | May also invade larynx |
| Respiratory syncytial virus | A and B | G protein on virus attaches to receptor on cell | May also invade lower respiratory tract |
| Adenovirus (41 types) | 5–10 | Penton fibre binds to cell receptor | Mainly pharyngitis; also conjunctivitis, bronchitis |

[a]A given type shows little or no neutralization by antibody against other types.
[b]ICAM-1, Intercellular adhesion molecule expressed on a wide variety of normal cells; member of immunoglobulin superfamily, coded on chromosome 19.

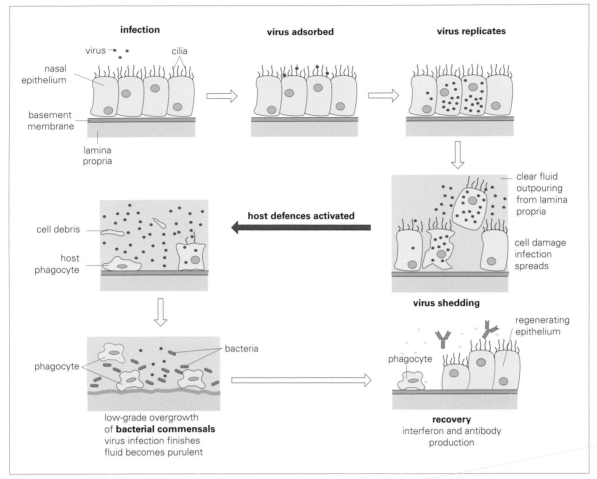

**Fig. 19.2** The pathogenesis of the common cold. For simplification, the epithelium is represented as one cell thick.

## Treatment of the common cold is symptomatic

Although there are many remedies to treat the *common cold* —a term for an amalgam of sore throat, headache, sneeze, cough, runny or blocked nose, muscle aches, usually due to rhinoviruses—few are helpful. Antibiotics are only indicated if there is a bacterial infection. Otherwise, drinking plenty of fluid, resting, decongestants and analgesics and antibiotics will help relieve some symptoms. There are no vaccines to protect against the common cold viruses as the vaccines would have to be polyvalent to cover this antigenically diverse group of viruses.

## PHARYNGITIS AND TONSILLITIS

### The majority of acute sore throats are caused by viruses

Microorganisms that cause sore throats, known as *acute pharyngitis*, are listed in Table 19.5. Those viruses that infect the upper respiratory tract inevitably encounter the submucosal lymphoid tissues that form a defensive ring around the oropharynx (see Fig. 19.1). The throat becomes sore either because the overlying mucosa is infected or because of inflammatory and immune responses in the lymphoid tissues. Sore throat is reported in influenza virus and SARS-CoV-2 infections (see Ch. 20). Adenoviruses are common causes, often infecting the conjunctiva as well as the pharynx to cause pharyngoconjunctival fever. EBV and CMV multiply locally in the pharynx

(Fig. 19.3), and herpes simplex virus (HSV) and certain enteroviruses (including coxsackie B, coxsackie A16, enterovirus 71) multiply in the oral mucosa to produce a painful local lesion or ulcer known as *herpangina*. Of these, coxsackie A16 is the most common cause of hand, foot and mouth disease presenting as vesicles on the hands and feet and in the mouth (Fig. 19.4).

## Cytomegalovirus infection

### Cytomegalovirus can be transmitted by saliva, urine, blood, semen and cervical secretions

CMV is the largest human herpesvirus (Fig. 19.5) and is species specific; humans are the natural hosts. CMV refers to the cells (*cyto*) being multinucleated (*megalo*, "large"), which, together with the intranuclear inclusions, are characteristic responses to CMV infection. It was originally called *salivary gland virus* and is transmitted by saliva and other secretions. In addition, it can be transmitted by sexual contact, as semen and cervical secretions may also contain this virus, and by blood transfusions (although leucodepletion reduces the risk significantly) and organ transplants from CMV antibody-positive donors. The CMV load will be extremely high in the urine from babies with congenital CMV infection, and careful hand washing and disposal of nappies will reduce the risk of transmission to susceptible individuals. CMV can be detected in breast milk, which is another route of transmission.

**Table 19.5** Microorganisms that cause acute pharyngitis

| Organisms | Examples | Comments |
|---|---|---|
| Viruses | Rhinoviruses<br>Coronaviruses | A mild symptom in the common cold<br>Seen with the three highly pathogenic and the four lower pathogenic HCoV |
| | Adenoviruses<br>(types 3, 4, 7, 14, 21) | Pharyngoconjunctival fever |
| | Parainfluenza viruses | More severe than common cold |
| | Influenza viruses | Often more severe in influenza A |
| | Coxsackie A and other enteroviruses | Small vesicles (herpangina) |
| | Epstein-Barr virus<br>Cytomegalovirus<br>Human immunodeficiency virus (HIV) | Occurs in 70–90% of glandular fever patients<br>Can occur in 50% of acute HIV infections |
| | Herpes simplex viruses | Can be severe, with palatal vesicles or ulcers |
| Bacteria | *Streptococcus pyogenes* | Causes 10–20% of cases of acute pharyngitis; sudden onset; mostly in 5–10-year-old children |
| | *Neisseria gonorrhoeae* | Often asymptomatic; usually via orogenital contact |
| | *Corynebacterium diphtheriae* | Pharyngitis often mild, but toxic illness can be severe |
| | *Haemophilus influenzae* | Epiglottis |
| | *Borrelia vincentii* plus fusiform bacilli | Vincent angina; commonest in adolescents and adults |

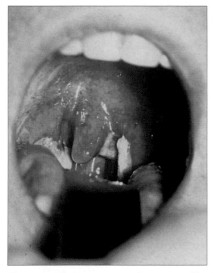

**Fig. 19.3** Infectious mononucleosis caused by Epstein-Barr virus. The tonsils and uvula are swollen and covered in white exudate. There are petechiae on the soft palate. (Courtesy J.A. Innes.)

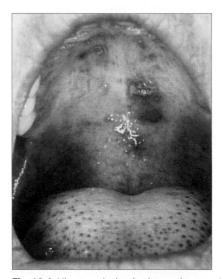

**Fig. 19.4** Ulcers on the hard palate and tongue in hand, foot and mouth disease due to coxsackie A virus. (Courtesy J.A. Innes.)

**Cytomegalovirus infection is often asymptomatic but can reactivate and cause disease when cell-mediated immunity defences are impaired**

After clinically silent infection in the upper respiratory tract, CMV spreads locally to lymphoid tissues and then systemically in circulating lymphocytes and monocytes to involve lymph nodes and the spleen. The infection then localizes in epithelial cells in salivary glands and kidney tubules and in the cervix, testes and epididymis from where the virus is shed to the outside world (Table 19.6).

Infected cells may be multinucleated or bear intranuclear inclusions, but pathologic changes are minor. The virus inhibits T-cell responses, and there is a temporary reduction in their immune reactivity to other antigens.

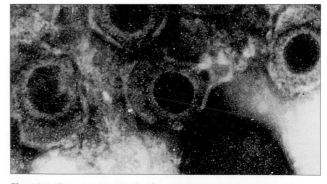

**Fig. 19.5** Electron micrograph of cytomegalovirus particles. This is the largest human herpesvirus, with a diameter of 150–200 nm and a dense DNA core. (Courtesy D.K. Banerjee.)

**Table 19.6** The effects of cytomegalovirus infection

| Site of infection | Result | Comment |
| --- | --- | --- |
| Salivary glands | Salivary transmission | Via kissing and contaminated hands |
| Tubular epithelium of kidney | Virus in urine | Probable role in transmission by contaminating environment |
| Cervix, testis/epididymis | Sexual transmission | CMV has been isolated and CMV DNA detected in cervical secretions and seminal fluid |
| Lymphocytes, macrophages | Virus spreads through body via infected cells Mononucleosis may occur Immunosuppressive effect | Probable site of persistent infection |
| Placenta, fetus | Congenital abnormalities | Greatest damage in fetus after primary maternal infection rather than reactivation |

Although specific antibodies and cell-mediated immunity (CMI) responses are generated, these fail to clear the virus (see Ch. 17), which often continues to be shed in saliva and urine for many months. The infection is, however, eventually controlled by CMI mechanisms, although infected cells remain in the body throughout life and can be a source of reactivation and disease when CMI defences are impaired.

CMV owes its success in our species to having a strategy of immune evasion by subverting many key pathways of innate and adaptive immunity, causing disease especially in immunocompromised hosts. For instance, it presents a poor target for cytotoxic T (Tc) cells by interfering with the transport of major histocompatibility complex (MHC) class I molecules to the cell surface (see Ch. 11), and it induces Fc receptors on infected cells (see Ch. 17). The cell surface display of MHC-I complexes recognized by CD8 T cells is regulated by viral regulators of antigen presentation. These immune evasion proteins limit CMV antigen display and protect against CMV disease by increasing the CD8 avidity threshold that recognizes infected cells. High avidity CD8 T cells protect against CMV infection and virus dissemination.

### Cytomegalovirus infection can cause pneumonia in immunodeficient individuals and fetal malformations

As with all infections there is a spectrum of clinical disease ranging from asymptomatic to severely ill. A glandular fever type illness can occur in adolescents that is similar to EBV infection with fever, lethargy, lymphocytosis or lymphopenia and abnormal lymphocytes in blood films. Primary infection during pregnancy allows the spread of virus from the blood to the placenta and then to the fetus, resulting in symptomatic CMV infection at birth in 18% and detection of other sequelae in 25% by <5 years of age, as described in Chapter 24. Reactivation of infection during pregnancy also occurs, and the baby may be asymptomatic at birth, but up to 8% of children will have symptoms by 5 years of age. CMV is second only to Down's syndrome as a cause of intellectual disability.

In immunodeficient patients such as bone marrow or solid organ transplant recipients (see Ch. 31), CMV infection can cause an interstitial pneumonitis with infiltrating infected mononuclear cells. Other sites affected include the central nervous system (CNS), with focal cerebral micronodular lesions with infected mononuclear cells, together with a variety of other complications including retinitis in individuals infected with human immunodeficiency virus (HIV) with acquired immunodeficiency syndrome (AIDS). This was a major complication before the advent of combined antiretroviral therapy. In addition, the gastrointestinal tract may be involved, with a colitis and hepatitis.

Clinical diagnosis of primary infection is rarely possible because it is often asymptomatic. However, in immunocompetent individuals who are symptomatic, the diagnosis is made by detecting CMV immunoglobulin M (IgM) in blood samples, together with the CMV IgG avidity being low. In those with possible CMV pneumonitis, a bronchoalveolar lavage sample is collected by passing a bronchoscope into the lungs and collecting washings; CMV DNA or CMV antigen detection methods are used to make the diagnosis. Multinucleated cells or cells with prominent intranuclear inclusions may be seen in lung biopsy material. CMV IgM and IgG serology is available but is unlikely to be of diagnostic help in patients who are immunosuppressed. The management of posttransplant recipients involves CMV DNA monitoring of whole blood or plasma samples and giving preemptive antiviral therapy, having detected a CMV viraemia (see Ch. 31).

### Antiviral treatment options in CMV infection

While ganciclovir, valganciclovir, foscarnet and cidofovir (although the latter is a third-line agent and used infrequently) are effective treatments, aciclovir is ineffective. Maribavir is another drug approved for treating posttransplant CMV infection/disease. These antiviral drugs reduce viral replication, do not eliminate the virus and can be used in specific clinical situations including preemptive therapy (see Ch. 31). Because CMV pneumonitis is an immunopathologic disease, CMV-specific or human normal immunoglobulin is given in addition to the antiviral agent to potentially block the Tc-cell response to pneumocytes expressing the target antigens.

### Primary prophylaxis of CMV is useful in specific bone marrow transplant recipients, but the wait for a vaccine to prevent CMV infection continues

Letermovir, a novel antiviral drug that is a nonnucleoside viral terminase complex inhibitor, is used for prophylaxis to prevent CMV reactivation and disease in adult CMV IgG-positive allogeneic hematopoietic stem cell transplant recipients. It is given orally for 100 days posttransplant.

There is no vaccine, but trials of live, inactivated, and recombinant vaccines have been carried out. Bearing in mind that it is the second most common cause of intellectual disability in babies, immunization is a major consideration once a number of practical issues have been resolved. The results of a recombinant CMV glycoprotein B vaccine trial reported in 2011 involving solid organ transplant recipients suggested that antibody levels generated in response to vaccine led to reduced viraemia and duration of antiviral use. In 2022 an evaluation of the safety and efficacy of a messenger RNA CMV vaccine was being carried out. Transmission can be reduced in various settings by avoiding contact between children who are congenitally infected and susceptible pregnant women or maintaining good hand hygiene if this is not possible. Blood for transfusion of newborns and solid organ and bone marrow transplant recipients should preferably come from CMV IgG-negative donors or be leucodepleted.

## Epstein-Barr virus infection

Mononucleosis classically presents with fever, lymphadenopathy and tonsillar pharyngitis. The term infectious mononucleosis was first used in the 1920s to describe an illness in a group of students with similar pharyngeal and blood laboratory findings of lymphocytosis and atypical mononuclear cells.

### EBV is transmitted in saliva

EBV, like CMV, is species specific. EBV is structurally and morphologically identical to other herpesviruses (see Ch. 3), but it is antigenically distinct. Major antigens include the viral capsid antigen (VCA) and the EBV-associated nuclear antigens (EBNA) that are used in diagnostic tests. Humans are the natural hosts, and lifelong infection is ubiquitous, with >90% of adults infected globally.

EBV is transmitted by the exchange of saliva, for instance, during kissing. In resource-poor countries, infection probably occurs via close contact in early childhood and is subclinical. Elsewhere, infection occurs in two peaks at 1–6 years of age and at 14–20 years of age, and in most cases it causes illness.

### The clinical features of EBV infection are immunologically mediated

Clinical and immunologic events in EBV infection are illustrated in Fig. 19.6. EBV replicates in B lymphocytes after making a specific attachment to the C3d receptor (CD21) on these cells as well as in certain epithelial cells. The pathogenesis of the disease and the clinical features can be accounted for on this basis. Virus is shed in saliva from infected oropharyngeal epithelial cells where it multiplies and then infects B cells within the oral cavity. There is clinically silent spread to B lymphocytes in local lymphoid tissues and elsewhere in the body, such as lymph nodes and spleen.

T lymphocytes respond immunologically to the infected B cells (outnumbering the latter by about 50 to 1) and appear in peripheral blood as atypical lymphocytes (Fig. 19.7). Much of the disease is attributable to an immunologic civil war, as specifically activated T cells respond to the infected B cells. In the naturally infected infant or small child there is generally no clinical disease, or it may be mild. It is thought that this may be because the EBV load they are exposed to is lower than in older children, and the immune response may, therefore, be weaker in the younger group. Human leucocyte antigen (HLA) type is also involved as a genetic risk factor. Older children, however, become unwell, and young adults develop infectious mononucleosis or glandular fever 4–7 weeks after initial infection. This is characterized by fever, sore throat, often with petechiae on the hard palate (see Fig. 19.3), lymphadenopathy and splenomegaly, with anorexia and lethargy as prominent features. Hepatitis may occur, with mild elevations of hepatocellular enzymes in 90% of cases and jaundice in 9%. Splenic rupture may occur.

Complications are seen in ~1% of acute EBV infections and may be due to virus invading the tissue or to immune-mediated damage. These include aseptic meningitis and encephalitis nearly always with complete recovery, haemolytic anaemia, airway obstruction due to oropharyngeal swelling, haemophagocytic syndrome and splenic rupture.

The symptoms are presumably due to the action of pro-inflammatory cytokines and chemokines released during the intense immunologic activity involving a strong Tc-cell response to the EBV-infected B cells. High levels of interferon gamma, produced by activated T cells and natural killer (NK) cells, are likely to contribute to the symptoms as it causes headache, tiredness and fever. The infected B cells are stimulated to differentiate and produce antibodies; this polyclonal activation of B cells is responsible for the production of heterophile antibodies and a variety of autoantibodies. Heterophile antibodies are, therefore, cross-reactive and bind to surface molecules on mammalian, but not human, red blood cells and are not EBV specific.

The autoantibodies produced in response to EBV infection include IgM antibodies to erythrocytes, referred to as cold agglutinins. These are antibodies that recognize antigens on red blood cells and agglutinate them at temperatures below the core body temperature. About 1% of those with EBV infections develop an autoimmune haemolytic anaemia, which subsides within 1–2 months.

Spontaneous recovery usually occurs in 2–3 weeks, but the symptoms may persist for a few months. The virus remains as a latent infection in spite of antibody and CMI responses, and saliva often remains infectious for months after clinical recovery.

### EBV remains latent in a small proportion of B lymphocytes

EBV is well equipped to evade immune defences (see Ch. 17). It acts against complement and interferon and produces a fake interleukin 10 (IL-10) molecule that interferes with the action of the host's own IL-10 (an important immunoregulatory cytokine). EBV also prevents apoptosis (lysis) of infected cells, and the boldness of its strategy has enabled it to take up permanent residence within the immune system. This is called *latency*, and it is established by a regulated set of viral proteins that are expressed in a complicated process. The two cycles of EBV infection are latency and the lytic stage. The latter produces infectious virions and is key to viral transmission between cells as well as hosts. In addition, there is evidence that lytic infection is important in the early development of EBV-associated tumours.

EBV DNA is present in episomal form in a small proportion of B lymphocytes, and a few copies may be integrated into the cell genome. Later in life, immunodeficiency can lead to reactivation of infection so that EBV reappears in the saliva, usually with no clinical symptoms.

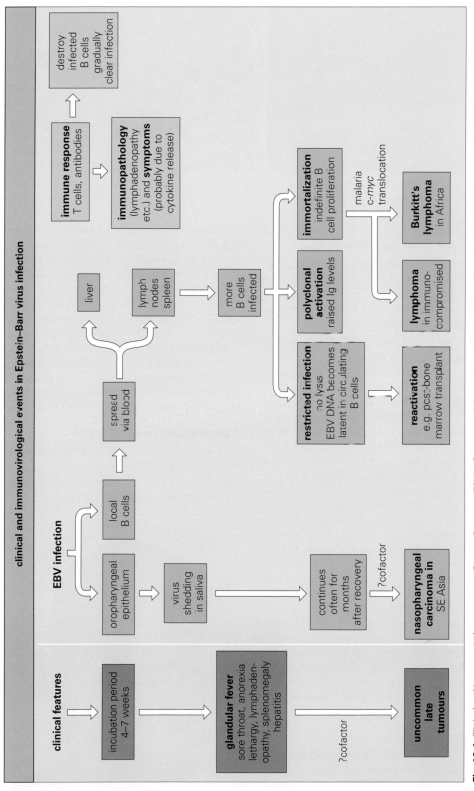

**Fig. 19.6** Clinical and immunovirologic events in Epstein–Barr virus (EBV) infection in adolescents or adults. A milder, often subclinical, infection occurs in children.

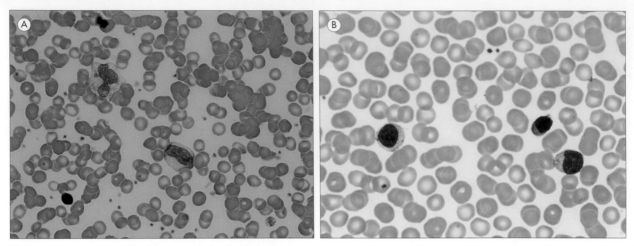

**Fig. 19.7** (A) Atypical lymphocytes characteristic of Epstein-Barr virus infection and (B) a normal lymphocyte for comparison. (Courtesy Dr. Sue Height, Paediatric Haematology, King's College Hospital NHS Foundation Trust, London.)

### Laboratory tests for diagnosing infectious mononucleosis should include viral capsid antigen IgM detection

Infectious mononucleosis is diagnosed clinically by the characteristic syndrome and the appearance of palatal petechiae in the throat. Laboratory diagnosis is made by detecting VCA IgM in the serum. However, there are other tests that help, and these include the following:

- Demonstrating atypical lymphocytes, comprising up to 30% of nucleated cells, in a blood film. However, a number of viral infections cause atypical lymphocytosis; therefore, this is not specific to EBV.
- Demonstrating heterophile antibodies to horse or sheep erythrocytes in the monospot test. These are present in 90% of EBV infections but may not be detected in those <14 years of age, and the response is also short lived.
- EBV-specific antibody is the mainstay of diagnosis; in particular, detecting VCA IgM indicates current infection. VCA IgG can be detected soon after VCA IgM, and EBNA IgG appears a few weeks later after symptom onset.
- EBV VCA IgG avidity is a key test as the antibody avidity is low in a recent infection. This is because the strength of the IgG binding to the virus antigen is low as the IgG has just been made and dissociates easily from the antigen. The test involves pipetting an aliquot of the patient's serum sample into an ELISA well coated with VCA antigen. This is then washed with buffer containing urea, a dissociating agent. That optical density value is compared with that of the sample when it was washed with just buffer alone, and an antibody index is measured as a percentage of the optical density values. Low avidity may be around 30%, for example, compared with 70% that would be high avidity and consistent with a previous, not recent, infection.

### Treatment of EBV infection is limited

Antiviral agents are not used to treat EBV-infected immunocompetent individuals. In immunosuppressed people in specific clinical settings, there are some in vitro data on using specific antivirals to reduce viral replication, but they are effective only in the lytic part of the life cycle. In addition, an anti-CD20 receptor humanized monoclonal antibody called *rituximab* has been used to target EBV-infected B cells in specific clinical settings.

There is no licensed vaccine, despite years of work, as the correlates of protection are undefined; improvements are needed with respect to appropriate animal models or the equivalent to determine vaccine efficacy; the ideal EBV vaccine antigen selection and combination is still unclear; and the optimal type of vaccine and delivery is not known. Placebo-controlled clinical trials have been carried out involving an envelope glycoprotein subunit vaccine and a CD8 T-cell peptide vaccine. The subunit vaccine was shown to have a significant effect on clinical disease but did not prevent infection. Other vaccines, including DNA vaccines, viral vector vaccines, and viruslike particles, did not induce optimal levels of protection and failed to prevent EBV infection.

## Cancers associated with EBV

### EBV is closely associated with Burkitt lymphoma in African children

Burkitt lymphoma (Fig. 19.8) can be classified into three subtypes (endemic, sporadic, HIV associated), but it is virtually

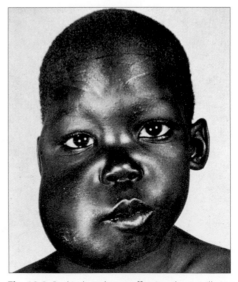

**Fig. 19.8** Burkitt lymphoma affecting the maxilla in an African child. (Courtesy I. Magrath, MD, Bethesda, MD. From Zitelli B., Davis H. *Atlas of Pediatric Physical Diagnosis*, Mosby Elsevier; 2007.)

restricted to parts of Africa and Papua New Guinea, so it is clear that EBV alone is not enough to cause the lymphoma. The endemic subtype also has the highest frequency of EBV detection. The most likely cocarcinogen is malaria, which acts by weakening T-cell control of EBV infection and perhaps by causing polyclonal activation of B cells, the increased turnover rendering them more susceptible to neoplastic transformation.

### EBV is closely associated with other B-cell lymphomas in immunodeficient patients

For example, B-cell lymphomas occur in 1–10% of solid organ transplant recipients, especially children, when primary EBV infection occurs posttransplantation. EBV DNA and RNA transcripts are found in the tumour cells, which also show a translocation of the *c-myc* oncogene on chromosome 8 to the immunoglobulin heavy chain locus on chromosome 14 (see Ch. 18). Posttransplant lymphoproliferative disorders are due to uncontrolled B-cell proliferation. In addition, there is the rare X-linked lymphoproliferative disease associated with EBV infection. This inherited disorder involves mutations in the *SH2D1A* gene that codes for the signalling lymphocyte activation-molecule–associated protein. The latter is key to B-cell activation of T cells and NK cells, which controls EBV-infected B cells. Therefore, individuals with this X-linked disorder can develop fatal infectious mononucleosis and lymphomas, and these can be prevented only by having an allogeneic bone marrow transplant.

### EBV infection is also closely associated with nasopharyngeal carcinoma

Nasopharyngeal carcinoma (NPC) is a very common cancer in China and Southeast Asia. EBV DNA is detectable in the tumour cells, and a cocarcinogen is likely, possibly ingested nitrosamines from preserved fish. Host genetic factors controlling HLA and immune responses may confer susceptibility to NPC.

### EBV-associated oral carcinomas

It is still unclear if EBV is implicated in the development of oral squamous cell carcinomas, which constitute >90% of oral cancers. However, EBV is associated with lymphoepitheliomas of the salivary glands and causes benign, hyperplastic, elevated, white, shaggy (hairy) patches mostly on the back and sides of the tongue, called *oral hairy leucoplakia (OHL)*. OHL is found in individuals with severe immunodeficiency due to HIV infection or organ transplantation and after chemotherapy. It is due to unregulated EBV lytic replication in oral epithelial cells.

### EBV associated with multiple sclerosis

With globally, 36/100,000 individuals were reported to have multiple sclerosis (MS) in 2020, making it the most common chronic inflammatory neurodegenerative disease of the CNS. The aetiology has always been complicated by an interplay of factors, including genetic susceptibility involving immune response genes and multiple environmental factors, including infection. EBV was shown to be highly associated with MS after the results of a 20-year serologic follow-up study were published in 2022 involving >10 million US army personnel. There was a 32-fold increased risk of MS in those who developed antibodies to EBV compared with those who remained antibody negative. The pathogenesis seems to involve the initial immune response to infection and the severity of and

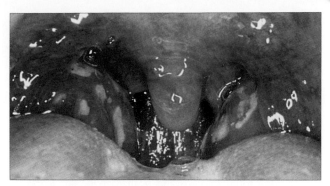

**Fig. 19.9** Streptococcal tonsillitis due to group A beta haemolytic *Streptococcus pyogenes* with intense erythema of the tonsils and a creamy-yellow exudate. (Courtesy J.A. Innes.)

inability to control the primary infection. Latently infected resident memory B cells may continually present viral antigens, resulting in cytotoxic T lymphocyte (CTL) autoreactivity to neuronal tissue, damaging the CNS through molecular mimicry. This discovery opened up further ways to treat individuals with MS, such as allogeneic EBV CTL therapy and autologous haematopoietic stem cell transplantation.

## Bacterial infections

Bacteria responsible for pharyngitis include:

- *Streptococcus pyogenes* (Fig. 19.9), which is a group A streptococcus (GAS), is beta haemolytic and colonizes the throat, skin, and anogenital tract. It is a common infection transmitted by respiratory droplets and direct skin contact, and diagnosis is important because it can lead to complications (see later), but it can be readily treated with penicillin
- *Corynebacterium diphtheriae*
- *Haemophilus influenzae* type B (Hib), which occasionally causes severe epiglottitis with obstruction of the airways, especially in young children
- *Borrelia vincentii* (also known as *Treponema vincentii*) together with certain fusiform bacilli, which can cause throat or gingival ulcers
- *Neisseria gonorrhoeae.*

Each of these types of bacteria attach to the mucosal surface, sometimes invading local tissues.

### Complications of *Streptococcus pyogenes* infection

**Complications of *S. pyogenes* throat infection include quinsy, scarlet fever and (rarely) rheumatic fever, rheumatic heart disease and glomerulonephritis**

These complications are important enough to be listed separately and can be associated with streptococcal toxic shock syndrome, although most are uncommon in resource-rich countries where there is good access to medical care and probably less exposure to streptococci. Invasive GAS (iGAS) is a severe infection in which the streptococci are isolated in sterile sites, including the bloodstream. In 2022 the World Health Organization reported an increase in iGAS disease and an increase in mortality in children <10 years old. This was reported in the United Kingdom, the Netherlands, France, Sweden, and Ireland and occurred at the same time as a rise in respiratory virus detection and possible viral coinfections. It was thought that this was a result of the lockdowns during the previous 2 years of the COVID-19 pandemic, reduced numbers of all infections, followed by increased population mixing in a background of a more susceptible population. Enhanced surveillance was implemented to ensure early recognition and immediate treatment of anyone with GAS infection. The complications include the following:

- Peritonsillar abscess (quinsy) is an uncommon complication of untreated streptococcal sore throat.
- Otitis media, sinusitis and mastoiditis (see later) are caused by local spread of *S. pyogenes*.
- Scarlet fever—certain strains of *S. pyogenes* produce an erythrogenic toxin coded for by a lysogenic phage. The toxin spreads through the body and localizes in the skin to induce a punctate erythematous rash (scarlet fever; Fig. 19.10). The tongue is initially furred but later red. Symptoms include a rash, sore throat, red cheeks and swollen tongue. It is a notifiable disease and is highly contagious. The rash begins as facial erythema and then spreads to involve most of the body except the palms and soles. The face is generally flushed with circumoral pallor. The rash fades over the course of 1 week and is followed by extensive desquamation. The skin lesions themselves are not serious, but they signal infection by a potentially harmful streptococcus, which, in preantibiotic days, could sometimes spread through the body to cause cellulitis and septicaemia.
- Impetigo, erysipelas and cellulitis (see Ch. 27).

- Pneumonia.
- Rheumatic fever as an indirect complication. Antibodies formed to antigens in the streptococcal cell wall cross-react with the sarcolemma of the heart and with tissues elsewhere. Granulomas are formed in the heart, called *Aschoff nodules*, and 2–4 weeks after the sore throat, the patient, usually a child, develops myocarditis or pericarditis, which may be associated with subcutaneous nodules, polyarthritis and (rarely) chorea. Chorea is an involuntary movement disorder and disease of the CNS resulting from streptococcal antibodies reacting with neurones. Dr T. Duckett-Jones produced the Jones criteria for the diagnosis of rheumatic fever with major and minor manifestations and evidence of a recent GAS infection as an essential criterion. These were modified by the American Heart Association in 2015 (Table 19.7).

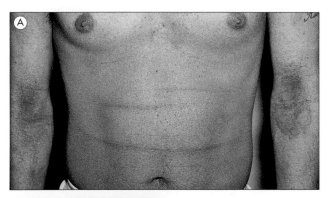

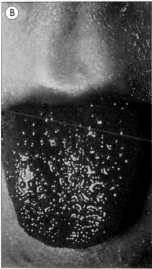

**Fig. 19.10** Scarlet fever. (A) Punctate erythema is followed by peeling for 2–3 weeks. (B) The tongue is furred at first and then becomes raw with prominent papillae. (A, From James WD, Berger T. *Andrews' Diseases of the Skin*, Saunders Elsevier; 2006; B, Courtesy W.E. Farrar.)

**Table 19.7** Revised Jones criteria for the diagnosis of rheumatic fever (RF) in people with evidence of a preceding group A streptococcus infection

| Acute RF | 2 major manifestations or 1 major plus 2 minor manifestations |
| --- | --- |
| Recurrent RF | 2 major or 1 major and 2 minor or 3 minor |

| Major criteria | |
| --- | --- |
| **Low-risk populations**[a] | **Moderate- and high-risk populations** |
| Carditis<br>• Clinical and/or subclinical | Carditis<br>• Clinical and/or subclinical |
| Arthritis<br>• Polyarthritis only | Arthritis<br>• Monoarthritis or polyarthritis<br>• Polyarthralgia |
| Chorea | Chorea |
| Erythema marginatum | Erythema marginatum |
| Subcutaneous nodules | Subcutaneous nodules |

| Minor criteria | |
| --- | --- |
| **Low-risk populations** | **Moderate- and high-risk populations** |
| Polyarthralgia | Monoarthralgia |
| Fever (≥38.5°C) | Fever (≥38°C) |
| ESR ≥60 mm in the first hour and/or CRP ≥3 mg/dL | ESR ≥30 mm/hr and/or CRP ≥3 mg/dL |
| Prolonged PR interval, after accounting for age variability (unless carditis is a major criterion) | Prolonged PR interval, after accounting for age variability (unless carditis is a major criterion) |

[a]Low-risk populations are those with acute rheumatic fever incidence ≤2/100,000 school-aged children or all-age rheumatic heart disease prevalence of ≤1/1000 population per year.

Reprinted with permission from the American Heart Association. Gewitz MH, Baltimore RS, Tani LY, et al. Revision of the Jones criteria for the diagnosis of acute rheumatic fever in the era of Doppler echocardiography. *Circulation.* 2015;131:1806–1818.

CRP, C-reactive protein; ESR, erythrocyte sedimentation rate.

- Rheumatic heart disease—repeated attacks of *S. pyogenes* with different M types can lead to heart valve damage. Certain children have a genetic predisposition to this immune-mediated disease. If a primary attack is accompanied by rising or high antistreptolysin O (ASO) antibody levels, future attacks must be prevented by penicillin prophylaxis throughout childhood. In many resource-poor countries, rheumatic heart disease is the most common type of heart disease, seen where there is poverty and overcrowding.
- Acute glomerulonephritis. This is an immune complex–mediated disease in which antibodies to streptococcal components combine with them to form circulating immune complexes, which are then deposited in glomeruli. Immune cells are recruited and cytokines and chemical mediators produced, together with local complement and coagulation systems being activated, resulting in inflammation in the glomeruli. Blood appears in the urine (red cells, protein), and there are signs of an acute nephritis syndrome, including oedema and hypertension 1–2 weeks after the sore throat. ASO antibodies are usually elevated. There are 7 of at least 80 M types of *S. pyogenes* that give rise to this condition, this being a protein that is a primary virulent factor, but nephritis may also follow group C streptococcal infection. Penicillin prophylaxis is therefore not given. In contrast to rheumatic fever, second attacks are rare.

### Diagnosis

**A laboratory diagnosis is not generally necessary for pharyngitis and tonsillitis**

There are many possible viral causes of pharyngitis and tonsillitis, and the clinical condition is generally not serious enough to seek laboratory help. The diagnosis of EBV or CMV infection is helped by detection of a lymphocytosis and atypical lymphocytes in a blood film. EBV is distinguished from CMV by detection of the VCA IgM, although the less specific tests such as the Paul-Bunnell, or monospot, test may be used in some laboratories, whereas CMV diagnosis is made by detection of CMV IgM. HSV DNA is detected in swabs from the lesions sent to the laboratory, but clinical diagnosis is usually adequate. Bacteria are identified by culture of throat swabs (see Ch. 32). It is especially important to diagnose *S. pyogenes* infection by culture because of the possible complications (see earlier) and because, unlike *Streptococcus pneumoniae*, it remains susceptible to penicillin. Resistance to erythromycin and tetracycline, however, is increasing. Although during the winter months up to 16% of schoolchildren carry GAS in the throat without symptoms, treatment is recommended.

## PAROTITIS

**Mumps virus is spread by airborne droplets and infects the salivary glands**

There is only one serotype of this single-stranded RNA paramyxovirus. It spreads by airborne droplets, salivary secretions and possibly urine. Close contact is necessary (e.g. at school) as the peak incidence is at 5–14 years of age. However, susceptible adults are at risk of complications of mumps such as orchitis.

After entering the body, the primary site of replication is the epithelium of the upper respiratory tract or eye. The virus spreads, undergoing further multiplication in local lymphoid tissues (lymphocytes and monocytes) and reticuloendothelial cells. After ~7–10 days the virus enters the blood, a primary viraemia, and localizes in salivary and other glands and body sites, including the CNS, testis, pancreas and ovary (Fig. 19.11), and is excreted in the urine. Infected cells lining the parotid ducts degenerate and finally, after an incubation period of 16–18 days that can range from 12–25 days, the inflammation, with lymphocyte infiltration and often oedema, results in disease. After a prodromal

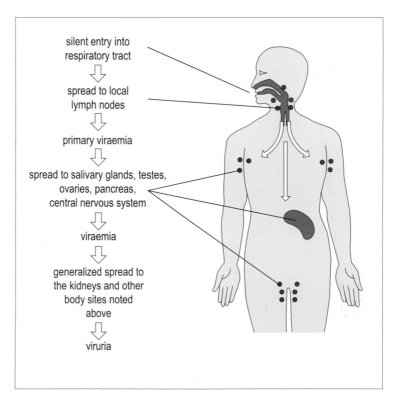

**Fig. 19.11** The pathogenesis of mumps. Understanding the pathogenesis of this infection helps to explain the disease picture, sites of shedding, and the complications that can arise.

silent entry into respiratory tract

spread to local lymph nodes

primary viraemia

spread to salivary glands, testes, ovaries, pancreas, central nervous system

viraemia

generalized spread to the kidneys and other body sites noted above

viruria

period of malaise and anorexia lasting 1–2 days, the parotid gland becomes painful, tender, and swollen and is sometimes accompanied by submandibular gland involvement (Fig. 19.12). This is the classic sign of mumps, and parotitis is the most common clinical sign. Other sites may be invaded, with clinical consequences such as inflammation of the testis and pancreas, resulting respectively in orchitis and pancreatitis (Table 19.8). CMI as well as antibody responses appear, and the patient usually recovers within 1 week. Mumps

reinfection can occur after both natural infection or having received the mumps, measles, and rubella (MMR) vaccine.

Laboratory diagnosis is made by detecting:

- viral RNA in throat swabs, cerebrospinal fluid, or urine or by isolating virus in cell culture
- mumps-specific IgM antibody.

**Treatment and prevention**

There is no specific treatment, but mumps is prevented by using the attenuated live virus vaccine, which is safe and effective. This is usually given in combination with the MMR vaccine.

Combined MMR has been a controversial issue in the United Kingdom after autism and bowel disorders were reported as being possibly associated with immunization. However, despite a series of epidemiologic studies showing no association with immunization, there was a fall in MMR uptake rates and subsequent outbreaks of mumps and measles around the country. These rates had improved by 2017: In the United Kingdom the coverage was >90%. However, outbreaks of measles were being reported in other parts of Europe.

## OTITIS AND SINUSITIS

### Otitis and sinusitis can be caused by many viruses and a range of secondary bacterial invaders

Many viruses are capable of invading the air spaces associated with the upper respiratory tract such as the sinuses, middle ear and mastoid. Mumps virus or RSV, for instance, can cause vestibulitis or deafness, which is generally temporary. The range of secondary bacterial invaders is the same as for other upper respiratory tract infections (i.e. *S. pneumoniae*, *H. influenzae*, *Moraxella catarrhalis* and sometimes anaerobes such as *Bacteroides fragilis*). Brain abscess is a major

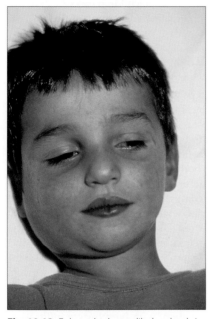

**Fig. 19.12** Enlarged submandibular glands in a child with mumps. (From Heumann et al. *Klinische Infektiologie*, Elsevier; 2008.)

**Table 19.8** Clinical consequences of mumps virus invasion of different body tissues

| Site of growth | Result | Comment |
|---|---|---|
| Salivary glands | Inflammation, parotitis<br>Virus shed in saliva (from 3 days before to 6 days after symptoms) | Parotitis can be unilateral |
| Meninges<br>Brain | Meningitis<br>Encephalitis | Central nervous system infection is common (~10% symptomatic)<br>Less common; complete recovery is the rule, deafness is a rare complication<br>Both may occur up to 7 days after parotitis |
| Kidney | Virus present in urine | No clinical consequences |
| Testis<br>Ovary | Epididymoorchitis: rigid tunica albuginea around testis make orchitis more painful and more damaging<br>Oophoritis | 25–50% in postpubertal males<br>Around 70% unilateral<br>Rare cause of sterility<br>Around 5% of postpubertal females |
| Pancreas | Pancreatitis | Rare complication and may see transient hyperglycaemia |
| Mammary gland | Virus detectable in milk<br>Mastitis in 10% postpubertal females | |
| Thyroid | Thyroiditis | Rare |
| Myocardium | Myocarditis | Rare |
| Joints | Arthritis | Rare |

complication (see Ch. 25). Blockage of the eustachian (auditory) tube or the opening of sinuses caused by allergic swelling of the mucosa, prevents mucociliary clearance of infection, and the local accumulation of inflammatory bacterial products causes further swelling and blockage.

## Acute otitis media

### Common causes of acute otitis media are viruses, *Streptococcus pneumoniae* and *Haemophilus influenzae*

This condition is extremely common in infants and small children, partly because the eustachian (auditory) tube is open more widely at this age. A study in Boston showed that 83% of 3-year-olds have had at least one episode, and 46% have had three or more episodes since birth. At least 50% of the attacks are viral in origin (especially RSV), and the bacterial invaders are nasopharyngeal residents, most commonly *S. pneumoniae, H. influenzae, M. catarrhalis* and sometimes *S. pyogenes* or *Staphylococcus aureus*. There may be general symptoms, and acute otitis media should be considered in any child with unexplained fever, diarrhoea or vomiting. The ear drum shows dilated vessels with bulging of the drum at a later stage (Fig. 19.13). Fluid often persists in the middle ear for weeks or months and is called *glue ear*, and, regardless of therapy, it contributes to impaired hearing and learning difficulties in infants and small children. Most uncomplicated infections resolve with oral analgesics, but if there is no improvement then systemic antibiotics should be started.

If acute attacks are inadequately treated, there may be continued infection with a chronic discharge through a perforated drum and impaired hearing. This is chronic suppurative otitis media.

## Otitis externa

### Causes of otitis externa are *Staphylococcus aureus*, *Candida albicans*, and gram-negative opportunists

Infections of the outer ear can cause irritation and pain, and they must be distinguished from otitis media. In contrast to the middle ear, the external canal has a bacterial flora similar to that of the skin (staphylococci, corynebacterial and, to a lesser extent, propionibacteria), and the pathogens responsible for otitis media are rarely found in otitis externa. The warm moist environment favours *S. aureus, C. albicans* and

gram-negative opportunists such as *Proteus* and *Pseudomonas aeruginosa*.

Ear drops containing neomycin or chloramphenicol are usually an effective treatment.

## Acute sinusitis

The aetiology and pathogenesis of acute sinusitis are similar to those of otitis media. Clinical features include facial pain and localized tenderness. It may be possible to identify the causative bacteria by microscopy and culture of pus aspirated from the sinus, but sinus puncture is not often carried out. In addition, the patient can be treated empirically with amoxicillin or coamoxiclav to deal with beta-lactamase–producing organisms.

## ACUTE EPIGLOTTITIS

### Acute epiglottitis is generally due to *Haemophilus influenzae* capsular type B infection

Acute epiglottitis is most often seen in young children. *H. influenzae* capsular type B can spread from the nasopharynx to the epiglottis, causing severe inflammation and oedema. There is usually a bacteraemia.

### Acute epiglottitis is an emergency and necessitates intubation and treatment with antibiotics

Acute epiglottitis is characterized by difficulty in breathing because of respiratory obstruction, and, until the airway has been secured by intubation, extreme care must be taken when examining the throat in case the swollen epiglottis is sucked into the oedematous airway and causes total obstruction. Treatment is begun immediately with antibiotics effective against *H. influenzae* such as third-generation cephalosporins that include cefotaxime. The clinical diagnosis is confirmed by isolating bacteria from the blood and possibly the epiglottis once breathing is stable and the airway secure. The Hib vaccine greatly reduces the frequency of this and other infections due to Hib.

Respiratory obstruction due to diphtheria (see later) is rare in resource-rich countries, but the characteristic false membrane and local swelling can extend from the pharynx to involve the uvula.

## ORAL CAVITY INFECTIONS

### Saliva flushes the mouth and contains a variety of antibacterial substances

The oral cavity is continuous with the pharynx but is dealt with separately because of the presence of teeth, which are subject to a particular set of microbiologic problems. The normal mouth contains commensal microorganisms, some of which are to a large extent restricted to the mouth (see Table 19.1). Most of them make specific attachments to teeth or mucosal surfaces and are shed into the saliva as they multiply. The litre or so of saliva secreted each day mechanically flushes the mouth. It also contains secretory antibodies, polymorphs, desquamated mucosal cells and antibacterial substances such as lysozyme and lactoperoxidase. When salivary flow is decreased for a few hours, as between meals, there is a fourfold increase in the number of bacteria in saliva, and in dehydrated patients or in severe illnesses such

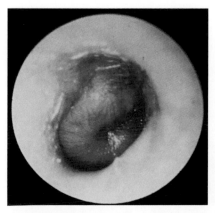

**Fig. 19.13** Acute otitis media with bulging ear drum. (Courtesy M. Chaput de Saintonge.)

as typhoid or pneumonia, the mouth becomes foul smelling because of microbial overgrowth.

## Oral candidiasis

### Changes in the oral flora produced by broad-spectrum antibiotics and impaired immunity predispose to thrush

The presence of commensal bacteria in the mouth makes it difficult for invading microorganisms to become established, but changes in oral flora upset this balance. For instance, prolonged administration of broad-spectrum antibiotics allows the normally harmless *C. albicans* to flourish, penetrating the epithelium with its pseudomycelia and causing thrush. Oral thrush (candidiasis, Fig. 19.14) is also seen when immunity is impaired, as in HIV infection and after cytotoxic chemotherapy to treat various cancers, and occasionally in newborns and the elderly. It sometimes spreads to involve the oesophagus. The diagnosis is readily confirmed by Gram stain and culture of scraped material, which shows large gram-positive budding yeasts.

Topical antifungal agents such as nystatin, clotrimazole or oral fluconazole (see Ch. 34) are effective treatments for thrush, together with attention to any predisposing factors.

Another example of the shifting boundary between harmless coexistence and tissue invasion by resident microbes is seen with vitamin C deficiency, which reduces mucosal resistance and allows oral residents to cause gum infections.

## Caries

### In the United States and Western Europe, 80–90% of people are colonized by *Streptococcus mutans*, which causes dental caries

The microorganisms specifically adapted for life on teeth form a film called dental plaque on the tooth surface. This is a complex mass containing about $10^9$/g of bacteria embedded in a polysaccharide matrix (Fig. 19.15). The film, visible as a red layer when a dye such as erythrosine is given as a mouth rinse, is largely removed by thorough brushing but reestablishes itself within a few hours. The clean teeth become covered with salivary glycoproteins to which certain streptococci (especially *S. mutans* and *S. sobrinus*) become attached and multiply. In the United States and Western Europe, 80–90% of people are colonized by *S. mutans*, which itself synthesizes glucan, a sticky high molecular weight polysaccharide, from sucrose and forms a matrix between these streptococci. Certain other bacteria, including anaerobic filamentous fusobacteria and actinomycetes, are also present. When the teeth are not cleaned for several days, plaque becomes thicker and more extensive — a tangled forest of microorganisms.

The bacteria in plaque use dietary sugar and form lactic acid, which decalcifies the tooth locally. Proteolytic enzymes from the bacteria help to break down other components of the enamel to give rise to painful cavities in the teeth, known as dental caries. Infection may then spread into the pulp of the tooth to form a pulp or root abscess and from here to the maxillary or mandibular spaces.

The pH in an active caries lesion may be as low as 4. Therefore caries usually develop in crevices on the tooth when bacteria such as *S. mutans* are in the plaque and there is a regular supply of sucrose. Acid tolerance is a primary ecologic advantage for the bacteria involved in caries. *S. mutans*, lactobacilli and *Bifidobacteria* spp. are very acid tolerant and break down carbohydrates in the diet to a pH far lower than that in which the commensal bacteria are able to survive. In addition, the commensals do not have a chance as the competitive advantage is bolstered even more by the bacteriocins that are produced by *S. mutans*, which are active against bacteria associated with oral health. It may legitimately be regarded as an infectious disease — one of the most prevalent infectious diseases in resource-rich countries due to closely placed bacteria-coated teeth and a sugary, often fluoride-deficient diet.

## Periodontal disease

### *Actinomyces viscosus*, *Actinobacillus* and *Bacteroides* spp. are commonly involved in periodontal disease

A space known as the gingival crevice readily forms between the gums and tooth margin, and it may be considered as an oral backwater. It contains polymorphs, complement and IgG and IgM antibodies, and it easily becomes infected. Gingival crevices normally contain microbes at an average of $2.7 \times 10^{11}$/g, and 75% of them are anaerobes. The oral microbiome contains hundreds of bacterial species of which a smaller number is associated with progressive periodontal disease, with gram-negative anaerobic rods and spirochetes predominant. Bacteria such as *Actinomyces viscosus*, *Actinobacillus*, *Porphyromonas gingivalis*, *Fusobacterium* spp. and *Bacteroides*

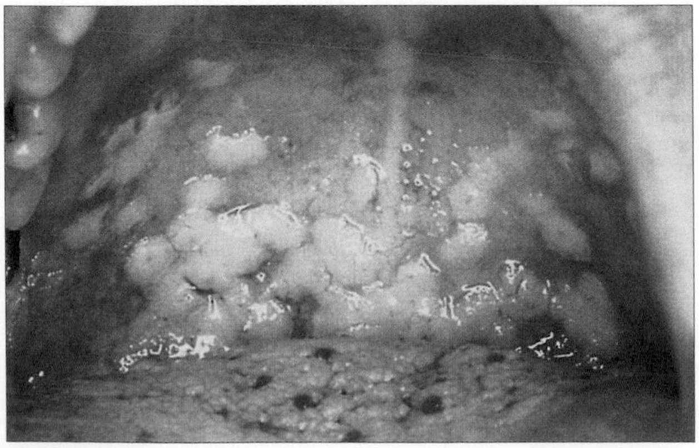

**Fig. 19.14** Oral candidiasis. (Courtesy J.A. Innes.)

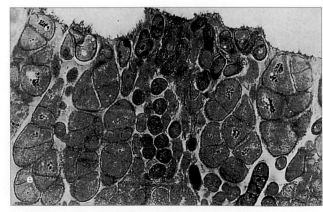

**Fig. 19.15** Dental plaque on the deep surface of a child's tooth. e, Enamel (× 20,000). (Courtesy H.N. Newman.)

spp. are commonly involved. In periodontal disease, the space enlarges to become a pocket with local inflammation, an increasing number of polymorphs, and a serum exudate. The inflamed gum bleeds readily and later recedes, while the multiplying bacteria cause halitosis. Finally, the structures supporting the teeth are affected, with reabsorption of ligaments and weakening of bone, causing the teeth to loosen. The interplay between bacterial factors and host response, once again, is key as bacterial lipopolysaccharides activate macrophages to produce cytokines that include interleukins and tumor necrosis factor. These cytokines activate periodontal fibroblasts and matrix metalloproteinases, inducing collagen degradation. This is a local disaster as collagen is the main constituent of the periodontal matrix, and the result is bone resorption. Periodontal disease with gingivitis is highly prevalent, although its severity varies greatly. It is a major cause of tooth loss in adults. Periodontal disease is multifactorial as there are other risk factors, including genetic risk factors, diet, smoking and diabetes.

## KEY FACTS

- The respiratory tract from the nose to the alveoli is a continuum, and any given pathogen can cause disease in more than one segment.

- Some respiratory infections, including influenza, diphtheria and pertussis, are restricted to the surface epithelium, whereas measles, rubella, mumps, CMV and EBV enter via the respiratory tract, causing local symptoms such as pharyngitis, but then spread throughout the body and are associated with a range of nonrespiratory symptoms.

- Professional invaders, including common cold viruses, coronaviruses, influenza viruses, mumps, CMV, EBV and *M. tuberculosis*, infect the healthy respiratory tract, whereas secondary invaders such as *S. aureus*, *Pneumocystis jirovecii* and *Pseudomonas* cause disease only when host defences are impaired.

- Common diseases of the teeth and neighbouring structures (caries, periodontal disease) are of microbial aetiology.

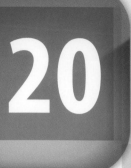

# 20

# Lower respiratory tract infections

## Introduction

Although the respiratory tract is continuous from the nose to the alveoli, it is convenient to distinguish between infections of the upper and lower respiratory tracts even though the same microorganisms might be implicated in infections of both. Infections of the upper respiratory tract and associated structures are the subject of Ch. 19. Here we discuss infections of the lower respiratory tract. These infections tend to be more severe than infections of the upper respiratory tract, and the choice of appropriate antimicrobial therapy is important and may be life saving. In addition, immunization is important to protect those at particular risk of complications.

All these aspects were encapsulated in the coronavirus disease 2019 (COVID-19) pandemic. The usual suspects are not always involved in pandemics as was seen when another novel coronavirus emerged. Unlike its predecessors, it was highly transmissible and was a global wakeup call about how populations can be affected in many ways by an infectious agent.

## LARYNGITIS AND TRACHEITIS

### Parainfluenza viruses are common causes of laryngitis

Laryngeal infection (laryngitis) and tracheitis cause hoarseness and a burning retrosternal pain. The larynx and trachea have nonexpandable rings of cartilage in the wall and are easily obstructed in children due to their narrow passages, leading to hospital admission. Swelling of the mucous membrane may lead to a dry cough and inspiratory stridor (*crowing*, a term for noisy breathing) known as *croup*. Viral infections of the upper respiratory tract may spread downward to involve the larynx and trachea. Molecular diagnostic tests detect a broader range of viruses causing laryngitis and tracheitis, including rhinovirus, parainfluenza virus, influenza virus, adenovirus and respiratory syncytial virus (RSV) infections. Diphtheria (see later) may involve the larynx or trachea.

Bacteria such as group A streptococci, *Haemophilus influenzae* and *Staphylococcus aureus* are less common causes of laryngitis and tracheitis.

## DIPHTHERIA

### Diphtheria is mostly caused by toxin-producing strains of *Corynebacterium diphtheriae* and can cause life-threatening respiratory obstruction due to a pseudomembrane forming in the throat

Diphtheria is now rare in resource-rich countries owing to widespread immunization with toxoid; as a result, it may be difficult to diagnose clinically but is still common in resource-poor countries. It can be respiratory or cutaneous in nature due to the exotoxin-producing *C. diphtheriae* and *C. ulcerans*, respectively. *C. pseudotuberculosis* is also toxigenic and, together with *C. ulcerans*, is zoonotic, transmitted by domestic and wild mammals, with *C. pseudotuberculosis* being associated with lymphadenitis. The diphtheria toxin is encoded by the *tox* gene carried by a bacteriophage that integrates into specific sites of the *Corynebacterium* chromosome. Nontoxigenic strains occur in the normal pharynx

and can cause severe disease that cannot be prevented by vaccination.

*Corynebacterium* spp. can colonize the pharynx (especially the tonsillar regions), the larynx, the nose and occasionally the genital tract. In the tropics or in indigent people with poor skin hygiene, it can colonize the skin.

Adhesion is mediated by pili or fimbriae covalently attached to the bacterial cell wall. The bacteria multiply locally without invading deeper tissues or spreading through the body. The toxin destroys epithelial cells and polymorphs and an ulcer forms, which is covered with a necrotic exudate forming a false membrane. This soon becomes dark and malodorous, and bleeding occurs on attempting to remove it. The onset of membranous pharyngitis and fever is accompanied by extensive inflammation and swelling of the soft tissue (Fig. 20.1) and enlarged cervical lymph nodes giving a bull-neck appearance. The pathogenesis is attributed

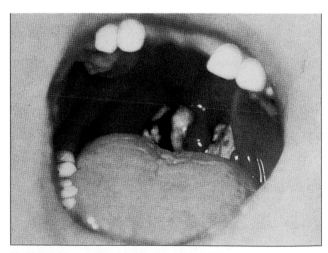

**Fig. 20.1** Pharyngeal diphtheria. Characteristic diphtheria false membrane in a child with local inflammation. (Courtesy Norman Begg.)

## Box 20.1    Lessons in Microbiology

### Diphtheria toxin

The genes encoding toxin production are carried by a temperate bacteriophage which, during the lysogenic phase, is integrated into the bacterial chromosome. The toxin is synthesized as a single polypeptide (molecular weight 62,000; 535 amino acids) consisting of:

- fragment B (binding) at the carboxy terminal end, which attaches the toxin to the host cells (or to any eukaryotic cell)
- fragment A (active) at the amino terminal end, which is the toxic fragment.

Toxic fragment A is formed only by protease cleavage and reduction of disulphide bonds after cellular uptake of the toxin. Fragment A inactivates elongation factor 2 (EF-2) by adenosine diphosphate ribosylation and thereby inhibits protein synthesis (see Fig. 20.2). Prokaryotic and mitochondrial protein synthesis is not affected because a different EF is involved. A single bacterium can produce 5000 toxin molecules/h, and the toxic fragment is so stable within the cell that a single molecule can kill a cell. Myocardial and peripheral nerve cells are particularly susceptible.

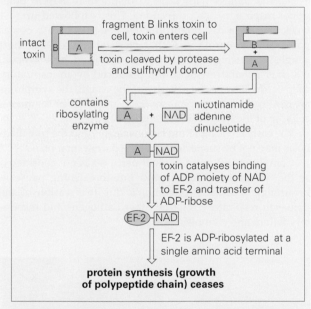

**Fig. 20.2** Mechanism of action of diphtheria toxin. ADP, Adenosine diphosphate; EF-2, elongation factor-2.

less well absorbed from this site, and a nasal discharge may be the main symptom. However, the patient will be highly infectious.

The incubation period is 2–5 days but may be up to 10 days. It is most commonly spread by droplets, but direct contact with cutaneous diphtheria lesions or infected secretions can also result in transmission. People can be infectious to others for up to 4 weeks.

### Diphtheria toxin can cause fatal heart failure and a polyneuritis

Although there are four biovars of *C. diphtheria*, the management from both a clinical and a public health perspective is the same. The exotoxin prevents protein synthesis, leading to cell death and causing local tissue necrosis, and has several effects when absorbed into the lymphatics and blood (Box 20.1 and Fig. 20.2):

- Constitutional upset with fever, pallor and exhaustion
- Myocarditis, usually within the first 2 weeks, as cardiac myocytes have the HB-EGF receptor (Electrocardiographic changes are common with a variety of arrhythmias, and cardiac failure can occur. If this is not lethal, complete recovery is usual.)
- Polyneuritis, which may occur after the onset of illness due to demyelination (Neurones have the HB-EGF receptor. Cranial nerve 9 may be affected, resulting in paralysis of the soft palate and regurgitation of fluids.)

### Diphtheria is managed by immediate treatment with antitoxin and antibiotics

Diphtheria is a life-threatening disease, and clinical diagnosis is a matter of urgency. As soon as the diagnosis is suspected clinically, the patient is isolated to reduce the risk of the toxigenic strain spreading to other susceptible individuals, and antitoxin and antibiotic treatment are started. The antitoxin is produced in horses, and tests for hypersensitivity to horse serum should be carried out. Until the patient can swallow properly, parenteral benzylpenicillin or erythromycin is also given. Laryngeal diphtheria may result in an obstructed airway and require a tracheotomy to assist with respiration. Patients should also be immunized with a diphtheria-toxoid–containing vaccine once they have recovered because the antitoxin level may be inadequate postinfection.

Two nasopharyngeal and throat swab sets are collected 24 hours after stopping the antibiotic treatment and then 24 hours after that. If both are negative, then the patient has been cleared of the infection. If the pathogen is still grown, then a further 10 days of antibiotics are given.

The diagnosis is confirmed in the laboratory by culture on standard agar and identification by biochemical tests or, depending on availability, matrix-assisted laser desorption/ionization–time of flight (MALDI-TOF) analysis. Polymerase chain reaction (PCR) can be carried out in some reference laboratories to detect the *tox* gene responsible for producing the toxin, and toxin production is demonstrated by a gel-diffusion precipitin reaction (Elek test).

There are some reports of *C. diphtheriae* antimicrobial resistance in a few countries, but it is not a major issue unlike the multidrug-resistant *C. ulcerans* and *C. pseudotuberculosis*.

to both the diphtheria toxin and adhesins, haemagglutinins and nonfimbrial proteins that help the bacteria enter the host cell. The diphtheria toxin secreted by the bacteria binds to the proheparin-binding epidermal growth factor (HB-EGF)–like growth factor receptor on epithelial cells that acts as the toxin receptor.

Nasopharyngeal diphtheria is the most severe form of the disease. When the larynx is involved, increasing hoarseness and stridor can result in life-threatening respiratory obstruction. Anterior nasal diphtheria is a mild form of the disease if it occurs on its own because the toxin is

### Contacts may need chemoprophylaxis or immunization

Close contacts of diphtheria patients should have a naso-pharyngeal and throat swab collected and tested for carriage of toxigenic *C. diphtheriae* before chemoprophylaxis to see if they are asymptomatic carriers. They should then be given antibiotic prophylaxis with erythromycin and be immunized. Toxigenic bacteria may be carried and transmitted by asymptomatic convalescents or by apparently healthy individuals.

### Diphtheria is prevented by immunization

Diphtheria has almost disappeared from resource-rich countries as a result of the immunization of children with a safe, effective toxoid vaccine; however, the disease reappears when immunization is neglected. Worldwide in 2021 the World Health Organization (WHO) reported there were 8638 cases, and the childhood immunization coverage globally was ~81%.

## WHOOPING COUGH

### Whooping cough is caused by the bacterium *Bordetella pertussis*

Whooping cough or pertussis is a severe disease of childhood. Infants, especially if not immunized, are at the highest risk of severe complications. *B. pertussis*, first isolated by Bordet and Gengou in 1906, is confined to humans and is very contagious, spreading from person to person by airborne droplets. *B. parapertussis* can also cause a less severe whooping coughlike illness. The bacteria attach to and multiply in the ciliated respiratory mucosa but do not invade deeper structures. Surface components such as filamentous haemagglutinin and fimbriae play an important role in specific attachment to respiratory epithelium and/or suppressing the initial inflammatory response to infection, helping persistence.

### *B. pertussis* infection is associated with the production of a variety of toxic factors

Some of these virulence factors affect inflammatory processes, whereas others damage ciliary epithelium. They are:

- Pertussis toxin, sometimes called *lymphocytosis-promoting factor* as it induces lymphocytosis, resembles diphtheria and other toxins in being a subunit toxin with an active (A) catalytic subunit and membrane-binding (B) subunits. The A unit is an adenosine diphosphate (ADP) ribosyl transferase, which catalyses the transfer of ADP-ribose from nicotinamide adenine dinucleotide to the host cell inhibitory G proteins. The functional consequence of this is a disruption of signal transduction to the affected cell as the modification stops the G proteins, inhibiting adenylate cyclase activity, thereby increasing the cyclic adenosine monophosphate (cAMP) levels in the cell, causing dysregulation of the immune response in addition to other effects the toxin has on the cell surface.
- Adenylate cyclase toxin has a C-terminal domain that mediates binding to target cells and forms pores in the plasma membrane and an N-terminal domain, which is adenylate cyclase that converts adenosine triphosphate (ATP) to cAMP. It affects host cells on entry by causing ion permeability and increased cAMP levels, the latter of which has an effect on cell signalling, and reducing

intracellular ATP. In neutrophils, this results in an inhibition of defence functions such as chemotaxis, phagocytosis and bactericidal killing. This toxin may also be responsible for the haemolytic properties of *B. pertussis*.
- Dermonecrotic toxin, which differs from the classic endotoxin of other gram-negative rods, has functional similarities and may play a role in the pathogenesis of infection.
- Tracheal cytotoxin, which is a cell wall component derived from the peptidoglycan of *B. pertussis*, specifically kills tracheal epithelial cells.

Apart from these toxins, other factors influencing virulence and whose expression is positively controlled by the *bvg*AS genes include surface structures, such as filamentous hemagglutinin, fimbriae, pertactin and a number of metabolic proteins.

### *B. pertussis* infection is characterized by paroxysms of coughs followed by a whoop

Although most often presenting as whooping cough, there is a spectrum of signs and symptoms varying from mildly symptomatic upper respiratory tract infection to severe, persistent and worsening cough. There are three phases (catarrhal, paroxysmal, and convalescent), and each one can last 1–3 weeks. After an incubation period of 7–10 days (range 5–21 days), *B. pertussis* infection is manifest first as a catarrhal illness with little to distinguish it from other upper respiratory tract infections. This is followed up to 1 week later by a dry nonproductive cough, which becomes paroxysmal. A paroxysm is characterized by a series of short coughs producing copious mucus, followed by a whoop, which is a characteristic sound produced by an inspiratory gasp of air. Despite the severity of the cough, the symptoms are confined to the respiratory tract, and lobar or segmental collapse of the lungs can occur (Fig. 20.3).

The early clinical picture is nonspecific, and the true diagnosis may not be suspected until the paroxysmal phase.

Complications, more likely if pertussis is not considered as the diagnosis, include apnea (life-threatening pause in breathing), secondary pneumonia due to invasion of the damaged respiratory tract by other pathogens and respiratory failure and convulsions.

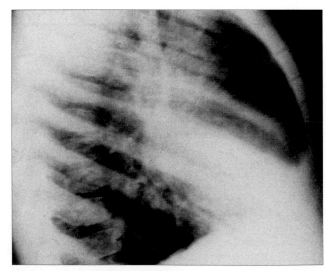

**Fig. 20.3** Chest radiograph showing patchy consolidation and collapse of the right middle lobe in whooping cough. (Courtesy J.A. Innes.)

The organisms can be isolated on suitable media from nasopharyngeal or per nasal swabs—not throat swabs because the bacteria are most likely to be found on the posterior wall of the nasopharynx or on cough plates—but they are fastidious and do not survive well outside the host. PCR is usually more sensitive than culture but may not be positive if the symptoms have lasted >3 weeks.

### Whooping cough is managed with supportive care and erythromycin

Supportive care is of prime importance. Infants are at greatest risk of complications, and admission to hospital should be considered for children <1 year of age. For specific antibacterial treatment to be effective, it must penetrate the respiratory mucosa and inhibit or kill the infecting organism. Treatment with macrolide antibiotics such as erythromycin, clarithromycin or azithromycin is recommended. Although the treatment is often started only when the disease is recognized in the paroxysmal phase, it does appear to reduce its severity and duration. It also reduces the bacterial load in the throat, thereby helping to reduce both the infectivity of the patient and the risk of secondary infections.

Prophylaxis with macrolide antibiotics of close contacts of active cases is helpful in controlling the spread of infection.

### Whooping cough can be prevented by active immunization

For many years, a whole cell vaccine comprising a killed suspension of *B. pertussis* cells was used, combined with purified diphtheria and tetanus toxoids and administered as DPT or triple vaccine. Although an effective vaccine, there were major concerns about side effects. These included fever, malaise and pain at the site of administration in up to 20% of infants; convulsions, thought to be associated with the vaccine in ~0.5% of vaccinees; and encephalopathy and permanent neurologic sequelae associated with vaccination, with an estimated rate of 1 in 100,000 vaccinations (<0.001%).

Concern about side effects led to a marked fall in uptake of the vaccine and subsequently to a marked increase in the incidence of whooping cough.

Acellular pertussis vaccines became the dominant vaccine preparation as they provide the same or better protection against whooping cough and cause fewer side effects as they are highly purified with much reduced levels of endotoxin compared with whole cell vaccines. The acellular vaccines contain pertussis toxoid and other bacterial components, including the filamentous haemagglutinin and fimbriae, and are given in combination with other vaccines such as diphtheria, tetanus and inactivated polio. In 2012 surveillance in the United Kingdom detected the highest rise in pertussis infections in 20 years. These were seen in young adults and adolescents, but morbidity and mortality occurred in unimmunized infants. Pertussis immunization in pregnancy was introduced that year as 83% of deaths due to pertussis since 2000 had been in infants <3 months old, and babies born to immunized mothers were 90% less likely to develop pertussis than were those born to unimmunized mothers. This was due to passively transferred maternal antibody to the baby. In 2021 ~81% of all infants worldwide received three doses of pertussis vaccine. WHO estimated there were >29,623 reported infections worldwide in 2021.

## ACUTE BRONCHITIS

### Acute bronchitis is an inflammatory condition of the tracheobronchial tree usually due to infection

Causative agents include rhinoviruses and the seasonal human coronaviruses (e.g. OC43, NL63, HKU1, 229E), which also infect the upper respiratory tract and lower tract pathogens such as influenza viruses, adenoviruses and *Mycoplasma pneumoniae*. Secondary bacterial infection with *Streptococcus pneumoniae* and *H. influenzae* may also play a role in pathogenesis. The degree of damage to the respiratory epithelium varies with the infecting agent:

- With influenza virus infection, it may be extensive and leave the host prone to secondary bacterial invasion (postinfluenza pneumonia; see later).
- With *M. pneumoniae* infection, a cause of community-acquired pneumonia, there is specific attachment of the organism to receptors on the bronchial mucosal epithelium, evading the host's attempts at mucociliary clearance (Fig. 20.4), and the release of community-acquired respiratory distress toxin that causes airway inflammation and sloughing of affected cells. It was considered an atypical bacterium due to the pneumonia not responding to antibiotics that act on the cell wall—a result of it not having a cell wall! There is a 4-year epidemic cycle that normally occurs 2 years after the Olympic Games. A dry cough is the most prominent presentation, with fever, and treatment is largely symptomatic. However, it can cause pneumonia and complications involving other organs, such as hepatitis, encephalitis, arthralgia, haemolytic anaemia, skin lesions known as erythema multiforme and Stevens-Johnson syndrome, which is a toxic epidermal necrolysis. Treatment involves antibiotics such as macrolides or tetracyclines.

## ACUTE EXACERBATIONS OF CHRONIC BRONCHITIS

### Infection is only one component of chronic bronchitis

Chronic bronchitis is a condition characterized by cough and excessive mucous secretion in the tracheobronchial tree that is not attributable to specific diseases (bronchiectasis, asthma, tuberculosis). Infection appears to be only one component of the syndrome, the others being cigarette smoking and inhalation of dust or fumes from the workplace.

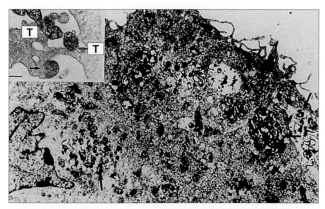

**Fig. 20.4** Opsonized *Mycoplasma pneumoniae* cells *(arrowed)* phagocytosed by an alveolar macrophage (bar, 2 µm). The insert shows *M. pneumoniae* cells adhering with the tip organelle *(T)* to macrophage surfaces. (From Jacobs E. Mycoplasma pneumoniae virulence factors and the immune response. *Rev Med Microbiology* 1991;2:83–90.)

Bacterial infection does not appear to initiate the disease but is probably significant in perpetuating it and in producing the characteristic acute exacerbations. *S. pneumoniae* and unencapsulated strains of *H. influenzae* are the organisms most frequently isolated, but interpretation of the significance of their presence in sputum is difficult because they are also commonly found in the normal throat flora and can therefore contaminate expectorated sputum. Other bacteria such as *S. aureus* and *M. pneumoniae* are less commonly associated with infection and exacerbation. Viruses are frequent causes of acute infection and cause the initial damage that results in secondary bacterial infections.

Antibiotic therapy may be helpful in the treatment of acute exacerbations, although its efficacy is difficult to assess.

## BRONCHIOLITIS

Bronchiolitis is a disease restricted to childhood, usually to children <2 years of age. The bronchioles of a young child have such a fine bore that if the child's lining cells are swollen by inflammation, the passage of air to and from the alveoli can be severely restricted. Infection results in necrosis of the epithelial cells lining the bronchioles and leads to peribronchial infiltration, which may spread into the lung fields to give an interstitial pneumonia (see later). As many as 75% of these infections are caused by RSV; the rest are of viral aetiology, including parainfluenza viruses, human metapneumovirus (hMPV) and influenza viruses.

## RESPIRATORY SYNCYTIAL VIRUS INFECTION

### RSV is the most important cause of bronchiolitis and pneumonia in infants

RSV is a typical paramyxovirus, and two major strains have been identified: group A and group B. Its surface spikes bear G protein (not haemagglutinin or neuraminidase) for attachment to the cell and fusion (F) protein. The latter initiates viral entry by fusing the viral envelope to the cell membrane and fuses host cells to form syncytia.

RSV infection is transmitted by droplets and, to some extent, by hands. Outbreaks occur each winter and, during the RSV season, infection can spread in hospitals as well as in the community. Nearly all individuals have been infected by 2 years of age. About 1 in every 100 infants with RSV bronchiolitis or pneumonia requires admission to hospital.

### RSV infection can be particularly severe in young infants but also in older adults

After inhalation, the virus establishes infection in the nasopharynx and lower respiratory tract. Clinical illness appears after an incubation period of 4–5 days. The illness can be particularly severe in babies, with peak mortality at 3 months of age, the virus invading the lower respiratory tract by direct surface spread to cause bronchiolitis or pneumonia. They develop a cough, rapid respiratory rate and cyanosis. In young children and adults, however, the virus may be restricted to the upper respiratory tract, causing a less severe common cold-type illness. Otitis media is quite common. Secondary bacterial infection is thought to be rare, but with more sensitive diagnostic tests, over time it may become apparent that it is more frequent than was recognized previously. Adults >65 years old, those with chronic heart or lung disease and those immunocompromised are also at risk of severe RSV infection. The US Centers for Disease Control and Prevention (CDC) estimated that 60,000–160,000 older adults with RSV infection are admitted to hospital annually.

### The manifestations of RSV infection appear to have an immunopathologic basis

Maternal antibodies in the infant react with virus antigens, perhaps with the liberation of histamine and other mediators from the host's cells. In early trials, a killed vaccine was used, and during subsequent natural RSV infection, the vaccinees had more frequent and severe lower respiratory tract disease compared with unimmunized children, supporting an immune-mediated pathogenesis.

Neutralizing antibodies are formed at lower levels in younger infants, but cell-mediated immunity (CMI) is needed to terminate the infection. The virus continues to be shed from the lungs of children lacking CMI for many months. Apparently healthy children may continue to show depressed pulmonary function or wheeze even 1–2 years after apparent recovery.

Recurrent infections are common but are less severe. The reason for recurrence, which is also a feature of parainfluenza virus infection, is unknown.

### RSV RNA is detectable in throat swab specimens, and ribavirin is indicated for severe disease

Molecular methods, such as PCR, detect RSV RNA in throat swab specimens and have a higher diagnostic sensitivity than the older diagnostic tests such as immunofluorescence (Fig. 20.5) and virus isolation.

In most children, treatment is supportive, involving rehydration, bronchodilators and, if needing admission to hospital, oxygen. The antiviral agent ribavirin, given as an aerosol or orally, has been used successfully in a number of clinical settings, including children with severe infection and immunosuppressed individuals at risk of severe disease. A recombinant humanized monoclonal antibody that binds to the RSV fusion protein, palivizumab, can be used as prophylaxis to prevent RSV infection in children <2 years of age who are at risk of severe disease such as those with chronic lung disease, congenital heart disease or those born <32 weeks of gestational age.

Nirsevimab is a recombinant human IgG1-kappa monoclonal antibody that binds the F1 and F2 subunits of the RSV fusion protein and locks it, blocking viral entry into the host cell. In 2022 it was shown to reduce hospital admissions due to RSV lower respiratory tract infection in healthy late preterm and term babies over a period of 150 days after the nirsevimab injection.

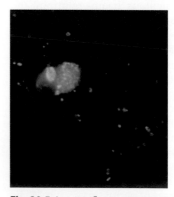

**Fig. 20.5** Immunofluorescent preparation from the nasopharynx showing respiratory syncytial virus–infected cells *(bright green)*. (Courtesy H. Stern.)

As of 2023 RSV vaccine candidates included live attenuated, protein, recombinant vector and nucleic acid based vaccines. In May 2023 a recombinant protein adjuvanted vaccine (Arexvy) was the first RSV vaccine to be approved for use by the US Food and Drug Administration (FDA) for people age ≥60 years. Others were expected to be licensed, and the messenger RNA (mRNA)–based vaccines were looking promising in clinical trials.

## HANTAVIRUS PULMONARY SYNDROME

The reservoir host for Sin Nombre virus (SNV), a New World hantavirus, is the deer mouse found commonly in North America. In 1993 individuals were infected in the southwestern United States and developed severe cardiopulmonary disease. Hantavirus pulmonary syndrome (HPS) followed flulike symptoms, such as fever and myalgia, followed ~10 days later by cough and dyspnoea as viral invasion of the pulmonary capillary endothelium results in fluid pouring into the lungs, owing to increased vascular permeability. At least 26 deaths were reported secondary to pulmonary oedema, hypotension and cardiogenic shock.

The route of transmission is by inhaling SNV-infected rodent faeces, saliva or urine with symptoms occurring 2–4 weeks after exposure. The Old World hantaviruses cause haemorrhagic fever with renal syndrome. The pathogenesis of both diseases involves exaggerated immune responses by SNV-infected endothelial cells that are also involved in regulating vascular permeability. Highly activated immune responses involving proinflammatory cytokines that may activate cytotoxic T-cell responses are associated with more severe disease. Between 1993, when hantavirus disease surveillance was started, and 2020, 807 individuals with HPS had been reported in the United States by the CDC, with a 35% mortality rate. HPS has also been reported in South America. There are other hantaviruses that cause HPS in other areas of the United States, with different rodent hosts (white-footed mouse, cotton rat). Infection usually occurs in rural areas where the rodent hosts may be found. Limited person-to-person transmission has been reported in Argentina. Treatment is mainly supportive in an intensive care unit (ICU) setting. Ribavirin treatment has not been shown to be effective despite success treating patients with haemorrhagic fever with renal syndrome.

## PNEUMONIA

Pneumonia is the most common cause of infection-related death in the elderly in the United States and Europe. It is caused by a wide range of microorganisms, and the challenge lies not in the clinical diagnosis of pneumonia, except perhaps in children in whom it may be more difficult to diagnose, but in the laboratory identification of the microbial cause.

### Microorganisms reach the lungs by inhalation, aspiration or via the blood

Microorganisms gain access to the lower respiratory tract by inhalation of aerosolized material or by aspiration of the normal flora of the upper respiratory tract. The size of inhaled particles is important in determining how far they travel down the respiratory tract; only those <5 mm in diameter reach the alveoli. Less frequently, the lungs become seeded with organisms as a result of spread via the blood from other infected sites. Healthy individuals are susceptible to infection by a range of pathogens possessing adhesins, which allow the pathogens to attach specifically to the respiratory epithelium. In addition, people with impaired defences (e.g. immunocompromised, preceding viral damage, cystic fibrosis) may develop infections with organisms that do not cause infections in healthy individuals. An example is *Pneumocystis jirovecii*, a fungal infection that is an important cause of pneumonia in individuals with acquired immunodeficiency syndrome (AIDS).

### The respiratory tract has a limited number of ways in which it can respond to infection

The host's response can be defined by pathologic and radiologic findings. Four descriptive terms are in common use (Fig. 20.6):

- *Lobar pneumonia* refers to involvement of a lobe, a distinct region of the lung. The polymorph exudate formed in response to infection clots in the alveoli and renders them solid. Infection may spread to adjacent alveoli until constrained by anatomic barriers between segments or lobes of the lung. Thus one lobe may show complete consolidation.
- *Bronchopneumonia* refers to a more diffuse patchy consolidation, which may spread throughout the lung as a result of the original pathologic process in the small airways.
- *Interstitial pneumonia*, or *pneumonitis*, involves invasion of the lung interstitium and is particularly characteristic of viral infections of the lungs but is also seen in atypical bacterial causes of pneumonia and *Pneumocystis* infection.
- *Lung abscess*, sometimes referred to as *necrotizing pneumonia*, is a condition in which there is cavitation and destruction of the lung parenchyma.

The outcomes common to all these conditions are respiratory distress resulting from the interference with air exchange in the lungs and systemic effects as a result of infection in any part of the body.

### A wide range of microorganisms can cause pneumonia

Age is an important determinant:

- Most childhood pneumonia is caused either by viruses or by bacteria invading the respiratory tract secondary to a viral infection, such as influenza. Neonates born to mothers with genital *Chlamydia trachomatis* infection may develop a chlamydial interstitial pneumonitis resulting from colonization of the respiratory tract during birth.
- In the absence of an underlying disorder such as cystic fibrosis, pneumonia is unusual in older children. Children and young adults with cystic fibrosis are very prone to lower respiratory tract infection caused characteristically by *S. aureus*, *H. influenzae* and *Pseudomonas aeruginosa*.
- The cause of pneumonia in adults depends on a number of risk factors such as older age, underlying disease and exposure to pathogens through occupation, travel or contact with animals.

Pneumonia acquired in hospital tends to be caused by a different spectrum of organisms, particularly gram-negative bacteria. The causative agents of community-acquired pneumonia in different age groups in China from 2009–2020 are summarized in Fig. 20.7 (parts 1–4).

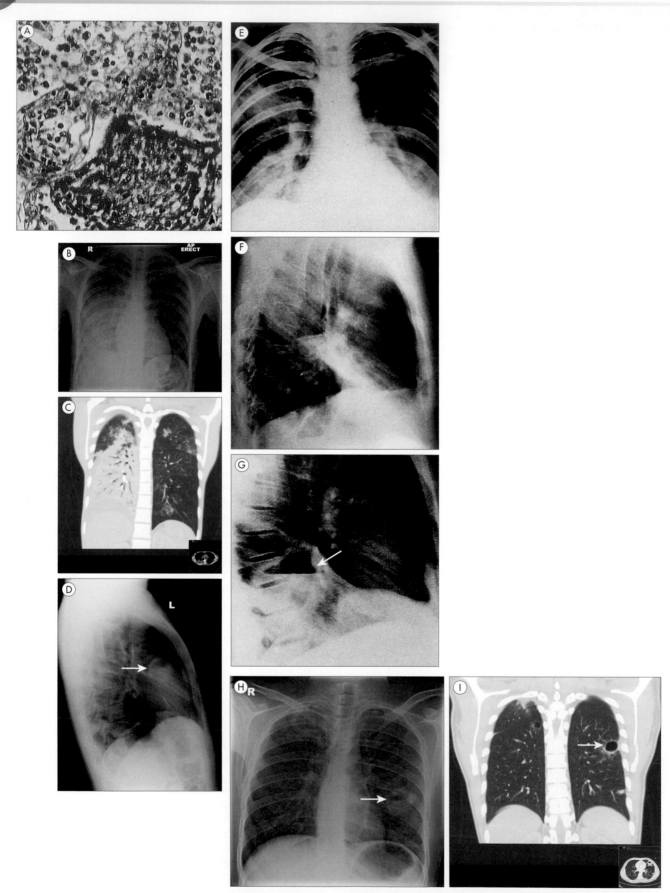

**Fig. 20.6** Four types of pneumonia. (A) Pneumococcal lobar pneumonia showing consolidated alveoli filled with neutrophils and fibrin (H&E stain). Right lower lobe pneumonia—white out on chest x-ray (B) and (C) chest computed tomography (CT). (E) Mycoplasma bronchopneumonia with patchy consolidation in several areas of both lungs. (F) Interstitial pneumonia due to influenza virus. (G) Lung abscess showing an abscess cavity *(arrowed)* on lateral chest X ray (D), chest x-ray (H) and chest CT (I). (A and F, Courtesy I.D. Starke and M.E. Hodson; B–D and G–I, courtesy G. Bain, London North West Healthcare Trust; E, courtesy J.A. Innes.)

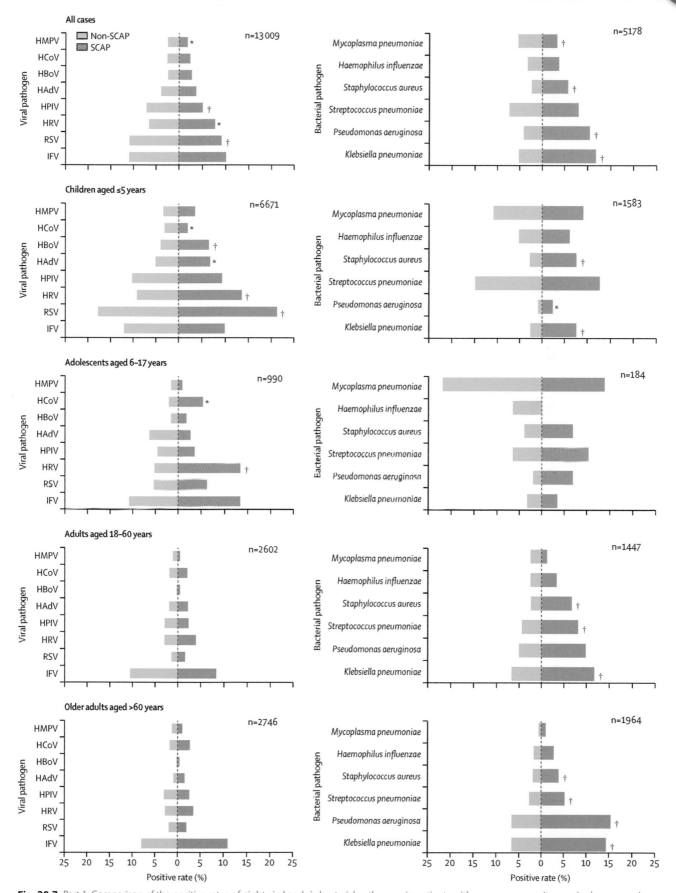

**Fig. 20.7** Part 1. Comparison of the positive rates of eight viral and six bacterial pathogens in patients with severe community acquired pneumonia (SCAP) and non-SCAP in mainland China, 2009–2020. *HAdV*, Human adenovirus; *HBoV*, human bocavirus; *HCoV*, seasonal human coronavirus; *HMPV*, human metapneumovirus; *HPIV*, human parainfluenza virus; *HRV*, human rhinovirus, *IFV*, influenza virus; *RSV*, respiratory syncytial virus; *SCAP*, severe community acquired pneumonia. *p < 005. †p < 001.

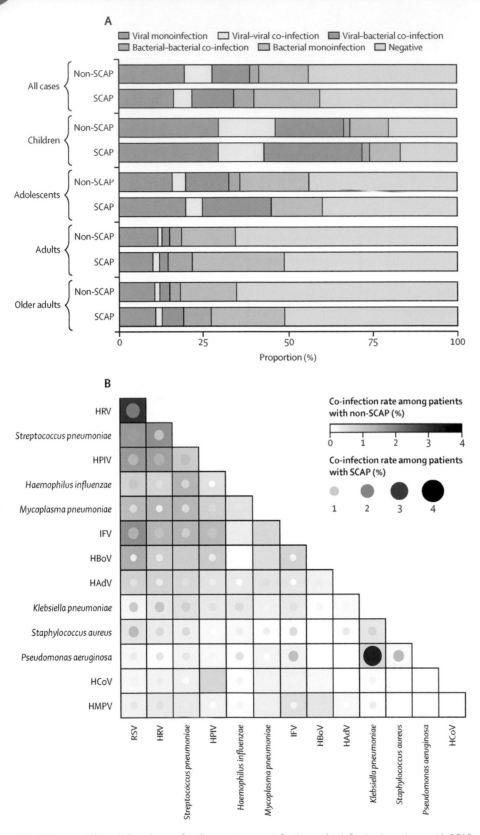

**Fig. 20.7—cont'd** Part 2. Prevalence of pathogens in monoinfection and coinfection in patients with SCAP and non-SCAP in mainland China, 2009–2020. (A) Positive proportion of viruses, viral–viral coinfections, viral–bacteria coinfections, bacterial–bacterial coinfections, and bacteria in different age groups. (B) Heatmap of the coinfection rate of respiratory pathogens.

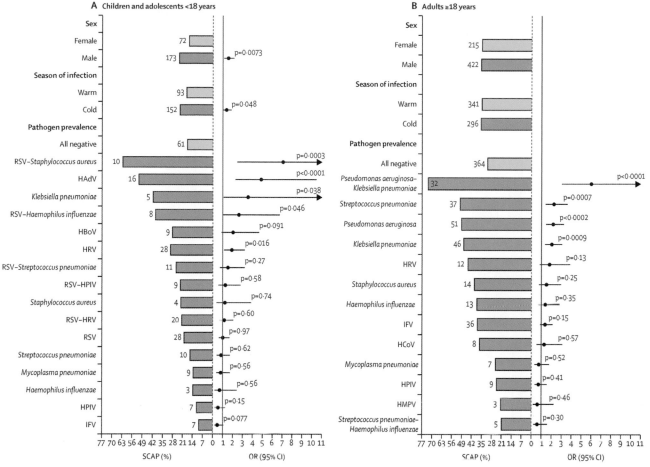

**Fig. 20.7—cont'd** Part 3. Adjusted odds ratios (ORs) for SCAP.
The black points are the adjusted ORs for SCAP, the black error bars are the 95% CIs, and the arrow indicates that the 95% CI is out of the graph.

Although clinical and epidemiologic clues help to suggest the likely cause, microbiologic investigations are essential to confirm the diagnosis and ensure optimal antimicrobial therapy.

Viral pneumonias show a characteristic interstitial pneumonia on chest radiography more often than bacterial pneumonias (see Fig. 20.6F), and for the sake of clarity, they are described separately later. Infections with RSV have been described earlier in this chapter; opportunist pathogens, such as *P. jirovecii*, associated specifically with pneumonia in the immunocompromised, are described in Ch. 31.

## BACTERIAL PNEUMONIA

*Streptococcus pneumoniae* **is the classic bacterial cause of acute community-acquired pneumonia**

In the past, 50–90% of pneumonias were caused by *S. pneumoniae* (the pneumococcus), and it is still the most common cause of bacterial pneumonia in children worldwide, with *H. influenzae* being the second most common cause. WHO reported that pneumonia causes 14% of all deaths of children age <5 years, accounting for ~740,000 deaths in 2019. Between 2009 and 2020, a national surveillance study of community acquired pneumonia was carried out in hospitals in 30 provinces in China. Nearly 19,000 children and

adults were enrolled and divided into those with severe community-acquired pneumonia (SCAP) and non-SCAP (see Fig. 20.7A–D).

RSV was the main viral infection in children with viral CAP and SCAP groups. The main bacterial pathogen in children was *S. pneumoniae*, *M. pneumoniae* for adolescents, *K. pneumoniae* for adults and *P. aeruginosa* for older adults.

Adults with CAP were more likely to have bacterial (24%) than viral (20%) infections, whereas children were more likely to have viral (52%) than bacterial (34%) infections.

Higher rates of viral-bacterial coinfection were found in children and older adults with SCAP, but this was mostly bacterial-bacterial coinfection in adults.

There was an age difference in coinfection patterns in the SCAP group. In children there was a higher coinfection rate with RSV-rhinovirus infections, but in adults and older adults the higher rate was with *K. pneumoniae*–*P. aeruginosa*. In children and adolescents there were more coinfections with RSV–*H. influenzae* and RSV–*S. aureus*; in adults age ≥18 years, the coinfections were *P. aeruginosa*–*K. pneumoniae*.

**A variety of bacteria causes primary atypical pneumonia**

When penicillin, an effective antibiotic treatment for pneumococcal infection, became widely available, a significant

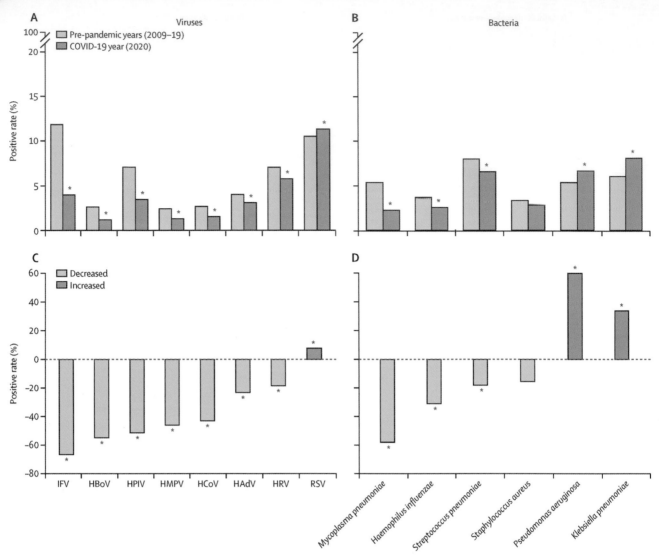

**Fig. 20.7—cont'd** Part 4. Comparison of age-standardized test positive rates of pathogens and their percent changes between the prepandemic years (2009–2019) and the first COVID-19 pandemic year (2020). Statistic significance was based on χ2 test or Fisher's exact test. *p<0·01. (From Liu Y-N, Zhang Y-F, Xu Q, et al. Infection and coinfection patterns of community-acquired pneumonia in patients of different ages in China from 2009–2020: A national surveillance study. *Lancet Microbe* 2023;4:e330–e339.)

proportion of patients with pneumonia failed to respond to this treatment and were labelled primary atypical pneumonia. *Primary* referred to pneumonia occurring as a new event (e.g. not secondary to influenza), and atypical to the fact that *S. pneumoniae* was not isolated from sputum from such patients, the symptoms often general as well as respiratory and the pneumonia did not to respond to penicillin or ampicillin. The causes of atypical pneumonia include *M. pneumoniae, Chlamydophila pneumoniae* and *C. psittaci, Legionella pneumophila* and *Coxiella burnetii. M. pneumoniae* and *C. pneumoniae* appear to be solely human pathogens, whereas *C. psittaci* and *C. burnetii* are acquired from infected animals and *L. pneumophila* from contaminated environmental sources (Fig. 20.8).

*Moraxella catarrhalis* can cause pneumonia particularly in patients with carcinoma of the lung or other underlying lung disease. Other aetiologic agents of pneumonia associated with particular underlying diseases, occupations or exposure to animals and travel are summarized in Fig. 20.8

and described in other chapters. It is important to note that a causative organism is not isolated in up to 35% of lower respiratory tract infections.

### Patients with pneumonia usually present feeling unwell and with a fever

Signs and symptoms of a chest infection include:

- chest pain, which may be pleuritic in nature (pain on inspiration)
- a cough, which may produce sputum
- shortness of breath (dyspnoea).

Some infections result in symptoms confined mainly to the chest, whereas others such as Legionnaires' disease caused by *L. pneumophila* have a much wider systemic involvement, and the patient may present with confusion, diarrhoea and evidence of renal or liver dysfunction. However, the distinction between localized and systemic symptoms is not usually reliable enough for an accurate diagnosis.

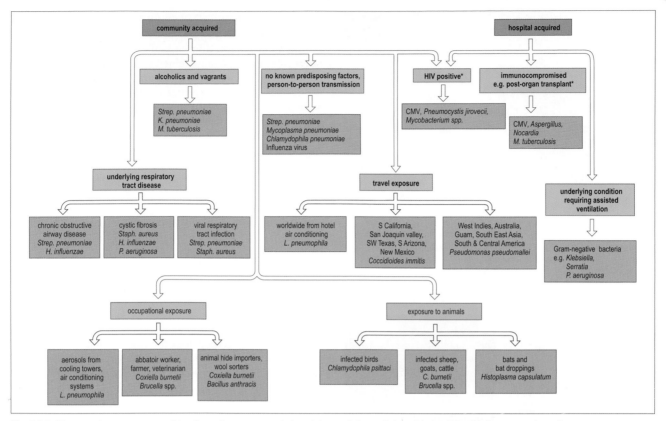

**Fig. 20.8** Many pathogens are capable of causing pneumonia in adults, and the aetiology is related to risk factors such as the exposure to pathogens through occupation, travel and contact with animals. The elderly are more likely to be infected and tend to have a more severe illness than young adults. *These infections are often reactivating endogenous infections rather than community or hospital acquired. CMV, Cytomegalovirus.

Chest examination may reveal abnormal crackling sounds (rales) and evidence of consolidation even before changes become evident on radiography.

### Patients with pneumonia usually have shadows in one or more areas of the lung

Imaging the chest with chest x-rays, computed tomography (CT) and magnetic resonance imaging is an important adjunct to the clinical diagnosis. Patients with pneumonia usually have shadows indicating consolidation (see earlier for descriptions of lobar, broncho- and interstitial pneumonia). However, careful interpretation is required to differentiate between infection and noninfective processes such as tumours.

### Pneumonia is the most common cause of death from infection in the elderly

It is also an important cause of death in the young and previously healthy. Complications of infection include spread of the infecting organisms:

- directly, to extrapulmonary sites such as the pleural space, giving rise to empyema (see later)
- indirectly, via the blood to other parts of the body.

For example, the majority of patients with pneumococcal pneumonia have positive blood cultures, and pneumococcal meningitis may follow pneumonia in the elderly.

### Sputum samples are best collected in the morning and before breakfast

Microscopic examination and culture of expectorated sputum remain the mainstays of respiratory bacteriology despite doubts about the value of these procedures. Collection of sputum is noninvasive, but more invasive techniques, such as transtracheal aspiration, bronchoscopy and bronchoalveolar lavage and open lung biopsy, may yield more useful results.

Sputum samples are best collected in the morning because sputum tends to accumulate while the patient is lying in bed, and before breakfast to reduce contamination by food particles and bacteria from food. It is important that the specimen submitted for examination is truly sputum and not simply saliva. A physiotherapist can be of great assistance to ill patients who may be unable to cough unaided.

### The usual laboratory procedures carried out on sputum specimens from patients with pneumonia are Gram stain and culture

Examination of the Gram-stained sputum can give a presumptive diagnosis within minutes if the film reveals a host response in the form of abundant polymorphs and the putative pathogen (e.g. gram-positive diplococci characteristic of *S. pneumoniae*) (Fig. 20.9). The presence of organisms in the absence of polymorphs is suggestive of contamination of the specimen rather than infection, but it is important

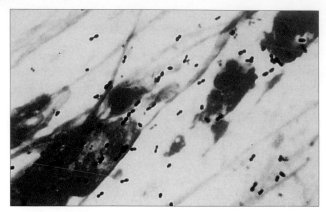

**Fig. 20.9** Gram-stained smears of sputum can help the physician make a rapid diagnosis if, like this, they contain abundant gram-positive diplococci characteristic of pneumococci, as well as polymorphs. However, many of the important causes of pneumonia will not be stained by Gram stain.

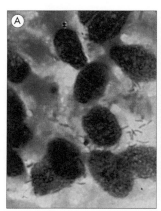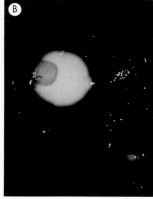

**Fig. 20.10** *Legionella pneumophila*. (A) Gram stain of a bronchial biopsy specimen in a patient with fulminant Legionnaires' disease. (B) Culture plate showing white colonies on buffered charcoal yeast extract medium. (A, Courtesy S. Fisher-Hoch; B, courtesy I. Farrell.)

to remember that immunocompromised patients may not be able to mount a polymorph leukocyte response. Also remember that the causative agents of atypical pneumonia, with the exception of *L. pneumophila* (Fig. 20.10A), will not be seen in Gram-stained smears.

Standard culture techniques will allow the growth of the bacterial pathogens such as *S. pneumoniae*, *S. aureus*, *H. influenzae* and *K. pneumoniae* and other nonfastidious gram-negative rods. Special media or conditions are required for the causative agents of atypical pneumonia, including *L. pneumophila* (see Fig. 20.10B).

Rapid noncultural techniques have been applied successfully to the diagnosis of pneumococcal pneumonia. Detection of pneumococcal antigen by agglutination of antibody-coated latex particles can be used with both sputum and urine specimens, as antigen is excreted in the urine. Use of this technique means the result is available within 1 h of receipt of the specimen, but antibiotic susceptibility tests cannot be performed unless the organisms are isolated.

### Microbiologic diagnosis of atypical pneumonia can be difficult and involves molecular assays

As mentioned, several important causes of pneumonia will not be revealed in Gram-stained sputum smears and cannot be grown on simple routine culture media. Molecular diagnostic tests and urinary antigen detection for *L. pneumophila* are more helpful in confirming a diagnosis of atypical pneumonia. Serologic antibody tests lack sensitivity and specificity, and the classic techniques involving detection of a single high titre of specific antibodies, or preferably demonstration of a rising titre between the acute and convalescent phase of the disease, making a diagnosis retrospectively, are now historical.

### Pneumonia is treated with appropriate antimicrobial therapy

Once the cause of the pneumonia has been identified, appropriate antimicrobial therapy can be given, although there are different guidelines around the world, and the incidence of penicillin and other antibiotic resistance in pneumococci has increased in some countries (Table 20.1).

The choice of treatment is more difficult when sputum is not produced or does not reveal the pathogen. It is, therefore, important to take a full history and use invasive diagnostic techniques if appropriate to help establish the cause.

### Prevention of pneumonia involves measures to minimize exposure and pneumococcal immunization postsplenectomy and for those with sickle cell disease

Respiratory infections are usually transmitted by airborne droplets, so person-to-person spread is virtually impossible to prevent, although less crowding and better ventilation help to reduce the chances of acquiring infection. Infections acquired from sources other than humans may be more amenable to prevention, for example, by avoiding contact with sick animals (Q fever) or birds (psittacosis). Contamination of cooling systems and hot-water supplies by *Legionella* is well recognized, and regulations provide guidance for maintenance engineers.

Immunization is available for a few respiratory pathogens. A pneumococcal vaccine incorporating the polysaccharide capsular antigens of the most common types of *S. pneumoniae* is recommended for those at particular risk (e.g. postsplenectomy or individuals with sickle cell disease who are unable to deal effectively with capsulate organisms).

## VIRAL PNEUMONIA

Many viruses cause pneumonia (Table 20.2) in the face of normal host defences. Healthy individuals are susceptible, and most of these viruses have surface molecules that attach specifically to the respiratory epithelium.

Even when viruses of this group do not themselves cause pneumonia, they may damage respiratory defences, laying the ground for secondary bacterial pneumonia. Sometimes the virus fails to spread significantly to air spaces but remains in interstitial tissues to cause interstitial pneumonitis. An example is cytomegalovirus (CMV) pneumonitis in immunodeficient patients, particularly allogeneic bone marrow transplant recipients.

**Table 20.1** Antibiotic treatment for bacterial pneumonia

| Initial treatment of community-acquired pneumonia | |
|---|---|
| First choice | Amoxicillin[a] or co-amoxiclav + doxycycline |
| Pneumonia secondary to viral respiratory tract infection | Co-amoxiclav |
| Pneumonia in chronic bronchitis | Co-amoxiclav or cefuroxime |
| Pneumonia in an alcoholic, drug user or patient who may have aspirated | Co-amoxiclav + gentamicin |
| **Treatment of choice when pathogen has been identified** | |
| *Streptococcus pneumoniae* | Amoxicillin[a] (erythromycin if allergic to beta-lactams) |
| *Mycoplasma pneumonia* <br> *Legionella pneumonia* <br> *Chlamydophila pneumonia* <br> *Chlamydophila psittaci* <br> *Coxiella burnetii* | Doxycycline |
| *Staphylococcus aureus* | Flucloxacillin |
| *Haemophilus influenzae* | Co-amoxiclav or cefuroxime |
| *Klebsiella pneumoniae* | Gentamicin, chloramphenicol or ciprofloxacin |

Amoxicillin remains the agent of choice for pneumococcal infections as long as the isolates are susceptible. Penicillin-resistant pneumococci now occur in many countries, and in some it is no longer safe to assume susceptibility to amoxicillin. Many of the resistant strains are still susceptible to cephalosporins, and in countries with a high incidence of resistance these agents may replace amoxicillin, at least until the results of antibiotic susceptibility are known. It is important to recognize that amoxicillin and cephalosporins are not active against the other common causes of pneumonia. Therefore a combination is often recommended for initial therapy.
[a]If non–beta-lactamase producer.

**Table 20.2** Viral pneumonia

| Virus | Clinical condition | Comments |
|---|---|---|
| Influenza A or B | Primary viral pneumonia or pneumonia associated with secondary bacterial infection | Pandemics (type A) and epidemics (type A or B); increased susceptibility in elderly or in certain chronic diseases; antivirals and vaccine available |
| SARS-CoV <br> MERS <br> SARS-CoV-2 | Primary viral pneumonia | No treatment available for SARS-CoV and MERS infections SARS-CoV-2 pandemic started in December 2019; antivirals, immunomodulators and vaccines available |
| Parainfluenza (types 1–4) | Croup, pneumonia in children <5 years of age; upper respiratory illness (often subclinical) in older children and adults | No treatment available (no published evidence of ribavirin being effective), supportive care, vaccines not available |
| Measles | Secondary bacterial pneumonia common; primary viral (giant cell) pneumonia in those with immunodeficiency | Adult infection rare but severe; ribavirin may be used as treatment, the king and queen of Hawaii both died of measles when they visited London in 1824; vaccine available |
| Respiratory syncytial virus | Bronchiolitis (infants); common cold syndrome (adults) | Peak mortality in 3 to 4-month-old infants; ribavirin treatment available, palivizumab and nirsevimab prophylaxis if at high risk; first vaccine approved for use in 2023 |
| Adenovirus | Pharyngoconjunctival fever, pharyngitis, atypical pneumonia (military recruits) | Cidofovir or ribavirin could be used in specific clinical settings, vaccine available for military |
| Cytomegalovirus | Interstitial pneumonitis | In immunocompromised patients (e.g. bone marrow transplant recipients); antivirals (e.g. ganciclovir, valganciclovir, foscarnet, cidofovir) and immunoglobulin available |
| Herpes simplex | Interstitial pneumonitis | In immunocompromised patients; antivirals (e.g. aciclovir, valacyclovir, foscarnet) |
| Varicella-zoster virus | Pneumonia in young adults with chickenpox | Uncommon; recognized 1–6 days after rash; lung lesions may eventually calcify; antivirals (e.g. aciclovir, valacyclovir, foscarnet) and vaccine available |

Several different groups of viruses cause infection of the lower respiratory tract, particularly in children. Some, such as influenza and measles, leave the patient particularly susceptible to secondary bacterial infection. Since polymerase chain reaction (PCR) assays have been used to make a diagnosis, more viral coinfections have been detected and more secondary bacterial infections, too.

## HUMAN CORONAVIRUS INFECTIONS

**If a pandemic was to occur in the 21st century, it was thought most likely to involve an avian influenza virus— and many still do—but then a new coronavirus emerged at the end of 2019**

The early warnings of new emerging viruses that could cause severe respiratory infections appeared in 2002 and 2012 with the identification of severe acute respiratory syndrome coronavirus (SARS-CoV) and Middle East respiratory syndrome coronavirus (MERS-CoV), respectively, both highly pathogenic and zoonotic in origin.

In December 2019, clusters of individuals with pneumonia of unknown aetiology were reported in Wuhan, China. After public health investigations of the first patients admitted to hospital found they were linked to a seafood and live animals market in Wuhan, another emerging virus infection was suspected. In 2002 the initial identification of the new coronavirus named SARS-CoV was made by electron microscopic analysis of lung tissue from a patient with pneumonia. In 2019 virus isolation, direct PCR and genome sequencing was carried out on bronchoalveolar lavage fluid samples from patients in Wuhan. These tests led to the identification of a new beta-coronavirus named severe acute respiratory syndrome coronavirus 2 (SARS-CoV-2) that caused coronavirus disease 2019 (COVID-19). By January 30, 2020 WHO declared the novel coronavirus a public health emergency of international concern and by March 11, 2020 COVID-19 was declared a pandemic.

### There is a large animal reservoir for a variety of coronaviruses that includes bats and wild birds that infect intermediate hosts

The *Coronaviridae* family is made up of the subfamily *Orthocoronavirinae* that has four genera and various subgenera. Recombination events can occur between all of these, and bats have been the reservoir identified as having infected intermediate hosts such as camels (MERS-CoV) and palm civets (SARS-CoV). Other human coronaviruses (HCoV) include HCoV-229E, -OC43, -NL63 and -HKU1 and cause mild upper respiratory tract illness, in general. Repeat infections can occur as a protective, short-lived immune response.

There are a number of animal coronaviruses, including infectious bronchitis virus, a severe respiratory disease in young chicks, feline infectious peritonitis coronavirus and transmissible gastroenteritis virus that causes diarrhoea in piglets.

Coronaviruses are enveloped, single-stranded, nonsegmented, positive sense RNA viruses. The envelope is studded with surface spike glycoproteins that give it the electron microscopic appearance of a crown; hence the name corona (Latin for crown) (Fig. 20.11).

The CoV genomic structure, replication cycles, protein functions and host receptor to which they bind are similar. However, the key viral glycoprotein is the spike that contains the receptor binding domain (RBD) and that differs between CoVs. The spike (S) glycoprotein determines the specific host and cell tropism. The three other structural proteins are the envelope (E), membrane (M) and nucleoprotein (N), which have roles in virulence, assembly, transcription and packaging.

### The predecessor of SARS-CoV crossed species barriers over the years when changes in the viral reservoir and eating habits of humans resulted in virus transmission

In China the quality of the food is considered to be best if it is prepared freshly from live animals in wet markets found close to residential areas. In addition, eating a range of exotic wild animals, including bats and civet cats, is popular in South China as it is thought to improve both health and sexual performance. A number of SARS-CoV–like viruses were detected in various wildlife species, including an eclectic mix of Himalayan masked palm civet cats, Chinese ferret badgers, raccoon dogs and horseshoe bats. The animals were

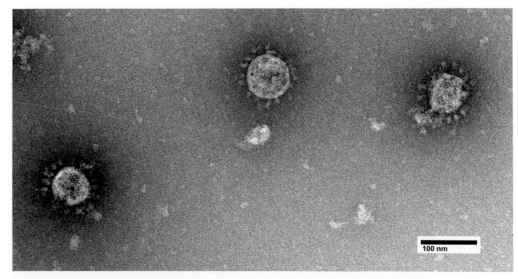

**Fig. 20.11** Severe acute respiratory syndrome coronavirus 2 (SARS-CoV-2) was grown in culture, fixed and inactivated with formaldehyde and negatively stained for transmission electron microscopy with ammonium molybdate. (Courtesy Matthew Hannah, UK Health Security Agency.)

incidental hosts, and bats were found to be the reservoir of not only SARS-CoV but also other coronaviruses (Fig. 20.12).

How SARS-CoV-2 emerged was still a matter of debate in 2023. The two theories were either the virus came from an animal in the wet market in Wuhan or from the Wuhan Institute of Virology where coronavirus research had been carried out.

With molecular clock analyses, one can answer the question about whether these viruses had been around for ages or had just appeared. The analysis, based on sequencing the genome, showed that SARS-CoV crossed the species barrier into masked palm civets and other animals in the markets of China in late 2002. The same was true of MERS-CoV, except it infected dromedary camels around the mid-1980s. As humans and camels are in close contact, MERS-CoV infections are still happening, in contrast to SARS-CoV.

## SARS-CoV, MERS-CoV, SARS-CoV-2 infections

### SARS-CoV

Over the first 12 years of the 21st century, two previously unknown coronaviruses had been identified as causes of severe respiratory infections. An outbreak of severe respiratory disease with no identifiable cause was reported from Guangdong Province in the People's Republic of China in November 2002. The agent spread to mainly parts of East and Southeast Asia as well as Toronto in Canada, and it was eventually reported in 30 countries. WHO issued a global health alert in March 2003 concerning severe acute respiratory syndrome. The main symptoms were high fever (>38°C), cough, shortness of breath and difficulty in breathing. Chest x-ray images were consistent with pneumonia. Close contact with someone infected with SARS-CoV was the highest risk of the infection spreading from person to person and occurred mostly in family members and hospital staff caring for patients with SARS. The incubation period was generally 2–7 days, with a 10-day maximum.

SARS-CoV was a new member of the coronavirus family, identified by virus isolation in cell culture and electron microscopy in conjunction with molecular methods. Diagnostic methods included PCR detection and serology. A global standard for investigating disease outbreaks was set as:

- rapid identification of SARS-CoV
- implementation of infection control on a scale not seen previously involving:
  - face masks
  - checking for fever in the community and at airports
  - rapid isolation on detecting symptom onset
  - international scientific networking and immediate availability of data.

By July 2003, just slightly more than 4 months since the virus began moving between countries via international air travel, WHO reported that all known chains of person-to-person transmission of the SARS virus had been broken. The largest outbreaks had occurred in mainland China and Hong Kong, with reports of 5327 infections and 348 deaths, and 1755 infections

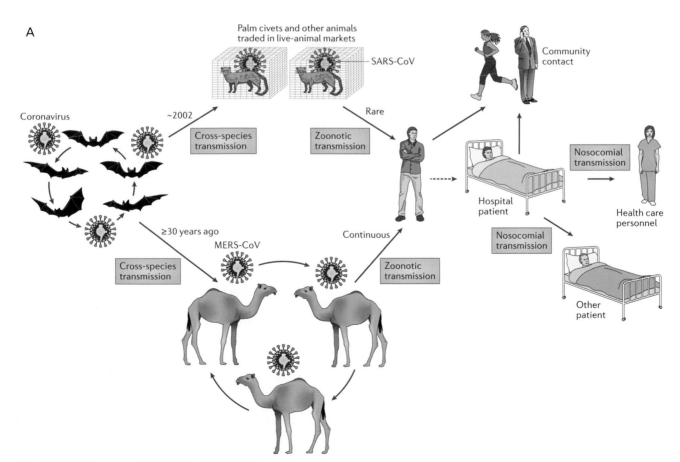

**Fig. 20.12** (A) Emergence of SARS-CoV and MERS-CoV.

B

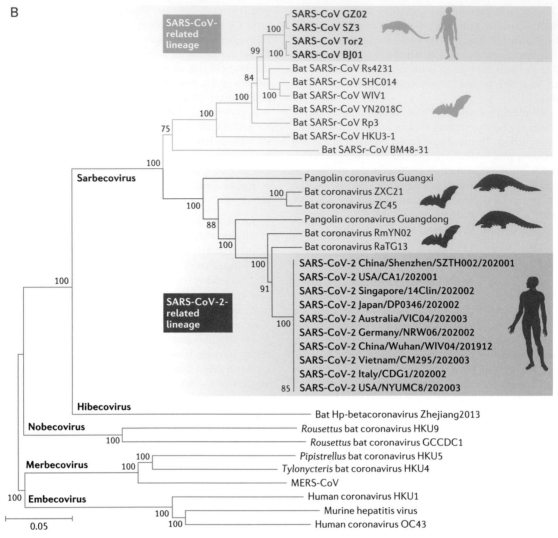

**Fig. 20.12—Cont'd** (B) Phylogenetic tree of the full-length genome sequences of SARS-CoV-2, SARSr-CoVs and other betacoronaviruses. The construction was performed by the neighbour joining method with use of the program MEGA6 with bootstrap values being calculated from 1000 trees. Severe acute respiratory syndrome coronavirus 2 (SARS-CoV-2) clusters with closely related viruses in bats and pangolins and together with SARS-CoV and bat SARS-related coronaviruses (SARSr-CoVs) forms the sarbecoviruses. The sequences were downloaded from the GISAID database and GenBank. *MERS-CoV*, Middle East respiratory syndrome coronavirus. (A, From de Wit F, van Doremalen N, Falzarano D, et al. SARS and MERS: recent insights into emerging coronaviruses. *Nat Rev Microbiol* 2016;14[8]:523-534; B, from Hu B, Guo H, Zhou P, et al. Characteristics of SARS-CoV-2 and COVID-19. *Nat Rev Microbiol.* 2021;19:141–154.)

and 298 deaths, respectively. Overall, there were 8437 SARS diagnoses in 29 countries with a ~10% case fatality rate.

### Pathogenesis and transmissibility of SARS-CoV infection

Angiotensin-converting enzyme 2 (ACE2) is the SARS-CoV receptor on host cells that binds the viral spike protein. Once bound, the receptor is downregulated, resulting in lung injury due to massive production of angiotensin-2, which may stimulate angiotensin-2 receptors that then increase lung blood vessel permeability and lead to respiratory distress.

Immune mechanisms may play a part as it was shown that the SARS-CoV RNA load fell whilst there was a clinical deterioration. Increases in proinflammatory cytokines and chemokines had also been noted in patients with SARS-CoV acute respiratory distress syndrome. However, if those

levels dropped due to an adaptive immune response, then patients were more likely to survive.

With respect to transmissibility, it is interesting to note the large difference in the binding affinity of the palm civet strain and human SARS-CoV strain spike proteins to the human ACE2 receptor despite there being only four amino acid differences between them. Sequencing studies showed that during the outbreaks various genes evolved quite rapidly in the animal reservoirs, which would have improved the transmissibility between animals and humans and between humans as well (Fig. 20.13).

From a management perspective, the relatively poor transmissibility of the virus spreading mainly by respiratory droplets over a short distance was helpful in controlling infections. However, transmission also occurred by direct and indirect contact with respiratory secretions, faeces or

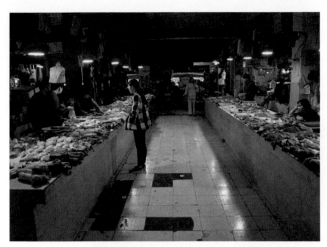

**Fig. 20.13** Chinese wet markets and severe acute respiratory syndrome (SARS). (From Xin-Lei G, Shao M-F, Luo Y, et al. Airborne bacterial contaminations in typical Chinese wet market with live poultry trade. *Sci Total Environ*. 2016;572:681–687.)

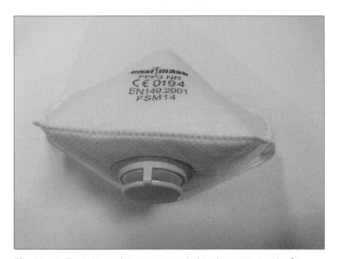

**Fig. 20.14** The N95 mask is recommended in this setting and is fit tested to ensure maximum protection to that individual. (Courtesy A Letters, King's College Hospital, London.)

infected animals. The virus was shown to be stable at room temperature, surviving up to 2 days on surfaces and up to 4 days in faeces. Protection was afforded by face masks, including the N95 masks (Fig. 20.14). SARS-CoV spread more efficiently in hospitals, especially in ICU settings, and clusters of cases occurred in hotel and apartment buildings in Hong Kong. Attack rates as high as ≥50% were seen. Isolation of infected individuals and stringent infection control measures were observed. By 2016 no other people were infected with SARS-CoV.

### PCR is the key diagnostic test, but no specific antiviral therapy has proven efficacy

Laboratory diagnosis involves SARS-CoV RNA detection by PCR in clinical specimens, including respiratory samples and faeces.

No specific antiviral treatment is available. Ribavirin was used to treat some individuals, although little effect was seen in vitro unless ribavirin was used at a high concentration. Corticosteroids damped down the effect of virally induced cytokine responses that could damage lung tissue. Interferons were reported to inhibit the virus in vitro. Protease inhibitors, used to treat human immunodeficiency virus (HIV) infections, were shown to improve the outcome of patients with SARS-CoV infection when combined with ribavirin, but there were no clinical trials to provide an evidence base.

Finally, with regard to potential vaccines and the correlates of protection, neutralizing antibodies were found in convalescent human serum. Passive immunotherapy for SARS demonstrated a reduction in mortality when convalescent plasma containing neutralizing antibodies was used. These antibodies to the viral spike protein prevent virus entry and neutralize virus infectivity in vitro. Whole inactivated virus and recombinant protein vaccines were developed that stimulate neutralizing antibody responses and prevent SARS, although CMI may also assist viral clearance and disease resolution.

### MERS-CoV

In June 2012 another new coronavirus, MERS-CoV, was isolated from a sputum sample collected from a man in Saudi Arabia who died of acute pneumonia and kidney failure. By April there was a report of a cluster of patients with a severe respiratory disease in Jordan, diagnosed as MERS-CoV infections, that spread after travel to other countries. The largest nosocomial outbreak was reported in South Korea after someone with MERS-CoV infection travelled from Saudi Arabia and resulted in 186 patients being infected in 16 hospitals over 1 month. By April 2023, 27 countries had reported 2604 patients with MERS-CoV infections (nearly 2200 of whom were from Saudi Arabia), of whom 936 had died. WHO reported that 50 to 59-year-olds were at the highest risk for acquiring infection. Pneumonia is the most common finding, although gastrointestinal symptoms have also been reported.

### Dromedary camels are the intermediate host

Most infections have been due to person-to-person transmission. It is a zoonosis, and camels are the major reservoir host, but their exact role and route of transmission is still not known. However, direct contact with infected camel upper respiratory secretions is a likely route of transmission to humans.

The incubation period is 2–14 days, with median ~5 days. A survey found a high prevalence of MERS-CoV antibodies in dromedary camels together with MERS-CoV RNA in respiratory swabs collected from camels in a farm in Qatar linked to human infections.

### The MERS-CoV receptor is present in deeper parts of the lungs as well as other organs

MERS-CoV binds to the transmembrane dipeptidyl peptidase 4 (DPP-4 or CD26) receptor. It is mostly found in the epithelial cells of the lower parts of the lungs, including the bronchioles and alveoli, less so in the upper respiratory tract. DPP-4 can also be found in the kidney, intestines and liver, so MERS-CoV has a wider tissue tropism. Pathogenesis is both viral and immunologic as MERS-CoV can evade innate immune responses leading to immune dysregulation with cytokine activation.

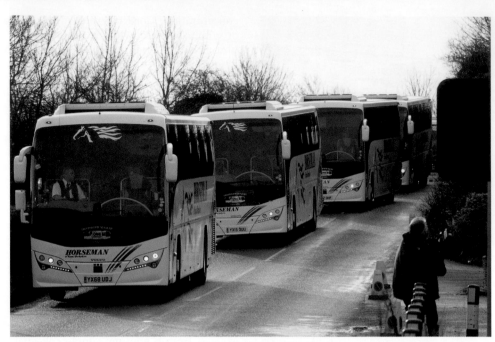

**Fig. 20.15** Coaches ready to transport passengers to quarantine. (Courtesy Tom Maddick/SWNS.)

Laboratory diagnosis involves detecting MERS-CoV RNA by PCR in clinical specimens, including respiratory samples and faeces.

No specific antiviral treatment is available. Ribavirin was shown to have little effect in vitro, and corticosteroid treatment did not affect mortality when used as treatment.

Protease inhibitors are in clinical trial, and convalescent plasma was difficult to prepare as antibody levels were low, so monoclonal antibodies against the spike protein are being developed. Finally, there are no licensed vaccines, but clinical trials are taking place.

### SARS-CoV-2

The COVID-19 outbreak started in China, and the frst wave peaked there in February 2020 at >3000 new infections per day after implementing the strictest public health measures. Initial symptoms included fever, dry cough, shortness of breath, fatigue, nasal congestion, sore throat and diarrhoea. In a report of 45,000 confirmed SARS-CoV-2 infections in China from February 2020, 81% were classed as mild and the rest severe, requiring ventilation in an ICU. Those in the severe group had dyspnea (shortness of breath), tachypnea (increased frequency of breathing), low blood oxygen saturation (<93%) and lung infitrates on chest imaging. A little later when the virus had spread to other countries, loss of taste and smell was another defining symptom. The mortality rate was 8% in the 70–79-year-old group and 49% among those with critical infections (i.e. respiratory failure, multiple organ failure). Those age >70 years and/or with preexisting comorbidities were at particular risk of severe infection.

#### Infection prevention measures included reducing the movement of populations and introducing strict public health measures around the world

Wuhan was locked down on January 23, 2020, and global concern increased with the news agencies reporting that a 4000-bed hospital had been built within 10 days for COVID-19 admissions. Strict public health measures were put in place around China, including reduced travel; shutting shops, restaurants, schools and entertainment venues; stopping outdoor activities and gatherings (including all Lunar New Year celebrations); and advising people to observe hand hygiene measures, wear face masks and stay at home. International flights continued, however, and returning travellers received flyers alerting them to watch for symptoms. The potential for asymptomatic infections had been discussed but had yet to be demonstrated, so possible transmission in that setting was considered theoretical. In the United Kingdom an unintentional image of a potentially apocalyptic future was seen when returning travellers from China were driven to a quarantine complex by four coaches belonging to a company called Horseman (Fig. 20.15).

COVID-19 spread internationally with clusters of infection in Italy, Iran, Korea and Japan. The high transmission efficiency of SARS-CoV-2, together with international travel, enabled rapid global spread. In Europe the news from Italy of hospital ICUs being overwhelmed by patients with COVID-19 spread rapidly, and countries prepared themselves as the pandemic struck. Italy was the first country in Europe to report a COVID-19 outbreak that started in the north on February 21, 2020. By March 3, the CDC reported 60 individuals with COVID-19 in 11 states (21 travel related, 11 person-to-person transmission and the rest unknown). By March 11, WHO declared COVID-19 a pandemic. The world became accustomed to new terms, including personal protective equipment (PPE), different types of face masks, social distancing, contact tracing, PCR COVID-19 tests, combined nose and throat swabs, herd immunity (or lack of), hand hygiene, room ventilation, lockdowns and self-isolation. Virologists did not need to explain virology anymore as everyone became a virologist. The focus was on:

- reducing transmission
- identifying risk factors

**Table 20.3** Factors associated with increased transmission

| Factors | |
| --- | --- |
| Environmental | Poor ventilation indoors<br>Crowding and close contact (i.e. superspreader events: family and religious gatherings, cruise ships, nightclubs, choirs)<br>Cold temperature and low humidity<br>Fomites—viable virus on surfaces |
| Viral | Variants being more transmissible<br>Viral load: acute infection—highest in upper respiratory tract; later—increases in lower respiratory tract<br>Higher in severe COVID-19 |
| Host | Acute infection<br>Immunocompromised and higher viral load for a longer time |
| Behavioural | Hand hygiene<br>Length of contact time and type of contact (shaking hands, hugging)<br>Aerosolization—coughing, sneeezing, singing, loud talking |

- rapid diagnostic test provision
- supportive care and management of severely ill individuals in hospital
- understanding the pathogenesis of COVID-19 to develop treatments
- the race to develop and mass produce vaccines.

Travel bans were announced around the world. By April 10, 2020 nearly 19,000 deaths and >500,000 individuals with COVID-19 had been reported in the United States.

By August 11, 2020, 216 countries and regions from all six continents had reported >20 million individuals with COVID-19 of whom >733,000 had died. By November 22, 2021, ~257 million SARS-CoV-2 infections had been recorded with >5 million deaths globally.

### Understanding transmission to reduce spread of infection and identifying risk factors for severe disease

Airborne transmission is the main route via respiratory droplets, sneezing, coughing and close contact between people. Close contacts were more likely to develop COVID-19 if they had been exposed 2–3 days before the index patient developed symptoms and it was shown that the peak SARS-CoV-2 viral load in the upper respiratory tract was at a median of 3 days. Factors leading to increased transmission are shown in Table 20.3.

People with mild disease were infectious for a median of 5 days, the range being 3–7 days. On July 9, 2020 WHO announced that the virus could not only be transmitted through the air but was also likely to be spread by asymptomatic individuals. SARS-CoV-2 could survive on various surfaces with a half-life of ~5 h, and transmission by fomites (inanimate objects exposed to an infectious agent) could occur. This is why hand hygiene was so important. Nosocomial transmission or hospital-acquired infection was reported at ~16% by May 2020 and was higher in community care hospitals at ~62%, However, transmission was negligible when PPE was worn by health care workers. School and university settings were shown to be lower infection settings, which was an area of much discussion when schools were shut.

The length of viral shedding is another factor as it is longer in symptomatic infection at ~17 days in the upper respiratory tract and in the faeces. It was found to be longer in immunocompromised and shorter in immunized individuals. Virus isolation studies demonstrated it was unusual to find viable virus after ~10 days in those with mild symptoms, ~20 days in those severely ill, and a rough guide in terms of semiquantitative assessment of SARS-CoV-2 load by PCR was that viable virus could be isolated in ~4% of respiratory samples with a cycle threshold (Ct) value of 36—in other words, a low viral load.

Early in 2020 it was quickly recognized that older age, ethnic origin, male sex, having chronic lung disease, diabetes, high blood pressure, being immunosuppressed were all risk factors for severe disease. Host genetic makeup influenced susceptibility and severity, and a gene cluster on chromosome 3 was strongly linked. Polymorphisms in genes, including the ACE2 receptor, could be involved in specific ethnic groups being more at risk.

### A cytokine storm involves a cascade of immune activation events resulting in severe COVID-19

The S glycoprotein of SARS-CoV-2 is key to entering the host cell. It has two subunits, S1 and S2, with S1 housing the RBD that binds to the ACE2 receptor on the host cell. S2 is involved in fusion and the virus genome entering the host cell (Fig. 20.16). The ACE receptor is found in many cell

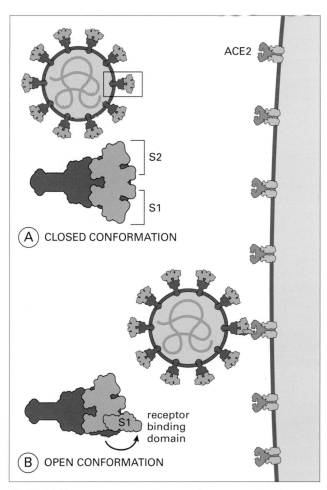

**Fig. 20.16** The severe acute respiratory syndrome coronavirus 2 (SARS-CoV-2) spike protein S1 and S2 subunits (A) closed and (B) open conformation allowing binding with the host cell ACE2 receptor, which allows viral entry.

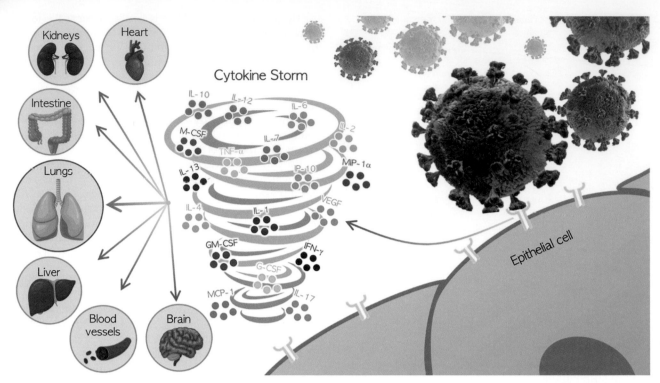

**Fig. 20.17** Cytokine storm leading to organ damage. G-CSF, Granulocyte colony-stimulating factor; GM-CSF, Granulocyte-macrophage colony-stimulating factor; IFN, Interferon; IL, Interleukin; IP, Interferon-gamma induced protein; M-CSF, Macrophage colony-stimulating factor; MCP, Monocyte chemotactic protein; MIP, Macrophage inflammatory proteins; TNF, Tumor necrosis factor; VEGF, Vascular endothelial growth factor. (From Costela-Ruiz V, Illescas-Montes R, Puerta-Puerta J, et al. SARS-CoV-2 infection: the role of cytokines in COVID-19 disease. *Cytokine Growth Factor Rev*. 2020;54:62–75.)

types, explaining the multisystem symptomatology, including oral and nasal mucosa, lungs, heart, gastrointestinal tract, kidneys, liver, spleen and brain.

SARS-CoV-2 infects the upper respiratory tract where the first line of defence involves mucosal epithelial cells secreting mucins and host defence amphipathic peptides called defensins. These trap and eliminate microbes but, when breached, innate immune sensors release immune proteins. Endosomal Toll-like receptors (TLR), including TLR-2, TLR-3 and TLR-7, detect SARS-CoV-2 as does cyclic guanosine monophosphate–AMP synthase stimulator of interferon gene pathways. The cascade involves various transcription factors being activated resulting in proinflammatory chemokines and cytokines focusing on the site of infection. These include tumour necrosis factor alpha, interleukin 1 (IL-1) and IL-6 secreted by monocytes, macrophages, neutrophils and dendritic cells. They stimulate natural killer (NK) cells that are appropriately named as they directly kill virus-infected cells. All of this is augmented by stimulation of type I interferons and, as a result, other interferon-stimulated genes.

The cytokine storm seen in severe COVID-19 is a result of a lowered type 1 interferon response and high cytokine levels. Organ damage to the lungs, heart and kidneys is a result of the hyperinflammatory response secondary to the activation of these immune sytem cells (Fig. 20.17).

### The adaptive immune response, cellular and humoral arms, is then activated by the innate system

Dendritic cells, monocytes and macrophages mature into antigen presenting cells (APCs) as a result of type I interferon responses. APCs display viral antigenic peptides complexed with major histocompatibility complex class II and are involved in activating T cells, including CD4 ($T_H$), CD8 ($T_S$) and regulatory T lymphocytes (Treg).

In patients with severe COVID-19 disease there are low numbers of APCs and NK cells leading to suppression of antigen presentation. In severe COVID-19, T-cell lymphopenia, especially CD4 $T_H$ cells, together with increased inflammation, is most likely due to the interferon type 1 response being suppressed by the virus and an uninhibited cytokine response leading to inflammatory activation of innate effector cells. Furthermore, CD8 $T_S$ cells directly kill virus-infected cells by releasing soluble cytotoxic factors called *perforin* and *granzymes*.

The humoral immune response to SARS-CoV-2 infection is mediated by neutralizing antibodies against the RBD of the S protein. The respiratory tract mucosal lymphoid tissue secretes IgA that stops SARS-CoV-2 binding to mucosal epithelium.

The response of the innate and adaptive immune systems to SARS-CoV-2 infection plays a key part in COVID-19 pathogenesis.

### Microangiopathy and hypercoagulability cause thromboembolic disease

Microthrombi, blood clots or plugs made up of red blood cells, platelets and fibrin can form and may be widespread, affecting blood capillaries, veins and arteries. They block vessels and lead to end-organ damage, including the lungs, heart and kidney.

Clinical presentations varied during the pandemic, with differences between adults and children.

The COVID-19 clinical features in adults in 2020 varied widely, from asymptomatic infection to mild to moderate disease in ~80%, to ~14% with severe pneumonia with respiratory failure of whom around half would require intensive care support. Acute kidney injury and cardiac dysfunction, including arrhythmias, myocardial injury probably due to myocarditis and other factors were also prominent features. Children and adolescents had more mild infections and rarely developed severe disease; however, some presented ~4 weeks after infection with fever, conjunctivitis, rash, cardiac dysfunction and abdominal pain that was called paediatric inflammatory multisystem syndrome. The inflammatory markers were raised, and management was mostly supportive, often in intensive care, with steroid treatment. The prognosis was generally good, resolving after ~6 months.

### Management of individuals with COVID-19 was initially supportive, then rapid developments were reported based on understanding the pathogenesis

Intensive and high-dependency care units became full very quickly around the world, and many hospitals turned operating theatres into makeshift ICUs. Invasive mechanical ventilation was required, and treating people in the prone position (lying on the abdomen) was beneficial in improving breathing and oxygenation. Extracorporeal membrane oxygenation (ECMO) was another option where available. The Randomised Evaluation of COVID-19 Therapy (RECOVERY) clinical trial in the United Kingdom was the world's largest COVID-19 treatment study involving the National Health Service (NHS), gaining unique access to >40,000 individuals across 185 hospital sites. The study was the first to report in June 2020 that the steroid dexamethasone reduced COVID-19 mortality by ~30%. The group also showed in February 2021 the antiinflammatory IL-6 receptor inhibitor tocilizumab reduced mortality and time to discharge from hospital and need for mechanical ventilation. Similarly, the Janus kinase inhibitor baricitinib, another antiinflammatory drug, was shown in March 2022 to reduce mortality. Other treatments that were thought to be helpful were shown not to be, including the antimalarial hydroxychloroquine and the protease inhibitor lopinavir. The Adaptive COVID-19 Treatment Trial (ACTT-1) Study Group, a collaboration involving medical centers in North America, Europe and Asia funded by the United States, sent a preliminary report in May 2020 that the antiviral drug remdesivir, an inhibitor of the viral RNA dependent RNA polymerase and shown to have in vitro activity against SARS-CoV-1, MERS-CoV and SARS-CoV-2, reduced the recovery time in adults admitted to hospital with COVID-19 compared with placebo. That all this was carried out early on in a pandemic at multiple centers globally when the pathogenesis was not fully elucidated was an incredible achievement.

Coinfections and viral reactivations were also seen in ~20% of patients. The most common bacteria detected were *Klebsiella pneumonia*, *S. pneumoniae* and *S. aureus* and the fungus *Aspergillus*. CMV viraemias were seen in severe COVID-19 probably due to the lymphopenia and reduced T-cell surveillance.

Low–molecular-weight heparin as a prophylactic anticoagulant was found to be very effective at preventing thromboembolic events. Investigations key to managing individuals with COVID-19 are set out in Table 20.4.

**Table 20.4** Investigations guiding management of someone with COVID-19 and markers of infection severity

| Investigation | Marker of severity |
|---|---|
| Real-time polymerase chain reaction for SARS-CoV-2 RNA Combined nose and throat swab | |
| Pulse oximetry | Hypoxia |
| Full blood count | Lymphopenia and thrombocytopenia Neutrophil to lymphocyte ratio: high |
| Arterial blood gas | High $pCO_2$ Low $pO_2$ |
| Liver function tests | Hepatitis |
| Renal function tests Urea and electrolytes | Acute kidney injury |
| Cardiac function tests: | |
| Creatine kinase | High |
| B-type natriuretic peptide (BNP) | High |
| N-terminal proBNP | High |
| Troponin | High |
| Coagulation screen: | |
| D-dimers | High: thrombosis risk |
| Fibrinogen | High |
| Prothrombin time | Prolonged |
| International normalised ratio (INR) | Prolonged |
| Serum C-reactive protein | High |
| Serum lactate dehydrogenase | High |
| Serum interleukin-6 (also IL-1, 2, 4, 8, 10, 18) | High |
| Serum procalcitonin | High |
| Serum ferritin | High |
| Imaging: | |
| Chest x-ray | Ground glass shadowing Consolidation |
| Chest computed tomography scan | Ground glass shadowing Consolidation |

### The therapeutic armamentarium increased over a short time to include other antiviral drugs and neutralizing monoclonal antibody treatments

See more details in Ch. 34. By the end of 2021 a number of antiviral drugs were available, with remdesivir reducing the risk of hospitalization or death by 87% compared with placebo in high-risk adults. Molnupiravir given within 5 days of symptom onset reduced the same parameters by 33% in the 29 days after being given, but nirmatrelvir-ritonavir (Paxlovid) given within 5 days of symptom onset was found to reduce the risk of hospitalization or death by 88% in high-risk adults.

Single and combination monoclonal antibodies (mAbs) had been developed that:

- targeted, bound and neutralized the RBD and other domains of the S protein

- prevented binding to the host cell ACE2 receptor
- lead to antibody-dependent cellular phagocytosis, antibody-dependent cell-mediated cytotoxicity or complement activation.

These mAbs could be offered to individuals at high risk of severe disease due to immunodeficiency and/or immunocompromise either exposed to or infected by SARS-CoV-2. They included casirivimab-imdevimab (Ronapreve) that reduced risk of hospital admission or death and improved 28-day mortality in those admitted to hospital. Bamlanivimab-etesevimab reduced hospital admission or death if given within 3 days of symptom onset. By 2022 sotrovimab and tixagevimab-cilgavimab (Evusheld) had been shown to be effective, but the choice of mAb depended on the circulating SARS-CoV-2 variant as some reduced mAb efficacy. For example, the Omicron lineages BA.4 and BA.5 had specific RBD amino acid substitutions leading to mutations resulting in *in vitro* resistance to the mAb treatments.

There was an unprecedented use of the word *unprecedented*. However, clinical trials demonstrating the efficacy of a number of treatments in such a short a timescale was unprecedented as were the global collaborations resulting in the rapid production and clinical trials of COVID-19 vaccines.

### Outbreaks of guidelines and treatment algorithms

As the pandemic continued there were daily surveillance reports and news bulletins, guidelines about reducing transmission, social distancing, wearing PPE, clinical care pathways in hospitals (e.g. PCR tests, infection prevention, control guidance), treatment algorithms and regular updates on all aspects of management of individuals in contact with those with COVID-19. Once lockdowns were eased, guidance about travel and needing to have a SARS-CoV-2 RNA PCR test negative result before travel, on return and then when vaccines were available, having a vaccine certificate, made travel arrangements complicated.

By 2023 a lot of guidance in terms of screening and treatment had been simplified.

### SARS-CoV-2 variants identified by surveillance and nucleotide sequencing analysis

Viral variation has been recognized in many RNA viruses due to nucleotide substitutions that occur naturally during viral replication. Error-prone replication, lack of proofreading and recombination events can all lead to variation, some of which may be an advantage to the virus and others a disadvantage. *Viral fitness* is the term used to describe the extent to which the virus has adapted. Selection pressure can be driven by use of antiviral drugs, immunization responses and antibody-driven escape after receiving convalescent plasma or monoclonal antibody treatments.

SARS-CoV-2 variants were classified by the WHO into two types: variants of concern (VOC) and variants of interest (VOI) (Table 20.5).

A VOC is defined by one or more characteristics, including being more transmissible or more virulent, causing reinfection by escaping natural and vaccine-induced immunity, and by being may be less easy to detect by PCR and other tests.

Since the original wild-type virus appeared in December 2019, changes in the S protein were seen. An example was the aspartate glycine substitution at codon 614 (D614G substitution) that was rare before March 2020 but was seen in >74% of viruses sequenced by June 2020, the earliest VOC that swept the world. It was more infectious but could be neutralized by antibody in convalescent serum. Transmissibility could be increased by changes in the S protein, resulting in higher binding affinity for the ACE2 receptor (Fig. 20.18).

The incubation period changed between the wild-type virus (median 5–7 days, range 1–14 days) and the succeeding virus waves. The Alpha, Beta, Delta and Omicron variants median incubation periods were 5, 4.5, 4.4 and 3.4 days, respectively. The $R_O$ value (see Ch. 33) in 2020 was ~2.7 for the wild type, ~5 for Delta and ~8 for Omicron; however, these $R_O$ values varied between countries and at different times but demonstrated increased transmissibility.

**Table 20.5** SARS-CoV-2 variants of concern (VOC) and receptor binding domain (RBD) amino acid substitutions

| RBD amino acid substitutions | | | N501Y | E484K/Q/A | K417T/N | L452R |
|---|---|---|---|---|---|---|
| VOC | | First seen | | | | |
| Alpha | B.1.1.7 | Sep 2020, predominant strain in United Kingdom | + | − | − | − |
| Beta | B.1.1.351 | Oct 2020, predominant strain in South Africa | + | + | + | − |
| Gamma | P.1 | Jan 2021, predominant strain in Brazil | + | + | + | − |
| Delta | B.1.617.2 | Dec 2020, predominant strain in India | − | − | − | + |
| Omicron | B.1.1.529 | Nov 2021, predominant strain in South Africa then the world | + | + | + | − |

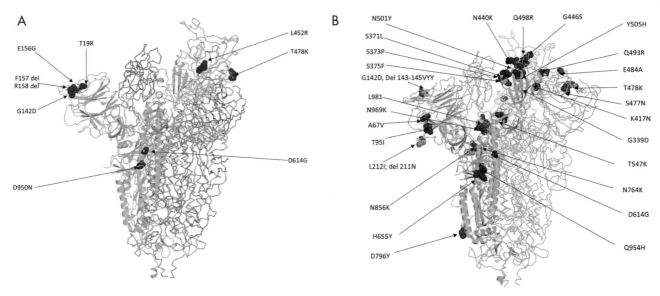

**Fig. 20.18** (A) Ribbon representation of Spike protein substitution in Delta variant (PDB ID 7W92), red spheres indicate amino acid substitution. (B) Ribbon representation of Spike protein substitution in Omicron variant (PB ID 7TGW), red spheres indicate amino acid substitution. (From Shrestha L, Foster C, Rawlinson W, et al. Evolution of the SARS-CoV-2 omicron variants BA.1 to BA.5: implications for immune escape and transmission. *Rev Med Virol.* 2022;32:e2381.)

By 2023 the Omicron variant and subvariants dominated globally and exhibited a high number of mutations. This distinguished it from its predecessors, and it was more transmissible. However, Omicron infections were less severe, with lower mortality and less likely to affect the lower respiratory tract cells. Recombinant variants (i.e. between Omicron and Delta) had been reported but had not been found to cause more severe infection, and others were only seen over a short period.

### Diagnostic tests included standard and rapid PCR tests, antigen-based tests and antibody detection

What do you do when there are no commercially available diagnostic tests for a novel pathogen? Diagnostic laboratories around the world initially received instructions, reagents and controls from reference laboratories in their countries that had started testing samples for SARS-CoV-2 RNA to standardize and validate the test on their sites. Real-time (RT) PCR tests were run using combined nose and throat swabs, initially with targets such as RNA-dependent RNA polymerase that has no host homologue, as well as other targets such as the S, N and E genes. Dual targets were used in most assays in case there were gene variations that could lead to false-negative results. Other samples tested included saliva, lower respiratory tract bronchoalveolar lavage, whole blood, cerebrospinal fluid and faeces. However, combined nose and throat swabs were universally tested.

As more rapid diagnostic tests were needed, point-of-care PCR-based tests were developed together with rapid antigen–based tests that could also be carried out at home, called lateral flow tests (LFTs). The method involves placing a combined nose and throat swab in a plastic tube with liquid and squeezing it to get an extract of the swab material that is then pipetted onto a strip. It migrates from the initial pipetting site, which contains antibodies specific to the target analyte that are conjugated to coloured particles, and travels by capillary action along the nitrocellulose strip into the detection area. This has specific antibodies immobilized in a line that react with the analyte bound to the conjugated antibody. A line appears (a positive result) as does a control line, demonstrating the liquid flow through the strip.

LFTs are easy to carry out and results can be read within 15–30 minutes, but they are not as sensitive in making a diagnosis of COVID-19 as PCR tests. For example, the Ct value of a PCR is a semiquantitative measure of the viral load. The Ct is the point at which the target is detected and the threshold line broken by the exponential phase of the sigmoid curve. If the target is detected after 10 PCR cycles, the Ct is 10—a high viral load. Detection at cycle 13 means there is one $\log_{10}$ less target in the sample. Depending on the assay sensitivity, which can vary, generally a Ct of ~37 is the limit of detection. The limit of detection of a line on an LFT would equate to a PCR Ct ~28; however, LFTs gave rapid results, were easier to carry out, could be done at home and were less expensive.

A plethora of different tests, many not fully optimised nor validated as they were being rushed into potential service, were made available; careful thought had to be given about the type of test and its use in which setting (e.g. emergency departments, care homes, at home where different factors were involved in ease of use, technical experience, how quickly results were available, level of accuracy, test costs).

### Interpretation of the test results were sometimes difficult

Having explained the term Ct value, one can see the problem when nucleic acid is detected by the presence of a sigmoid curve seen at the limit of detection of the assay. That is determined by testing a dilution series of a known amount of nucleic acid in triplicate until not all three tests at the highest dilution are positive. This may be a Ct of 37 or 38. That sample may have been collected early in infection, late in infection or the swab had been wafted around the nose and throat and so neither was adequately sampled. The only way of assessing this is by collecting a second sample. In the hospital setting this caused some difficulty to ensure best infection control and prevention practices were observed and to reduce nosocomial transmission. Furthermore, at the limit of assay detection it is much less likely the virus is viable and infectious to others if at the end of an infection.

RT-PCR sensitivity and specificity for combined nose and throat swabs was reported as 88% and 88–100%, respectively. Finally, if LFTs were used, the level of sensitivity of detection was lowered by at least 20%. However, if someone was symptomatic with a high SARS-CoV-2 RNA load, the LFT reliability was high. In general, at a Ct <25 and >25, the LFT sensitivity of detection was 95% and 41%, respectively. Some considered this as a laterally flawed test.

### N and S antibody detection differentiated between a natural infection and a postimmunization response

The first serology tests developed in China involved RBD as the target and included IgM and IgG tests. RBD IgG could be detected after a natural infection or immunization. Nucleoprotein (N) antibody assays were helpful once the vaccine had been developed as the vaccine was based on Spike protein. If you needed to know if someone had been infected in the past, N antibody as well as RBD/S antibody would be detected. If uninfected in the past but immunized, only RBD/S antibody would be found, not N antibody.

Early on, before the waves of VOC appeared, S antibody levels were helpful in guiding the use of mAbs. However, as a reduction in neutralization was seen in vitro, this test was not so helpful.

### Diagnostic testing in a pandemic: lighthouses, flotillas and commercial opportunities

As PCR tests and LFT became available, the opportunity to build mass diagnostic test centres and drive-through screening centres as well as tests that could be carried out by post in the high street and at home became very broad.

In the United Kingdom, lighthouse laboratories were set up as mass SARS-CoV-2 RNA PCR test facilities. These were not named to warn travellers about dangerous hazards ahead but because the PCR test used light fluorescence to detect the virus. Initially they could carry out 2000 tests/day, but eventually the capacity was 750,000 tests/day. There were questions about quality control and regulation especially over analysis of results and the test process even though it only involved one test to detect SARS-CoV-2 RNA. Two high-profile incidents in the United Kingdom included 45,000 people with positive LFTs being mistakenly given negative PCR results, and the UK Department of Health settling out of court for £2 million having chosen a PCR software analysis system that initially missed some PCR-positive results as well as giving a result for samples that were reported as invalid during a test evaluation.

Another option would have been to upgrade the flotilla of NHS and private laboratories to carry out more testing as they were already linked into the public health system. An array of test options could be found online and in the high street, commercial opportunities to help with travelling and providing a test certificate.

### Complications include postacute COVID-19 (long COVID)

It was reported that a number of people developed chronic sequelae having had mild or moderate COVID-19, as well as those with severe infection. These sequelae were similar to those chronic illnesses triggered by other infections, many of which have yet to be proven, but one feels it is only a matter of time. These postacute infection syndromes are well recognized, most often occur in females and include chronic fatigue, muscle and joint pain, neurocognitive and sensory impairment, flulike symptoms and exercise intolerance. Examples of infections associated with these syndromes include Epstein-Barr virus (EBV), influenza, dengue, enterovirus, Q fever (*Coxiella burnetii*) and Lyme disease (*Borrelia burgdorferi*). The pathogenesis is mostly unclear and hypotheses include:

- Persistent infection that may be undetected, possibly in sanctuary sites, that cause pathogen-associated molecular patterns involving viral RNA that engage host pattern recognition receptors leading to innate and cellular immune activation. If the T and B cells cannot clear the infection, chronic activation can result in inflammation in the sanctuary site (i.e. chronic eye pain after Ebola virus infection)
- Autoimmune activation due to the immune system targeting the pathogen antigen that is seen as self-antigen (molecular mimicry see Ch. 17) or is set off as part of a bystander action
- Immune dysregulation that can involve herpesvirus reactivation especially EBV
- Dysregulation of the microbiome/virome/mycobiome induced by the infection or as a result of the immune response. Translocation from the gastrointestinal tract to other tissues and organs can link in to autoimmune activation
- Defects in tissue repair after immunopathologic effects such as microthrombi and cytokine storms.

A number of organizations defined long COVID, and an amalgamation of these definitions included signs and symptoms that develop after probable or confirmed SARS-CoV-2 infection. These usually occurred 3 months from the onset of symptoms and lasted for at least 2 months, and they could not be explained by an alternative diagnosis.

By 2023 it was recognised that the number of people with long COVID was ~10% (estimated 65 million people), the majority of whom would have been admitted to hospital, with ~10–30% in the community and 10% in the postimmunization group. Risk factors included being older or younger, female sex, minority ethnic group, smoking, symptom severity, comorbidities (e.g. obesity, type 2 diabetes) and hospital admission. Various studies reported half of the clinic attendees still had one of more symptoms at 2–5 months and half had one or more symptoms at ≥6 months post–COVID-19. Fatigue and muscle weakness were prominent symptoms. The risk of developing long COVID may be variant dependent, lower with the Omicron than Delta variant. The chronic sequelae are multisystemic (Fig. 20.19) and mainly associated with immune responses and inflammation:

- Circulatory system: endothelial dysfunction, venous thrombosis, pulmonary emboli, microclots
- Cardiovascular disease: cardiac failure, arrhythmias, stroke (cardiac impairment in nearly 60% in one large study of long COVID)
- Respiratory: lung damage due to pneumonia, acute respiratory distress syndrome causing dyspnoea and persistent cough, reduced lung function

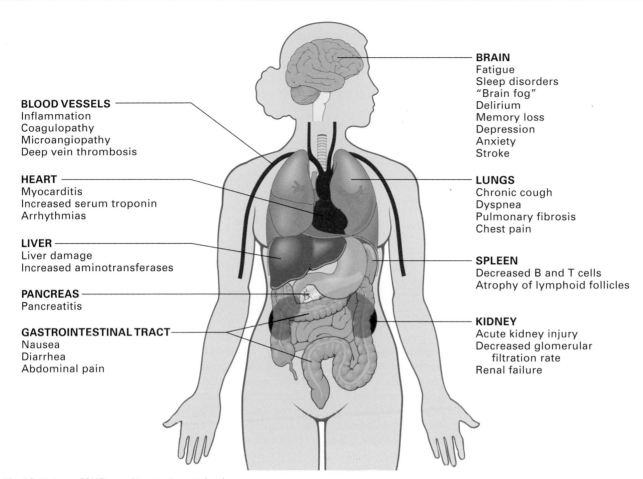

**BRAIN**
Fatigue
Sleep disorders
"Brain fog"
Delirium
Memory loss
Depression
Anxiety
Stroke

**BLOOD VESSELS**
Inflammation
Coagulopathy
Microangiopathy
Deep vein thrombosis

**HEART**
Myocarditis
Increased serum troponin
Arrhythmias

**LIVER**
Liver damage
Increased aminotransferases

**PANCREAS**
Pancreatitis

**GASTROINTESTINAL TRACT**
Nausea
Diarrhea
Abdominal pain

**LUNGS**
Chronic cough
Dyspnea
Pulmonary fibrosis
Chest pain

**SPLEEN**
Decreased B and T cells
Atrophy of lymphoid follicles

**KIDNEY**
Acute kidney injury
Decreased glomerular
  filtration rate
Renal failure

**Fig. 20.19** Long COVID—multisystemic complications.

- Neurologic and sensorimotor system: exercise intolerance, chronic fatigue, neurocognitive and sensory impairment, including memory loss, loss of smell and/or taste, headaches, myalgia, arthralgia, autonomic dysfunction
- Gastrointestinal system: nausea, abdominal pain, appetite loss, constipation possibly due to changes in the gastrointestinal tract microbiome
- Mental health: post-ICU syndrome, post-traumatic stress

### Long COVID management and diagnosis needs a multidisciplinary approach

Specific outpatient clinics have been developed to diagnose, investigate and treat individuals with long COVID. Diagnosis involves collating a full clinical history and assessing physical and cognitive/psychological symptoms. An integrated multidisciplinary approach is required. The most common symptoms reported 12 months post–COVID-19 were fatigue, sweating, chest tightness, anxiety and myalgia.

Laboratory blood test investigations will cover all organ systems, but immunologic tests include markers of inflammation and cytokines. Chest imaging and lung function tests are key as nearly half of all patients will have pulmonary fibrosis; 33% still had residual CT abnormalities after 1 year.

Management again involves a multidisciplinary rehabilitation plan that covers physical and psychological aspects of rehabilitation with input from specialists in the relevant fields. Treatment for specific components of long COVID is available, but there is no overarching treatment in 2023. Examples are anticoagulant use, intravenous immunoglobulin for immune dysfunction and apheresis, which has shown promise by removing microclots and reducing autoantibodies, but physical exercise is harmful. An active global research programme is key to developing new treatments (see Ch. 35).

Early in the pandemic, the term herd immunity was discussed as lockdowns loomed. The idea was that as more of the population became exposed to COVID-19 and were infected, the less likely the virus would continue circulating as people would be protected and incident infections would fall. The concept collapsed once the morbidity and mortality in the infected population was seen. However, the urgency and global drive to produce effective vaccines was the holy grail of long-term protection and herd immunity postimmunization. Several vaccines were produced in various countries using different methods (Table 20.6). The novel approach involved nucleoside-modified mRNA vaccines, BNT162b2 (Pfizer/Biontech) and mRNA-1273 (Moderna). The first vaccine given was BNT162b2 in December 2020. Vector-based vaccines included a replication-deficient chimpanzee adenoviral vector, ChAdOx1 nCoV-19 (AstraZeneca/Oxford University); Gam-COVID-Vac vaccine (Sputnik V) and Ad26.COV2.S (Johnson & Johnson). The protein subunit vaccine developed was NVX-CoV2373 (Novavax), and the inactivated virus vaccine was CoronaVac (Sinovac Life Sciences). By 2021 WHO had reported 44 potential vaccines in clinical and 151 in preclinical development, respectively.

The ease of administration, availability and efficacy varied between vaccines and countries, and as more doses were

**Table 20.6** COVID-19 vaccine manufacturers and types

| Type of vaccine | Vaccine and manufacturer |
|---|---|
| Nucleoside-modified mRNA lipid nanoparticle mRNA encoding the full-length S protein. | Pfizer/Biontech BNT162b2 |
| Nucleoside-modified mRNA lipid nanoparticle mRNA encoding the full-length S protein. | Moderna mRNA-1273 |
| Adenovirus recombinant vector a replication-deficient chimpanzee adenoviral vector vaccine containing the SARS-CoV-2 structural surface glycoprotein antigen gene | Oxford-AstraZeneca AZD1222(ChAdOx1nCoV19) |
| Adenovirus recombinant vector (Ad26) a recombinant and replication-incompetent adenovirus serotype 26 vector encoding a full-length, stabilized S protein | Johnson and Johnson Ad26.COV2.S |
| Inactivated SARS-CoV-2 (vero cells) | Sinovac, Sinopharm COVID-19 Vaccine (Vero Cell), Inactivated/CoronaVac |
| Adenovirus vector (recombinant Ad5 and Ad26) a heterologous recombinant adenovirus-based vaccine carrying the gene for SARS-CoV-2 full-length glycoprotein S | Gam-COVID-Vac Sputnik V |
| Recombinant spike glycoprotein nanoparticle vaccine composed of trimeric full-length SARS-CoV-2 spike glycoproteins and matrix-M1 adjuvant | Novavax NVX-CoV2373/Covovax |

administered rare complications were reported leading to scares around the world and vaccine uptake hesitancy. By May 2023, 13 billion doses of vaccine had been given globally, 70% of the world's population had received at least one dose and in the United States 69%, China 90% and India 67% of the population had completed the initial course. Pfizer, Moderna and Oxford/Astrazeneca vaccines were the most administered with 666 million, 152 million and 67 million doses, respectively.

Efficacy data varied between vaccines with ~95% for the mRNA and 76–91% for the vector-based vaccines.

As VOC became evident, studies reported mixing the vaccines and boosters could result in better immune responses and efficacy. This was called the mix and match approach using heterologous vaccines.

**When developing vaccines the key question is which end point defines efficacy?**

This pivots around the pathogen, associated morbidity/mortality and transmissibility. Often randomized controlled vaccine trial data are presented as the amount of disease reduction between immunized participants and unimmunized controls. The aims for vaccine effectiveness include:

- reducing infection due to vaccine response and protection
- reducing disease severity
- reducing duration of infectivity
- preventing or attenuating infection and disease
- minimizing the effect of high levels of admission to hospital and intensive care
- relieving stress on health care systems
- leading to protection and interrupting transmission of the infection.

Furthermore, the duration of protection is important given what is known about seasonal coronavirus infections and waning antibody levels.

**Complications postimmunization, eventually found to be rare, were detected as more people were immunized**

At the same time as social media–based unfounded scares concerning a misunderstanding about potential female infertility circulated leading to vaccine hesitancy, in March 2021 AstraZeneca vaccine was associated with a thrombo-embolic complication known as vaccine-induced immune thrombotic thrombocytopenia (VITT). By 2023 the incidence was estimated as 10–20 VITT events/million doses depending on the age of the vaccinee.

Myocarditis or pericarditis was reported postimmunization with mRNA vaccines and more rarely with adenovirus vector vaccines and protein subunit vaccines. Myocarditis occurred mostly in males between 12 and 29 years old, more likely after the second dose (less if given >31 days after the first dose) and was rare. The pooled incidence rate for myocarditis was 1.4/million doses. Generally, symptoms including chest pain, tachycardia, palpitations, tachypnoea, dyspnoea and dizziness developed 2–4 days, sometimes within 10 days, postimmunization. Most were admitted to hospital, 25% of whom went to intensive care, but the majority had recovered by 3 months.

## PARAINFLUENZA VIRUS INFECTION

As with RSV, parainfluenza viruses are most likely to cause lower respiratory tract disease, croup and pneumonia in children.

The surface spikes of parainfluenza viruses are composed of haemagglutinin plus neuraminidase on one type of spike and fusion proteins on another. The four types of virus have different antigens. After infection by respiratory droplets, these viruses spread locally on respiratory epithelium.

Parainfluenza viruses 1–3 cause pharyngitis, croup, otitis media, bronchiolitis and pneumonia. Croup is seen in children <5 years old and consists of acute laryngotracheobronchitis with a harsh cough and hoarseness. Parainfluenza virus 4 is less common and generally causes a common cold–type illness.

RT-PCR methods detecting parainfluenza RNA in throat swabs have revolutionized the diagnosis of these and other respiratory virus infections owing to the increased sensitivity and rapid diagnosis using these tests. Treatment involves supportive care as no antiviral drugs have been shown to be effective, and there is no vaccine.

## ADENOVIRUS INFECTION

### Adenoviruses cause ~5% of acute respiratory tract illness overall

There are >110 antigenic types of adenovirus, divided into seven species (A–G), some of which cause upper respiratory tract infections such as pharyngoconjunctival fever and sore throat (see Ch. 19) and lower respiratory tract infections. Adenovirus infections are ubiquitous and may be severe in immunocompromised individuals and children. Diagnosis involves detecting adenovirus DNA by PCR on combined nose and throat swabs. In immunocompromised individuals, especially transplant recipients, an adenoviraemia that can lead to viral dissemination may be seen. Reducing immunosuppression if possible, together with giving the antiviral drug cidofovir, are mainstays of treatment. Adenovirus specific T-cell therapy is another option if available.

Adenovirus types B3, B7 and E4 have caused outbreaks of respiratory illness ranging from pharyngitis to atypical pneumonia in military recruits, with crowding and stress as possible cofactors.

Recovery is generally uneventful, but adenoviruses may persist in the body as latent infections and in the 1950s were detected in tissue extracts from surgically removed tonsils and adenoids. An enteric-coated vaccine for types E4 and B7 has been used to prevent outbreaks of infection in military recruits. In 2011 the FDA approved a new version of this vaccine that is offered to all military trainees in the United States.

## HUMAN METAPNEUMOVIRUS INFECTION

Discovered in Holland in 2001, hMPV is a negative-strand RNA virus closely related to RSV; infection peaks in the winter and spring. It is associated with a spectrum of illness from mild infection to bronchiolitis and pneumonia in young children and elderly adults. Symptoms may include a fever, runny nose, cough, sore throat and wheeze. Infection occurs mostly in infants and young children, with ~1/1000 <5 years of age being admitted to hospital, with most being <2 years old. In addition, reinfections are common as hMPV has also been detected in older children and adults. Archived sera have been tested and demonstrated that humans have been exposed to hMPV for many decades. Detection is by PCR and treatment is supportive.

## HUMAN BOCAVIRUS INFECTION

Human bocavirus (hBoV), discovered in 2005, is a member of the *Parvoviridae* family. Of the four hBoV species, hBoV1 has been detected in respiratory samples from patients with upper and lower respiratory tract infections and hBoV2–4 in faecal specimens from patients with gastroenteritis. The clinical importance of hBoV has been difficult to determine especially as it can be detected in both ill and healthy control subjects. However, when quantifying the hBoV load in the upper respiratory tract, it has been shown to be significantly higher in those patients with hBoV alone compared with those coinfected. However, the hBoV pathogenic role is still unresolved.

## INFLUENZA VIRUS INFECTION

### Influenza viruses cause endemic, epidemic, pandemic influenza

The structure of a typical orthomyxovirus single-stranded RNA is shown in Fig. 20.20, and the budding process in Fig. 20.21.

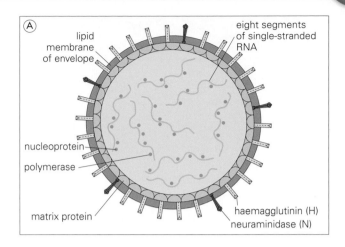

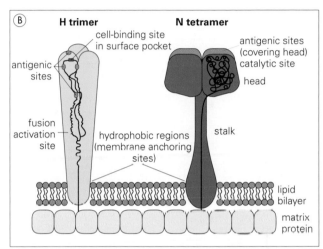

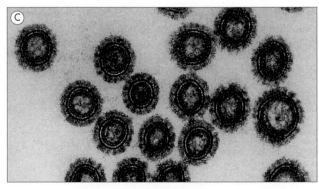

**Fig. 20.20** The influenza A virus particle (A), with detail enlarged (B) to show surface haemagglutinin (*H*) and neuraminidase (*N*). Each particle has ~500 H spikes, which bind to the host cell and fuse the viral envelope to the cell's plasma membrane to initiate infection, and ~100 N spikes, which release the virus from the cell surface. Nucleoprotein and polymerase proteins are closely associated with RNA segments to form ribonucleoprotein. The N tetramer is propeller shaped as viewed from the end. Detail of only one unit of H trimer and N tetramer is shown. The three-dimensional structure is known from x-ray crystallographic analysis. Electron micrograph (C) shows sectioned influenza virus particles (× 300,000). (C, Courtesy D. Hockley.)

### There are four types of influenza virus: A, B, C, D

Antigenic differences between the nucleocapsid and matrix proteins distinguishes influenza A, B, C and D viruses:

- Influenza A viruses cause epidemics and occasionally pandemics, and there is an animal reservoir, notably in birds.

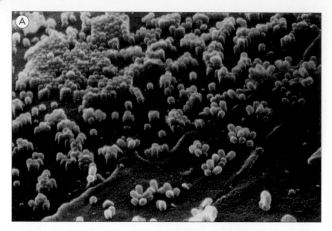

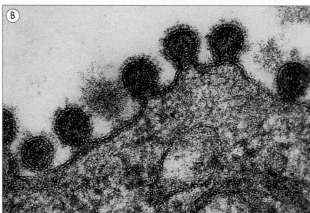

**Fig. 20.21** Influenza virus budding from the surface of an infected cell. (A) Scanning electron micrograph (× 27,000). (B) In section (× 350,000). (Courtesy D. Hockley.)

- Influenza B viruses can cause epidemics and do not involve animal hosts.
- Influenza C viruses do not cause epidemics and give rise to only minor respiratory illness.
- Influenza D viruses mostly affect cattle.

### The influenza virus envelope has haemagglutinin and neuraminidase spikes

These are shown in Fig. 20.20. In the case of influenza A, the haemagglutinin (H) and neuraminidase (N) are type-specific antigens and are used to characterize different strains of influenza A virus (Table 20.7). In 2023 the circulating influenza A viruses in humans were H3N2 and H1N1. In giving the full nomenclature, the influenza antigenic type, the host origin if not human, geographic origin, strain number and year of isolation are included (e.g. A / Philippines / 82 / H3N2).

The single-stranded RNA genome is segmented, and these eight segments can be reassorted during virus replication to give a progeny virus with a novel combination of H and N antigens when virus particles of more than one strain infect a cell simultaneously. Two different influenza A viruses can simultaneously infect one cell and reassort resulting in a new influenza virus strain.

### Influenza viruses undergo genetic change as they spread through the host species

These changes are of two types:

1. Antigenic drift (Fig. 35.10). Small mutations affecting the H and N antigens occur constantly. When changes in these antigens enable the virus to multiply significantly in individuals with immunity to preceding strains, the new subtype can reinfect the community. Antigenic drift is seen with all types of influenza.
2. Antigenic shift (Fig. 17.10). Less common, and only with influenza A, there is a sudden major change referred to as shift, in the antigenicity of the H or N antigens. This is based on recombination between different virus strains when they infect the same cell. The major change in H or N means that the new strain can spread through populations immune to preexisting strains, setting the stage for a new pandemic (see Table 20.7). Associated with the change in H and N are other genetic changes, which may or may not confer increased pathogenicity or change the ability to spread rapidly from person to person.

However, the H1N1 virus pandemic in 2009 demonstrated that antigen shift alone may not be required for a global outbreak. Epidemiologic data revealed that a younger age group (<35 years old) was more susceptible to infection than an older one (65 years). Therefore preexisting immunity and host factor adaptations can affect the pathologic potential of influenza A virus infections.

**Table 20.7** Pandemic human influenza viruses

| Type | Subtype[a] | Year | Clinical severity | Prototype virus |
|------|---------|------|-------------------|-----------------|
| A | H3N2 (?) | 1889 | Moderate | Designation based on serological studies |
| | H1N1 (avian)[b] | 1918 | Severe | H1N1 virus sequenced retrospectively |
| | H2N2 (Asian) | 1957 | Severe | A/Japan/57/H2N2 |
| | H3N2 (Hong Kong)[c] | 1968 | Moderate | A/Hong Kong/68/H3N2 |
| | H1N1 | 1977 | Mild | A/USSR/77 |
| | H1N1pdm09 | 2009 | Mild | H1N1 virus sequenced |

Novel strains of virus arising in one continent spread rapidly to other continents, causing outbreaks during appropriate times of the year (winter months in temperate climates). There is a World Health Organization global surveillance system for influenza.

[a]Antigenic shift in influenza A virus is shown by the appearance of a novel combination of H and N antigens.

[b]Reports suggest that this virus was derived from an avian source. In a remarkable experiment, viral RNA was extracted from the lung tissue of someone who died in the 1918 pandemic and was buried in the permafrost and from formalin-fixed lung tissue. This allowed the 1918 viral genome to be reconstructed.

[c]Amino acid and base sequence analysis suggest that recombination between H3N8 (from ducks) and H2N2 gave rise to H3N2.

Influenza is a highly infectious, acute viral infection that has affected both humans and animals over the centuries. It was so named after an outbreak of a respiratory disease in Italy in the 15th century that was thought to have developed under the influence (Italian, *influenza*) of the stars.

## Influenza A viruses can infect a wide variety of mammalian and avian species

The mixing vessel hypothesis for the production of new influenza strains came about as a result of influenza A viruses infecting pigs, horses, seals and other mammals, and the ability of the virus to reassort. For example, pigs in some countries live in the same dwellings as the farmers, allowing the potential mixing of influenza viruses and emergence of new strains.

The 1918 Spanish influenza pandemic (H1N1) was estimated to have led to 50–100 million deaths around the world and was followed in 1957 and 1968 by the less severe Asian (H2N2) and Hong Kong (H3N2) influenza pandemics, respectively. These were examples of antigenic shift, whereas antigenic drift resulted in frequent epidemics between the pandemic years. In 1976 there was a swine influenza scare at the US Fort Dix; in 1997 in Hong Kong, 18 people became ill having had an H5N1 avian influenza A virus infection. Six of the infected people subsequently died. The outbreak ceased after public health authorities ordered the slaughter of all live chickens in Hong Kong.

Five human infections were reported in 1999 in Hong Kong and South China with the avian influenza A virus H9N2. There was no evidence of wider spread nor of human-to-human transmission with either strain although it had circulated widely among birds in Hong Kong and China.

Another avian influenza virus, H7N7, is highly pathogenic in birds and may be more transmissible between humans. During an outbreak of highly pathogenic avian influenza in Holland in 2003, an H7N7 virus infected 86 poultry workers and three family members who had no contact with chickens. They developed conjunctivitis and/or flulike symptoms. A veterinarian who handled infected chickens died of pneumonia and acute respiratory distress.

## Avian influenza viruses can be of high and low pathogenicity, and their receptor-binding properties affect their infection and transmission ability

The 18 antigenically distinct H subtypes (H1–18) of influenza A virus reservoirs include wild birds, especially waterfowl. These include the H5 and H7 subtypes. There are nine N subtypes (N1–9). Avian influenza A viruses have been found in >100 wild bird species globally, including wild aquatic birds as well as other birds and poultry in farms. They mulitply in the intestinal and respiratory tracts and are shed in nasal secretions and feces, resulting in wider transmission. Avian influenza A viruses are classed as highly pathogenic and low pathogenic avian influenza, HPAI and LPAI, respectively. HPAI can cause severe disease and high mortality, whereas LPAI causes mild or no disease; both can spread rapidly in flocks, and LPAI viruses can change into HPAI types.

Human influenza A viruses preferentially bind to receptors with sialic acid linked to galactose by alpha-2,6 linkage found in the human upper respiratory tract. However, most avian influenza A viruses preferentially bind to sialic acid linked to galactose by alpha-2,3 receptor linkage found in avian intestinal mucosa but not to a great degree in the human upper respiratory tract. This alpha-2,6/-2,3 difference in receptor binding is thought to be key to avian viruses rarely infecting humans and human influenza viruses not being so able to infect birds.

Outbreaks of H5N1 avian influenza in migratory waterfowl, domestic poultry and humans in Asia have occurred (Fig. 20.22). Over time, the host range has increased, with infections in waterfowl, ferrets, members of the cat family and humans. The virus has become more virulent as seen by the mortality rate in the human population together with neurologic clinical features.

Descriptive molecular epidemiology has shown that the precursor of the 1997 Hong Kong H5N1 virus was first seen in geese in 1996 in Guangdong, China. In turn, the goose virus had RNA segments from influenza viruses found in quail and the N segment from a duck virus. Subsequent evolution of the goose virus resulted in a predecessor of the Z genotype that caused the death of many waterfowl in Hong Kong nature parks and infected humans in that area in 2002. The Z genotype then predominated and spread across Southeast Asia and killed, or resulted in culling of, millions of domestic fowl.

The 1918 pandemic H1N1 strain is believed to have resulted from spontaneous mutations in an avian H1N1 virus after sequence analysis was carried out on viral RNA recovered from people who had died and had been buried in the Scandinavian permafrost. However, the other pandemic viruses mentioned earlier, including the 2009 pandemic H1N1 strain, were due to genetic reassortment of the viral segmented RNA genomes after a host was infected by avian and human influenza A viruses at the same time. This is a key concern, that an avian influenza virus infects a person who already has a human influenza virus infection and becomes coinfected. The viruses can infect the same cells and reassort their gene segments. That could lead to a novel virus that could then be more infectious to humans.

## The concern about when the next influenza pandemic would happen was realized in 2009 with the H1N1 pandemic

In April 2009, Mexico and the southern United States (California) reported a respiratory illness caused by a novel swine influenza A H1N1 virus. These were worrying times as it was thought that this new influenza virus could cause a pandemic with high morbidity and mortality. Pandemic influenza response plans had been developed and refined in many countries for the expected and overdue influenza outbreak. Viral sequence analysis showed that it was composed of a combination of genes most closely related to North American and Eurasian swine-lineage H1N1 influenza viruses. Exposure to pigs was not seen when investigating those infected. In addition, the new virus was circulating among humans and not among pig herds. Within weeks there were reports of people with influenza in a number of US states as well as Canada and other parts of the world. The influenza pandemic alert was raised to phase 4 on the basis of human-to-human spread and outbreaks in the community. This became phase 5 by the end of April, and countries started to activate their pandemic response plans. Diagnostic RT-PCR tests were developed in days to confirm the diagnosis and a

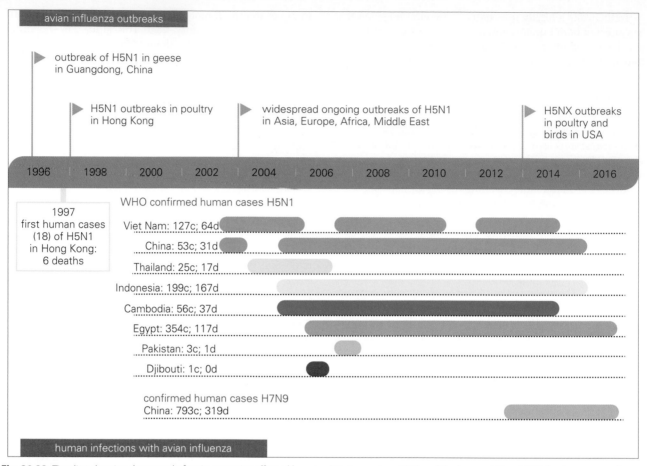

**Fig. 20.22** Timeline showing the spread of main countries affected by avian H5 viruses since 1996 and the human H5 and H7 infections reported to the World Health Organization. *c*, Cases; *d*, deaths. (From Barr I, Wong F. Avian influenza. Why the concern? *Microbiol Today*. 2016, November. https://microbiologysociety.org/publication/past-issues/the-mobile-microbe/article/avian-influenza-why-the-concern-mobile-microbe.html.)

vaccine virus chosen for high-yield preparation in case it was needed. National stockpiles of antiviral drugs (oseltamivir and zanamivir) and PPE were activated.

By June 2009 WHO changed its alert level to pandemic phase 6 as pandemic H1N1 was reported in >70 countries, and community outbreaks were happening globally. This virus contained gene reassortments from Eurasian and North American swine influenza, North American avian influenza and North American human influenza virus infections. The seasonal aspect of testing for influenza virus infections had altered as laboratories experienced huge workloads over the Northern Hemisphere summer months.

Confirmed and probable infections occurred mainly among 5- to 24-year-olds. Mostly older children and young adults were admitted to hospital as well as those in the at-risk groups identified in previous influenza pandemics, including women who were pregnant. In addition, increased risk of complications was seen in obese people and those with chronic neurologic conditions. There were few influenza infections seen in the ≥65-year-old group, which was unusual. Studies showed that children and young adults had no preexisting cross-reactive antibody to the 2009 H1N1 influenza virus compared with >30% of adults age ≥60 years who had been exposed previously.

Networks were set up worldwide to ensure that the experiences managing influenza-infected individuals in critical care facilities and elsewhere in the Southern Hemisphere were shared and lessons learnt. In addition, the circulating influenza viruses were monitored closely for any antigenic variation as well as the development of antiviral resistance. Influenza-infected patients on critical care units in acute respiratory failure received mechanical ventilation with intermittent positive-pressure ventilation in which the lungs receive air enriched with oxygen at high pressure. However, ECMO treatment improved recovery by providing gas exchange outside the body using heart-lung bypass equipment and obviating the deleterious effects of providing direct oxygenation at high pressure.

Across the Northern Hemisphere, the 2009 H1N1 influenza A summer activity peaked and declined during the summer, but levels of influenza activity remained above normal with small community outbreaks. On August 10, 2010 the WHO International Health Regulations Emergency Committee declared an end to the 2009 H1N1 pandemic globally.

There was concern about a second wave of infection, and preparations were made to offer the recently prepared vaccine to specific groups of individuals: those at risk and health care workers. The anticipated second wave started in the autumn, and the amount of influenza activity fell quite quickly and remained at lower levels until the spring. By 2016 H1N1 and H3N2 viruses were circulating around the world.

**The WHO Global Influenza Surveillance and Response System and the Tool for Influenza Pandemic Risk Assessment provide the early warning systems for novel influenza virus strains**

The WHO system for monitoring circulating influenza viruses detected an avian influenza A H5N1 virus that was reported as H5N1 clade 2.3.2.1 that circulated in poultry in parts of Asia in February 2011. This was not detected in humans and was not seen as a public health threat but as a marker of the continual evolution of these viruses.

Between 2003 and March 2023, 873 human infections with H5N1 from 22 countries were reported to WHO of whom 458 (53%) died. Most infections were reported in Egypt, Indonesia, Vietnam and Cambodia. In addition, by March 2023 there had been 83 human infections in China with avian influenza A H5N6 and 1 infection in Laos with a 35% mortality rate.

Epidemics and pandemics are due to the appearance of new strains of viruses so that a given individual is regularly reinfected with different strains. This is in contrast to viruses that undergo minimal antigenic variation (monotypic viruses), such as hepatitis A. Monitoring avian influenza viruses such as H5N1 and H7N7 is therefore critical in determining their potential to become more pathogenic and spread. Reassortment between H5N1 or H7N7 and human H1N1 or H3N2 influenza viruses may result in efficient transmissibility together with retention of viral pathogenicity. An influenza pandemic could then evolve.

**A new subclade of H5 avian influenza A started sweeping the world in 2022**

There are different clades of H5 viruses that have reassorted with other avian influenza viruses N genes leading to H5N2, H5N6 and H5N8, often referred to as H5NX. They were seen in migrating birds in North America in 2014, and then a new subclade appeared in 2020 spreading across Africa and Eurasia. This appeared, via Europe, in the Americas in 2022 (Fig. 20.23A) and resulted in a huge global infection control crisis in poultry farms and wild birds. Over 58 million birds in ~300 affected farms were culled between 2022 and 2023 in the United States. In Europe the HPAI A (H5N1) virus, clade 2.3.4.4b, was found in 24 countries, in residential/captive and wild birds, especially black-headed gulls (see Fig. 20.23). Although human-to-human transmission was not reported, human infections occurred after close contact with infected chickens. Mammals that ate infected dead bird carcasses also became infected but had not been shown to transmit to each other. However, reports in 2022 from an H5N1 outbreak in a mink farm in Spain demonstrated that spread between mink had occurred.

**Prevention strategies in response to the HPAI situation**

The Tool for Influenza Pandemic Risk Assessment started in 2016 and is a global structured approach to assessing whether a novel virus might emerge with pandemic potential. The framework includes:

- enhanced virologic and serologic surveillance of wild birds as well as wild and farmed mammals, especially in areas where HPAI is reported in wild birds and poultry
- preparedness and prevention strategies in poultry farms

- biosecurity and good farming practices to prevent exposure to infected wild birds
- immunization of poultry and developing new candidate vaccine viruses (including mRNA vaccines)
- culling birds and poultry that devastated these populations around the world and affects local economies.

Individuals were advised to wear PPE when in contact with potentially infected birds and animals. Antiviral prophylaxis was considered for anyone exposed to infected mammals together with monitoring to identify transmission.

**Transmission of influenza is by droplet inhalation**

Influenza infections occur throughout the world. Except in the tropics, the infection is almost entirely restricted to the coldest months of the year. This is largely because, during cold weather, people spend more time inside buildings with limited air space, which favours transmission by droplet inhalation, and perhaps also because of decreased host resistance. Influenza activity within a community is reflected not only in the numbers of people becoming ill and consulting doctors but also in excess mortality due to acute respiratory disease, such as pneumonia, which particularly affects the elderly (Fig. 20.24).

With respect to the avian influenza viruses, they are spread by movement of poultry and poultry products, live poultry markets, unhygienic practices and backyard flocks that are not controlled.

The initial symptoms of influenza are due to direct viral damage and associated inflammatory responses. The virus enters the respiratory tract in droplets and attaches to sialic acid receptors on epithelial cells via the H glycoprotein of the virus envelope. Just 1–3 days after infection, the cytokines liberated from damaged cells and from infiltrating leukocytes cause symptoms such as chills, malaise, fever and muscular aches. There are also respiratory symptoms such as a runny nose and cough. Most people feel better within 1 week. The direct viral damage and associated inflammatory responses can be severe enough to cause bronchitis and interstitial pneumonia.

**Influenzal damage to the respiratory epithelium predisposes to secondary bacterial infection**

Secondary bacterial invaders include staphylococci, pneumococci and *H. influenzae*. Life-threatening influenza is often due to secondary bacterial infection, especially with *S. aureus*, the viral infection being brought under control by antibody and cell-mediated immune responses to the infecting virus. Although antiviral antibodies may not be detected within the serum for 1–2 weeks, they are produced at an earlier stage but complexed with viral antigens in the respiratory tract.

Mortality due to secondary bacterial pneumonia is higher in apparently healthy individuals age >60 years and in those with impaired resistance due to, for example, chronic cardiorespiratory disease or renal disease. Women who are pregnant are also more vulnerable.

**Rarely, influenza causes neurologic complications**

Central nervous system (CNS) complications include meningitis, encephalomyelitis and polyneuritis. These appear to be indirect immunopathologic complications rather than due

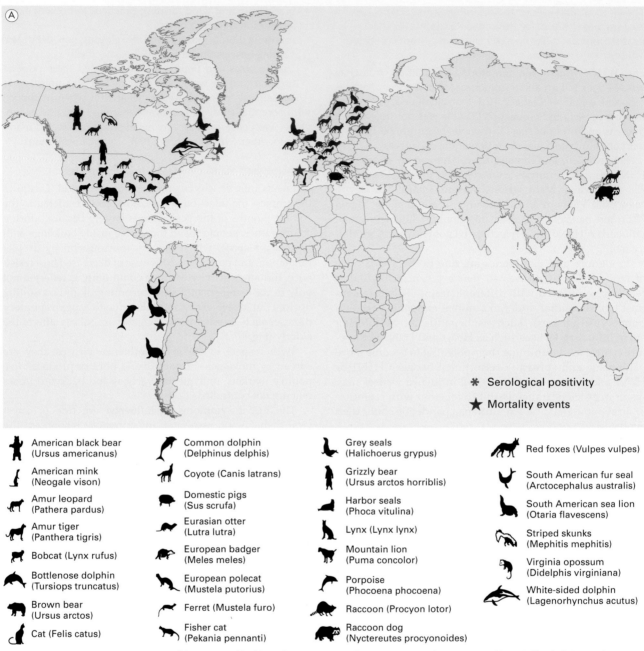

Fig. 20.23 (A) Geographic distribution of detections of highly pathogenic avian influenza in mammals since 2016. (From Adlhoch C, Fusaro A, Gonzales J, et al. Avian influenza overview May-September 2021. European Food Safety Authority. 2021. https://www.ecdc.europa.eu/sites/default/files/documents/avian-influenza-overview-march-2023.pdf.)

to CNS invasion by the virus. Guillain-Barré syndrome, a polyneuropathy with proximal, distal or generalized motor weakness, occurred as a significant but rare (1/100,000) sequel to the widespread immunization of those in the United States with inactivated H3N2 influenza virus in 1976. However, subsequent vaccines have not been associated with this syndrome.

### During influenza epidemics a diagnosis can generally be made clinically

Rapid diagnosis can be made by collecting samples from the respiratory tract, such as throat swabs that can be tested by RT-PCR for influenza viral RNA, and the viruses can

be typed simultaneously. Antiviral resistance can also be detected using PCR and sequence analysis.

### Vaccines can be used to prevent influenza

The aim of immunization is to help prevent infection, and those at risk of complications from influenza infection should be offered vaccine before the flu season. The vaccines may be trivalent or quadrivalent and the viruses inactivated or live attenuated. However, it is often said that pandemics can accelerate certain aspects of daily life, and the innovative vaccine development programme driven by the COVID-19 pandemic included nucleic acid-based mRNA vaccines in which the stabilized mRNA sits within

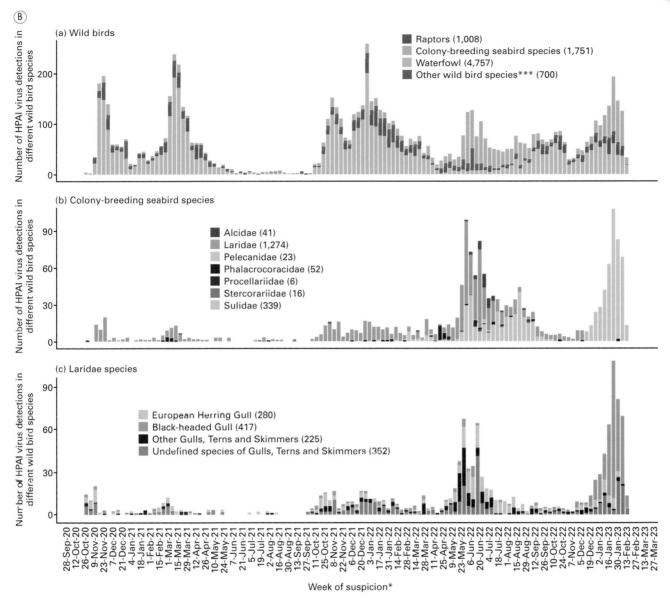

(B)

(a) Wild birds

Raptors (1,008)
Colony-breeding seabird species (1,751)
Waterfowl (4,757)
Other wild bird species*** (700)

(b) Colony-breeding seabird species

Alcidae (41)
Laridae (1,274)
Pelecanidae (23)
Phalacrocoracidae (52)
Procellariidae (6)
Stercorariidae (16)
Sulidae (339)

(c) Laridae species

European Herring Gull (280)
Black-headed Gull (417)
Other Gulls, Terns and Skimmers (225)
Undefined species of Gulls, Terns and Skimmers (352)

Week of suspicion*

**Fig. 20.23—Cont'd** (B) Distribution of total number of highly pathogenic avian influenza virus detections reported in Europe by week of suspicion (dates indicate the first day of the week) and (a) affected wild bird categories (8216), (b) affected colony-breeding seabird families (1751), (c) affected Laridae species (1274) from October 2020 to March 2023. (From Adlhoch C, Fusaro A, Gonzales J, et al. Avian influenza overview December 2022 to March 2023. European Food Safety Authority. 2021. https://www.ecdc.europa.eu/sites/default/files/documents/avian-influenza-overview-march-2023.pdf.)

a lipid nanoparticle. The first step to a universal influenza vaccine that could be immunogenic and rapidly produced was reported in 2022. A multivalent mRNA-based vaccine that included the 20 influenza A and B virus HA subtypes was given to ferrets, an animal model when investigating influenza vaccine responses. Multistrain-specific antibodies were detected as well as modified disease severity, and the ferrets were protected when challenged with a mismatched H1N1 virus.

Influenza virus vaccines in regular use are:

- those consisting of egg-grown virus, which are then purified, formalin-inactivated and extracted with ether
- the less reactogenic purified H and N antigens prepared from virus that has been disrupted (split) by lipid solvents
- live attenuated egg-grown virus.

Studies investigating the protective efficacy of cell culture–derived influenza virus vaccines have demonstrated similar results to the egg-grown vaccine. A cell-based quadrivalent inactivated influenza vaccine was approved for use in the United States in 2016.

Influenza A (H3N2 and H1N1 strains) and influenza B are included in the vaccine. The exact virus strains are reviewed annually in relation to the viruses circulating the previous year. The vaccines are given by parenteral injection and provide protection against disease in up to 70% of individuals for ~1 year. Vaccination of individuals at high risk, especially those >65 years old and those with chronic cardiopulmonary disease, is recommended. It might be expected that the respiratory route would be a better way of inducing respiratory immunity, and on this basis live attenuated virus vaccines were developed and

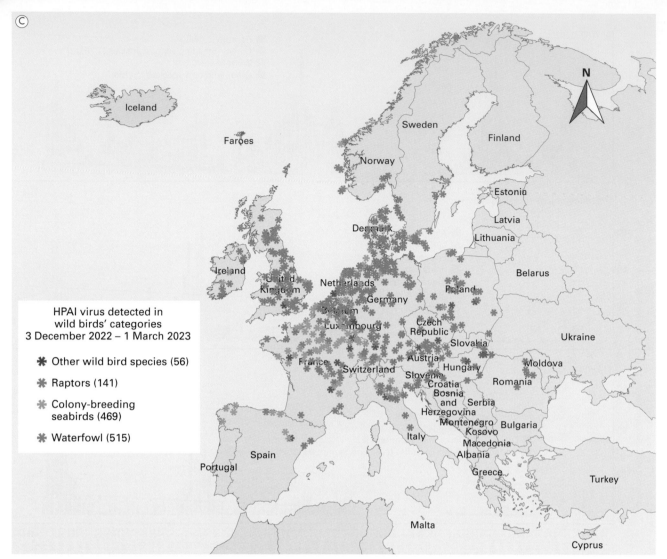

**Fig. 20.23—Cont'd** (C) Geographic distribution based on available geocoordinates of highly pathogenic avian influenza infections in wild birds categories in Europe, by species category, from December 2022 to March 2023.(From Adlhoch C, Fusaro A, Gonzales J, et al. Avian influenza overview December 2022 to March 2023. European Food Safety Authority. 2021. https://www.ecdc.europa.eu/sites/default/files/documents/avian-influenza-overview-march-2023.pdf.)

are administered intranasally. They are offered to specific age groups of children providing there are no contraindications as part of the annual immunization programme.

### Antiviral drugs can be used to treat and prevent influenza

Oseltamivir and zanamivir are neuraminidase inhibitor antiviral agents that act on both influenza A and B viruses (see Ch. 34). They superseded rimantadine and amantadine, M2 ion channel blockers that stop hydrogen ion efflux by altering the pH as they are basic compounds and affect intracellular viral uncoating. They inhibit only the replication of influenza A viruses. Oseltamivir (Tamiflu) is easier to administer as it is given orally, as opposed to zanamivir that is given by inhaler. These antivirals can reduce the severity of the infection but should be given within 1–2 days of disease onset. They have also been shown to be effective when used for prophylaxis if given within 48 hours of symptom onset.

Oseltamivir resistance has been widely reported, and transmission of oseltamivir resistance has occurred without direct selective drug pressure. This did not affect virulence or viral replication. During the 2009 influenza A H1N1 pandemic, intravenous oseltamivir and zanamivir preparations were made available together with other neuraminidase inhibitors, peramivir and laninamivir. Since then baloxavir, an influenza cap-dependent endonuclease inhibitor, has been shown to be effective in alleviating influenza symptoms in individuals with uncomplicated influenza A and B virus infections. In addition, favipiravir, a nucleoside analogue targeting the influenza polymerase, is active against influenza A and B viruses, including strains that are resistant to other antiviral drugs.

Finally, another therapeutic option from last century involved using hyperimmune plasma made from blood collected from human donors who had recovered from the 1918 Spanish influenza pandemic. This was given to patients with severe influenza infections who subsequently recovered. Some individuals with severe pandemic H1N1 infections recovered, having received hyperimmune plasma infusions

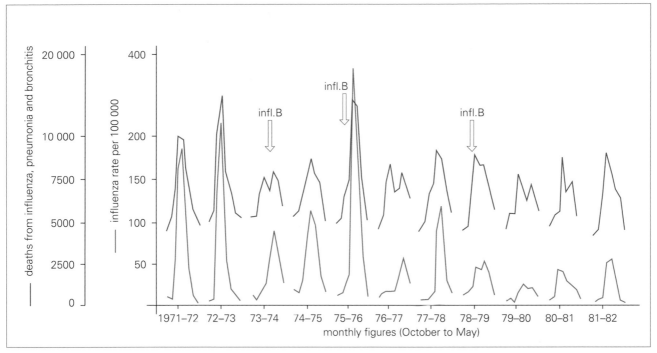

**Fig. 20.24** Outbreaks of influenza within a community are reflected by a general increase in deaths from acute respiratory disease. Notifications of new cases of clinical influenza are paralleled by an increase in deaths attributed to influenza, pneumonia and bronchitis. Monthly figures from October to May for England and Wales (1971–1983) are shown. The peaks are due to the spread of different strains of influenza A (H3N2 and H1N1) and influenza B (*infl. B; arrows*) viruses in the community. (From Office of Population, Censuses and Surveys.)

collected from individuals with pandemic H1N1 infection or from vaccinated donors.

With an eye to a future pandemic, nations developed stockpiles of antiinfluenza drugs. New approaches included developing drug targets focusing on entry, replication and maturation as well as novel approaches to rapid vaccine production.

Culling domestic poultry has contained the spread of the H5N1 virus as well as other avian influenza viruses, including H5N8 and H7N9. However, rapid detection and increased biosecurity together with the use of vaccines are critical in controlling the infection. In addition, there are questions as to what lessons have been learnt for any future influenza or other respiratory virus epidemic or pandemic.

## MEASLES VIRUS INFECTION

### Secondary bacterial pneumonia is a frequent complication of measles in developing countries

Measles is dealt with in detail as a multisystem infection in Ch. 27. It is mentioned here because:

- it can cause giant cell pneumonia in those with impaired immune responses
- the virus replicates in the lower respiratory tract and, under certain circumstances, causes sufficient damage to lead to secondary bacterial pneumonia.

Secondary bacterial pneumonia is now uncommon in resource-rich countries but is a frequent complication among children in resource-poor countries, and measles remains a major cause of death in childhood. Depressed immune responsiveness, inadequate vaccination programmes, malnutrition (especially vitamin A) and poor medical care to deal with complications tip the host-parasite balance markedly in favour of the virus.

After an incubation period of 10–14 days, symptoms include fever, a runny nose, conjunctivitis and cough. Koplik spots and then the characteristic rash appear 1–2 days later.

The virus replicates in the epithelium of the nasopharynx, middle ear and lung, interfering with host defences and enabling bacteria such as pneumococci, staphylococci and meningococci to establish infection. Pneumonia generally results in those with measles being admitted to hospital, but otitis media is also common. Virus replication continues unchecked in children with severely impaired cell-mediated immune responses, giving rise to a giant cell pneumonia, which is a rare and usually fatal manifestation (Fig. 20.25). Other complications are referred to in Ch. 27 and neurologic complications in Ch. 25.

Measles is diagnosed clinically, but detection of specific IgM responses and measles viral RNA detection and

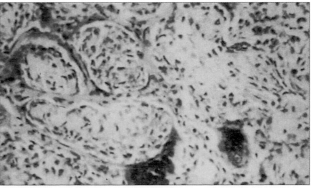

**Fig. 20.25** Lung biopsy in measles pneumonia showing inflammatory cell infiltrate, proliferation of the alveolar lining cells and large, darkly staining, multinucleate giant cells (H&E stain). (Courtesy I.D. Starke and M.E. Hodson.)

sequence analysis are important to confirm the diagnosis and for surveillance purposes.

### Antibiotics are needed for secondary bacterial complications of measles, but the disease can be prevented or attenuated by immunization

If severe, ribavirin treatment is available, but antibiotics are needed for bacterial complications. Children with severe measles in resource-poor countries generally have very low levels of serum retinol, the predominant circulating form of vitamin A in the blood. Therefore, vitamin A supplements improve clinical outcome reducing the number of deaths from measles by half.

Measles is prevented by a highly effective, live attenuated vaccine given with mumps and rubella vaccines (MMR; see Ch. 35). Since immunization began, the number of infections has declined by 70%. In the United States, after a rise to nearly 30,000 cases in 1990, the number fell to 488 (47 of them imported) in 1996. It was planned to eliminate the disease in the Americas by the year 2000, by which time a group of scientists convened by the CDC decided that measles was no longer endemic in the United States. Due to an unfounded MMR vaccine scare in the United Kingdom, the number of individuals with measles rose considerably owing to a fall in vaccine uptake. By 2016 vaccine uptake had improved to 95%, and the number of notifications of measles infection had dropped.

Before the vaccine was available in the 1960s, there were 135 million infections and 7–8 million deaths each year worldwide. Between 2000 and 2018 there was a 73% reduction in deaths globally; in 2018, however, >140,000 deaths were reported worldwide in mostly <5-year-olds. Improved vaccine coverage meant that 86% of 1-year-olds worldwide had received one dose of vaccine. WHO estimated that measles vaccine had prevented ~23 million deaths between 2000 and 2018, a remarkable achievement; however, measles elimination or eradication was still proving difficult in 2023.

## CYTOMEGALOVIRUS INFECTION

### CMV infection can cause an interstitial pneumonitis in patients who are immunocompromised

CMV does not normally replicate in respiratory epithelium or cause respiratory illness; however, in immunocompromised patients and in certain allogeneic bone marrow transplant recipients it can give rise to an interstitial pneumonia. Monitoring CMV DNA levels in blood in specific groups of immunosuppressed patients is critical especially in the first few months posttransplantation. However, compartmentalization may be seen with CMV viraemia not being detected despite causing end-organ damage. Therefore if suspecting a CMV pneumonitis, a bronchoscopy may need to be carried out unless contraindicated and the bronchoalveolar lavage tested for CMV DNA load. Characteristic owl's-eye inclusions may be demonstrated if a lung biopsy is carried out (Fig. 20.26).

## TUBERCULOSIS

### Tuberculosis is one of the most serious infectious diseases of the resource-poor world

*Mycobacterium tuberculosis* (*Mtb*) causes tuberculosis (TB), one of the top 10 causes of death globally. In 2021 WHO

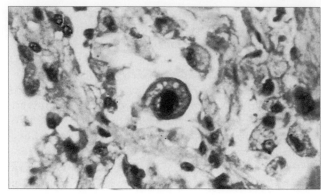

**Fig. 20.26** Owl's-eye inclusion body in cytomegalovirus infection. Large numbers of virus particles accumulate in the nucleus of the enlarged infected cell to produce a single dense inclusion (H&E stain). (Courtesy I.D. Starke and M.E. Hodson.)

estimated 10.6 million people were infected with TB and 1.6 million died, with >95% of deaths occurring in low- and middle-income countries, wherever poverty, malnutrition and poor housing prevail. The COVID-19 pandemic did affect global TB reporting, but it was getting back on track by 2023. It affects the apparently healthy as well as being a serious disease of the immunocompromised and is an AIDS-defining illness in HIV-positive individuals. TB is primarily a disease of the lungs but may spread to other sites or proceed to a disseminated infection (miliary TB).

Other species of mycobacteria, referred to as atypical mycobacteria, mycobacteria other than tuberculosis or non-tuberculous mycobacteria also cause infection in the lungs (Table 20.8).

Infection is acquired by inhalation of *Mtb* in aerosols and dust. Airborne transmission of TB is efficient because infected people cough up enormous numbers of mycobacteria, projecting them into the environment, where their waxy outer coat allows them to withstand drying and therefore survive for long periods in air and house dust.

### The pathogenesis of TB depends on the history of previous exposure to the organism

In primary infection, in individuals encountering *Mtb* for the first time, the organisms are engulfed by the alveolar macrophages, in which they can both survive and multiply. Nonresident macrophages are attracted to the site where they ingest the mycobacteria, inducing the macrophage differentiation into dendritic cells (DCs). These cells then migrate via the lymphatics to the pulmonary hilar lymph nodes. Once the DC arrive in the lymph nodes, they localize to T-cell–rich zones where they present antigen to T cells triggering a T-cell mediated immune response. This T-cell response can be detected in the tuberculin skin test, also called the Mantoux test, 4–6 weeks after infection by injecting a small amount of purified protein derivative of *Mtb* into the skin to assess whether someone is sensitive to *Mtb* antigens. A positive result is shown by local induration and erythema 48–72 h later. However, as with the interferon-gamma release assay (IGRA), a blood test for TB, a positive response could mean that the person has been infected previously, has latent TB infection or has an active TB infection. A strong skin test reaction would lead to referral to a respiratory clinic for further assessment and treatment.

**Table 20.8** Mycobacteria associated with human disease

| Species | Clinical disease |
| --- | --- |
| Slow growers[a] | |
| M. tuberculosis | Tuberculosis |
| M. bovis | Bovine tuberculosis |
| M. leprae | Leprosy |
| M. avium[b]<br>M. intracellulare[b] | Disseminated infection in AIDS patients M. avium complex (MAC) |
| M. kansasii | Lung infections |
| M. marinum | Skin infections and deeper infections (e.g. arthritis, osteomyelitis) associated with aquatic activity |
| M. scrofulaceum | Cervical adenitis in children |
| M. simiae | Lung, bone and kidney infections |
| M. szulgai | Lung, skin and bone infections |
| M. ulcerans | Skin infections |
| M. xenopi | Lung infections |
| M. paratuberculosis | ? Association with Crohn disease |
| Rapid growers[a] | |
| M. fortuitum<br>M. chelonae | Opportunist infections with introduction of organisms into deep subcutaneous tissues; usually associated with trauma or invasive procedures |

Many species of mycobacteria are associated with occasional disease, but the major pathogens of the genus are M. tuberculosis, M. bovis and M. leprae.
[a]Slow growers require >7 days for visible growth from a dilute inoculum; rapid growers require <7 days from a dilute inoculum
[b]M. avium complex; the two species are distinct. Of the M. avium complex, serotypes 1–6 and 8–11 are assigned to M. avium, serotypes 7, 12–17, 19, 20 and 25 are assigned to M. intracellulare.

### The CMI response helps to curb further spread of *M. tuberculosis*

However, some *Mtb* organisms may have already escaped to set up foci of infection in other body sites. Sensitized T cells

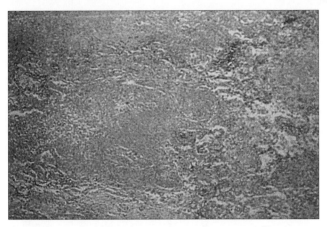

**Fig. 20.27** Histopathology showing dense inflammatory infiltration, granuloma formation and caseous necrosis in pulmonary tuberculosis. (Courtesy R. Bryan.)

release lymphokines that activate macrophages and increase their ability to destroy the mycobacteria. The body reacts to contain the organisms within tubercles, which are small granulomas consisting of epithelioid cells and giant cells (Fig. 20.27). The lung lesion plus the enlarged pulmonary hilar lymph nodes (Fig. 20.28) is often called the Ghon or primary complex. After a time, the material within the granulomas becomes necrotic and caseous or cheesy in appearance.

The tubercles may heal spontaneously, become fibrotic or calcified and persist as such for a lifetime in people who are otherwise healthy. They will show up on a chest x-ray as radiopaque nodules. However, in a small percentage of people with primary infection, and particularly in the immunocompromised, the mycobacteria are not contained within the tubercles but invade the bloodstream and cause disseminated disease (miliary TB) (Fig. 20.29A).

Secondary TB is due to reactivation of dormant mycobacteria and is usually a consequence of impaired immune function resulting from some other cause such as malnutrition, infection (e.g. advanced HIV and AIDS), chemotherapy for treatment of malignancy or corticosteroids for the treatment of inflammatory diseases.

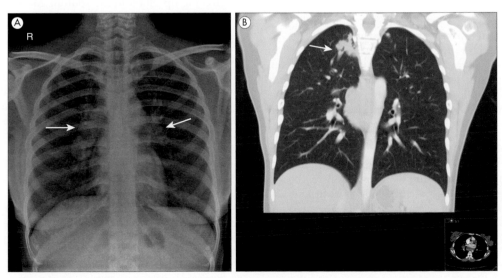

**Fig. 20.28** (A) Chest radiograph showing bilateral hilar and paratracheal lymphadenopathy (*arrowed*). (B) Computed tomography scan of patchy parenchymal consolidation in both upper lobes. (Courtesy G. Bain, London North West Healthcare Trust.)

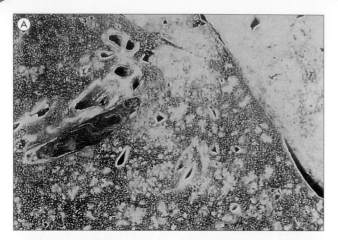

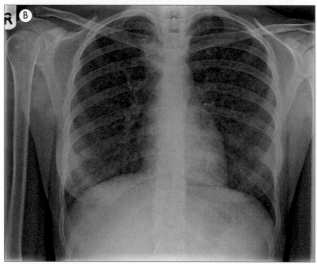

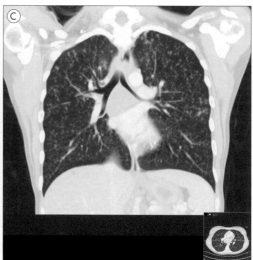

**Fig. 20.29** Miliary tuberculosis (TB). (A) Gross specimen of lung showing the cut surface covered with white nodules, which are the miliary foci of TB. (B) Miliary TB chest x-ray and (C) computed tomography. (A, Courtesy J.A. Innes; B and C, courtesy G. Bain, London North West Healthcare Trust.)

### TB illustrates the dual role of the immune response in infectious disease

On the one hand, the CMI response controls the *Mtb* infection and, when it is inadequate, the infection disseminates or reactivates. On the other hand, nearly all TB pathology and disease is a consequence of this CMI response, as *Mtb* causes little or no direct or toxin-mediated damage.

Reactivation occurs most commonly in the apex of the lungs. This site is more highly oxygenated than elsewhere, allowing the mycobacteria to multiply more rapidly to produce caseous necrotic lesions, which spill over into other sites in the lung, and from where organisms spread to more distant sites in the body.

### Primary TB is often asymptomatic

In contrast to pneumonia, which is usually an acute infection, the onset of TB is insidious, the infection proceeding for some time before the patient becomes sufficiently ill to seek medical attention. Primary TB is usually mild and asymptomatic and in 90% of infections does not proceed further. However, clinical disease develops in the remaining 10%.

Mycobacteria have the ability to colonize almost any site in the body. The clinical manifestations are variable: Fatigue, weight loss, weakness and fever are all associated with TB.

Infection in the lungs characteristically causes a chronic productive cough, and the sputum may be blood stained as a result of tissue destruction. Necrosis may erode blood vessels, which can rupture and cause haemoptysis, which is coughing up blood in the sputum. Massive haemoptysis may cause death through haemorrhage.

### Complications of *M. tuberculosis* infection arise from local spread or dissemination

The organism may disseminate via the lymphatics and bloodstream to other parts of the body. This usually occurs at the time of primary infection, and in this way chronic foci are established, which may proceed to necrosis and destruction in, for example, the kidney. Alternatively, spread may be by extension to a neighbouring part of the lung—for instance, when a tubercle erodes into a bronchus and discharges its contents or into the pleural cavity, resulting in a pleural effusion.

Although the number of cases of pulmonary TB has been declining in resource-rich countries since the beginning of the 20th century, hastened by the advent of specific antimicrobial drugs the incidence of extrapulmonary TB has stayed roughly constant for many years and therefore makes up a greater proportion of the TB case load in resource-rich countries than in resource-poor countries. For reasons still not

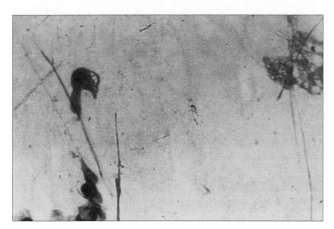

**Fig. 20.30** Pulmonary tuberculosis. Sputum preparation showing pink-stained, acid-fast tubercle bacilli (Ziehl-Neelsen stain). (Courtesy J.A. Innes.)

well understood, extrapulmonary TB numbers in resource-rich countries are higher amongst the migrant population.

### Ziehl-Neelsen staining of a sputum smear can provide a diagnosis of TB within an hour, whereas culture can take 6 weeks

A diagnosis of TB is suggested by the clinical signs and symptoms referred to earlier, supported by characteristic changes on chest radiography (see Fig. 20.29B and C) and positive antigen reactive tests such as skin test reactivity in the tuberculin (Mantoux) test or IGRA. These tests are confirmed by microscopic demonstration of acid-fast rods and culture of *Mtb*. Microscopic examination of a smear of sputum stained by the Ziehl-Neelsen method or by auramine often reveals acid-fast rods (Fig. 20.30). This result can be obtained within 1 h of receipt of the specimen in the laboratory. This is important because *Mtb* can take up to 6 weeks to grow in culture and therefore confirmation of the diagnosis is delayed. Rapid nonculture tests to detect *Mtb* are PCR, such as the automated Xpert MTB-RIF Ultra and Truenat molecular tests that detect TB and rifampicin resistance in sputum samples. Other molecular tests, such as whole genome sequencing, can identify the mycobacteria to species level and genotypic susceptibility to anti-TB drugs.

### Specific anti-TB drugs and prolonged therapy are needed to treat TB

Mycobacteria are innately resistant to most antibacterial agents, and specific anti-TB drugs must be used; these are reviewed in Ch. 34. The key features of treatment are the use of:

- combination therapy — usually four drugs such as isoniazid, rifampicin, ethambutol and pyrazinamide to prevent emergence of resistance
- prolonged therapy — minimum 6-month duration, which is necessary to eradicate these slow-growing intracellular organisms.

The number of strains resistant to the first-line anti-TB drugs has increased as these antibiotics have been used for decades. Resistance may appear if there are compliance problems due to the number of drugs and lengthy treatment period. Other factors can include variable quality of the drugs and poor prescribing practices. Treatment

is monitored carefully with directly observed treatment. Multidrug-resistant TB (MDR-TB) and rifampicin-resistant TB (RR-TB) occurs when there is little response to the first-line drugs isoniazid and rifampicin. In 2021 the estimated number of people worldwide with MDR/RR-TB was 3.6% among new infections and 18% in those previously treated. Of these, 42% were reported in India, the Russian Federation, China and Pakistan. Treatment for MDR-TB requires using other drugs such as fluoroquinolones and second-line injectable drugs. Extremely drug-resistant TB (XDR-TB) does not respond to isoniazid, rifampicin, the fluoroquinolones or second-line injectable drugs. Both MDR-TB and XDR-TB increase TB mortality, and the Global Burden of Disease Study reported in 2019 that there were just over 25,000 new XDR-TB infections globally that year. By 2021 TB incidence and mortality had fallen by 11% and 9%, respectively, but the global strategy to reduce TB burden aimed for higher falls. Drug resistance will have contributed to the slower decline in numbers. In 2022 WHO prioritized a new 6-month oral regime for treating adults with MDR-TB or XDR-TB known as the BPaLM/BPal regime (i.e. bedaquiline, a diarylquinoline targeting the ATP synthase of mycobacteria; pretomanid, a novel compound and member of the nitroimidazooxazines; linezolid, an oxazolidinone protein synthesis inhibitor; moxifloxacin, a fluoroquinolone targeting the bacterial DNA gyrase and topoisomerase intravenous enzymes).

### TB is prevented by improved social conditions, immunization, chemoprophylaxis

The steady decline in incidence of TB since the beginning of the 20th century, and before specific preventive measures were available, underlines the importance of improvements in social conditions in the prevention of this and many other infectious diseases. However, the fall in TB incidence rate based on new infections/100,000 people/year of ~2% for most of the years between 2000 and 2019 was reversed during the COVID-19 pandemic. Between 2020 and 2021, the incidence rate was estimated to have risen by 3.6% due to service disruptions over that period. The likelihood of developing TB is 18 times higher in HIV-positive individuals and causes ~33% of AIDS-related mortality worldwide. In 2021 there were ~187,000 deaths due to TB in this group. The highest TB burden in HIV-positive individuals was in the WHO African region.

Immunization with a live attenuated bacille Calmette-Guérin (BCG) vaccine has been used effectively in situations where TB is prevalent, although its effectiveness is variable and mainly associated with prevention of disseminated disease in chidren. It was introduced in the United Kingdom in 1953, and the programme changed along sociodemographic lines as it was initially targeted at 14-year-olds as most TB was seen in young adults. This was subsequently modified to a selective neonatal immunization programme aimed at infants born to parents who had emigrated from high-prevalence countries as those groups were found to have higher rates of TB than those born in the United Kingdom. Immunization, which confers positive skin test reactivity, does not prevent infection but it does allow the body to react quickly to limit proliferation of the organisms. In areas where there is a low prevalence of disease, immunization has been largely replaced by chemoprophylaxis. Those immunized have been reported to be up to 8% less likely to develop the most severe complications of TB.

In the United Kingdom prophylaxis with rifampicin and isoniazid for 3 months is recommended for people who have had close contact with someone with TB (unless isoniazid resistant). It is also advocated for individuals who show recent conversion to skin test positivity when it is essentially early treatment of subclinical infection rather than prophylaxis. A 6-month course with isoniazid may be an option in patients who cannot receive rifampicin due to intolerance, toxicity or drug-drug interactions.

## CYSTIC FIBROSIS

### Individuals with cystic fibrosis are predisposed to develop lower respiratory tract infections

Cystic fibrosis is the most common lethal inherited disorder among those of European descent, with an incidence of ~1/2500 live births. The disease is characterized by pancreatic insufficiency, abnormal sweat electrolyte concentrations and production of highly viscid bronchial secretions. The latter tend to lead to stasis in the lungs, which predisposes to infection.

### *P. aeruginosa* colonizes the lungs of almost all 15- to 20-year-olds with cystic fibrosis

The respiratory mucosa of individuals with cystic fibrosis presents a different environment for potential pathogens from that found in healthy individuals, and the common infecting organisms and the nature of infections differ from other lung infections. These invaders include:

- *S. aureus*, which causes respiratory distress and lung damage but can be well controlled by specific antistaphylococcal chemotherapy
- *P. aeruginosa*, which is the main pathogen
- *Burkholderia cepacia*, which is aggressive and hard to treat
- *H. influenzae*, typically nonencapsulated strains, which may be found in association with *S. aureus* and *P. aeruginosa*; their pathogenic significance is unclear, but they appear to contribute to respiratory exacerbations
- *Aspergillus fumigatus*, which is a fungus in the environment that may cause symptoms
- nontuberculous mycobacteria, which may also cause symptoms.

*P. aeruginosa* infection is uncommon in those <5 years of age but colonizes the lungs of almost all patients aged 15–20 years, often encouraged by its intrinsic resistance to antistaphylococcal agents. Early in the course of infection normal colony types are grown from sputum cultures, but as infection progresses the organism changes to a highly mucoid form, almost mimicking the mucoid secretions of the patient (Fig. 20.31). These mucoid forms are thought to grow in microcolonies in the lung, but most of the lung damage is due to immunologic responses to the organisms and to the alginate, which forms the mucoid material (Fig. 20.32). *P. aeruginosa* rarely invades beyond the lung even in the most severely infected individuals. Inhaled antibiotics are recommended for bacterial eradication and to prevent chronic infection.

Although specific antibacterial chemotherapy can reduce the symptoms of infection and improve the quality of life, infections particularly with *P. aeruginosa* and *B. cepacia* are

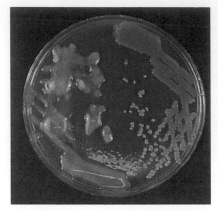

**Fig. 20.31** *Pseudomonas aeruginosa* isolated from the sputum of patients with cystic fibrosis characteristically grows in a very mucoid colonial form, shown here on the left of the picture, with the normal colonial form on the right for comparison.

difficult to eradicate and are still a major cause of morbidity and mortality.

## LUNG ABSCESS

### Lung abscesses usually contain a mixture of bacteria, including anaerobes

This is a suppurative infection of the lung sometimes referred to as necrotizing pneumonia. The most common predisposing cause is aspiration of respiratory or gastric secretions as a result of altered consciousness. The infection is therefore endogenous in origin, and cultures often reveal a mixture of bacteria with anaerobes such as *Bacteroides* and *Fusobacterium* playing an important role (Fig. 20.33).

Patients with lung abscesses may be ill for at least 2 weeks before presentation, with possible swinging fever, and usually produce large amounts of sputum, which if foul smelling gives a strong hint of the presence of anaerobes and often suggests the diagnosis. Most diagnoses are made from chest radiographs (see Fig. 20.6G) and the cause confirmed by microbiologic investigation.

### Treatment of lung abscess should include an antianaerobic drug and last 2–4 months

Because of the likely presence of anaerobes, a suitable antianaerobic agent such as metronidazole should be part of the treatment regimen and treatment may be needed for 2–4 months to prevent relapse. If diagnosis and treatment are delayed, infection may spread to the pleural space, giving rise to empyema (see later).

### Pleural effusion and empyema

#### Up to 50% of patients with pneumonia have a pleural effusion

Pleural effusions arise in a variety of different diseases. Sometimes the organisms infecting the lung spread to the pleural space and give rise to a purulent exudate or empyema.

Pleural effusions can be demonstrated radiologically, but detection of empyema can be difficult particularly in a patient with extensive pneumonia.

Aspiration of pleural fluid provides material for microbiologic examination, and *S. aureus*, gram-negative rods and anaerobes are commonly involved.

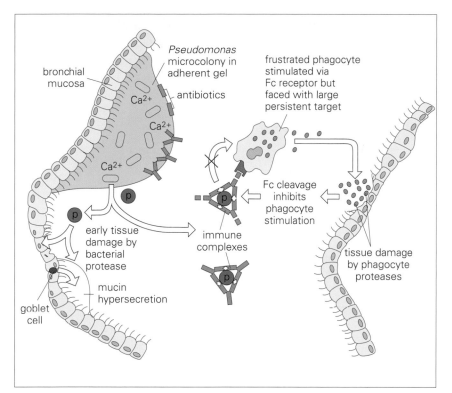

**Fig. 20.32** *Pseudomonas* infection in the lung of cystic fibrosis is chronic but rarely invasive beyond the bronchial mucosa. The organisms are thought to grow in microcolonies embedded in a calcium ($Ca^{2+}$)–dependent mucoid alginate gel, which contains DNA and tracheobronchial mucin and attaches to the bronchial mucosa. This protects the organisms from the host defences and provides a physical and electrolyte barrier to antibiotics. Much of the damage to tissue is thought to be due to the slow release of bacterial proteases, which disrupt the mucosa and cause mucin hypersecretion, immunopathologic mechanisms exacerbated by the size, antigenicity and persistence of the alginate matrix and the indirect action of immune complexes associated with *Pseudomonas* antigens (P). Tissue damage is also caused by phagocyte proteases. Intermittent exacerbations can be explained by the cleavage of the Fc of immune complexes by these proteases and consequent inhibition of further phagocyte stimulation. (From Govan JRW and Glass S. The microbiology and therapy of cystic fibrosis lung infections. *Rev Med Microbiol.* 1990;1:19–28.)

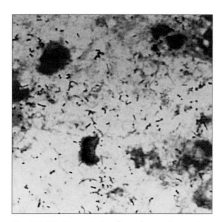

**Fig. 20.33** Gram stain of pus from a lung abscess showing gram-positive cocci and both gram-negative and gram-positive rods. (Courtesy J.R. Cantey.)

Treatment should be directed at drainage of pus, eradication of infection and expansion of the lung.

## FUNGAL INFECTIONS

Disease associated with fungal infection is most seen in patients with defective immunity as a consequence either of immune suppressive treatment or of concomitant disease. A number of species can cause opportunistic infections, and two are of particular importance: *A. fumigatus* and *P. jirovecii*.

### *Aspergillus*

The most important species are *A. fumigatus* and *A. flavus.*

#### *Aspergillus* can cause allergic bronchopulmonary aspergillosis, aspergilloma, disseminated aspergillosis

The genus *Aspergillus* contains many species, and these are ubiquitous in the environment. They do not form part of the normal flora. Their spores are regularly inhaled without harmful consequences, but some species, notably *A. fumigatus*, are able to cause a range of diseases:

- Allergic bronchopulmonary aspergillosis (ABPA), which is, as its name suggests, an allergic response to the presence of *Aspergillus* antigen in the lungs and occurs in patients with asthma. ABPA occurs in some 10% of patients with cystic fibrosis.
- Aspergilloma in patients with preexisting lung cavities or chronic pulmonary disorders. *Aspergillus* colonizes a cavity and grows to produce a fungal ball, a mass of entangled hyphae—the aspergilloma (Fig. 20.34). In this case, fungi do not invade the lung tissue, but the presence of a large aspergilloma can cause respiratory problems such as cough and haemoptysis. Aspergillomas can be related, however, to chronic pulmonary aspergillosis where invasion of lung tissue does occur.
- Disseminated disease in the immunosuppressed patient when the fungus spreads from the lungs.

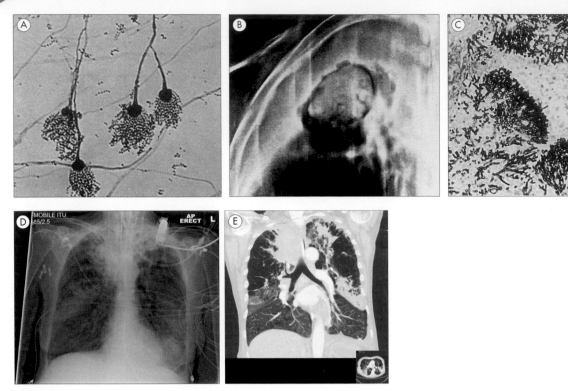

**Fig. 20.34** (A) *Aspergillus fumigatus*. Lactophenol cotton blue–stained preparation showing the characteristic conidiophores. (B) Aspergilloma. Tomogram showing fungus ball contained within the lung cavity, outlined by air space. Invasive aspergillosis: (C) histologic section showing fungal hyphae invading the lung parenchyma and blood vessels (Grocott stain); (D) chest x-ray and (E) chest computed tomography scan. (A and B, Courtesy J.A. Innes; C, courtesy C. Kibbler; D and E, courtesy G. Bain, London North West Healthcare Trust.)

Invasive aspergillosis carries a high mortality as treatment is very difficult owing to the limited number and toxic nature of antifungal agents active against *Aspergillus* plus the lack of functional host defences. Treatment is with voriconazole. Isavuconazole or an intravenous lipid formulation of amphotericin B are alternatives. Where possible, steps should be taken to reduce immunosuppression and improve the neutrophil count.

### *Pneumocystis jirovecii* (formerly *P. carinii*)

**Pneumocystis pneumonia is an important opportunistic infection in AIDS**

*P. jirovecii* is a fungus commonly found in immunocompetent humans and in rodents. In contrast to other pathogenic fungi, there is strong host specificity, so *Pneumocystis* infection of humans is not a zoonosis. Infection probably spreads by inhalation, though airborne transmission has been directly demonstrated only in animal models. Disease occurs in debilitated and immune-deficient individuals. Before the advent of combined active antiretroviral therapy, a high proportion of patients with advanced HIV infection developed *Pneumocystis* pneumonia, which could be fatal.

*Pneumocystis* occurs as three developmental forms: a trophozoite, 2–10 μm in diameter, a precyst and a cyst (ascus) containing eight spores. Spores released when the cysts rupture are the infective stage, which new hosts acquire by inhalation. Disease is associated with an interstitial pneumonitis (Fig. 20.35) with plasma cell infiltration. Infections of internal organs other than the lung (e.g. lymph nodes, spleen, liver) have also been reported at postmortem examination.

Treatment is with co-trimoxazole or pentamidine. Adjunctive corticosteroids are given in moderate to severe disease.

## PARASITIC INFECTIONS

**A variety of parasites localize to the lung or involves the lung at some stage in their development**

These include the following:

- Nematodes such as *Ascaris*, *Strongyloides* and hookworm (see Chs. 6 and 23), which migrate through the lungs as they move to the small intestine, breaking out of the capillaries around the alveoli to enter the bronchioles. The damage caused by this process and the development of inflammatory responses can lead to transient pneumonitis with cough, wheeze, dyspnoea and pulmonary infiltrates.

- Schistosome larvae (schistosomulae), which may cause mild respiratory symptoms as they migrate through the lungs. Heavy acute infections may produce pneumonitis with poorly defined nodular lesions or reticulonodular appearances.

- The microfilariae of filarial nematodes such as *Wuchereria* or *Brugia*, which appear in the peripheral circulation, normally with a regular nocturnal periodicity, their appearance coinciding with the time at which the vector mosquitoes are likely to feed. Outside these periods, the larvae become sequestered in the capillaries of the lung. The precise mechanism for sequestration is as yet undefined but thought to include C3-dependent adherence of microfilariae to vascular endothelial cells, pulmonary

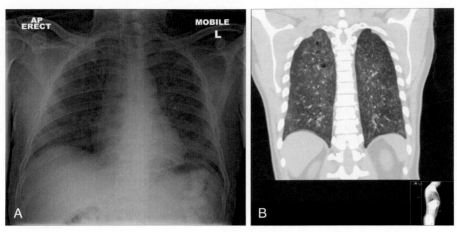

**Fig. 20.35** (A) Chest x-ray and (B) chest computed tomography scan of *Pneumocystis* pneumonia. (Courtesy G. Bain, London North West Healthcare Trust.)

vascular tone, plus the effects of host oxygen tension and temperature. Under certain conditions, as yet undefined and in certain individuals representing <1% of filarial infections, the presence of the larvae triggers a hypersensitivity reaction resulting in a condition known as tropical pulmonary eosinophilia (TPE or Weingarten syndrome). This is characterized by the onset over several months of cough, dyspnoea and wheeze, which is worse at night, and marked peripheral blood eosinophilia of >3000/µL. Microfilariae are absent from the peripheral blood. Antifilarial antibody tests are strongly positive. Chest x-ray examination shows bilateral fine nodular or reticulonodular shadowing, more so in the mid to lower zones. Miliary mottling may be present, leading to confusion with miliary TB.

- Hookworm, *Ascaris* and *Strongyloides* infections, which may also trigger pulmonary eosinophilia, although the condition is distinct from TPE.

- *Echinococcus granulosus* infection, which leads to the development of echinococcal (hydatid) cysts in 20–30% of cases owing to localization of the larvae of this tapeworm in the lungs. These cysts may reach a considerable size, causing respiratory distress, largely as a consequence of the mechanical pressure exerted on lung tissue. Spontaneous rupture may occur and result in acute anaphylaxis.

- *Entamoeba histolytica* infection, which may involve the lung as a complication of amoebic liver abscess.

- *Paragonimus westermani*, the oriental lung fluke, which is the most important example of one of the very few adult parasites that live in the lung, infecting an estimated 22 million people mainly in Asia. Infection is acquired by

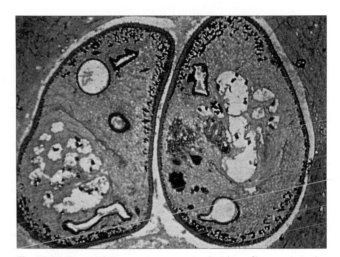

**Fig. 20.36** Two adult *Paragonimus* contained within a fibrous cyst in the lung. (Courtesy H. Zaiman.)

eating crustaceans containing the infective metacercariae. These hatch and migrate from the intestine across the body cavity and penetrate into the lungs. The adults are found, usually as pairs, within fibrous cysts, which connect with the bronchi, thus providing an exit for the eggs, which can be found in sputum and faeces (Fig. 20.36). Infections cause pleuritic chest pain, haemoptysis, chronic cough and fever. Bronchopneumonia can occur when large numbers of parasites are present. Single lesions can be confused with lung cancer, TB and fungal lesions. Praziquantel is an efficient anthelmintic for paragonimiasis.

## KEY FACTS

- Although continuous from nose to alveoli, the respiratory tract is divided into the upper and lower from the viewpoint of infection.
- Infections in the lower respiratory tract are spread by the airborne route (except parasites), are acute or chronic, tend to be severe and may be fatal without correct treatment. They are caused by a wide range of organisms: usually bacteria or viruses but also fungi and parasites.
- Bronchitis, an inflammatory condition of the tracheobronchial tree, is usually chronic with acute exacerbations associated with infection by viruses and bacteria. The disease is characterized by cough and excessive mucous production, and the diagnosis is clinical. Antibiotics are often given, but their efficacy is uncertain.
- Bronchiolitis, usually caused by RSV, is especially acute and severe in infants. RSV causes outbreaks in the community and in hospitals. The disease has an immunopathologic basis, and specific prophylaxis with monoclonal antibodies and treatment with the antiviral drug ribavirin can be given. The first step to prevention by immunization was made in May 2023 when a recombinant protein vaccine was approved for use in specific groups in the United States.
- Pneumonia is caused by a variety of pathogens depending on the individual's age, previous or underlying disease, occupational and geographical factors. Correct microbiologic diagnosis is essential to optimize therapy. Mortality from pneumonia remains significant.
- *B. pertussis* colonizes the ciliated respiratory epithelium causing the specifically human infection whooping cough. Pertussis toxin and other toxic factors are important for virulence. Diagnosis is clinical, alerted by the characteristic paroxysmal cough. Supportive care is paramount; antibiotics play a peripheral role. Prevention by immunization is effective, and new safer vaccines are becoming available.
- Influenza viruses cause endemic, epidemic and pandemic infections as a result of the capacity of the virus for antigenic drift and shift. The disease is acute in onset and can be clinically severe. Viral damage to the respiratory mucosa predisposes to secondary bacterial pneumonia. Antiviral agents are available. Immunization is important, but regular global surveillance and viral sequence analysis are required owing to the frequent antigenic changes in the circulating virus.

- The usual suspects are not always involved in pandemics as was seen in 2019, when another novel coronavirus emerged. Unlike its predecessors, it was highly transmissible and was a global wakeup call about how populations can be affected in many ways by an infectious agent.
- The COVID-19 pandemic triggered a succession of innovations with respect to rapid development of novel vaccines, antiviral and monoclonal antibody treatments, clinical trials of potential treatments and development of molecular diagnostic techniques.
- In addition, controlling the COVID-19 pandemic whilst those developments took place involved extraordinary public health measures, including lockdowns, isolation, stopping travel, tracking and tracing infected individuals and closing down society (including work and school). The effects of some of these measures are still being considered for the future.
- Although the number of TB deaths and the TB incidence rate fell globally up to 2019, the COVID-19 pandemic disrupted this progress, but by 2023 the situation had improved. TB was the second most common cause of death due to infectious diseases worldwide in 2022, the first being SARS-CoV-2.
- Primary infection with *M. tuberculosis* results in a localized pulmonary lesion, whereas secondary disease arises from reactivation as a result of an impairment of immune function. Clinical diagnosis is supported by demonstrating the acid-fast *M. tuberculosis* in sputum. Effective treatment is available, but long courses of drug combinations are essential. Chemoprophylaxis and BCG immunoprophylaxis are important in prevention.
- *Aspergillus* causes disease in the lung ranging from invasive disease in the immunocompromised to allergic conditions in the otherwise healthy. Effective treatment is difficult because of the limited number of active antifungals and lack of host defences.
- Cystic fibrosis is an inherited disease that predisposes to a particular pattern of lung disease characterized by infection with *P. aeruginosa*. Infection can be controlled by antibacterials but is rarely eradicated.
- Various species of parasites pass through or localize in the lungs at some stage in their life cycle. Damage is limited unless the parasite load is high and is usually immunopathologic in nature.

# Urinary tract infections

# 21

## Introduction

### Urinary tract infections are common, especially among women

The urinary tract is one of the most common sites of bacterial infection, particularly in females; 40–60% of women have recurrent urinary tract infections (UTIs) at some time in their life. UTIs in men are less common and primarily occur after 50 years of age. Although the majority of infections are acute and short lived, they contribute to a significant amount of morbidity in the population. Severe infections result in a loss of renal function and serious long-term sequelae. In females, a distinction is made between cystitis, urethritis and vaginitis, but the genitourinary tract is a continuum and symptoms often overlap.

## ACQUISITION AND AETIOLOGY

### Bacterial infection is usually acquired by the ascending route from the urethra to the bladder

The infection may then proceed to the kidney. Occasionally, bacteria infecting the urinary tract invade the bloodstream to cause septicaemia. Less commonly, infection may result from haematogenous spread of an organism to the kidney, with the renal tissue being the first part of the tract to be infected.

From a clinical viewpoint, UTIs are classified as uncomplicated or complicated. Uncomplicated UTIs are usually seen in individuals who are generally healthy and who have no urinary tract abnormalities. These UTIs are further categorized as lower (involving the bladder; cystitis) or upper (kidney infection; pyelonephritis). Complicated UTIs are associated with issues affecting the urinary tract or host response (e.g. urinary obstruction or retention, immune suppression, indwelling catheters).

From an epidemiologic viewpoint, UTIs occur in two general settings: community acquired and health care (nosocomially) acquired, the latter most often being associated with catheterization. Thus complicated UTIs are most often seen in a health care setting.

### The gram-negative rod, *Escherichia coli*, is the commonest cause of all ascending UTIs

Other common gram-negative species include *Klebsiella pneumoniae*, *Pseudomonas aeruginosa* and *Proteus mirabilis* (Table 21.1). *Proteus mirabilis* is also associated with urinary stones (calculi) probably because this organism produces a potent urease, which acts on urea to produce ammonia, rendering the urine alkaline.

Gram-positive species causing infection include *Enterococcus*, group B *Streptococcus*, *Staphylococcus aureus* and *Staphylococcus saprophyticus*, the latter exhibiting a particular propensity for causing infections, especially in young women who are sexually active. UTIs in patients who are

hospitalized (especially those with acquired immunodeficiency syndrome) commonly involve strains exhibiting multiple antibiotic resistance complicating treatment strategies (see Ch. 34). In some instances, capnophilic species (organisms that grow better in air enriched with carbon dioxide), including corynebacteria and lactobacilli, have been implicated as possible causes of UTI. Obligate anaerobes are very rarely involved.

When there has been haematogenous spread to the urinary tract, other species may be found (e.g. *Salmonella typhi*, *S. aureus*, *Mycobacterium tuberculosis* [renal tuberculosis]).

**Table 21.1** Common causes of urinary tract infection (UTI)

| | Uncomplicated UTI (%) | Complicated UTI (%) |
|---|---|---|
| UPEC | 75 | 65 |
| *Klebsiella pneumoniae* | 6 | 8 |
| *Staphylococcus saprophyticus* | 6 | – |
| *Enterococcus* | 5 | 11 |
| Group B *Streptococcus* | 3 | 2 |
| *Proteus mirabilis* | 2 | 2 |
| *Pseudomonas aeruginosa* | 1 | 2 |
| *Staphylococcus aureus* | 1 | 3 |
| *Candida* | 1 | 7 |

UPEC, Uropathogenic *Escherichia coli*.
The approximate percentages of infections caused by different bacteria in uncomplicated and complicated UTIs are shown. *E. coli* is by far the commonest isolate in both groups of patients, but note the difference in the percentage of infections caused by other organisms. These isolates often carry multiple antibiotic resistance and colonize patients in the hospital, especially those receiving antibiotics. (Data taken from Flores-Mireles AL, et al. Urinary tract infections: epidemiology, mechanisms of infection and treatment options. *Nat Rev Microbiol.* 2015;13:269–284.)

The fungus (yeast) *Candida* is also a potential cause of UTIs. However, because the organism is considered an opportunistic pathogen, its presence should spur investigation for more systemic issues (e.g. diabetes, immunosuppression) predisposing to infection (see Ch. 31).

**Viral causes of UTI appear to be rare, although there are associations with haemorrhagic cystitis and other renal syndromes**

Certain viruses may be recovered from the urine in the absence of urinary tract disease and include the following:

* The human polyomaviruses, JC and BK, enter the body via the respiratory tract, spread through the body, and infect epithelial cells in the kidney tubules and ureter, where they establish latency with persistence of the viral genome. The viruses may reactivate asymptomatically, with high viral load detected in the urine due to persistence in the urinary tract. Reactivation may occur in immunocompromised patients, especially transplant recipients (see Ch. 31) and may lead to haemorrhagic cystitis. Polyomavirus-associated nephropathy (PVAN) is an important cause of graft dysfunction and graft loss. PVAN diagnosis is made by carrying out a renal biopsy that shows intranuclear viral inclusions within tubular epithelial cells and immunohistochemical staining for viral antigen. Most renal transplant recipients with PVAN will have a BK virus infection. Less than 1% of recipients may have a JC virus infection that is rarely associated with PVAN.
* High levels of cytomegalovirus DNA and rubella virus RNA may be shed asymptomatically in the urine of congenitally infected infants (see Ch. 24).
* In contrast to asymptomatic shedding, some serotypes of adenovirus have been implicated as a cause of haemorrhagic cystitis.
* The rodent-borne hantaviruses responsible for haemorrhagic fever and renal syndrome, mainly in Europe and Asia, infect capillary blood vessels in the kidney and can cause a renal syndrome with proteinuria.
* Finally, a number of other viruses can infect the kidneys, including mumps and human immunodeficiency virus (HIV).

Urine samples are commonly investigated by molecular detection methods.

**Very few parasites cause UTIs**

Potential causes of UTI include:

* the fungi *Candida* spp. (more common in complicated UTIs), *Cryptococcus* and *Histoplasma capsulatum* (especially in immunocompromised patients)
* the protozoan *Trichomonas vaginalis* (see Ch. 22), which can cause urethritis in both males and females but is most often thought of in the context of vaginitis. Importantly, *T. vaginalis* infection is strongly linked to an increased risk of acquisition and transmission of HIV.
* infections with *Schistosoma haematobium* (see Ch. 28), which result in inflammation of the bladder and commonly haematuria. The eggs penetrate the bladder wall, and in severe infections, large granulomatous reactions and bladder fibrosis can occur and the eggs may become

calcified. The World Health Organization classifies *S. haematobium* as a class 1 carcinogen. The causative mechanism responsible for squamous cell bladder cancer is unclear at present, but actions of the parasite, the host immune response, tissue regeneration, coinfections, and environmental exposure to carcinogens are all thought to play a part. Obstruction of the ureter as a result of egg-induced inflammatory changes can also lead to hydronephrosis.

## PATHOGENESIS

### A variety of mechanical factors predispose to UTI

Anything that disrupts normal urine flow or complete emptying of the bladder or facilitates access of organisms to the bladder will predispose an individual to infection (Fig. 21.1). The shorter female urethra is a less effective deterrent to infection than the male urethra (see Ch. 14). Sexual intercourse facilitates the movement of organisms up the urethra, particularly in females, so the incidence of UTI is higher among women who are sexually active than celibate. Preceding bacterial colonization of the periurethral area of the vagina is perhaps important (see later).

In male infants, UTIs are more common in those who are uncircumcised, and this is associated with colonization of the inside of the prepuce and urethra with faecal organisms.

**Pregnancy, prostatic hypertrophy, renal calculi, tumours and strictures are the main causes of obstruction to complete bladder emptying**

Increased volumes of postvoid residual urine are associated with a greater likelihood of infection. Infection superimposed on urinary tract obstruction may lead to ascent of infection to the kidney and rapid destruction of renal tissue.

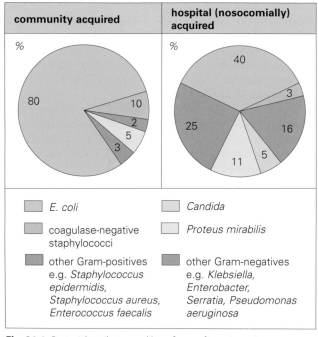

**Fig. 21.1** Bacterial attributes and host factors favouring urinary tract infection (UTI). Abnormalities of the urinary tract tend to predispose to infection. Bacterial adherence factors have been studied in detail, but relatively little is known about other bacterial virulence factors in UTI.

Loss of neurologic control of the bladder and sphincters (e.g. in spina bifida, paraplegia, multiple sclerosis) and the resultant large residual volume of urine in the bladder cause a functional obstruction to urine flow, and such patients are particularly prone to recurrent infections.

Vesicoureteral reflux (reflux of urine from the bladder cavity up the ureters, sometimes into the renal pelvis or parenchyma) is common in children with anatomic abnormalities of the urinary tract and may predispose to ascending infection and kidney damage. Reflux may also occur in association with infection in children without underlying abnormalities but tends to disappear with age.

Clinical studies indicate an increased propensity for UTI in individuals with diabetes mellitus. People with diabetes mellitus may have more severe UTIs, and if diabetic neuropathy interferes with normal bladder function, then persistent UTIs are common.

### Catheterization is a major predisposing factor for UTI

During insertion of the catheter, bacteria may be carried directly into the bladder; while in situ, the catheter facilitates bacterial access to the bladder either via the lumen of the catheter or by tracking up between the outside of the catheter and the urethral wall. The catheter disrupts the normal bladder's protective function action and allows bacterial introduction into the bladder as the catheter is inserted; while the catheter is in place, bacteria reach the bladder by tracking up between the outside of the catheter and the urethra. Contamination of the catheter drainage system by bacteria from other sources can also result in infection. The duration of catheterization (e.g. ≥2 days) is directly associated with increased probability of infection due, in part, to the formation of biofilms (see Ch. 2), which protect the organisms from antimicrobials and host defence mechanisms. Thus the risk of UTI increases by about 3–10% each day of catheterization.

### A variety of virulence factors are present in the causative organisms

The conflict between host and parasite in the urinary tract has been discussed in Chapter 14. Most urinary tract pathogens originate in the faecal flora, but only the aerobic and facultative species such as *E. coli* possess the attributes required to colonize and infect the urinary tract. The ability to cause infection of the urinary tract is associated with certain serogroups of *E. coli* such as O (semantic) serotypes (e.g. O1, O2, O4, O6, O7, O8, O75) and K (capsular) serotypes (e.g. K1, K2, K3, K5, K12, K13). These serotypes differ from those associated with gastrointestinal tract infection (see Ch. 23), which has led to use of the term *uropathogenic E. coli (UPEC)*. The success of these strains is attributable to a variety of genes in chromosomal pathogenicity islands (see Ch. 2), which are not found in faecal *E. coli*. For example, UPEC typically contains genes associated with colonization of the periurethral areas. A prime example is the adhesion known as *P fimbriae* (pyelonephritis-associated pili), which allows UPEC to adhere specifically to urethral and bladder epithelium. Studies with other species of urinary tract pathogens have confirmed the presence of similar adhesins for uroepithelial cells (Fig. 21.2).

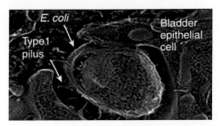

**Fig. 21.2** High-resolution deep-etch electron micrograph showing attachment of Enteropathogenic *E. coli* (EPEC) to bladder epithelial cells. (Reprinted with permission from American Association for the Advancement of Science. Mulvey MA, Lopez-Boado YS, Wilson CL, et al. Introduction and evasion of host defenses by type 1-piliated uropathogenic *Escherichia coli. Science.* 1998;282:1494–1497.)

Other features of *E. coli* that appear to assist in the localization of organisms in the kidney and in renal damage include the following:

- The capsular acid polysaccharide (K) antigens are associated with the ability to cause pyelonephritis and are known to enable *E. coli* strains to resist host defences by inhibiting phagocytosis.
- Haemolysin production by *E. coli* is linked with the capacity to cause kidney damage; many haemolysins act more generally as membrane-damaging toxins.

The production of urease by organisms such as *Proteus* spp. has been correlated with their ability to cause pyelonephritis and stones.

### The healthy urinary tract is resistant to bacterial colonization

With the exception of the urethral mucosa, the urinary tract usually eliminates microorganisms rapidly and efficiently (see Ch. 14). The pH, chemical content, and flushing mechanism of urine help dispose of organisms in the urethra. Although urine is a good culture medium for most bacteria, it is inhibitory to some, and anaerobes and other species (non-haemolytic streptococci, corynebacterial, staphylococci) that comprise most of the normal urethral flora do not readily multiply in urine.

Although the inflammatory response to UTI involves leukocytic, chemokine and cytokine response, the role of humoral immunity in the host's defence against infection of the urinary tract is poorly understood. After infection of the kidney, immunoglobulin G (IgG) and secretory IgA antibodies can be detected in urine but do not appear to protect against subsequent infection. Infection of the lower urinary tract is usually associated with a low serologic response, reflecting the superficial nature of the infection.

## CLINICAL FEATURES AND COMPLICATIONS

### Acute lower UTIs cause dysuria, urgency and frequency

Acute infections of the lower urinary tract are characterized by a rapid onset of:

- dysuria (burning pain on passing urine)
- urgency (the urgent need to pass urine)
- frequency of micturition.

However, UTIs in the elderly and those with indwelling catheters are usually asymptomatic.

The urine is cloudy, owing to the presence of pus cells (pyuria) and bacteria (bacteriuria), and may contain blood (haematuria). Examination of urine specimens in the laboratory is essential to confirm diagnosis. Patients with genital tract infections such as vaginal thrush or chlamydial urethritis may present with similar symptoms (see Ch. 22).

Pyuria in the absence of positive urine cultures can be due to chlamydiae or tuberculosis and is seen in patients receiving antibacterial therapy for UTI, as the bacteria are inhibited or killed by the antibacterial agent before the inflammatory response dies away.

Recurrent infections of the lower urinary tract occur in a significant proportion of patients. They may be:

- relapses caused by the same strain of organism
- reinfections by different organisms.

Recurrent infections can result in chronic inflammatory changes in the bladder, prostate and periurethral glands.

### Acute bacterial prostatitis causes systemic symptoms (fever) and local symptoms (perineal and low back pain, dysuria, frequency)

Acute bacterial prostatitis may arise from ascending or haematogenous infection, and people lacking the antibacterial substances normally present in prostatic fluid are perhaps more susceptible. Chronic bacterial prostatitis, however, although usually caused by *E. coli*, is difficult to cure and can be a source of relapsing infection within the urinary tract.

## Upper UTIs

Although it may be important to know whether an infection is restricted to the bladder (lower urinary tract) or has ascended to the upper urinary tract and kidney, distinguishing the two can be difficult (e.g. examining urine directly from the ureter by ureteric catheterization).

### Pyelonephritis causes a fever and lower urinary tract symptoms

Patients with pyelonephritis (infection of the kidney) present with lower urinary tract symptoms and usually have a fever. UPEC is the common cause, and renal abscesses may be present. Recurrent episodes of pyelonephritis result in a loss of function of renal tissue, which may, in turn, cause hypertension, itself a cause of renal damage. Infection associated with stone formation can result in obstruction of the renal tract and septicaemia.

Haematuria is a feature of endocarditis and a manifestation of immune complex disease, as well as a result of infections of the kidney, and its presence warrants careful investigation. Pyuria may be associated with kidney infection by *M. tuberculosis*. This organism cannot be grown by normal urine culture methods, and, therefore, the patient may appear to have sterile pyuria.

Asymptomatic infection (i.e. significant numbers of bacteria in the urine in the absence of symptoms; see later) can be detected only by screening urine samples in the laboratory. It is important in instances such as:

- pregnant women and young children in whom failure to treat may result in chronic renal damage
- people undergoing instrumentation of the urinary tract in whom bacteriuria may proceed to bacteraemia
- the elderly and those with diabetes (both risk factors for asymptomatic bacteriuria).

## LABORATORY DIAGNOSIS

A key feature is the detection of significant bacteriuria.

### Infection can be distinguished from contamination by quantitative culture methods

Historically, the urinary tract has been considered to be sterile; however, modern molecular methods indicate that low levels of harmless organisms may be present. The distal region of the urethra is colonized with commensal organisms, which may include periurethral and faecal organisms. Because urine specimens are usually collected by voiding a specimen into a sterile container, they may become contaminated with the periurethral flora during collection. However, infection is traditionally distinguished from contamination by quantitative culture methods. Bacteriuria is defined as significant when a properly collected midstream urine (MSU) specimen is shown to contain over $10^5$ organisms/mL. Infected urine usually contains a single predominant bacterial species. Contaminated urine usually has <$10^4$ organisms/mL and often contains more than one bacterial species (Fig. 21.3). Distinguishing infection from contamination when counts are $10^4$–$10^5$ organisms/mL can be difficult. Careful collection and rapid transport of urine specimens to the laboratory are essential (see later).

It is important to recognize that the criteria for significant bacteriuria do not apply to urine specimens collected from catheters or nephrostomy tubes or by suprapubic aspiration directly from the bladder in which any number of organisms may be significant because the specimen is not contaminated by periurethral flora. In addition, infection of sites in the urinary tract below the bladder and by organisms that are not members of the normal faecal flora may not lead to the presence of significant numbers in the urine.

### The usual urine specimen for microbiologic examination is an MSU sample

An MSU sample should be collected into a sterile wide-mouthed container after careful cleansing of the labia or glans with soap (not antiseptic) and water and after allowing

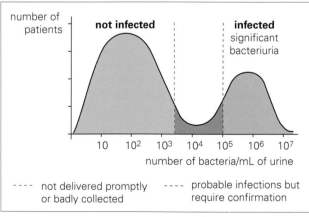

**Fig. 21.3** Significant bacteriuria. Voided specimens of urine are rarely sterile because the urine is contaminated with organisms from the periurethral area during collection. Even well-collected specimens from healthy individuals may contain up to $10^3$ bacteria/mL of urine. A count of $10^5$ bacteria/mL is considered a reliable indicator of infection. However, there are various reasons why lower counts may sometimes be significant (acute dysuria, ureteral obstruction, etc.).

the first part of the urine stream to be voided, as this helps to wash out contaminants in the lower urethra. After suitable instruction, the majority of adult patients can collect satisfactory samples with minimum supervision, although collection may be difficult for elderly and bedridden patients; consideration should be given to these difficulties when interpreting results.

Collection of MSU samples from babies and young children is difficult. Bag urine may be collected by sticking a plastic bag to the perineum in girls or to the penis in boys, but such specimens are frequently heavily contaminated with faecal organisms. These problems can be overcome by suprapubic aspiration of urine directly from the bladder.

Urine specimens should be transported to the laboratory with minimum delay because urine is a good growth medium for many bacteria and multiplication of organisms in the specimen between collection and culture will distort the results, giving much greater numbers than those present in the patient.

Ideally, samples should be collected before antimicrobial therapy is started. If the patient is receiving or has received therapy within the previous 48 hours, this should be stated clearly on the request form.

### For patients with a catheter, a catheter specimen of urine is used for microbiologic examination

Patients should not be catheterized simply to obtain a urine sample. Urine is obtained from patients who have a catheter in situ by withdrawing a sample with a syringe and needle from the catheter tube.

### Special urine samples are required to detect *Mycobacterium tuberculosis* and *Schistosoma haematobium*

These include the following:

- Three early-morning urine samples on consecutive days for *M. tuberculosis*; these do not require the same precautions during collection as an MSU sample because the culture technique prohibits the growth of organisms other than mycobacteria. Molecular tests (e.g. polymerase chain reaction) are now widely used to expedite *M. tuberculosis* diagnosis.
- The last few millilitres of a urine sample are collected early in the afternoon after exercise for detection of *S. haematobium* eggs.

## Laboratory investigations

Urine specimens should be examined macroscopically and microscopically and should be cultured by quantitative or semiquantitative methods (see Ch. 32).

### Microscopic examination of urine allows a rapid preliminary report

Bacteria may be seen on microscopy when present in the specimen in large numbers. However, they are not necessarily indicative of infection but may indicate that the specimen has been poorly collected or left at room temperature for a prolonged time.

The presence of red and white blood cells, although abnormal, is not necessarily indicative of UTI. Haematuria may be present in association with:

- infection of the urinary tract and elsewhere (e.g. bacterial endocarditis)
- renal trauma
- calculi
- urinary tract carcinomas
- clotting disorders
- thrombocytopenia.

Occasionally red blood cells may contaminate urine specimens in women who are menstruating.

White blood cells are present in the urine in very small numbers (e.g. <5 per high power microscopic field) in healthy individuals; a higher count is considered abnormal but is not always associated with bacteriuria. Sterile pyuria is an important finding and may reflect:

- concurrent antibiotic therapy
- other diseases such as neoplasms or urinary calculi
- infection with organisms not detected by routine urine culture methods.
- renal tubular cells seen in the urine of aspirin misusers that may be confused with white blood cells. Urinary casts are also indicative of renal tubular damage.

### A laboratory diagnosis of significant bacteriuria requires quantification of the bacteria

Conventional culture methods produce results within 18–24 hours, but rapid methods (e.g. dipstick tests for leukocyte esterase/nitrate reductase; white blood cells and nitrate-reducing bacteria, respectively) are also available. In some laboratories, direct antibiotic susceptibility tests may be initiated upon detection of abnormal numbers of white blood cells or bacteria on microscopy so that both culture and susceptibility results are available within 24 hours.

### Interpretation of the significance of bacterial culture results depends on a variety of factors

These factors relate to:

- *collection* — the specimen collection must be carried out properly
- *storage* — the urine must be cultured within 2 hours of collection or held at 4°C for ≤24 hours before culture
- *antibiotic treatment* — in a patient receiving antibiotics, smaller numbers of organisms may be significant and may represent an emerging resistant population; laboratory methods are available to detect antibacterial substances
- *fluid intake* — the patient may be taking more or less fluid than usual, and this will clearly influence the quantitative result
- *the specimen* — the quantitative guidelines are valid for MSU specimens; they do not apply to catheter specimens, suprapubic aspirates or nephrostomy samples.

## TREATMENT

### Depending on clinical evaluation of the patient and local antimicrobial resistance trends, uncomplicated UTI is typically treated with an oral antibacterial (e.g. for 3 days)

Uncomplicated UTI (cystitis) generally resolves spontaneously within 4–6 weeks in up to 40% of patients; however, treatment with antibacterial agents reduces symptoms and ensures bacterial eradication. Administration of oral

**Table 21.2** Examples of oral antibacterials for urinary tract infections (UTIs)

| Common oral antibacterials for UTIs | | |
|---|---|---|
| **Antibacterial** | **Class of agent** | **Comments** |
| Trimethoprim | Antimetabolite/nucleic acid synthesis inhibitor | Incidence of resistant strains increasing |
| Trimethoprim-sulphamethoxazole | Combination of trimethoprim with sulphamethoxazole (also antimetabolite nucleic acid synthesis inhibitor) | One of the most common first-line therapeutic approaches; may be useful in blind treatment but more toxic than trimethoprim alone; resistance is also an issue |
| Nitrofurantoin | Urinary antiseptic | For uncomplicated UTI caused by *Escherichia coli* and *Staphylococcus saprophyticus*; not active in alkaline pH, therefore, not useful for *Proteus* infections |
| Ciprofloxacin, levofloxacin, ofloxacin, etc. | Fluoroquinolone | Very broad spectrum; not highly active against enterococci; increasing resistance an issue |

Several different classes of antibacterial are available in oral formulations and suitable for treatment of UTI. Nitrofurantoin is useful only for lower UTIs as it does not achieve adequate serum and tissue concentrations to treat upper UTIs.

antimicrobial chemotherapy depends on the drug and the clinical evaluation of the patient. Examples of commonly prescribed agents are shown in Table 21.2. The choice of agent should be based on the results of susceptibility tests. However, for uncomplicated UTIs in patients in the community, therapy is often best guess at least until laboratory results are available. This requires knowledge of the likely pathogens, their antibiotic susceptibility patterns in the locality and predisposing patient host factors. Follow-up cultures should be carried out after treatment for complicated UTIs or where symptoms have not resolved. In addition to antibacterial therapy, the patient should be advised to drink large volumes of fluid to help the normal flushing process.

Children and pregnant women with asymptomatic bacteriuria should be treated with antibacterials and followed up with to check for eradication of the infection. Instrumentation of the urinary tract should be delayed in patients with significant bacteriuria until appropriate treatment has eliminated the infection.

### Initial treatment of complicated UTI (pyelonephritis) usually involves a longer period of treatment (e.g. 10–14 days)

Hospital-acquired infections or recurrent infections, particularly in catheterized patients, may be caused by antibiotic-resistant organisms, and the agent of choice will depend on the antibacterial susceptibility pattern. If possible, the catheter should be removed, as eradication of infection is extremely difficult to achieve in catheterized patients, and some would advocate treatment only when the patient complains of symptoms or before invasive procedures. Guidelines for catheter care and for the prevention of catheter-associated UTIs are shown in Box 21.1.

Infections acquired by haematogenous spread require specific antibacterial therapy as described in Chapter 34 for tuberculosis, Chapter 23 for *S. typhi*, Chapter 27 for *S. aureus* and Chapter 28 for schistosomiasis.

---

**Box 21.1    Guidelines for catheter care**

- Avoid catheterization whenever possible.
- Keep duration of catheterization to a minimum.
- Use intermittent rather than continuous catheterization when feasible.
- Insert catheters with good aseptic technique.
- Use a closed sterile drainage system.
- Maintain a gravity drain.
- Use topical antiseptics around the meatus in women.
- Wash hands before and after inserting catheters and collecting specimens and after emptying drainage bags.
- Catheters that drain into open collecting vessels are highly conducive to infection. Thus closed drainage systems are now used in most hospitals; even then, bacteriuria occurs in a significant number of patients.

### PREVENTION

**Many of the features of the pathogenesis of UTI and host predispositions are not clearly understood**

Recurrent infections in otherwise healthy women can be prevented by regularly emptying the bladder. This washes bacteria out of the urinary tract and is particularly important following intercourse. The prophylactic use of antibiotics may also prevent recurrent infections, but in the presence of underlying abnormalities, there is a tendency to select antibiotic-resistant strains, which subsequently cause infections that are more difficult to treat.

Infection in catheterized patients is very common but can be reduced by good catheter care procedures (see Box 21.1; also see Ch. 37). Catheterization should be avoided if possible or kept to a minimum duration because, as noted earlier, the risk of UTI increases by about 3–10% each day of catheterization.

## KEY FACTS

- UTIs are among the commonest bacterial infections, especially in women.

- Most UTIs are acute episodes without sequelae.

- UTIs are usually endogenously acquired, with colonizing bacteria ascending the urinary tract from the periurethral area. *E. coli* is the predominant pathogen; other gram-negative rods are also responsible, especially in patients who are hospitalized. Viruses are not important causes of UTI.

- Structural or mechanical factors in the host, or catheterization, predispose to infection.

- Bacterial attributes such as adhesions and capsular polysaccharides may be important in the development of UTI. Specific toxins are not implicated, but haemolysins (cytotoxins) may be.

- Lower UTI usually presents with acute frequency and dysuria. Asymptomatic infection is common in pregnancy and in children. Infection is recurrent in a significant proportion of people.

- Pyelonephritis (upper UTI) has a more severe presentation than does lower UTI, with fever and loin pain; recurrent infection results in renal damage.

- Bacteriologic confirmation of the diagnosis requires quantitative methods. Pyuria also implies infection.

- Short-course treatment with oral antibacterials is effective for lower UTI; pyelonephritis needs longer treatment.

- Hospital-acquired UTI is often caused by multiple-resistant gram-negative bacteria, and treatment should be based on the results of antibiotic susceptibility tests.

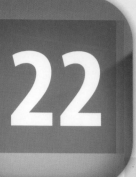

# Sexually transmitted infections

## Introduction

### Sexually transmitted infections usually cause diseases

In some instances, sexually transmitted infections (STIs) may not result in overt disease symptoms, such as in the early stages of human immunodeficiency virus (HIV) infection and asymptomatic gonorrhoea in females. This is particularly concerning as people with asymptomatic or unreported STIs are unlikely to receive treatment, thus facilitating further cycles of infection and spread. While STIs are of major medical importance throughout the world, HIV infection has had the greatest global impact, estimated to affect >38 million people in 2021. In addition to HIV, new cases of other STIs occur globally with alarming frequency (hundreds of millions of new cases) each year.

### STIs are difficult to control

This is typified by the situation in the United Kingdom where there were 311,604 new STI cases reported by genitourinary medicine clinics in 2021. A similar situation exists in other countries, including the United States. The reasons for this increase include:

- increasing density and mobility of human populations
- the difficulty of engineering changes in human sexual behaviour
- the absence of vaccines for almost all STIs, except for the human papillomavirus (HPV) vaccine.

HIV infection, syphilis, gonorrhoea, chlamydia and genital wart infections are some of the STIs included in national and global surveillance programmes.

The most common STIs are listed in Table 22.1. Table 22.2 gives examples of the strategies used by the pathogens to overcome host defences.

### STIs AND SEXUAL BEHAVIOUR

The general principles of entry, exit and transmission of the pathogens that cause STIs are set out in Chapter 14.

#### The spread of STIs is inextricably linked with sexual behaviour

There are therefore many more opportunities for controlling STIs than, for instance, respiratory infections. Infected but asymptomatic individuals play an important role, and important determinants are promiscuity and sexual practices involving contact between different orifices and mucosal surfaces (see Ch. 14). For example, transmission between heterosexuals or men who have sex with men (MSM) can take place following oral or anal intercourse. The gonococcus, for instance, causes pharyngitis and proctitis, although it infects stratified squamous epithelium less readily than columnar epithelium. As described more fully in Chapter 33, calculations regarding the number of infected secondary cases resulting from each primary STI case depends on a variety of behavioural factors since the number of sexual partners acquired by a given individual

(i.e. the level of promiscuity) varies considerably. Those who have many sexual partners are both more likely to acquire and to transmit infection and play a key role in the persistence of such infections in the community of sexually active individuals. People with many sexual partners are therefore an obvious target for treatment and education about safer sex practices such as condom use.

#### Various host factors influence the risk of acquiring an STI

It is not surprising that the type of sexual activity is important or that genital lesions or ulcers increase the risk of acquiring infections such as HIV. In addition, it is well reported that uncircumcised men have a higher risk of infection.

STIs do not necessarily occur singly, and the possibility of multiple infections must always be borne in mind. For instance, syphilis can accompany gonorrhoea, and there is evidence that genital herpes may be reactivated during an attack of gonorrhoea.

### SYPHILIS

#### Syphilis is caused by the spirochete *Treponema pallidum*

*T. pallidum* is closely related to the treponemes that cause the nonvenereal infections of pinta and yaws (Table 22.3; Fig. 22.1). *T. pallidum* has a worldwide distribution, and syphilis remains a serious problem not only in resource-rich countries but also especially in resource-poor areas due to the serious sequelae and the risk of congenital infection. In the United States during 2020–2021 the rate of syphilis increased by almost 30%, and congenital syphilis increased by 15%, a trend that continues currently and has also been seen in the United Kingdom.

*T. pallidum* enters the body through minute abrasions on the skin or mucous membranes. Transmission of *T. pallidum* requires close personal contact because the organism does not survive well outside the body and is very sensitive to drying, heat and disinfectants. Horizontal spread (see Ch. 14) occurs through sexual contact, and vertical spread occurs via transplacental infection of the fetus (see Ch. 24).

**Table 22.1** The most common sexually transmitted infections (STIs)

| Organism | Disease | Comment | Treatment |
|---|---|---|---|
| Papillomaviruses (types 6, 11, 16, 18) | Genital warts, dysplasias | Vaccines available; most common STI in the United States | Podophyllin Imiquimod Cryotherapy Cidofovir gel |
| Chlamydia trachomatis | D-K serotypes (nonspecific urethritis); L serotypes (lymphogranuloma venereum) | Most common easily cured STI in the United States; urethritis very common; lymphogranuloma venereum primarily in resource-poor countries | Azithromycin, doxycycline |
| Candida albicans | Vaginal thrush | Predisposing factors | Clotrimazole, fluconazole |
| Trichomonas vaginalis | Vaginitis, urethritis | Often asymptomatic; causes ~50% of curable vaginal infections worldwide | Metronidazole, tinidazole |
| Herpes simplex virus types 1 and 2 | Genital herpes | Problem of latency and reactivation | Acyclovir, valacyclovir, famciclovir |
| Neisseria gonorrhoeae | Gonorrhoea | Second most commonly reported notifiable disease in the United States; quinolone resistance common | Cephalosporin (e.g. ceftriaxone) |
| Human immunodeficiency virus (HIV) | Acquired immunodeficiency syndrome | Number of new HIV infections was falling by 2021 in most countries worldwide | Antiretroviral drugs |
| Treponema pallidum | Syphilis | Incidence increasing in the United States | Penicillin |
| Hepatitis B virus | Hepatitis B | Vaccine available | Antivirals include tenofovir, entecavir, lamivudine, interferon alpha |
| Haemophilus ducreyi | Chancroid | Mainly tropical | Azithromycin, ceftriaxone |
| Sarcoptes scabiei | Genital scabies | Human mite burrows into upper skin layer | Permethrin cream |
| Phthirus pubis | Pubic lice | Number 1 louse infestation in US adults | Permethrin cream |

**Table 22.2** Strategies adopted by sexually transmitted microorganisms to combat host defences

| Host defences | Microbial strategies | Examples |
|---|---|---|
| Integrity of mucosal surface | Specific attachment mechanism | Gonococcus or chlamydia to urethral epithelium |
| Urine flow (for urethral infection) | Specific attachment; induce own uptake and transport across urethral epithelial surface in phagocytic vacuole | Gonococcus |
| | Infection of urethral epithelial or subepithelial cells | Herpes simplex virus (HSV), chlamydia |
| Phagocytes (especially polymorphs) | Induce negligible inflammation | Treponema pallidum, mechanism unclear, perhaps poorly activates alternative complement pathway due to sialic acid coating |
| | Resist phagocytosis | Gonococcus (capsule), T. pallidum (absorbed fibronectin) |
| Complement | C3d receptor on pathogen binds C3b/d and reduces C3b/d-mediated polymorph phagocytosis | Candida albicans |
| Inflammation | Induce strong inflammatory response, yet evade consequences | Gonococcus, C. albicans, HSV, chlamydia |
| Antibodies (especially IgA) | Produce IgA protease | Gonococcus |
| Cell-mediated immune response (T cells, lymphokines, natural killer cells, etc.) | Antigenic variation; allows reinfection of a given individual with an antigenic variant | Gonococcus, chlamydia |
| | Poorly understood factors cause ineffective cell-mediated immune response | T. pallidum, human immunodeficiency virus |

**Table 22.3** Spiral organisms of medical importance

| Family | Genus | Species | Subspecies | Disease |
|---|---|---|---|---|
| Spirochaetaceae | *Treponema* | *pallidum* | *pallidum* | Syphilis |
| | | *pallidum* | *pertenue* | Yaws |
| | | *carateum* | | Pinta |
| | *Borrelia* | *recurrentis* | | Relapsing fever |
| | | *burgdorferi* | | Lyme disease |
| Leptospiraceae | *Leptospira* | *interrogans* | (serovar) Icterohaemorrhagiae | Leptospirosis (Weil disease) |

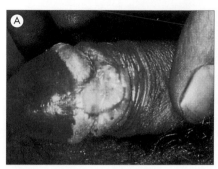
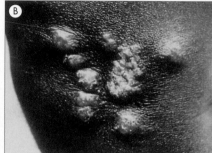
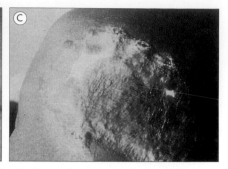

**Fig. 22.1** (A) Typical penile chancre of primary syphilis. (B) Yaws and (C) pinta are endemic in tropical and subtropical countries and are spread by direct contact. (A, Courtesy R.D. Catterall; B and C, courtesy P.J. Cooper and G. Griffin.)

Local multiplication leads to plasma cell, polymorph and macrophage infiltration, with later endarteritis. The bacteria multiply very slowly, and the average incubation period is 3 weeks.

### Classically, *T. pallidum* infection is divided into three stages

The three classical stages of syphilis are primary, secondary and tertiary syphilis (Table 22.4). However, not all patients go through all three stages; a substantial proportion remains permanently free of disease after suffering the primary or secondary stages of infection. The lesion of primary syphilis is illustrated in Fig. 22.1. The secondary stage may be followed by a latent period of some 3–30 years, after which the disease may recur (tertiary stage). Unlike most bacterial pathogens, *T. pallidum* can survive in the body for many years despite a vigorous immune response. It has been suggested that the healthy treponeme evades recognition and elimination by the host by maintaining a cell surface rich in lipid. This layer is antigenically unreactive, and the antigens are uncovered only in dead and dying organisms when the host is then able to respond. Tissue damage is mostly due to the host response.

Despite many years of effort, *T. pallidum* still cannot be cultivated in the laboratory in artificial media. It has therefore been difficult to study possible virulence factors at a molecular level although more recent advances in whole genome sequencing, will allow better molecular characterization.

### An infected woman can transmit *T. pallidum* to her baby in utero

Congenital syphilis is acquired after the first 3 months of pregnancy. The disease may manifest as:

- serious infection resulting in intrauterine death
- congenital abnormalities, which may be obvious at birth
- silent infection, which may not be apparent until about 2 years of age (facial and tooth deformities).

## Laboratory diagnosis of syphilis

As *T. pallidum* cannot be grown in vitro, laboratory diagnosis hinges on microscopy and serology.

### Microscopy

Exudate from the primary chancre should be examined by either dark field microscopy immediately after collection or ultraviolet (UV) microscopy after staining with fluorescein-labelled antitreponemal antibodies.

The organisms have tightly wound, slender coils with pointed ends and are sluggishly motile in unstained preparations. *T. pallidum* is very thin (~0.2 mm in diameter, compared with *Escherichia coli*, which is ~1 mm) and cannot be seen in Gram-stained preparations. Silver impregnation stains can be used to demonstrate the organisms in biopsy material.

### Serology

Serologic tests for syphilis are the mainstay of diagnosis. They are divided into nonspecific and specific tests for the detection of antibodies in patients' serum.

### Nonspecific tests (nontreponemal tests) for syphilis

The term *nonspecific* is used because the antigens are not treponemal in origin but are from extracts of normal mammalian tissues. Cardiolipin, from beef heart, allows the detection of antilipid immunoglobulin G (IgG) and IgM formed in the patient in response to lipoidal material released from cells damaged by the infection, as well as to lipids in the surface of *T. pallidum*. Two tests in common use today are the Venereal Disease Research Laboratory test and the rapid plasma reagin test. Both are available in kit form.

Nonspecific tests show up as positive within 4–6 weeks of infection (or 1–2 weeks after the primary chancre appears) and decline in positivity in tertiary syphilis or after effective antibiotic treatment of primary or secondary disease.

**Table 22.4** The pathogenesis of syphilis

| Stage of disease | Signs and symptoms | Pathogenesis |
|---|---|---|
| Initial contact<br><br>↓<br><br>2–10 weeks (depends on inoculum size) | Primary chancre[a] at site of infection | Multiplication of treponemas at site of infection; associated host response |
| ↓<br>Primary syphilis<br>↓<br>1–3 months | Enlarged inguinal nodes, spontaneous healing | Proliferation of treponemas in regional lymph nodes |
| ↓<br>Secondary syphilis<br>↓<br>2–6 weeks | Flulike illness; myalgia, headache, fever; mucocutaneous rash[a]; spontaneous resolution | Multiplication and production of lesion in lymph nodes, liver, joints, muscles, skin and mucous membranes |
| ↓<br><br>Latent syphilis<br><br>↓<br>3–30 years | | Treponemas dormant in liver or spleen<br><br><br><br>Reawakening and multiplication of treponemas |
| Tertiary syphilis | Neurosyphilis; "general paralysis of the insane," tabes dorsalis<br>Cardiovascular syphilis; aortic lesions, heart failure<br>Progressive destructor disease | Further dissemination and invasion and host response (cell-mediated hypersensitivity)<br><br><br>Gummas in skin, bones, testis |

A feature of *Treponema pallidum* infection is its chronic nature, which seems to involve a delicately balanced relationship between pathogen and host.
[a]Chancre: initially a papule; forms a painless ulcer; heals without treatment within 2 months. Live treponemas can be seen in dark-ground microscopy of fluid from lesions; patient highly infectious.

Therefore these tests are useful for screening. However, they are nonspecific and may give positive results in conditions other than syphilis (biologic false positives) (Table 22.5). All positive results should therefore be confirmed by a specific test. However, treatment (e.g. especially during the primary and secondary stages) tends to result in seroreversion to these tests. Thus with confirmed disease (see later), these tests can provide at least an indication of therapeutic efficacy.

### Commonly used specific tests for syphilis

These tests use recombinant proteins or treponemal antigens extracted from *T. pallidum*. Tests in common use include:

- the enzyme-linked immunosorbent assay, which detects IgM and IgG
- the fluorescent treponemal antibody absorption test (Fig. 22.2) in which the patient's serum is first absorbed with nonpathogenic treponemes to remove cross-reacting antibodies before reaction with *T. pallidum* antigens
- the microhaemagglutination assay for *T. pallidum*.

These tests should be used to confirm that a positive result with a nonspecific test is truly due to syphilis. Also, because they become positive earlier in the course of the disease, they can be used for confirmation when the clinical picture is strongly indicative of syphilis. They tend to remain positive for many years and may be the only positive test in patients with late syphilis. However, they remain positive

**Table 22.5** Serologic tests for syphilis and conditions associated with false-positive results

| Test | Conditions associated with false-positive results |
|---|---|
| Nonspecific (nontreponemal)<br>VDRL<br>RPR | Viral infection, collagen vascular disease, acute febrile disease, postimmunisation, pregnancy, leprosy, malaria, drug misuse |
| Specific (nontreponemal)<br>FTA-ABS<br>TP-PA<br>TPHA | Diseases associated with increased or abnormal globulins, lupus erythematosus, Lyme disease, autoimmune disease, diabetes mellitus, alcoholic cirrhosis, viral infections, drug misuse, pregnancy |

FTA-ABS, Fluorescent treponemal antibody absorption test; MHA-TP, microhaemagglutination assay for *T. pallidum*; RPR, rapid plasma reagin test; TPHA, *T. pallidum* haemagglutination test; TP-PA, *T. pallidum* particle agglutination test; VDRL, Venereal Disease Research Laboratory test.

after appropriate antibiotic treatment and therefore cannot be used as indicators of therapeutic response. They can also give false-positive reactions (see Table 22.5).

### Confirmation of a diagnosis of syphilis depends upon several serologic tests

Positive serologic test results for babies born to infected mothers may represent passive transfer of maternal antibody

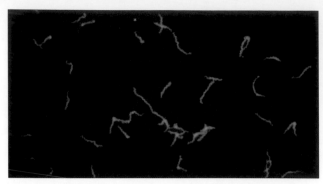

**Fig. 22.2** The fluorescent treponemal antibody absorption test for syphilis. Antibody in the patient's serum binds to bacteria and is visualized by a fluorescent dye.

or the baby's own response to infection. These two possibilities can be distinguished by testing for IgM and retesting at 6 months of age, by which time maternal antibody levels have waned. Antibody titres remain elevated in babies with congenital syphilis.

At present, several serologic tests are needed to confirm a diagnosis of syphilis. None of these tests distinguishes syphilis from the nonsexually transmitted treponematoses, yaws and pinta. Western blot assays for *T. pallidum* are also a potential confirmatory test.

### Treatment

#### Penicillin is the drug of choice for treating people with syphilis and their contacts

Penicillin is very active against *T. pallidum* (see Table 22.1). For patients who are allergic to penicillin, treatment with doxycycline should be given. Only penicillin therapy reliably treats the fetus when administered to a pregnant mother.

Prevention of secondary and tertiary disease depends upon early diagnosis and adequate treatment. Contact tracing with screening and treatment are also important. Several STIs may be present in one patient concurrently, and patients with other STIs should be screened for syphilis.

Congenital syphilis is completely preventable if women are screened serologically early in pregnancy (<3 months) and if those who are positive are treated with penicillin.

## GONORRHOEA

#### Gonorrhoea is caused by the gram-negative coccus *Neisseria gonorrhoeae* (the gonococcus)

This bacterium is a human pathogen and does not cause natural infection in other animals. Therefore its reservoir is human and transmission is direct, usually through sexual contact from person to person. The organism is sensitive to drying and does not survive well outside the human host, so intimate contact is required for transmission. It is thought that a woman has a 50% chance of becoming infected after a single sexual intercourse with an infected man, whereas a man has a 20% chance of acquiring infection from an infected woman.

Asymptomatically infected individuals (almost always women, see later) form the major reservoir of infection. Infection may also be transmitted vertically from an infected mother to her baby during childbirth. Infection in babies usually manifests as ophthalmia neonatorum (see Ch. 24).

#### The gonococcus has special mechanisms to attach itself to mucosal cells

The usual site of entry of gonococci into the body is via the vagina or the urethral mucosa of the penis, but other sexual practices may result in the deposition of organisms in the throat or on the rectal mucosa. Special adhesive mechanisms (Fig. 22.3) prevent the bacteria from being washed away by urine or vaginal discharges. Following attachment the gonococci rapidly multiply and spread through the cervix in women and up the urethra in men. Spread is facilitated by various virulence factors (see Fig. 22.3), although the organisms do not possess flagella and are nonmotile. Production of an IgA protease helps to protect them from the host's secretory antibodies.

#### Host damage in gonorrhoea results from gonococcal-induced inflammatory responses

The gonococci invade nonciliated epithelial cells, which internalize the bacteria and allow them to multiply within intracellular vacuoles that are protected from phagocytes and antibodies. These vacuoles move down through the cell and fuse with the basement membrane, discharging their bacterial contents into the subepithelial connective tissues. *N. gonorrhoeae* does not produce a recognized exotoxin. Damage to the host results from inflammatory responses elicited by the organism (e.g. lipopolysaccharide and other cell wall components; see Ch. 2). Persistent untreated infection can result in chronic inflammation and fibrosis.

Infection is usually localized, but in some cases bacteria isolates (e.g. resistant to the bactericidal action of serum, etc.) can invade the bloodstream and so spread to other parts of the body.

#### Gonorrhoea is initially asymptomatic in many women but can later cause infertility

Symptoms develop within 2–7 days of infection and are characterized:

- in the male by urethral discharge (Fig. 22.4) and pain on passing urine (dysuria)
- in the female by vaginal discharge.

At least 50% of all infected women have only mild symptoms or are completely asymptomatic. They do not therefore seek treatment and will continue to infect others. Asymptomatic infection, however, is not the usual course of events in men. Women may not be alerted to their infection unless or until complications arise, such as:

- pelvic inflammatory disease (PID)
- chronic pelvic pain
- infertility resulting from damage to the fallopian tubes.

Ophthalmia neonatorum is characterized by a sticky discharge (see Fig. 24.6).

Gonococcal infection of the throat may result in a sore throat (see Ch. 19), and infection of the rectum also results in a purulent discharge.

In men, local complications of urethral infection are rare (Fig. 22.5). Invasive gonococcal disease is much more common in infected women than in men, but prompt treatment is important in containing local infection. The common occurrence of asymptomatic infection in women is an important factor in the occurrence of complications (i.e. the infection

**Fig. 22.3** The spread of *Neisseria gonorrhoeae* is facilitated by various virulence factors. Changes in the surface structure of the gonococcus render the organism avirulent.

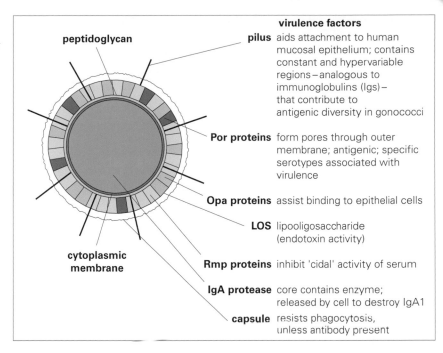

**virulence factors**

**pilus** aids attachment to human mucosal epithelium; contains constant and hypervariable regions – analogous to immunoglobulins (Igs) – that contribute to antigenic diversity in gonococci

**Por proteins** form pores through outer membrane; antigenic; specific serotypes associated with virulence

**Opa proteins** assist binding to epithelial cells

**LOS** lipooligosaccharide (endotoxin activity)

**Rmp proteins** inhibit 'cidal' activity of serum

**IgA protease** core contains enzyme; released by cell to destroy IgA1

**capsule** resists phagocytosis, unless antibody present

peptidoglycan

cytoplasmic membrane

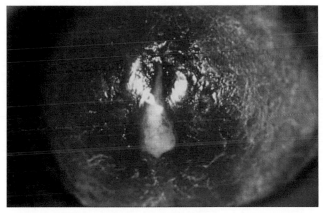

**Fig. 22.4** Gonococcal urethritis. Typical purulent meatal discharge with inflammation of the glans. (Courtesy J. Clay.)

is unrecognized and untreated). In 10–20% of untreated women, infection spreads up the genital tract to cause PID and damage to the fallopian tubes.

Disseminated infection occurs in 1–3% of women, but is less common in men (see earlier) (Fig. 22.6). It is a function not only of the strain of gonococcus (see earlier), but also host factors (e.g. ~5% of people with disseminated infection have deficiencies in the late-acting components of complement [C5–C8]).

### A diagnosis of gonorrhoea is made from microscopy and culture of appropriate specimens

Urethral and vaginal discharges and other specimens where indicated are used for microscopy and culture. Although a purulent discharge is characteristic of local gonococcal infection, it is not possible to distinguish reliably between gonococcal discharge and that caused by other pathogens such as *Chlamydia trachomatis* on clinical examination.

With experience, the finding of gram-negative intracellular diplococci in a smear of urethral discharge from a symptomatic male patient is a highly sensitive and specific test for the diagnosis of gonorrhoea.

Culture is essential in the investigation of infection in women and asymptomatic men and for specimens taken from sites other than the urethra. Specimens from symptomatic men should also be cultured:

- to confirm the identity of the isolate; misinterpretation of microscopy or culture results can cause severe distress and may result in litigation
- to perform antibiotic susceptibility tests (see Ch. 34)
- to aid in the distinction between treatment failure and reinfection.

Because of the organism's sensitivity to drying, cultures should be made on warmed selective (i.e. modified Thayer Martin) and nonselective (chocolate blood agar) medium to ensure recovery. Inoculation into appropriate transport medium is required if transfer to the laboratory will be delayed (≤48 h). Blood cultures should be collected if disseminated disease is suspected, and joint aspirates may yield positive cultures.

Serologic tests are unsatisfactory. Commercial molecular approaches (specific probes, amplification, etc.) provide reliable results within a few hours.

### Antibacterials used to treat gonorrhoea are cefixime or ceftriaxone

The antibacterial agents of choice are shown in Table 22.1. Penicillinase-producing *N. gonorrhoeae* were first observed in 1976 with increasing resistance that has severely compromised the effective treatment of gonorrhoea in many parts of the world, especially Southeast Asia. Resistance to fluoroquinolones has also occurred, leading to recommendation of dual therapy (ceftriaxone and azithromycin), which has the added benefit of targeting chlamydia (see later), which may also be infecting the patient. Early treatment of a significant proportion of sexually promiscuous patients achieves a striking reduction in the duration of infectiousness and transmission rates. Prophylactic use of antibacterials has no

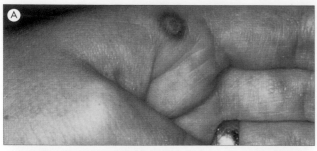

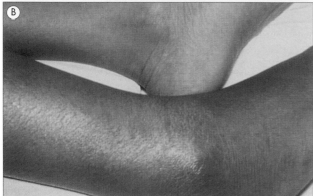

**Fig. 22.5** Local and systemic complications of gonococcal infection. (A) Skin lesions start as erythematous papules, which often become pustular and haemorrhagic with necrotic centres. (B) Septic arthritis of the ankle with marked erythema and swelling of the ankle and leg. (A, Courtesy J.S. Bingham; B, courtesy T.F. Sellers, Jr.)

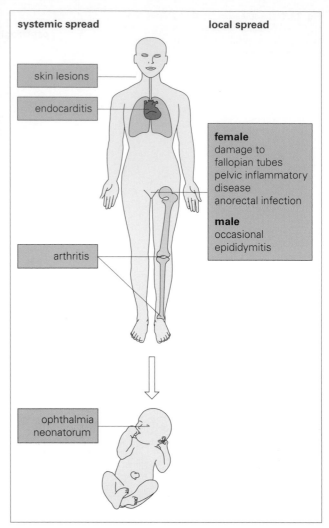

**Fig. 22.6** Local and systemic spread of gonococcal infection and complications.

effect in preventing sexually acquired gonorrhoea, but the application of antibacterial eye drops to babies born to mothers with gonorrhoea or suspected gonorrhoea is effective. Infection can be prevented by the use of condoms.

Follow-up of patients and contact tracing are vital to control the spread of gonorrhoea. At present, effective vaccines are not available, but the possibility of using some of the pilus proteins or other outer membrane components of the gonococcal cell as antigens has been under investigation. However, immunisation may prevent symptomatic disease without preventing infection, and the dangers of asymptomatic infection have been discussed earlier.

Repeat infections can occur with strains of bacteria with different pilin proteins (e.g. antigenic variation; see Ch. 17).

## CHLAMYDIAL INFECTION

### *C. trachomatis* serotypes D–K cause sexually transmitted genital infections

The chlamydiae are very small bacteria that are obligate intracellular parasites. They have a more complicated life cycle than free-living bacteria because they can exist in different forms:

- The elementary body (EB) is adapted for extracellular survival and for initiation of infection.
- The reticulate body (RB) is adapted for intracellular multiplication (Fig. 22.7).

Three species of *Chlamydia* are recognized: *C. trachomatis, C. psittaci* and *C. pneumonia* (Table 22.6). *C. psittaci* and *C. pneumoniae* infect the respiratory tract (see Ch. 20). The species *C. trachomatis* can be subdivided into different serotypes (also known as *serovars*), and these have been shown to be linked characteristically with different infections:

- Serotypes A–C are the causes of the serious eye infection trachoma (see Ch. 26).
- Serotypes D–K are the cause of genital infection and associated ocular and respiratory infections (Table 22.7).
- Serotypes L1–L3 cause the systemic disease lymphogranuloma venereum (LGV) (see later).

*C. trachomatis* serotypes D–K have a worldwide distribution, whereas the distribution of LGV serotypes is more restricted.

Most infections are genital and are acquired during sexual intercourse. Asymptomatic infection is common, especially in women. Ocular infections in adults are probably acquired by autoinoculation from infected genitalia or by ocular–genital contact. Ocular infections in neonates are acquired during passage through an infected maternal birth canal, and the infant is also at risk of developing *C. trachomatis* pneumonia (see Ch. 20).

### Chlamydiae enter the host through minute abrasions in the mucosal surface

They bind to specific receptors on the host cells and enter the cells by parasite-induced endocytosis (see Ch. 14). Once inside the cell, fusion of the chlamydia-containing vesicle with lysosomes is inhibited by an incompletely understood

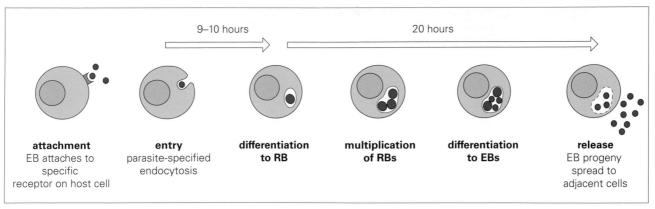

**Fig. 22.7** The life cycle of *Chlamydia*. EB, Elementary body; RB, reticulate body.

**Table 22.6** Medically important species of Chlamydiaceae

| Species | Serotype | Natural host | Disease in humans |
|---|---|---|---|
| *Chlamydia trachomatis* | A–C | Humans | Trachoma |
| | D–K | Humans | Cervicitis, urethritis, proctitis, conjunctivitis, pneumonia (in neonates) |
| | L1–L3 | Humans | Lymphogranuloma venereum |
| *C. psittaci* | Primarily A | Birds and nonhuman mammals | Pneumonia |
| *C. pneumoniae* | ? | Humans | Acute respiratory disease |

*C. trachomatis* is the species associated with sexually transmitted disease.

mechanism, and the EB begins its developmental cycle (see Fig. 22.7). Within 9–10 h of cell invasion, the EBs differentiate into metabolically active RBs, which divide by binary fission and produce fresh EB progeny. These are then released into the extracellular environment within a further 20 h.

### The clinical effects of *C. trachomatis* infection appear to result from cell destruction and the host's inflammatory response

The released EBs invade adjacent cells or cells distant from the site of infection if carried in lymph or blood.

Growth of *C. trachomatis* serotypes D–K seems to be restricted to columnar and transitional epithelial cells, but serotypes L1–L3 cause systemic disease (LGV). The site of infection determines the nature of clinical disease (see Table 22.7). Genital tract infection with serotypes D–K is locally asymptomatic in most women but usually symptomatic in men.

### *C. trachomatis* can be detected directly on microscopy using the direct fluorescent antibody test

*C. trachomatis* can be detected directly in smears of clinical specimens made on microscope slides stained with fluorescein conjugated monoclonal antibodies and viewed by UV microscopy—the direct fluorescent antibody test. The EBs stain as bright yellow-green dots (Fig. 22.8). Results can be obtained within a few hours, but this method is not sensitive enough for asymptomatic infections.

### A variety of nucleic acid–based tests are commercially available for chlamydial detection

Chlamydial urethritis and cervicitis cannot be reliably distinguished from other causes of these conditions on clinical

**Table 22.7** Clinical syndromes and complications caused by *Chlamydia trachomatis*, serotypes D–K

| Infection in | Clinical syndromes | Complications |
|---|---|---|
| Men | Urethritis, epididymitis, proctitis, conjunctivitis | Systemic spread, Reiter syndrome[a] |
| Women | Urethritis, cervicitis, bartholinitis, salpingitis, conjunctivitis | Ectopic pregnancy, infertility, systemic spread: perihepatitis, arthritis, dermatitis |
| Neonates | Conjunctivitis | Interstitial pneumonitis |

[a]Urethritis, conjunctivitis, polyarthritis, mucocutaneous lesions.

grounds alone. Traditional methods of detection (e.g. cell culture and direct antigen detection) have been largely replaced by rapid molecular tests.

Nucleic acid probe and amplification-based tests are capable of directly detecting *C. trachomatis* in specimens from infected individuals (e.g. cervix, urethra, urine). As mentioned, these commercially available kits can provide rapid (within 2–4 h) and specific detection of both *N. gonorrhoeae* and *Chlamydia* DNA, which is important as patients are often coinfected with both organisms.

### Chlamydial infection is treated or prevented with doxycycline or azithromycin

It is important to remember that chlamydiae are not susceptible to the beta-lactam antibiotics, which are important for the treatment of gonorrhoea and syphilis. It is recommended that patients receiving treatment for gonorrhoea also be treated with azithromycin for possible concurrent chlamydial infection (see Table 22.1). In addition, patients

**Fig. 22.8** Direct fluorescent antibody test for *Chlamydia trachomatis*. Elementary bodies can be seen as bright yellow-green dots under the ultraviolet microscope. (Courtesy J.D. Treharne.)

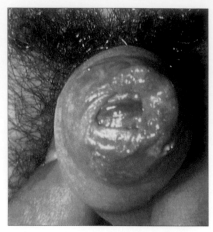

**Fig. 22.10** Chancroid. Several irregular ulcers on the prepuce. (Courtesy L. Parish.)

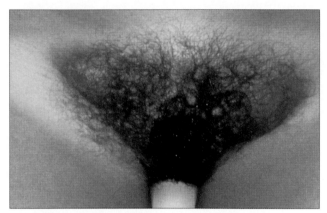

**Fig. 22.9** Lymphogranuloma venereum. Bilateral enlargement of inguinal glands. (Courtesy J.S. Bingham.)

with clinically diagnosed chlamydial genital infections, their sexual contacts and babies born to infected mothers should be treated. Erythromycin should be used for babies.

Prevention depends upon recognizing the importance of asymptomatic infections. Early diagnosis and treatment of cases and of their sexual partners is important to avoid complications and reduce opportunities for transmission. Remember that STIs are not mutually exclusive, and patients may have concurrent infections with quite different pathogens.

## OTHER CAUSES OF INGUINAL LYMPHADENOPATHY

Genital infections are common causes of inguinal lymphadenopathy (swelling of lymph nodes in the groin) among sexually active people. Syphilis and gonorrhoea have been discussed already. LGV, chancroid and donovanosis are more common in tropical and subtropical countries than in Europe and the United States but may be imported by travellers who have acquired the disease through sexual contact in these areas.

### Lymphogranuloma venereum

**LGV is caused by *C. trachomatis* serotypes L1–L3**

LGV is a serious disease especially common in Africa, Asia and South America. It occurs sporadically in Europe,

Australia and North America, particularly among MSM. The prevalence appears to be higher among males than females probably because symptomatic infection is more common in men.

**LGV is a systemic infection involving lymphoid tissue and is treated with doxycycline or erythromycin**

The clinical picture can be contrasted with the more restricted infection seen with *C. trachomatis* serotypes (see earlier). The primary lesion is an ulcerating papule at the site of inoculation (after an incubation period of 1–4 weeks) that may be accompanied by fever, headache and myalgia. The lesion heals rapidly, but the chlamydiae proceed to infect the draining lymph nodes, causing characteristic inguinal buboes (Fig. 22.9), which gradually enlarge. Chlamydiae may disseminate from the lymph nodes via the lymphatics to the tissues of the rectum to cause proctitis. Other systemic complications include fever, hepatitis, pneumonitis and meningoencephalitis. The infection may resolve untreated, but:

- abscesses may form in lymph nodes, which suppurate and discharge through the skin
- chronic granulomatous reactions in lymphatics and neighbouring tissues can eventually give rise to fistula in ano or genital elephantiasis.

Cell culture methods, immunofluorescence or nucleic acid–based tests are used for diagnosis. Treatment with doxycycline or erythromycin (see Table 22.1) is recommended. Pregnant women and children <9 years of age should be treated with erythromycin.

### Chancroid (soft chancre)

**Chancroid is caused by *Haemophilus ducreyi* and is characterized by painful genital ulcers**

Infection by the gram-negative bacterium *H. ducreyi* is manifest as painful nonindurated genital ulcers and local lymphadenitis (Fig. 22.10). Note the difference between this and the chancre of primary syphilis, which is painless. The ulcers may be confused with those of genital herpes, although they are usually larger and have a more ragged appearance. While the disease is endemic in some areas of the United States, cases generally tend to occur in distinct outbreaks. However, in Africa and Asia the chancroid is a common cause of genital ulcers. Epidemiologic information is important because the diagnosis is usually clinical as the organism is difficult to grow in the laboratory. Chancroid may also be confused with donovanosis (see later).

### Chancroid is diagnosed by microscopy and culture and treated with azithromycin, ceftriaxone, erythromycin or ciprofloxacin

Gram-stained smears of aspirates from the ulcer margin or enlarged lymph node characteristically show large numbers of short gram-negative rods and chains, often described as having a "school of fish" appearance within or outside polymorphs. Aspirates should be cultured on a rich medium (GC agar with 1–2% haemoglobin, 5% fetal bovine serum, 10% CVA and vancomycin 3 μg/mL) at 33°C in 5–10% carbon dioxide. *H. ducreyi* will not tolerate higher temperatures. Growth is slow, and it may take 2–9 days for colonies to appear. However, efforts to develop rapid molecular (e.g. polymerase chain reaction [PCR]) diagnostics are promising. Treatment with a macrolide (e.g. erythromycin or azithromycin) or ceftriaxone (see Table 22.1) is generally recommended.

### Donovanosis

#### Donovanosis is caused by *Klebsiella granulomatis* and is characterized by genital nodules and ulcers

Donovanosis (granuloma inguinale or granuloma venereum) is rare in temperate climates but common in tropical and subtropical regions such as the Caribbean, New Guinea, India and central Australia. The infection is characterized by nodules, almost always on the genitalia, which erode to form granulomatous ulcers that bleed readily on contact. The infection may extend, and the ulcers may become secondarily infected. The pathogen is a gram-negative rod previously called *Calymmatobacterium granulomatis* but now known as *K. granulomatis* on the basis of genomic analysis. The bacteria invade and multiply within mononuclear cells and are liberated when the cells rupture.

#### Donovanosis is diagnosed by microscopy and treated with doxycycline

The diagnosis of donovanosis is made by examining a smear from the lesion stained with Wright or Giemsa stain. Donovan bodies appear as clusters of blue- or black-stained organisms in the cytoplasm of mononuclear cells. Treatment with doxycycline, azithromycin or co-trimoxazole is recommended.

### MYCOPLASMAS AND NONGONOCOCCAL URETHRITIS

#### *Mycoplasma hominis, M. genitalium* and *Ureaplasma urealyticum* may be causes of genital tract infection

Although *M. pneumoniae* has a proven role in the causation of pneumonia (see Ch. 20), the role of *M. hominis, M. genitalium* and *U. urealyticum* (which metabolizes urea; also called *T strains*) in STIs is less certain. These organisms frequently colonize the genital tracts of healthy sexually active men and women. They are less common in sexually inactive populations, which supports the view that they are sexually transmitted. *M. genitalium* may cause nongonococcal urethritis; *M. hominis* may cause PID, postabortal and postpartum fevers and pyelonephritis; *U. urealyticum* has been associated with nongonococcal urethritis and prostatitis.

*M. hominis, M. genitalium* and *U. urealyticum* are commonly treated with doxycycline or azithromycin (depending on susceptibility testing), which is also the treatment for chlamydial infections.

### OTHER CAUSES OF VAGINITIS AND URETHRITIS

### *Candida* infection

#### *Candida albicans* causes a range of genital tract diseases, which are treated with oral or topical antifungals

Clinical features of candidiasis vary from mild, superficial, localized infections in an otherwise healthy individual to disseminated, often fatal infections in immunocompromised people. *Candida* is a normal inhabitant of the female vagina, and vulvovaginal candidal infection has been estimated to affect ~75% of women at least once in their lifetime. So whilst it can be transmitted sexually, the presence of vulvovaginal candidiasis does not necessarily imply sexual transmission. Other risk factors for vulvovaginal candidiasis are the use of antibiotics, corticosteroid therapy, pregnancy, use of sodium glucose cotransporter 2 inhibitors and poorly controlled diabetes mellitus. Symptomatic infections result from fungal overgrowth in the vagina, epithelial invasion and mucosal inflammation driven by the innate immune system, thus producing an intensely irritant vaginitis with a cheesy vaginal discharge. This may be accompanied by urethritis and dysuria and may present as a urinary tract infection (see Ch. 21). The diagnosis can be confirmed by microscopy and culture of the discharge (Fig. 22.11).

Treatment is with a topical antifungal such as clotrimazole or with an oral antifungal such as fluconazole. Approximately 8% of women experience troublesome recurrence.

Balanitis (inflammation of the glans penis) is seen in ~10% of male partners of females with vulvovaginal candidiasis, but urethritis is uncommon in men and is rarely symptomatic. Factors for candidal balanitis include immunosuppression, diabetes mellitus and being uncircumcised.

### *Trichomonas* infection

#### *Trichomonas vaginalis* is a protozoan parasite and causes vaginitis with copious discharge

*T. vaginalis* inhabits the vagina in women and the urethra (and sometimes the prostate) in men. It is transmitted during sexual intercourse and is one of the most prevalent nonviral STIs in the United States. Incidence is higher in HIV-infected people, and in HIV-infected women its presence is significantly associated with PID. In pregnancy, *T. vaginalis* infection is associated with preterm delivery. In women, heavy infections cause vaginitis with a characteristic copious foul-smelling discharge, although the infection may be asymptomatic in some females. There is an associated increase in the vaginal pH. *Trichomonas* is known to host an endosymbiont, *M. hominis*, and it has been suggested that this association could modulate the virulence of *T. vaginalis*.

Trichomoniasis should be distinguished from bacterial vaginosis (see later) by microscopic examination of the discharge, which shows actively motile trophozoites if sufficient numbers are present (Fig. 22.12). *Trichomonas* may be detected by wet preparation microscopy of vaginal secretions, but sensitivity is low, or it may be cultured from a vaginal swab. Rapid point-of-care immunochromatographic tests are available. Nucleic acid

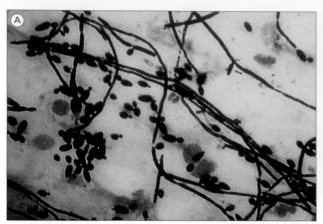 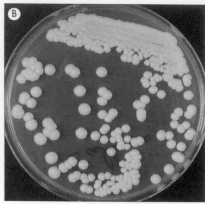

**Fig. 22.11** *Candida albicans*. (A) Light microscopic appearance and (B) culture of vaginal discharge.

detection tests are much more sensitive than wet preparation microscopy; both PCR and loop-mediated isothermal amplification assays are available.

The nitroimidazoles, metronidazole or tinidazole are recommended treatment of *T. vaginalis* infections. Resistance to the nitroimidazoles (higher with metronidazole than with tinidazole) is well documented, so there is a clear need for orally active alternative compounds.

In men, *T. vaginalis* is frequently asymptomatic but sometimes causes a mild urethritis. In addition, it is associated with nongonococcal urethritis, prostatitis, impaired sperm function and increased viral shedding in the seminal fluid of HIV-positive individuals.

Sexual partners of those infected should be treated at the same time to prevent reinfection, reduce transmission and prevent new cases in the community.

### Bacterial vaginosis

**Bacterial vaginosis is associated with *Gardnerella vaginalis* plus anaerobic infection and a fishy-smelling vaginal discharge**

This nonspecific vaginitis is a syndrome in women characterized by at least three of the following signs and symptoms:

- excessive malodorous vaginal discharge
- vaginal pH >4.5
- presence of clue cells (vaginal epithelial cells coated with bacteria; Fig. 22.13)
- a fishy amine-like odour.

There is a significant increase in the numbers of *G. vaginalis* in the vaginal flora and a concomitant increase in the numbers of obligate anaerobes such as *Bacteroides*.

*G. vaginalis* is consistently found in association with vaginosis but is also found in 20–40% of healthy women. It is generally present in the urethra of male partners of women with vaginosis, indicating that it can be sexually transmitted. *G. vaginalis* has also been isolated from blood cultures from women with postpartum fever.

*G. vaginalis* has had a chequered taxonomic history, being first classified as a haemophilus and then as a corynebacterium, reflecting the fact that it tends to be gram variable (sometimes appearing gram negative, sometimes gram positive). It grows in the laboratory on human blood agar in a moist atmosphere enriched with carbon dioxide. The organism is commonly treated with oral metronidazole. Species of

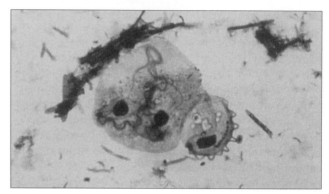

**Fig. 22.12** Trophozoites in vaginal discharge in *Trichomonas vaginalis* infection (Giemsa stain). (Courtesy R. Muller.)

the genus *Mobiluncus* (also gram variable and rod shaped) appear to be related to *G. vaginalis* and have been implicated in vaginosis.

The pathogenesis of bacterial vaginosis is still unclear but appears to be related to factors that disrupt the normal acidity of the vagina and the equilibrium between the different constituents of the normal vaginal flora. Whether any of these or other unknown factors are sexually transmissible is unclear.

### GENITAL HERPES

**Herpes simplex virus 2 is the most common cause of genital herpes, but herpes simplex virus 1 is detected frequently**

Herpes simplex virus (HSV) is a ubiquitous infection of humans worldwide. HSV-1 is generally transmitted via saliva, causing primary oropharyngeal infection in children, and cold sores occur after virus reactivation. However, HSV-2 emerged as a result of independent transmission by sexual intercourse. HSV-2 shows biologic and antigenic differences from HSV-1 and can be distinguished by molecular typing methods as well as older techniques such as immunofluorescence. There is little cross-immunity. Although originally recovered from separate sites, orogenital sexual practices have obscured the topographic difference between the strains so that HSV-1 and HSV-2 can be recovered from oral and genital sites. Most recurrent genital herpes is due to HSV-2, and between 2015 and 2016 the Centers for Disease Control and Prevention's National Health and Nutritional

Examination Survey reported that nearly 12% of the 14- to 49-year-old group had had an HSV-2 infection and 48% had HSV-1 in the United States. The age-adjusted prevalence of both HSV-1 and HSV-2 infections had fallen over time, by 11% and 6%, respectively, from 1999 to 2000. More anogenital herpetic infections were due to HSV-1, especially among young women and MSM. It was also shown that as people grew older, the prevalence of both HSV types increased, and the HSV-2 prevalence was higher among females.

HSV-2 is one of the most common STIs, and it has been estimated that there are >500 million individuals with HSV-2 globally. It is estimated there are ~800,000 newly infected individuals in the United States annually. One of the worrying aspects surrounding HSV-2 is that most people do not know that they have been infected, as up to 75% may not have symptoms and therefore will not realize that they may transmit this infection. Finally, HSV-2 infection can result in a twofold increased risk of developing HIV infection. This is likely to be due to breaches in the mucosal barrier as a result of the HSV ulcers.

### Genital herpes is characterized by ulcerating vesicles that can take up to 2 weeks to heal

The primary genital lesion on the penis or vulva is seen 3–7 days after infection. It consists of vesicles that soon break down to form painful shallow ulcers (Fig. 22.14). Local lymph nodes are swollen, and there may be constitutional symptoms, including fever, headache and malaise. The lesions can also be urethral, causing dysuria or pain on micturition. Healing takes up to 2 weeks, but the virus in the lesion travels up sensory nerve endings to establish latent infection in dorsal root ganglion neurones (see Ch. 25). From this site it can reactivate, travel down nerves to the same area and cause recurrent genital lesions.

Aseptic meningitis occurs in adults, HSV being the most common viral cause; HSV encephalitis is a rare complication. Spread of infection from mother to infant at the time of delivery can give rise to neonatal disseminated herpes and/or encephalitis.

### Genital herpes is generally diagnosed from the clinical appearance, and acyclovir can be used for treatment and prophylaxis

HSV DNA can be detected and typed in vesicle fluid or ulcer swabs using PCR. Typing is helpful in terms of prognosis as recurrent genital infection is more frequent with HSV-2. Older, less sensitive diagnostic methods involved virus isolation and subsequently typing the isolate by immunofluorescence using type-specific monoclonal antibodies. The cytopathic effect is characteristic and is generally seen within 1–2 days postinoculation, with ballooning degenerating cells and multinucleate giant cells. A number of antivirals, including oral acyclovir, valacyclovir and famciclovir, can be used for treatment of severe or early lesions, and acyclovir may need to be given intravenously if there are systemic complications. Recurrent attacks are distressing, and treatment options include starting an antiviral when prodromal symptoms occur or alternatively taking low-dose acyclovir for 6–12 months, or taking one of the alternative agents to stop or at least reduce the frequency of recurrences.

## HUMAN PAPILLOMAVIRUS INFECTION

There are >120 distinct types of HPV, all infecting skin or mucosal surfaces and the DNA of each showing <50% cross-hybridization with that of others. These are evidently ancient viral associates of humans that have evolved extensively, and many of the different types are adapted to specific regions of the body.

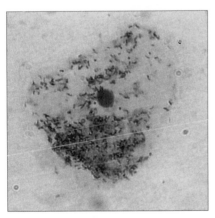

**Fig. 22.13** Clue cells in bacterial vaginosis.

**Fig. 22.14** Genital herpes. Vesicles (A) on the penis and (B) in the perianal area and vulva. Those on the labia minora and fourchette have ruptured to reveal characteristic herpetic erosions. (Courtesy J.S. Bingham.)

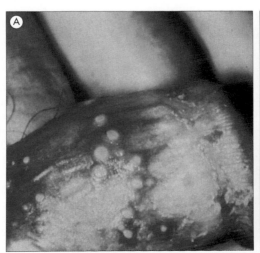

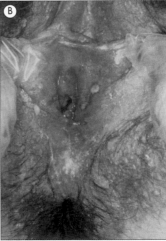

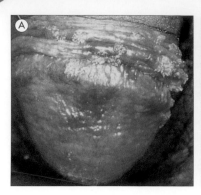

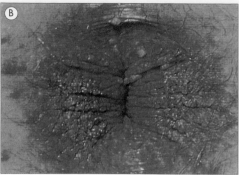

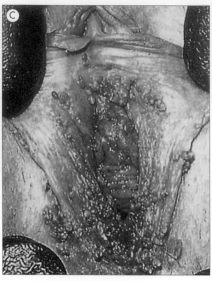

**Fig. 22.15** Genital warts. (A) Warts on the penis are usually multiple and on the shaft are often flat and keratinized. (B) Warts in the perianal area often extend into the anal canal. (C) Warts in the vulvoperineal area can enlarge dramatically and extend into the vagina. (Courtesy J.S. Bingham.)

### Many papillomavirus types are transmitted sexually and cause genital warts

The European Centre for Disease Prevention and Control estimated that ~33,000 women develop cervical cancer mostly due to persistent genital tract infection by high-risk HPV types and 15,000 deaths annually. HPV-associated warts (condylomata acuminata) appear on the penis, vulva and perianal regions (Fig. 22.15) after an incubation period of 1–6 months (see Ch. 27). There are >100 HPV types, >40 of which affect the anogenital regions, of which 90% are caused by the low-risk types 6 and 11. They may not regress for many months and can be treated with podophyllin, imiquimod or cryotherapy. The lesion on the cervix is a flat area of dysplasia visible by colposcopy as a white plaque (Fig. 22.16) after the local application of 5% acetic acid. Because of their association with cervical cancer, especially types 16 and 18 that cause ~70% of cervical cancer, cervical lesions are best removed by laser or loop excision.

Three HPV vaccines include a bivalent, a quadrivalent and a 9-valent vaccine that all afford protection against HPV types 16 and 18, with the 9-valent vaccine including antigens to HPV type 31, 33, 45, 52 and 58.

## MONKEYPOX, PREVIOUSLY A RARE VIRAL ZOONOSIS, EMERGED IN 2022 AS AN STI

Monkeypox, now known as *mpox*, is caused by the monkeypox virus, a member of the Poxviridae family. This virus was first detected in monkeys in a laboratory in Denmark in 1958, and the first human infection was seen in a baby in the Democratic Republic of the Congo (DRC) in 1970. Mpox spread to mainly Central and West Africa, and the first infection outside Africa was reported in 2003. In the DRC the number of suspected mpox infections increased from >10,000 between 2000 and 2009 to >18,000 between 2010 and 2019. Mpox outbreaks were then seen in 10 African countries and 4 outside Africa, including one in the United States (see Ch. 14 and Box 14.2). There are two genetic clades: Clade 1 is endemic in Central Africa and clade 2 in West Africa.

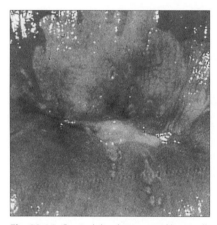

**Fig. 22.16** Cervical dysplasia caused by papillomavirus should be removed by laser. (Courtesy A. Goodman.)

### Eradication of smallpox and stopping the vaccine programme led to waning herd immunity

Transmission via contact with lesions or fluids of an infected source occurred in Africa from animal-to-animal and animal-to-human contact. This was then seen outside Africa in people travelling to other countries, having had contact with infected animals and then from human to human contact in household transmission. The reason for the increasing incidence of mpox was thought mostly to be due to stopping the routine smallpox vaccination programme after the World Health Organization (WHO) declared smallpox eradicated in 1980. Smallpox vaccination gave ~85% protection against the related mpox. Therefore, by 2018, only 9% of the population had been vaccinated previously, the estimated population immunity was ~2% and most of those with mpox had not been vaccinated. In addition, deforestation may have been a factor as well as mpox genome diversity and evolution.

On July 23, 2022, WHO declared a global health emergency after unlinked mpox infections were reported in the United Kingdom, then Portugal and then the United States in individuals with no recent travel to mpox endemic countries. By February 2023, 85,645 laboratory-confirmed infections and 1381

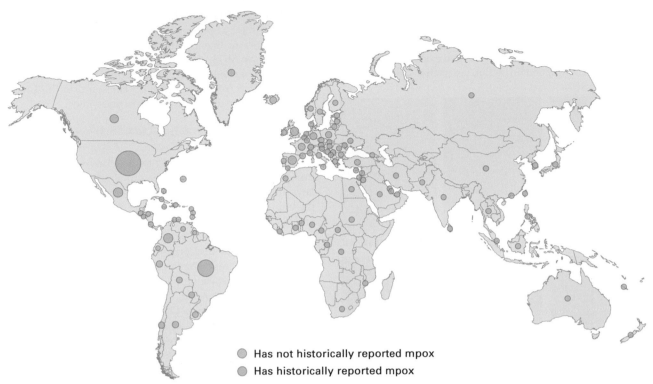

○ Has not historically reported mpox

○ Has historically reported mpox

**Fig. 22.17** A 2022 mpox outbreak global map. (From Centers for Disease Control and Prevention. 2022 Mpox Outbreak Global Map. Author; 2023.)

probable infections, including 92 deaths, had been reported to WHO from 110 member states across all six WHO regions. However, by March 2023, the number of mpox infections was continuing to decline due to preventative measures, including education, awareness and vaccination. Human infections and sustained chains of transmission had not been reported in most countries without epidemiologic travel links involving Africa. Moreover, the mpox infections mostly affected MSM, with most infections reported in the United States, Brazil and Spain (Fig. 22.17). Transmission was linked to sexual contact in most of those infected, especially in those with multiple sexual partners, and mpox DNA was detected in semen. The lesions were mostly in the genital, perianal and anal areas (Fig. 22.18). In addition, transmission can occur through large respiratory droplets, contact with a skin lesion and fomites (such as clothes and bed linen).

### Clinical features were completely different to mpox infections seen previously in Africa and those associated with travel

The features of mpox include a variable incubation period from 5–21 days (mean 9 days), fever, tiredness, headache, myalgia, sore throat, lymphadenopathy and skin lesions. The skin lesions evolve from macules and papules to vesicles and pustules that ulcerate and crust before healing over several weeks. The skin lesions usually occur in crops. The initial lesions are usually at the site of inoculation. In addition, individuals presented with proctitis and pharyngitis.

Diagnosis is made by collecting lesion swabs and testing for mpox DNA by PCR.

### Treatment is available, and prevention includes source isolation and immunisation

Two antiviral drugs used to treat mpox infection are tecovirimat, which blocks cell–cell viral transmission by inhibiting the viral p37 protein that mediates the formation and exit of enveloped virions from infected cells, and brincidofovir, a viral DNA polymerase inhibitor. Brincidofovir has gastrointestinal and hepatic side effects.

Vaccines for smallpox prevention were made available that also covered mpox. These included modified vaccinia Ankara–Bavarian Nordic (MVA-BN), a live attenuated, replication incompetent, modified vaccinia vaccine that was offered to those at high risk of infection. Vaccines can be used as before or after exposure to prevent infection and disease or to attenuate infection and disease, respectively.

Globally, awareness and education were key in preventing and reducing transmission together with diagnostic tests. Those with mpox infection were advised to self-isolate at home for the duration of the illness and until the rash had healed.

## HUMAN IMMUNODEFICIENCY VIRUS

HIV is a retrovirus (Table 22.8), so-called because this single-stranded RNA virus contains a *pol* gene that codes for a reverse transcriptase (Latin: *retro*, "backwards"). Looking back to the start of the HIV pandemic, by 2021 new HIV infections had fallen by 54% to ~1.5 million, having peaked in 1996. Acquired immunodeficiency syndrome (AIDS)–related deaths had fallen by 68% to ~650,000 having peaked in 2004. The following sections give some perspective to the changes over the decades.

### AIDS was first recognized in 1981 in the United States

In 1981 the US Communicable Disease Center noted an increase in requests to use pentamidine to treat *Pneumocystis carinii* (now classified as *P. jirovecii*) infection in previously well individuals who also suffered severe infections by other microorganisms that were mainly seen in immunocompromised individuals. These included *C. albicans* oesophagitis, mucocutaneous HSV, toxoplasma central nervous system (CNS) infection or pneumonia, cryptosporidial enteritis and Kaposi sarcoma skin lesions. These individuals had evidence of impaired immune function, as shown by skin test anergies, and depletion

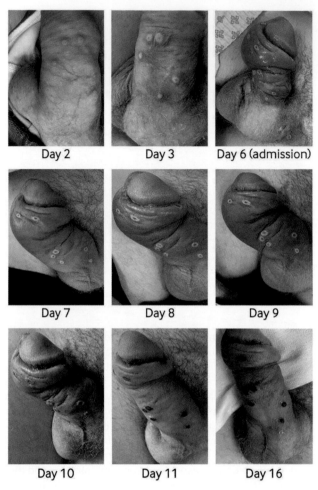

**Fig. 22.18** Progression of penile lesions and penile oedema. (From Patel A, et al. Clinical features and novel presentations of human monkeypox in a central London centre during the 2022 outbreak: descriptive case series. *BMJ*. 2022;378.)

of CD4-positive T-helper (Th) lymphocytes. This immunodeficiency syndrome appearing in an individual without a known cause such as treatment with immunosuppressive drugs was referred to as AIDS. An internationally agreed definition of AIDS soon followed. Epidemics subsequently occurred in San Francisco, New York and other US cities and in the United Kingdom and the rest of Europe a few years later.

### HIV that causes AIDS was isolated from blood lymphocytes in 1983

It was recognized as belonging to the lentivirus (slow virus) group of retroviruses and related to similar agents in monkeys and to visnavirus in sheep and goats. The structure of the viral particle and its genome are illustrated in Fig. 22.19 and its replication mechanism in Figs. 22.20 and 22.19.

Three genes (*gag, pol, env*) encode the matrix, capsid and nucleocapsid structural proteins, reverse transcriptase, proteases and integrase enzymes and gp120 and gp41 envelope proteins, respectively. The regulatory and accessory proteins Tat and Rev, Vif, Vpr, Vpu / x and Nef are coded by their respective genes. Overall there are 16 proteins that are involved in a variety of pairwise interactions, ensuring efficient viral replication at key parts of the HIV life cycle, such as virus entry, reverse transcription, virus integration, transcription and translation, virus assembly, budding and maturation (see Fig. 22.20).

### HIV infection started in Africa between 1910 and 1930

The molecular biologic evidence based on nucleic acid sequencing studies demonstrated that both HIV-1 and the closely related HIV-2 seen in West Africa arose from closely related primate viruses. HIV-1 is separated into four groups, namely M (major), N (new), O (outlier) and P. The latter was reported in 2009 after identifying an HIV strain closely related to a gorilla simian immunodeficiency virus (SIV) in a Cameroonian woman, the only person in whom it has been found. By 2023 group M, the most widespread group, comprised nine HIV-1 subtypes A–K as well as 19 circulating recombinant forms (CRF), which were due to recombination events between those subtypes, with the N and O groups focused in West and Central Africa. The geographic prevalence of the subtypes differs, with

**Table 22.8** Human retroviruses

| Virus | Comment |
|---|---|
| HTLV-1 | Endemic in West Indies and Southwest Japan; transmission via blood, sexual intercourse, vertical transmission, breast milk transmission; can cause adult T-cell leukaemia, and HTLV1-associated myelopathy, also known as *tropical spastic paraparesis* |
| HTLV-2 | Uncommon, sporadic occurrence; transmission via blood, sexual intercourse, vertical transmission; can cause hairy T-cell leukaemia and neurologic disease |
| HIV-1, HIV-2 | Transmission via blood, sexual intercourse; responsible for AIDS. HIV-2 West African in origin, closely related to HIV-1 but antigenically distinct |
| Human foamy virus | Causes foamy vacuolation in infected cells; little is known of its occurrence or pathogenic potential |
| Human placental virus(es) | Detected in placental tissue by electron microscopy and by presence of reverse transcriptase |
| Human genome viruses | Nucleic acid sequences representing endogenous retroviruses are common in the vertebrate genome, often in well-defined genetic loci; acquired during evolutionary history; not expressed as infectious virus; function unknown; perhaps should be regarded as mere parasitic DNA |

HTLV-1, HTLV-2, HIV-1 and HIV-2 have been cultivated in human T cells in vitro. The human placental and genome viruses are not known as infectious agents. Retroviruses are also common in cats (FAIDS), monkeys (MAIDS), mice (mouse leukaemia) and other vertebrates. AIDS, Acquired immunodeficiency syndrome; HIV, human immunodeficiency virus; HTLV, human T-cell lymphotropic virus.

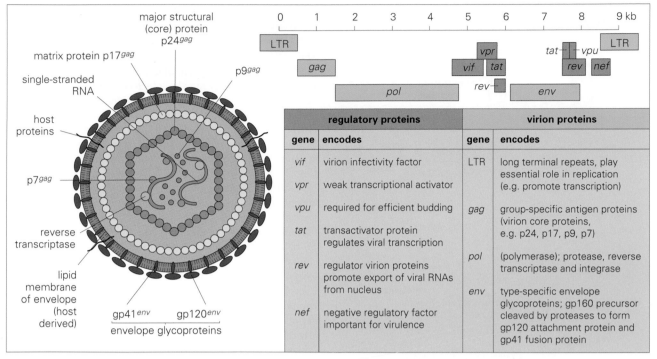

**Fig. 22.19** The structure and genetic map of human immunodeficiency virus (HIV). The *rev* and *tat* genes are divided into noncontiguous pieces, and the gene segments are spliced together in the RNA transcript. Occasional host proteins such as major histocompatibility complex molecules are present in the envelope. (p) is protein and (gp) is glycoprotein. About $10^9$ HIV-1 particles are produced each day at the peak of infection, and this, together with the low fidelity of reverse transcriptase, means that new virus variants are always appearing. Mutations are seen especially in *env* and *nef* genes. Any one patient contains many variants, and drug-resistant and immune-resistant mutants emerge.

subtype B being most common in North America, Australia and Europe and the non-B strains such as A and C being found more frequently in Africa and Russia and Africa and India, respectively. The genetic distance within a subtype is ~15–20% and 25–35% between subtypes. However, with increasing travel, the subtype distribution is changing and, together with the potential for mixed or superinfections (i.e. an HIV-infected individual becoming infected with another strain), and viral recombination events, other subtypes are being seen such as the CRFs. The M–P groups resulted from independent cross-species human and ape contact in West and Central Africa. Transmission events were most likely to have occurred through skin and mucous membrane exposure to infected ape blood and body fluids, probably when hunting. Group M was found first and is the pandemic form as it comprises the majority of HIV infections globally. This has been the subject of molecular clock analyses, a method used in evolutionary biology. The molecular clock hypothesis is that DNA and protein sequences evolve at a rate that is relatively constant over time. Due to this fact, the genetic difference between two species is proportional to the time since they shared a common ancestor.

On analyzing the HIV pandemic, the onset of the HIV-1 group M infections was in the early 20th century. Having emerged between 1910 and 1930 in West and Central Africa, HIV spread for the next 50+ years, having diversified around Kinshasa, formerly Leopoldville, the capital and largest city of the DRC. Moreover, the rivers that serve as routes for travel and commerce would have been a link between the chimpanzee reservoir on the banks of the Congo. In addition, the four groups cluster with a particular lineage of SIV cpz (cpz = chimpanzees), the original reservoir of human and gorilla infections. HIV-2 originated from sooty mangabeys and is mostly seen in West Africa but also in Portugal, France, India and the United States.

HIV-1 may have been present in humans in Central Africa for many years, but in the late 1970s it began to spread rapidly (Fig. 22.21), possibly with changed biologic properties as a result of increased transmission following major socioeconomic upheavals and migration of people from Central to East Africa. Female prostitutes and male soldiers and workers travelling around the country played a major part in transmission. The migration pathways of the different subtypes have been charted; subtype B, which predominates in Europe and the Americas, originated from one African strain that spread to Haiti in the 1960s and then to the United States and Europe.

In the late 1980s HIV began to appear in Asian countries, beginning with Thailand, and by 1995 explosive spread was based on heterosexual transmission, with high infection rates in female sex workers and transmission among users of injected drugs in Asia.

Worldwide by 2021, around 38.4 million people were living with HIV, including:

- 20.6 million in East and South Africa and 5 million in West and Central Africa
- 6 million in Asia and the Pacific
- 1.8 million in Eastern Europe and Central Asia
- 2.3 million in North America, Western and Central Europe
- 2.2 million in Latin America

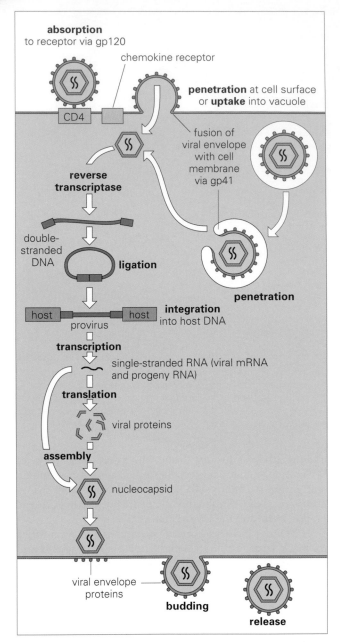

**Fig. 22.20** The human immunodeficiency virus replication cycle. The virus enters the cell either by fusion with the cell membrane at the cell surface or via uptake into a vacuole and release within the cell.

In 2021 nearly 1.5 million people were newly infected (almost a 50% fall since 2009) and 650,000 died (almost 66% fall since 2009) as a result of HIV infection that year.

By 2021 the UNAIDS global report stated that 28.7 million people were accessing antiretroviral therapy (ART) compared with 7.8 million in 2010. AIDS-related deaths had fallen to 650,000 from 1.4 million in 2010. The global percentage of all people living with HIV accessing ART by 2021 was 75%, compared with 46% by the end of 2015. This included 78% in Africa where 25.6 million people were living with HIV.

Since the start of the HIV epidemic it is estimated that 84.2 million (range 64–113 million) people became HIV positive and 40.1 million (range 33.6–48.6 million) people have died from AIDS-related illnesses.

## HIV mainly infects cells bearing the CD4 glycoprotein on the cell surface and requires chemokine coreceptors CCR5 and CXCR4

The HIV transmission route for >80% of adults involves mucosal surfaces, in particular cervicovaginal, penile and rectal. The remainder may be infected by intravenous or percutaneous routes. The window period for detecting the virus is 7–21 days, as HIV multiplies in the mucosa and draining lymphoreticular tissues. The first targets are CD4 receptor-bearing cells that include Th cells, monocytes, Langerhans cells and other dendritic cells, macrophages and microglia (Fig. 22.22; see also Fig. 22.21). The CD4 molecule acts as a high-affinity binding site for the viral gp120 envelope glycoprotein. This interacts with the gp41 transmembrane protein and leads to a conformational change that produces a fusion pore for viral entry. Productive replication and cell destruction does not occur until the Th cell is activated. Th cell activation is greatly enhanced not only in attempts to respond to HIV antigens but also as a result of the secondary microbial infections seen in patients. Monocytes and macrophages, Langerhans cells and follicular dendritic cells also express the CD4 molecule and are infected but are not generally destroyed, potentially acting as a reservoir for infection. Langerhans cells (e.g. dendritic cells in the skin and genital mucosa) may be the first cells infected. Later in the disease there is a remarkable disruption of histologic pattern in lymphoid follicles as a result of the breakdown of follicular dendritic cells.

HIV-1 enters host cells by binding the viral gp120 to the CD4 receptor and a chemokine coreceptor on the host cell surface. The CCR5 beta-chemokine receptor is important in establishing the infection. Those people with CCR5 gene deletions are resistant to infection. On the other hand, disease progression has been associated with HIV variants using the CXCR4 alpha-chemokine receptor. Cell susceptibility to infection is therefore affected by the levels of these chemokine coreceptors (e.g. their expression may be upregulated by opportunistic infections).

Productive infection of resting CD4 T cells in the lymphoreticular system of the gastrointestinal tract occurs. These cells express integrin receptors, viral attachment molecules and Th cell surface markers, and HIV-1 infection rapidly expands with a rise in HIV-1 RNA levels at the same time as the irreversible depletion of reservoirs of Th cells as well as induction of an inflammatory cytokine and chemokine response. A latency state is soon established with the formation of persistent lymphoid tissue viral reservoirs.

## At first the immune system fights back against HIV infection, but then it begins to fail

During the first few months virus-specific CD8-positive T cells are formed and reduce the viraemia, which is referred to as the HIV load. Innate and adaptive immune responses to HIV infection lead to this set-point of HIV replication (see Fig. 22.22). This is followed by the appearance of neutralizing antibodies at ~3 months postinfection, and viral escape mutants develop. Up to $10^{10}$ infectious virus particles and up to $10^{9}$ infected lymphocytes are produced daily. Then the immune system begins to suffer gradual damage, and the number of circulating CD4-positive T cells steadily falls and the HIV load rises. In addition to the loss of total CD4 T cells, T-cell subsets change,

**Fig. 22.21** Early spread of human immunodeficiency virus (HIV) infection (now worldwide). HIV-1 may have been present in Central Africa for many years before increased migration and socioeconomic upheaval caused it to begin spreading in the late 1970s. Outside Africa, most infections occurred in men.

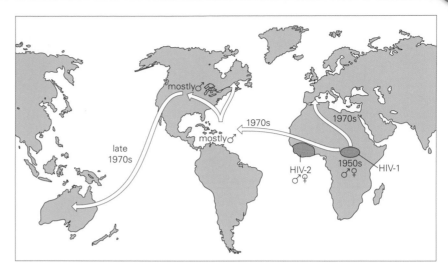

including those involved in defence against bacteria. Nearly all infected CD4-positive T cells are in lymph nodes. The cell-mediated immune responses to viral antigens, as judged by lymphoproliferation, weaken, whereas responses to other antigens are normal. Perhaps the virus initially engineers a specific suppression of protective responses to itself. Eventually the patient loses the battle to replace lost T cells, and the number falls more rapidly. Skin test delayed-type hypersensitivity responses are absent, natural killer cell and cytotoxic T-cell activity is reduced and there are various other immunologic abnormalities, including polyclonal activation of B cells. Functional changes in T lymphocytes—reduced responses to mitogens, reduced interleukin 2 and interferon gamma production—are also seen. As AIDS develops, responses to HIV and unrelated antigens are further depressed. The immune system has lost control. Plasma HIV-1 RNA load measurements predict clinical outcome and are used in clinical management to help determine disease stage and progression as well as ART response.

The following factors need to be considered in the development of immune suppression:

- Th cells directly killed by virus
- Th cells induced to commit suicide (apoptosis, programmed cell death) by virus
- Th cells made vulnerable to immune attack by cytotoxic T cells
- T-cell replenishment impaired by damage to the thymus and lymph nodes and by infection of stem cells
- defects in antigen presentation associated with infection of dendritic cells
- immunosuppressive virus-coded molecules (gp120, gp41).

The host response is further handicapped by the high rate of viral evolution assisted by the lack of a reverse transcriptase proofreading function. The virus exists as a quasispecies—in other words, the infection comprises a number of heterogeneous strains. Some are immune escape variants and others show increased pathogenicity.

Before the advent of combined ART (cART), the immunosuppression was permanent, the patient remained infectious, the virus persisted in the body and death was due to opportunist infections and tumours.

HIV-2 appears to be transmitted less easily than HIV-1 probably because the viral load is lower and the progression to AIDS is slower.

## Routes of transmission

In resource-rich countries, such as western and central Europe and North America, the main route of transmission involves the MSM group. This is due to the higher risk of transmission by receptive anal intercourse and sex networks. Infection is transmitted primarily from male to male and from male to female although not very efficiently compared with other STIs. Transmission from female to male, however, is a common and well-established feature of HIV in Africa and Asia.

### Heterosexual transmission in resource-rich as well as in resource-poor countries is due to a number of factors, including unprotected sexual intercourse and other STIs

One explanation for the greater heterosexual spread in resource-poor countries is that other STIs are more common, causing ulcers and discharges, which are sources of infected lymphocytes and monocytes. Genital ulcers are associated with a fourfold increase in the risk of infection. As with other STIs, uncircumcised males are more likely to be infected.

Mother-to-child transmission (MTCT) of HIV can occur in utero, at delivery and by breastfeeding. Breast milk transmission is involved in >40% of MTCT. Preventing transmission has been a global programme that involves antenatal HIV screening, offering antiretroviral drugs during pregnancy, caesarean section delivery, avoiding breastfeeding and giving prophylactic antiretroviral drugs to the newborn infant. The MTCT rate without prevention programmes in resource-rich countries is 15–25% and 25–45% in resource-poor countries. In sub-Saharan Africa, a fall in the MTCT rate from 28% in 2009 to 18% in 2013 was seen when interventions were introduced. In 2013 WHO produced guidelines for offering ART to all pregnant women living with HIV. By the end of 2021 there were ~160,000 new HIV infections in children aged 0–14 years compared to 320,000 in 2010.

Haemophiliacs and others who received unidentified contaminated blood products were infected in the 1980s. As with other bloodborne virus infections, using contaminated needles can lead to infection (i.e. in injecting drug use, tattooing, body piercing, acupuncture).

Finally, health care workers are at risk of HIV infection after sustaining needlestick or mucous membrane splash injuries involving an HIV-infected source. The risk of infection is ~1 in 400 and is dependent on a number of factors, including depth of the injury and amount of blood to which

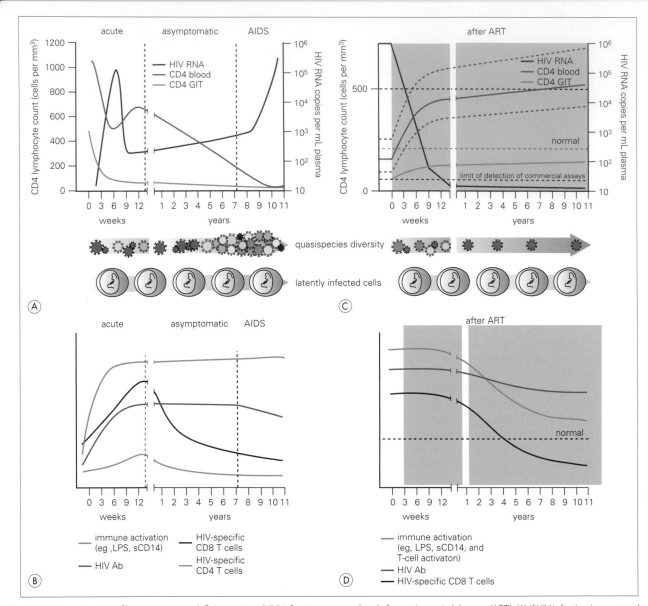

**Fig. 22.22** A comparison of human immunodeficiency virus *(HIV)* infection untreated and after antiretroviral therapy (ART). (A) If HIV infection is untreated, CD4 T cells progressively decrease in blood and are rapidly depleted early on in the gastrointestinal tract. (B) The immediate result of HIV infection is the activation of the immune response, including production of nonneutralizing antibodies and HIV-specific CD4 and CD8 T cells, resulting in a temporal decrease in HIV RNA in blood. (C) Antiretroviral therapy significantly decreases HIV RNA with CD4 T-cell recovery varying with the individual *(panel)*. Conversely, there is reduced recovery of CD4 T cells in the gastrointestinal tract. (D) Antiretroviral therapy is associated with decreased HIV RNA and viral antigen and a decrease in HIV-specific T cells, although antibody persists in all patients. Immune activation also decreases but remains significantly increased in most patients compared with healthy controls. AIDS, Acquired immunodeficiency syndrome; ART, antiretroviral therapy; GIT, gastrointestinal tract; LPS, lipopolysaccharide. (From Maartens G, Celum C, Lewin SR. HIV infection: epidemiology, pathogenesis, treatment, and prevention. *Lancet.* 2014;384:258–271.)

the recipient has been exposed. Wearing protective clothing such as gloves and goggles is part of universal precautions to avoid exposure. Postexposure prophylaxis with the antiretroviral drug combination raltegravir and emtricitabine/tenofovir (Truvada) is available in many centres.

## Clinical features

**Primary HIV infection may be accompanied by a mild mononucleosis-type illness**

Signs and symptoms of the mild mononucleosis-type illness associated with HIV infection include fever, malaise, maculopapular rash and lymphadenopathy. The acute infection and rapid, widespread viral dissemination are followed by a chronic asymptomatic stage. Viral replication is reduced

in line with the immune response, and the individual usually remains well. The duration of this stage is dependent on a number of factors, including the viral phenotype, host immune response and use of ART (Fig. 22.23). Infected cells are, however, still present, and at a later stage the infected individual may develop weight loss, fever, persistent lymphadenopathy, oral candidiasis and diarrhoea. Further viral replication takes place until finally, some years after initial infection, full-blown AIDS develops (Fig. 22.24).

### Progression to AIDS

Viral invasion of the CNS, with self-limiting aseptic meningoencephalitis as the most common neurologic picture, occurs in early infection.

**Fig. 22.23** Kinetics of immunologic and virologic events associated with human immunodeficiency virus (HIV) infection during acute and early chronic phases. The schematic represents the sequence of events, including the appearance of viral antigens, HIV-specific antibodies, and HIV-specific CD8 T cells during the acute and early chronic phases of infection. HIV reservoirs are established during the acute phase of infection soon after emergence of plasma viraemia. Throughout the acute phase of infection, characterized by massive virus replication and high levels of plasma viraemia, an acute HIV syndrome develops in the majority of infected individuals, and the virus rapidly spreads to various lymphoid organs, causing extensive depletion of CD4 T cells. Although anti-HIV immunity, including virus-specific CD8 T cells and antibodies, develops during the acute phase of infection, escaped viral mutants rapidly emerge. CD, Cluster of differentiation; ELISA, enzyme-linked immunosorbent assay; PCR, polymerase chain reaction. (Modified from Moir S, Chun TW, Fauci AS. Pathogenic mechanisms of HIV disease. *Ann Rev Pathol Mech Dis.* 2011;6:223–248.)

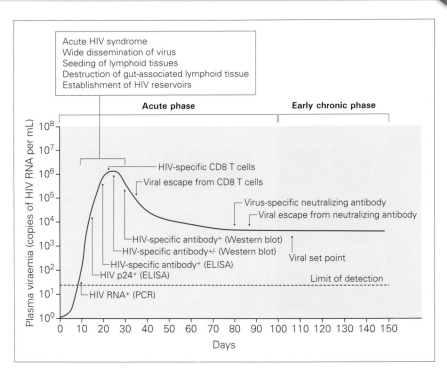

A progressive HIV-associated encephalopathy is seen in individuals with AIDS and is characterized by multiple small nodules of inflammatory cells; most of the infected cells appear to be microglia or infiltrating macrophages. These cells express the CD4 antigen, and it has been suggested that infected monocytes carry the virus into the brain, but the picture is complicated by the various persistent infections that are activated and give rise to their own CNS pathology. These include infections by *Cryptococcus neoformans, Toxoplasma gondii*, cytomegalovirus (CMV), Epstein-Barr virus, JC virus (progressive multifocal leukoencephalopathy) and (more rarely) HSV and varicella-zoster virus.

HIV exercises complex control over its own replication (see Fig. 22.20). Replication is also affected by responses to other infections, which act as antigenic stimuli, and some of them directly as transactivating agents.

AIDS, a symptomatic disease, consists of a large spectrum of microbial diseases acquired or reactivated as a result of the underlying immunosuppression due to HIV (Fig. 22.25; Table 22.9). The disease picture of AIDS is therefore an indirect result of infection with HIV.

Before the advent of ART, one study in New York reported a mortality rate of 80%, 5 years after the onset of the disease, and the average survival time after hospital admission was 242 days.

## Treatment

### ART results in a dramatic improvement in disease prognosis

In the 1990s a range of ART was introduced, which included the nucleoside reverse transcriptase inhibitors (NRTIs), non-nucleoside reverse transcriptase inhibitors (NNRTIs) and protease inhibitors (PIs). These were developed further over the next 2 decades in terms of new drugs in all classes and combinations. In 2003 a fusion inhibitor was added to the list, and by 2009 two other classes were available, an integrase inhibitor and chemokine receptor antagonist (see Ch. 34 for more detail). In combination with two NRTIs, the NNRTI or PI drugs had a dramatic effect on progression to AIDS, and the term *highly active ART* had changed by 2016 to *cART*. Side effects of the drugs included mitochondrial toxicity and altered fat distribution known as lipodystrophy. Treatment compliance was a problem because of the side effects and the number and frequency of pills taken each day. Missing doses can lead to the development of drug resistance, thus limiting treatment options. However, treatment has been simplified by combining not just individual classes of up to three drugs in one tablet but also combinations of classes (see Ch. 34). Improved monitoring using plasma HIV load measurements and CD4 counts and percentages has shown the success of cART, with rapid falls in plasma HIV load and rises in CD4 cells seen after initiating therapy.

However, HIV can be detected in various compartments of the body, including the cerebrospinal fluid and genital tract. Antiretroviral drugs may not penetrate these sites, resulting in a high viral load detectable in semen despite suppression of the plasma HIV load.

As a result of improved diagnosis, surveillance, prevention and use of cART, the number of AIDS-related deaths among children and adults worldwide had fallen from 1.1 million in 2015 to ~650,000 in 2021.

### Antiretroviral drug resistance and improved treatment options

Plasma HIV-1 RNA load is a good indicator of viral replication, and failure of ART is seen by a rise in viral load. Antiretroviral resistance testing and therapeutic drug monitoring are part of clinical management. Drug resistance testing may be carried out when the plasma HIV-1 load is not suppressed whilst on ART. Specific mutations in the HIV reverse transcriptase, protease and integrase regions associated with reduced susceptibility to one or more antiretroviral drugs have been identified by nucleic acid sequencing, known as *genotypic analysis*.

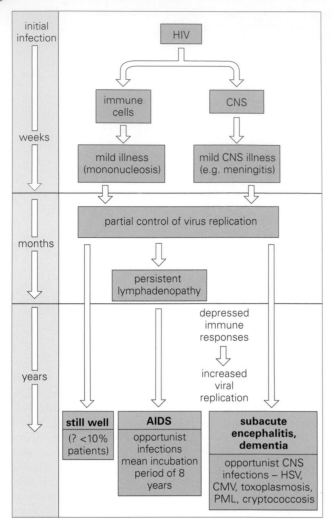

**Fig. 22.24** The clinical features and progression of untreated human immunodeficiency virus (HIV) infection. AIDS, Acquired immunodeficiency syndrome; CMV, cytomegalovirus; CNS, central nervous system; HSV, herpes simplex virus; PML, progressive multifocal leukoencephalopathy.

HIV-1 genetic variability is due to reverse transcriptase processing errors, and proviral variants occur over time. Variation is also due to

- infection involving one or a few viral clones
- the number of virions, which can increase exponentially each day, leading to viral diversity if the individual is not on cART
- the mutation rate, with one nucleotide mutation per replication cycle
- variants that can infect the same cell, causing a high HIV-1 recombination rate.

Drug resistance can be acquired in individuals on cART, and others can become infected with HIV-resistant strains, known as *transmitted drug resistance*. Drug resistance can develop whilst on cART due to suboptimal drug treatment and selection of drug-resistant viruses as replication of drug-resistant viruses in this setting can increase the mutation rate.

There are often high levels of cross-resistance within each drug class. Most drug resistance mutations in a specific antiretroviral class will mean reduced susceptibility to one

or more of those drugs. However, the virus will be susceptible to drugs of other classes, although occasionally cross-resistance between drug classes is seen.

Transmission of drug-resistant HIV is an important issue. The WHO HIV drug resistance report in 2021 reported results from 38 countries, many of which had NNRTIs as first-line treatment, and >10% of adults starting treatment had NNRTI resistance, which rose to 30% in those who had received antiretroviral drugs. In the United Kingdom a study of 1000 new HIV infections with no previous exposure to antiretroviral drugs in 2019 reported a 6% resistance prevalence made up of 3.4% NRTIs, 3.1% PIs and 2.2% NNRTIs. The figure was 7.8% in 2015, and the fall probably reflected the introduction of improved combinations of ART both in terms of drug classes and reduced pill burden improving compliance. The prevalence of drug-resistant viruses in newly infected individuals will depend on factors such as changes in testing guidance, more individuals virologically suppressed on cART and whether the individual was infected by someone failing on ART. Furthermore, a huge reduction was seen in the prevalence of drug resistance mutations in ART experienced individuals from 72% in 2002 to 33% in 2013 for reasons noted earlier.

Baseline antiretroviral drug resistance testing is part of the management guidelines in many countries before starting treatment, as infection with a drug-resistant virus may affect the efficacy of subsequent therapy.

### Treatment of AIDS involves use of prophylaxis for treatment of opportunistic infections as well as antiretroviral drugs

Depending on the CD4 count, prophylaxis is given for specific opportunistic infections such as *P. jirovecii* and *C. neoformans*. When opportunist infections are diagnosed, they are treated appropriately (e.g. co-trimoxazole or pentamidine with or without steroids for *P. jirovecii* infection, ganciclovir for CMV, and fluconazole or amphotericin for *C. neoformans* infection).

### Laboratory tests

#### Laboratory tests for HIV infection involve both serologic and molecular analysis

AIDS is a clinical definition; in the presence of antibodies to HIV, any of the conditions listed in Table 22.9, regardless of the presence of other causes of immunodeficiency, indicate AIDS. The range and complexity of tests used for HIV-1 and HIV-2 screening, diagnosis of infection, and monitoring disease progression and response to therapy have increased dramatically over time.

Viral replication occurs during the incubation period, during which time the viral genome and, briefly, viral p24 antigen, but not the host's antibody response, may be detected. HIV-1 and HIV-2 diagnostic tests can be divided into combined antibody and antigen detection, antigen detection, antibody detection alone (although this is a less sensitive test) and genome detection. The last can be divided into qualitative HIV-1 or HIV-2 proviral DNA and quantitative HIV-1 or HIV-2 RNA detection. In addition, antiretroviral drug resistance and tropism assays are part of standard management.

Initially, an HIV-1 and HIV-2 antibody/antigen combination assay, which includes antibody and p24 antigen, is carried out. These assays have been developed to reduce the diagnostic window period. Assay reactivity is confirmed

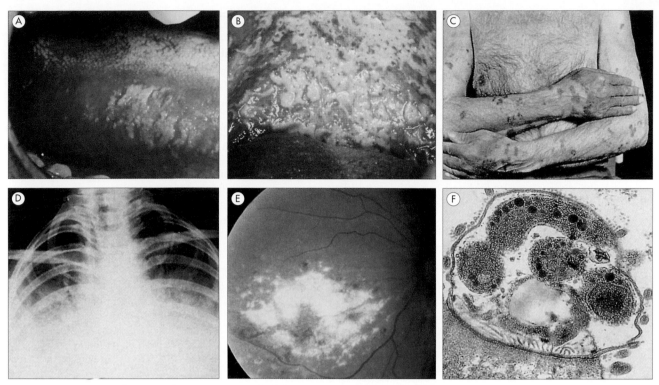

**Fig. 22.25** Opportunist infections and tumours associated with human immunodeficiency virus (HIV) infection. (A) Hairy leukoplakia—raised white lesions of oral mucosa, predominantly along the lateral aspect of the tongue, due to Epstein-Barr virus infection. (B) Extensive oral candidiasis. (C) Kaposi sarcoma—brown pigmented lesions on the upper extremities. (D) *Pneumocystis* pneumonia, with extensive infiltrates in both lungs. (E) Cytomegalovirus retinitis showing scattered exudates and haemorrhages, with sheathing of vessels. (F) Cryptosporidiosis—electron micrograph showing mature schizont with several merozoites attached to intestinal epithelium. (A, Courtesy H.P. Holley; B and F, courtesy W.E. Farrar; C, courtesy E. Sahn; D, courtesy J.A. Innes; E, courtesy C.J. Ellis.)

**Table 22.9** Opportunist infections and tumours in AIDS

| Viruses | Disseminated CMV (including retina, brain, peripheral nervous system, gastrointestinal tract)<br>HHV-8 (Kaposi sarcoma)[b]<br>JC virus (brain—PML)<br>EBV (hairy leukoplakia, primary cerebral lymphoma)<br>HSV (lungs, gastrointestinal tract, CNS, skin) |
|---|---|
| Bacteria[a] | Mycobacteria (e.g. *Mycoplasma avium*, *M. tuberculosis*—disseminated, extrapulmonary)<br>*Salmonella* (recurrent, disseminated) septicaemia |
| Protozoa | *Toxoplasma gondii* (disseminated, including CNS) |
| Fungi | *Cryptococcus neoformans* (CNS)<br>Histoplasmosis (disseminated, extrapulmonary)<br>*Coccidioides* (disseminated, extrapulmonary) |
| Other | Wasting disease (cause unknown)<br>HIV encephalopathy |

[a]Also pyogenic bacteria (e.g. *Haemophilus, Streptococcus, Pneumococcus*) causing septicaemia, pneumonia, meningitis, osteomyelitis, arthritis, abscesses, etc.; multiple or recurrent infections, especially in children.

[b]Associated with HHV-8, an independently transmitted agent; 300 times as frequent in AIDS as in other immunodeficiencies. AIDS is defined as the presence of antibodies to HIV plus one of the conditions in this table.

AIDS, Acquired immunodeficiency syndrome; CMV, cytomegalovirus; CNS, central nervous system; EBV, Epstein-Barr virus; HHV, human herpesvirus; HSV, herpes simplex virus; PML, progressive multifocal leukoencephalopathy.

using an alternative HIV test format on the original unseparated sample stored in the laboratory to ensure that a specimen separation error has not occurred. HIV type differentiation may be carried out using a number of assays that may include an immunoblot in which the antigens are coated on nitrocellulose strips. A positive result is confirmed on a further blood sample to ensure that the original sample had not been mislabelled at collection.

HIV-1 RNA or proviral DNA tests may be carried out on plasma and whole blood samples, respectively, if it is difficult to make a diagnosis because low level assay reactivity is detected when the serum sample is tested and the result is indeterminate, or the patient may have a seroconversion illness and the screening tests are negative.

Part of monitoring individuals infected with HIV-1 on or off ART involves measuring the plasma HIV-1 RNA load, which can be quantified using several commercial or in-house assays using different methods. The main assay formats are based on reverse transcription PCR (RT-PCR), branched DNA signal amplification and RNA transcription isothermal amplification.

In addition, part of the laboratory portfolio involves antiretroviral resistance genotypic analysis by automated DNA sequencing. This is a more specialized test, and the interpretation of the results may be complicated.

Diagnosis of HIV infection in newborn infants can be difficult because passively acquired maternal IgG will be detected in the first 12 months after birth. Reference laboratories may have virus-specific IgM and IgA in-house tests, which would signify in utero infection (see Ch. 24) as part of their test portfolio. Samples from infants are tested at various time intervals up to 12–24 months for p24 antigen, HIV-1 RNA and/or HIV-1 proviral DNA and HIV antibody to assess their HIV status.

## Measures to control spread

*There are a number of preventative measures to reduce the spread of HIV*

In resource-rich countries such as the United Kingdom, new diagnoses in 2021 had fallen to 2955; although highest in the MSM group, the number had almost halved since 2017 (Fig. 22.26A and B). The estimated annual number of new HIV infections in all ages had substantially changed from ~2.2 million in 2010 to ~1.5 million in 2021 (see Fig 22.26B). The largest fall in new adult HIV infections was seen in sub-Saharan Africa, from 1.4 million in 2014 to 860,000 in 2021.

Much smaller reductions occurred in the Asia and Pacific region (340,000 in 2014 to 260,000 in 2021), West and Central

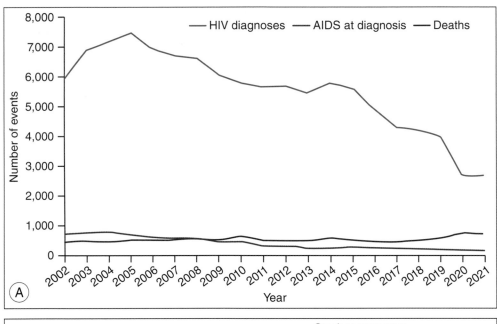

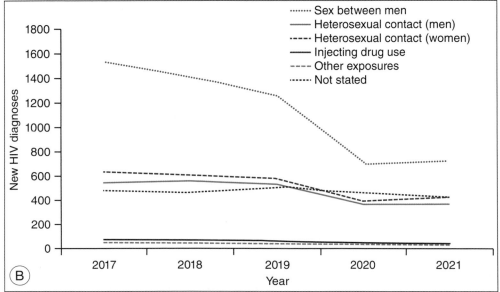

**Fig. 22.26** (A) New human immunodeficiency virus *(HIV)* diagnoses, acquired immunodeficiency syndrome (AIDS) at diagnosis and all-cause deaths in people with HIV: England, 2002–2021. (B) New HIV diagnoses among people first diagnosed in England by probable route of exposure: England, 2017–2021. (Modified from HIV Testing, PrEP, New HIV Diagnoses, and Care Outcomes for People Accessing HIV Services: 2022 Report, GOV.UK; 2022.)

Europe and North America (85,000 in 2014 to 63,000 in 2021) and the Middle East and North Africa (22,000 in 2014 to 14,000 in 2021). Although increases were seen in Latin America (87,000 in 2014 to 110,000 in 2021), the Caribbean (13,000 in 2014 to 14,000 in 2021) and Eastern Europe and Central Asia (140,000 in 2014 to 160,000 in 2021), the ranges were quite broad for these estimates according to the UNAIDS global AIDS update in 2021 (e.g. the range for Latin America was 68,000–150,000).

Prevention measures include reducing mother-to-child HIV transmission, where transmission may be seen in ~25% at delivery if no interventions are used. cART is a key intervention, and reducing plasma HIV load to below detection means vaginal delivery may be carried out instead of caesarean section delivery and may reduce transmission by breastfeeding in countries where infant mortality may be higher if breastfeeding is avoided. Reducing sexual transmission by modifying sexual behaviour and condom use is a major public health effort, but preexposure prophylaxis with daily antiretroviral use has been shown to reduce HIV transmission. Treating genital herpes simplex infections is another intervention.

The risk of transmitting HIV via blood and blood products is reduced considerably by donor screening programmes, pathogen reduction and inactivation technology, including heat treatment, organic solvents and detergents, nanofiltration, methylene blue and UVA light with a psoralen compound, respectively. Those at risk of infection are advised not to donate. Heat treatment of factor VIII is a further precaution before this product is used to treat haemophiliac patients. HIV has a delicate outer envelope and is highly susceptible to heat and chemical agents. HIV is inactivated under pasteurization conditions and by hypochlorites even at concentrations as low as 1 in 10,000 ppm; 2.5% glutaraldehyde and ethyl alcohol are also effective against the virus.

The problem of transmission between injecting drug users is reduced by freely distributing clean needles and syringes.

Public health educational programmes are key in reducing the incidence of all STIs.

## Vaccination

### There are a number of challenges in developing a successful vaccine against HIV infection

More than 50 vaccine regimens have undergone clinical trials since 1999. The fact that there is a successful killed virus vaccine for a feline retrovirus (feline leukaemia) and that a similar vaccine protects monkeys from simian AIDS gave some hope for the development of an HIV vaccine. The prospects are limited for a number of reasons, including viral antigenic variation and sequence diversity, slow neutralizing antibody response to HIV infection, viral evasion of immune responses and establishment of latent viral reservoirs. Various subunit envelope glycoproteins, whole killed virus vaccines, plasmid DNA vaccines and virus vectors to carry HIV antigens have been investigated and tested. Trials have been carried out in animal (monkey) models and humans.

The aim is to prevent infection or reduce the HIV load and clinical progression postinfection. The immune correlates of protection have yet to be well defined and are critical to protect against infection. Two vaccine candidates involved in efficacy studies were an envelope gp120 protein vaccine that resulted in type-specific but not broadly reactive neutralizing antibody responses and a replication-incompetent adenovirus vector expressing HIV-1 *gag*, *pol* and *nef* gene products. The latter resulted in cellular immune responses in most recipients. However, the vaccine was neither protective nor reduced HIV loads postinfection. In the 2009 RV144 Thai HIV vaccine trial involving a recombinant canarypox vector vaccine ALVAC-HIV and two booster injections of the recombinant gp 120 subunit vaccine, the estimated vaccine efficacy was ~31%, and it was thought that antibody generated against the V1V2 loop of the envelope glycoprotein may have contributed to protection. In 2016 the South African Uhambo HVTN 702 vaccine trial used the same vaccine with a different booster but was unsuccessful. Subsequently, an adenovirus vector vaccine that was thought to be more immunogenic went into trial but did not show significant efficacy. Passively transferred neutralizing antibodies in sera or monoclonal broadly neutralizing antibodies have been shown to be protective in preventing SIV infection in macaques. Broadly neutralizing antibodies (bnAbs) could act by blocking cells from getting infected. The IAVI G001 phase 1 vaccine trial results were promising, and a bnAb precursor response was seen in 97% of vaccinees. The idea behind the vaccine was that the immunogen would stimulate the precursor B cells that produce bnAbs. Immunogens could also be delivered using mRNA vaccines, a successful approach when COVID vaccines were developed.

To prevent sexual transmission, mucosal immunity is needed, and this is likely to come from a mucosally administered vaccine. The major route of HIV-1 transmission is via mucosal surfaces. Penile foreskin increases the risk of HIV transmission, owing to the high density of HIV target Langerhans cells in addition to the inner mucosal surface not being keratinized. Circumcision has been shown to reduce the risk of transmission. Macaque SIV infection models have shown additional mucosal routes of entry, suggesting that HIV infection might also be transmitted through oropharyngeal and upper gastrointestinal mucosa. A T-cell vaccine would need to induce a long-lasting mucosal immune response that includes mucosal neutralizing IgA and IgG antibody and T-cell responses. Mucosal CD8 cytotoxic T lymphocytes would limit infection and subsequent HIV viraemia as well as clearance of viral reservoirs in the gut mucosa.

Finally, epitope-based vaccine design could focus the immune response on the viral fusion peptide that is key to viral entry and produce fusion peptide antibodies that neutralize diverse HIV-1 strains.

### Allogeneic bone marrow transplantation leading to HIV cure

HIV entry into CD4 T cells by R5 tropic virus can be inhibited if the homozygous deletion CCR5Δ32 is present in the CCR5 receptor gene. The result is HIV cannot infect these cells.

The variant allele is homozygous in ~1% of Caucasians and even less in other ethnic groups. In 2006 an HIV-positive individual in Berlin had acute myeloid leukaemia and needed an allogeneic bone marrow transplant as treatment. An HLA-identical donor with the CCR5Δ32 deletion was selected, the transplantation procedure was successful and the patient remained in remission and was not taking cART. Donor-derived peripheral CD4 T cells were then detected in peripheral blood and in gut mucosa. There were no signs of HIV infection as HIV-1 RNA was undetectable in peripheral blood mononuclear cells and in plasma. In addition, the patient became HIV negative on serologic testing.

After this success, another HIV-positive individual with Hodgkin lymphoma was transplanted in London with a CCR5Δ32 homozygous donor.

Although these two individuals were cured of HIV infection, it is rare to find HLA-matched donors with this deletion, but it demonstrated that HIV could be cured.

## OPPORTUNIST STIs

### Opportunist STIs include salmonellae, shigellae, hepatitis A, *Giardia duodenalis* and *Entamoeba histolytica* infections

Although STIs are classically transmitted during heterosexual intercourse, they can also be transmitted whenever two mucosal surfaces are brought together. Anal intercourse allows the transfer of microorganisms from penis to rectal mucosa or to anal and perianal regions. Gonococcal or papillomavirus lesions, for instance, may occur in any of these sites. A few microorganisms (hepatitis B, HIV) are transmitted more often across rectal mucosa. If there is oral–anal contact, a variety of intestinal pathogens are given the opportunity to spread as STIs and can then be regarded as opportunistic STIs. These include salmonellae, shigellae, hepatitis A virus, *G. duodenalis* and *E. histolytica* (also see Ch. 23). Together with chronic infections such as CMV and cryptosporidiosis, they contribute to intestinal symptoms and diarrhoea in AIDS patients.

### Hepatitis B virus is often transmitted sexually

Hepatitis B virus (HBV) is detectable in semen, saliva and vaginal secretions. HBV transmission, like HIV, is more likely when genital areas are ulcerated or contaminated with blood. Combined immunisation against hepatitis A and B is a key preventative measure for at-risk groups. Hepatitis C is less commonly transmitted sexually; <5% of long-term sexual partners are infected.

## ARTHROPOD INFESTATIONS

### Infection with the pubic or crab louse causes itching and is treated with permethrin shampoo

The crab louse (*Pthirus pubis*) is distinct from the other human lice (*Pediculus humanus humanus* and *P. h. capitis*). The crab louse is well adapted for life in the genital region, clinging tightly to the pubic hairs (see Ch. 6), but it can infest any hair-bearing area so hairs on the eyebrows, eyelashes or in the axilla are occasionally colonized. *P. pubis* takes up to 10 blood feeds a day, which results in itching at the site of the bites. Eggs known as nits are seen attached to the affected hairs, and the characteristic lice, up to 2 mm long, are visible (often at the base of a hair) by dermoscopy, under a hand lens or by microscopy of a detached hair. Infestation is estimated to affect 1–2% of the world population, but in some regions the incidence has fallen in parallel to an increase in the practice of pubic hair removal, which destroys the preferred habitat of the lice.

Treatment is by the application of permethrin cream or malathion lotion.

### Genital scabies is also treated with permethrin cream

*Sarcoptes scabiei* (see Ch. 27) can be sexually transmitted and cause local lesions on the genitalia, particularly the penis and scrotum in males. In females it usually spares the vulva, but pruritus vulvae and vulvar nodules have been reported. Patients may have evidence of scabies elsewhere on the body, with burrows between the fingers or toes. Crusted (Norwegian) scabies has been reported in males and females. Genital scabies is treated with permethrin cream. Oral ivermectin may be required in immunocompromised patients.

## KEY FACTS

- Microorganisms transmitted by the sexual route in humans include representatives from all groups apart from the rickettsiae and helminths.

- STIs are found in the general community rather than being confined only to high-risk groups.

- Genital herpes, warts, chlamydial urethritis, and gonorrhoea are by far the most common of all the STIs, but HIV infection has had a major impact, although it is now considered as a long-term, chronic infection compared with the clinical situation in the late 1980s and early 1990s.

- Except for hepatitis A and B and HPV infections, there are no vaccines for these other STIs, but antimicrobial chemotherapy is often available.

- At present, the best method of control is prevention.

- Transmission depends upon human behaviour, which is notoriously difficult to influence.

- Long intervals between the onset of infectiousness and disease increase the chances of transmission.

# Gastrointestinal tract infections

**23**

## Introduction

### Ingested pathogens may cause disease confined to the gut or involve other parts of the body

Ingestion of pathogens can cause many different infections. These may be confined to the gastrointestinal tract or are initiated there before spreading to other parts of the body. In this chapter we consider the bacterial causes of diarrhoeal disease and summarize the other bacterial causes of food-associated infection and food poisoning. Viral and parasitic causes of diarrhoeal disease are discussed, as well as infections acquired via the gastrointestinal tract and causing disease in other body systems, including typhoid and paratyphoid fevers, listeriosis and viral hepatitis. For clarity, all types of viral hepatitis are included in this chapter, despite the fact that some are transmitted by other routes of infection. Infections of the liver can also result in liver abscesses, and several parasitic infections cause liver disease. Peritonitis and intraabdominal abscesses can arise from seeding of the abdominal cavity by organisms from the gastrointestinal tract. Several different terms are used to describe infections of the gastrointestinal tract; those in common use are shown in Box 23.1.

A wide range of microbial pathogens can infect the gastrointestinal tract, and the main bacterial and viral pathogens are listed in Table 23.1. They are acquired by the faecal–oral route, from faecally contaminated food, fluids or fingers.

For an infection to occur, the pathogen must be ingested in sufficient numbers or possess attributes to elude the host defences of the upper gastrointestinal tract and reach the intestine (Fig. 23.1; see also Ch. 14). Here they remain localized and cause disease as a result of multiplication and/or toxin production, or they may invade through the intestinal mucosa to reach the lymphatics or the bloodstream (Fig. 23.2). The damaging effects resulting from infection of the gastrointestinal tract are summarized in Box 23.2.

---

### Box 23.1    Terms Used to Describe Gastrointestinal Tract Infections

As well as many colloquial expressions, several different clinical terms are used to describe infections of the gastrointestinal tract. Diarrhoea without blood and pus is usually the result of enterotoxin production, whereas the presence of blood and/or pus cells in the faeces indicates an invasive infection with mucosal destruction.

**Gastroenteritis**

- A syndrome characterized by gastrointestinal symptoms, including nausea, vomiting, diarrhoea and abdominal discomfort

**Diarrhoea**

- Abnormal faecal discharge characterized by frequent and/or fluid stool; usually resulting from disease of the small intestine and involving increased fluid and electrolyte loss

**Dysentery**

- An inflammatory disorder of the gastrointestinal tract often associated with blood and pus in the faeces and accompanied by symptoms of pain, fever and abdominal cramps; usually resulting from disease of the large intestine

**Enterocolitis**

- Inflammation involving the mucosa of both the small and large intestines

---

### Food-associated infection versus food poisoning

Infection associated with consumption of contaminated food is often termed *food poisoning*, but *food-associated infection* is a better term. True food poisoning occurs after consumption of food containing toxins, which may be chemical, such as heavy metals, or bacterial in origin, associated with *Clostridium botulinum* or *Staphylococcus aureus*. The bacteria multiply and produce toxins within contaminated food. The organisms may be destroyed during food preparation, but the toxin is unaffected, consumed and acts within hours. In food-associated infections, the food may simply act as a vehicle for the pathogen, *Campylobacter* being an example, or provide conditions in which the pathogen, such as *Salmonella*, can multiply to produce numbers large enough to cause disease.

**Table 23.1** Important bacterial and viral pathogens of the gastrointestinal tract

| Pathogen | Animal reservoir | Foodborne | Waterborne |
|---|---|---|---|
| **Bacteria** | | | |
| *Escherichia coli* | +? | + (EHEC) | + (ETEC) |
| *Salmonella* | + | + + + | + |
| *Campylobacter* | + | + + + | + |
| *Vibrio cholerae* | − | + | + + + |
| *Shigella* | − | + | − |
| *Clostridium perfringens* | + | + + + | − |
| *Bacillus cereus* | − | + + | − |
| *Vibrio parahaemolyticus* | − | + + | − |
| *Yersinia enterocolitica* | + | + | − |
| **Viruses** | | | |
| Rotavirus | − | − | − |
| Noroviruses (previously known as SRSV or Norwalk-like viruses) | − | + + | + |

Many different pathogens cause infections of the gastrointestinal tract. Some are found in both humans and animals, while others are strictly human parasites. This difference has important implications for control and prevention. EHEC, Enterohaemorrhagic (verotoxin-producing) *E. coli*; ETEC, enterotoxigenic *E. coli*; SRSV, small round structured viruses.

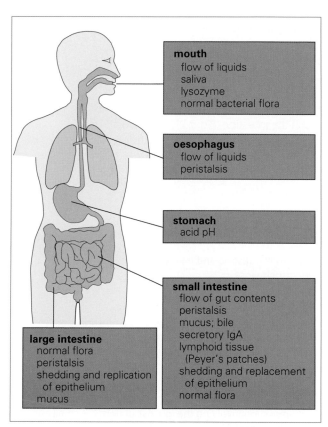

**mouth**
flow of liquids
saliva
lysozyme
normal bacterial flora

**oesophagus**
flow of liquids
peristalsis

**stomach**
acid pH

**small intestine**
flow of gut contents
peristalsis
mucus; bile
secretory IgA
lymphoid tissue
(Peyer's patches)
shedding and replacement
of epithelium
normal flora

**large intestine**
normal flora
peristalsis
shedding and replication
of epithelium
mucus

**Fig. 23.1** Every day we swallow large numbers of microorganisms. Because of the body's defence mechanisms, however, they rarely succeed in surviving the passage to the intestine in sufficient numbers to cause infection. IgA, Immunoglobulin A.

## DIARRHOEAL DISEASES CAUSED BY BACTERIAL OR VIRAL INFECTION

**Diarrhoea is the most common outcome of gastrointestinal tract infection**

Infections of the gastrointestinal tract range in their effects from a mild self-limiting attack of the so-called runs to severe

**Box 23.2 ■ Damage Resulting From Infection of the Gastrointestinal Tract**

- Pharmacologic action of bacterial toxins that are local or distant to site of infection (e.g. cholera, staphylococcal food poisoning)
- Local inflammation in response to superficial microbial invasion (e.g. shigellosis, amoebiasis)
- Deep invasion to blood or lymphatics; dissemination to other body sites (e.g. hepatitis A, enteric fevers)
- Perforation of mucosal epithelium after infection, surgery or accidental trauma (e.g. peritonitis, intraabdominal abscesses)

Infection of the gastrointestinal tract can cause damage locally or at distant sites.

and sometimes fatal diarrhoea. There may be associated vomiting, fever and malaise. Diarrhoea is the result of an increase in fluid and electrolyte loss into the gastrointestinal tract lumen, leading to the production of unformed or liquid faeces, and can be thought of as the method by which the host forcibly expels the pathogen and, in doing so, aids its dissemination. However, diarrhoea also occurs in many noninfectious conditions, and an infectious cause should not be assumed.

**In the resource-poor world, diarrhoeal disease is a major cause of mortality in children**

In the resource-poor world, diarrhoeal disease is a major cause of morbidity and mortality, particularly in young children (Fig. 23.3). The Global Burden of Diseases study of 2016 reported the burden of diarrhoea measured in disability-adjusted life-years (DALYs) that included morbidity and mortality. Around 85% of long-term DALYs, amounting to 15 652 300 episodes, are due to infectious diseases as a consequence of undernutrition.

In the resource-rich world, it remains a very common complaint but is usually mild and self-limiting except in the

**Fig. 23.2** Infections of the gastrointestinal tract can be grouped into those that remain localized in the gut and those that invade beyond the gut to cause infection in other sites in the body. To spread to a new host, pathogens are excreted in large numbers in the faeces and must survive in the environment for long enough to infect another person directly or indirectly through contaminated food or fluids. (From World Health Organization (WHO). World health statistics 2012. Geneva, Switzerland: Author; 2012.)

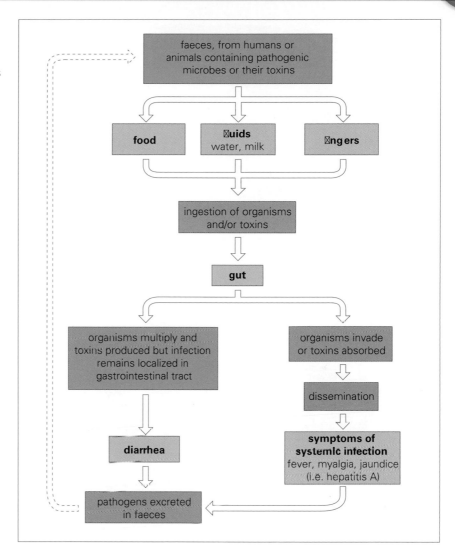

very young, the elderly and immunocompromised patients. Most of the pathogens listed in Table 23.1 are found throughout the world, but some, such as *Vibrio cholerae*, have a more limited geographic distribution. However, such infections can be acquired by travellers to these areas and imported into their home countries.

Data from the Global Enteric Multi-Center Study, a large case control investigation set up to determine the burden of paediatric diarrhoeal disease in South Asia and sub-Saharan Africa, showed that enterotoxigenic *Escherichia coli* and *Shigella* are in the top four causes of moderate to severe diarrhoea and therefore mortality in children in these areas.

Many cases of diarrhoeal disease are not diagnosed either because they are mild and self-limiting and the patient does not seek medical attention or because medical and laboratory facilities are unavailable. It is generally impossible to distinguish on clinical grounds between infections caused by the different pathogens. However information about the patient's recent food and travel history and macroscopic and microscopic examination of the faeces for blood and pus can provide helpful clues. A precise diagnosis can be achieved only by laboratory investigations. This is especially important in outbreaks because of the need to instigate appropriate epidemiologic investigations and control measures.

## Bacterial causes of diarrhoea

### Escherichia coli

*E. coli* is one of the most versatile of all bacterial pathogens. It was named in the 1950s after Theodor Escherich, who isolated and characterized the short rods from an infant's faecal sample in 1885. Some strains are important members of the normal intestinal flora of humans and animals, whereas others possess virulence factors that enable them to cause infections in the intestinal tract or at other sites, particularly the urinary tract, bloodstream and central nervous system. Strains that cause diarrhoeal disease do so by several distinct pathogenic mechanisms and differ in their epidemiology (Table 23.2).

**There are six distinct pathotypes of E. coli with different pathogenetic mechanisms.** Initially, all diarrhoea-associated *E. coli* pathotypes were termed enteropathogenic *E. coli* (EPEC). However, greater insight into mechanisms of pathogenicity has led to specific group designations: EPEC, enterotoxigenic *E. coli* (ETEC), Shiga toxin–producing *E. coli* (STEC; also called enterohaemorrhagic *E. coli* [EHEC] or verocytotoxin-producing *E. coli*), enteroinvasive *E. coli* (EIEC), enteroaggregative *E. coli* (EAEC) and diffusely aggregative *E. coli* (DAEC).

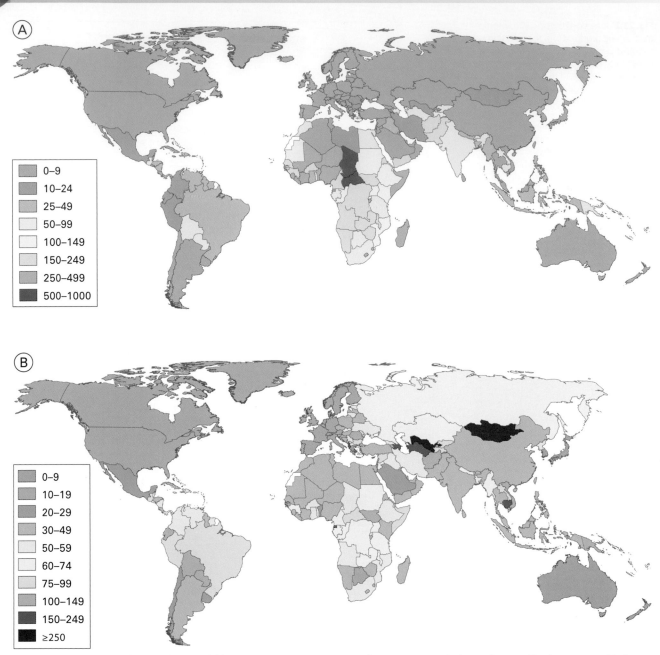

**Fig. 23.3** Global mortality from diarrhoea in children age <5 years in 2016. Many infectious causes, including pathogenic *E. coli*, are responsible for diarrhoea-related mortality in these children. The total diarrhoea DALYs is reached by adding the acute and long-term sequelae DALYs per 1000 children age <5 years in 2016. (A) The sum of the acute DALYs (diarrhoea incidence and mortality) and long-term sequelae diarrhoea DALYs due to growth impairment per 1000 children age <5 years in 2016. (B) The relative percentage increase in the total number of DALYs due to diarrhoeal diseases in 2016 among children age <5 years after including long-term sequelae diarrhoea DALYs compared with the acute diarrhoea DALYs only. (Reprinted with permission from Elsevier. Troeger C, Colombara DV, Rao PC, et al. Global disability-adjusted life-year estimates of long-term health burden and undernutrition attributable to diarrhoeal diseases in children younger than 5 years. *Lancet Glob Health*. 2018;6: e255–269.)

***EPEC pathogens do not make any toxins.*** They are attaching and effacing pathogens that form distinct lesions on the surfaces of intestinal epithelial cells in the small intestine. They are classified as typical and atypical subtypes based on whether they have the adherence factor plasmid and produce bundle-forming pili, intimin (an adhesin) and an associated protein (translocated intimin receptor). These virulence factors allow bacterial attachment to epithelial cells of the small intestine, leading to disruption of the microvillus

(an attaching–effacing mechanism of action; see Table 23.2, Fig. 23.4) leading to diarrhoea (Table 23.3).

***ETEC pathogens possess colonization factors (fimbrial adhesins).*** These bind the bacteria to specific receptors on the cell membrane of the small intestine (Fig. 23.5). They are a major cause of traveller's diarrhoea as well as ETEC-induced diarrhoea in the swine industry. ETEC produce powerful plasmid-associated enterotoxins, which are characterized as being either heat labile (LT) or heat stable (ST):

**Table 23.2** General overview of enteric *Escherichia coli* pathotypes

| Pathotype | Host(s) | Site of colonization | Disease(s) | Known reservoir(s)/source(s) of contamination | Treatment | Adhesion | Genetic identifiers |
|---|---|---|---|---|---|---|---|
| tEPEC | Children <5 yr, adults at high inocula | Small intestine | Profuse watery diarrhoea | Humans | Oral rehydration, antibiotics for persistent cases | Attaching and effacing | *eae*+, *bfp*+, *stx*- |
| aEPEC | | | | Humans, animals | | | *eae*+, *stx*- |
| STEC | Adults, children | Distal ileum, colon | Watery diarrhoea, hemorrhagic colitis, HUS | Humans, animals, food, water | Hydration, supportive for HUS | Attaching and effacing[a] | *eae*+/-, *stx*+ |
| EIEC/Shigella | Children <5 yr, adults, travellers, immunocompromised individuals | Colon | Shigellosis/bacillary dysentery, potential HUS | Humans, animals, food, water | Oral rehydration, antibiotics | NA (invasive) | *ipaH*+, *ial*+, *stx*+ (*S. dysenteriae*) |
| EAEC | Adults | Small intestine and/or colon | Traveller's diarrhoea, HUS (*stx*+) | Food, occasionally adult carriers | Antibiotics, oral rehydration | Stacked brick and/or invasive | *aatA*+, *aaiC*+, other candidates |
| | Children | | Persistent diarrhoea | | Antibiotics, oral rehydration, potentially probiotics | | |
| | Immunocompromised individuals | | Persistent diarrhoea | | Fluoroquinolones | | |
| ETEC | Children <5 yr, travellers | Small intestine | Watery diarrhoea | Food, water, humans, animals | Rehydration, antibiotics | CF mediated | CFs, LT, ST |
| DAEC | Children (increasing in severity from 18 months to 5 yr), adults | Intestine (uncharacterized location) | Persistent watery diarrhoea in children, speculated to contribute to Crohn disease in adults | Unknown | Rehydration | Diffuse adherent and/or invasive | No uniform markers |
| AIEC | Adults, children | Small intestine | Crohn disease | Unknown | Antibiotics, surgical resection | NA (invasive) | Uncharacterized |

[a]Only for LEE-positive STEC, not for LEE-negative STEC.

AIEC, Adherent invasive *E. coli*; aEPEC, atypical enteropathogenic *E. coli*; CF, colonization factor; DAEC, diffusely adherent *E. coli*; EAEC, enteroaggregative *E. coli*; EIEC, Shigella/enteroinvasive *E. coli*; EPEC, enteropathogenic *E. coli*; ETEC, enterotoxigenic *E. coli*; HUS, haemolytic uraemic syndrome; LT, heat-labile enterotoxin; NA, not applicable; ST, heat-stable enterotoxin; TEC, Shiga toxin–producing *E. coli* (e.g. enterohaemorrhagic *E. coli* [EHEC]); tEPEC, typical EPEC.

From Croxen MA, Law RJ, Scholz R, et al. Recent advances in understanding enteric pathogenic *Escherichia coli*. *Clin Mic Rev.* 2013;26:822–880, table 1.

- Heat-labile enterotoxin LT-I is very similar in structure and mode of action to cholera toxin produced by *V. cholerae*, and infections with strains producing LT-I can mimic cholera, particularly in young and malnourished children (see Table 23.3).
- Other ETEC strains produce heat-stable enterotoxins in addition to or instead of LT. STs have a similar but distinct mode of action to that of LT. $ST_a$ activates guanylate cyclase activity, causing an increase in cyclic guanosine monophosphate, which results in increased fluid secretion. Immunoassays are commercially available for the identification of ETEC, but multiplex polymerase chain reaction (PCR) methods for detecting enterotoxin have been developed.

***EHEC isolates produce a verotoxin.*** EHEC is a subset of STEC, and the verotoxin (i.e. toxic to tissue cultures of vero cells) is essentially identical to Shiga (*Shigella*) toxin (Stx). After attachment to the mucosa of the large intestine by the attaching–effacing mechanism also seen in EPEC, the produced toxin has a direct effect on intestinal epithelium, resulting in diarrhoea (see Table 23.3). EHEC causes haemorrhagic colitis (HC) and haemolytic uraemic syndrome (HUS). In HC there is destruction of the mucosa and consequent haemorrhage; this may be followed by HUS. The Stx receptor is the glycosphingolipid globotriaosylceramide (known as Gb3), and it is found on the surface of renal epithelial cells accounting for kidney involvement. While there are many serotypes of EHEC, the most common is O157:H7, and there are many reports worldwide of its association with severe illness. Cattle are major reservoirs for pathogenic STEC, and human illness occurs after exposure to faecal material via contaminated water and food and is associated with poor hand hygiene after visiting petting farms. STEC can survive in soil for months.

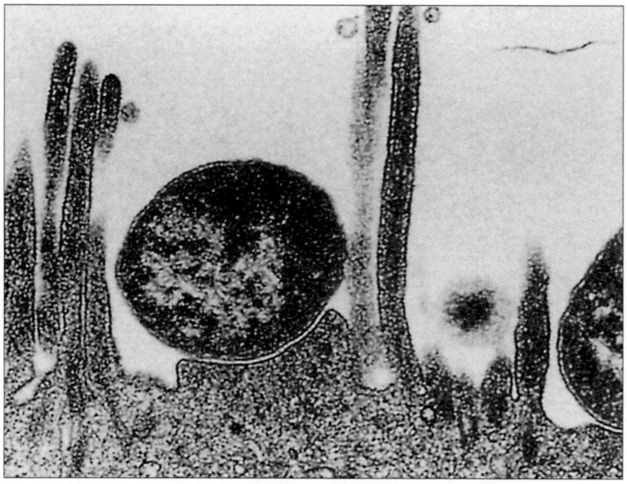

**Fig. 23.4** Electron micrograph of enteropathogenic *Escherichia coli* adhering to the brush border of intestinal mucosal cells with localized destruction of microvilli. (Courtesy S. Knutton.)

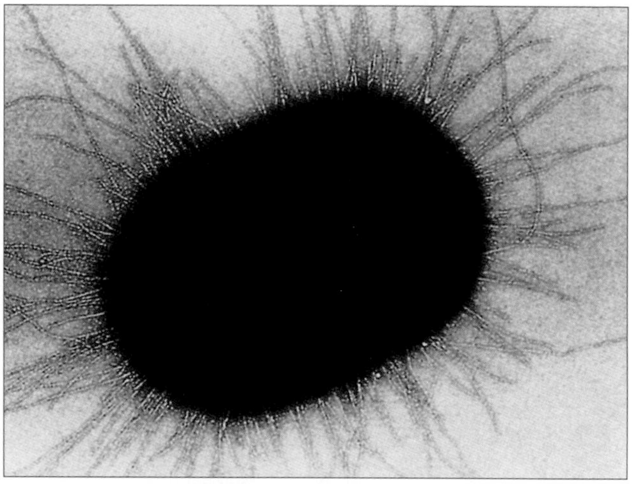

**Fig. 23.5** Electron micrograph of enterotoxin *Escherichia coli* showing pili necessary for adherence to mucosal epithelial cells. (Courtesy S. Knutton.)

**Table 23.3** The clinical features of bacterial diarrhoeal infection

| Pathogen | Incubation period | Duration | Symptoms: Diarrhoea | Vomiting | Abdominal cramps | Fever |
|---|---|---|---|---|---|---|
| *Salmonella* | 6 h–2 days | 48 h–7 days | Watery | + | + | + |
| *Campylobacter* | 2–11 days | 3 days–3 weeks | Bloody | – | + | + |
| *Shigella* | 1–4 days | 2–3 days | Bloody | – | + | + |
| *Vibrio cholerae* | 2–3 days | Up to 7 days | Watery | + | + | – |
| *Clostridium perfringens* | 8 h–1 day | 12 h–1 day | Watery | – | + | – |
| *Bacillus cereus* | | | | | | |
| Diarrhoeal | 8 h–12 h | 12 h–1 day | Watery | – | + | – |
| Emetic | 15 min–4 h | 12 h–2 days | Watery | + | + | – |
| *Yersinia enterocolitica* | 4–7 days | 1–2 weeks | Bloody | – | + | + |
| Enteropathogenic *Escherichia coli* (EPEC) | 1–2 days | Weeks | Watery | + | + | + |
| Enterotoxigenic *E. coli* (ETEC) | 1–7 days | 2–6 days | Watery | + | + | – |
| Enterohaemorrhagic *E. coli* (EHEC) | 3–4 days | 5–10 days | Bloody | + | + | – |
| Enteroinvasive *E. coli* (EIEC) | 1–3 days | 7–10 days | Bloody | + | + | + |

It is difficult, if not impossible, to determine the likely cause of a diarrhoeal illness on the basis of clinical features alone, and laboratory investigations are essential to identify the pathogen.

*EIEC pathogens attach specifically to the mucosa of the large intestine.* They invade the cells by endocytosis by using plasmid-associated genes. Inside the cell they lyse the endocytic vacuole, multiply and spread to adjacent cells, causing tissue destruction, inflammation, necrosis and ulceration and resulting in blood and mucus in stools (see Table 23.3).

*EAEC pathogens are named after their characteristic attachment pattern to tissue culture cells.* The pattern is an aggregative or stacked brick formation. These organisms adhere to the small intestinal mucosa to cause persistent diarrhoea, especially in children in resource-poor countries. Their aggregative adherence ability is due to plasmid-associated fimbrial adhesins. EAEC pathogens also produce heat-labile (LT) toxins (an enterotoxin and a toxin related to *E. coli* haemolysin), but their role in diarrhoeal disease is uncertain. The last stage of the EAEC pathogenesis model involves the host innate immune mechanism and strain of EAEC influencing the amount of inflammation. EAEC has caused many large outbreaks of diarrhoea across the world and is associated with traveller's diarrhoea via contaminated water and food.

*DAEC pathogens produce an alpha haemolysin and cytotoxic necrotizing factor 1.* They attach to cells but are not classified under localized adherence or attachment/effacing. Their role in diarrhoeal disease, especially in young children, is incompletely understood and somewhat controversial, with some studies reporting no association as DAEC was detected in healthy age-matched controls.

*EPEC and ETEC are the most important contributors to global incidence of diarrhoea, whereas EHEC is more important in resource-rich countries.* The diarrhoea produced by *E. coli* varies from mild to severe, depending on the strain and the underlying health of the host. ETEC diarrhoea in children in resource-poor countries may be clinically indistinguishable from cholera. EIEC and EHEC strains both cause bloody diarrhoea (see Table 23.3). Following EHEC infection, HUS is characterized by acute renal failure (Fig. 23.6), anaemia and thrombocytopenia, and there may be neurologic complications. HUS is the most common cause of acute renal failure in children in the United Kingdom and United States. Although *E. coli* O157:H7

is the most commonly recognized serotype involved in HUS, *E. coli* 0104:H4, which had not been reported as causing an outbreak previously, caused a significant outbreak of HUS and bloody diarrhoea in 15 countries across Europe in 2011. Over several months starting in May 2011, 860 individuals with HUS and >3000 with bloody diarrhoea were reported in Germany, many of whom had laboratory-confirmed *E. coli* 0104:H4 infection. More than 50 people died, and the likely vehicle was sprouted beans imported from the Middle East. Detecting *E. coli* O157:H7 is a key focus; non-0157:H7 is a major contributor to both sporadic cases and outbreaks in North America, Australia and Europe. In the United States the Foodborne Diseases Active Surveillance Network (FoodNet) has been reporting trends for infections transmitted via food since 1996. In 2014 the incidence rate of *E. coli* O157:H7 was 0.91 per 100000 people, highest in <5-year-old children, and 16% of infections were associated with outbreaks. Non-0157 had an incidence of 1.43 per 100000 people in mostly the same age group, and 6% of infections were associated with outbreaks. Between 2016 and 2019, the incidence of HUS per 100000 people <18 years old in the US population was ~0.5 but fell, presumably due to the coronavirus disease 2019 (COVID-19) pandemic, to 0.34 in 2020. Over the same period, STEC 0157 incidence fell from 2.5 in 2016 to 1.6 in 2019 and to 1.3 in 2020. Finally, the STEC non-0157 rose from 7–9 between 2016 and 2019 and dropped to 5/100000 in 2020 (Fig. 23.7).

*Specific tests are needed to identify strains of pathogenic* **E. coli.** Because *E. coli* is a member of the normal gastrointestinal flora, specific tests are required to identify strains that may be responsible for diarrhoeal disease. Infections are more common in children and are often travel associated, and these factors should be considered when samples are received in the laboratory. It is important to note that specialized tests beyond routine stool cultures are required to identify specific diarrhoea-associated *E. coli* types. Such tests are not ordinarily performed with uncomplicated diarrhoea, which is usually self-limiting. However, concern regarding EHEC (e.g. bloody diarrhoea) has led most laboratories in resource-rich countries to screen for *E. coli* O157:H7.

*Antibiotic therapy is not indicated for* **E. coli** *diarrhoea.* Specific antibacterial therapy is not indicated. Fluid replacement may be necessary, especially in young children. Treatment of HUS is urgent and may involve dialysis.

Provision of a clean water supply and adequate systems for sewage disposal are fundamental to the prevention of disease. Food and unpasteurized milk can be important vehicles of infection, especially for EIEC and EHEC, but there is no evidence of an animal or environmental reservoir.

### Salmonella

*Salmonellae are the most common cause of food-associated diarrhoea in many resource-rich countries.* In some countries such as the United States and United Kingdom, however, they have been relegated to second place by *Campylobacter*. FoodNet reported that, in 2019 in the United States, the incidence rate was 13.3/100000 population, mostly in those <5 years old. The majority of serotypes were *Salmonella enteritidis* (16%), *S. typhimurium* (14%) and *S. newport* (10%), and 6% of infections were associated with an outbreak. Like *E. coli*, the salmonellae belong to the family Enterobacteriaceae. Historically, salmonella nomenclature has been

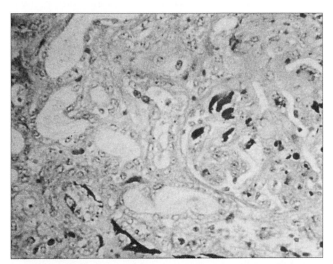

**Fig. 23.6** Verotoxin-producing *Escherichia coli* infection showing fibrin thrombi in glomerular capillaries in haemolytic uraemic syndrome (Weigert stain). (Courtesy H.R. Powell.)

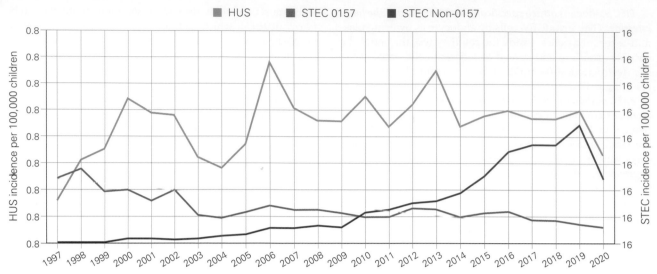

**Fig. 23.7** Incidence of haemolytic uraemic syndrome (HUS), Shiga toxin–producing *Escherichia coli* (*STEC*) 0157 and STEC non-0157, respectively, per 100 000 younger than age 18. (From FoodNet Fast. HUS surveillance tool. Centers for Disease Control and Prevention, Atlanta, GA; 2023.)

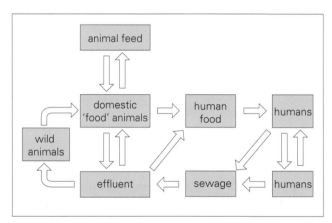

**Fig. 23.8** The recycling of salmonellae. With the exception of *Salmonella typhi*, salmonellae are widely distributed in animals, providing a constant source of infection for humans. Excretion of large numbers of salmonellae from infected individuals and carriers allows the organisms to be recycled.

somewhat confusing, with >2000 serotypes defined based on differences in the cell wall (O) and flagellar (H) antigens (Kauffmann–White scheme). However, DNA hybridization studies indicate there are only two species, the most important of which for human infection is *S. enterica*. *S. enterica* serovars Typhi, Paratyphi A–C are known as typhoidal *Salmonella*, which are restricted to humans and cause typhoid and paratyphoid fever, together called *enteric fever*. The rest are known as nontyphoidal *Salmonella*. To simplify discussion and comparison, past convention has been to replace this species name with the serotype designation. While technically incorrect (the serotype is not a species), this practice is helpful when discussing interrelationships between different isolates (e.g. in epidemiologic analysis when tracing the source of an outbreak). This convention is thus followed here to maintain continuity with other scientific literature.

All salmonellae except *S. typhi* and *S. paratyphi* are found in animals as well as humans. There is a large animal reservoir of infection, which is transmitted to humans via contaminated food, especially poultry and dairy products

(Fig. 23.8). Waterborne infection is less frequent. Salmonella infection is also transmitted from person to person, and secondary spread can therefore occur (e.g. within a family after one member has become infected after consuming contaminated food). In 2018 the World Health Organization (WHO) estimated that 11–20 million people had typhoid fever, and between 128 000 and 161 000 people die annually as a result in low- and middle-income countries.

***Salmonellae are almost always acquired orally in food or drink that is contaminated with human faeces.*** The host barrier to infection involves gastric acid secretion, safe in the knowledge that the bacterium is acid susceptible. However, keeping one step (or fluid movement) ahead, gastric acid secretion has been shown to be suppressed during the acute infection. Diarrhoea is produced as a result of invasion by the salmonellae of epithelial cells in the terminal portion of the small intestine (Fig. 23.9). Initial entry is probably through uptake by M cells (the antigenic samplers of the bowel) with subsequent spread to epithelial cells. A similar route of invasion occurs in *Shigella*, *Yersinia* and reovirus infections. The bacteria migrate to the lamina propria layer of the ileocaecal region, where their multiplication stimulates the production and release of proinflammatory cytokines, both of which confine the infection to the gastrointestinal tract and mediate the release of prostaglandins. These, in turn, activate cyclic adenosine monophosphate (cAMP) and fluid secretion, resulting in diarrhoea.

Species of *Salmonella* that normally cause diarrhoea (e.g. *S. enteritidis*, *S. choleraesuis*) may become invasive in patients with particular predispositions, including children, immunocompromised patients or those with sickle cell anaemia. The organisms are not contained within the gastrointestinal tract, but they invade the body to cause septicaemia; consequently, many organs become seeded with salmonellae, sometimes leading to osteomyelitis, pneumonia or meningitis.

In the vast majority of cases, *Salmonella* spp. cause an acute but self-limiting diarrhoea, although in the young and the elderly the symptoms may be more severe. Vomiting is also common with enterocolitis, while fever is usually a sign

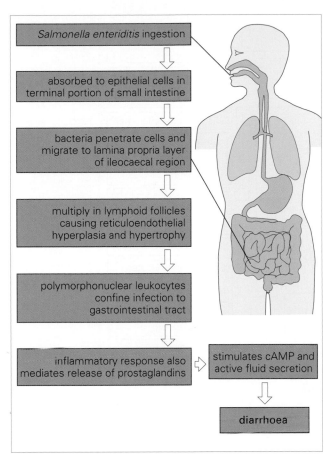

| |
|---|
| *Salmonella enteriditis* ingestion |
| ⇩ |
| absorbed to epithelial cells in terminal portion of small intestine |
| ⇩ |
| bacteria penetrate cells and migrate to lamina propria layer of ileocaecal region |
| ⇩ |
| multiply in lymphoid follicles causing reticuloendothelial hyperplasia and hypertrophy |
| ⇩ |
| polymorphonuclear leukocytes confine infection to gastrointestinal tract |
| ⇩ |
| inflammatory response also mediates release of prostaglandins ⇨ stimulates cAMP and active fluid secretion |
| ⇩ |
| diarrhoea |

**Fig. 23.9** The passage of salmonellae through the body. The vast majority of salmonellae cause infection localized to the gastrointestinal tract and do not invade beyond the gut mucosa. cAMP, Cyclic adenosine monophosphate.

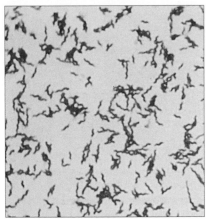

**Fig. 23.10** *Campylobacter jejuni* infection. Gram stain showing gram-negative, S-shaped bacilli. (Courtesy I. Farrell.)

of invasive disease (see Table 23.3). *S. typhi* and *S. paratyphi* invade the body from the gastrointestinal tract to cause systemic illness (see later).

Salmonella *diarrhoea can be diagnosed by culture on selective media.* The organisms are not fastidious and can usually be isolated within 24 h, although small numbers may require enrichment in selenite broth before culture. The best time to detect the bacteria in the bloodstream is in the first or second week of illness. Culture is diagnostic, and the isolate is then tested for antibiotic sensitivity and can be typed and characterized using molecular techniques for epidemiologic purposes. Isolates must be dealt with carefully as they have been a common cause of laboratory-acquired infection.

The classic antibody detection method is called the *Widal test,* an agglutination assay carried out on serum samples, detecting antibodies against the lipopolysaccharide (O) and flagella (H) antigens of *S. typhi.* There are time delay issues as it involves testing acute and convalescent sera collected 10 days apart, looking for a fourfold rise in titre. Commercially available serologic tests have been developed, as have molecular assays to make a rapid diagnosis.

*Fluid and electrolyte replacement may be needed for* Salmonella *diarrhoea.* Diarrhoea is usually self-limiting and resolves without treatment. Fluid and electrolyte replacement may be required, particularly in the very young and the elderly. Unless there is evidence of invasion and septicaemia,

antibiotics should be positively discouraged because they do not reduce the symptoms or shorten the illness and may prolong excretion of salmonellae in the faeces. There is some evidence that symptomatic treatment with drugs that reduce diarrhoea has the same adverse effect.

*Salmonellae may be excreted in the faeces for several weeks after a* Salmonella *infection.* Fig. 23.8 illustrates the problems associated with the prevention of *Salmonella* infections. The large animal reservoir makes it impossible to eliminate the organisms, and preventive measures must therefore be aimed at breaking the chain between animals and humans and from person to person. Such measures include:

- maintaining adequate standards of public health such as clean drinking water and proper sewage disposal
- education programmes on hygienic food preparation.

Following an episode of *Salmonella* diarrhoea, an individual can continue to carry and excrete organisms in the faeces for several weeks. Although in the absence of symptoms the organisms will not be dispersed so liberally into the environment, thorough hand washing before food handling is essential. People employed as food handlers are excluded from work until three specimens of faeces have failed to grow *Salmonella.*

### Campylobacter

Campylobacter *infections are among the most common causes of diarrhoea.* *Campylobacter* spp. are curved or S-shaped gram-negative rods (Fig. 23.10). They have long been known to cause diarrhoeal disease in animals but are also one of the most common causes of diarrhoea in humans. The delay in recognizing the importance of these organisms was due to their cultural requirements, which differ from those of the enterobacteria as they are microaerophilic and thermophilic (growing well at 42°C); they do not therefore grow on the media used for isolating *E. coli* and salmonellae. Several species of the genus *Campylobacter* are associated with human disease, but *Campylobacter jejuni* is by far the most common, together with *E. coli,* and is a major cause of gastroenteritis worldwide. It may also result in Guillain-Barré syndrome (GBS), an autoimmune condition (Fig. 23.11).

As with salmonellae, there is a large animal reservoir of *Campylobacter* in cattle, sheep, rodents, poultry and wild birds. Infections are acquired by consumption of undercooked or

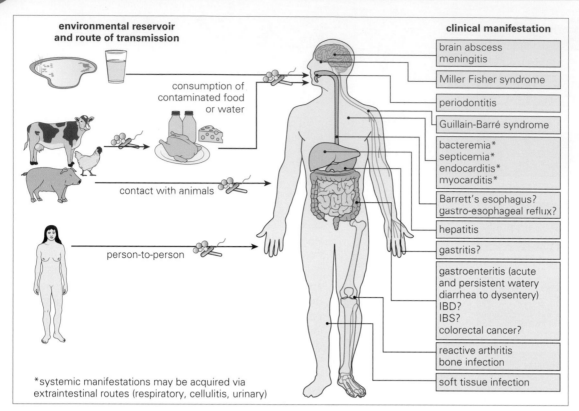

**Fig. 23.11** Environmental reservoirs, routes of transmission, and clinical manifestations associated with *Campylobacter* spp. IBD, Inflammatory bowel diseases; IBS, irritable bowel syndrome. Infection is implicated in some conditions and these are marked by a question mark. (From Kaakoush NO, Castaño-Rodríguez N, Mitchell HM, et al. Global epidemiology of *Campylobacter* infection. *Clin Micro Rev.* 2015;28[3]:687–720, fig 1.)

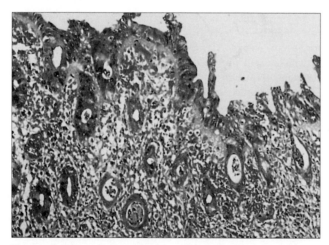

**Fig. 23.12** Inflammatory enteritis caused by *Campylobacter jejuni*, involving the entire mucosa, with flattened atrophic villi, necrotic debris in the crypts and thickening of the basement membrane (Cresyl-fast violet stain). (Courtesy J. Newman.)

contaminated food, especially poultry, milk or water. Studies have shown an association between infection and consumption of milk from bottles with tops that have been pecked by wild birds. Household pets such as dogs and cats can become infected and provide a source for human infection, particularly for young children. Person-to-person spread by the faecal–oral route is rare, as is transmission from food handlers.

*Campylobacter diarrhoea is clinically similar to that caused by other bacteria such as* **Salmonella** *and* **Shigella.** The gross pathology and histologic appearances of ulceration and inflamed bleeding mucosal surfaces in the jejunum, ileum and colon (Fig. 23.12) are compatible with invasion of the bacteria, but the production of cytotoxins by *C. jejuni* has also been demonstrated. Invasion and bacteraemia are not uncommon, particularly in neonates and debilitated adults.

The clinical presentation is similar to that of diarrhoea caused by salmonellae and *Shigella*, although the disease may have a longer incubation period and a longer duration. The key features are summarized in Table 23.3.

*Cultures for* **Campylobacter** *should be set up routinely in every investigation of a diarrhoeal illness.* *Campylobacter*-selective media and conditions for growth differ from those required for the enterobacteria. Growth is often somewhat slow compared with that of the enterobacteria, but a presumptive identification should be available within 48 h of culture.

*Azithromycin is used for severe* **Campylobacter** *diarrhoea.* Most people with *Campylobacter* infections recover without antibiotic treatment. Macrolide antibiotics such as clarithromycin and azithromycin can be used in severe diarrhoeal disease or in immunocompromised individuals. Invasive infections may require treatment with an additional antibiotic such as a fluoroquinolone (e.g. ciprofloxacin), but resistance is common.

The preventive measures for *Salmonella* infections described earlier are equally applicable to the prevention of *Campylobacter* infections, but there are no requirements for the screening of food handlers because contamination of food by this route is very uncommon.

### Cholera

Cholera is an acute infection of the gastrointestinal tract caused by the comma-shaped gram-negative bacterium *V. cholerae* (Fig. 23.13). The disease has a long history characterized by epidemics and pandemics. The last cases of cholera acquired in the United Kingdom were in the 19th century following the introduction of the bacterium by sailors arriving from Europe, and in 1849 Snow published his historic essay *On the Mode of Communication of Cholera*, proposing that it was a communicable disease and that infectious material was contained in the faeces.

***Cholera flourishes in communities with inadequate clean drinking water and sewage disposal.*** The disease remains endemic in >50 countries, especially Southeast Asia and

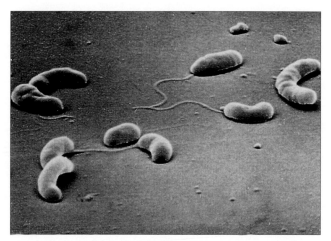

**Fig. 23.13** Scanning electron micrograph of *Vibrio cholerae* showing comma-shaped rods with a single polar flagellum (× 13 000). (Courtesy D.K. Banerjee.)

parts of Africa and South America. It is estimated there are 3–5 million people infected annually. Unlike salmonellae and *Campylobacter*, *V. cholerae* is a free-living inhabitant of fresh water but causes infection only in humans. Asymptomatic human carriers are believed to be a major reservoir. The disease is spread via contaminated food; shellfish grown in fresh and estuarine waters have also been implicated. Direct person-to-person spread is thought to be uncommon. Therefore cholera continues to flourish in communities where there is absent or unreliable provision of clean drinking water and sewage disposal. Natural disasters, such as floods and earthquakes, can result in a breakdown of public health facilities and cause cholera epidemics. In 2010, after a devastating earthquake in Haiti, >7000 people died of cholera; by 2014 >750 000 people had been infected.

***V. cholerae is classified into >200 serogroups based on the somatic (O) antigens of the lipopolysaccharide.*** Only O1 and O139 serogroups cause epidemic cholera. O1 is the most important and is further divided into two biotypes: classic and El Tor (Fig. 23.14). The El Tor biotype, named after the quarantine camp where it was first isolated from pilgrims returning from Mecca, differs from classic *V. cholerae* in several ways. In particular, it causes only mild diarrhoea and has a higher ratio of carriers to cases than classic cholera; carriage is also more prolonged, and the organisms survive better in the environment. The El Tor biotype, which was responsible for the seventh pandemic, spread throughout the world and largely displaced the classic biotype.

In 1992 a new strain, O139, arose in southern India. It spread rapidly, infected O1-immune individuals, caused epidemics and was the eighth pandemic strain of cholera. *V. cholerae* O139 appeared to have originated from the El Tor O1 biotype when the latter acquired a new O (capsular) antigen by horizontal gene transfer from a non-O1 strain, but it is almost identical to O1 El Tor. This provided the recipient strain with a selective advantage in a region where a large part of the population was immune to O1 strains. These hybrid strains dominated and included a number of mutations in the gene encoding the cholera toxin B subunit, ctxB.

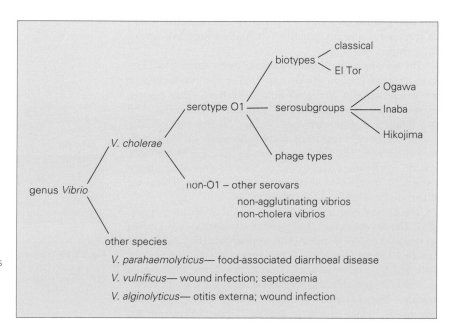

**Fig. 23.14** *Vibrio cholerae* serotype O1, the cause of cholera, can be subdivided into different biotypes with different epidemiologic features and into sero subgroups and phage types for the purposes of investigating outbreaks of infection. Although *V. cholerae* is the most important pathogen of the genus, other species can also cause infections of both the gastrointestinal tract and other sites.

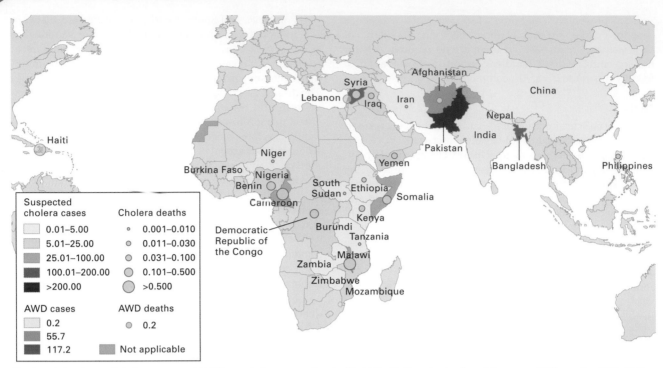

**Fig. 23.15** Incidence of cholera cases per 100 000 population reported to the World Health Organization from 1 January to 30 November 2022. AWD, acute watery diarrhoea. (From World Health Organization (WHO). Cholera—global situation. Geneva, Switzerland: WHO Disease Outbreak News; 2022.)

At least 10 ctxB alleles have been reported, with ctxB1 being the classic O1 biotype; ctxB3 (the El Tor biotype) and ctxB7 (the recent El Tor variants) are a concern as they secrete more cholera toxin than the original El Tor.

Since 2021 cholera infections and their global distribution have increased. In 2022 WHO reported outbreaks in at least 29 countries, mainly in Africa and the Eastern Mediterranean (Fig. 23.15), with higher numbers and mortality than before. There were outbreaks in 13 countries where cholera had not been reported for many years, demonstrating a resurgence of the ongoing seventh cholera pandemic of circa 1961.

Other species of *Vibrio* cause a variety of infections in humans (see Fig. 23.14). *V. parahaemolyticus* is another cause of diarrhoeal disease, but this is usually much less severe than cholera (see later).

***The symptoms of cholera are caused by an enterotoxin.*** The symptoms of cholera are entirely due to the production of an enterotoxin in the gastrointestinal tract. This protein exotoxin has an A subunit and pentameric B subunit. The A subunit activates adenylate cyclase, causing intracellular cAMP to rise and resulting in chloride secretion and secretory diarrhoea. The B subunit binds to the ganglioside GM1 site on eukaryotic cells. *V. cholerae* has additional virulence factors to enable it to survive the host defences. These are illustrated in Fig. 23.16 (see also Ch. 14).

The clinical features of cholera are summarized in Table 23.3. The severe watery but nonbloody diarrhoea is known as rice water stool because of its appearance (Fig. 23.17) and can result in the loss of 1 L of fluid every hour. It is this fluid loss and the consequent electrolyte imbalance that results in marked dehydration, metabolic acidosis (loss of bicarbonate), hypokalaemia (potassium loss) and hypovolaemic shock, which results in cardiac failure. Untreated, the

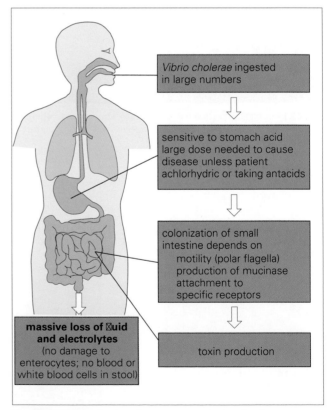

**Fig. 23.16** The production of an enterotoxin is central to the pathogenesis of cholera, but the organisms must possess other virulence factors to allow them to reach the small intestine and to adhere to the mucosal cells.

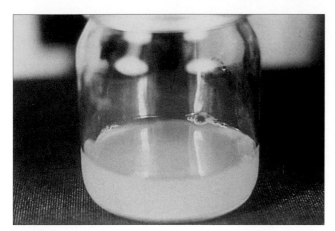

**Fig. 23.17** Rice water stool in cholera. (Courtesy A.M. Geddes.)

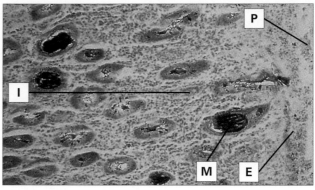

**Fig. 23.18** Shigellosis. Histology of the colon showing disrupted epithelium covered by pseudomembrane and interstitial infiltration. Mucin glands have discharged their contents, and the goblet cells are empty. *E*, Epithelium; *I*, interstitial infiltration; *M*, mucin in glands; *P*, pseudomembrane (colloidal iron stain). (Courtesy R.H. Gilman.)

mortality from cholera is 40–60%; rapidly instituted fluid and electrolyte replacement reduce the mortality to <1%.

*Culture is necessary to diagnose sporadic or imported cases of cholera and carriers.* In countries where cholera is prevalent, diagnosis is based on clinical grounds, and laboratory confirmation is rarely sought. It is worth remembering that ETEC infection can resemble cholera in both its severity and the management of infected individuals, as fluid and electrolyte replacement are of paramount importance.

*Prompt rehydration with fluids and electrolytes is central to the treatment of cholera.* Oral or intravenous rehydration is critical in the management of those affected. Antibiotics are helpful in moderate to severe dehydration as they reduce the duration of excretion of *V. cholerae* thereby reducing the risk of transmission as well as shortening the duration and volume of diarrhoea. The antibiotics must be chosen on the basis of antimicrobial resistance patterns locally. Tetracycline-resistant *V. cholerae* has been reported, but most strains are susceptible. Quinolones and macrolides (azithromycin and erythromycin) may be effective. However, azithromycin resistance, as well as ciprofloxacin and ceftriaxone resistance, has been reported. Doxycycline is generally the antibiotic of choice.

As with other diarrhoeal disease, a clean drinking water supply and adequate sewage disposal are fundamental to the prevention of cholera. As there is no animal reservoir, it should in theory be possible to eliminate the disease. However, carriage in humans, albeit for only a few weeks, occurs in 1–20% of previously infected patients, making eradication difficult to achieve.

*Cholera vaccines are not recommended for most travellers.* A killed whole-cell oral vaccine is available but is effective in only ~50% of those vaccinated, with protection lasting for only 3–6 months. It is no longer recommended by the WHO for travellers to cholera-endemic areas, although it may be required in certain countries. By 2022 a number of live attenuated oral vaccines had been developed and were being evaluated; however, all were still prototypes, and further validation was required.

### Shigellosis

*Symptoms of **Shigella** infection range from mild to severe gastroenteritis, depending on the infecting species.* *Shigella* and *E. coli* are similar genetically and are gram-negative rods. *Shigellosis* is also known as bacillary dysentery (in contrast to amoebic

dysentery; see later) because in its more severe form it is characterized by an invasive infection of the mucosa of the large intestine, causing inflammation and resulting in the presence of pus and blood in the diarrhoeal stool. However, symptoms range from mild to severe depending on the species of *Shigella* involved and on the underlying state of health of the host. There are four species (also referred to as subgroups):

- *Shigella sonnei* causes most infections at the mild end of the spectrum.
- *S. flexneri* and *S. boydii* usually produce more severe disease.
- *S. dysenteriae* is the most serious.

*Shigellosis* is primarily a paediatric disease. Globally, the incidence of shigellosis is estimated annually by WHO at ~80 million individuals with bloody diarrhoea, but there has been a significant reduction in the mortality rate over the last 30 years and is now ~700000. Many of these infections are in resource-poor countries and mostly affect <5-year-olds. When associated with severe malnutrition, it may precipitate complications such as the protein deficiency syndrome kwashiorkor. Like *V. cholerae*, shigellae are human pathogens without an animal reservoir, but, unlike the vibrios, they are not found in the environment and they are spread from person to person by the faecal–oral route and less frequently by contaminated food and water. Shigellae appear to be able to initiate infection from a small infective dose of only 10–100 organisms, therefore spread is easy in situations where sanitation or personal hygiene may be poor. These include refugee camps, nurseries, day care centres and other residential institutions.

*Shigella diarrhoea is usually watery at first, but later contains mucus and blood.* *Shigella* has a large virulence plasmid that encodes secreted proteins acting on colonic epithelial cells that damage the epithelial lining as well as acting on the host immune response. Shigellae attach to and invade the mucosal epithelium of the distal ileum and colon, causing inflammation and ulceration (Fig. 23.18). However, they rarely invade through the gut wall to the bloodstream. *S. dysenteriae* produce a Shiga toxin similar to that associated with EHEC (see earlier), which can cause damage to the intestinal epithelium and glomerular endothelial cells, the latter leading to kidney failure (HUS; see *E. coli* section).

The main features of *Shigella* infection are summarized in Table 23.3. Diarrhoea is usually watery initially, but later contains mucus and blood. Lower abdominal cramps can be severe. The disease is usually self-limiting, but dehydration can occur especially in the young and elderly. Complications can be associated with malnutrition, and extraintestinal manifestations can occur.

*Culture and serologic typing are helpful in distinguishing Shigella from E. coli.* This is critical for both diagnosis and epidemiologic and public health purposes. The four subgroups (A–D) include *S. dysenteriae* (A), *S. flexneri* (B), *S. boydii* (C) and *S. sonnei* (D).

*Antibiotics should be given only for severe Shigella diarrhoea, but extensive and multidrug resistance has increased.* Once again, rehydration is critical, and antibiotics, especially those that also decrease intestinal motility, should not be given except in severe cases. Plasmid-mediated resistance is common, and antibiotic susceptibility tests should be performed on *Shigella* isolates if treatment is required.

Education in personal hygiene and proper sewage disposal are important. Infected individuals may continue to excrete shigellae for a few weeks, but longer-term carriage is unusual; therefore, with adequate public health measures and no animal reservoir, the disease is potentially eradicable.

In February 2022, the WHO was notified about a high number of extensive drug-resistant (XDR) *S. sonnei* infections in a cluster of 84 individuals in the United Kingdom as well as reports from nine countries in the European region, with similar resistance profiles. The route of transmission was direct, person-to-person, sexual transmission between men who have sex with men.

### Other bacterial causes of diarrhoeal disease

The pathogens described in the previous sections are the major bacterial causes of diarrhoeal disease. *Salmonella* and *Campylobacter* infections and some types of *E. coli* infections are most often food associated, whereas cholera is more often waterborne, and shigellosis is usually spread by direct faecal–oral contact.

From a diagnostic perspective (see Ch. 32), although culture, biochemical identification and serologic typing are the classical techniques, molecular methods such as mass spectrometry and multiplex PCR panels are being added to the diagnostic armamentarium.

Other bacterial pathogens that cause food-associated infection or food poisoning are described next.

*V. parahaemolyticus and Yersinia enterocolitica are foodborne gram-negative causes of diarrhoea.* *V. parahaemolyticus* is a halophilic (salt-loving) vibrio found in estuarine, marine and coastal environments and can contaminate seafood and fish. If these foods are consumed uncooked, diarrhoeal disease can result. These bacteria have a number of different virulence factors, including adhesins and haemolysins. After binding to the host cell, most strains associated with infection are haemolytic owing to production of a heat-stable cytotoxin and have been shown to invade intestinal cells (in contrast to *V. cholerae*, which is noninvasive and produces cholera toxin, which is not cytotoxic).

The clinical features of infection are summarized in Table 23.3. The methods used for the laboratory diagnosis of *V. parahaemolyticus* infection involve special media for

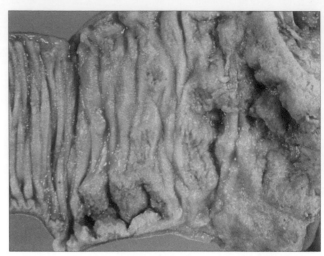

**Fig. 23.19** *Yersinia enterocolitica* infection of the ileum, showing superficial necrosis of the mucosa and ulceration. (Courtesy J. Newman.)

culture. Prevention of infection depends on cooking fish and seafood properly.

*Y. enterocolitica* is a member of the Enterobacteriaceae family and is a cause of food-associated infection especially among infants and particularly in the winter months possibly because the organism can multiply at refrigerator temperatures. *Y. enterocolitica* is a zoonosis and is found in a variety of animal hosts, including rodents, rabbits, pigs, sheep, cattle, horses and domestic pets. Transmission to humans from household dogs has been reported. The organism survives and multiplies, albeit more slowly, at low temperatures and has been implicated in outbreaks of infection associated with contaminated milk as well as other foods.

The virulence factors include proteins promoting adhesion and epithelial cell invasion as well as the production of an enterotoxin, but the clinical features of the disease result from invasion of the terminal ileum, necrosis in Peyer's patches and an associated inflammation of the mesenteric lymph nodes (Fig. 23.19). The presentation, with enterocolitis and often mesenteric adenitis, can easily be confused with acute appendicitis, particularly in children. The clinical features are summarized in Table 23.3. As with *V. parahaemolyticus*, an indication of a suspicion of *Yersinia* infection is useful so that the laboratory staff can process the specimen appropriately.

*Clostridium perfringens and Bacillus cereus are spore-forming gram-positive rods that cause diarrhoea.* The gram-negative organisms described in the previous sections invade the intestinal mucosa or produce enterotoxins, which cause diarrhoea. None of these organisms produces spores. Two gram-positive species are important causes of diarrhoeal disease, particularly in association with spore-contaminated food. These are *C. perfringens* and *B. cereus* and are discussed in the next section.

## FOOD POISONING: BACTERIAL TOXIN–ASSOCIATED DIARRHOEA

Toxins elaborated by contaminating bacteria in food before it is consumed include the emetic toxin of *B. cereus*, *S. aureus* enterotoxin, *C. botulinum* and *C. perfringens* toxin.

**Table 23.4** Staphylococcal enterotoxins

| Enterotoxin | | |
|---|---|---|
| A | Most commonly associated with food poisoning | |
| B | Associated with staphylococcal enterocolitis (rare) | |
| C | Rare | |
| D | Second most common | Associated with contaminated milk products |
| E | Alone or in combination with A | |
| | Rare | |
| TSST-1 | Toxic shock syndrome toxin, not food-associated | |

*Staphylococcus aureus* produces at least eight immunologically distinct enterotoxins, the most important of which are listed here. Strains may produce one or more of the toxins simultaneously. Enterotoxin A is by far the most common in food-associated disease.

## Staphylococcus aureus

### Enterotoxigenic strains of *S. aureus* are associated with foodborne illness

More than 20 distinct enterotoxin and enterotoxin-like molecules have been reported to be produced by strains of *S. aureus*, the classic serotypes are enterotoxins A–E (Table 23.4). All are heat stable and resistant to destruction by enzymes in the stomach and small intestine. Their mechanism of action is incompletely understood; however, similar to the toxic shock syndrome toxin (TSST-1; see Ch. 27), they generally behave as superantigens (see Ch. 17), binding to major histocompatibility complex (MHC) class II molecules, which results in immune system activation and intense T-cell stimulation and proliferation resulting in the production of proinflammatory mediators. Their effect on the central nervous system results in severe vomiting within 3–6 h of consumption. Diarrhoea is not a feature, and recovery within 24 h is usual. In addition, the enterotoxins are implicated in autoimmune dysregulation and may be involved in the pathogenesis of inflammatory bowel diseases.

Up to 50% of *S. aureus* strains produce enterotoxin, and food, especially processed meats, may be contaminated by human carriers; up to 50% of healthy people carry the bacteria on their skin and in their nose. The bacteria grow at room temperature and release toxin. Subsequent heating may kill the organisms, but the toxin is stable, and nanogram quantities are sufficient to cause illness. Often there are no viable organisms detectable in the food consumed, but enterotoxin can be detected by a latex agglutination test, but immunoassays are more sensitive.

## Botulism

### Exotoxins produced by *C. botulinum* cause botulism, which has a mortality rate of ~10%

Botulism is a rare but serious disease caused by the exotoxin of *C. botulinum*. The organism is widespread in the environment, is mesophilic with a minimum and optimum temperature for growth of 12°C and 37°C, respectively, and spores can be isolated readily from soil samples and from various animals, including fish. There are seven major botulinum neurotoxins (BoNTs), products of the BoNT genes labelled A–G, but only four (A, B, E and less frequently F) are associated with human disease. While not destroyed by digestive enzymes, the toxins are inactivated after 30 min at 80°C. The toxins are ingested in food (often canned or reheated) or produced in the gut after ingestion of the organism; they

are absorbed from the gut into the bloodstream and then reach their site of action: the peripheral nerve synapses. A person need ingest only 30–100 ng of neurotoxin to develop botulism. Botulism is characterized by a symmetric descending flaccid muscle paralysis affecting proximal before distal limbs and starts with the cranial nerves causing blurred vision, swallowing difficulty and slurred speech. Then the respiratory and cardiac muscles are affected if it is not treated quickly. The amount and severity of paralysis is proportional to the toxin dose. Acetylcholine (ACh) release from presynaptic motor neurone terminals is inhibited by the BoNT blocking ACh transmission across the neuromuscular junction (see Ch. 17).

### Infant botulism is the most common form of botulism

There are three forms of botulism: foodborne, infant and wound botulism. In foodborne botulism, toxin is elaborated by organisms in food, which is then ingested. Often caused by eating home-canned foods that have undergone inadequate heat processing, the aim is to reach 121°C for 3 minutes. In infant and wound botulism, the organisms are, respectively, ingested or implanted in a wound and multiply and elaborate toxin in vivo. Infant botulism has been associated with feeding babies honey contaminated with *C. botulinum* spores.

The clinical disease is the same in all three forms and is characterized by flaccid paralysis leading to progressive muscle weakness and respiratory arrest. Intensive supportive treatment is urgently required, and complete recovery may take many months. Improvements in supportive care have reduced the mortality from ~70% to ~10%, but the disease, although rare, remains life threatening. In addition, since botulinum toxin is one of the most potent biologic toxins known, there is concern regarding its potential use as an agent of biowarfare.

### Considering botulism in the differential diagnosis is key and then confirming by laboratory diagnosis

Laboratory diagnosis involves demonstrating

- the presence of neurotoxin in clinical specimens, including serum, faeces, gastric fluid or food
- neurotoxin-producing *Clostridial* species in faecal or wound bacterial culture.

A mouse bioassay is the gold standard method to detect neurotoxin if serum is available. The serum is injected intraperitoneally into mice that have been protected with botulinum antitoxin or left unprotected. This is carried out in reference centres with staff experienced in looking for signs of botulism over 96 h.

Toxin detection by real-time PCR-based assays detecting BoNT A–G gene targets is another reference centre test and detects the DNA but not the neurotoxin, which is why a confirmatory test is needed such as the mouse bioassay and enzyme-linked immunosorbent assay (ELISA; see Ch. 32) to test for functional toxin activity.

### Polyvalent antitoxin is recommended as an adjunct to intensive supportive therapy for botulism

Since botulinum toxins are antigenic they can be inactivated and used to produce antitoxin in animals. When botulism is suspected, antitoxin should be promptly administered along with supportive care, which may include mechanical ventilation due to difficulty in breathing and intravenous and nasogastric nutritional support due to difficulty in swallowing. Antibiotics are generally used only for treatment of secondary infections.

It is not practical to prevent food becoming contaminated with botulinum spores, so prevention of disease depends on preventing the germination of spores in food by:

- maintaining food at an acid pH
- storing food at <4°C
- inactivating spores by heating at 121°C for 3 min before storage
- inactivating toxin by heating for 5 min at 80°C.

Two gram-positive species, *C. perfringens* and *B. cereus,* are enterotoxin producers and important causes of diarrhoeal disease, particularly in association with spore-contaminated food. However, much more rarely, *C. perfringens* can also be present in inadequately cooked food and multiply, and beta toxin–producing strains produce an acute necrotizing disease of the small intestine, accompanied by abdominal pain and diarrhoea. The pathogenesis is summarized in Fig. 23.20. This form occurs after the consumption of contaminated meat by people who are unaccustomed to a high-protein diet and do not have sufficient intestinal trypsin to destroy the toxin. It is traditionally associated with the orgiastic pig feasts enjoyed by the natives of New Guinea, but it also occurred in people released from prisoner-of-war camps.

The clinical features of the more common enterotoxin type of infection are shown in Table 23.3. *C. perfringens* is an anaerobe and grows readily on routine laboratory media. Enterotoxin production can be demonstrated by a latex agglutination method, but more sensitive tests include an ELISA carried out on faecal material and PCR detection.

Antibacterial treatment of *C. perfringens* diarrhoea is rarely required. Prevention depends on thorough reheating of food before serving or preferably avoiding cooking food too long before consumption.

*C. perfringens* is also an important cause of wound and soft tissue infections (see Ch. 27).

*B. cereus* is widely distributed in the environment, especially in soil and the spores, and vegetative cells contaminate many foods. Food-associated infection takes one of two forms:

- diarrhoea resulting from the production of enterotoxin in the gut
- vomiting due to the ingestion of enterotoxin in food.

Two different toxins are involved in pathogenicity and cause exoenzymes that destroy tissue, as illustrated in Fig. 23.21. In the small intestine, having ingested the spores, the vegetative cells secrete an enterotoxin causing diarrhoea. However, the emetic toxin, which is plasmid encoded, is produced in food products and ingested preformed. The clinical features of the infections are summarized in Table 23.3. *B. cereus* is very serious and can cause a spectrum of infections, including meningitis, brain abscesses, endophthalmitis and pneumonia. Laboratory confirmation of the diagnosis requires specific media. The emetic type of disease may be difficult to assign to *B. cereus* unless the incriminated food is cultured.

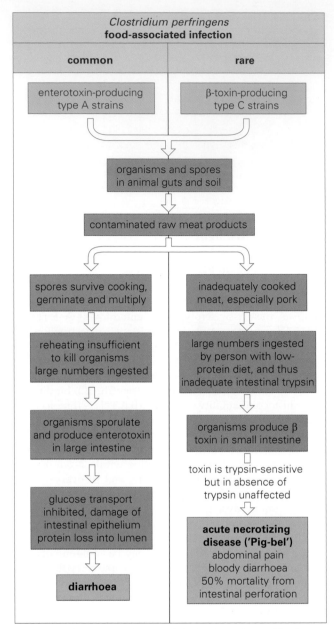

**Fig. 23.20** *Clostridium perfringens* is linked with two forms of food-associated infection. The common, enterotoxin-mediated infection (*left*) is usually acquired by eating meat or poultry that has been cooked enough to kill vegetative cells but not spores. As the food cools, the spores germinate. If reheating before consumption is inadequate (as it often is in mass catering outlets), large numbers of organisms are ingested. The rare form associated with β-toxin–producing strains (*right*) causes a severe necrotizing disease.

As with *C. perfringens,* prevention of *B. cereus* food-associated infection depends on proper cooking and rapid consumption of food. Specific antibacterial treatment is not indicated in this setting.

### Antibiotic-associated diarrhoea—*Clostridioides difficile* (formerly *Clostridium difficile*)

*C. difficile* infection is the most commonly diagnosed bacterial cause of hospital-acquired infectious diarrhoea in resource-rich countries. In the United States the Centers for Disease Control and Prevention estimated there were

**Bacillus cereus food-associated infection**

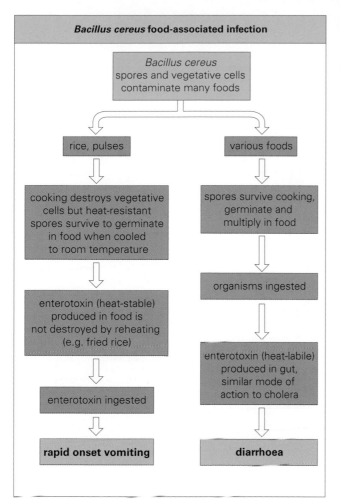

**Fig. 23.21** *Bacillus cereus* can cause two different forms of food-associated infection. Both involve toxins.

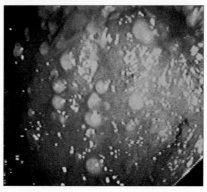

**Fig. 23.22** Antibiotic-associated colitis due to *Clostridioides difficile*. Sigmoidoscopic view showing multiple pseudomembranous lesions. (Courtesy J. Cunningham.)

former and survives in the environment as it is resistant to heat and acid. The spores contaminate the environment and become vegetative bacteria that can be transmitted between patients on the wards.

In common with other clostridia, *C. difficile* produces exotoxins. Toxin A, an enterotoxin, causes increased intestinal permeability and secretion of fluids; toxin B, a cytotoxin, causes colonic inflammation, haemostasis and tissue necrosis in the colon resulting in diarrhoea.

Toxins A and B are encoded by the *tcdA* and *tcdB* genes (Fig. 23.23) within a short chromosomal segment carried by pathogenic strains of *C. difficile*, referred to as the pathogenicity locus. Some strains may produce a binary toxin called *C. difficile* transferase (CDT), and its role is not clear as the symptoms are not as severe, and the incidence of *C. difficile* infections involving strains that produce only CDT is low.

An epidemic of a *C. difficile* variant strain was a true millennial starting in 2000; it was called *C. difficile* ribotype NAP1/B1/027 (short for North American pulsed-field gel electrophoresis type 1, restriction endonuclease analysis type B1, PCR ribotype 027). This fully formed verbal diarrhoea version was shown to produce much more of toxins A and B. Toxin production is related to spore production, so this is a highly sporulating strain that therefore dominates the environment it inhabits. The increased toxin production causes a number of direct and indirect cytopathic effects causing colonocyte death, the loss of the intestinal barrier function and colitis. This strain detected in the United States, Canada, the United Kingdom and other parts of Europe is not only highly transmissible but causes more severe disease in individuals in both hospitals and the community. It has been associated with higher case fatality rates, with some infected individuals requiring a colectomy and intensive care unit support, and has been shown to be more resistant to the fluoroquinolone antibiotics than other strains. Increasingly severe *C. difficile* infections have been reported and, as mentioned earlier, the result of disturbing the gut microbiota can lead to *C. difficile* colonisation. Populations of gut bacteria can affect the severity of *C. difficile* infection, in addition to the effects of the host and *C. difficile* subtype.

Although initially associated with clindamycin, *C. difficile* diarrhoea has since been shown to follow therapy with many other broad-spectrum antibiotics—hence the term antibiotic-associated diarrhoea or colitis. The infection is often severe

224000 *C. difficile* infections and 12,800 deaths in 2017. It is the most common cause of healthcare-associated infections in US hospitals.

### Treatment with broad-spectrum antibiotics can be complicated by antibiotic-associated *C. difficile* diarrhoea

All the infections described so far arise from the ingestion of organisms or their toxins. However, diarrhoea can also arise from disruption of the normal gut flora. Even in the early days of antibiotic use it was recognized that these agents affected the normal flora of the body as well as attacking the pathogens. For example, orally administered tetracycline disrupts the normal gut flora, and patients sometimes become recolonized not with the usual facultative gram-negative anaerobes but with *S. aureus*, causing enterocolitis, or with yeasts such as *Candida*. Soon after clindamycin was introduced for therapeutic use it was found to be associated with severe diarrhoea in which the colonic mucosa became covered with a characteristic fibrinous pseudomembrane (pseudomembranous colitis; Fig. 23.22). However, clindamycin is not the cause of the condition; it merely inhibits the normal gut flora and allows *C. difficile* to multiply. This organism is commonly found in the gut of children and to a lesser extent in adults, but it can also be acquired from other patients in hospital by cross-infection. *C. difficile* is a spore

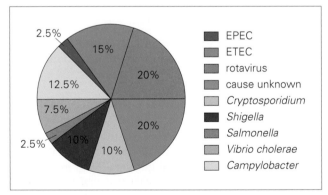

**Fig. 23.23** Toxin delivery into the host cell cytosol can be divided into seven main steps: (1) toxin binding to the host cell surface receptor, (2) toxin internalization through a receptor-mediated endocytosis, (3) endosome acidification, (4) pore formation, (5) GTD release from the endosome to the host cell cytoplasm, (6) rho GTPases inactivation by glucosylation; and (7) downstream effects within the host cell (i.e. toxin-induced cytopathic and cytotoxic effects). ADP, Adenosine diphosphate; ATP, adenosine triphosphate; CPD, cysteine protease domain (*cyan*); DD, delivery domain (*yellow*); GTD, *N*-terminal glucosyltransferase domain (*red*). TcdA, *C. difficile* Toxin A; TcdB, *C. difficile* Toxin B; ROS, reactive oxygen; UDP, Uridine Diphosphate. (From Di Bella S, Ascenzi P, Siarakas S, et al. *Clostridium difficile* toxins A and B: insights into pathogenic properties and extraintestinal effects. *Toxins.* 2016;8[5]:134, fig 2.)

and may require treatment with the antianaerobic agent metronidazole or with oral vancomycin. However, the emergence of vancomycin-resistant enterococci, probably originating in the gut flora, led to the recommendation that oral vancomycin be avoided wherever possible (see Ch. 34).

Hopefully you are not reading and eating at the same time, as an alternative therapeutic approach, faecal microbiota transplantation, is about to be summarized. This is the ingestion of a faecal suspension from a donor in order to reset the diversity of the normal gastrointestinal flora, referred to as the microbiome within the colon. Studies have shown that this is a safe and effective way to treat *C. difficile*–associated diarrhoea. Just in case you are wondering, the routes of administration involve either a nasogastric or naso-jejunal tube approach or a rectal tube or colonoscope, but the optimal route is still unclear.

## VIRAL CAUSES OF DIARRHOEA

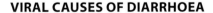

**Huge reductions have been seen in diarrhoeal deaths, especially in <5-year-olds**

Nonbacterial gastroenteritis and diarrhoea are usually caused by viruses, and infection appears in all parts of the world especially in infants and young children (Fig. 23.24). The bacterial and parasitic infections have reduced as a result of improved sanitation and hygiene. Diarrhoeal

**Fig. 23.24** Diarrhoeal disease is a major cause of illness and death in children in resource-poor countries. This illustration shows the proportion of infections caused by different pathogens. Note that in as many as 20% of infections a cause is not identified, but many of these are likely to be viral. EPEC, Enteropathogenic *Escherichia coli*; ETEC, enterotoxigenic *E. coli*. (Data from World Health Organization.)

infections were the eighth most common cause of deaths in all ages and fourth in <5-year-olds globally in 2016. World-wide, annual deaths in all age groups due to diarrhoea have fallen considerably to ~1.6 million in 2017 compared with an estimated 2.6 million in 1990. This is particularly seen in the <5-year-old age group, where mortality had fallen to 370 000 by 2019. However, it is the second most common cause of morbidity in that group.

Although viruses appear to be the most common causes of gastroenteritis in infants and young children, viral gastroenteritis is not distinguishable clinically from other types of gastroenteritis. The viruses are specific to humans, and infection follows the general rules for faecal–oral transmission. Oral transmission of nonbacterial gastroenteritis was first demonstrated experimentally in 1945, but it was not until 1972 that viral particles were identified in faeces by electron microscopy. It has been difficult or impossible to cultivate most of these viruses in cell culture.

## Noroviruses

### The most common cause of diarrhoea worldwide, causing nearly 20% of all diarrhoea episodes

Noroviruses, previously known as small round structured viruses or Norwalk-like viruses, cause winter vomiting disease and diarrhoea. They are part of the *Caliciviridae* family and are 27 nm in diameter, unenveloped, single-stranded RNA viruses. Three of the six genogroups affect humans, namely GI, GII and GIV, and there is much genetic diversity, which is driven by immune selection. Cultivation in vitro has been problematic; cofactors are probably needed and were shown to cause gastroenteritis when fed to adult volunteers. One of the first identified norovirus outbreaks was in a school in Norwalk, Ohio, in 1969. Infection is common in older children and adults. These viruses are highly infectious, spread rapidly and nosocomial infection is common. The incubation period is 12–72 h. In up to 50% of cases there may be chills, headache, myalgia or fever as well as nausea, abdominal pain, vomiting and diarrhoea. Recovery may occur within 24–48 h but may take longer.

Noroviruses bind to cell surface carbohydrates of the histo-blood group antigens, and some strains have different binding affinities for different patterns of these antigens. These are complex glycans expressed on the surface of red blood cells and mucosal surfaces of secretor individuals. They can also be found as free antigens in saliva, milk and intestinal contents of secretor individuals. In humans, most G1 noroviruses bind to H- and A-histo-blood group antigens and Lewis antigens important for a productive norovirus infection. GII noroviruses have a more varied histo-blood group antigen binding pattern, including H, A and B types. In addition, these antigens are expressed to varying degrees in different individuals, resulting in some people being resistant to infection with specific norovirus strains.

Laboratory diagnosis, important in outbreaks and for epidemiologic studies, is usually by PCR, but electron microscopy or ELISA methods may still be used in some laboratories. Viruses in this group are often implicated in diarrhoea associated with food- or waterborne routes occurring after eating sewage-contaminated shellfish such as cockles or mussels. In particular, noroviruses are a major cause of gastroenteritis in healthcare settings, and many outbreaks have been reported in crowded environments such as cruise ships. Noroviruses show a high level of variability resulting in both limited cross-protection between strains and reduced immunity in the population. In addition, due to this diversity diagnostic assays must be modified to optimize detection, and vaccine design either must involve a cross-protective component or the development of a multivalent vaccine.

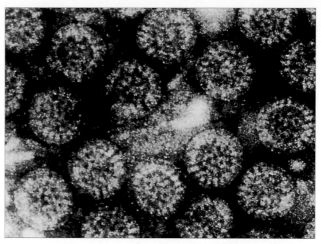

**Fig. 23.25** Rotavirus. The virus particles (65 nm in diameter) have a well-defined outer margin and capsules radiating from an inner core to give the particle a wheel-like (hence *rota*) appearance. (Courtesy J.E. Banatvala.)

Viruslike particles are potential vaccines, and antibody that blocks their binding to histo-blood group antigens may be a key model as a correlate of protection.

## Rotaviruses

These are morphologically characteristic viruses (Fig. 23.25) named after the Latin *rota* ("wheel"), with a genome consisting of 11 separate segments of double-stranded RNA.

The capsid contains the proteins VP7 and VP4, key in stimulating neutralising antibodies. Human rotaviruses have at least 12 different VP7 antigens (G types) and 15 different VP4 antigens (P types). By 2022 90% of all human rotavirus infections involved five dominant G-P combinations (G1P[8], G2P[4], G3P[8], G4P[8]), G9P[8]). Surveillance is important when deciding on vaccine composition as it is with influenza virus vaccines.

Different rotaviruses infect the young of many mammals, including children, kittens, puppies, calves, foals and piglets. This varied host range in different human and animal populations is determined by host histo-blood group antigen receptor (see norovirus section, earlier) polymorphisms.

### Replicating rotavirus causes diarrhoea by damaging transport mechanisms in the gut

The incubation period is 1–2 days. After virus replication in intestinal epithelial cells there is an acute onset of vomiting, which is sometimes projectile, and diarrhoea that lasts 4–7 days. The replicating virus damages transport mechanisms in the gut, and loss of water, salt and glucose causes diarrhoea (Fig. 23.26). Infected cells in the intestine are destroyed, resulting in villous atrophy. The villi (long fingerlike projections) become flattened, resulting in the loss of both the surface area for absorption and the digestive enzymes, and raised osmotic pressure in the gut lumen causes diarrhoea. There is no inflammation or loss of blood. Exceedingly large numbers ($10^{10}$–$10^{11}$/g) of virus particles appear in the faeces. For unknown reasons respiratory symptoms such as cough and coryza are quite common. The disease is more severe in infants in resource-poor countries.

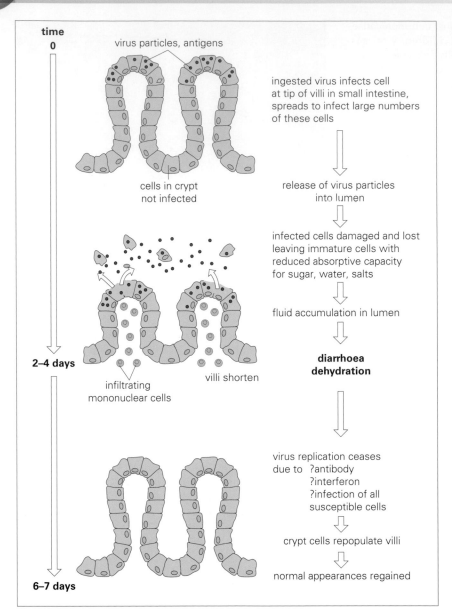

**Fig. 23.26** The pathogenesis of rotavirus diarrhoea. This may differ from other viral infections of the gastrointestinal tract.

Infection is most common in children <2 years of age and has a seasonal pattern, being most frequent in the cooler winter months of the year in resource-rich countries with temperate climates. However, in resource-poor countries in Asia and Africa periods of high viral circulation occur within a background of year-round transmission.

IgA antibodies in colostrum give protection during the first 6 months of life.

The Global Burden of Disease Study 2016 estimated there were ~129 000 deaths among <5-year-olds globally due to rotavirus infection compared with 500 000 in 2000, a significant decline.

Globally in 2019 rotavirus infection caused 19.1% of diarrhoeal-related deaths, with the highest mortality in African, Oceanian, and South Asian countries since 1990 (Fig. 23.27). The rotavirus age standardised death rate fell from 11.4/100 000 people in 1990 to 3.4/100 000 people in 2019. The death rate was the highest among children <5 years worldwide and individuals age >70 years in relatively resource-rich regions.

Outbreaks are sometimes seen in nurseries. Older children are less susceptible to infection, nearly all of them having developed antibodies, but occasional infections occur in adults.

Rotaviruses are well-adapted intestinal infectious agents. As few as 10 ingested particles can cause infection, and by generating diarrhoea laden with enormous quantities of infectious particles, together with their stability in the environment, these organisms have ensured their continued transmission and survival.

### Rotavirus infection is confirmed by viral RNA or antigen detection

Laboratory diagnosis may not be available in resource-poor countries but is made by detecting viral RNA or antigen using PCR or ELISA methods, respectively. The characteristic 65-nm particles can be seen in faecal samples by electron microscopy. They show cubic symmetry and an outer capsid coat arranged like the spokes of a wheel (see Fig. 23.25).

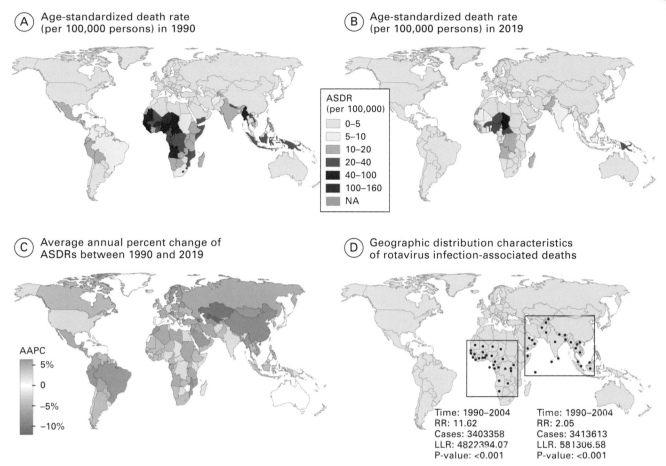

Ⓐ Age-standardized death rate (per 100,000 persons) in 1990

Ⓑ Age-standardized death rate (per 100,000 persons) in 2019

ASDR (per 100,000)
- 0–5
- 5–10
- 10–20
- 20–40
- 40–100
- 100–160
- NA

Ⓒ Average annual percent change of ASDRs between 1990 and 2019

AAPC
- 5%
- 0
- –5%
- –10%

Ⓓ Geographic distribution characteristics of rotavirus infection-associated deaths

Time: 1990–2004
RR: 11.62
Cases: 3403358
LLR: 4822394.07
P-value: <0.001

Time: 1990–2004
RR: 2.05
Cases: 3413613
LLR: 581306.58
P-value: <0.001

**Fig. 23.27** Mortality figures for rotavirus infections in individuals living in 204 countries and territories in (A) 1990, (B) 2019, (C) 1990–2019, and (D) spatial and temporal aggregation 1990–2019. AAPC, average annual percentage changes; ASDRs, age-standardized death rate; LLR, logarithmic likelihood ratios; NA, not available; RR, relative risk. (From Du Y et al. Global burden and trends of rotavirus infection-associated deaths from 1990 to 2019: an observational trend study. *Virol Jogy Journal*. 2022;19;166, fig 1.)

## Prevention by immunization with oral vaccines and fluid and salt replacement can be life saving in rotavirus diarrhoea

Dehydration occurs readily in infants, and fluid and salt replacement orally or intravenously can be life saving. There are no antiviral agents available, but a variety of live attenuated oral vaccines have undergone successful trials. In 2006 the US Food and Drug Administration announced the approval of a live oral vaccine for use in preventing rotavirus gastroenteritis in infants.

Rotavirus vaccines are live, oral, attenuated rotavirus strains of human and/or animal origin that multiply in the human intestine. The first two rotavirus vaccines prequalified by WHO were RotaTeq in 2008 and Rotarix in 2009. In 2018 two additional vaccines were added, and the vaccine efficacy was ~95% against severe disease in countries with low mortality and 44–70% efficacy for high-mortality countries. It is thought that this might be due to no cross-protection between rotavirus genotypes that are more common in resource-rich countries and other P-type rotaviruses more common in resource-poor countries.

Intussusception — where a section of the intestine slides into another section, like a telescope, resulting in obstruction with severe abdominal pain, vomiting and blood in the faeces — has been associated with rotavirus vaccines.

The WHO position was that rotavirus vaccines should be included in all national immunization programmes as part of a comprehensive preventive strategy to control diarrhoeal diseases. This included early breastfeeding, hand washing, improved water supply and sanitation as well as treating those infected with low osmolarity oral rehydration solutions and zinc.

By the start of 2022 the vaccine was introduced in 118 countries, and the global coverage was ~50%. The WHO recommended the first dose of rotavirus vaccine be given after 6 weeks of age, with 4 weeks between doses (3 doses for three-vaccine type and 2 doses for the Rotarix vaccine).

## Other viruses causing diarrhoea in humans include sapoviruses, astroviruses, adenoviruses and coronaviruses

Sapoviruses, also members of the Caliciviridae family, were first detected in an outbreak of diarrhoea in an orphanage in Sapporo, Japan. Astroviruses are 28 nm single-stranded RNA viruses and have characteristic five- or six-pointed star patterns. Most infections occur in childhood and are mild. Both sapoviruses and astroviruses are each thought to account for ~10% of gastroenteritis globally. Adenoviruses are unenveloped, 70–80 nm double-stranded DNA viruses of which types 40 and 41 are associated with ~5% of gastroenteritis. Types 40 and 41 can be grown only in specialized cell culture lines, so molecular diagnostic methods have revolutionised detection. They are often used as multiplexes involving panels of microbial pathogens causing gastroenteritis that can be refined into, for example, the most common viral causes. The role of coronaviruses, human bocavirus and a number of newly identified viral infections in causing gastroenteritis is uncertain.

Although outbreaks of gastroenteritis often have a viral aetiology, it may be difficult to be sure about the exact role of a given virus when it is identified in faeces as there are a number of viruses that replicate in the gastrointestinal tract (e.g. enteroviruses), which are not associated with acute diarrhoeal illness.

## HELICOBACTER PYLORI AND GASTRIC ULCER DISEASE

### H. pylori is associated with most duodenal and gastric ulcers

The gram-negative spiral bacterium *H. pylori* infects the stomach of half the world's population (~4 billion people) and is associated with >90% of duodenal ulcers and 70–80% of gastric ulcers (Fig. 23.28). Marshall and Warren were awarded a Nobel Prize for discovering the bacterium and its role. Marshall bravely ingested an *H. pylori* culture having had a normal endoscopy, developed nausea and vomiting a few days later, a repeat endoscopy demonstrated gastritis and *H. pylori* was grown from the biopsy, showing cause and effect. *H. pylori* was the first bacterium proven to cause malignancy, gastric cancer, and is the cause of 25% of all infection-associated cancers. The most common presentation is with persistent or recurrent pain in the upper abdomen in the absence of structural evidence of disease.

*H. pylori* colonizes the host for life, but eradication can be achieved by antibiotics, although resistant strains are being detected more frequently and treatment failure follows. Persistence is due to the production of urease that breaks down urea to ammonia and $CO_2$, increasing the pH and providing protection against gastric acid. In addition, *H. pylori* has various surface attributes that help evade the immune response. Outcome of infection depends on a mix of bacterial genotype and host polymorphisms together with the various *H. pylori* virulence factors encoded by *cagA* (cytotoxin-associated gene A [CagA]), *vacA* (vacuolating toxin A [VacA]), *babA* (blood

antigen–binding adhesin [BabA]), *sabA* (sialic acid–binding adhesin) and *oipA* (outer inflammatory protein adhesion [OipA]). CagA, a cytotoxin, affects cell signalling, reduces cell adhesion and changes the cell phenotype from epithelial to mesenchymal cells, which is associated with carcinogenesis. VacA induces large vacuoles in host cells and forms porelike structures that result in osmotic swelling. In addition, it causes mitochondrial dysfunction and apoptosis, disrupts the epithelial cell barrier and improves the ability of *H. pylori* to colonize the gastric epithelium. BabA binds to the Lewis b ABO blood group antigen on red blood cells and some epithelial cells. SabA also promotes cell-to-cell adhesion, as well as stimulates a neutrophil response. This adhesion activity causes double-stranded DNA breaks in gastric epithelial cells and may lead to cancer-associated gene mutation. It may also improve adherence to those cells, and OipA is an outer membrane protein that acts as an adhesin and is associated with carcinogenesis. As it can also stick to mucins, the cumulative effect is to keep its position in the mucous gel layer despite the gastric churning motion.

*H. pylori* infection is associated with dyspepsia, stomach or upper abdominal pain due to gastric ulcers, acute and chronic gastritis in ~15% of people infected and gastric adenocarcinoma and mucosa-associated lymphoid tissue lymphoma in ~2% of people. The International Agency for Research on Cancer classified *H. pylori* as a group 1 carcinogen (the other groups are possible, probable or not carcinogenic). In addition, *H. pylori* has been found in other sites of the body and associated with extragastric diseases.

Rapid diagnosis may be made by using either the noninvasive urea breath test or faecal *H. pylori* antigen testing. For the breath test, a person ingests carbon-radiolabelled urea and, as *H. pylori* produces large amounts of urease, it is broken down into ammonia and carbon dioxide. The latter is absorbed into the bloodstream, and the radiolabelled carbon is detected in the expired air. The sensitivity and specificity is ~95%, but false-negative results can be seen if the person is taking antibiotics and/or proton pump inhibitor (PPI) drugs. Both tests are more sensitive and specific than ELISA-based serology tests with values that vary between 55% and 96%. In addition, *H. pylori* IgG can be detected for years, making it difficult to know whether the infection is recent or past.

Invasive methods involve endoscopy, with a diagnosis made on the basis of histologic examination of biopsy specimens. It also allows a direct assessment of inflammation in the stomach, and there is an updated Sydney grading system for chronic gastritis with mild, moderate or severe for the intensity of the inflammatory cell infiltrates. Rapid urease testing can be carried out on gastric biopsy material, and this time, when urea is added to the sample, the ammonia produced increases the pH detected in the test device. Biopsies can also be tested by PCR. *H. pylori* can be cultured in the laboratory, but is difficult to grow, taking >1 week in selective blood agar and is usually used when testing the sensitivity to specific antibiotics. Testing for antibiotic resistance is becoming more necessary, and so culture and PCR are critical tests.

Eradication of *H. pylori* to promote the remission and healing of ulcers requires combination therapy involving quadruple, triple or concomitant drugs. Quadruple therapy involves a PPI, bismuth salts and two antibiotics such as metronidazole and amoxicillin. Triple therapy includes a PPI

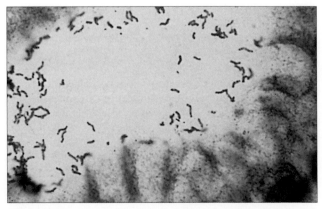

**Fig. 23.28** *Helicobacter pylori* gastritis, showing numerous spiral-shaped organisms adhering to the mucosal surface (silver stain). (Courtesy A.M. Geddes.)

and two antibiotics, clarithromycin and either amoxicillin or metronidazole. Concomitant treatment includes a PPI and triple antibiotic therapy with clarithromycin, amoxicillin and metronidazole (see Ch. 34). There are second-line and rescue treatments, too. Treatment duration is up to 14 days, and management is dictated by local antibiotic resistance rates. Since 2010 increasing resistance to clarithromycin resulted in <80% efficacy in many countries. Moreover, rates of primary and secondary resistance to clarithromycin, metronidazole and levofloxacin are >15% globally.

Vaccines have been developed, but the clinical trial results have been disappointing.

## PARASITES AND THE GASTROINTESTINAL TRACT

Many species of protozoan and helminth (worm) parasites live in the gastrointestinal tract, infecting some 3.5 billion people worldwide and resulting in >200 000 deaths each year. Only a few commonly cause serious pathology (Fig. 23.29), and these will form the focus of this part of the chapter.

### Transmission of intestinal parasites is maintained by the release of life cycle stages in faeces

The different life cycle stages include cysts, eggs and larvae. In most cases, new infections depend either directly or indirectly on contact with faecally derived material, infection rates therefore reflecting standards of hygiene and levels of sanitation. In general, the stages of protozoan parasites passed in faeces are either already infective or become infective within days. These parasites are therefore usually acquired by swallowing infective stages in faecally contaminated food or water. Worm parasites, with two major

exceptions, threadworm (also known as pinworm) and the dwarf tapeworm, produce eggs or larvae that require a period of development outside the host before they become infective. Some species are acquired through food or water contaminated with infective eggs or larvae, or they are picked up directly via contaminated fingers.

- Some have larvae that can actively penetrate through the skin, migrating eventually to the intestine.
- Others are acquired by eating animals or animal products containing infective stages.

The symptoms of intestinal infection range from very mild, through acute or chronic diarrhoeal conditions associated with parasite-related inflammation, to life-threatening diseases caused by spread of the parasites into other organs of the body. Most infections fall into the first of these categories.

### Protozoan infections

Three species are of particular importance:

- *Entamoeba histolytica*
- *Giardia duodenalis* (also known as *G. intestinalis* or *G. lamblia*)
- *Cryptosporidium hominis.*

All three can give rise to diarrhoeal illnesses, but the parasites have distinctive morphologic features that allow a precise diagnosis to be made easily by an experienced microscopist (Fig. 23.30). Other intestinal protozoa of concern, particularly in immunosuppressed patients, include *Cyclospora cayetanensis* and *Cystoisospora belli* (previously known as *Isospora belli*).

**Fig. 23.29** Gastrointestinal parasites of humans. The majority of these infections are found in resource-poor countries, but all species may also present in the resource-rich world, and some have come to prominence because of their association with acquired immunodeficiency syndrome. The most important parasite species are highlighted in bold type.

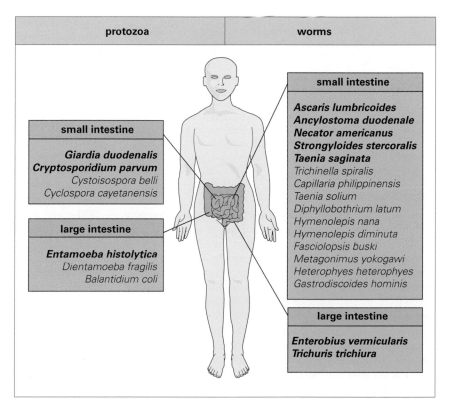

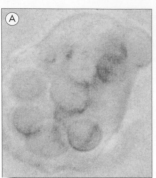

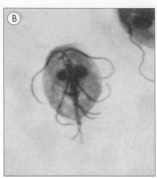

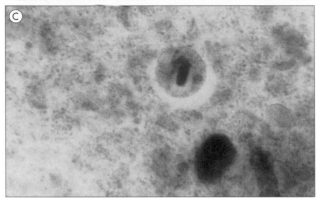

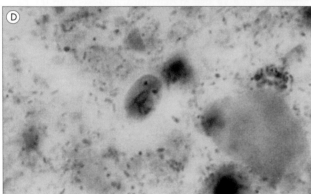

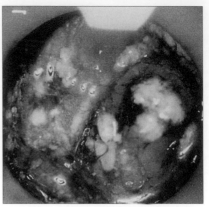

**Fig. 23.31** Amoebic colitis. Sigmoidoscopic view showing deep ulcers and overlying purulent exudate. (Courtesy R.H. Gilman.)

**Fig. 23.30** Protozoan infections of the gastrointestinal tract. (A) *Entamoeba histolytica*. Trophozoite found in the acute stage of the disease, which often contains ingested red blood cells. (B) *Giardia duodenalis* trophozoite associated with acute infection in humans. (C) Cyst of *E. histolytica*, with only one of the four nuclei visible. The broad chromidial bar is a semicrystalline aggregation of ribosomes (H&E stain). (D) Oval cyst of *G. duodenalis* showing two of the four nuclei (iron haematoxylin stain). (B, Courtesy D.K. Banerjee; D, courtesy R. Muller and J.R. Baker.)

### Entamoeba histolytica

**E. histolytica *infection is particularly common in subtropical and tropical climate zones.*** For many years it was considered that infections with *E. histolytica* could be asymptomatic or pathogenic, with dysentery a key symptom when the amoebae invaded the mucosa. In fact, rather than a single species behaving differently, the explanation is that two species are involved: *E. histolytica* is invasive and *E. dispar* is nonpathogenic and noninvasive. *E. histolytica* occurs worldwide, but it is most often found in subtropical and tropical climate zones where seroprevalence rates may exceed 40%. *E. histolytica* is responsible for ~55,000 deaths per year worldwide. The trophozoite stages of the amoebae live in the large intestine on the mucosal surface. Reproduction of these stages is by simple binary fission, and there is periodic formation of resistant encysted forms, which pass out of the body. These cysts can survive in the external environment (for up to 30 days in water) and act as the infective stages. Infection occurs when food or drink is contaminated either by infected food handlers or as a result of inadequate sanitation. Transmission can also take place as a result of oral–anal and anal sexual activity. Men who have sex with men are at greater risk of sexually transmitted *E. histolytica* infection in some of the more resource-rich countries in East Asia as well as Europe. Many may be asymptomatic; in those presenting with acute abdominal pain, the diagnosis may not be considered in the differential diagnosis.

The cysts pass intact through the stomach when swallowed and excyst in the small intestine, each giving rise to four progeny. These adhere to the epithelial cells using a combination of adhesins and lectins and damage them via amoebapore-, phospholipase- and cysteine protease-induced cytolysis accompanied by phagocytosis. Intruigingly, *E. histolytica* also use trogocytosis, a process by which they "nibble" host cells and display surface antigens from host cells on their own surface, thus protecting themselves from lysis by human serum—yet another mechanism of immune evasion. Via a combination of all these processes, amoebae are able to invade the mucosa and feed on host tissues, including red blood cells, resulting in amoebic colitis.

**E. histolytica *infection may cause mild diarrhoea or severe dysentery.*** Infections with *E. dispar* are asymptomatic, and this protozoan does not cause illness in humans. In contrast, invasion of the mucosa by *E. histolytica* may produce small localized superficial ulcers or involve the entire colonic mucosa with the formation of deep confluent ulcers (Fig. 23.31). The former causes mild diarrhoea, whereas more severe invasion leads to amoebic dysentery, which is characterized by mucus and blood in the stools. All *E. histolytica* are regarded as pathogenic, but the outcome of infection with this parasite can vary, with isolates from different geographic areas displaying different virulence patterns. Much work on genotyping is underway to unravel the underlying mechanisms (e.g. single nucleotide polymorphisms in the *kerp2* gene of *E. histolytica* have been suggested as potential markers linked to a high risk of amoebic liver abscess occurring in individuals with persistent intestinal infection).

Dysenteries of amoebic and bacillary origin can be distinguished by a number of features (Table 23.5).

Complications include perforation of the intestine, leading to peritonitis, and extraintestinal invasion. Trophozoites can spread via the blood to the liver, with the formation of an abscess, and may secondarily extend to the lung and other organs. Rarely, abscesses spread directly and involve the overlying skin. *E. histolytica* is able to evade the immune response by a variety of methods, including immunomodulation, protease-based destruction of soluble immune mediators, apoptosis, phagocytosis and trogocytosis, as mentioned earlier. Antibody detection by IgG ELISA is the mainstay of diagnosis for an amoebic liver abscess and is ~95% sensitive.

**E. histolytica *infection can be diagnosed in asymptomatic patients from the presence of characteristic four-nucleate cysts in the stool followed by ELISA or PCR confirmation.*** These cysts may be infrequent in light infections, and repeated stool examination is necessary. Care must be taken to differentiate *E. histolytica* from other nonpathogenic species that might be present, especially as the cysts of *E. dispar* (nonpathogenic) are morphologically identical to those of *E. histolytica* (Fig. 23.32). Differentiation of *E. histolytica* from *E. dispar* requires antigen detection tests or species-specific PCR.

***Diagnosis of amoebic dysentery is made by detection of trophozoites in fresh stools, antigen detection ELISA or PCR.*** Motile, haematophagous trophozoites of *E. histolytica* can be found in cases of dysentery (when the stools are loose and wet), but they are fragile and deteriorate rapidly; specimens should therefore either be examined within 20 min of being passed, when the amoebae will still be active or be preserved before examination of a stained preparation. Antigen detection ELISA tests for *E. histolytica* are available, as is a triage panel ELISA assay that can distinguish between *E. histolytica*/*E. dispar*, *Cryptosporidium* spp. and *G. duodenalis*.

**Acute E. histolytica *infection can be treated with metronidazole or tinidazole.*** If infection is treated early, recovery is expected, and there is some immunity to reinfection associated with the secretory IgA response. Metronidazole or tinidazole kills amoebic trophozoites in both intestinal and extraintestinal sites of infection and results in rapid clinical improvement, but relapse of the infection may occur unless a second antiamoebic agent (e.g. paromomycin) is given to eradicate amoebae from the gut lumen. Prevention of amoebiasis in the community requires the same approaches to hygiene and sanitation as those adopted for bacterial infections of the intestine. A vaccine directed against the Lec A fragment of the Gal/GalNAC lectin, which mediates attachment of *E. histolytica* to the colonic mucosa, is being developed.

## Giardia duodenalis

*Giardia* was the first intestinal microorganism to be observed under a microscope. It was discovered in 1681 by Antonie van Leeuwenhoek, who used the microscope he had invented to examine specimens of his own faeces. There have been changes in nomenclature, and the species infecting humans is also commonly referred to as *G. intestinalis* or *G. lamblia*.

It has a global distribution with ~280 million infections annually and is a frequent cause of travellers' diarrhoea. *Giardia* is the most diagnosed intestinal parasite in the United States, where it is reported to cause >1 million cases a year, having been detected in both drinking and recreational water.

***Like* Entamoeba, Giardia *has only two life cycle stages.*** The two life cycle stages are the flagellate (four pairs of flagella) binucleate trophozoite and the resistant four-nucleate cyst. The trophozoites live in the upper portion of the small intestine, adhering closely to the brush border of the epithelial cells by specialized attachment regions (Fig. 23.33). They divide by binary fission and can occur in such numbers that

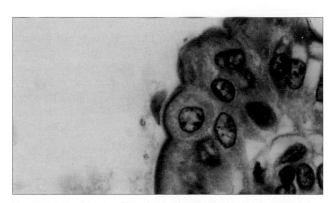

**Fig. 23.33** Trophozoite of *Giardia duodenalis* attached to the mucosal surface of the small intestine (iron haematoxylin stain). (Courtesy R. Muller and J.R. Baker.)

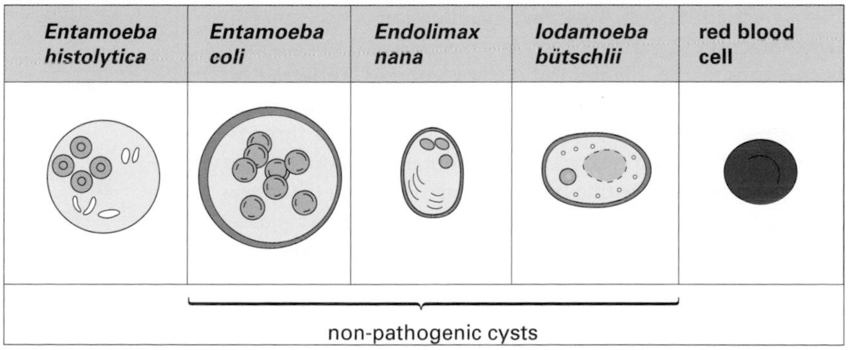

**Table 23.5** Features of bacillary and amoebic dysentery

|  | Bacillary | Amoebic |
|---|---|---|
| Organism | Shigella | Entamoeba |
| Polymorphs and macrophages in faeces | Many | Few |
| Eosinophils and Charcot–Leyden crystals in faeces | Few or absent | Often present |
| Organisms in faeces | Many | Few |
| Blood and mucus in faeces | Yes | Yes |

**Fig. 23.32** Characteristics of cysts (size and number of nuclei) are used to differentiate pathogenic from nonpathogenic protozoa. A red blood cell is shown for comparison.

| Entamoeba histolytica | Entamoeba coli | Endolimax nana | Iodamoeba bütschlii | red blood cell |
|---|---|---|---|---|
|  | non-pathogenic cysts | | | |

they cover large areas of the mucosal surface. Cyst formation occurs at regular intervals, each cyst being formed as one trophozoite rounds up and produces a resistant wall. Cysts pass out in the stools and can survive for several weeks under optimum conditions. Infection occurs when the cysts are swallowed, usually as a result of drinking contaminated water. Each cyst releases two trophozoites on hatching, and the minimum infective dose is very small (10–25 cysts).

Epidemics of giardiasis have occurred when public drinking supplies have become contaminated, but smaller outbreaks have been traced to drinking from rivers and streams that have been contaminated by animals. Apart from waterborne transmission, *Giardia* can be passed from person to person, especially within families and child care facilities, with foodborne transmission being rare. *Giardia* may also be transmitted sexually as a result of oral–anal contact. Genotyping has demonstrated that *Giardia* consists of eight different assemblages (A–H). Assemblages A and B are the main assemblages that infect humans. In addition, assemblage A can infect dogs, cats and cattle; B can infect dogs and cattle, so human infection with these genotypes can also be zoonotically acquired.

*Mild* Giardia *infections are asymptomatic; more severe infections cause diarrhoea.* The diarrhoea may be:

- self-limiting, with 7–10 days being the usual course
- chronic, and develop into a debilitating condition, particularly in patients with deficient or compromised immunologic defences. Characteristically, the stools are loose, foul smelling and often fatty.

The different clinical presentations of *Giardia* infection are the result of differences in the host immune response, the parasite itself and its interaction with the intestinal microbiota.

*Giardia* trophozoites adhere to the small bowel mucosa and release excretory secretory products, the most important of which are thought to be cysteine proteases. These substances interact with intestinal tight junctions, induce cellular apoptosis, damage intestinal villi and may adversely affect intestinal mucus. The ability of *Giardia* to exhibit antigenic variation in its variant-specific surface proteins is felt to play a part in immune evasion.

*Diagnosis of* Giardia *infection is based on identifying cysts or trophozoites in the stool.* Trophozoites can be detected by direct microscopy of a wet preparation or microscopy of a fixed, stained faecal smear but are not visualized in concentration methods. Cysts can be detected in wet preparations and by direct immunofluorescence microscopy of faecal smears, which has high specificity. Formalin ethyl acetate concentration is superior to direct wet film microscopy for the detection of cysts. Repeated examination is necessary in light infections, so if giardiasis is suspected and microscopy is the only test available, three stool samples, collected on separate days, should be examined. Duodenal intubation or the use of recoverable swallowed capsules and threads, known as the string test, may aid in obtaining trophozoites directly from the intestine but is seldom used now that alternatives to microscopic methods are increasingly available. These include faecal antigen-detecting ELISA tests with good specificity, immunochromatographic tests in cassette form and PCR. Multiplex PCR assays detecting *Giardia*, *Cryptosporidium* and *E. histolytica* in faecal specimens, some of them multiplexed with bacterial and viral pathogens, are now widely deployed. PCR is more sensitive than microscopy, so where it is available, examination of one stool by PCR is likely to replace microscopy of three separate faecal samples. Assemblage genotyping and sequence analysis can be deployed in outbreak investigations.

Giardia *infection can be treated with a variety of drugs.* The nitroimidazole compounds metronidazole and tinidazole are commonly used. Increasing numbers of nitroimidazole treatment failures have occurred in the last 10 years however, especially in giardiasis acquired in the Indian subcontinent, and nitazoxanide, albendazole or mepacrine (also known as quinacrine) are alternatives. Community measures for prevention include the usual concerns with hygiene and sanitation, and improved treatment of drinking water supplies (largely filtration and chlorination) where these are suspected as a source. Avoiding drinking from potentially contaminated natural waters is also important.

## Cryptosporidium hominis *and* C. parvum

*The protozoan genus* Cryptosporidium *is widely distributed in many animals.* Awareness of *Cryptosporidium* as an important cause of diarrhoea in humans was established during the early years of the acquired immunodeficiency syndrome (AIDS) epidemic, although similar parasites were known to be widely distributed in many animals. Although there are 26 species of *Cryptosporidium*, a very high proportion of human infection is due to *C. hominis*, which is specific to humans, and *C. parvum*, which has a wide host range, including livestock such as calves, but is also capable of causing disease in humans. Outbreaks of *C. parvum* have been associated with animal and environmental contact and with foodborne outbreaks. Outbreaks of *C. hominis* are strongly associated with person-to-person spread, but both species have been responsible for drinking water outbreaks, and these two species are responsible for >90% of cases of human cryptosporidiosis. Identification of subtypes of the *gp60* gene is a valuable tool in the investigation of cryptosporidial outbreaks. The parasite has a complex life cycle, going through both asexual and sexual phases of development in the same host. Transmission requires ingestion of a minimum of 10 of the resistant oocysts (4–5 μm in diameter) in faecally contaminated material (Fig. 23.34). In the small intestine, the oocyst releases infective sporozoites, which invade the epithelial cells, remaining closely associated with the apical plasma membrane such that they are intracellular but extracytoplasmic.

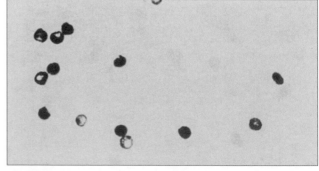

**Fig. 23.34** *Cryptosporidium* oocysts in faecal specimen. (Courtesy S. Tzipori.)

Here they form meronts, which produce and release merozoites, and these then reinvade further epithelial cells. A second type of meront produces sexual stages known as gamonts. Fertilization occurs, and thick-walled oocysts are released in the faeces. The major risk factors for developing cryptosporidiosis are ingesting contaminated drinking or recreational water, contact with infected people or animals and travel to areas with poor sanitation. Most outbreaks are waterborne, and *Cryptosporidium* first came to prominence in the public health arena in 1993 when it caused a massive outbreak of watery diarrhoea affecting 403 000 people in Milwaukee, Wisconsin. It was transmitted through the public water supply. It continues to be a formidable adversary, and *Cryptosporidium* is estimated to cause >8 million foodborne cases per year worldwide.

*Cryptosporidial diarrhoea ranges from moderate to severe.* Symptoms of infection with *Cryptosporidium* range from moderate diarrhoea to more severe profuse diarrhoea that is self-limiting in 15–40 days in immunocompetent individuals, but it can become chronic in immunocompromised patients, including those with advanced human immunodeficiency virus (HIV) infection. In individuals with CD4 T-cell counts $<100/\text{mm}^3$, diarrhoea is prolonged, may become irreversible in the absence of immune reconstitution and can be life threatening.

*Routine faecal wet preparation examinations are inadequate for diagnosing cryptosporidial diarrhoea.* Fluorescence microscopy (e.g. with auramine) or modified Ziehl–Neelsen staining can be used to demonstrate oocysts in thin faecal smears. Direct immunofluorescence microscopy of faecal smears using monoclonal antibodies to oocyst wall antigen is highly specific for detection of oocysts. Antigen detection ELISA assays, which are capable of high throughput and immunochromatographic lateral flow cassette tests, are also deployed. PCR is both sensitive and highly specific. It is now widely available, commonly as a multiplex assay detecting *Cryptosporidium*, *Giardia* and *E. histolytica*, plus bacterial and viral pathogens.

*Antiparasitic treatment for cryptosporidial diarrhoea is suboptimal.* Symptomatic therapy is an important part of management. Combination antiretroviral therapy (cART) in individuals with advanced HIV infection and cryptosporidiosis has been reported to improve the diarrhoea symptoms. This may be due to the protease inhibitors used in combination therapy interfering directly with the cryptosporidial proteases involved in the protozoal life cycle. In addition, cART results in lowering the plasma HIV load and promotes immune reconstitution. Paromomycin reduces oocyst output but does not clear infection. Nitazoxanide is effective in individuals who are HIV negative but is only partially active in those coinfected with HIV. Public health measures are similar to those outlined for controlling giardiasis, although *Cryptosporidium* is more resistant to chlorination. Various filtration methods are in use, and some water treatment facilities deploy an additional ozonation step to inactivate cryptosporidia.

### Cyclospora and Cystoisospora

*Cyclospora*, like *C. belli* and *Cryptosporidium*, is a coccidian parasite in which life cycle stages take place in epithelial cells of the mucosa. *Cyclospora* and *Cystoisospora* have only been found in humans, unlike other coccidia that are zoonotic.

*C. cayetanensis*, named in 1994, is one cause of travellers' diarrhoea, but it can also be acquired from contaminated imported food such as soft fruits (e.g. Guatemalan raspberries were thought to be the cause of five diarrhoeal outbreaks in the United States in 1995–2000). Outbreaks have also been associated with consumption of vegetables (e.g mesclun lettuce) or herbs such as basil or cilantro. In 2015 and 2016 outbreaks of cyclosporiasis occurred in UK travellers having returned from Mexico. More recently, in 2020 an outbreak of cyclosporiasis occurred in the United States involving 701 people in 14 states. The likely source was bagged mixed salad, possibly contaminated by a regional water management canal supplying irrigation water to a farm identified in the outbreak investigation.

Diarrhoea in cyclosporiasis can be prolonged and is severe in immunosuppressed individuals. Diagnosis is similar to methods mentioned previously, such as modified acid-fast staining and ultraviolet fluorescence microscopy, but concentration methods are more sensitive. Regarding prevention, unlike *Cryptosporidium*, the *Cyclospora* oocyst is noninfective when passed in the faeces and takes 1–2 weeks in the environment to sporulate and become infective, so direct person-to-person spread is not feasible. Treatment with trimethoprim-sulphamethoxazole (co-trimoxazole) is effective. Ciprofloxacin is partially effective.

People living with advanced HIV infection coinfected with *Cystoisospora belli* may show particularly severe symptoms, with persistent diarrhoea causing weight loss and even death. Treatment is with co-trimoxazole.

## MICROSPORIDIA

Microsporidia are now regarded as fungi, but they are mentioned here as traditionally they have been discussed with the protozoa. Infections with this unusual group have also become recognized as a cause of diarrhoea in advanced HIV infection, usually with a CD4 count $<100/\text{mm}^3$, and in other immunosuppressed patients. *Enterocytozoon bieneusi* is the commonest cause, although *Encephalitozoon intestinalis* also occurs. Transmission appears to be direct. Albendazole treatment is effective against *E. intestinalis* but has disappointing activity against *E. bieneusi*. Where possible, immune reconstitution is the mainstay of treatment.

## OTHER INTESTINAL PROTOZOA

The human intestine may harbour a large number of protozoa, many of which appear to be quite harmless, such as *Entamoeba coli*. Some have a questionable role in intestinal disease (e.g. *Blastocystis hominis*).

### Worm infections

**The most important intestinal worms clinically are the nematodes known as the soil-transmitted helminths**

Soil-transmitted helminths (STHs) fall into two distinct groups:

- *Ascaris lumbricoides* (large roundworm) and *Trichuris trichiura* (whipworm), in which infection occurs by swallowing the infective eggs
- *Ancylostoma duodenale* and *Necator americanus* (hookworm) and *Strongyloides stercoralis*, which infect via active skin penetration by infective larvae, which then undertake a systemic migration through the lungs to the intestine

Except for *Trichuris* all the soil-transmitted nematodes inhabit the small bowel.

The pinworm or threadworm *Enterobius vermicularis* is probably the commonest intestinal nematode in resource-rich countries and is the least pathogenic. The females of this species, which live in the large bowel, release infective eggs onto the perianal skin. This causes itching, and transmission usually occurs directly from contaminated fingers, but the eggs are also light enough to be carried in dust.

The STHs are commonest in warmer resource-poor countries. About one-quarter of the world's population carry these worms, children being the most heavily infected group. They result in a considerable burden of morbidity, including anaemia and malnutrition, and their effects on physical and cognitive development. Transmission is favoured where there is inadequate disposal of faeces, contamination of water supplies, use of faeces (night-soil) as fertilizer or low standards of hygiene (see later). Vast numbers of eggs are released in the lifetime of each female worm (tens of thousands by *Trichuris* and *Ancylostoma* and hundreds of thousands by *Ascaris*).

### Life cycle and transmission

*Female* Ascaris *and* Trichuris *lay thick-shelled eggs in the intestine, which are expelled with faeces and hatch after being swallowed by another host.* The thick-shelled eggs of *Ascaris* and *Trichuris* are shown in Fig. 23.35. The eggs require incubation for several days at optimum conditions (warm temperature, high humidity) for the infective larvae to develop. Once this occurs, the eggs remain infective for many weeks or months, depending upon the local microclimate, and *Ascaris* eggs can survive in moist soil for up to 10 years. After being swallowed, the eggs hatch in the intestine, releasing the larvae. Those of *Ascaris* penetrate the bowel wall and are

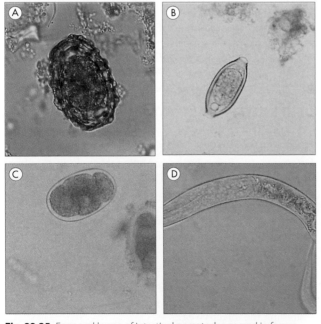

**Fig. 23.35** Eggs and larvae of intestinal nematodes passed in faeces. (A) Egg of *Ascaris* (fertile). (B) Egg of *Trichuris*. (C) Egg of hookworm. The embryo continues to divide in the faecal sample and may be at the 16- or 32-cell stage by the time the sample is examined. (D) Larva of *Strongyloides stercoralis*. (Courtesy J.H. Cross.)

carried in the blood through the liver to the lungs, migrating up the bronchi and trachea before being swallowed and once again reaching the intestine. The adult worms live freely in the gut lumen, feeding on intestinal contents. In contrast, *Trichuris* larvae remain within the large bowel, penetrating into the mucosa, where they remain as they mature.

*Adult female hookworm lay thin-shelled eggs that hatch in the faeces shortly after leaving the host.* A hookworm egg is shown in Fig. 23.35C. The larvae of these hookworms (*A. duodenale* and *N. americanus*) feed on bacteria until infective, and then migrate away from the faecal mass. Infection takes place when larvae come into contact with unprotected skin (or additionally, in the case of *Ancylostoma*, are swallowed). They penetrate the skin, migrate via the bloodstream to the lungs, ascend the trachea and are swallowed. Adult worms attach by their enlarged mouths to the intestinal mucosa, ingest a plug of tissue, rupture capillaries and suck blood.

*The adult female* Strongyloides *lays eggs that hatch in the intestine.* The life cycle of *Strongyloides* is broadly similar to that of hookworms but shows some important differences. Humans harbour only parthenogenetic females that lay eggs into the mucosa. These eggs hatch in the intestine, and the released rhabditiform larvae usually pass out in the faeces (see Fig. 23.35D). Development outside the host can follow the hookworm pattern, with the direct production of skin-penetrating filariform larvae, or may be diverted into the production of a complete free-living generation, including adult males and females, which then produce infective larvae. Under certain conditions, and particularly when the host is immunocompromised, instead of being voided in the faeces, *Strongyloides* larvae can develop to the filariform stage and reinvade through the intestinal mucosa. This process of auto-infection can give rise to the severe clinical condition known as disseminated strongyloidiasis, also called hyperinfection, which is often complicated by gram-negative bacterial septicaemia. All soil-transmitted helminths (STHs) are relatively long lived (several months to years), but authenticated cases show that *Strongyloides* infections can persist for >30 years presumably through continuous internal autoinfection.

### Clinical features

In most individuals, worm infections produce chronic mild intestinal discomfort rather than severe diarrhoea or other conditions. Infections may lead to hypersensitivity responses and can reduce responses to vaccination. Each parasite has a number of characteristic pathologic conditions linked with it.

*Large numbers of adult* Ascaris *worms can cause intestinal obstruction.* The migration of *Ascaris* larvae through the lungs can cause severe respiratory distress due to pneumonitis; ascariasis is one of the causes of Löffler syndrome. This stage is often associated with pronounced eosinophilia. Worms in the intestine can cause abdominal pain, nausea and digestive disturbances. In children with a suboptimal nutritional intake, these disturbances can contribute to clinical malnutrition. Large numbers of adult *Ascaris* can cause a physical blockage in the intestine, and this may occur as worms die following antiparasitic chemotherapy. Intestinal worms tend to migrate out of the intestine, often up the common bile duct, causing cholangitis or liver abscess. Perforation of the intestinal wall can also occur. Worms have occasionally been reported in unusual locations, including

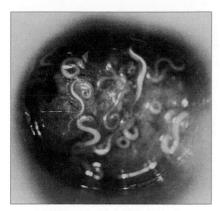

**Fig. 23.36** Trichuriasis in a healthy, infected child. Proctoscopic view showing numerous adult *Trichuris trichiura* attached to the intestinal mucosa. (Courtesy R.H. Gilman.)

the orbit of the eye and the male urethra. *Ascaris* is highly allergenic, and infections often give rise to symptoms of hypersensitivity, which may persist for many years after the infection has been cleared.

*Moderate to severe* **Trichuris** *infection can cause chronic diarrhoea.* As with all intestinal worms, children are the members of the community most heavily infected with *Trichuris*. Although previously regarded as of little clinical significance, research has shown that moderate to heavy infections in children can cause chronic mucoid diarrhoea with rectal bleeding (Fig. 23.36), the *Trichuris* dysentery syndrome resulting in impaired nutrition and retarded growth. Occasionally heavy infections lead to rectal prolapse.

*Hookworm disease can result in iron-deficiency anaemia.* Migration of hookworm larvae through the skin and lungs can cause dermatitis and pneumonitis, respectively. The blood-feeding activities of the intestinal worms can lead to iron-deficiency anaemia if the diet is inadequate. Heavy infections cause marked debility and growth retardation.

*Strongyloidiasis can be fatal in immunosuppressed people.* Heavy intestinal infection with strongyloidiasis causes persistent and profuse diarrhoea with dehydration and electrolyte imbalance. Profound mucosal changes can also lead to a malabsorption syndrome, which is sometimes confused with tropical sprue. People with human lymphotropic virus type 1 infection, diseases that suppress immune function such as advanced HIV infection and cancer, or who are being treated with immunosuppressive drugs, are susceptible to the development of disseminated strongyloidiasis. This parasite is a remarkable opportunist, and the use of dexamethasone therapy in the treatment of COVID-19 has resulted in dissemination of underlying *Strongyloides* infection. In this and other examples of disseminated infection, invasion of the body by many thousands of autoinfective *Strongyloides* larvae can be fatal. Gram-negative bacterial septicaemia or meningitis, which can be polymicrobial in both cases, can ensue.

The most common sign of pinworm (threadworm) infection is anal pruritus. Occasionally this is accompanied by mild diarrhoea. *Enterobius* are sometimes found in the appendix, but their role in appendicitis is controversial. Having emerged onto the perianal skin, adult female worms occasionally enter the vagina in women and produce local irritation.

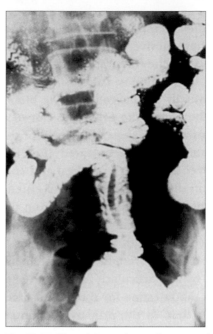

**Fig. 23.37** Filling defect in the small intestine due to the presence of *Ascaris*, seen on a radiograph after a barium meal. (Courtesy W. Peters.)

### Laboratory diagnosis

All five of the soil-transmitted species can be diagnosed by finding eggs or larvae in a fresh stool. Although these stages may be detected in direct faecal smears in heavy infections, concentration techniques are significantly more sensitive. A charcoal or agar plate culture of faeces is added if *Strongyloides* is suspected. Faecal PCR for *Strongyloides* is now entering service in specialist laboratories. Acute infections with *Ascaris*, hookworm and *Strongyloides* are often accompanied by a marked blood eosinophilia. Although this is not diagnostic, it is a strong indication to suspect a helminth infection. An enzyme immunoassay can be used to detect *Strongyloides* antibody and has ~90% sensitivity of detection. However, there is some cross-reactivity with IgG made against other nematode infections, and one cannot determine whether the *Strongyloides* infection occurred recently or in the past. Duodenal aspiration and biopsy may be required to make the diagnosis.

*The eggs of* **Ascaris**, **Trichuris** *and hookworm are characteristic.* These eggs are shown in Fig. 23.35 and are easily recognizable. Identification of the species of hookworm requires charcoal culture of the stool to allow the eggs to hatch and the larvae to mature into the infective third stage and is not routinely performed in clinical practice. The presence of adult *Ascaris* is sometimes demonstrated incidentally by radiography (Fig. 23.37).

The presence of characteristic rhabditiform larvae in fresh stools is diagnostic of *Strongyloides* infection. Filariform larvae detected by charcoal or agar plate culture need to be distinguished morphologically from those of hookworm.

*Pinworm (threadworm) infection is diagnosed by finding eggs on perianal skin.* Although adult pinworms sometimes appear in the stools, the eggs are seldom seen in faecal concentrates because they are laid directly onto the perianal skin (Fig. 23.38). They can be found by pressing this area with a piece of clear adhesive tape (the Scotch tape test) and

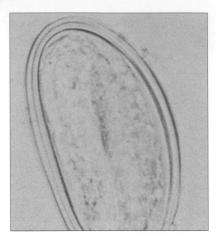

**Fig. 23.38** Egg of *Enterobius* on perianal skin. (Courtesy J.H. Cross.)

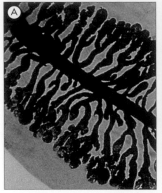
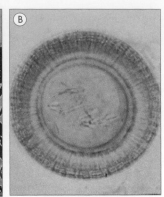

**Fig. 23.39** *Taenia saginata*. (A) Gravid proglottid stained with India ink to show numerous side branches. (B) Egg containing six hooked (hexacanth) larva. (Courtesy R. Muller and J.R. Baker.)

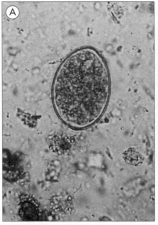
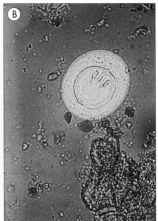

**Fig. 23.40** Eggs of (A) *Diphyllobothrium latum* and (B) *Hymenolepis nana*. (Courtesy R. Muller and J.R. Baker.)

examining the tape mounted sticky side down on a microscope slide.

### Treatment and prevention

*Enterobius* is treated with mebendazole, albendazole or pyrantel pamoate, but treatment failures are becoming more frequent. *Ascaris* is treated with mebendazole or albendazole; hookworm with albendazole or mebendazole; and *Trichuris* with mebendazole or albendazole. *Strongyloides* requires treatment with ivermectin; thiabendazole is also effective but is less well tolerated by the patient and is no longer available in most health systems; albendazole is less effective than ivermectin or thiabendazole.

To control STHs at the community level, mass drug administration (MDA) is used to reduce morbidity, but very high rates of treatment coverage would be required for MDA alone to achieve eradication. In the long term, given sufficient resources, prevention can be achieved through improved hygiene and sanitation, making sure that faecal material is disposed of properly.

### Other intestinal worms

***Many other worm species can infect the intestine, but most are uncommon in resource-rich countries.*** Of the human tapeworms:

- the beef tapeworm *Taenia saginata*, transmitted through eating undercooked or raw infected beef, is the most widely distributed. However, infection is usually asymptomatic, apart from revulsion felt on passing the large segments. Diagnosis involves finding these segments or the characteristic eggs in the stool (Fig. 23.39). Particularly dangerous is the pork tapeworm, *T. solium,* acquired from eating raw or undercooked infected pork. Although its intestinal stage is often asymptomatic like the beef tapeworm, infection with *T. solium* can produce cerebral cysticercosis. This is because *T. solium* eggs are infective to humans as well as pigs. Cysticerci in the brain are a common cause of epilepsy in endemic areas.
- *Diphyllobothrium latum*, the fish tapeworm, is widely distributed geographically, but infection is restricted to individuals eating raw or undercooked fish carrying the infective larvae. Prolonged infection can produce

vitamin B12 deficiency in the human host. The eggs of this species have a terminal lidlike structure known as an operculum and are the diagnostic stage in the stool (Fig. 23.40A).

- *Hymenolepis nana*, the dwarf tapeworm, occurs primarily in children, infection occurring directly by swallowing eggs (see Fig. 23.40B). This worm has the ability to initiate autoinfection within the host's intestine so that a large number of worms can build up, leading to diarrhoea and some abdominal discomfort.

All these tapeworms can be treated with praziquantel or niclosamide.

Intestinal symptoms (predominantly diarrhoea and abdominal pain) are associated with infection by the nematode *Trichinella spiralis*, which is better known clinically for the pathology caused by the bloodborne muscle phase (see Chs. 27 and 29). Infection with species of schistosomes situated in mesenteric blood vessels (*Schistosoma japonicum* and *S. mansoni*) can also cause symptoms of intestinal disease. As the eggs pass through the intestinal wall, they cause marked inflammatory responses, granulomatous lesions form and diarrhoea may occur in the early acute phase. Heavy, chronic *S. mansoni* infection is associated with inflammatory polyps in the colon, whereas severe involvement of the small bowel is more common with *S. japonicum*.

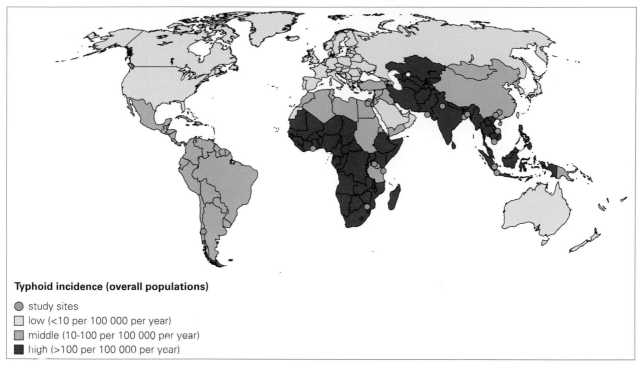

**Fig. 23.41** Typhoid incidence in low-income and middle-income countries. (Reprinted with permission from Elsevier. Mogasale V, Maskery B, Ochiai RL, et al. Burden of typhoid fever in low-income and middle-income countries: a systematic, literature-based update with risk-factor adjustment. *Lancet Glob Health*. 2014;2:e570–580.)

## SYSTEMIC INFECTION INITIATED IN THE GASTROINTESTINAL TRACT

We opened this chapter by noting that infections acquired by the ingestion of pathogens could remain localized in the gastrointestinal tract or could disseminate to other organs and body systems. Important examples of disseminated infection are the enteric fevers and viral hepatitis types A and E. Listeriosis can also be acquired via the gastrointestinal tract. For the sake of clarity and convenience, other types of viral hepatitis will also be discussed in this chapter.

### Enteric fevers: typhoid and paratyphoid

The term *enteric fever* was introduced in the last century to clarify the distinction between typhus (see Ch. 28) and typhoid. For many years these two diseases had been confused, as the common root of their names suggests (typhus, a fever with delirium; typhoid, resembling typhus), but even before the causative agents were isolated, typhoid caused by *S. typhi* and typhus caused by *Rickettsia* spp., it was pointed out that it was "just as impossible to confuse the intestinal lesions of typhoid with the pathologic findings of typhus as it was to confuse the eruptions of measles with the pustules of smallpox." In fact, enteric fevers can be caused by *S. typhi* and three additional *Salmonella* spp., but the name typhoid has stuck.

### *S. typhi* and paratyphi types *S. paratyphi A*, *S. schottmuelleri* (previously named *S. paratyphi B*) and *S. hirschfeldii* (previously named *S. paratyphi C*) cause enteric fevers

These species of *Salmonella* are restricted to humans and do not have a reservoir in animals. Therefore spread of the infection is from person to person, usually through contaminated food or water (Fig. 23.41). After infection, people can carry the organism for months or years, providing a continuing source from which others may become infected. Typhoid Mary, a cook in New York City in the early 1900s, is one such example. She was a long-term carrier who succeeded in initiating at least 10 outbreaks of the disease (see Ch. 17, Box 17.1).

### The salmonellae multiply within and are transported around the body in macrophages

After ingestion, the salmonellae that survive the antibacterial defences of the stomach and small intestine penetrate the gut mucosa through the Peyer's patches, probably in the jejunum or distal ileum (Fig. 23.42). Once through the mucosal barrier, the bacteria reach the intestinal lymph nodes, where they survive and multiply within macrophages. They are transported in the macrophages to the mesenteric lymph nodes and thence to the thoracic duct and are eventually discharged into the bloodstream. Circulating in the blood, the organisms can seed many organs, most importantly in areas where cells of the reticuloendothelial system are concentrated, such as the spleen, bone marrow, liver and Peyer's patches. In the liver they multiply in Kupffer cells. From the reticuloendothelial system, the bacteria reinvade the blood to reach other organs (e.g. kidney). The gallbladder is infected either from the blood or from the liver via the biliary tract, the bacterium being particularly resistant to bile. As a result, *S. typhi* enters the intestine for a second time in much larger numbers than on the primary encounter and causes a strong inflammatory response in Peyer's patches, leading to ulceration with the danger of intestinal perforation.

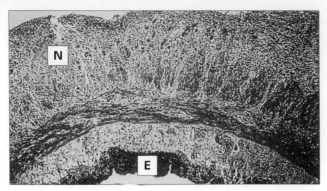

**Fig. 23.42** Typhoid. Section of ileum showing a typhoid ulcer with a transmural inflammatory reaction, focal areas of necrosis (*N*) and a fibrinous exudate (*E*) on the serosal surface (H&E stain). (Courtesy M.S.R. Hutt.)

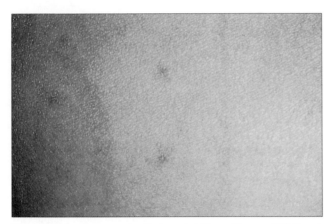

**Fig. 23.43** Rose spots on the skin in typhoid fever. (Courtesy W.E. Farrar.)

### Rose spots on the upper abdomen are characteristic, but absent in up to half of patients with enteric fever

After an incubation period of 10–14 days (range 7–21 days), the disease has an insidious onset with nonspecific symptoms of fever and malaise accompanied by aches and respiratory symptoms, and may resemble a flulike illness. Diarrhoea may be present, but constipation is just as likely. At this stage, the patient often presents with a fever of unknown origin. In the absence of treatment, the fever increases and the patient becomes acutely ill. Rose spots (erythematous maculopapular lesions that blanch on pressure [Fig. 23.43]) are characteristic on the upper abdomen but may be absent in up to half of patients. They are transient and disappear within hours to days. Without treatment, an uncomplicated infection lasts 4–6 weeks.

### Before antibiotics, 12–16% of patients with enteric fever died, usually of complications

The complications can be classified into:

- those secondary to the local gastrointestinal lesions (e.g. haemorrhage and perforation; Fig. 23.44)
- those associated with toxaemia (e.g. myocarditis, hepatic and bone marrow damage)
- those secondary to a prolonged serious illness
- those resulting from multiplication of the organisms in other sites, causing meningitis, osteomyelitis or endocarditis.

Before antibiotics became available, 12–16% of patients died, usually of complications occurring in the third or fourth week of the disease. Relapse after an initial recovery was also common.

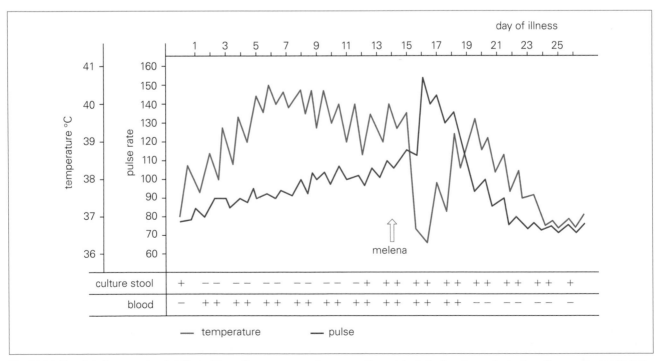

**Fig. 23.44** The clinical course of typhoid fever. Chart of temperature, pulse rate and bacteriologic findings in a patient whose illness was complicated by massive haemorrhage. Melena: dark black, tarry faeces due to upper gastrointestinal blood loss colour due to altered blood. (Courtesy H.L. DuPont.)

## 1–3% of patients with enteric fever become chronic carriers

Patients usually continue to excrete *S. typhi* in the faeces for several weeks after recovery, and 1–3% become chronic carriers, which is defined as *S. typhi* excretion in faeces or urine for 1 year after infection. Chronic carriage is more common in women, in older patients and in those with underlying disease of the gallbladder (e.g. stones) or urinary bladder (e.g. schistosomiasis).

## Diagnosis of enteric fever depends on isolating *S. typhi* or paratyphi types using selective media

Diagnosis cannot be made on clinical grounds alone, although the presence of rose spots in a febrile patient is highly suggestive. Samples of blood and faeces/rectal swab should be cultured on selective media. Two sets of blood cultures and three faecal samples are collected at different times. *Salmonella* serotyping is a phenotypic subtyping method and is still used for screening positive cultures in many laboratories. Specific Salmonella antisera are used to agglutinate the somatic O and flagellar H antigens of the isolate, which is then classified using the Kauffman–White–LeMinor scheme. Other laboratories use matrix-assisted laser desorption-ionization time-of-flight mass spectrometry, which is a faster method for bacterial identification with a high sensitivity and specificity. Whole genome sequencing will be carried out in reference laboratories.

Laboratories once used the Widal test, an agglutination test that detected an antibody response to infection, but nonspecific cross-reaction with other enterobacteria may also cause an increase in H and O antibody levels. Interpretation of the results was complicated and depended on knowing the normal antibody titres in the population and whether the patient had been vaccinated.

## Antibiotic treatment should be started as soon as enteric fever is diagnosed

In the United Kingdom, a 7-day course of oral azithromycin treatment is given unless the infection is complicated and intravenous ceftriaxone would be used. For returning travellers to the United Kingdom from South Asia, ciprofloxacin would not be used before the antibiotic susceptibility is known as most will have a resistant infection. If shown to be sensitive to ciprofloxacin, the antibiotic can be changed if necessary. XDR *S. typhi* or *S. paratyphi* infections have been reported in Pakistan since 2016. Azithromycin or meropenem would be the antibiotics of choice in XDR infection.

Some antibiotics appear active in vitro but do not achieve a clinical cure presumably because they do not reach the bacteria in their intracellular location.

## Prevention of enteric fever involves public health measures, treating carriers and vaccination

Breaking the chain of spread of infection from person to person depends upon good personal hygiene, adequate sewage disposal and a clean water supply. These conditions exist in the resource-rich world where outbreaks of enteric fever are rare but still occur.

Typhoid carriers are a public health concern and should be excluded from employment involving food handling. Every effort should be made to eradicate carriage by antibiotic treatment; if this is unsuccessful, removal of the gallbladder (the most common site of carriage) should be considered.

A single-dose injectable vaccine (Typhim Vi), which contains capsular polysaccharide antigen, and an oral live attenuated vaccine (strain Ty21a) are available and recommended for travellers to resource-poor countries. However, with both vaccines there is complete protection in only 50–80% of recipients.

## Listeriosis

### *Listeria* infection is associated with pregnancy and reduced immunity

*Listeria monocytogenes* is a gram-positive coccobacillus that is widespread among animals and in the environment. It is a foodborne pathogen associated particularly with uncooked foods such as pâté, contaminated milk, soft cheeses and coleslaw. Studies involving unpasteurized milk suggest that <1000 organisms may cause disease, and the ability of the organism to multiply, albeit slowly, at refrigeration temperatures allows an infective dose to accumulate in goods stored in this way. Even then, the population at risk primarily appears to be:

- pregnant women with the possibility of infection of the baby in the uterus or during birth
- immunocompromised individuals, including those with cancer or AIDS or those taking immunosuppressive drugs
- elderly individuals.

The disease usually presents as meningitis (see Ch. 25).

### Parasitic infections affecting the liver

Few protozoa affect the liver. Some worms live there as adults and others migrate through the liver to reach other locations.

### Inflammatory responses to the eggs of *S. mansoni* result in severe liver damage

Liver pathology in parasitic infections is most severe in *S. mansoni* infection. Although the worms spend only a relatively short time in the liver before moving to the mesenteric vessels, eggs released by the females can be swept by the bloodstream into the hepatic portal circulation and be filtered out in the hepatic sinusoids. The inflammatory response to these trapped eggs is the primary cause of the complex changes that result in hepatomegaly, pipe-stem fibrosis, portal hypertension and the formation of oesophageal varices (Fig. 23.45).

Whereas schistosomiasis is widespread in tropical and subtropical regions, other parasitic infections affecting the liver are more restricted in their distribution (e.g. clonorchiasis and alveolar echinococcosis [alveolar hydatid disease]).

In Asia, infections with the human liver fluke *Clonorchis sinensis* are acquired by eating freshwater fish infected with the metacercarial stage. Juvenile flukes released in the intestine move up the bile duct and attach to the duct epithelium where they are capable of living for 20 years, feeding on the cells, blood and tissue fluids. In heavy infections there is a pronounced inflammatory response, with proliferation and hyperplasia of the biliary epithelium. Cholangitis, jaundice and liver enlargement are possible consequences, but many people are asymptomatic in the early stages or experience

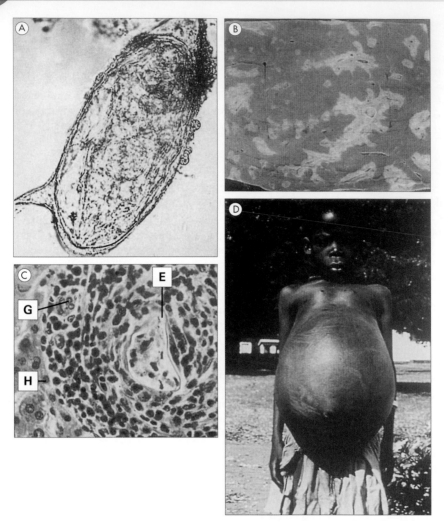

**Fig. 23.45** The portal fibrosis of *Schistosoma mansoni* is the end result of large numbers of granulomas formed around worm eggs deposited in the liver. In the related *S. haematobium* infection, a similar process occurs in the wall of the bladder. (A) Egg of *S. mansoni* (× 400). (B) Pipe-stem fibrosis in the liver as a result of coalescent calcified granulomas. (C) Cellular reaction around an egg in the liver. *E*, Egg containing miracidium; *G*, giant cell; *H*, hepatic cell. (D) Advanced clinical schistosomiasis with massive hepatosplenomegaly and ascites due to portal obstruction. (A–C, Courtesy R. Muller; D, courtesy G. Webbe.)

nonspecific symptoms. Chronic infection with *C. sinensis* or *Opisthorchis viverrini* is a recognized cause of intrahepatic cholangiocarcinoma, and *C. sinensis* is classified as a group 1 biocarcinogen.

A number of animal liver flukes can also establish themselves in humans. These include species of *Opisthorchis* (in Asia and Eastern Europe) and the common liver fluke *Fasciola hepatica*. In general, the symptoms associated with these infections are similar to those described for *C. sinensis*.

The larval stages of the dog tapeworm *Echinococcus granulosus* can develop in humans when the eggs are swallowed. Larvae from the eggs move from the intestine into the portal circulation and develop into large cysts (cystic echinococcosis, previously termed cystic hydatid disease). They are found in the liver in around two-thirds of cases, in the lungs in 20–30% and occasionally other organs. They can be seen on ultrasound or cross-sectional imaging as large cysts. Apart from pressure damage to surrounding tissues, rupture of the cysts leads to secondary spread and may cause anaphylaxis. Treatment strategy is determined by cyst size, site and type. Options include treatment with

benzimidazole drugs alone (usually albendazole or mebendazole) for small unilocular cysts, percutaneous aspiration injection and reaspiration (PAIR) plus a benzimidazole drug for larger unilocular cysts and open operation plus a benzimidazole drug for large cysts with daughter cysts. *E. multilocularis*, acquired from eggs passed by wild carnivores, usually foxes, behaves very differently and develops in the liver not as cysts but as a ramifying mass resembling a carcinoma (alveolar echinococcosis). *E. multilocularis* is treated by radical excision plus benzimidazole therapy. Inoperable cysts require lifelong drug therapy. Liver transplantation is sometimes used.

Other parasitic infections associated with liver pathology are malaria, leishmaniasis, ascariasis and extraintestinal amoebiasis, which causes liver abscesses.

### Liver abscesses

**Despite the name, an amoebic liver abscess does not consist of pus**

*E. histolytica* can move from the gastrointestinal tract and cause disease in other sites, including the liver (see earlier).

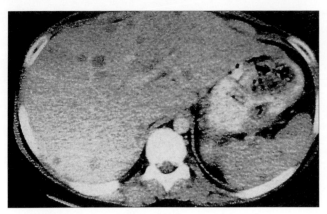

**Fig. 23.46** Multiple pyogenic liver abscesses due to *Pseudomonas aeruginosa*. (Courtesy N. Holland.)

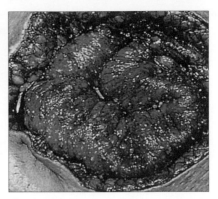

**Fig. 23.47** Tuberculous peritonitis. Oedematous bowel with multiple lesions on the peritoneal surface. (Courtesy M. Goldman.)

However, the term amoebic liver abscess is not strictly accurate because the lesion formed in the liver consists of necrotic liver tissue rather than pus. True liver abscesses (walled-off lesions containing organisms and dead or dying polymorphs [pus]) are frequently polymicrobial, containing a mixed flora of aerobic and anaerobic bacteria (Fig. 23.46). Lesions caused by both types of hydatid disease can become secondarily infected with bacteria. The source of infection may be local to the lesion or another body site but is usually undiagnosed. Antibacterial therapy is required to cover both aerobes and anaerobes.

## Biliary tract infections

### Infection is a common complication of biliary tract disease

Although infection is not often the primary cause of disease in the biliary tract, it is a common complication. Many patients with gallstones obstructing the biliary system develop infective complications caused by organisms from the normal gastrointestinal flora such as enterobacteria and anaerobes. Local infection can result in cholangitis and subsequent liver abscesses or invade the bloodstream to cause septicaemia and generalized infection. Removing the underlying obstruction in the biliary tree is a prerequisite to successful therapy. Antibacterial therapy is usually broad spectrum, covering both aerobes and anaerobes.

## Peritonitis and intraabdominal sepsis

The peritoneal cavity is normally sterile but is in constant danger of becoming contaminated by bacteria discharged through perforations in the gut wall arising from trauma (accidental or surgical) or infection. The outcome of peritoneal contamination depends upon the volume of the inoculum (1 mL of gut contents contains many millions of microorganisms) and the ability of the local defences to wall off and destroy the microorganisms.

### Peritonitis is generally classified as primary (without apparent source of infection) or secondary (e.g. due to perforated appendicitis, ulcer, colon)

Peritonitis usually begins as an acute inflammation in the abdomen, which may progress to the formation of localized intraabdominal abscesses. In general, the aetiologic agents responsible for primary and secondary peritonitis and intraperitoneal abscesses are different. Spontaneous bacterial peritonitis (SBP) is most commonly associated with cirrhosis of the liver. SBP is typically due to gram-negative enteric bacteria, most commonly *E. coli*. Secondary peritonitis and intraabdominal abscesses are often polymicrobial, especially involving the gram-negative anaerobe *Bacteroides fragilis*. *Mycobacterium tuberculosis* and *Actinomyces* can also cause intraperitoneal infection (Fig. 23.47). In the absence of appropriate antibiotic therapy, infections are frequently fatal, and even with appropriate treatment the mortality remains at 1–5%. Empiric antibiotic therapy for SBP commonly involves third-generation cephalosporins, such as ceftriaxone (see Ch. 34), with re-evaluation when culture results are available.

If a hospital-acquired infection and/or risk of an antibiotic-resistant organism occurs, then treatment options include piperacillin/tazobactam or carbapenem (e.g. meropenem). Vancomycin should be added if requiring wider action against gram-positive cocci.

Initial antimicrobial treatment of secondary peritonitis must especially target the gram-negative anaerobe *B. fragilis* (e.g. metronidazole) and gram-negative aerobic pathogens as well as taking steps to eliminate the source of contamination. Mycobacterial infection requires specific antituberculosis therapy (see Ch. 34), while actinomycosis responds well to prolonged treatment with penicillin.

## Viral hepatitis

### An alphabetic litany of viruses directly target the liver, from hepatitis A to E

Hepatitis means inflammation and damage to the liver and has differing aetiologies, including noninfectious multisystemic conditions and drug toxicity as well as infectious agents. The latter include viruses and less commonly bacteria (e.g. *Leptospira* spp.) and other microorganisms. There is a broad spectrum of clinical illness ranging from asymptomatic through symptomatic with malaise, anorexia, nausea, abdominal pain and jaundice, to acute life-threatening liver failure, which is rare.

Jaundice is a clinical term for the yellow tinge to the skin, sclera and mucous membranes. This is a result of liver cell damage, which means that the liver cannot transport bilirubin into the bile, causing increased bilirubin levels in the body fluids. More than half of the liver must be damaged or destroyed before liver function fails. Regeneration of liver cells is rapid, but fibrous repair, especially when infection

**Table 23.6** The main viruses causing hepatitis in humans

| Virus | Virus classification | Type of virus | Mode of infection | Incubation period | Other comments |
|---|---|---|---|---|---|
| Hepatitis A (HAV) | *Hepatovirus* | ssRNA | Faecal–oral | 2–4 weeks | No chronic infection |
| Hepatitis B (HBV) | *Hepadnavirus* | dsDNA | Bloodborne, sexual | 6 weeks–6 months | Chronic infection associated with liver cancer |
| Hepatitis C (HCV) | *Flavivirus* | ssRNA | Bloodborne | 2 months | Chronic infection associated with liver cancer |
| Hepatitis D (HDV) | *Deltavirus* | ssRNA | Bloodborne | 2–12 weeks | Needs concurrent HBV infection |
| Hepatitis E (HEV) | *Paslahepevirus* | ssRNA | Faecal–oral | 2–6 weeks | Sporadic infection, large outbreaks in Asia, foodborne, can cause persistent infection in immunosuppressed individuals |
| Yellow fever | *Flavivirus* | ssRNA | Mosquito | 3–6 days | No person-to-person spread, no chronic infection |

Other viruses causing hepatitis include Epstein-Barr virus (mild hepatitis in 15% of infected adults and adolescents), cytomegalovirus (CMV), adenovirus and rarely herpes simplex virus, while intrauterine infection with rubella or CMV causes hepatitis in the newborn. ds, Double-stranded; ss, single-stranded.

persists, can lead to permanent damage called cirrhosis. Cirrhosis results in a small, shrunken liver with poor function.

At least six different viruses are referred to as hepatitis viruses (Table 23.6), and generally they cannot be distinguished clinically. However, hepatitis A and E viruses (HAVs and HEVs) are transmitted by the faecal–oral route and generally do not result in a chronic infection; both resolve, although chronic HEV infection can occur in immunocompromised individuals. In contrast, hepatitis B, D (delta) and C are transmitted by similar routes involving blood-contaminated equipment, although sexual transmission of hepatitis B is much more common than in hepatitis C, and all can lead to chronic infection.

Some agents have been reported that were thought to be involved in the spectrum of what is referred to as non-A–E hepatitis. However, there is no evidence that the GB, hepatitis G and TT viruses infect the liver directly, the liver being affected as a bystander. Other viruses also cause hepatitis as part of a disease syndrome and are dealt with in other chapters.

Dramatic elevations of serum aminotransferase concentration (i.e. alanine aminotransferase [ALT], aspartate aminotransferase [AST]) are characteristic of acute viral hepatitis. Specific laboratory tests to make the serologic diagnosis of hepatitis A–E virus infections are available, as are PCR tests to detect and quantify the hepatitis B, C and E virus load in those with chronic infections. With the exception of hepatitis A and B there are no licensed vaccines, and specific antiviral treatments with and without immunomodulators are available for hepatitis B, C and E.

## Hepatitis A

This infection is caused by hepatitis A virus (HAV), a single-stranded unenveloped RNA virus that has its own genus *Hepatovirus* in the *Picornaviridae* family. There is only one serotype despite the identification of five genotypes of which genotypes I, II and III infect humans, and the virus is endemic worldwide infecting an estimated 1.5 million people annually.

### HAV is transmitted by the faecal–oral route

Virus is excreted in large amounts in faeces ($10^8$ infectious doses per gram) and spreads from person to person by the faecal–oral route involving close contact (poor hand hygiene), by sexual contact (men who have sex with men) or by contamination of food or water. Being unenveloped, it is a hardy, robust virus that can withstand temperature extremes and acidity in the stomach. The incubation period is 3–5 weeks, with a mean of 4 weeks; virus is present in faeces 1–2 weeks before symptoms appear and during the first week (sometimes also the second and third week) of the illness. Person-to-person transmission can lead to outbreaks in places such as schools and camps, and viral contamination of water or food is a common source of infection (Fig. 23.48). In resource-poor countries, up to 90% of children have been infected by 5 years of age, whereas in resource-rich countries up to 20% of young adults have been infected. The latter figure used to be higher but is mostly a result of improved sanitation and less overcrowding.

### Clinically, hepatitis A is milder in young children than in older children and adults

After infection, the virus enters the blood from the gastrointestinal tract, where it may replicate. It then infects liver cells, passing into the biliary tract to reach the intestine and appears in faeces (Fig. 23.49). Relatively small amounts of virus enter the blood at this stage. Events during the rather lengthy incubation period are poorly understood, but liver cells are damaged, and this is thought to be due to direct viral action. Common clinical manifestations are fever, anorexia, nausea and vomiting; jaundice is more common in adults. HAV does not cause chronic infection and rarely causes extrahepatic manifestations.

The best laboratory method for the diagnosis of an acute infection is to detect HAV IgM in serum, but a careful history must be taken as this may also be detected postimmunization. HAV RNA detection can be used to confirm infection if there is a doubt about the diagnosis and sequencing carried out as part of surveillance as well as phylogenetic analysis in an outbreak.

Pooled human normal immunoglobulin (HNIG) is no longer the mainstay of protecting contacts, having been replaced by vaccine. HNIG contains antibody to HAV and

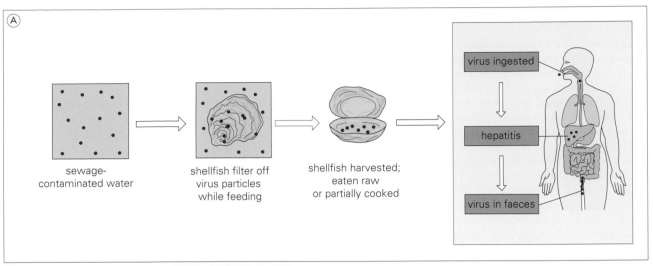

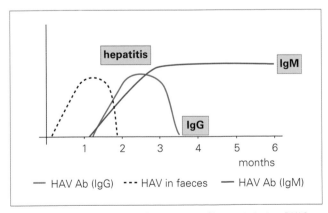

**Fig. 23.48** (A) Contamination of shellfish by hepatitis A virus (HAV) can lead to human infection. (B) HAV in a faeces sample from a patient with acute HAV infection. Electron micrograph (× 170 000). (From Zuckerman AJ, Banatvala JE, Pattison JR. Principles and practice of clinical virology. Chichester, UK: John Wiley & Sons; 1987.)

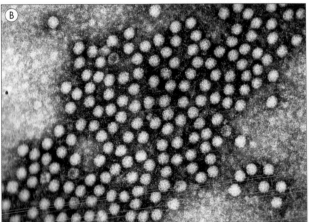

**Fig. 23.49** The clinical and virologic course of hepatitis A virus (HAV). Ab, Antibody; Ig, immunoglobulin.

will prevent or attenuate infection if given as pre- or post-exposure prophylaxis. It is used in exposed immunocompromised individuals less able to mount a response to vaccine and in babies <1 year old where maternal antibody may affect their response and those allergic.

There is no antiviral therapy, but there is interest in developing these to treat severe infections. Effective inactivated

hepatitis A vaccines have been available since the 1990s and are part of a prevention strategy. Groups at particular risk of infection include travellers to HAV endemic countries, sewage workers, child day care centre staff, institutional care workers, men who have sex with men, injecting drug users, and individuals with chronic liver disease and those with haemophilia. The vaccine is used alone or together with HNIG in certain situations, mostly if the contact is immunosuppressed, in the postexposure setting providing it can be given to contacts within 14 days of the onset of jaundice in the infected individual. If the exposure was 2–4 weeks previously, HNIG may be offered alone to contacts at risk of severe complications such as those with chronic liver disease.

## Hepatitis E

Hepatitis E virus (HEV) is an unenveloped single-stranded RNA virus that shares similarities with the caliciviruses. It has been classified in the genus *Paslahepevirus* in the family *Hepeviridae*, with eight genotypes, of which HEV-1 to HEV-4 and HEV-7 infect humans and one serotype. It has been estimated that there are ~20 million HEV infections annually worldwide.

### HEV spreads mainly by the faecal–oral route and is a zoonosis

Genotypes 1 and 2 have been involved in large outbreaks in resource-poor countries, transmitted between humans via the faecal–oral route. Genotypes 3 and 4, detected mainly in Europe and North America, infect humans and other animals in both resource-rich and -poor settings and are zoonoses. The virus is excreted in faeces and spreads by the faecal–oral route. It is the major cause of sporadic, up to 60%, as well as epidemic hepatitis in Asia, in the latter due to waterborne routes of transmission. In Europe, highest prevalence has been reported in the Netherlands, France and Germany. In addition, there are increasingly identified sporadic infections in resource-rich countries.

HEV has been identified in a variety of animals, especially pigs, rabbits, wild boar, chickens and sika deer, and they constitute a reservoir for infection. Pigs are the major animal reservoir, and they are asymptomatic. Zoonotic transmission is mainly due to eating undercooked pork or game meat, although direct contact with infected animals may be important as vets and swine handlers are more likely to have serologic evidence of infection compared with the general population. HEV RNA has also been detected in seafood as well as untreated water. Reports of blood transfusion–transmitted HEV infections in the United Kingdom in 2014 resulted in providing HEV RNA-screened negative blood products to transplant recipients as well as advice on cooking pork and pork products properly. HEV RNA had been detected in 1 in 2848 blood donations collected in South East England and 42% of the recipients who could be followed up had been infected.

### HEV can cause chronic hepatitis in immunocompromised individuals

The incubation period is 2–9 weeks, with a mean of 6 weeks, and the acute infection is usually self-limiting and mild, lasting a few weeks. The diagnosis is made using serologic tests to detect HEV IgM, and confirmation can be carried out by HEV RNA testing.

HEV infection may be severe in pregnant women, with a high mortality of ~20% during the third trimester in endemic countries due to fulminant hepatitis. Chronic HEV infection is well reported in immunosuppressed individuals, including transplant recipients and those receiving immunomodulators. Rapid development of cirrhosis can occur. These patients are monitored by carrying out blood and faecal HEV RNA load tests. If detected, the aim is to clear the infection by reducing the immunosuppressive treatment where possible, in conjunction with antiviral treatment using ribavirin or the immunomodulator drug pegylated interferon alpha (IFNα) unless contraindicated. Other antiviral drugs are under investigation, together with immunotherapies.

### HEV infection can lead to extrahepatic manifestations

HEV multiplies in hepatic tissue as well as in the brain, kidney and spleen and, together with cross-reactive immunologic responses, can lead to extrahepatic manifestations. These include neurologic conditions such as GBS, neuralgic amyotrophy, encephalitis and myelitis; kidney injury includes membranoproliferative glomerulonephritis, and haematologic disorders include anaemia and thrombocytopaenia.

### Prevention is the main focus as vaccine development continues

Exposure to HEV can be reduced by ensuring the quality of the water supply, appropriate disposal of human waste, cooking meat thoroughly and maintaining standard hygiene practices.

A number of HEV vaccines have been developed targeting the open reading frame 2 (ORF2) structural capsid protein and are in preclinical trials. A recombinant ORF2-based vaccine has been licensed in China but is not yet available elsewhere.

## Hepatitis B

Hepatitis B virus (HBV) is a member of the *Hepadnaviridae* family (Box 23.3), and it has been estimated that >2 billion people have been exposed to HBV, of whom nearly 300 million have a chronic infection. The prevalence of chronic HBV infection is estimated to be up to 0.5% in North, West and Central Europe, North America and Australia; up to 0.7% in East Europe, the Mediterranean littoral, Central and South America, Russia and Southwest Asia; up to 20% in South East Asia, sub-Saharan Africa and China. In countries where infant and childhood infection is common (possibly because more mothers have a chronic infection), overall rates are higher.

The global annual mortality is ~800 000 due to the complications of chronic infection that include cirrhosis and liver cancer. Liver cancer is the sixth most common tumour worldwide, and the most common risk factor is chronic hepatitis B and C viral infections. WHO targeted 2030 as the year when new HBV infections would have been reduced by 90% and deaths by 65% compared with 2015, but by 2023 only 1 in 10 countries were on track (Table 23.7). This is despite the effective hepatitis B vaccines that have been available for 4 decades.

HBV is enveloped and contains a partially double-stranded circular DNA genome and three principal antigens: HB surface antigen, HB core antigen and HBe antigen (Fig. 23.50; Table 23.8). HBe antigen is a soluble component secreted by the virus core, is expressed on the hepatocyte surface and seems to modulate the host immune system.

Infection with a given strain of HBV confers resistance to all strains, but antigenic variation occurs. The four classical serologic subtypes all of which include the immunogenic *a* determinant (*adw, adr, ayw* and *ayr*) have been superseded by the genotypic classification in which eight genotypes A–H have been determined. These can influence the clinical outcome of infection and response to antiviral treatment and are useful in epidemiologic studies.

### HB surface antigen can be found in blood and other body fluids

HBV can be transmitted by various routes, including:

- sexual intercourse
- vertically from mother to child: intrauterine, perinatal and postnatal infection
- via blood and blood products, blood-contaminated needles and equipment that may be used by injecting drug users
- in association with tattooing, body piercing and acupuncture, again due to reusing needles that may be contaminated by blood.

## Box 23.3  Lessons in Microbiology

### Hepatitis A

In August 1988 the Florida Department of Health and Rehabilitation Services traced 61 people who had suffered serologically confirmed infection with HAV. These individuals resided in five different states, but 59 of them had eaten raw oysters from the same growing areas in Bay County coastal waters. The oysters had been gathered illegally from outside the approved harvesting areas and were contaminated with HAV. The mean incubation period of the disease was 29 days (range 16–48 days). Probable sources of faecal contamination near the oyster beds included boats with inappropriate sewage disposal systems and discharge from a local sewage treatment plant that contained a high concentration of faecal coliforms.

### Hepatitis B

One of the largest outbreaks of hepatitis B virus infections in Europe occurred in London in 1998. A patient went to an alternative medicine clinic and was treated with a technique called autohaemotherapy. This involved mixing a small sample of the patient's blood with saline, then injecting the blood and saline mixture into her buttocks or acupuncture points. She subsequently developed acute hepatitis B, and the public health doctors were contacted and an investigation started having identified the practices in the clinic that could have resulted in her becoming jaundiced.

A lookback exercise was carried out involving 352 patients who had attended the clinic between January 1997 and February 1998 and four staff. Evidence of

exposure to hepatitis B was found in samples from 57 (16%) of this group. Hepatitis B surface antigen (HBsAg) was detected in blood samples collected from 33 patients and staff, 23 of whom had acute hepatitis B. Molecular analysis revealed that 30 (91%) samples had identical nucleotide sequences and were part of a large community outbreak of hepatitis B. Five patients had chronic hepatitis B infections, one of whom was the likely source of infection, with the vehicle being the contaminated saline in a vial that was used to mix the blood on a number of occasions for the other patients involved in the outbreak.

This demonstrated once again that only single-use vials must be used in healthcare settings, together with the benefits in those countries that offer universal immunization against hepatitis B to their populations.

### Hepadnaviruses

Hepadnaviruses are also found in woodchucks, ground squirrels and Peking ducks. In each case, the infection persists in the body, with HBsAg-like particles in the blood and chronic hepatitis and liver cancer as sequelae. These viruses often infect nonhepatic cells. In North East United States, for instance, 30% of woodchucks carry their own type of hepadnavirus and most develop liver cancer by later life. The virus replicates not only in liver cells but also in lymphoid cells in the spleen, peripheral blood and thymus and in pancreatic acinar cells and bile duct epithelium.

**Table 23.7** WHO Global Health Sector Strategy for hepatitis B for the period 2022–2030

|  | Baseline 2020 | Target 2025 | Target 2030 |
|---|---|---|---|
| HBsAg prevalence among children 0–4 years old | 0.94% | 0.5% | 0.1% |
| Number of new hepatitis B virus infections per year | 1.5 million 20/100 000 | 850 000 11/100 000 | 170 000 2/100 000 |
| Number deaths from hepatitis B per year | 820 000 10/100 000 | 530 000 7/100 000 | 310 000 4/100 000 |

HBsAg, Hepatitis B surface antigen. Modified from World Health Organization (WHO). Global progress report on HIV, viral hepatitis and sexually transmitted infections, 2021. Geneva, Switzerland: Author; 2021.

Transmission has been reported in healthcare settings such as renal units and has been associated with blood-contaminated haemodialysis equipment. This has been reduced dramatically since the introduction of regular hepatitis B surface antigen (HBsAg) monitoring of patients and disposable dialysis cartridges. In addition, incidents have been reported involving HBV transmission from hepatitis B carrier healthcare workers (HCWs) to their patients while carrying out exposure-prone procedures, such as cardiothoracic surgery, from intraoperative needlestick injuries resulting in blood-to-blood contact. Hepatitis B immunization and HBsAg screening of HCWs reduces the incidence of these transmission events. Blood and organ donors are also screened for HBsAg and HB core antibody in many countries worldwide, reducing the potential for transmission to recipients.

### HBV is not directly cytopathic for liver cells, and liver damage is largely immune mediated

After entering the body, the virus reaches the blood, then the liver, where the result is inflammation and necrosis. Much of the pathology is immune mediated, as infected liver cells are attacked by virus-specific cytotoxic T cells. The incubation period ranges from 6 weeks to 6 months, the median being 2.5 months.

### Complex interplay between molecular and immune mechanisms underpin infection and disease

People with a more vigorous immune response to the infection clear the virus more rapidly but tend to suffer a more severe illness. However, ~10% of infected adults fail to eliminate the virus from the body and become chronically infected; they are referred to as carriers. The HBV viraemia

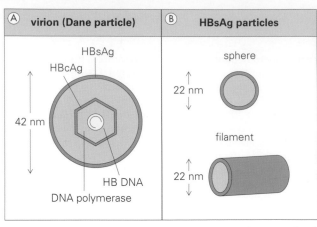

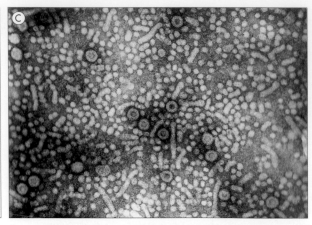

**Fig. 23.50** During acute infection, and in some carriers, there are $10^6$–$10^7$ infectious (Dane) particles per milliliter of serum (A), and as many as $10^{12}$ hepatitis B surface antigen (HBsAg), hepatitis B core antigen (HBcAg) particles per milliliter (B). (C) Electron micrograph showing Dane particles and HBsAg particles. (From Zuckerman AJ, Banatvala JE, Pattison JR. Principles and practice of clinical virology. Chichester, UK: John Wiley & Sons; 1987.)

**Table 23.8** Characteristics of hepatitis B virus (HBV) antigens (Ag) and antibodies (Ab)

| | |
|---|---|
| HBsAg | Envelope (surface) antigen of HBV particle also occurs as free particles (spheres and filaments) in blood; indicates infectivity of blood |
| HBsAb | Antibody to HBsAg; posthepatitis B vaccine response; appears late after resolved HBV infection (not in carriers) |
| HBcAb (total) | Antibody to hepatitis B core antigen; appears early; includes HB core IgM |
| HBc IgM | Appears in acute HBV infection; can last for 3 months and is a marker of acute HBV infection if it has resolved; seen in HBeAg-positive carriers with high viral replication; seen in HBeAg HBeAb reversion |
| HBeAg | Antigen derived from HBV core; indicates high transmissibility |
| HBeAb | Antibody to the HBV core |

HBsAg, Hepatitis B surface antigen; HBsAb, Hepatitis B surface antibody; HBcAb, Hepatitis B core antibody; HBc IgM, Hepatitis B core IgM; HBeAg, Hepatitis B e antigen; HBeAb, Hepatitis B e antibody.

means the person is infectious often for life, but sometimes spontaneous clearance occurs. Although continuing liver damage can cause chronic hepatitis, the damage may be minimal, and the carrier remains in good health. In general, after chronic infection is established, there can be clinical variation moving through the immune-tolerant, immune-active and inactive phases. The phases, defined by HBV DNA viraemia, HBe antigen and ALT levels, differ in the levels of viral replication and amount of infected hepatocyte damage due to the immune response.

The first phase, immune-tolerant is characterised by very high levels of HBV replication, HBV DNA, HBsAg and HBeAg levels are high, with persistently normal ALT levels and little to no inflammatory activity. Due to the latter, hepatologists in different countries refer to the phases in different ways. In Europe, immune-tolerant phase is referred to as HBeAg-positive chronic HBV infection, but as normal ALT levels do not exclude inflammation and fibrosis, the cut-off levels for raised ALT were adjusted in different countries.

The same is true for HBV DNA levels defining the phases, and appropriate cutoffs of the ALT and HBV DNA levels used to predict prognosis and treatment recommendations are still being evaluated.

The second phase is the immune-active, or HBeAg-positive immune-active, phase. The HBV DNA level remains high but may fluctuate. High ALT suggests liver inflammation and can be associated with liver damage, and antiviral therapy is recommended.

The third phase is the immune inactive phase, also called HBeAg-negative chronic HBV infection and low replicative phase. There is minimal intrahepatic inflammation and low HBV DNA levels with a normal ALT level. There is generally a good prognosis when remaining in this phase, but low-level persistent viraemia can be associated with liver disease progression and transition to the HBeAg-negative immune-active phase.

The fourth phase is the HBeAg-negative immune-active phase, previously known as the immune escape phase or reactivation phase. This phase consists of moderate to high levels of HBV DNA in conjunction with no HBeAg production due to mutations in the precore or core promoter regions. This is the HBV Trojan horse ploy as HBe antigen is a marker of high levels of replication, but despite these mutations resulting in no HBe antigen production there can still be high levels of HBV DNA replication as the mutations do not affect viral replication. Prolonged viral replication and liver inflammation seen in this phase can lead to liver cirrhosis and/or liver cancer.

Finally, phase 5 is the HBsAg-negative phase. HBsAg can clear spontaneously in ~0.5% of chronic infections annually. Although the risk of disease progression falls, liver cancer monitoring continues if it happens when patients are 40–50 years old (Fig. 23.51).

Certain groups of people are more or less likely to become carriers:

- Immunodeficient patients may have few if any symptoms due to the effect of reducing the host response to the infection but are more likely to become carriers.
- There is a marked age-related effect (e.g. in a study carried out in Taiwan, 90–95% of infants who were perinatally infected became carriers, compared with 23% of those infected at 1–3 years of age and only 3% of those infected as university students).

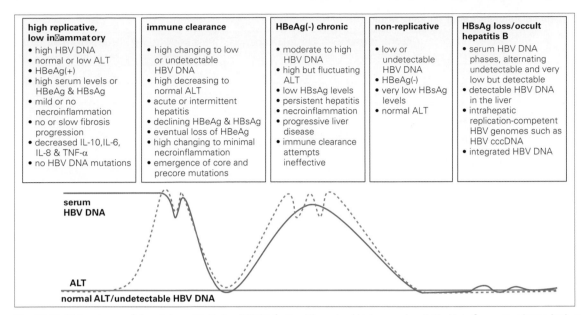

| high replicative, low inflammatory | immune clearance | HBeAg(-) chronic | non-replicative | HBsAg loss/occult hepatitis B |
|---|---|---|---|---|
| • high HBV DNA<br>• normal or low ALT<br>• HBeAg(+)<br>• high serum levels or HBeAg & HBsAg<br>• mild or no necroinflammation<br>• no or slow fibrosis progression<br>• decreased IL-10,IL-6, IL-8 & TNF-α<br>• no HBV DNA mutations | • high changing to low or undetectable HBV DNA<br>• high decreasing to normal ALT<br>• acute or intermittent hepatitis<br>• declining HBeAg & HBsAg<br>• eventual loss of HBeAg<br>• high changing to minimal necroinflammation<br>• emergence of core and precore mutations | • moderate to high HBV DNA<br>• high but fluctuating ALT<br>• low HBsAg levels<br>• persistent hepatitis<br>• necroinflammation<br>• progressive liver disease<br>• immune clearance attempts ineffective | • low or undetectable HBV DNA<br>• HBeAg(-)<br>• very low HBsAg levels<br>• normal ALT | • serum HBV DNA phases, alternating undetectable and very low but detectable<br>• detectable HBV DNA in the liver<br>• intrahepatic replication-competent HBV genomes such as HBV cccDNA<br>• integrated HBV DNA |

**Fig. 23.51** Major phases of chronic hepatitis B virus (HBV) infection. The natural history can be divided into five major phases: high-replicative, low-inflammatory; immune clearance; HBeAg(−) chronic hepatitis; nonreplicative; and hepatitis B surface antigen (HBsAg) loss/occult hepatitis. These phases do not occur in all patients, and transitions between them are dynamic and can be nonconsecutive. Ag, Antigen; ALT, alternating; IL, interleukin; TNF, tumour necrosis factor. (From Ghish RG, Given BD, Lai C-L., et al. Chronic hepatitis B; virology, natural history, current management and a glimpse at future opportunities. *Antivir Rcs.* 2015;121:47–58, fig 4.)

• Sex is another factor, with males being more likely to develop chronic infection.

### The HBV life cycle and host immune response to hepatocyte infection demonstrate the pathogen-host conflict

Viral entry starts with attachment to the hepatocyte surface, most likely followed by endocytosis. Once the virus is uncoated, the partially double-stranded relaxed circular (rc) DNA is released and transported to the nucleus. Host cellular enzymes repair the rcDNA to form the covalently closed circular (ccc) DNA. cccDNA is the template for all messenger RNA transcription that is, together with translation, controlled by viral promoters and enhancers. In the cytoplasm, core proteins self-assemble, become encapsidated, packaging the pregenomic RNA and viral polymerase to form the nucleocapsid. In the endoplasmic reticulum, the rcDNA containing capsids are then enveloped with the surface proteins and secreted from the infected cell as intact, infectious virions, known as Dane particles.

After this has occurred, the innate part of the immune response is involved early on and type III interferon, together with natural killer and Kupffer cell activation, can affect viral replication and viral spread. The adaptive side of the immune system involves the T cells, of which the CD8 T cells kill the hepatocytes expressing HB surface antigen epitopes on class I MHC. The CD4 component provides help.

Viral clearance and a resolved acute infection are the result of these responses together with the B-cell neutralising antibody activity. On the other hand, the interplay between viral factors and host immune response, in particular dysfunction of the innate and adaptive responses, can lead to chronic infection. This uncontrolled viral replication and buildup of unregulated inflammatory infiltrates lead to hepatocyte damage and tissue fibrosis.

These clinical outcomes have multifactorial causes, including age at infection, sex, ethnicity, host and viral genotype, other medical conditions including immunosuppression and coinfections.

### Complications of hepatitis B are cirrhosis and hepatocellular carcinoma

Complications of hepatitis B include:

• cirrhosis, as a result of chronic active hepatitis; this is an irreversible form of liver injury that may lead to primary hepatocellular carcinoma
• hepatocellular carcinoma, which is one of the 10 most common cancers worldwide. Hepatitis B carriers are 200 times more likely than noncarriers to develop liver cancer. This is not seen until 20–30 years after the infection. The cancer cells contain multiple integrated copies of HBV DNA (see Ch. 18).

### Serologic tests are used in the diagnosis of HBV infection

HBsAg appears in the serum during the incubation period in the form of infectious Dane particles, named after David Dane who detected the 42 nm virions by electron microscopy (Fig. 23.52). The characteristic serologic picture in an acute HBV infection includes the detection of HBsAg, HB core IgM and HBe antigen. If the acute infection leads to jaundice, the HBsAg concentration generally falls and finally disappears during recovery and convalescence. As HBsAg disappears, the HB core IgM level wanes over the next 3 months, HB core total antibody (IgM and IgG) is detected but is almost all IgG by this stage and HB surface antibody becomes detectable. Therefore evidence of past infection will give the following serologic profile (Table 23.9): HBsAg negative, HB core total antibody positive and HB surface antibody positive. HBV carriage is defined by detecting HBsAg in blood for 6 months after the acute infection. When HBe antigen is detected, there

**Table 23.9** Interpretation of hepatitis B virus serologic results

|  | Acute hepatitis B | Chronic hepatitis B infection | Chronic hepatitis B infection | Past hepatitis B virus infection[b] | Hepatitis B vaccine response |
|---|---|---|---|---|---|
| HBsAg[a] | + | + | + | − | − |
| HB core antibody (total) | + | + | + | + | − |
| HB core IgM | + | − | − | − | − |
| HBe antibody | − | + | − | + | − |
| HBe antigen | + | − | + | − | − |
| HB surface antibody | − | − | − | + | + |

[a]Always confirm by neutralization if positive.
[b]Or passively acquired antibody having received blood products from someone with a history of past hepatitis B virus (HBV) infection.

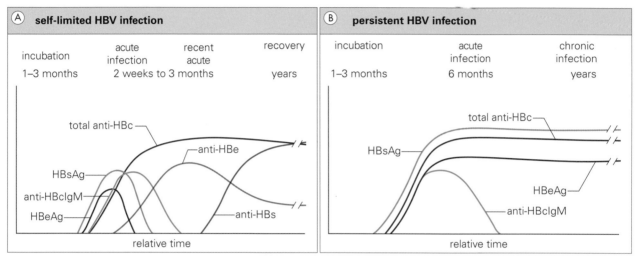

**Fig. 23.52** (A) Clinical and virologic course of hepatitis B virus (HBV) infection with recovery. (B) Clinical and virologic course in a carrier of hepatitis B. (From Farrar WE, Wood MJ, Innes JA, et al. *Infectious diseases*, ed 2, London: Mosby International; 1992.)

are large amounts of virus in the blood, and the carrier is of high infectivity; when it disappears, HBe antibody may become detectable. HBe antibody-positive carriers are of low infectivity; however, HBV DNA load is a more useful marker of infectivity as mutations have been detected in the region encoding the e antigen, which result in absence of e antigen production yet infectious virus is still assembled. Analagous to the famous Trojan horse, as mentioned previously, all seems normal, but that is not the case. They are known as precore mutant viruses. Therefore these patients will be HBe antigen negative and HBe antibody positive but could be highly infectious with high HBV DNA loads found in the blood.

### Treatment is guided by viral monitoring as well as HBV genotype and disease stage

The main aim of treatment is to prevent disease progression, the complications of which include cirrhosis and liver cancer, and improve survival. Suppressing HBV replication is the main endpoint, preferably with HBsAg loss.

The two treatment options for chronic hepatitis B by 2023 were a nucleos(t)ide analogue antiviral drug such as entecavir and tenofovir, where antiviral resistance is rare and pegylated IFNα. Other antivirals approved in Europe include lamivudine, adefovir and telbivudine, but they have a low barrier against resistance. Pegylated IFN may be used in mild or moderate chronic hepatitis B, leading to fixed-duration long-term immunologic control. Unfortunately

the response to treatment is variable, and there are a few adverse effects.

The decision to treat is guided by HBV DNA, HBsAg and HBeAg levels, disease activity, HBV genotype and disease stage.

Regular assessment is important, given the movement between phases, to assess whether treatment is required in a variety of settings. One of these, for example, is with individuals with HBeAg-positive infection and normal ALT over a long period. If their HBV DNA load is >20,000 IU/mL and ALT levels under 2 times the upper limit of normal, a liver biopsy is carried out to assess fibrosis and inflammation and treatment started if they are significant and moderate/severe, respectively. Noninvasive tests to investigate fibrosis include a FibroScan that uses ultrasound and an electric wave or vibration that, together, measure liver stiffness.

Individuals with inactive chronic HBV are assessed each year to see if HBsAg is still detectable in a blood sample. If HBsAg is negative and they have cirrhosis, the individuals are still regularly assessed for liver cancer.

### Tests include measuring HBV DNA load in blood, HBsAg quantification and genotype detection

- Serum HBV DNA load testing guides treatment.
- HBsAg quantitation can help in following the response to pegylated IFN treatment. This is an additional

biomarker, together with HBV RNA and HBV core-related antigen, that may be used as markers of cccDNA activity and therefore monitoring antiviral drug response, predicting relapse after stopping treatment or estimating liver cancer risk.

- HBV genotyping and subgenotyping are key guides to prognosis and treatment responses in specific settings. The 10 genotypes (A–J) can be found in varied global locations:
  - A is prevalent in Northern Europe, West and sub-Saharan Africa, United States
  - B and C in Asia
  - D in Europe, Africa, the Mediterranean and India
  - E in West and Central Africa
  - F in South America
  - G in the United States, France and Germany
  - H in the United States, Central and South America
  - I in Vietnam and Laos
  - J in the Ryuku islands in Japan

It is interesting that this genotype distribution may be influenced by route of exposure, migration and sociodemographic reasons.

With respect to pegylated IFN therapy, genotype A is associated with significantly higher rates of HBeAg and HBsAg loss, followed by individuals with B, C and D.

With regard to prognosis and clinical disease, genotype B is associated with HBeAg seroconversion at an earlier age, more sustained remission after HBeAg seroconversion, less active liver inflammation, a slower and lower rate of progression to cirrhosis and liver cancer compared with genotype C. HBeAg seroconversion occurs later, together with cirrhosis and liver cancer in genotype C. Furthermore, genotype A is more common in chronic hepatitis B and genotype D in those with acute hepatitis and acute liver failure.

Finally, antiviral resistance testing can help guide treatment in patients with past treatment experience and those in whom HBV DNA is detected on treatment.

A sustained virologic response (SVR) involves the absence of HBsAg and HBV DNA in the blood in individuals having stopped antiviral therapy, with the caveat that HBV DNA is integrated in the hepatocytes and can reactivate owing to immune senescence; as we get older the immune response also feels the years of active duty and immunosuppression.

The two classes of drugs used to treat HBV infections are pegylated IFN and nucleotide/nucleoside analogues (NAs) (see Ch. 34). There are differences in management of individuals with chronic hepatitis B in terms of the liver enzyme level criteria between American and European guidelines. Antiviral treatment approved in Europe includes lamivudine, adefovir, telbivudine, entecavir and two types of tenofovir. As the first three have a low and the last three a high barrier to resistance, the latter are more effective as development of antiviral resistance is rare.

NAs are also used to prevent HBV reactivation in immunocompromised individuals with past HBV infection.

Pegylated IFN is an option for those with mild to moderate chronic HBV and is given for a set time (48 weeks). The main disadvantages of pegylated IFNα treatment are the variable response and the adverse effects, but it can result in long-term immunologic control.

Other direct- and indirect-acting antiviral drugs targeting multiple stages of the viral life cycle and interfering with the host immune function, respectively, are being investigated.

### Hepatitis B infection can be prevented by immunization

The original vaccine was produced in 1981 and consisted of purified HBsAg, prepared from the plasma of carriers, which was chemically treated to kill any contaminating viruses. The current vaccine is genetically engineered HBsAg produced in yeast or mammalian cells. Three injections of vaccine over a 6-month period will lead to a response and protection in >90% of healthy adults. Immunization is recommended especially for those who may be exposed to blood or blood products, such as receiving multiple transfusions or dialysis patients, all HCWs, sexual contacts of individuals with acute or chronic hepatitis B and injecting drug users. One problem is that up to 10% of healthy individuals may not respond to the vaccine, even when reimmunised. This could be due to genetically determined defects in the immune repertoire or because of the induction of immune suppressor cells.

The global prevalence of HBV infections fell after the vaccine was introduced in 1982. The WHO global hepatitis report of 2017 revealed an estimate that 4.5 million HBV childhood infections were prevented annually. By December 2019, 50 of 53 countries in the WHO European Region provided routine universal hepatitis B immunization programmes to all 1–12-year-olds. In 23 of those countries the vaccine is offered at birth to newborns. Universal hepatitis B immunization programmes for newborns or babies are conducted worldwide in at least 187 countries.

After accidental exposure to infection, hepatitis B immunoglobulin can be used to provide immediate passive protection to unimmunised people. This is prepared from the serum of individuals with high titres of HB surface antibody. It may also be used together with hepatitis B vaccine to prevent transmission to babies born to mothers with chronic HBV and are highly infectious.

## Hepatitis C

### Hepatitis C virus was the most common cause of transfusion-associated non-A–non-B viral hepatitis in the 1970s and 1980s

Hepatitis C virus (HCV) was discovered in 1989 as the cause of 90–95% of cases of transfusion-associated non-A–non-B hepatitis. It is an enveloped single-stranded RNA virus in the *Hepacivirus* genus in the *Flaviviridae* family. The discovery of HCV was a tour de force in molecular virology. The viral RNA was extracted from blood, a complementary DNA (cDNA) clone was made and viral antigen produced. Serum from individuals with non-A–non-B hepatitis was then tested for the presence of antibody to the viral antigen. The introduction of first-generation HCV antibody-screening tests between 1990 and 1992 and subsequent improvement in sensitivity and specificity of these assays and genome detection methods have resulted in a massive reduction in transfusion-associated HCV infection. It is estimated that >177 million people worldwide are infected with HCV, ~58 million of whom have a chronic infection and ~1.5 million new infections occur annually. WHO targeted 2030 as the year when new HCV infections and HCV-related deaths would have been reduced by 80% and 65% compared with 2015 (Table 23.10). By 2020 only 9 of 45 high-income countries were on target. In 2019 ~290000 people had died from HCV-related cirrhosis or liver cancer.

**Table 23.10** WHO Global Health Sector Strategy for hepatitis C for the period 2022–2030

| | Baseline 2020 | Target 2025 | Target 2030 |
|---|---|---|---|
| Number of new hepatitis C infections per year | 1.575 million<br>20/100 000 | 1 million<br>13/100 000 | 350 000<br>5/100 000 |
| Number of new hepatitis C infections among persons who inject drugs per year | 8/100 | 3/100 | 2/100 |
| Number of people dying from hepatitis C per year | 290 000<br>5/100 000 | 240 000<br>3/100 000 | 140 000<br>2/100 000 |

Modified from World Health Organization (WHO). Global progress report on HIV, viral hepatitis and sexually transmitted infections, 2021. Geneva, Switzerland: Author; 2021.

## HCV transmission routes share similarities with hepatitis B

HCV is present in blood, and transmission routes include blood and blood products, blood-contaminated needles and equipment that may be used by injecting drug users. It is also associated with tattooing, body piercing and acupuncture, again due to reusing potentially blood-contaminated needles from other clients. Transmission has been reported in healthcare settings such as renal units because of contaminated dialysis equipment and other fomites, including gloves. Although the introduction of regular HCV monitoring of patients and disposable dialysis cartridges has helped in infection control, transmission has also occurred by other routes, probably often involving contaminated gloves worn by HCWs, which may not have been changed between patients. In addition, there have been incidents involving HCV transmission from HCV carrier HCWs carrying out exposure-prone procedures on their patients, such as intra-operative needlestick injuries resulting in blood-to-blood contact during cardiothoracic surgery. Unlike hepatitis B, HCV transmission is uncommon vertically, from mother to infant, and by sexual intercourse. There may be other methods of spread, as the route of transmission is unknown in up to 40% of infected individuals.

The HCV envelope binds to the hepatocyte cell surface membrane allowing viral entry through a number of host cell receptors. It involves a multistep entry process with host lipoproteins and viral envelope glycoproteins interacting together with host factors at the hepatocyte surface that include CD81, scavenger receptor class B type 1, claudin-1 and occludin. The latter act as viral receptors and interact with each other, making a complex that is key to viral internalization. Some of the HCV proteins interfere with the host response, and other evasive measures include the high degree of genetic diversity due to the high error rate of RNA replication.

By 2023, eight major HCV genotypes and ~90 subtypes had been identified. There is a global distribution, but genotypes 1, 3 and 4 are most common. Genotype 1 was most prevalent in high and upper/middle-income countries, 3 in lower/middle-income countries and 4 in low-income countries. Around 90% of HCV infections are genotypes 1, 2 and 3 in Europe, whereas in the Americas mostly genotype 1 is seen, and the rest are genotypes 2 and 3. Genotype 4 is found mostly in Northeast and Central Africa, and subtype 4a in Egypt particularly after syringe needles were reused during a schistosomiasis treatment national campaign. Genotype 6 is found mostly in East and Southeast Asia.

Genotype determination is predictive of antiviral therapy response. Viral and host factors affect the disease progression rate, with high HCV load in blood, genotype and the degree of viral heterogeneity referred to as the quasispecies, being associated with more rapid progression. Viral clearance is associated with both the development and persistence of strong HCV-specific cytotoxic T-cell and helper T-cell responses.

Being infected with one genotype does not protect against the others; therefore multiple infections are possible, making the production of a cross-protective vaccine more difficult.

### About 75–85% of HCV-infected individuals develop chronic HCV

The incubation period is 2–4 months, with a mean of 7 weeks. Subclinical infection is the rule, with ~25% of individuals developing jaundice in the acute infection, in contrast to the 90% seen in acute HBV infection. This makes the diagnosis of HCV infection more difficult as many individuals do not know they have been infected. Virus is often detectable in the blood after recovery from the acute illness, and carriers are a source of infection. Up to 2% of apparently healthy individuals in the United States have HCV antibody, and as a result between 2.7 and 3.9 million people have an active infection. About 75–85% of HCV-infected individuals will develop chronic HCV, and 10–15% will progress to cirrhosis within the first 20 years, with a resultant 1–4% risk per year of liver cancer in those with established cirrhosis. It is also a leading indication for liver transplantation. The rate of chronic HCV infection depends on the infected individual's age, gender, ethnicity and immune response.

Diagnostic tests for HCV infection involve serologic assays to detect HCV antibody or combined HCV antibody and antigen assays, qualitative and quantitative HCV RNA detection methods and genotype analysis. HCV RNA is present in ~70% of HCV antibody-positive individuals.

Assessing liver disease severity pretreatment involves noninvasive methods such as a FibroScan to determine liver stiffness, a measure of portal hypertension and liver fibrosis. There are biomarkers too, including the AST to platelet ratio index and fibrosis-4 index. Liver biopsy may be needed if there are comorbidities.

### Direct-acting antiviral agents revolutionized HCV treatment in a short time

The aim of treatment is a sustained virologic response (SVR), which means that HCV RNA cannot be detected at 3 or 6 months after completing a course of treatment (see Ch. 34). Beyond 6 months of monitoring having completed a treatment course, ~0.2% of individuals have a late relapse. In those with cirrhosis and having cleared the infection, there is still a risk of liver cancer.

It is worth just spending a moment to consider the brief history that rapidly changed the HCV treatment landscape.

Pegylated IFNα and ribavirin was the standard of care. Originally, IFNα monotherapy resulted in up to 40% initial response rates, but <20% were sustained responses. Treatment with pegylated IFNα in which polyethylene glycol is attached to IFN extended the half-life and duration of activity, and ribavirin resulted in an SVR in 45% of patients with genotype 1 or 4 infections (48-week treatment) with 80% of those with genotype 2 or 3 (24-week treatment).

Since 2011, after determining the crystal structure of the nonstructural (NS) protein domains, numerous direct-acting antiviral agents (DAAs), which were a new generation of drugs that interfered directly with specific viral proteins that are key for replication, and combinations of these agents were licensed. Targeting the viral NS3 protease and NS5 polymerase, the DAAs eradicated chronic HCV RNA viraemias within 8–24 weeks of starting oral treatment. But monotherapy led to viral breakthrough due to resistance-associated substitutions developing, and triple therapy regimens were introduced. Combining pegylated IFN and ribavirin with some DAAs improved the SVR rates in the more difficult to treat HCV infections.

Pharmaceutical companies have been competing with one another to come up with a more tongue-twisting drug name than previously. The NS3 protease inhibitor drugs started with the protease inhibitors telaprevir and boceprevir, replaced by simeprevir, asunaprevir and paritaprevir. The NS5A and B polymerase inhibitors included daclatasvir, elbasvir, ledipasvir, ombitasvir, sofosbuvir and velpatasvir. By January 2014, the HCV treatment field changed completely with sofosbuvir having a high barrier of resistance. Simeprevir and daclatasvir added options for treating those with genotype 1 and 3 infections. Then fixed-dose DAA combinations changed the landscape, with >95% SVR rates in individuals with genotype 1 infections. This was followed by pan-genotypic regimens, including sofosbuvir-velpatasvir where a 3-month course resulted in 99% SVR almost irrespective of genotype. By 2023 the further development of pan-genotypic HCV treatment included sofosbuvir-velpatasvir and glecaprevir-pibrentasvir as combinations for individuals without carrying out either HCV genotype or subtype. However, genotype and subtype identification before starting treatment is useful as some HCV subtypes can contain natural polymorphisms that result in NS5A inhibitor resistance and treatment failure. This is an evolving and complex topic, especially when considering chronic HCV infection in patients with cirrhosis and if being considered for liver transplantation, in relapses and recurrent infection.

In summary, HCV is another RNA virus that continuously evolves as a quasispecies. As a result, it has the advantage of evading host immune responses, the action of antivirals and makes vaccine development a massive challenge. The success of the pan-genotypic antiviral drugs, improving screening and treatment uptake programmes around the world and reducing new infections are all critical to achieve the aim to eliminate HCV infections.

## Hepatitis D (Delta)

### Hepatitis D virus can multiply only in a cell infected with HBV

Hepatitis D (HD) is caused by hepatitis D virus (HDV, or delta virus), which has the smallest genome among animal viruses, a circular, single-stranded RNA genome. It is the only member of the *Kolmioviridae* family, genus *Deltavirus*. It is a defective virus, so-named because it can successfully

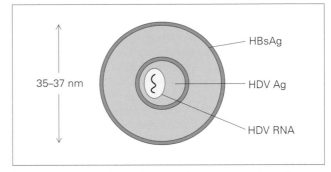

**Fig. 23.53** Structure of hepatitis D virus (HDV) in serum. Ag, Antigen.

multiply in a cell only when the cell is infected with HBV at the same time. When HDV buds from the surface of a liver cell it acquires an envelope consisting of HBsAg (Fig. 23.53). HDV needs the HBV capsid only to enter hepatocytes and once inside it replicates using host cell RNA polymerases.

### Spread of HDV is similar to that of HBV

Infected blood contains very large amounts of virus (up to $10^{10}$ infectious doses per milliliter in experimentally infected chimpanzees), and spread is similar to that of the other parenterally transmitted hepatitis viruses.

HDV infection may occur at the same time as an HBV infection, and the resulting disease is often more severe than with HBV alone. Moreover, HDV superinfection in someone with chronic HBV infection may occur, which may accelerate the course of the chronic hepatitis B–related liver disease, with higher rates of cirrhosis, liver cancer and mortality at a younger age. It was estimated that 15 million people globally had an HDV infection and 5% of HBV-infected individuals had an HDV coinfection. Over the last 2 decades, the epidemiology of HDV infection has changed owing to universal hepatitis B immunization and changes in immigration patterns from higher prevalence countries. These included the Mediterranean, Middle East, Pakistan, Central and North Asia and parts of Africa, South America and the Pacific region. In 2019 reports estimated a much higher worldwide prevalence of HDV/HBV coinfection exists at 62–72 million people. Suboptimal testing worldwide has also resulted in underestimating infection prevalence.

The diagnosis is made by serologic tests for HDV IgM and IgG as well as HD (delta) antigen and HDV RNA. HBsAg will also be present.

### Antiviral treatments are looking promising targeting entry, assembly and export

Antiviral treatment is limited by the fact that antivirals used to treat HBV infection have no effect on HDV, although pegylated IFNα was shown to be effective in small numbers of infected individuals in whom HDV RNA became negative and ALT became normal. However, >50% of these individuals had a late relapse having stopped treatment. IFNλ is a novel type 3 IFN being investigated, which binds to a unique receptor highly expressed on mostly hepatocytes and so has fewer side effects.

In 2020, bulevirtide was shown to reduce HDV load significantly. The drug is a virion entry inhibitor that stops HDV and HBV entering hepatocytes by blocking the bile acid transporter, sodium taurocholate cotransporting polypeptide, a transmembrane protein that is highly expressed in human hepatocytes. Clinical trials as monotherapy, with pegylated IFNα and NAs, reported promising results.

Prenylation is a posttranslational modification of HDAg required for it to interact with HBsAg, which is catalyzed by the cellular enzyme farnesyltransferase. This leads to delta virion assembly. Lonafarnib is a farnesyltransferase inhibitor that can inhibit HDV resulting in significant falls in HDV RNA levels.

Finally, nucleic acid polymers can stop HBsAg being secreted from hepatocytes and stop virion entry. These drugs could prevent HDV particles being exported.

There is no HDV-specific vaccine, but successful hepatitis B immunization prevents infection with hepatitis D.

## Viral hepatitis, the rest of the alphabet

After the discovery of HCV, a small percentage of hepatitis infections known to be transmitted by blood transfusion have yet to be attributed to a virus infection, although hepatitis G virus, referred to as GB virus C, transfusion-transmitted virus or Torque Teno virus (TTV) and SENV 25–28 have been detected in individuals with posttransfusion hepatitis. There are even more human hepatitis viruses waiting to be discovered.

## KEY FACTS

- Diarrhoeal disease is a major cause of morbidity and mortality in the resource-poor world. A wide range of diverse pathogens cause infections of the gastrointestinal tract. Diarrhoea, the most common symptom, ranges from mild and self-limiting to severe with consequent dehydration and death.

- Gastrointestinal pathogens are transmitted by the faecal–oral route. They may invade the gut, causing systemic disease (e.g. typhoid), or multiply and produce locally acting toxins and damage only the gastrointestinal tract (e.g. cholera). The number of organisms ingested and their virulence attributes are critical factors in determining whether infection becomes established.

- Microbiologic diagnosis is usually impossible without laboratory investigations, but the patient's history, including food and travel history, provides useful pointers.

- The major bacterial causes of diarrhoea are *E. coli*, salmonellae, *Campylobacter*, *V. cholerae* and shigellae. Other less common causes include *C. perfringens*, *B. cereus*, *V. parahaemolyticus* and *Y. enterocolitica*. Food poisoning (i.e. the ingestion of bacterial toxins in food) is caused by *S. aureus* and *C. botulinum*.

- *E. coli* is the major bacterial cause of diarrhoea in resource-poor countries and of traveller's diarrhoea. Distinct groups within the species (ETEC, EHEC, EPEC, EIEC) have different pathogenic mechanisms—some are invasive, others toxigenic.

- Salmonellae and *Campylobacter* are common in resource-rich countries, have large animal reservoirs and spread via the food chain. Both cause disease by multiplication in the gut and the production of locally acting toxins.

- *V. cholerae* and shigellae have no animal reservoirs, and the diseases are potentially eradicable. Transmission is prevented by good hygiene, clean drinking water and hygienic disposal of faeces. The pathogenesis of cholera depends upon production of cholera enterotoxin, which acts on the gastrointestinal mucosal cells. In contrast, *Shigella* invades the mucosa, causing ulceration and bloody diarrhoea, symptoms similar to those of amoebic dysentery.

- *H. pylori* is associated with gastritis and duodenal ulcers. Removal of the bacterium by combination treatment with antibiotics and PPIs reduces symptoms and encourages healing.

- Disruption of the normal bacterial flora of the gut (usually due to antibiotic treatment) allows organisms normally absent or present in small numbers (e.g. *C. difficile*) to multiply and cause antibiotic-associated diarrhoea.

- Although viruses appear to be the most common causes of gastroenteritis in infants and young children, viral gastroenteritis is not distinguishable clinically from other types of gastroenteritis. The chief culprits are norovirus and rotavirus infections, although rotavirus immunization programmes will reduce the incidence of infections.

- Ingestion of food or water contaminated with *S. typhi* or *S. paratyphi* types can result in the systemic infection enteric (typhoid) fever. These pathogens invade the gut mucosa and are ingested by and survive in macrophages. They are transported via the lymphatics to the bloodstream from whence they seed many organs and give the characteristic multisystem disease. Positive diagnosis depends upon culture of the organism. Specific antibiotic therapy is required, and specific prevention is achievable through immunization.

- Hepatitis is usually caused by viruses, especially hepatitis A–E viral infections. Hepatitis A and E are transmitted by the faecal–oral route and the rest by contaminated blood or the sexual route. Infection with HBV and HCV often leads to chronic hepatitis and can result in liver cancer. Antiviral treatments have been developed for both HBV and HCV, which are highly effective. In particular, the oral DAAs for treating HCV infection could potentially eliminate this infection with high SVR. Vaccines can prevent HAV and HBV infections.

- Many protozoa and worms live in the intestine, but relatively few cause severe diarrhoea. Important protozoa are *E. histolytica*, *G. intestinalis* and *Cryptosporidium*, which are acquired by ingestion of infective cysts in faecally contaminated food or water. Important worms are *Ascaris*, *Trichuris*, *Strongyloides* and hookworm. They have more complex routes of transmission, with the eggs or larvae requiring a development period outside the human host.

- Parasitic infections involving the liver include infections by *S. mansoni* in the tropics and subtropics, and *C. sinensis*, the human liver fluke, in Asia. Other parasitic infections with important liver pathology include malaria, leishmaniasis, extraintestinal amoebiasis, echinococcosis (hydatid disease) and ascariasis.

- Infection of the biliary tree is usually secondary to obstruction. The normal intestinal flora causes mixed infections, which may extend to produce liver abscesses and septicaemia.

- Peritonitis and intraabdominal sepsis follow contamination of the normally sterile abdominal cavity with intestinal pathogens. The presentation is acute, and infection can be fatal. Antibiotic therapy against both aerobic and anaerobic bacteria is essential.

# Obstetric and perinatal infections

# 24

## Introduction

During pregnancy a novel set of tissues potentially susceptible to infection appears, including the fetus, the placenta and the lactating mammary glands. The placenta acts as an effective barrier, protecting the fetus from most circulating microorganisms, and the fetal membranes shield the fetus from microorganisms in the genital tract. Perforation of the amniotic sac, for instance, at a late stage of pregnancy often results in fetal infection.

During pregnancy certain infections in the mother can be more severe than usual, including malaria and viral hepatitis, or latent viruses such as herpes simplex virus (HSV) and cytomegalovirus (CMV) can reactivate and infect the fetus, and after delivery the raw uterine tissue is susceptible to streptococcal and other pathogens, causing puerperal sepsis.

The fetus, once infected via the placenta, is highly susceptible but may survive certain pathogens and develop congenital abnormalities; examples include rubella, CMV, Zika virus, *Toxoplasma gondii* and *Treponema pallidum*. However, not all babies become infected after a maternal primary infection, and there is an important distinction between babies being infected and, as a result, affected. Bacteria from the vagina such as group B streptococci can cause neonatal septicaemia, meningitis and death, and a birth canal infected with *Neisseria gonorrhoeae* or *Chlamydia trachomatis* inoculates the infant to cause neonatal conjunctivitis. Maternal genital HSV infection can cause more serious neonatal disease and is underreported.

Maternal human immunodeficiency virus (HIV) infection in resource-poor countries or where maternal infection is undiagnosed can lead to 40% of infants infected, about one-third in utero, causing abortion, prematurity and low birth weight and two-thirds perinatally from maternal viraemia or milk. Maternal chronic hepatitis B virus (HBV) infection can be transmitted in utero as well as during delivery, and breast milk can be a source of human T-cell lymphotropic virus type 1 (HTLV-1) infection.

Here we describe infections that occur during pregnancy and around the time of birth, and we discuss their effects on the mother, the fetus and the neonate. Congenital infections are transmitted from mother to baby before or during pregnancy, perinatal infections occur during labour and delivery and postnatal infections can occur after receiving breast milk, for example.

The way in which the virus interacts with the maternal immune system, the maternal–fetal interface and the placenta explain these results and the differences that are observed from time to time in the fetal-neonatal outcomes of maternal infections. The maternal immune system undergoes functional adaptation during pregnancy, once thought as physiologic immunosuppression. This adaptation, crucial for generating a balance between maternal immunity and fetus, is necessary to promote and support the pregnancy itself and the growth of the fetus. When this adaptation is upset by the viral infection, the balance is broken, and the infection can spread and lead to the adverse outcomes previously described. In this review we will describe the main viral harmful infections in pregnancy and the potential mechanisms of the damages on the fetus and newborn.

## INFECTIONS OCCURRING IN PREGNANCY

### Immune and hormonal changes during pregnancy worsen or reactivate certain infections

The fetus may be considered as an immunologically incompatible implant that must not be rejected by the mother. Reasons for failure to reject the fetus include:

- the absence or low density of major histocompatibility complex antigens on placental cells
- a covering of antigens with blocking antibody
- subtle defects in the maternal immune responses.

A severe or generalized immunosuppression in the mother would be undesirable because it would mean potentially disastrous susceptibility to infectious disease. Certain infections, however, are known to be more severe (Table 24.1), and certain persistent infections reactivate during pregnancy. The hormonal changes that accompany pregnancy can also increase susceptibility. The picture is further complicated

**Table 24.1** The effect of pregnancy on the severity of infectious disease

| Infection | Comments |
|---|---|
| Malaria | ? Depressed cell-mediated immunity |
| Viral hepatitis | The viral load may fluctuate owing to immunomodulation in pregnancy |
| Influenza COVID-19 | Higher morbidity and mortality |
| Poliomyelitis | Paralysis more common |
| Urinary tract infection | Cystitis; pyelonephritis more common; atony of bladder and ureter leads to less-effective flushing, emptying |
| Candidiasis | Vulvovaginitis |
| Listeriosis | Influenza-like illness |
| Coccidioidomycosis | Leading cause of maternal mortality in endemic areas in southwest United States and Latin America |

when there is malnutrition, which in itself impairs host defences by weakening immune responses, decreasing metabolic reserves and interfering with the integrity of epithelial surfaces.

### The fetus has poor immune defences

Once the fetus is infected, it is exquisitely susceptible because:

- immunoglobulin M (IgM) and IgA antibodies are not produced in significant amounts until the second half of pregnancy
- there is no IgG antibody synthesis
- cell-mediated immune responses are poorly developed or absent, with inadequate production of the necessary cytokines.

Indeed, if the fetus were able to generate a vigorous response to maternal antigens, a troublesome 'graft-versus-host' reaction could be unleashed.

Most microorganisms have sufficient destructive activity to kill the fetus once it is infected, leading to spontaneous abortion or stillbirth. Here our interests focus on the few microorganisms that are capable of subtler, nonlethal effects. They overcome the placental barrier by infecting it so that the infection then spreads to the fetus. They can then interfere with fetal development or cause lesions so that a live but damaged baby is born.

## CONGENITAL INFECTIONS

### Intrauterine infection may result in death of the fetus or congenital malformations

After primary infection during pregnancy, certain microorganisms enter the blood, establish infection in the placenta, then invade the fetus. The fetus sometimes dies, leading to spontaneous abortion, but when the infection is less severe, as in the case of a relatively noncytopathic virus, or when it is partially controlled by the maternal IgG response, the fetus survives and there may be intrauterine growth retardation. The baby may then be born with a congenital infection, often showing malformations or other pathologic changes. The infant is generally small and fails to thrive. Virus-specific antibodies may be produced, but often, for instance with cytomegalovirus (CMV), the fetus fails to generate an adequate virus-specific cell-mediated immune response, remaining infected for a long period. Hence the lesions may progress after birth. It is a striking feature of these infections that they are generally mild or unnoticed by the mother.

Important causes of congenital infections are shown in Table 24.2. Viruses that induce fetal malformations (i.e. act as teratogens) share certain characteristics with other teratogens such as drugs or radiation. The fetus tends to show similar responses, including hepatosplenomegaly, encephalitis, eye lesions and low birth weight to different

**Table 24.2** Maternal infections that are transmitted to the fetus

| Microorganism | Effects |
|---|---|
| Rubella virus | Congenital rubella |
| Cytomegalovirus (CMV) | Congenital CMV, deafness, mental retardation |
| Human immunodeficiency virus | Congenital infection, childhood acquired immunodeficiency syndrome |
| Zika virus (ZIKV) | Microcephaly, facial disproportionality, cutis verticis gyrata[a] |
| Varicella-zoster virus | Skin lesions; musculoskeletal, central nervous system abnormalities when fetus infected <20 wk |
| Herpes simplex virus (HSV) | Neonatal HSV infection, often disseminated. Much higher risk when maternal infection primary rather than recurrent, infection in utero is rare |
| Hepatitis B virus | Congenital hepatitis B, persistent infection |
| Parvovirus B19 | After maternal infection 5–10% fetuses lost (abortion, hydrops fetalis) |
| *Treponema pallidum* | Congenital syphilis, classical syndrome |
| *Toxoplasma gondii* | Congenital toxoplasmosis |
| *Trypanosoma cruzi* | Congenital Chagas disease |
| *Listeria monocytogenes* | Congenital listeriosis, pneumonia, septicaemia, meningitis |
| *Mycobacterium leprae* | Congenital infection common in mothers with lepromatous leprosy |

[a]This term describes the overgrowth of scalp skin that looks like the cerebral sulci and gyri (folds and furrows of the surface of the brain).

infectious agents, and the diagnosis is difficult on purely clinical grounds. Most of these infections, such as rubella, CMV, parvovirus B19, Zika virus and syphilis, can also lead to fetal death. They generally follow primary infection of the mother during pregnancy so their incidence depends upon the proportion of nonimmune females of childbearing age.

The factors that influence transmission include:

- which stage of the pregnancy the infection occurs
- whether the infection was a primary infection, reactivation, reinfection or chronic infection
- how long the membranes (amniotic sac) had been ruptured before delivery
- type of delivery: vaginal or caesarean
- whether the delivery involved instrumentation (i.e. forceps, ventouse [vacuum cup] suction)
- breastfeeding.

Routine antenatal screening for rubella antibody, treponemal antibody (which includes syphilis, yaws, pinta or bejel, which cannot be identified individually by serology), hepatitis B surface antigen and human immunodeficiency virus (HIV) combination antibody and antigen assays are being carried out to differing degrees worldwide. These tests help identify women who are infected with hepatitis B or HIV, infected or have been exposed in the past to treponemal infections (the most important of which is syphilis in this setting) or are susceptible to rubella.

Routine screening programmes lead to clinical management issues for both the mother and the child. For example, an HIV-positive diagnosis will lead to health care staff discussing antiretroviral therapy for the mother and, immediately on birth, the child, planning a vaginal delivery unless a caesarean section is indicated and advising against breastfeeding to reduce the risk of vertical transmission. In addition, the child will then be followed up for 3–6 months using molecular diagnostic tests to determine whether HIV has been transmitted vertically.

Diagnosis of chronic hepatitis B virus (HBV) infection will result in determination of the maternal level of infectivity and the baby subsequently being offered an accelerated course of hepatitis B vaccine alone or, if the mother is highly infectious, vaccine and HBV-specific immunoglobulin to the baby. In addition, there are antiviral drugs for chronic hepatitis B that might be offered, together with long-term follow-up, to the mother.

Rubella-susceptible women are offered immunization post-natally, although in the United Kingdom rubella antibody testing was removed from the antenatal screening programme in 2016. This was because it did not meet the criteria for a screening programme on the basis that the incidence of rubella infection in the United Kingdom was so low that it was within the World Health Organization's (WHO's) definition of having been eliminated, that rubella infection in pregnancy was very rare, and that the measles, mumps and rubella (MMR) vaccine uptake had improved considerably. This had dropped in previous years, but by 2016 it was deemed to be more effective in protecting women against rubella in pregnancy, before becoming pregnant, as the screening test used could potentially be interpreted incorrectly in women with an acute rubella infection.

Women found to have been exposed to treponemal infection in pregnancy are offered antibiotic treatment, and the baby is followed up for the first year using serology to identify active infection as congenital syphilis can result from earlier untreated infection of the mother. In the case of CMV, which is not part of routine antenatal screening in the United Kingdom and United States, for example, a primary infection, reinfection or reactivation of the latent virus during pregnancy can lead to fetal infection (see next section).

The likelihood of fetal infection is increased in a primary maternal infection and when the mother has a chronic infection, although there are a number of factors that result in varying risks of fetal infection.

There is no good evidence to suggest that maternal mumps, influenza or poliovirus infection during pregnancy leads to harmful effects in the fetus, but with human parvovirus B19 infection (see Ch. 27), the risk of intrauterine infection is ~15% at 5–16 weeks of pregnancy and 25–70% after 16 weeks gestation, with a risk of fetal death around 9% in the first 20 weeks. The infected fetus develops hydrops fetalis due to severe anaemia, with ascites and hepatosplenomegaly in 3% as the virus infects progenitor erythroid stem cells. Intrauterine exchange blood transfusion is used to manage hydrops fetalis.

In terms of emerging infectious diseases, a Zika virus outbreak in Brazil, which by 2016 had emerged in South, Central and North America and the Caribbean, resulted in reports of neonatal microcephaly and neurologic illness, including Guillain-Barré syndrome (GBS).

## Congenital rubella

### The fetus is particularly susceptible to rubella virus infection when maternal infection occurs during the first 3 months of pregnancy

At this time, the heart, brain, eyes and ears are being formed, and the infecting virus interferes with their development. If the fetus survives, it may show characteristic abnormalities (Fig. 24.1). Not all fetuses are affected despite the risk of intrauterine infection being 90% at <11 weeks, 55% at 11–16 weeks and 45% at >16 weeks. The risk of an adverse fetal outcome was seen in 90% of babies when maternal rubella occurred in the first 11 weeks of pregnancy, 20% when it occurred between 11 and 16 weeks, by 16–20 weeks there was a minimal risk of deafness and no increased risk at >20 weeks.

### Congenital rubella can affect the eyes, heart, brain and ears

Clinical manifestations of congenital rubella include low birth weight and eye (Fig. 24.2) and heart lesions. Effects on the brain and ears may not become detectable until later in childhood in the form of mental retardation and deafness. Up to 80% of infected infants eventually suffer from deafness. About 25% of congenitally infected children develop insulin-dependent diabetes mellitus later in life (the virus replicates in the pancreas), but rubella is a very uncommon cause of this disease. There is 15% mortality in infants showing signs of infection at birth, often associated with hypogammaglobulinaemia.

### Fetal rubella IgM is found in cord and infant blood

Infected fetuses produce their own IgM antibody to rubella virus, which can be detected in cord and infant blood.

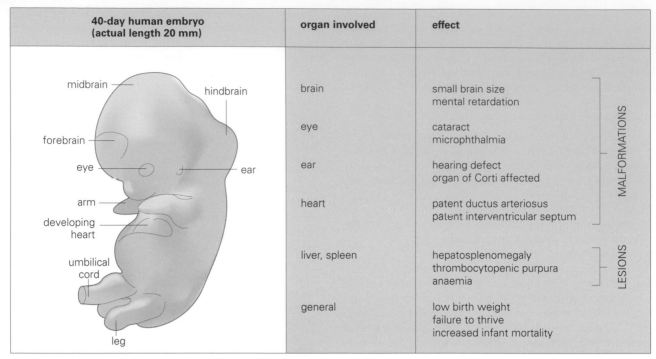

| 40-day human embryo (actual length 20 mm) | organ involved | effect | |
|---|---|---|---|
| | brain | small brain size<br>mental retardation | MALFORMATIONS |
| | eye | cataract<br>microphthalmia | |
| | ear | hearing defect<br>organ of Corti affected | |
| | heart | patent ductus arteriosus<br>patent interventricular septum | |
| | liver, spleen | hepatosplenomegaly<br>thrombocytopenic purpura<br>anaemia | LESIONS |
| | general | low birth weight<br>failure to thrive<br>increased infant mortality | |

**Fig. 24.1** Organ involvement and effects in congenital rubella.

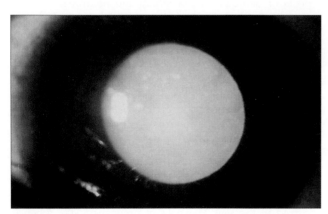

**Fig. 24.2** Cataract in congenital rubella. (Courtesy R.J. Marsh and S. Ford.)

Maternal IgG antibodies are also present and, together with interferons, help to control the spread of infection in the fetus. Virus can be isolated from the infant's throat or urine. The infant sheds virus into the throat and urine for several months and can infect susceptible individuals. Rubella virus RNA detection may be carried out in mostly reference centres to assist with the diagnosis.

**Congenital rubella can be prevented by immunization**

Immunization with live attenuated rubella virus is given during childhood usually as the combined MMR vaccine. Pregnancy is a contraindication to immunization as it is a live vaccine, and the only safe time during reproductive life is the immediate postpartum period. This is an interesting example of a vaccine that is given to protect an as yet nonexistent individual (the future fetus), the infection being only subclinical or mild in the mother. Until effective vaccines became available in the late 1960s (Box 24.1), rubella was an

important cause of congenital heart disease, deafness, blindness, and mental retardation. The virus continues to circulate in the community and damage fetuses in countries with less extensive rubella immunization programmes.

**Congenital CMV infection**

**Mothers with a poor T-cell proliferative response to CMV antigens are more likely to infect their fetus**

After primary maternal infection during pregnancy, ~40% of fetuses are infected, and 5% of these show signs at birth. It is not known whether the fetus is especially vulnerable at certain stages of pregnancy. The fetus is also infected following CMV reactivation during pregnancy in women with previous CMV exposure, but fetal damage is then uncommon. As many as 1–2% of infants born in the United States are infected, and up to ~10% of these are symptomatic, with up to 1 million infectious doses of virus present per millilitre of urine. However, the incidence of congenital CMV infection is likely to be an underestimate worldwide. In large cohorts of pregnant women studied, it was shown that 2% developed a primary CMV infection, but over 95% were asymptomatic. Of those women with a primary infection in the first trimester, up to 30% of babies may develop central nervous system (CNS) sequelae, including sensorineural hearing loss. Although the percentage is much reduced if the maternal infection is later in pregnancy, a degree of CNS damage still occurs. However, the relationship between a first-trimester infection and outcome is much clearer in rubella infections than with CMV. In CMV reactivation or reinfection, partial control of the infection by maternal antibody under these circumstances means that the baby may be infected but not affected, although a small percentage become symptomatic over the next couple of years. The frequency and outcome of congenital CMV infections in reactivation or reinfection in pregnancy are still not well understood. However, the

## Box 24.1    Lessons in Microbiology

### Rubella and the fetus

Dr. Norman McAllister Gregg (1892–1966) was ophthalmic surgeon to the Royal Alexandra Hospital for Children in Sydney, and during the Second World War he noticed what he called an "epidemic" of congenital cataract in infants. He went further and made the astute observation that all the mothers had suffered from rubella during early pregnancy. There were 78 infants with cataract, and 68 of the mothers had a history of rubella in early pregnancy. Many of the infants had heart defects, were small, and two-thirds had microphthalmia. He published his findings in 1941, providing the first clear demonstration that an environmental factor could cause congenital malformations. It is a striking feature of the infection that, whereas the fetus suffers cruel malformations, the mother shows little or no signs of illness. We now know that several other viruses, notably cytomegalovirus, can do this, as well as factors such as thalidomide and folate deficiency. Later studies on rubella revealed that congenitally infected infants also developed deafness and brain defects. Survivors were followed up until 1991 when they were 50, and other abnormalities had been observed, including the development of diabetes by the age of 25 years and certain vascular abnormalities.

It was not until 1962 that the causative virus was isolated and grown in cell culture. A rubella epidemic in the United States in 1964–1965 left in its wake 20,000 infants with congenital rubella syndrome. By the late 1960s an effective live virus vaccine was available, and congenital rubella is now seen only when vaccination cover is poor. The fetus is exquisitely vulnerable to rubella during the first trimester of pregnancy. This is the critical stage in embryonic development when key organs (heart, ears, eyes, and brain) are being formed and, although the virus does no damage to the cells in which it grows, it interferes with mitosis. Interference with programmed mitosis in these major organs causes the malformations, vasculitis playing a part. The fetus is good at repairing damage but it cannot at a later stage compensate for the failure in basic organ development. The antimitotic action of the virus also means that the total number of cells in the body is reduced, and this is why the rubella-infected infants are smaller. The rubella virus remains in infected organs such as the lens and brain for less than 1 year, but eventually there is an adequate cell-mediated immune response, and the virus is eliminated.

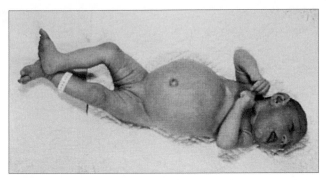

**Fig. 24.3** Microcephaly with associated severe psychomotor retardation and hepatosplenomegaly in congenital cytomegalovirus infection. (Courtesy W.E. Farrar.)

(AD169 and Towne strains), and in preliminary studies, no one who became pregnant after immunization transmitted the virus to the infant. Novel vaccine types are under investigation.

Antiviral drugs such as ganciclovir and valganciclovir can be considered in managing symptomatic babies with congenital CMV infection.

### Zika virus

Zika virus is a single-stranded virus belonging to the Flaviviridae family, which includes dengue virus, West Nile virus and yellow fever virus. Isolated as long ago as 1947 in a monkey in the Zika Forest of Uganda and reported to cause human infection in 1954, it rose to prominence in 2015 after an outbreak in Central and South America, the Caribbean, Oceania and parts of Asia. In 2016 WHO declared Zika-related microcephaly a public health emergency of international concern (PHEIC) but ended the PHEIC in 2017. Zika virus is transmitted by a variety of *Aedes* mosquitoes, especially *Aedes aegypti*. Approximately 80% of those who become infected are asymptomatic, and in those who do develop symptoms, the illness is relatively mild in most cases, although it can cause GBS in some instances. However, Zika virus can cross the placenta, and maternal infection contracted during pregnancy can result in fetal malformations and congenital microcephaly (Fig. 24.4). Infections were diagnosed in people who travelled to areas with established *A. aegypti* mosquitoes, and sexual transmission was confirmed as another route of transmission. However, almost as quickly as it appeared, numbers declined precipitously in 2017 across the world. By 2023 Zika virus transmission was reported at very low levels in the Americas and a few other regions. A few local infections were seen in Europe, and an outbreak occurred in 2021 in India. Overall, 89 countries and territories had reported individuals with Zika virus infection.

An active programme is underway to develop a vaccine against Zika virus, but in the meantime, until a vaccine becomes available, prevention of infection depends heavily on mosquito bite prevention. The virus has been detected in semen and in the female genital tract. Sexual transmission of Zika virus has occurred in a small minority of infections and has been reported to occur female to male or male to female. Females who are pregnant or planning to become pregnant and who might become exposed to the risk of Zika virus infection or whose sexual partner might become exposed

incidence of symptomatic congenital CMV infections has been reported to be similar in pregnant women with primary infections and reactivations or reinfections.

Clinical features of congenital CMV include mental retardation, chorioretinitis and optic atrophy, hearing defects, hepatosplenomegaly, thrombocytopenic purpura and anaemia (Fig. 24.3). Deafness and mental retardation may not be detectable until later in childhood.

Diagnosis is made by detecting CMV-specific IgM in infant blood within 3 weeks of delivery and by detecting and quantifying CMV DNA in the blood or urine during this period. Live attenuated vaccines have been investigated

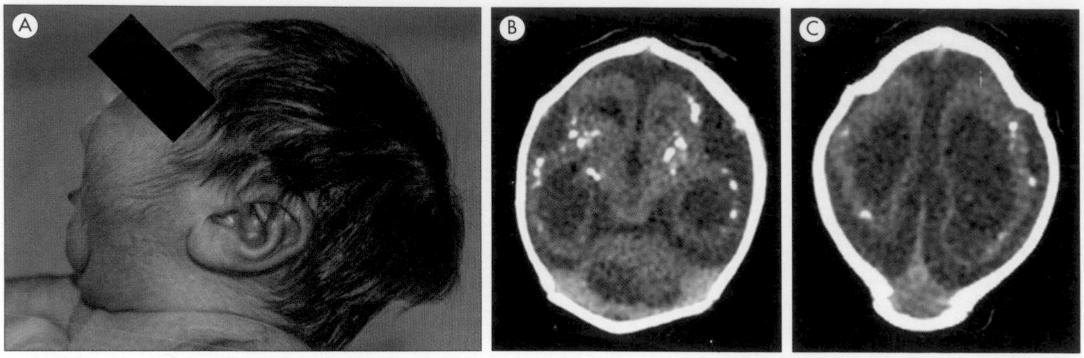

**Fig. 24.4** (A) Newborn baby with microcephaly with laboratory-confirmed Zika virus infection. (B, C) Abnormalities detected on computed tomography (CT) scan. The neonate shows phenotypic features previously described during the microcephaly epidemic, including craniofacial disproportion, prominent external occipital protuberance, and excessive scalp skin. Radiologic features found on brain CT imaging include reduced volume of cortical brain parenchyma, cortical and subcortical calcifications, simplified gyral pattern, and ventriculomegaly. (Reproduced with permission from Barreto de Araújo TV, et al. Association between Zika virus infection and microcephaly in Brazil, January to May 2016: preliminary report of a case–control study. *Lancet Infect Dis* 2016;16[12]:1356–1363.)

should consult their health care provider for individual assessment. Guidance is available from websites of the US Centers for Disease Control and Prevention, the European Centre for Disease Prevention and Control and the UK National Travel Health Network and Centre.

## Congenital syphilis

As a result of routine serologic screening for syphilis, a treponemal infection, in antenatal clinics and treatment with penicillin, congenital syphilis is now rare but is more common in resource-poor countries. Clinical features in the infant include rhinitis (a runny nose), skin and mucosal lesions, hepatosplenomegaly, lymphadenopathy, and abnormalities of bones, teeth and cartilage (saddle-shaped nose). Pregnancy often masks the early signs of syphilis, but the mother will have serologic evidence of treponemal infection, and treponemal IgM will be detected in the fetal blood. Vertical transmission most commonly takes place after 4 months of gestation; therefore treatment of the mother before the fourth month of pregnancy should prevent fetal infection.

## Congenital toxoplasmosis

### Acute asymptomatic infection by *Toxoplasma gondii* during pregnancy can cause fetal malformation

*Toxoplasma* is a ubiquitous parasitic infection worldwide. Depending on the country concerned, ~10–80% of healthy adults have serologic evidence of previous *T. gondii* infection, but the risk factor for congenital toxoplasmosis is primary infection of the mother acquired during pregnancy. The incidence of fetal infection increases from 14% when maternal infection is in the first trimester to 59% when in the third trimester. In contrast, damage to the fetus is more severe the earlier in pregnancy infection is contracted. At birth, most infants are asymptomatic, and there are often no detectable abnormalities at that time, but signs such as chorioretinitis generally appear within a few years.

In severely affected infants the clinical features of congenital toxoplasmosis include convulsions, microcephaly, chorioretinitis, hepatosplenomegaly and jaundice, with later hydrocephaly, mental retardation and defective vision. Some countries undertake serologic screening of pregnant women for toxoplasma-specific antibodies, including IgM. If

the serologic profile indicates maternal infection acquired in pregnancy, treatment of the mother is started with spiramycin to try to prevent transmission to the fetus. Amniotic fluid is tested by polymerase chain reaction (PCR) for toxoplasma DNA; if it confirms fetal infection, treatment with sulphadiazine plus pyrimethamine plus folinic acid is given instead of spiramycin.

There is no vaccine. Prevention is by avoidance of primary infection, which occurs via ingesting cysts from cat faeces or raw or lightly cooked meat during pregnancy.

## Congenital Chagas disease

Chagas disease (American trypanosomiasis) is endemic to parts of North, Central and South America. The causative agent is the protozoan *Trypanosoma cruzi*, which is transmitted by insect vectors known as reduviid bugs. Other routes of transmission include oral via food or drink contaminated by reduviid bugs in endemic areas, congenital or blood transfusion and organ transplantation.

The bugs bite animals and humans, often at night. The parasite is excreted in bug faeces and enters humans at the site of the bite or via mucous membranes.

Chagas disease has an acute and a chronic phase. Most infections are asymptomatic or oligosymptomatic, but ~10% produce more specific symptoms. These may be mild in the acute period with fever, tiredness, rash, diarrhoea and vomiting. Signs may include swollen eyelids (Romaña sign) due to a local bite or rubbing bug faeces accidentally into the eye. About 30% of those who have a chronic infection can suffer complications of the cardiac (heart failure, arrhythmias, cardiomegaly), gastrointestinal (megaoesophagus, megacolon), or less commonly peripheral nervous system.

As a result of vector control programmes, vertical transmission now accounts for ~20% of new infections. This is concerning because it permits continuing transmission even in the absence of a competent insect vector.

Congenital *T. cruzi* infection occurs in 5–10% of births from infected mothers. It is commonly asymptomatic or mild, but it can result in spontaneous abortion, prematurity, low birth weight, neonatal death, fever, myocarditis, features anaemia, thrombocytopenia, meningoencephalitis, hepatosplenomegaly and respiratory distress. Survivors of congenital infection left untreated progress to the chronic stage, with a risk of developing cardiac or gastrointestinal complications 20–30 years later. Treatment of infected infants in the first year of life with benznidazole or nifurtimox is very effective. In contrast to the situation with adults who commonly experience adverse effects, these drugs are well tolerated in infants.

Prevention of congenital Chagas disease depends on serologic screening of females born in endemic areas or females whose mother was born in an endemic area. After birth to a seropositive female, the infant is monitored at birth and in subsequent weeks for the presence of vertical infection by blood film and PCR. Serology is checked 9–12 months after birth to look for disappearance of maternal antibody from the baby. Antiparasitic treatment is offered if there is evidence that the baby has a *T. cruzi* parasitaemia.

### Congenital and perinatal HIV infection

**In resource-poor countries there has been a ~50% fall in new HIV infections in <5-year-olds**

In 2021 the United Nations International Children's Emergency Fund estimated that, in 35 HIV priority countries, there had been ~130,000 new HIV infections in <5-year-olds compared with 230,000 in 2010. The 2011 global plan to achieve this had focused on more access to prevention of mother-to-child transmission services and more pregnant women starting combination antiretroviral therapy.

Clinically, congenital HIV infection manifests as poor weight gain, susceptibility to sepsis, developmental delays, lymphocytic pneumonitis, oral thrush, enlarged lymph nodes, hepatosplenomegaly, diarrhoea and pneumonia, and some infants develop encephalopathy and acquired immunodeficiency syndrome by 1 year of age. As most infections take place during late pregnancy or during delivery, transmission rates are reduced by lowering the HIV load by offering antiretroviral drugs during pregnancy, during the last trimester or during labour if not started previously, carrying out an elective caesarean section where indicated (if the HIV load is suppressed, vaginal delivery is recommended) and avoiding breastfeeding.

IgG antibodies present in the neonatal blood sample may be maternal in origin and can persist for 9–12 months. The mainstay of laboratory diagnosis, therefore, involves detection of HIV-1 proviral DNA or HIV-1 RNA by PCR, although these tests may not be positive until several months after birth, in conjunction with testing by HIV antibody and antigen combination assays once maternal antibody has waned. As post-exposure prophylaxis (PEP) is offered to the baby, usually 2 weeks of zidovudine monotherapy in very low-risk settings to 4 weeks in low-risk settings and combination PEP in high-risk settings, a definitive result for the HIV test is not available until ~3 months of age.

### Congenital and neonatal listeriosis

**Maternal exposure to animals or foods infected with *Listeria* can lead to fetal death or malformations**

*Listeria monocytogenes* is a small gram-positive rod that is motile and beta-haemolytic. It is distributed worldwide in a great variety of animals, including cattle, pigs, rodents and birds; the bacteria also occur in plants and in soil. *Listeria* can grow at regular refrigeration temperatures (e.g. 3–4°C). Transmission to humans is by:

- contact with infected animals and their faeces
- consumption of unpasteurized milk or soft cheeses or contaminated vegetables.

In the United States there are ~2000 reported cases of listeriosis each year, about one-third of them in newborn infants. Molecular studies have shown that, while influenced by the gut microbiota, faecal carriage is more common than previously thought.

*L. monocytogenes* in the pregnant woman causes a mild influenza-like illness or is asymptomatic, but there is a bacteraemia that leads to infection of the placenta and then the fetus. This may cause abortion, premature delivery, neonatal septicaemia, or pneumonia with abscesses or granulomas. The infant can also be infected shortly after birth (for instance, from other babies or from hospital staff), and this may lead to a meningitic illness.

*L. monocytogenes* is isolated from blood cultures, cerebrospinal fluid (CSF) or newborn skin lesions.

Treatment is with amoxicillin, which may need to be combined with gentamicin to achieve a bactericidal effect. There are no vaccines.

Pregnant women should avoid exposure to infected material, but the exact source of infection is generally unknown.

## INFECTIONS OCCURRING AROUND THE TIME OF BIRTH

### Effects on the fetus and neonate

**The routes of infection in the fetus and neonate are shown in Fig. 24.5**

Viral infections such as rubella and CMV are generally less damaging to the fetus when the maternal infection occurs late in pregnancy. Primary infection with varicella-zoster virus in the first 20 weeks of pregnancy can lead to limb deformities and other severe lesions in the newborn. Herpes simplex viurus (HSV) infection in this setting is underdiagnosed and can lead to neonatal morbidity and mortality.

Bacterial infections originating from the vagina and perineum late in pregnancy, especially those occurring when the fetal membranes have been ruptured for >1–2 days, may result in chorioamnionitis, maternal fever, premature delivery, and stillbirth. Infants of low birth weight (<1500 g) tend to be more severely affected. Bacteria involved include:

- group B haemolytic streptococci; 10–30% of pregnant women are colonized in the rectum or vagina
- *Escherichia coli*
- *Klebsiella*
- *Proteus*
- *Bacteroides*
- *Staphylococcus*
- *Mycoplasma hominis*.

These infections may also be acquired after delivery to give later-onset disease.

**Neonatal septicaemia often progresses to meningitis**

Bacterial meningitis (Table 24.3) is frequently fatal unless treated. Clinical diagnosis is difficult because the infant shows generalized signs such as respiratory distress, poor feeding, diarrhoea and vomiting, but early diagnosis is essential, and emergency treatment is required. Blind

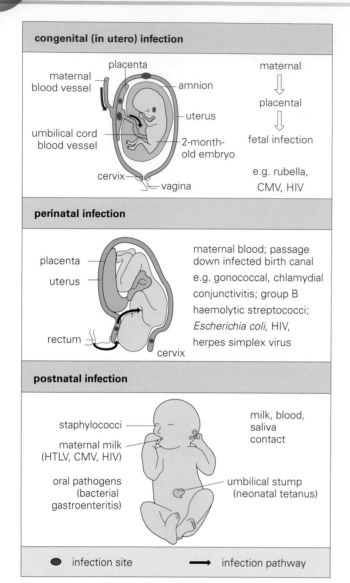

**congenital (in utero) infection**

maternal blood vessel — placenta — amnion — uterus — 2-month-old embryo — umbilical cord blood vessel — cervix — vagina

maternal ⇓ placental ⇓ fetal infection

e.g. rubella, CMV, HIV

**perinatal infection**

placenta — uterus — rectum — cervix

maternal blood; passage down infected birth canal e.g. gonococcal, chlamydial conjunctivitis; group B haemolytic streptococci; *Escherichia coli*, HIV, herpes simplex virus

**postnatal infection**

staphylococci — maternal milk (HTLV, CMV, HIV) — oral pathogens (bacterial gastroenteritis) — umbilical stump (neonatal tetanus)

milk, blood, saliva contact

● infection site ⟶ infection pathway

**Fig. 24.5** Routes of infection in the fetus and neonate. CMV, Cytomegalovirus; HIV, human immunodeficiency virus; HTLV, human T-cell lymphotropic virus.

antibiotic treatment should be started as soon as possible, preferably after CSF and blood culture samples have been collected, otherwise it may be difficult to make a diagnosis.

If, however, these are difficult to carry out immediately, then treatment must be started.

### Fetal infection with HSV must be considered in a baby who is acutely ill within a few days or weeks of birth

Fetal infection during labour results from direct contact with the infecting microorganism as the fetus passes down an infected birth canal (see Table 24.3). For instance, a vesicular skin rash due to HSV may develop 1 week after delivery, with generalized infection and severe CNS involvement. Approximately 80% of mothers with primary HSV infection (but only ~10% with recurrent HSV) have cervical lesions, and about a third of their infants are infected. Babies <4 weeks of age may present with neonatal HSV as acutely ill and septic, but classically there are three well-defined clinical presentations: (1) those with infection affecting the skin, eyes, and/or mouth (SEM); (2) encephalitis with or without skin involvement; (3) disseminated disease involving the lungs, liver, CNS, adrenal glands and SEM. The diagnosis may be missed as neonatal HSV infection may present without skin lesions in up to 39% of babies, some of whom may present with acute liver failure, for example. Therefore there must be a low threshold for considering this diagnosis, and intravenous aciclovir therapy must be started as soon as possible. Treatment could be started at the same time as samples are collected for HSV DNA detection that include swabs of the SEM and vesicles, if present, whole blood samples, and CSF. Morbidity and mortality rates are higher in those with encephalitis and disseminated disease.

Gonococci (Fig. 24.6), chlamydia or staphylococci can infect the eye to cause ophthalmia neonatorum. Infection with group B streptococci generally occurs at this time.

In countries with high rates of chronic HBV infection, maternal blood is a major source of infection during or shortly after birth. More than 90% of infants of mothers with chronic HBV may become infected and go on to chronic infection. Hepatitis B immunization at birth, plus specific hepatitis B immunoglobulin if the mother is highly infectious with a high HBV DNA load in the blood and detectable HBe antigen, are given to prevent mother-to-baby transmission. Hepatitis C, in contrast, is not usually transmitted in this way, and the risk is higher if the mother is immunocompromised as this is likely to lead to a higher maternal hepatitis C viraemia.

Human milk may contain rubella virus, CMV, human t-cell lymphotropic virus (HTLV), and, HIV as these viruses

**Table 24.3** Neonatal infections acquired during passage down an infected birth canal

| Infectious agent | Site of infection | Effects |
|---|---|---|
| *Neisseria gonorrhoeae* | Conjunctiva | Neonatal conjunctivitis (ophthalmia neonatorum) |
| *Chlamydia trachomatis* | Conjunctiva, respiratory tract | Neonatal conjunctivitis (ophthalmia neonatorum), neonatal pneumonia |
| Herpes simplex virus | Skin, eye, mouth | Neonatal herpetic infection[a] |
| Genital papillomavirus | Respiratory tract | Laryngeal warts in young children |
| Group B streptococci,[b] gram-negative bacilli (*Escherichia coli*, etc.) | Respiratory tract | Septicaemia; death if not treated |
| *Candida albicans* | Oral cavity | Neonatal oral thrush |

[a]Although preventable by caesarean section, it may be difficult to detect maternal genital infection; infants can be screened for HSV infecion at delivery and treated prophylactically with aciclovir, if clinically indicated, while awaiting the results.
[b]Up to 30% of women carry these bacteria in the vagina or rectum.

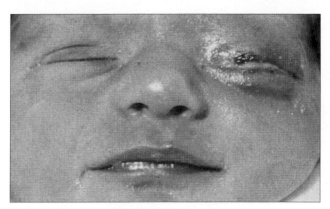

**Fig. 24.6** Gonococcal ophthalmia neonatorum. Signs appear 2–5 days after birth. The inflammation and oedema are more severe than with *Chlamydia* infection. (Courtesy J.S. Bingham.)

are cell associated. The amount of virus detectable in milk is low, and, except in the case of HTLV and HIV, milk is not thought to be an important source of infection. However, it makes sense to pasteurize milk in human milk banks just as we pasteurize cow milk.

### Effects on the mother

#### Puerperal sepsis is prevented by aseptic techniques

After delivery, a large area of damaged vulnerable uterine tissue is exposed to infection. Puerperal sepsis (childbed fever) was a major cause of maternal death in Europe in the 19th century. In 1843 Oliver Wendell Holmes made the unpopular suggestion that it was carried on the hands of doctors, and 4 years later Ignaz Semmelweiss in Vienna showed how it could be prevented if doctors and midwives washed their hands before attending a woman in labour and practiced aseptic techniques. This is because:

- group A beta-haemolytic streptococci were the major culprits and came from the nose, throat or skin of hospital attendants
- other possible organisms include anaerobes such as *Clostridium perfringens* or *Bacteroides*, E. coli and group B streptococci and originate from the mother's own faecal flora.

Puerperal sepsis carried a mortality rate of up to 10% until the 1930s but, like septic abortion, is now uncommon in resource-rich countries. Predisposing factors include premature rupture of the membranes, instrumentation, and retained fragments of membrane or placenta. High vaginal swabs and blood cultures should be collected if there is post-natal pyrexia or an offensive discharge.

### Other neonatal infections

Infection may be transmitted to the newborn infant during the first 1–2 weeks after birth, rather than during delivery as follows:

- Group B beta-haemolytic streptococci and gram-negative bacilli (see earlier) acquired by cross-infection in the nursery can still cause serious infection at this time, often with meningitis.
- HSV from facial cold sores or herpetic whitlows of attending adults can infect the infant.
- Staphylococci from the noses and fingers of adult carriers may cause staphylococcal conjunctivitis or sticky eye,

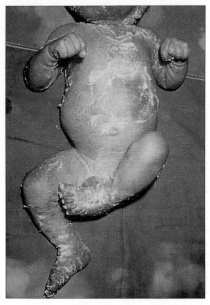

**Fig. 24.7** Staphylococcal scalded skin syndrome. There are large areas of epidermal loss where bullae have burst. (Courtesy L. Brown.)

skin sepsis in the neonate and sometimes the staphylococcal scalded skin syndrome (Fig. 24.7) due to a specific epidermolytic staphylococcal toxin.

During the first 1–2 weeks of life the nose of the neonate becomes colonized with *Staphylococcus aureus*, which can enter the nipple during feeding to cause a breast abscess. These infections are preventable if hospital staff members pay vigorous attention to hand washing and aseptic techniques.

If hygienic practices are poor, the umbilical stump, especially in resource-poor countries, may be infected with *Clostridium tetani* usually because instruments used to cut the cord are contaminated with bacterial spores, resulting in neonatal tetanus (Fig. 24.8). It can be prevented by immunization of mothers with tetanus toxoid.

In resource-poor countries, gastroenteritis is an important problem during the neonatal period as well as during infancy.

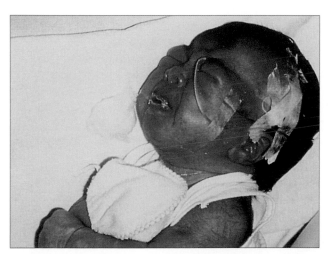

**Fig. 24.8** Tetanus. Risus sardonicus in a newborn infant. (Courtesy W.E. Farrar.)

Diarrhoea leading to water and electrolyte depletion is particularly serious in low–birth-weight infants. Causative agents include strains of *E. coli* and salmonellae rather than rotaviruses. Breastfeeding gives some protection by supplying specific antibodies and other less well-characterized protective factors.

## KEY FACTS

- During pregnancy certain infections (coccidioidomycosis, influenza) can be more severe than usual, and there can be reactivation of certain latent infections (HSV, CMV).

- A few infections are able to pass to the fetus via the placenta and cause damage. These infections are generally mild or subclinical in the mother (rubella, CMV, Zika virus, toxoplasmosis, American trypanosomiasis), but this is not always the case (syphilis).

- Once infected, the fetus may die, but if the baby survives it may be born with the infection (HIV, toxoplasmosis), often showing characteristic malformations (rubella, syphilis).

- Infection of the infant during birth or shortly afterward can cause local disease (conjunctivitis due to gonococci or chlamydia) or occasionally severe life-threatening illness (*E. coli* meningitis, HSV, or group B streptococcal infection).

- Life-threatening bacterial infection of the mother via the post-partum uterus (puerperal sepsis) used to be common but is now rare in resource-rich countries.

# Central nervous system infections

## 25

## Introduction

**Central nervous system (CNS) infections are usually bloodborne or infectious agents invading via peripheral nerves**

The brain and spinal cord are protected from mechanical pressure or deformation by enclosure in rigid containers, the skull and vertebral column, which also act as barriers to the spread of infection. The blood vessels and nerves that traverse the walls of the skull and vertebral column are the main routes of invasion. However, cellular barriers such as the blood-brain barrier and blood–cerebrospinal fluid (CSF) barrier protect against pathogen invasion. Bloodborne invasion is the most common route of infection (e.g. by polioviruses or *Neisseria meningitidis*). Invasion via peripheral nerves is less common (e.g. herpes simplex, varicella-zoster, and rabies viruses). Local invasion from infected ears or sinuses, local injury or congenital defects such as spina bifida also occur, whereas invasion from the olfactory tract leading to amoebic meningitis is rare.

Here we discuss the main routes of CNS invasion by pathogens and the body's response, followed by a more detailed discussion of the diseases that result. In particular, meningitis, inflammation of the meninges surrounding the brain, encephalitis, inflammation of the white matter substance of the brain, meningoencephalitis and focal CNS syndromes encompass the clinical presentations of these infections.

## INVASION OF THE CENTRAL NERVOUS SYSTEM

### Natural barriers act to prevent bloodborne invasion

Bloodborne invasion takes place across:

- the blood-brain barrier to cause encephalitis
- the blood-CSF barrier to cause meningitis (Fig. 25.1).

The blood-brain barrier consists of tightly joined endothelial cells surrounded by glial processes, whereas the blood-CSF barrier at the choroid plexus consists of endothelium with fenestrations and tightly joined choroid plexus epithelial cells. Pathogens can traverse these barriers by:

- growing across, infecting the cells that comprise the barrier
- being passively transported across in intracellular vacuoles
- being carried across by infected white blood cells.

Examples of each route are seen in viral infections. The clinical presentation may be headache and neck stiffness in meningitis, inflammation of the meninges surrounding the brain or a confusional state in encephalitis, inflammation of the white matter substance of the brain or a mixture of both in a meningoencephalitis. Poliovirus, for instance, invades the CNS across the blood-brain barrier. After the virus gains entry via oral ingestion, a complex stepwise series of events leads to CNS invasion (Fig. 25.2). Poliovirus also invades the meninges after localizing in vascular endothelial cells and can cross the blood-CSF barrier. Mumps virus behaves in the same way, as do circulating *Haemophilus influenzae*, meningococci and pneumococci. Once infection has reached

the meninges and CSF, the brain substance can, in turn, be invaded if the infection crosses the pia. In poliomyelitis, for instance, a meningitic phase often precedes encephalitis and paralysis.

CNS invasion, however, is a rare event because most microorganisms fail to pass from blood to the CNS across the natural barriers. A large variety of viruses can multiply and cause disease if introduced directly into the brain, but circulating viruses generally fail to invade, and CNS involvement by polio, mumps, rubella or measles viruses is seen in only a very small proportion of infected individuals. Other neurotropic viruses include enteroviruses, herpes simplex virus (HSV), varicella-zoster virus (VZV), cytomegalovirus (CMV), Epstein-Barr virus (EBV), John Cunningham (JC) virus, human immunodeficiency virus (HIV), human T-cell lymphotropic virus (HTLV), Japanese encephalitis (JE) virus and those that have emerged since 1999, including Zika virus and West Nile virus (WNV).

### Invasion of the CNS via peripheral nerves is a feature of herpes simplex, varicella-zoster, and rabies virus infections

HSV and VZV present in skin or mucosal lesions and travel up axons using the normal retrograde transport mechanisms that can move virus particles (as well as foreign molecules such as tetanus toxin) at a rate of ~200 mm/day to reach the dorsal root ganglia. Rabies virus, introduced into muscle or subcutaneous tissues by, for example, the bite of a rabid animal, infects muscle fibres and muscle spindles after the virus

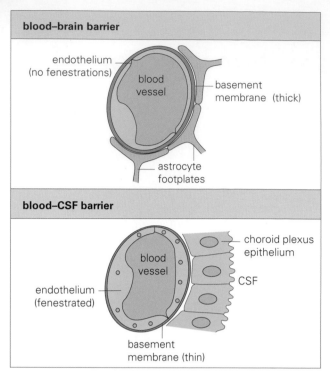

**blood–brain barrier**

endothelium
(no fenestrations)

blood vessel

basement membrane (thick)

astrocyte footplates

**blood–CSF barrier**

choroid plexus epithelium

blood vessel

CSF

endothelium (fenestrated)

basement membrane (thin)

**Fig. 25.1** Structures of the blood-brain and blood–cerebrospinal fluid (CSF) barriers.

binds to the nicotinic acetylcholine receptor. It then enters peripheral nerves and travels to the CNS to reach glial cells and neurones, where it multiplies.

## THE BODY'S RESPONSE TO INVASION

### CSF cell counts increase in response to infection

The response to invading viruses is reflected by an increase in lymphocytes, mostly T cells, and monocytes in the CSF (Table 25.1). A slight increase in protein also occurs, the CSF remaining clear. This condition is termed *aseptic meningitis*. The response to pyogenic bacteria shows a more spectacular and more rapid increase in polymorphonuclear leukocytes and proteins (Fig. 25.3) so that the CSF becomes visibly turbid. This condition is termed *septic meningitis*. Certain slower growing or less pyogenic microorganisms induce less dramatic changes, such as in tuberculous or listerial meningitis.

### The pathologic consequences of CNS infection depend upon the microorganism

In the CNS itself, viruses can infect neural cells, sometimes showing a marked preference. Polio and rabies viruses, for instance, invade neurones, whereas JC virus invades oligodendrocytes. The latter are myelin-producing cells of the CNS, and the viral infection leads to cell lysis. The axons lose their myelin sheath, rendering them dysfunctional, and demyelinated lesions appear. Because there is very little extracellular space, spread is mostly direct from cell to

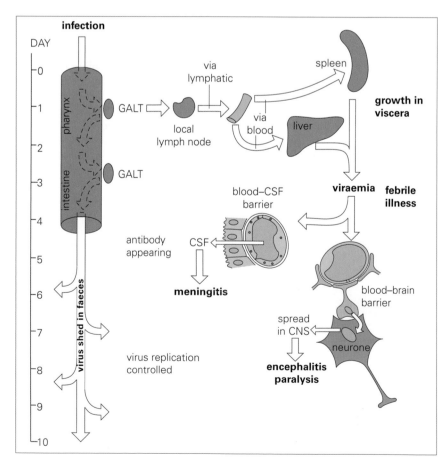

**infection**

DAY

0

pharynx

via lymphatic

spleen

1

GALT

local lymph node

via blood

liver

**growth in viscera**

2

intestine

3

GALT

blood–CSF barrier

**viraemia**   **febrile illness**

4

antibody appearing

CSF

5

**meningitis**

blood–brain barrier

6

virus shed in faeces

spread in CNS

7

neurone

8

virus replication controlled

**encephalitis paralysis**

9

10

**Fig. 25.2** The mechanism of central nervous system (CNS) invasion by poliovirus. CSF, Cerebrospinal fluid; GALT, gut-associated lymphoid tissue.

**Table 25.1** Changes in cerebrospinal fluid (CSF) in response to invading pathogens

|  | cells/mL | Protein (mg/dL) | Glucose (mg/dL) | Causes |
|---|---|---|---|---|
| Normal | 0–5 | 15–45 | 45–85 |  |
| Septic (purulent) meningitis | 200–20,000 (mainly neutrophils) | High (>100) | Low (<45) | Bacteria, including tuberculosis and leptospira, fungi, amoebae, brain abscess |
| Aseptic[a] meningitis or meningoencephalitis | 100–1000 (mainly mononuclear) | Moderately high (50–100) | Normal | Viruses, tuberculosis, leptospira, fungi, brain abscess, partly treated bacterial meningitis |

[a]Aseptic because the CSF is sterile on regular bacteriologic culture.

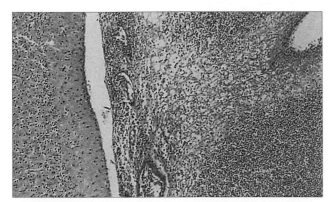

**Fig. 25.3** Bacterial meningitis. Exudate of acute inflammatory cells in the subarachnoid space (H&E stain). (Courtesy P. Garen.)

cell along established nervous pathways. Invading bacteria and protozoa generally induce more dramatic inflammatory events, which limit local spread so that infection is soon localized to form abscesses.

Viruses induce perivascular infiltration of lymphocytes and monocytes sometimes, as in the case of polio, with direct damage to infected cells. (The pathogenesis of viral encephalomyelitis is shown in Fig. 25.7.) Associated immune responses, not only to viral but also often to host CNS components, play a part in postvaccinial encephalitis. Infiltrating B cells produce antibody to the invading microorganism, and T cells react with microbial antigens to release cytokines that attract and activate other T cells and macrophages. The pathologic condition evolves over the course of several days and, occasionally, when partly controlled by host defences, over the course of years. Subacute sclerosing panencephalitis (SSPE) caused by measles is an example of this as it is has both a virologic (seen by defective, persistent viral replication) and an immunologic pathogenesis with high titres of neutralizing antibodies in the serum and CSF against viral structural proteins. The immune response is ineffective in clearing measles virus in the CNS. Bacteria cause more rapidly evolving pathologic changes, with local responses to bacterial antigens and toxins playing an important part.

In all cases a degree of inflammation and oedema that would be trivial in striated muscle, skin, or liver may be life-threatening when it occurs in the vulnerable closed box of the skull containing the leptomeninges, brain, and spinal cord. It may be several weeks after clinical recovery before cellular infiltrations are removed and histologic appearances are restored to normal.

### CNS invasion only rarely assists in the transmission of infection

From the point of view of a parasitic microorganism that needs to be transmitted to a fresh host, invasion of the CNS is generally foolish because it damages the host. The only occasions on which it makes sense are:

- when dorsal root ganglion neurones are invaded as an essential step in establishing latency (HSV and VZV); this gives a mechanism for reactivation and further episodes of shedding from mucosal or skin lesions.
- in the case of rabies (see later) in which CNS invasion in the animal host is necessary for two reasons. First, it enables the virus to spread from the CNS down peripheral nerves to the salivary glands, from where transmission takes place. Second, invasion of the limbic system of the brain causes a change in behaviour of the infected animal so that it becomes less retiring, more aggressive, and more likely to bite, thus transmitting the infection. Invasion of the limbic system can be regarded as a fiendish strategy on the part of rabies virus to promote its own transmission and survival.

## MENINGITIS

### Bacterial meningitis

#### Acute bacterial meningitis is a life-threatening infection, needing urgent specific treatment

Bacterial meningitis is more severe but less common than viral meningitis and may be caused by a variety of agents (Table 25.2). Prior to the 1990s, *H. influenzae* type b (Hib) was responsible for most cases of bacterial meningitis. However, the introduction of the Hib vaccine into childhood immunisation regimens has lowered overall Hib incidence in favour of *N. meningitidis* and *Streptococcus pneumoniae*, which are now responsible for most bacterial meningitis. These three pathogens have several virulence factors in common (Table 25.3), including possession of a polysaccharide capsule (Table 25.4).

#### Meningococcal meningitis

*Neisseria meningitidis* **is carried by about 20% of the population, but higher rates are seen in epidemics.** *N. meningitidis* is a gram-negative diplococcus that closely resembles *N. gonorrhoeae* in structure but with an additional polysaccharide capsule that is antigenic and by which the serotype of *N. meningitidis* can be recognized. The bacteria are carried asymptomatically in the population, up to 20% depending on geographic location, and are attached by their pili to the

**Table 25.2** The important causative agents of nonviral meningitis, their treatment and prevention

| Pathogen | Treatment[a] | Prevention |
|---|---|---|
| *Neisseria meningitidis* | Ceftriaxone (or chloramphenicol) | Ciprofloxacin prophylaxis for close contacts; polysaccharide vaccine |
| *Haemophilus influenzae* | Ceftriaxone or cefotaxime (or chloramphenicol) | Polysaccharide vaccine against type b (Hib) |
| *Streptococcus pneumoniae* | Ceftriaxone (or chloramphenicol) | Prompt treatment of otitis media and respiratory infections; polyvalent conjugate (13, 15, 20 serotypes) and polysaccharide (23 serotypes) vaccine |
| *Escherichia coli* (and other coliforms), group B streptococci | Gentamicin + cefotaxime or ceftriaxone (or chloramphenicol)[b] | No vaccines available |
| *Listeria monocytogenes* | Amoxicillin + gentamicin | No vaccines available |
| *Mycobacterium tuberculosis* | Isoniazid and rifampin and pyrazinamide ± streptomycin | Bacillus Calmette–Guérin (BCG) vaccination; isoniazid prophylaxis for contacts recommended in United States |
| *Cryptococcus neoformans* complex and *Cryptococcus gattii* complex | Amphotericin B, fluconazole, and flucytosine | No vaccines available |

[a]Treatment should be initiated immediately and the susceptibility of the infecting isolate confirmed in the laboratory.
[b]If isolate is shown to be susceptible (10–20% of isolates are resistant because they produce a plasmid coded beta-lactamase).

**Table 25.3** Virulence factors in bacterial meningitis

| Virulence factor | Bacterial pathogen | | |
|---|---|---|---|
| | *Neisseria meningitidis* | *Haemophilus influenzae* | *Streptococcus pneumoniae* |
| Capsule | + | + | + |
| IgA protease | + | + | + |
| Pili | + | + | − |
| Endotoxin | + | + | − |
| Outer membrane proteins | + | + | − |

IgA, Immunoglobulin A.

**Table 25.4** Polysaccharide capsules are important virulence factors in the pathogenesis of bacterial meningitis

| Pathogen | Capsule | Important type | Vaccine |
|---|---|---|---|
| *Neisseria meningitidis* | Polysaccharide | A, B, C, Y, W-135 | A, C, Y, W quadrivalent vaccine<br>B vaccine |
| *Haemophilus influenzae* | Polysaccharide | B | Hib vaccine for <1-yr-olds |
| *Streptococcus pneumoniae* | Polysaccharide | Many | Pneumovax: 23-valent most common types |
| Group B streptococcus | Polysaccharide rich in sialic acid | (Ia, Ib, II) III in neonatal meningitis | Multivalent protein–polysaccharide conjugate vaccines in clinical trial |
| *Escherichia coli* | Polysaccharide K antigen | KI in meningitis | No vaccine available |

epithelial cells in the nasopharynx. Invasion of the blood and meninges is a rare and poorly understood event. The known virulence factors are summarized in Table 25.3. People possessing specific complement-dependent bacterial antibodies to capsular antigens are protected against invasion. Those with C5–C9 complement deficiencies show increased susceptibility to bacteraemia (as they do to *N. gonorrhoeae* bacteraemia; see Ch. 22). Those most often infected include young children who have lost the antibodies passively acquired from their mother and adolescents who have not previously encountered the infecting serotype and, therefore, have no type-specific immunity.

Person-to-person spread takes place by droplet infection and is facilitated by other respiratory infections, often viral, that cause increased respiratory secretions. Thus conditions of overcrowding and confinement such as prisons, military barracks, and college dormitories contribute to the frequency of infection in populations. During outbreaks of meningococcal meningitis, which most frequently occur in late winter and early spring, the carrier rate may reach 60–80%. Specific serotypes associated with infection exhibit some geographic variation. However, serotypes B, W, Y and C, in that order, tend to predominate in more resource-rich countries, whereas serotypes A and W-135 are more common in less-developed regions. Available vaccines target serotypes A, B, C, Y and W-135 (see Table 25.4). The United Kingdom was the first country to introduce the meningitis C conjugate vaccine. It has been part of routine childhood immunisation since November 1999 and resulted in a 96% fall in incidence of meningitis C infections.

Group B meningococcal disease is diagnosed in >50% of meningitis cases, particularly in infants and toddlers. By 2023 meningitis B vaccine was being offered in the United Kingdom to 2-month-old babies, and the meningitis ACWY vaccine was offered to 14-year-olds and those age >25 years who had not had a meningitis C–containing vaccine. In the United States the Centers for Disease Control and Prevention (CDC) recommended meningitis B vaccine to those age ≥10 years at increased risk for meningococcal disease and meningitis ACWY to all 11- to 12-year-olds. Meningococcal immunisation programmes varied across Europe and other parts of the world, too.

*Clinical features of meningococcal meningitis include a haemorrhagic skin rash.* After an incubation period of 1–3 days, the onset of meningococcal meningitis is sudden with a sore throat, headache, drowsiness and signs of meningitis, which include fever, irritability, neck stiffness and photophobia. There is often a haemorrhagic skin rash with petechiae, reflecting the associated septicaemia (Fig. 25.4). In ~35% of patients, this septicaemia is fulminating, with complications due to disseminated intravascular coagulation, endotoxaemia and shock and renal failure. In the most severe cases there is an acute addisonian crisis, with bleeding into the brain and adrenal glands referred to as *Waterhouse-Friderichsen syndrome*. Mortality from meningococcal meningitis reaches 100% if untreated, but it remains at ~10% even if treated. In addition, serious sequelae such as permanent hearing loss may occur in some survivors (Table 25.5).

*A diagnosis of acute meningitis is usually suspected on clinical examination.* Laboratory identification of the bacterial cause of acute meningitis is essential so that appropriate antibiotic therapy can be given and prophylaxis of contacts initiated.

A **lumbar puncture** (LP) also called a spinal tap involves inserting a hollow needle into the **subarachnoid space** in the spinal canal. This space between the arachnoid and pia mater, two meningeal layers coveing the brain and spinal cord, contains the CSF.

Preliminary CSF microscopy results involving white cell counts and Gram staining for bacteria should be available as soon as possible. The CSF/plasma glucose ratio is also useful as bacteria break down glucose, and so a low CSF sugar compared with plasma glucose indicates a bacterial infection in the CSF (see Table 25.1). The normal level of CSF glucose should be ~60% of the plasma glucose level. Results of culture of CSF and blood should follow after 24 h. Molecular diagnosis of meningococcal infection can also be carried out and may be of clinical assistance as early treatment saves lives, but it makes culture of viable organisms from specimens more difficult.

Serology is not helpful in the diagnosis because the infection is too acute for an antibody response to be detectable. Bacterial meningitis is a medical emergency, and antibiotic therapy such as ceftriaxone or chloramphenicol if the patient is allergic to penicillin must be given immediately if the diagnosis is suspected (see Table 25.2) and is the treatment of choice if the diagnosis is confirmed.

Close contacts in the family, referred to as kissing contacts, should be given single-dose ciprofloxacin. Note that penicillin is not used for prophylaxis because it does not eliminate nasopharyngeal carriage of meningococci. Rifampicin used to be recommended, but it is associated with rapid induction of resistance, has to be taken for a longer time, and interacts with oral contraceptives.

### Haemophilus meningitis

*Type b H. influenzae causes meningitis in infants and young children.* H. influenzae is a gram-negative coccobacillus. *Haemophilus* means "blood-loving," and the name *influenzae* was given because it was originally thought to be the cause of influenza, but it is now known to be a common secondary invader in the lower respiratory tract. There are six types (a–f) of *H. influenzae*, distinguishable serologically by their capsular polysaccharides:

- Unencapsulated strains are common and are present in the throat of most healthy people.

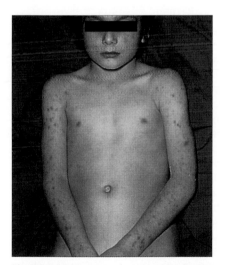

**Fig. 25.4** Meningococcal septicaemia showing a mixed petechial and maculopapular rash on the extremities and exterior surfaces. (Courtesy W.E. Farrar.)

**Table 25.5** Clinical features of bacterial meningitis

| Pathogen | Host (patient) | Important clinical features | Mortality[a] | Sequelae[a,b] |
|---|---|---|---|---|
| *Neisseria meningitidis* | Children and adolescents | Acute onset (6–24 h); skin rash | 7–10 | <1 |
| *Haemophilus influenzae* | Children age <5 yr | Onset often less acute (1–2 days) | 5 | 9 |
| *Streptococcus pneumoniae* | All ages, but especially children age <2 yr and elderly | Acute onset may follow pneumonia and/or septicaemia in elderly | 20–30 | 15–20 |

[a]As percentage of treated cases.
[b]Major central nervous system deficit; in addition, up to 10% of patients develop deafness.

- The capsulated type b, a common inhabitant of the respiratory tract of infants and young children (where it may cause infection: see Ch. 19), very occasionally invades the blood and reaches the meninges.

Maternal antibody protects infants up to 3–4 months of age, but as it wanes, there is a window of susceptibility until children produce their own antibody. Anticapsular antibodies are good opsonins, which allow the bacteria to be phagocytosed and killed, but children do not generally produce them until 2–3 years of age possibly because these antibodies are T cell independent. In addition to the capsule, *H. influenzae* has several other virulence factors, as shown in Table 25.3.

*Acute* **H. influenzae** *meningitis is commonly complicated by severe neurologic sequelae*. The incubation period of *H. influenzae* meningitis is 5–6 days, and the onset is often more insidious than that of meningococcal or pneumococcal meningitis (see Table 25.5). The condition is less frequently fatal, but, as with meningococcal infection, serious sequelae such as hearing loss, delayed language development and mental retardation and seizures may occur.

General diagnostic features are the same as for meningococcal meningitis, as explained earlier. It is important to note that the organisms may be difficult to see in gram-stained smears of CSF, particularly if they are present in small numbers. Ceftriaxone treatment is recommended.

**H. influenzae** *type b (Hib) vaccine is effective for children from 2 months of age*. General features of treatment are referred to earlier under meningococcal meningitis; details are summarized in Table 25.2. An effective Hib vaccine, suitable for children ≥2 months of age, is available. Conjugate Hib vaccines are made from the purified polyribosylribitol phosphate capsular polysaccharide of Hib linked to a carrier protein. Rifampicin prophylaxis is recommended for close contacts of patients with invasive Hib disease.

### Pneumococcal meningitis

**Streptococcus pneumoniae** *is a common cause of bacterial meningitis, particularly in children and the elderly*. *S. pneumoniae* was first isolated >100 years ago, but relatively little is known about its virulence attributes apart from its polysaccharide capsule (see Tables 25.3 and 25.4), and the pneumococcus remains a major cause of morbidity and mortality. (Pneumococcal respiratory tract infections are reviewed in Ch. 20.)

*S. pneumoniae* is a capsulate gram-positive coccus carried in the throats of many healthy individuals. Invasion of the blood and meninges is a rare event but is more common in the very young (<2 years of age), in the elderly, in those with sickle cell disease, in debilitated or splenectomized patients and following head trauma. Susceptibility to infection is associated with low levels of antibodies to capsular polysaccharide antigens: Antibody opsonizes the organism and promotes phagocytosis, thereby protecting the host from invasion. However, this protection is type specific, and there are >85 different capsular types of *S. pneumoniae*.

The clinical features of pneumococcal meningitis are generally worse than with *N. meningitidis* and *H. influenzae* and are summarized in Table 25.5. The general diagnostic features are the same as for meningococcal meningitis described earlier.

Treatment and prevention of pneumococcal meningitis are summarized in Table 25.2. Since penicillin-resistant pneumococci have been observed worldwide, attention must be paid to the antibiotic susceptibility of the infecting strain, and empiric chemotherapy usually involves a combination of vancomycin and either cefotaxime or ceftriaxone.

Two effective pneumococcal vaccines are the pneumococcal conjugate vaccine (PCV) containing polysaccharide from 13 common capsular types conjugated to protein (PCV13) and the pneumococcal polysaccharide vaccine PPV23 with 23 common capsular types. PCV13 is available and is recommended in the United Kingdom for all <1-year-olds (i.e. to be given with other recommended childhood vaccines) and for 2- to 64-year-olds at high risk (e.g. sickle cell disease, HIV infection, chronic illness, weakened immune systems) for serious pneumococcal infection. The older 23-valent PPV remains available for all adults age ≥65 years and individuals from 2–64 years of age at high risk (as earlier). This is because children age <2 years have poor antibody responses to PPV. The CDC has similar recommendations, but PCV15 and PCV20 vaccine formulations are included.

### Listeria monocytogenes meningitis

**L. monocytogenes** *causes meningitis in immunocompromised adults*. *L. monocytogenes* is a gram-positive coccobacillus and an important cause of meningitis in immunocompromised adults. It also causes intrauterine infections and infections of the newborn, as summarized in Chapter 24. *L. monocytogenes* is less susceptible than *S. pneumoniae* to penicillin, and the recommended treatment is a combination of ceftriaxone and amoxicillin.

### Neonatal meningitis

In general, neonates, especially those with low birth weight, are at increased risk for meningitis because of their immature immunologic status. This is illustrated by problems with, for example, humoral and cellular immunity, phagocytic capability and inefficient alternative complement pathway. This is especially true as a result of medical advances that have contributed to the increased survival of preterm infants.

*Although mortality rates due to neonatal meningitis in resource-rich countries are declining, the problem is still serious*. Neonatal meningitis can be caused by a wide range of bacteria, but the most frequent are group B haemolytic streptococci and *Escherichia coli* (Table 25.6; see also Ch. 24). This may occur by routes such as nosocomial infection; however, the infant may also be infected from the mother. For example, with women vaginally colonized by group B streptococci, the infant may swallow maternal secretions such as infected amniotic fluid during delivery.

Neonatal meningitis often leads to permanent neurologic sequelae such as cerebral or cranial nerve palsy, epilepsy, mental retardation or hydrocephalus. This is partly because the clinical diagnosis of meningitis in the neonate is difficult, perhaps with no more specific signs than fever, poor feeding, vomiting, respiratory distress or diarrhoea. In addition, due to the possible range of aetiologic agents, blind antibiotic therapy in the absence of susceptibility tests may not be optimal, and adequate penetration of the antibiotic into the CSF is an issue. Antibiotic treatment includes benzylpenicillin and gentamicin.

### Tuberculous meningitis

Patients with tuberculous meningitis always have a focus of infection elsewhere, but ~25% may have no clinical or historic

**Table 25.6** Group B streptococci are a major cause of neonatal meningitis

| Group B streptococci *(Streptococcus agalactiae)* are normal inhabitants of the female genital tract and may be acquired by the neonate | | |
|---|---|---|
| | **At or soon after birth** | **In the nursery** |
| | *Early onset disease* | *Late onset disease* |
| Age | <7 days | 1 wk–3 mo |
| Risk factors | Heavily colonized mother lacking specific antibody<br>Premature rupture of membranes<br>Preterm delivery<br>Prolonged labour, obstetric complications | Lack of maternal antibody<br>Exposure to cross-infection from heavily colonized babies<br>Poor hygiene in nursery |
| Type of disease | Generalized infection, including bacteraemia, pneumonia, meningitis | Predominantly meningitis |
| Type of group B streptococcus | All serotypes but meningitis mostly due to type III | 90% type III |
| Outcome | ~60% fatal; serious sequelae in many survivors | ~20% fatal |
| Treatment | Collect blood and CSF for culture | Treat on suspicion |
| | Treat on suspicion | Collect blood and CSF for culture |
| | Gentamicin and benzylpenicillin | Gentamicin and benzylpenicillin |
| Prevention | Antibiotic treatment does not reliably abolish carriage in mother, not recommended | Good hygiene practices in nursery |
| | Blind treatment of sick baby who has risk factors<br>Future: ? immunise antibody-negative females of childbearing age | Do not allow mothers to handle other babies |

CSF, Cerebrospinal fluid.

**Fig. 25.5** The association between acute miliary tuberculosis and meningitis. (* Leads to miliary tuberculosis [Latin: *milium*, millet seed—each tubercle resembles a millet seed]. Miliary tuberculosis also occurs in the lungs and elsewhere.)

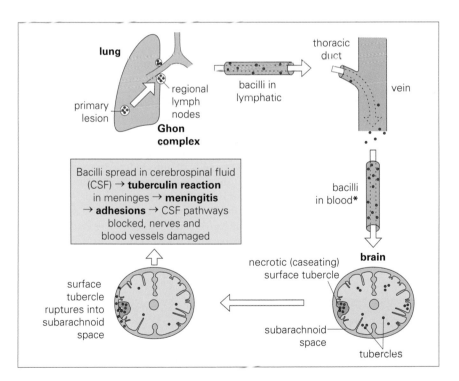

evidence of such an infection. In >50% of cases, meningitis is associated with acute miliary tuberculosis (Fig. 25.5). In areas with a high prevalence of tuberculosis, meningitis tends to be most commonly seen in children from 0–4 years of age. However, in areas where tuberculosis is less frequent, most meningitis cases are in adults.

***Tuberculous meningitis usually presents with a gradual onset over a few weeks***. There is a gradual onset of generalized illness beginning with malaise, apathy and anorexia and proceeding within a few weeks to photophobia, neck stiffness and impairment of consciousness. Occasionally the onset is much more rapid and may be mistaken for a subarachnoid haemorrhage. The variability of presentation means that the clinician needs to maintain an awareness of possible tuberculous meningitis to make the diagnosis. A delay in making the diagnosis and in starting appropriate antimicrobial therapy (see Table 25.2) results in serious complications and sequelae.

Spinal tuberculosis is more common in resource-poor countries; bacteria in the vertebrae destroy the intervertebral disks to form epidural abscesses. These compress the spinal cord and lead to paraplegia.

## Fungal meningitis

*Cryptococcus* spp. and *Coccidioides immitis* can invade the blood from a primary site of infection in the lungs and then travel to the brain to cause meningitis.

### Cryptococcosis

*Cryptococcus* has a marked tropism for the CNS and is the major cause of fungal meningitis.

*Cryptococcus* occurs as two species complexes, *C. neoformans* and *C. gattii*.

*C. neoformans* meningitis is seen in patients with depressed cell-mediated immunity. Therefore, it occurs in individuals with advanced HIV infection and other immunosuppressive conditions. *C. gattii* was first recognized in tropical and subtropical areas but has now been responsible for outbreaks of meningitis in the temperate zone. A significant proportion of *C. gattii* cases have occurred in immunocompetent individuals.

The onset of cryptococcal meningitis is usually slow, over days or weeks. The round, capsulate, budding yeasts of various sizes can be seen in Indian ink–stained preparations of CSF (Fig. 25.6) and can be cultured. Rapid cryptococcal antigen detection using a lateral flow assay on serum and CSF is also a useful diagnostic tool. Treatment with the antifungal drugs fluconazole, amphotericin B and flucytosine in combination is recommended, plus therapeutic lumbar puncture if the CSF pressure is elevated.

### *Coccidioides immitis* infection is common in particular geographic locations

These locations are notably the US southwest, Mexico, and South America. CNS infection occurs in <1% of infected individuals but is fatal unless treated. It may be part of generalized disease or may represent the only extrapulmonary site. The organisms are rarely visible in the CSF, and cultures are positive in <50% of cases, but the diagnosis can be made by antigen detection, polymerase chain reaction (PCR) and antibody detection in the CSF. Enzyme-linked immunosorbent assay (ELISA), immunodiffusion or complement fixation tests detect antibodies in the serum. Treatment with fluconazole or liposomal amphotericin B is recommended.

## Protozoal meningitis

The thermophilic free-living amoeba, *Naegleria fowleri*, lives in warm fresh water, especially in the sludge at the bottom of lakes and swimming pools where it feeds on bacteria. If inhaled, *N. fowleri* can reach the meninges via the olfactory tract and cribriform plate. Primary amoebic meningoencephalitis (PAM) caused by *Naegleria* affects healthy individuals with no obvious defect in immunity. The United States and Pakistan have reported the highest numbers of cases. The disease has a rapid onset, and the mortality rate is ~98%, with death occurring in <2 weeks.

*Acanthamoeba* spp. are widespread in the environment. They more commonly affect those who are already unwell, for example, with diabetes, or immunocompromised, including organ transplant recipients and people living with HIV. *Acanthamoeba* are thought to enter via the skin or the respiratory tract and go on to cause a chronic progressive condition, granulomatous amoebic encephalitis (GAE). Neuroimaging shows one or more hyperintense, rim-enhancing lesions, which need to be differentiated from those due to *Toxoplasma*. GAE is almost always fatal, although survival has been seen in patients diagnosed early and given combination therapy.

*Balamuthia mandrillaris* is found in soil or stagnant water as vegetative trophozoites and dormant cysts. Humans become infected by inhalation of cysts or direct contamination of skin. Several months may elapse between the appearance of cutaneous lesions and invasion of the CNS. Cases have been reported in patients with a variety of underlying medical conditions but also in immunocompetent individuals. Infection of the CNS produces GAE with raised protein, lymphocytic CSF and normal or low CSF glucose, but in the presence of severely compromised cellular immunity there may be little granuloma formation. Mortality from *Balamuthia* encephalitis is >90%, and death occurs in days to weeks.

Under the microscope, *N. fowleri* appears as slowly motile amoebae on careful examination of a fresh wet sample of CSF. *Acanthamoeba* spp. are rarely seen in the CSF but can be visualized in brain biopsies. They also grow well in cultures prepared from fresh tissue biopsies. PCR is available in specialist centres. Diagnosis of *Balamuthia* infection is by histopathology of biopsy samples and PCR on brain tissue or CSF.

Serology for *Acanthamoeba* and *Balamuthia* is available in some reference laboratories but is of limited value given the frequent exposure to amoebae in the healthy general population on the one hand and a greatly reduced antibody response in advanced immunosuppression on the other. Serology is of no value in the diagnosis of *Naegleria* infection given its fulminant progression.

Treatment for PAM and GAE is not fully satisfactory. There have been no randomized clinical trials, and recommendations for management are based on expert review of case reports. Treatment needs to be given as early as possible, and combination therapy is administered for all forms of amoebic encephalitis. The inclusion of miltefosine in the regimen is reported to be associated with a greater chance of survival in *Balamuthia* and *Acanthamoeba* cases.

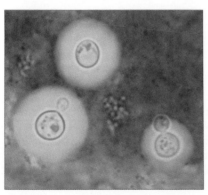

**Fig. 25.6** *Cryptococcus neoformans* in India ink–stained preparation of cerebrospinal fluid sediment. (Courtesy A.E. Prevost.)

## Viral meningitis

### Viral meningitis is the most common type of meningitis

The incidence of viral, compared with bacterial, meningitis in the United Kingdom is ~2.73/100,000 population compared with 1.24/100,000. Around 42,000 admissions annually to US hospitals are due to viral meningitis. It is a milder disease than bacterial meningitis, with headache, fever and photophobia but less neck stiffness. The CSF is clear in the absence of bacteria, and the cells are mainly lymphocytes, although polymorphonuclear leukocytes may be present in the early stages (see Table 25.1).

Enteroviral infections are the most common cause of meningitis in infants and young children. There are five groups of human enteroviruses, which include the echoviruses, coxsackie group A and B viruses and three types of polioviruses. The non-polio enteroviruses are the most common causes of seasonal aseptic meningitis, usually from late spring to autumn. HSV meningitis is seen in young and older adults. HSV type 2 is more common than type 1 and can be a benign recurrent aseptic meningitis; it is called *Mollaret meningitis* after the French neurologist who first described it in 1944. Mumps is another cause, mostly in those unimmunised. Otherwise, in specific parts of the world, tick or mosquitos are vectors for seasonal arboviral infections, and as the climate changes, these infections may emerge elsewhere.

PCR revolutionised viral detection in this clinical setting as virus isolation methods in cell culture resulted in a diagnosis of viral meningitis in <50% of samples. No specific antiviral treatment has been shown to affect the clinical course and so is not recommended. Pain relief and conservative management is the rule. In contrast to bacterial meningitis, viral meningitis usually has a benign course, and complete recovery is the rule.

## ENCEPHALITIS

### Encephalitis is usually caused by viruses, but there are many cases in which the infectious aetiology is not identified

The pathogenesis of viral encephalitis is shown in Fig. 25.7. The estimated incidence of encephalitis in a US study between 1998 and 2010 reported ~20,000 encephalitis-associated hospital admissions per year, with a 6% mortality rate and substantial morbidity, including physical, cognitive and behavioural difficulties. It is thought that the annual costs of illness caused by encephalitis to the US health service amounts to roughly US$630 million.

Characteristically, there are signs of cerebral dysfunction, as the substance of the brain is affected, unlike meningitis in which the lining of the brain is inflamed. Someone with an encephalitic illness will present with abnormal behaviour, headache, confusion, seizures and altered consciousness, often with nausea, vomiting and fever.

Up to 85% of individuals diagnosed with encephalitis globally are of unknown aetiology. The most common viral causes include HSV, enterovirus and mumps virus infections. Emerging viruses that can cause encephalitis include the

**Fig. 25.7** The pathogenesis of viral encephalomyelitis. Mφ, Macrophage; NK, natural killer cell.

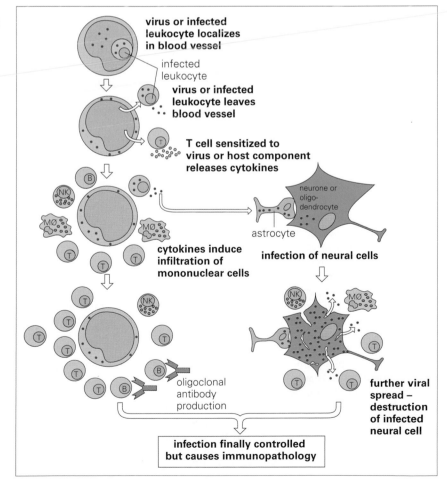

virus or infected leukocyte localizes in blood vessel

infected leukocyte

virus or infected leukocyte leaves blood vessel

T cell sensitized to virus or host component releases cytokines

neurone or oligo-dendrocyte

astrocyte

cytokines induce infiltration of mononuclear cells

infection of neural cells

oligoclonal antibody production

further viral spread – destruction of infected neural cell

infection finally controlled but causes immunopathology

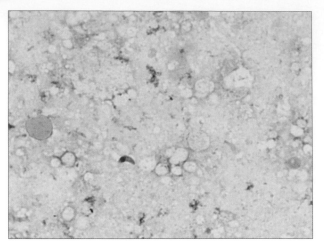

**Fig. 25.8** *Toxoplasma* tachyzoite in a brain biopsy smear. (Courtesy Peter Chiodini.)

Nipah virus and bat lyssaviruses. Immune-mediated forms of encephalitis, including voltage-gated potassium channel and *N*-methyl-D-aspartate (NMDA) receptor antibody-associated encephalitis, must be considered in the differential diagnosis as they have a presentation similar to that of infectious causes. This diagnosis is particularly important to consider as steroids can be used to treat the immune-mediated encephalitides, including acute disseminated encephalomyelitis (ADEM).

Antiviral drugs such as aciclovir are used to treat HSV and VZV encephalitis. Preventative measures include measles, mumps, and rubella immunisation.

*Toxoplasma gondii* and *C. neoformans* can also cause life-threatening encephalitis or meningoencephalitis (Fig. 25.8). This is particularly likely in those with defective cell-mediated immunity, and cerebral malaria as a complication of *Plasmodium falciparum* infection is frequently fatal. Encephalitis may occur in Lyme disease (*Borrelia burgdorferi*) and Legionnaires' disease (*Legionella pneumophila*), but the relative importance of bacterial invasion, bacterial toxins and immunopathology is unknown.

### HSV encephalitis (HSE) is the most common form of severe sporadic acute focal encephalitis, and early aciclovir treatment is critical

It is thought that the incidence of HSE in the United States is ~1/250,000–500,000 population per year. A distinction is made between HSV infections of the CNS during the neonatal period and those in older children and adults. Neonates may acquire a primary and disseminated infection with diffuse encephalitis after vaginal delivery from a mother shedding HSV-2 in the genital tract. Most HSE seen in older children and adults is due to HSV-1, of which most are due to virus reactivation in the trigeminal ganglia, the infection then passing back to the temporal lobe of the brain, and the minority are due to a primary infection. About 30% of HSE is seen in people <20 years old, and 50% in those >50 years.

Herpetic skin or mucosal lesions may be present. The diagnosis is indicated by finding temporal lobe enhancement using computed tomography (CT) and the more sensitive magnetic resonance imaging (MRI) scans of the head (Fig. 25.9). HSV DNA detection is carried out on a CSF sample using PCR. An electroencephalogram (EEG) may also

be helpful. The 70% mortality rate in untreated patients is greatly reduced by early and prolonged treatment with intravenous aciclovir. The 14- to 21-day treatment course is important, as relapse can occur. It is recommended that when HSV DNA is detected in the CSF, a further CSF is collected at 2 weeks and treatment is continued if the HSV DNA result is still positive.

### Other herpesviruses less commonly cause encephalitis

With VZV, encephalitis generally occurs as a sequel to reactivation and with CMV during either primary infection in utero or reactivation as a complication of immunosuppression. Human herpesvirus 6 (HHV-6) encephalitis has also been reported in immunosuppressed patients. Finally, B virus is a Cercopithecine herpesvirus of macaque monkeys that does not really affect the animal but can cause severe and fatal encephalitis in humans who are bitten or scratched by an infected monkey. The wound should be cleaned immediately, and aciclovir prophylaxis is recommended.

## Enteroviral infections

### Enterovirus 71–associated hand, foot, and mouth epidemic resulted in a high rate of neurologic complications

Other enteroviruses such as coxsackieviruses and echoviruses occasionally cause meningoencephalitis. However, in 1998 there was a large outbreak of enterovirus 71 (EV71) hand, foot and mouth disease (HFMD) infection in Taiwan in which most of the 405 patients were children age <5 years with a mortality rate of 19%. The most severely affected children had brainstem involvement, and many were left with permanent neurologic sequelae. Treatment is supportive, and there is no vaccine. Since then, EV71, having been identified in Guangdong province in the People's Republic of China and having caused epidemics in south China, then caused several epidemics reported in the middle or north of China. Overall, by August 2016, ~1,800,000 HFMD infections had been reported nationwide, including 172 deaths.

### Poliovirus used to be a common cause of encephalitis

In the great 1916 polio epidemic in New York City, 9000 cases of paralysis were reported, nearly all in children <5 years old. CNS disease occurs in <1% of those infected. After an initial 1–4 days of fever, sore throat and malaise, meningeal signs and symptoms appear, followed by involvement of motor neurones and paralysis (see Fig. 25.2).

There are effective vaccines; the structure (Fig. 25.10) and replication of the virus are better understood, and efforts to eradicate the disease by 2023 had driven the incidence of polio to its lowest point in history. The disease is completely preventable by vaccination (see Ch. 35) and has been disappearing in resource-rich countries since vaccination programmes were first carried out in the 1950s (Fig. 25.11). There are three polioviruses (types 1, 2, 3), and the Global Polio Eradication Initiative reduced the number of polio-endemic countries. The fall in poliovirus transmission in these countries was due to oral live attenuated polio vaccine and new ways of delivering the vaccine. However, in areas where vaccine coverage is low, the live attenuated vaccine could circulate and revert to wild type. Inactivated polio vaccines (IPVs) replaced oral polio vaccines (OPVs) in many countries in the late 1990s.

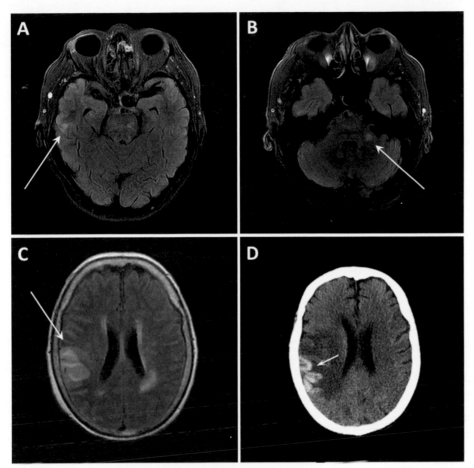

**Fig. 25.9** Brain imaging in a case of herpes simplex virus encephalitis. (A) and (B) demonstrate T2-weighted brain magnetic resonance imaging (MRI) 1 day after presentation, with *arrows* showing signal abnormalities in right temporal (A) and left middle cerebellar peduncle (B) regions. (C) Shows T2-weighted MRI signal abnormality in the right parietal region *(arrow)* 11 days after presentation. (D) Computed tomography head shows laminar necrosis *(arrow)* in the right parietal lesion 37 days after presentation. (From Niksefat M, et al. Third time's a charm: diagnosis of herpes simplex encephalitis after two negative polymerase chain reaction results. *Heliyon.* 2020;6(6):E04247. https://doi.org/10.1016/j.heliyon.2020.e04247.)

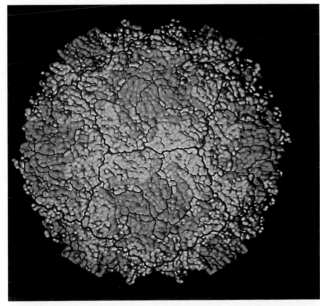

**Fig. 25.10** Computer graphic model of the surface of a poliovirus based on x-ray diffraction studies. The capsid protein subunits visible on the surface of the virus particle are viral protein 1 (VP1) in blue, VP2 in green and VP3 in grey. (Courtesy A.J. Olson, Research Institute of Scripps Clinic, La Jolla, CA.)

Wild poliovirus infections have fallen by >99% since 1988, from ~350,000 in >125 endemic countries to 6 reported infected individuals in 2021. Wild poliovirus types 2 and 3 were eradicated in 1999 and 2020, respectively. By 2022, however, endemic wild poliovirus type 1 transmission was still occurring in Pakistan and Afghanistan. In addition, emergence and spread of circulating vaccine-derived polioviruses led to 44 outbreaks between 2020 and 2021 in 37 countries with >90% of all vaccine-derived outbreaks involving the OPV type 2 strain. In 2022 there were environmental surveillance reports involving testing wastewater samples as the live attenuated vaccine virus is excreted in faeces, of mostly poliovirus type 2 detection, in IPV-only regions, including parts of Italy, the Netherlands, United Kingdom, Canada, United States, Israel, Argentina, Japan, Indonesia and Switzerland. Between February 8 and July 4, 2022, 118 genetically linked OPV type 2 polioviruses were detected in multiple sites in the London sewage network. After sequencing and phylogenetic analysis, these indicated local transmission and enhanced surveillance, thus an IPV immunisation programme in those areas was instituted.

The three serologic (antigenic) types of poliovirus have little cross-reaction between them so that antibody to each type is necessary for protection. At least 75% of paralytic cases are due to type 1 polioviruses.

357

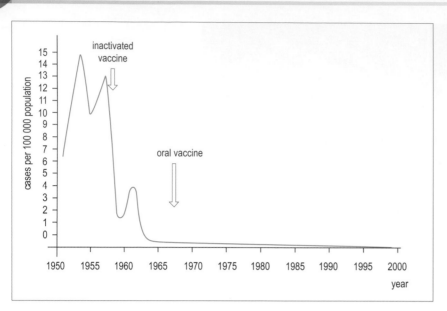

**Fig. 25.11** The incidence of paralytic poliomyelitis in the United States from 1951–2000.

## Paramyxoviral infections

### Mumps virus is a common cause of mild encephalitis

Asymptomatic CNS invasion may be common because there are increased numbers of cells in the CSF in ~50% of patients with parotitis. However, meningitis and encephalitis are often seen without parotitis.

### Four different types of encephalitis are associated with measles virus infection at different times after rash onset

Primary measles encephalitis and acute postinfectious measles encephalitis may occur ~7 days after the rash in 1/1000 individuals with measles. ADEM can also occur (see later). In immunocompromised patients, measles inclusion body encephalitis is very rare (Fig. 25.12) and can occur weeks to many months later. SSPE can occur 1–15 years after rash onset, and depending on the age at infection it can occur in 1/8000 if <2 years of age and 1/25,000 in older age groups.

### Nipah virus encephalitis, a zoonotic paramyxovirus infection

In 1998 an outbreak of encephalitis with a high mortality rate was reported among pig farm workers in Malaysia. In total, there were 105 deaths among 265 patients with Nipah virus encephalitis. Some patients had respiratory symptoms early on in the infection. At first attributed to JE, the clinical, epidemiologic and virologic characteristics showed that the virus was a paramyxovirus transmitted to humans by close contact with infected pigs, probably by aerosol. The outbreak was ended by culling >1 million infected or exposed pigs in the local and surrounding regions in Malaysia. The island flying fox, *Pteropus hypomelanus*, a fruit bat, is the natural reservoir for the virus, and the virus can be found in the urine and saliva of infected bats. The pigs were infected, having eaten food contaminated by fruit bat secretions. Human-to-human transmission can also play an important role in Nipah virus transmission. Further outbreaks were reported in 2001 in Bangladesh and India, where there were reports of human-to-human transmission in hospital settings. Since then there have been almost annual outbreaks in Bangladesh and occasionally in East India, with a mortality rate of 40–75%. By 2023 Nipah virus had been found in several bat species in other parts of the world, including Ghana, Cambodia, Thailand and the Philippines. The diagnosis is made by PCR and antibody detection. There are neither specific antiviral treatments nor vaccines available. Raising awareness and reducing potential exposure are key.

## Rabies encephalitis

### More than 55,000 people die of rabies worldwide each year

- Rabies occurs in >150 countries and territories.
- Wound cleansing and immunization within a few hours after contact with a suspect rabid animal can prevent the onset of rabies and death.
- Every year >29 million people worldwide receive a post-exposure preventive regimen to avert the disease, which is estimated to prevent hundreds of thousands of rabies-related deaths annually.

Rabies is caused by a rhabdovirus, an enveloped, bullet-shaped, single-stranded RNA virus. The *Lyssavirus* genus sits within the Rhabdoviridae family, and there are seven genotypes: Genotype 1 occurs worldwide and is the classic rabies virus; genotypes 2, 3 and 4 are the African Lagos, Mokola and Duvenhage bat viruses, respectively; genotypes 5 and 6 are the European bat Lyssaviruses (EBLV) 1 and 2, respectively; and genotype 7 is the Australian bat Lyssavirus.

The virus is excreted in the saliva of infected dogs, foxes, jackals, wolves, skunks, raccoons and vampire and other bats, and transmission to humans follows a bite or salivary contamination of other types of skin abrasions or wounds. The infection is eventually fatal, although the course of the disease varies considerably between species. If an apparently healthy dog is still healthy 15 days after biting a human, rabies infection in the dog is extremely unlikely. However, the virus may be excreted in the dog's saliva before the animal shows any clinical signs of disease.

The virus can infect all warm-blooded animals. Rabies from vampire bats causes >1 million deaths per year in cattle in Central and South America. Dogs are the source of >99% of

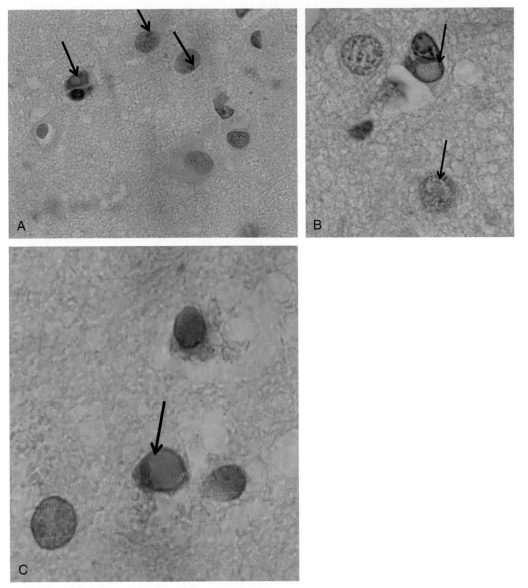

**Fig. 25.12** Measles inclusion body encephalitis. Brain biopsy showing many viral inclusion bodies *(shown by arrows)*, mild reactive changes and no significant inflammation (A–C low to higher power magnification). (Courtesy Dr. I. Bodi, King's College Hospital, London.)

human rabies deaths and are involved in most of the estimated 57,000 cases of human rabies that occur in the world each year. In all the mainland masses, the infection maintains itself in nonhuman mammalian hosts. Islands such as Australia, Great Britain, Japan, Hawaii, most of the Caribbean islands and Scandinavia are free of rabies because of strict controls over the importation of animals such as dogs and cats, although this is changing. Since the development of the Channel Tunnel linking the United Kingdom and the rest of Europe, a number of rabies infections occurred associated with contact with bats. Thirty different bat species have been identified in Europe, a number of which carry EBLV 1 or 2. They are distinct from rabies genotype 1 infections in foxes, dogs, and other terrestrial animals. In the United States the incidence of human rabies has been falling since the 1940s and 1950s, when most cases followed exposure to infected dogs. Since then, the source has more often been nondomesticated animals such as skunks, raccoons and bats or exposure to dogs in other countries.

Raccoon rabies spread slowly northwards from Florida in the 1950s and, in the 1980s, caused an explosive epidemic in Virginia, Maryland and the District of Columbia. This outbreak was due to the importation of raccoons from infected areas for sporting purposes.

The incubation period in humans is generally 4–13 weeks, although it may occasionally be as long as 6 months or more, possibly due to a delay in virus entry into peripheral nerves. The virus travels up peripheral nerves, and, in general, the further the bite is from the CNS, the longer the incubation period. For instance, a bite on the foot leads to a longer incubation period than a bite on the face.

While the virus is travelling up the axons of motor or sensory neurones, there is no detectable antibody or cell-mediated immune response possibly because antigen remains sequestered in infected muscle cells. Therefore, passive immunization using rabies-specific immunoglobulin may be given during the incubation period.

Once in the brain, the virus spreads from cell to cell until a large proportion of neurones are infected, but there is little cytopathic effect and almost no cellular infiltration. The striking symptoms of this disease are largely due to dysfunction rather than to visible damage to infected cells. The change in behaviour of infected animals results from virus invasion of the limbic system.

### Clinical features of rabies include muscle spasms, convulsions and hydrophobia

After developing discomfort at the site of the bite and a sore throat, headache and fever, the patient becomes excited, with muscle spasms and convulsions. Involvement of the muscles of swallowing when attempting to drink water gave the old name for rabies—hydrophobia—as the symptoms are sometimes precipitated by the mere sight of water.

Once rabies has developed, it is fatal, with rare exceptions (see below), and death occurs following cardiac or respiratory arrest. Paralysis is often a major feature of the disease.

### Rabies can be diagnosed by detecting viral antigen or RNA

Laboratory diagnosis can be made by the detection of viral antigen by immunofluorescence or using PCR to detect rabies viral RNA in skin biopsies, corneal impression smears or brain biopsy. Characteristic intracytoplasmic inclusions called *Negri bodies* are seen in neurones (Fig. 25.13). There is no treatment except supportive care. Five individuals have survived having received immunoprophylaxis before symptom onset. There was also a report in 2005 of a 15-year-old girl who was bitten by a bat and developed rabies. She had not received rabies immunoprophylaxis and was put into a medically induced coma to rest and protect the brain from injury and to allow the immune response to mature. The coma was induced using specific receptor antagonists and agonists that reduced brain metabolism, autonomic reactivity and excitotoxicity. Antivirals were given, too, and she survived. This was referred to as the *Milwaukee protocol*.

Many countries (e.g. France) have developed vaccination programmes for domestic dogs, and in Canada and elsewhere, wild foxes have been vaccinated by dropping food baited with live virus vaccine from the air. For the rabies-free countries, constant vigilance at borders and strict quarantine regulations are necessary to prevent the introduction of infected animals. In 1886 there were 36 human rabies deaths

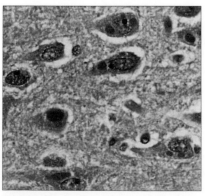

**Fig. 25.13** Multiple cytoplasmic Negri bodies in pyramidal neurones of the hippocampus in rabies. (Courtesy P. Garen.)

in England, 11 of them in London. As recently as 1906 rabies was still endemic in England, and there were deaths due to rabies in the deer in Hampton Court Park, London.

### After exposure to a possibly infected animal, immediate preventive action should be taken

This action includes:

- prompt cleaning of the wound (alcoholic iodine, debridement)
- confirmation of whether the animal is rabid (clinical observation of suspected dogs)
- administration of human rabies immunoglobulin (RIG) to ensure prompt passive immunization; RIG is infiltrated intramuscularly around the wound site
- active immunization with killed diploid cell-derived rabies virus (see Ch. 35). The chances of preventing the disease are greater when vaccination is started as early as possible after infection. Vaccine and RIG must never be administered at the same anatomic site.

## Togavirus meningitis and encephalitis

### Numerous arthropod-borne togaviruses can cause meningitis or encephalitis

These togaviruses sometimes cause outbreaks of infection. In different parts of the world, different mammals, birds or even reptiles act as reservoirs, and there are a variety of arthropod (mosquito and tick) vectors. Usually <1% of humans infected develop neurologic disease (see Ch. 28). There may be a febrile illness, but asymptomatic infection is common. In California, for instance, western equine encephalomyelitis (WEE) virus and St. Louis encephalitis (SLE) virus are prevalent and are transmitted by the mosquito *Culex tarsalis*; a WEE vaccine is available but only for horses.

## Flavivirus infections

### Japanese encephalitis virus infection is an important cause of encephalitis in Southeast Asia and mostly affects children

Japanese encephalitis (JE) virus, a flavivirus infection related to dengue, yellow fever and WNV, is (as you may have guessed) prevalent in Southeast Asia. The majority of reported JE infections (~70,000/yr) are in China and India. It is transmitted by *Culex* mosquitoes with pigs and wading birds as intermediate hosts. Many adults in endemic countries have been infected in childhood and are immune. Infection can result in a mortality of >30%. Inactivated and live attenuated vaccines have been developed, with immunisation programmes in endemic countries that are mostly using the live attenuated vaccine.

### West Nile virus infection swept rapidly through the United States after the initial reports

In 1999 a dramatic epidemic of viral encephalitis was reported in New York City, leading to 62 patients with encephalitis, 7 of whom died. Meningoencephalitis was rare in the younger age groups and more common in those >50 years of age. Originally thought to be due to SLE, once again the clinical, epidemiologic and virologic characteristics resulted in the correct identification of WNV infection, as there had been an epidemic of deaths among wild and other birds, which are the avian reservoir of SLE but are not usually killed by the virus. How the virus had been introduced into North America, having been circulating in Israel and Tunisia, was unclear. Israeli domestic geese had developed fatal WNV infections in 1997–1998, and human WNV infections occurred in August 1999 in both countries. Infected *Culex* spp. mosquitoes transmit WNV to birds, some of which develop high levels of viraemia, and other mosquitoes bite them and become infected, helping cycle WNV. In New York City an outbreak of infection in birds with a high mortality rate had been reported but not linked with the cluster of human infections. Extensive pathologic assessments were carried out, and genome sequencing demonstrated that the WNV strains were homologous. To illustrate the remarkable speed of WNV spread in North America, there were 21 human infections in 10 counties in the northeast in 2000; 66 human infections in 38 counties in 10 states by 2001, and by 2003 there were >4000 human infections with ~2500 cases of meningoencephalitis and 284 deaths. This was the largest outbreak of WNV meningoencephalitis ever recorded, with severe CNS disease seen in older people and milder, feverish illness in younger people. Bird death and mosquito pool surveillance was important to track from a public health perspective. Transmission was also reported due to untested WN viraemic blood transfusions and in four organ transplant recipients who had received organs from one donor who had West Nile viraemia antemortem.

WNV belongs to the JE serogroup of flaviviruses that includes SLE; it had not been seen in the Western Hemisphere but was well recognized in Africa and the Middle East. WNV is primarily an infection of birds and culicine mosquitoes, with humans and horses acting as incidental hosts. Since 1999 the virus has been successfully dispersed by migratory birds and has spread through most of the United States. At the start of the 2022 season, 965 WNV infections in humans were reported by the European Centre for Disease Prevention and Control in a host of European countries, including Italy, Greece, Romania, Hungary, Germany, Croatia, Austria, Spain, France and Slovakia.

The diagnosis can be made by detecting WNV RNA or an immunoglobulin M response in serum and/or CSF samples. Treatment is supportive; there is no vaccine, and prevention includes mosquito control programmes.

## HIV meningitis and encephalitis

### HIV can cause subacute encephalitis, often with dementia

HIV often invades the CNS shortly after initial infection by migration of HIV-infected monocytes across the blood-brain barrier mediated by increased chemokines and resulting in an increase in cells in the CSF and a mild meningitic illness. The monocytes may differentiate into perivascular macrophages that become long-lived reservoirs of HIV that release virus in the CNS and infect macrophages, microglia and astrocytes. These HIV-infected cells produce host and viral factors, activating nearby cells that release neurotoxic mediators and cytokines, leading to chronic neuroinflammation and neuronal damage. The CNS can be a sanctuary site where virus can persist despite combination antiretroviral therapy. A subacute encephalitis may develop, often with dementia. Early in the HIV epidemic, a number of opportunistic CNS infections were detected, part of acquired

immunodeficiency syndrome (AIDS)–defining diagnoses, and were a result of advanced HIV infection and immunosuppression. These included *T. gondii*, *C. neoformans*, CMV and JC virus infections. JC virus, a polyomavirus, occasionally invades oligodendrocytes in immunodeficient people, particularly in AIDS, and eventually gives rise to progressive multifocal leukoencephalopathy. In HIV-related dementia the brain is shrunken, with enlarged ventricles and vacuolation of myelin tracts.

Combined antiretroviral therapy has reduced the incidence of HIV-associated dementia, but neurologic effects of HIV are still seen as the population gets older and are reported as HIV-associated neurocognitive disorders (HAND). HAND is correlated with long-term CNS inflammation and neurotoxicity.

## Viral myelopathy

A number of viral infections can cause inflammation of the spinal cord, a myelitis. Acute myelitis may result in symmetric symptoms if it transverses the spinal cord. These will include motor weakness and sensory loss, for example. The symptoms will be asymmetric if only part of the spinal cord is involved. When the anterior horn cells of the cord are affected by polio, coxsackie, EV71 and WNV infection, the symptoms are motor and result in acute flaccid paralysis. A number of herpesviruses (HSV, CMV, EBV, VZV) have been associated with myelitis. Postinfectious causes have also been reported.

Chronic myelopathy can be caused by HTLV-1 infection, and patients present with tropical spastic paraparesis (TSP), also called *HTLV-1-associated myelopathy (HAM)*. HIV-1 infection is also part of the differential diagnosis.

### Guillain-Barré syndrome—an inflammatory demyelinating condition of the peripheral nervous system

Some 2–4 weeks before Guillain-Barré syndrome (GBS) develops, there is usually a history of an upper respiratory tract or other infection, leading to a rapidly evolving ascending muscle weakness with little sensory loss.

GBS can be classified into a demyelinating or axonal neuropathy, with viral infections more associated with the former and bacterial, especially *Campylobacter jejuni*, the latter. With respect to *C. jejuni*, the pathogenesis is an autoantibody-mediated immune process triggered by molecular mimicry between the Campylobacter lipooligosaccharides and the GM1 ganglioside, part of the plasma membrane of neurones.

GBS is the most common cause of acute flaccid paralysis globally. This can be severe, and patients can deteriorate rapidly, requiring mechanical ventilation to support their breathing. The mortality rate is 5%, and 20% of individuals may be left with mobility difficulties.

GBS has been associated with a variety of infections and with immunisation with noninfectious material. The viral infections include EBV, CMV, HIV, WNV, Zika virus and severe acute respiratory syndrome–associated coronavirus-2 (SARS-CoV-2), but the most common cause in ~30% of patients is bacterial—in particular, *C. jejuni*. *Mycoplasma pneumoniae* and *B. burgdorferi* are rare associations.

In 1976 most US adults were given inactivated influenza virus vaccine, which resulted in a small but highly significant number of cases of GBS.

Treatment is general supportive care, and plasma exchange, which directly removes immune complexes, cytokines, autoantibodies and other inflammatory mediators that may be involved in the pathogenesis, as well as intravenous immunoglobulin, have been shown to be effective.

## Postinfectious encephalitis

### Acute demyelinating encephalomyelitis often follows a viral infection or vaccination and has an autoimmune basis

Acute demyelinating encephalomyelitis (ADEM) is mostly seen in children and is a demyelinating disorder due to an autoimmune response involving antibody to myelin oligodendrocyte glycoprotein (MOG) that is on the surface of the nerve cell's myelin sheath often after an infection or vaccination.

ADEM is rare and has an incidence of ~0.2–0.4/100,000 children annually. It occurs 1–2 weeks after an uneventful measles virus infection and even less commonly after varicella. It may be seen after rubella, influenza, EBV, HSV, enterovirus and SARS-CoV-2 infections as well as *M. pneumoniae*, *B. burgdorferi* and beta-hemolytic Streptococcal infections. The infectious agent is generally neither detectable nor recoverable from the CNS, and the perivascular infiltration, sometimes with demyelination, is part of the autoimmune pathogenesis. A similar condition occurs after administration of brain-derived inactivated rabies vaccine, which is now obsolete, and after other immunisations with noninfectious materials. The clinical picture resembles experimental allergic encephalitis and is due to autoimmune responses triggered by the infection or by the injected material. ADEM is a diagnosis made clinically and by imaging the brain using MRI. Immunotherapeutic treatment includes high-dose intravenous steroids. Intravenous immunoglobulin and plasma exchange have also been given.

In addition, rubella or measles virus invades the CNS, but virus growth is slow, often incomplete, and partially controlled by host defences; clinical disease appears after an incubation period of up to 10 years. For instance:

- in otherwise uncomplicated measles, CNS invasion can take place and eventually result in SSPE
- rubella very occasionally causes a similar disease to SSPE but more commonly, like CMV, it invades the brain of the fetus, interfering with development to cause mental retardation.

## NEUROLOGIC DISEASES OF POSSIBLE VIRAL AETIOLOGY

It has often been suggested that certain neurologic diseases of unknown origin, including multiple sclerosis, amyotrophic lateral sclerosis, Parkinson's disease, schizophrenia and dementia, have a viral origin. These were made more tangible with the reports in 2022 of the epidemiologic association of EBV with multiple sclerosis followed by pathogenesis due to molecular mimicry between the EBV nuclear antigen 1 and the CNS protein glial cell adhesion molecule. Evidence for viruses and other infectious agents triggering autoimmune-type responses in the CNS is gaining ground; another example (mentioned earlier) involved *C. jejuni*.

## SPONGIFORM ENCEPHALOPATHIES CAUSED BY SCRAPIE-TYPE AGENTS

### Scrapie-type agents are closely associated with host-coded prion protein

Scrapie-type agents infect a variety of mammals, including humans, and are transmissible to laboratory rodents or primates. They show a number of remarkable biologic characteristics; their molecular biology is now well described, and experiments in laboratory mice have revealed much about their interaction with host tissues (see Ch. 8). Disease is characterized by the appearance of a spongiform appearance of nervous tissues caused by vacuolation and plaque formation. Infections in animals seem to have originated from sheep and goats with scrapie (see Fig. 8.5), which has been present in Europe for 200–300 years. Affected animals itch and scrape themselves against posts for relief.

## CNS DISEASE CAUSED BY PARASITES

### The CNS is an important target in toxoplasmosis

Although congenitally acquired infection with *T. gondii* is initially generalized, it may become localized in the eye or the CNS. Damage to the eye is the most common consequence (see Ch. 26), but the brain may also be affected, resulting in hydrocephalus and intracerebral calcification.

Most cases of *Toxoplasma* infection are acquired later in life, resulting in asymptomatic latent toxoplasmosis, affecting as much as a third of the world's population overall. In the presence of severe immunocompromise (e.g. due to organ transplantation, immunosuppressive medication, advanced HIV infection), reactivation of *Toxoplasma* present in dormant tissue cysts can occur, resulting in symptomatic disease. In the days before the advent of combined antiretroviral therapy, cerebral toxoplasmosis manifest as unifocal or multifocal necrotizing encephalitis was an important cause of death in patients with advanced HIV infection.

### Cerebral malaria is a major killer

The life cycle of *P. falciparum* shows an unusual feature in that red blood cells containing the asexual stages (asexual stages are in humans; sexual stages are in mosquitoes, see Ch. 28) adhere to the walls of capillaries, a processs known as *sequestration*. This leads to vascular congestion, hypoperfusion and localized hypoxia. When this occurs in the brain and is accompanied by a cytokine storm, cerebral malaria may result. Fever is accompanied by a variety of symptoms, including convulsions and progressive coma, which lead rapidly to death if not treated. Cerebral malaria is an important cause of mortality in African children. Even if they survive, almost a quarter of those children who recover from cerebral malaria with malarial retinopathy have persistent neurologic symptoms such as seizures, cerebral palsy and cognitive impairment. Intravenous artesunate followed by artemisinin combination therapy has replaced quinine as the treatment of choice as it has a clear survival advantage in severe and complicated malaria.

### *Toxocara* infection can result in granuloma formation in the brain and retina

The cat and dog roundworms, *Toxocara cati* and *Toxocara canis*, respectively, infect humans, usually children, when *Toxocara*

**Fig. 25.14** Echinococcosis. (A) Cerebral angiography showing displacement of vessels by a large frontal mass. (B) Cyst removed from patient in (A). (Courtesy H. Whitwell.)

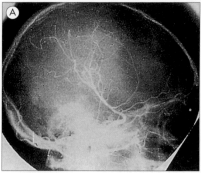
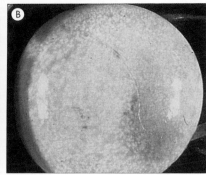

eggs derived from kitten or puppy faeces are ingested. The eggs are nonembryonated when first passed, taking a minimum of 2 weeks to mature in the soil and become infective. After ingestion by humans, the eggs hatch and larvae migrate from the gut via the bloodstream to the liver, lung, kidney, muscles, brain and eye. However, as humans are dead-end hosts for these parasites, they cannot reach full maturity. Granulomas, triggered by *Toxocara* excretory-secretory antigen, form around the larvae, which in the brain may cause convulsions and eosinophilic meningoencephalitis. In the eye it can present most commonly as a tumourlike granuloma in the peripheral retina, followed by a posterior pole granuloma or least commonly by endophthalmitis. Granulomas can cause retinal detachment, and blindness can ensue if the macula is involved. Peripheral blood eosinophilia is rarely seen in ocular toxocariasis.

Serum can be tested for antibodies to *Toxocara* excretory–secretory antigen by ELISA, confirmed by Western blot, but may give false-negative results in ocular toxocariasis. Antibody detection in ocular vitreous fluid samples is more sensitive. Albendazole, under corticosteroid cover, can be given for neurotoxocariasis. Anthelmintic therapy is not always given in ocular toxocariasis. Corticosteroids and appropriate ophthalmic surgery are the mainstays of therapy.

The disease can be prevented by deworming puppies and kittens and by reducing the contamination of children's play areas by dog excreta.

### Cystic echinococcosis (cystic hydatid disease) is characterized by cyst formation, potentially in any organ but most commonly in the liver

Cystic echinococcosis (cystic hydatid disease) is caused by the dog tapeworm *Echinococcus granulosus*, which has a worldwide distribution especially in sheep-rearing areas. When humans ingest eggs from infected dogs, the embryos emerge and migrate through the gut to the portal blood vessels. From there they are carried mainly to the liver, where they subsequently develop into echinococcal cysts. These may occur in any organ but are found especially in the liver and, less commonly, in the lungs, brain, and kidney. In highly endemic areas, cerebral echinococcosis can be found in 2% of humans with cysts in the liver, and it has been suggested that the G6 genotype of *E. granulosus* might have a higher affinity for the brain. Disease is caused by local pressure from the cyst and sometimes hypersensitivity reactions to hydatid antigens. Neurologic symptoms include nausea and vomiting, seizures and altered mental status.

Echinococcosis is diagnosed by detecting serum antibody to hydatid antigens using ELISA, with confirmation by Western blot and, specifically for CNS involvement, by CT or preferably MRI scanning to demonstrate the presence of cysts (Fig. 25.14). Echinococcal cysts in the CNS require surgical removal, with special care to avoid cyst rupture, plus adjunctive therapy with albendazole.

The disease is prevented by interrupting the natural dog–sheep, dog–goat, or other carnivore–herbivore transmission cycle. Deworming of dogs is particularly important.

### Cysticercosis is characterized by cyst formation in the brain and eye

Cysticercosis results from infection with eggs containing the larval stage of *Taenia solium*, the pork tapeworm. Eggs from the adult tapeworm present in human faeces normally infect pigs, which develop cysts in their muscles (measly pork) and are a source of further human infection if the meat is eaten raw or undercooked. However, humans can ingest *T. solium* eggs in material contaminated with human faeces, often from another person's tapeworm rather than from a tapeworm infection of their own, which explains why vegetarians can contract cysticercosis. After passing through the gut wall, larvae released from the eggs are carried in the circulation, usually to skeletal muscle, but also, and more importantly, to the brain (Fig. 25.15) or eye where they develop into cysts known as *cysticerci*. They may cause no symptoms at first if few in number, convulsions or, if very heavily infected, cysticercotic

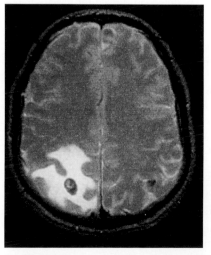

**Fig. 25.15** Cerebral cysticercosis. Magnetic resonance imaging head scan showing a cystic larva. (Courtesy J. Curé.)

encephalopathy. Diagnosis is by visualizing cysts, preferably by MRI scan, and detecting specific antibody using a Western blot and an antigen detection ELISA on serum and CSF where available. Treatment for parenchymal neurocysticercosis is generally with albendazole plus praziquantel under corticosteroid cover, which is superior to albendazole plus corticosteroids. Operative removal is the mainstay of treatment for intraocular cysticerci.

### Sleeping sickness is a trypanosomal infection that is being better controlled

There are two forms of the vector-borne protozoal disease human African trypanosomiasis (HAT; sleeping sickness).

Approximately 85–95% of HAT cases are due to *Trypanosoma brucei gambiense*, known as *West African trypanosomiasis*. They are transmitted to people in mostly rural areas after they have been bitten by the tsetse fly, the flies having acquired their infection from trypanosome-carrying humans, the main reservoir for this parasite.

A person infected with *T. b. gambiense* can be asymptomatic for a long time and only present at an advanced disease stage with CNS signs. Initially, the trypanosomes replicate in the bloodstream, lymphatic tissue and subcutaneous tissue, and symptoms include fever, headache and arthralgia. Then they can cross the blood-brain barrier, resulting in a meningoencephalitis, the hallmark of which is sleepiness, confusion and behavioural change.

Far fewer cases are due to *T. b. rhodesiense* infections, East African trypanosomiasis, which has a reservoir in domestic livestock and wild animals. It runs a shorter, more aggressive clinical course. Cases of imported *T. b. rhodesiense* HAT are occasionally seen in nonendemic areas in travellers returning from East African safari holidays.

### Diagnosis is made by microscopy carried out by skilled, experienced staff, and treatment is complex

Light microscopy is used to detect trypanosomes in peripheral blood for which concentration of samples is often needed. Lymph node aspirates and CSF must also be examined. Molecular-based methods such as PCR and loop-mediated isothermal amplification assays are available in some specialist laboratories. Antibody detection is used for initial screening and as an adjunct to diagnosis in *T. b. gambiense* HAT.

Treatment involves knowing which trypanosome is involved and the disease stage. The various drugs include fexinidazole, pentamidine, suramin, eflornithine, nifurtimox and melarsoprol.

There were huge epidemics in Africa in the 20th century, but sustained tsetse fly control efforts supported by case finding (in the case of *T. b. gambiense*) have been effective. In 2009 <10,000 cases were reported for the first time in 50 years, and in 2021 there were just over 800 cases.

## BRAIN ABSCESSES

### Brain abscesses are usually associated with predisposing factors

Since the development of antibiotics, brain abscesses have become rare and usually follow surgery or trauma, chronic osteomyelitis of neighbouring bone, septic embolism or chronic cerebral anoxia. They are also seen in children with

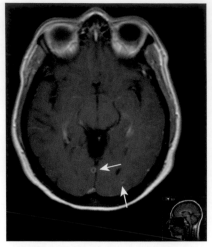

**Fig. 25.16** Magnetic resonance imaging head scan with two tuberculomas *(arrows)*. (Courtesy Dr. G. Bain, London North West Healthcare NHS Trust.)

congenital cyanotic heart disease in whom the lungs fail to filter off circulating bacteria. Acute abscesses are caused by various bacteria, generally of oropharyngeal origin, including anaerobes. There is usually a mixed bacterial flora. Chronic abscesses may be due to *Mycobacterium tuberculosis* (referred to as *tuberculomas*; Fig. 25.16) or *C. neoformans*. In immunosuppressed patients, opportunistic infection may occur with fungi and protozoan aetiologic agents.

Brain abscesses are diagnosed clinically and by CT and MRI brain scans. If an abscess is suspected, lumbar puncture is contraindicated due to potentially raised intracranial pressure and the possibility of coning, which involves cerebellar tonsillar herniation through the foramen magnum compressing the brainstem and death. If performed, it generally shows raised CSF cells and proteins (see Table 25.1). Treatment is by surgical drainage if the abscess is well encapsulated, and antibiotics should be given for at least 1 month. Other infections that may manifest as chronic meningitis or brain abscess are summarized in Table 25.7.

## TETANUS AND BOTULISM

Several bacteria release toxins that act on the nervous system but do not themselves invade the CNS. In the case of *Clostridium tetani* and *C. botulinum*, the major clinical impact is neurologic.

### Tetanus

#### *C. tetani* toxin is carried to the CNS in peripheral nerve axons

Tetanus spores are widespread in soil and originate from the faeces of domestic animals. The spores enter a wound, and if necrotic tissue or the presence of a foreign body permits local and anaerobic growth of bacteria, the toxin tetanospasmin (see Ch. 18) is produced. All strains of *C. tetani* produce the same toxin. The wound can be anything from a small gardener's scratch or cut to that seen in a large automobile or battlefield injury. However, in as many as 20% of cases there is no history of injury. Infection of the umbilical stump can cause neonatal tetanus, which killed ~25,000 newborns in 2018 worldwide (compared with the World Health Organization estimate of ~790,000 in 1989), especially in resource-poor countries.

**Table 25.7** Infections causing chronic meningitis or brain abscess

| Bacterial | |
|---|---|
| Tuberculosis | *Mycobacterium tuberculosis* |
| Syphilis | *Treponema pallidum* |
| Brucellosis | *Brucella abortus* |
| Lyme disease | *Borrelia burgdorferi* |
| Nocardiosis[a] | *Nocardia asteroides* |
| Actinomycosis[a] | *Actinomyces israelii* |
| **Fungal** | |
| Cryptococcosis | *Cryptococcus neoformans* complex *Cryptococcus gattii* |
| Coccidioidomycosis | *Coccidioides immitis* |
| Histoplasmosis | *Histoplasma capsulatum* |
| Candidiasis | *Candida albicans* Other *Candida* spp. (rare) |
| Blastomycosis[a] | *Blastomyces dermatitidis* |
| Aspergillosis | *Aspergillus fumigatus* Other *Aspergillus* spp. |
| Cerebral phaeohyphomycosis | *Cladophialophora bantiana* *Rhinocladiella mackenziei* *Exophiala* spp. Other neurotropic melanized yeasts and moulds |
| **Parasitic** | |
| Toxoplasmosis[a] | *Toxoplasma gondii* |
| Cysticercosis | *Taenia solium* |

[a]Disease manifests as necrotizing encephalitis.

The toxin is carried in peripheral nerve axons and probably in the blood to the CNS, where it binds to neurones and blocks the release of inhibitory mediators in spinal synapses, causing overactivity of motor neurones. It can also pass up sympathetic nerve axons and lead to overactivity of the sympathetic nervous system.

### Clinical features of tetanus include muscle rigidity and spasms

After a period of 3–21 days, but sometimes longer, there are exaggerated reflexes, muscle rigidity and uncontrolled muscle spasms. Lockjaw (trismus) is due to contraction of jaw muscles. Dysphagia, risus sardonicus (a sneering appearance), neck stiffness and opisthotonos (especially in neonatal tetanus) are also seen. Muscle spasms may lead to injury, and eventually there is respiratory failure. Tachycardia and sweating can result from effects on the sympathetic nervous system. Mortality is up to 50% depending on the severity and quality of treatment.

The diagnosis is clinical. Organisms are rarely isolated from the wound, and only a small number of bacteria are needed to form enough toxin to cause disease.

### Human antitetanus immunoglobulin should be given as soon as tetanus is suspected clinically

The wound should be excised if necessary and penicillin given to inhibit bacterial replication. Muscle relaxants are used and, if necessary, respiratory support in an intensive care unit.

Immunization with toxoid prevents tetanus, the effects of the vaccine lasting for 10 years after the last dose. Thus tetanus represents a vaccine-preventable disease that is unique in not being communicable but, instead, acquired from the environment as a result of exposure to *C. tetani* spores. Wounds should be cleaned, necrotic tissue and foreign bodies removed and a tetanus toxoid booster given. Those with badly contaminated wounds should also be given tetanus immunoglobulin and penicillin.

In resource-poor countries, routine immunization of women with tetanus toxoid and improved hygienic birth practices are having a significant impact in reducing the rates of neonatal tetanus.

## Botulism

Spores of *C. botulinum* are widespread in soil and contaminate vegetables, meat, and fish. When foods are canned or preserved without adequate sterilization (often at home), contaminating spores survive and can germinate in the anaerobic environment, leading to the formation of toxin.

### *C. botulinum* toxin blocks acetylcholine release from peripheral nerves

Preformed botulinus toxin is ingested and then absorbed from the gut into the blood. It acts on peripheral nerve synapses by blocking the release of acetylcholine. It is, therefore, a type of food poisoning that affects the motor and autonomic nervous systems. Sometimes spores contaminate a wound, and the toxin is then absorbed from this site. If the organism is ingested by infants, in the honey smeared on pacifiers, for instance, it can multiply in the gut and produce the toxin, causing infant botulism.

### Clinical features of botulism include weakness and paralysis

After an incubation period of 2–72 h there is descending weakness and paralysis, with dysphagia, diplopia, vomiting, vertigo and respiratory muscle failure. There is no abdominal pain, diarrhoea or fever. Infants develop generalized weakness (floppy babies), but they usually recover.

### Botulism is treated with antibodies and respiratory support

A diagnosis of botulism is mainly clinical. The toxin can be demonstrated in contaminated food and occasionally in the patient's serum.

Since the specific *C. botulinum* strain(s) responsible is(are) normally unknown, trivalent antitoxin (for type A, B, E toxins) must be given promptly together with respiratory support. The mortality is <20%, depending upon the success of the respiratory support.

Prevention is by avoiding imperfectly sterilized canned or preserved food. Contaminated cans are often swollen due to the release of gas by clostridial enzymes. Home-preserved foods are often incriminated, but fruit, with its acidic pH, usually prevents the development of the spores. The toxin is heat labile and is destroyed by adequate cooking (e.g. boiling for 10 min). The spores can, however, survive boiling for 3–5 h.

## KEY FACTS

- Microbial invasion of the CNS is uncommon, owing to the presence of the blood-brain and blood-CSF barriers, which limit the spread of infection.

- Once infectious agents have traversed these barriers, they generally cause neurologic disease by involving the meninges (meningitis) or the brain substance (encephalitis).

- Viral aetiology of meningitis is most common, followed by bacterial meningitis, with cerebral abscesses and viral encephalitis as rarities. The spinal cord (In myelitis) or peripheral nerves (in neuritis) are occasionally affected.

- Disease results from interference with the function of infected nerve cells (e.g. rabies), from direct damage to infected nerve cells (e.g. poliomyelitis), or from the inflammatory sequel to CNS invasion (e.g. bacterial meningitis, viral encephalitis).

- Herpes simplex encephalitis is a critical diagnosis to consider as aciclovir therapy must be given as soon as possible.

- Autoimmune causes of encephalitis may present with a fever, seemingly infectious in origin, but there is a good response to steroids and so a diagnosis must be made quickly.

- Because the anatomically defined compartments of the nervous system are adjacent or interconnected, more than one of them can be involved in a given infectious disease.

- CNS disease is sometimes seen in the helminth infections toxocariasis, echinococcosis (hydatid disease) and cysticercosis.

- CNS disease can also result when bacterial neurotoxins reach the CNS either from extraneural sites of growth (tetanus) or from contaminated food (botulism).

# Infections of the eye

# 26

## Introduction

The eye is composed of three layers (Fig. 26.1) and is contained within the orbit composed of bone, with superior and inferior eyelids. These anatomic structures are subject to infection. For example, the outer surface of the eye is exposed to the external world. Therefore it is easily accessible to infective organisms. The conjunctiva is particularly susceptible. Not only is it a vulnerable epithelial surface, it is covered by the eyelids, which create a warm, moist, enclosed environment in which contaminating organisms can quickly establish and set up a focus of infection. The eyelids and tears protect the external surfaces of the eye, both mechanically and biologically; any interference with their function increases the chance of a pathogen becoming established.

Eyelid infections are generally due to *Staphylococcus aureus*, *Streptococcus pneumoniae* or *Haemophilus influenzae*, with involvement of the lid margins causing blepharitis and eyelid glands or follicles causing styes or hordeolums.

Viruses are the most common cause of infectious conjunctivitis, especially adenoviral infections that do not usually need treatment. Bacterial conjunctivitis is the second most common cause and is treated with topical antibiotics.

The conjunctiva can be invaded by other routes such as the blood or nervous system. The deeper tissues of the eye can also be invaded from within, particularly by protozoan and worm parasites. Differentiating between the different causes of conjunctivitis on the basis of clinical signs and symptoms can be difficult.

## CONJUNCTIVITIS

A wide variety of viruses and bacteria can cause conjunctivitis or pinkeye (Table 26.1). Conjunctivitis can start in one eye and then progress to the other. The eye will be red, irritated and filled with tear fluid. A sticky discharge is likely to be secondary to a bacterial infection. Some infections are common in children and resolve quickly; others are potentially more serious. Keratoconjunctivitis from adenovirus, herpes simplex virus (HSV) or varicella-zoster virus (VZV) infection can result in severe damage. Acute haemorrhagic conjunctivitis is highly contagious, and outbreaks have been reported around the world. It presents as a pink eye, fast-onset eye pain with tear formation and light sensitivity or photophobia. It can follow infection with enterovirus 70 or coxsackievirus A24.

### Chlamydial infections

**Different serotypes of *Chlamydia trachomatis* cause inclusion conjunctivitis and trachoma**

To establish infection on the conjunctiva, microorganisms must avoid being rinsed and wiped away in tears. The best way of achieving this is to have a specific mechanism of attachment to conjunctival cells. *Chlamydia*, for example, has surface molecules that bind specifically to receptors on host cells. This is one of the reasons that, of all the organisms infecting the conjunctiva (see Table 26.1), they are among the

most successful. There are eight different serotypes of *C. trachomatis* responsible for inclusion conjunctivitis (D–K) (Fig. 26.2) and another four serotypes responsible for trachoma (A, B, Ba and C), which, globally, is the most important eye infection in the world.

**Two million people worldwide are visually impaired because of trachoma**

Over 200 million people in 42 countries are affected by trachoma. Of these, approximately 2 million have some degree of visual impairment, and the disease accounts for 1–2% of the world's blindness. Trachoma is endemic in resource-poor countries (Fig. 26.3) where prevalence rates in preschool children can reach 60–90%. Trachoma was known in ancient Egypt 4000 years ago, and tweezers to remove in-turned eyelashes have been found in royal tombs. Transmission of *C. trachomatis* is by contact, for example, by contaminated flies, fingers and towels.

Trachoma itself is the result of chronic repeated infections (Fig. 26.4), which are especially prevalent when there is poor access to water, preventing regular washing of the hands and face. Under these circumstances, chlamydial infection is frequently spread from one conjunctiva to another. Some chlamydial serotypes can infect the urogenital tract (see Ch. 22) as well as the conjunctiva, and the conjunctiva or lungs of a newborn infant may become infected after

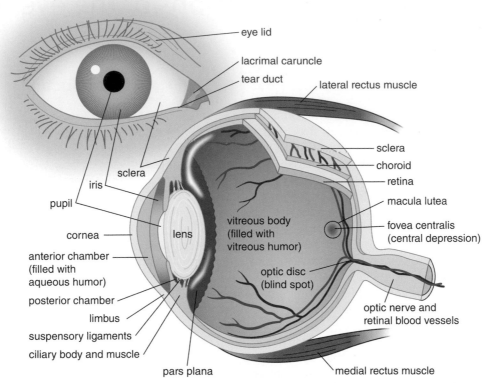

**Fig. 26.1** Horizontal schematic of the human eye demonstrating the three layers and their major components. (From Gropper MA. *Miller's Anesthesia*, ed 9, Elsevier; 2020.)

**Table 26.1** Examples of microbial infections of the conjunctiva

| Organism | Comments |
|---|---|
| Adenovirus | Very common, especially types 8 and 19 |
| Measles virus | Infection of conjunctiva via blood |
| Herpes simplex virus | Virus reactivating in ophthalmic division of trigeminal ganglia causes corneal lesion (dendritic ulcer) |
| Varicella-zoster virus | May involve conjunctiva |
| Enterovirus 70 Coxsackievirus A24 | Acute haemorrhagic conjunctivitis |
| Zika virus | May cause infections, including conjunctivitis and uveitis |
| *Chlamydia trachomatis* Types A–C Types D–K | Cause of trachoma and commonly blindness Cause of inclusion conjunctivitis; infection via fingers or in newborn via birth canal |
| *Neisseria gonorrhoeae* | Infection of newborn via birth canal |
| *Staphylococcus aureus* *Streptococcus pneumoniae* *Haemophilus influenzae* | Cause eyelid infection (styes) and sticky eye in neonates |

passage down an infected birth canal (see Ch. 24), requiring systemic treatment with erythromycin.

### Chlamydial infections are treated with antibiotic and prevented by face washing

Nucleic acid amplification tests (NAATs; e.g. polymerase chain reaction [PCR]) are the most accurate for laboratory diagnosis of chlamydial infections (see Chs. 22 and 32), although trachoma is most often diagnosed in endemic areas based on clinical symptoms as well as microscopic analysis of conjunctival fluid or scrapings. Treatment is with topical or oral antibiotics (e.g. azithromycin, doxycycline). Because infection and reinfection are facilitated by overcrowding, shortage of water and abundant fly populations, the disease can be prevented by improvements in standards of hygiene. In many areas with high rates of endemic trachoma, disease

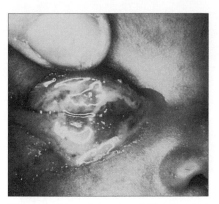

**Fig. 26.2** Chlamydial conjunctivitis is the most common form of neonatal conjunctivitis. (Courtesy G. Ridgway.)

leading to blindness has been sharply reduced or eliminated by socioeconomic development and specific intervention steps such as face washing. This has led the World Health Organization (WHO) to establish an international alliance for the global elimination of blinding trachoma by the year 2030. WHO aims to do this using the SAFE strategy: *s*urgery to treat trachomatous trichiasis (eyelashes scratch the cornea, which is unprotected due to the inward rolling of eyelids), *a*ntibiotics, *f*acial cleanliness, and *e*nvironment (improved access to water and sanitation).

Despite many decades of research, there are still no vaccines for chlamydial infections. This is partly because immunopathology itself makes a major contribution to the disease, and vaccine-induced immune responses could be harmful.

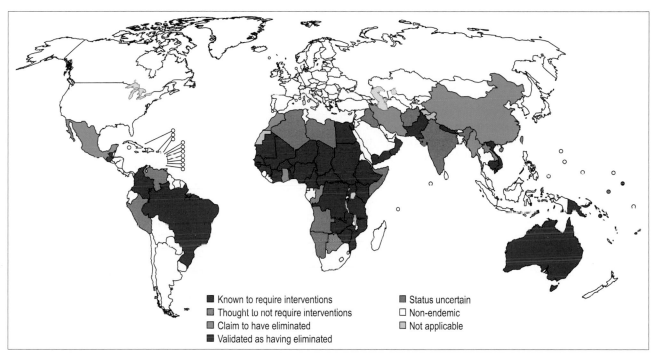

- ■ Known to require interventions
- ■ Thought to not require interventions
- ■ Claim to have eliminated
- ■ Validated as having eliminated
- ■ Status uncertain
- □ Non-endemic
- ■ Not applicable

**Fig. 26.3** Global trachoma incidence, 2016. (Modified from http://gamapserver.who.int/mapLibrary/Files/Maps/Trachoma_2016.png.)

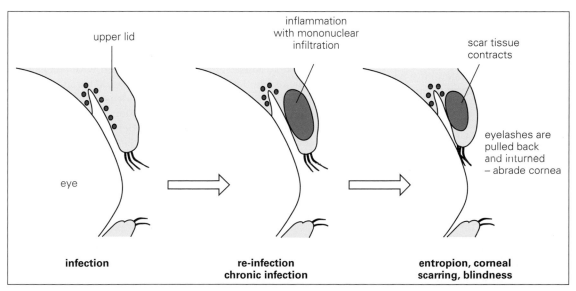

upper lid

inflammation with mononuclear infiltration

scar tissue contracts

eye

eyelashes are pulled back and inturned – abrade cornea

**infection**

**re-infection chronic infection**

**entropion, corneal scarring, blindness**

**Fig. 26.4** Steps in *Chlamydia trachomatis* pathogenesis leading to blindness.

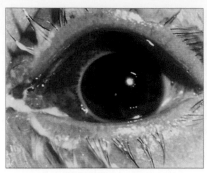

**Fig. 26.5** Purulent discharge in bacterial conjunctivitis is often associated with infections by *Streptococcus pneumoniae, Haemophilus influenzae* or *Staphylococcus aureus*. (Courtesy M. Tapert.)

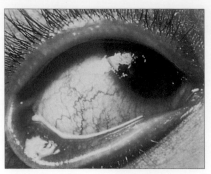

**Fig. 26.6** Herpes simplex virus (HSV) keratitis. Dendritic ulcers, seen here on the cornea, are common in recurrent HSV infections. (Courtesy M.J. Wood.)

## Other conjunctival infections

### In resource-rich countries, conjunctivitis is caused by a variety of bacteria

Several bacteria (especially *H. influenzae, S. aureus* and *S. pneumoniae*) can cause conjunctivitis (Fig. 26.5).

Infection by *Neisseria gonorrhoeae* is a hazard of birth through an infected birth canal and can result in a severe purulent condition. It is seen on the first or second day of life and called *ophthalmia neonatorum*. It requires urgent treatment with ceftriaxone as penicillin resistance is widespread. The eyes of infants may be invaded by this organism if the organism is transferred from the child's own body or from an infected adult. Conjunctivitis caused by *H. influenzae* has decreased in areas with available vaccine but can continue to be a problem for children with nontypeable (nonencapsulated) strains or in resource-poor areas.

### Direct infection of the eye (keratitis) may be associated with wearing contact lenses, and *Acanthamoeba* infection must always be kept in mind

Excessive wearing of contact lenses can lead to a reduction in the effectiveness of the eye's defence mechanisms, allowing pathogens to become established, but more likely hazards are the use of contaminated eye drops or cleaning solutions and the insertion of contaminated lenses. A number of bacteria can be transmitted directly in this way and lead to keratitis. Unlike conjunctivitis, a bacterial infection of the cornea can lead to blindness. A typical presentation will involve symptoms such as unilateral eye pain, photophobia and tearing up. The most common cause worldwide is *Pseudomonas aeruginosa*, which is strongly associated with extended contact lens wear. This bacterium can adhere to the contact lens and then the cornea and result in a liquefactive necrosis through the release of protease enzymes. Species of the free-living amoeba *Acanthamoeba* can multiply in some unchanged lens cleaning fluids (although newer products are more effective at killing) and be transferred when the lens is inserted, causing corneal ulceration. In noncontact wearers, the main risk factors for *Acanthamoeba* keratitis are trauma and exposure to contaminated water. The clinical features may be confused with herpes simplex or fungal keratitis, leading to a delay in receiving antiparasitic medication. Further to this, a delay in diagnosis can lead to difficulty in treatment as the amoebae

go deeper into the corneal stroma. Confocal microscopy may reveal *Acanthamoeba* cysts. Laboratory diagnosis is by microscopy and culture of corneal scrapings. PCR has a higher sensitivity than culture and is a well-established method. Molecular diagnostic tests can therefore be helpful if patients have been pretreated and the amoebae may not grow and are few in number. As acanthamoebae can encyst in the cornea, reinfection can occur, so it is important to monitor response to treatment, which is complicated. Combination therapy involves topical polyhexamethylene biguanide, a polymerized biguanide compound that is a broad-spectrum antiseptic that has antimicrobial activity, and chlorhexidine.

### Conjunctival infection may be transmitted by the blood or nervous system

Several organisms invade the superficial tissues of the eye after transport through the blood or, in the case of HSV, by movement along the trigeminal nerve. Reactivation of this latent virus can result in the development of a keratitis with the formation of dendritic ulcers (Fig. 26.6). The keratitis can lead to corneal scarring, with new blood vessel formation called *neovascularization* and stromal opacification, resulting in loss of sight. Of individuals with ocular HSV, 20% can develop keratitis. Diagnosis involves detecting HSV DNA by PCR in a conjunctival swab. Antiviral drugs such as aciclovir, valacyclovir and famciclovir, combined with steroid treatment, may be effective. However, if uncontrolled, corneal transplantation may be necessary. VZV may cause conjunctivitis associated with chickenpox or as a secondary infection. Overall, viral conjunctivitis is most commonly caused by adenovirus infections. Many years ago, due to the strong occupational association, shipyard eye was the name given to adenoviral conjunctivitis seen in shipbuilders and other workers exposed to the risk of eye injuries that could then result in an adenovirus infection. These viruses also cause pharyngoconjunctival fever, which includes, as one might expect, pharyngitis, fever and an acute follicular conjunctivitis that clears within a few weeks.

## INFECTION OF THE DEEPER LAYERS OF THE EYE

The deeper layers of the eye commonly subject to infection comprise the uvea (iris, ciliary body, choroid) and the retina (see Fig. 26.1). The spectrum of organisms causing disease

**Table 26.2** Examples of infections of the deep layers of the eye

| Organism | Disease | Route of infection |
|---|---|---|
| Rubella virus | Cataracts, microphthalmia | Infection in utero |
| Cytomegalovirus | Chorioretinitis | Infection in utero; may occur in AIDS and other immunocompromised individuals |
| Varicella-zoster virus Herpes simplex virus Cytomegalovirus Epstein-Barr virus | Necrotising retinopathy | Reactivation of latent virus in cranial nerve ganglia (VZV, HSV) |
| *Pseudomonas aeruginosa* | Serious inner eye infection | After trauma; foreign bodies in eye; eye operations; bacteria can contaminate eye drops |
| *Toxoplasma gondii* (toxoplasmosis) | Chorioretinitis | Infection in utero |
| *Echinococcus granulosus* (cystic hydatid disease) | Distortion of the eye by growth of larval tapeworm in hydatid cyst | Transmission by eggs passed by dogs |
| *Toxocara canis* (ocular toxocariasis) | Chorioretinitis, posterior pole granuloma, blindness | Transmission by eggs passed by dogs |
| *Onchocerca volvulus* (river blindness) | Sclerosing keratitis, chorioretinitis | Larvae transmitted by blood-feeding *Simulium* flies |

AIDS, Acquired immunodeficiency syndrome; HSV, herpes simplex virus; VZV, varicella-zoster virus.

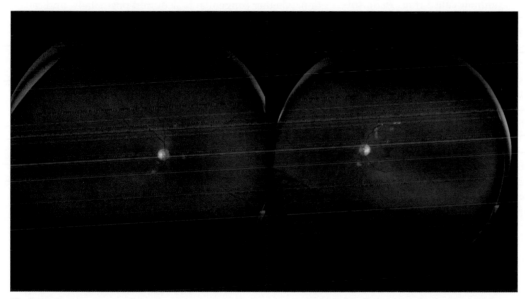

**Fig. 26.7** Human immunodeficiency virus retinopathy. (Courtesy Dr. T. Braithwaite.)

in the deeper layers of the eye, such as uveitis or chorioretinitis, is wider than that associated with the conjunctiva (Table 26.2).

### Entry into the deeper layers occurs by many routes

Trauma to the eye, which includes ocular surgery, may result in bacterial endophthalmitis. Coagulase-negative staphylococci such as S. *epidermidis* are common opportunistic invaders seeking to establish themselves within the deep ocular layers. Congenital syphilis produces a retinopathy with quiescent lesions, and keratitis may appear in later life. Secondary syphilis is also associated with ocular inflammation, typically posterior and panuveitis, but can present with an optic neuropathy and retinal vasculitis. Uveal and retinal inflammation is an established extrapulmonary manifestation of tuberculosis and can result in visual loss through irreversible intraocular tissue damage.

Rubella virus and cytomegalovirus (CMV) may invade the fetal eye in utero, the former causing cataracts and microphthalmia, the latter a severe chorioretinitis. CMV can also cause chorioretinitis in individuals with acquired immunodeficiency syndrome (AIDS), although antiretroviral therapy has resulted in a reduction of eye disease (see Fig. 22.26E). However, prior to the development of AIDS, human immunodeficiency virus can cause a retinal microvasculopathy, which can be viewed on fundal imaging (Fig. 26.7). Viral retinitis is a rare presentation; it can occur in immunocompetent and immunocompromised

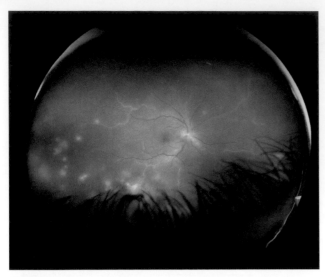

**Fig. 26.8** Acute retinal necrosis associated with varicella-zoster virus infection. (Courtesy Dr. T. Braithwaite.)

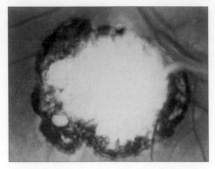

**Fig. 26.9** Congenital toxoplasmosis. Fundal photograph shows the scar of healed chorioretinitis. (Courtesy M.J. Wood.)

individuals. It can manifest as a spectrum of acute retinal necrosis, retinitis and progressive outer retinal necrosis. VZV infection is the most common cause (Fig. 26.8), followed by HSV, and rarely CMV or Epstein-Barr virus (EBV) is the cause. Symptoms include eye pain, redness, photophobia and blurred vision. Intraocular samples are tested by PCR for HSV, VZV, CMV and EBV DNA, with treatment involving intravitreal foscarnet alongside oral valacyclovir. This is initiated prior to getting the PCR results.

Ocular complications have been reported in patients with West Nile, dengue and Japanese encephalitis virus infections. Blindness due to anterior uveitis secondary to resurgent Ebola virus infection was identified in individuals who survived Ebola. Additionally, Zika virus can present with uveitis with ocular signs such as microphthalmia, iris colobomas, cataracts, intraocular calcification, optic disc hypoplasia as well as chorioretinal atrophy and scarring.

## Toxoplasmosis

### *Toxoplasma gondii* infection can cause retinochoroiditis leading to blindness

Infection with this protozoan is widespread in adults and children (see Ch. 5) and is normally acquired by swallowing oocysts released by infected cats (the definitive host) or by eating raw or undercooked meat containing tissue cysts. Ocular toxoplasmosis can be congenitally acquired and is increasingly recognised postnatally. Women who become infected in pregnancy may transmit the infection to the fetus, as tachyzoites can cross the placenta. Tissue cysts can form in the retina of the fetus and undergo continuous proliferation, producing progressive lesions particularly when levels of immunity are low. These lesions may also involve the choroid (Fig. 26.9), causing visual deterioration due to macular involvement and leading ultimately to blindness. One or both eyes may be affected. Acute ocular toxoplasmosis can present with diffuse inflammation in the choroid and retinal tissue (retinochoroiditis) with white focal lesions near pigmented scars, which are older lesions.

The severity of an individual episode of *Toxoplasma* infection is influenced by parasite genotype and host immune status. Toxoplasmosis is not usually serious unless:

- acquired in utero, when the organism invades all tissues, especially the central nervous system (CNS)
- acquired (or reactivated) under immunosuppression.

Damage to the eye occurs in both congenital and postnatally acquired toxoplasmosis and may present at any age. Ocular toxoplasmosis may present years after the initial infection, whether congenital or acquired postnatally, and can be more serious in the elderly population. Diagnosis is made on fundoscopy, together with blood tests involving toxoplasma immunoglobulin M (IgM), IgG and the dye test. PCR methods ae also available to identify *T. gondii* by PCR in aqueous and vitreous fluid.

Treatment usually involves pyrimethamine, sulfadiazine, folinic acid and prednisone, with spiramycin used in pregnancy in combination with some of the drugs mentioned earlier, depending on the trimester.

## Parasitic worm infections

### *Toxocara canis* larvae cause an intense inflammatory response and can lead to retinal detachment

Larval tapeworms (e.g. the cystic stage of *Echinococcus granulosus* [cystic echinococcosis, cystic hydatid disease]) transmitted by eggs passed from infected dogs occasionally enter the eye, with growth of the cysts causing severe mechanical damage. The larval form (cysticercus) of *Taenia solium* (the pork tapeworm) is acquired when humans ingest eggs of this tapeworm. Cysticerci develop mainly in skeletal muscle but can invade the nervous system or the eye. Ocular cysticerci are diagnosed by direct vision (e.g. seen as a translucent vesicle in the vitreous), ultrasonography (e.g. as a subretinal, subchoroidal cyst), cross-sectional imaging and serology. Treatment of intraocular cysticercosis is by surgical removal. Antiparasitic drugs are not given to avoid causing an inflammatory reaction. Corticosteroids are given if uveitis is present. Invasion by migratory larvae of the nematode *Toxocara canis* (commonly called *dog roundworm*) is more common. This parasite occurs naturally in the intestines of dogs, releasing thick-shelled resistant eggs into the environment. The eggs can hatch if swallowed by humans, the larvae initiating but failing to complete their customary migration through the tissues. In the canine host, migration results in the worms reentering the intestine where they mature. In humans, larvae can enter almost any organ, especially

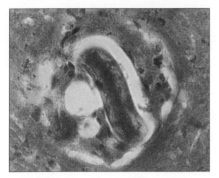

**Fig. 26.10** *Toxocara.* Granuloma in the posterior pole of an infected eye. The larval nematode is clearly visible in the centre of the granuloma. (Courtesy D. Spalton.)

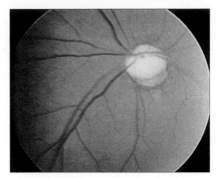

**Fig. 26.11** Onchocerciasis. Sclerosis of the choroidal vessels caused by invading microfilaria of *Onchocerca volvulus*. (Courtesy J. Anderson.)

the liver, and often the CNS or eye (Fig. 26.10), triggering an intense eosinophilic inflammatory response. In the eye, *Toxocara* larvae may lead to posterior uveitis, localized retinal granuloma, traction bands and retinal detachment. The misdiagnosis of retinal granuloma as retinoblastoma has led to enucleation. Serology by enzyme-linked immunosorbent assay and Western blot on vitreous samples is preferable to serum samples in diagnosing ocular toxocariasis. Treatment requires joint management with an ophthalmology team. Corticosteroids are given to suppress ocular inflammation. Anthelmintic treatment is not routinely given because, if given alone, it might lead to worsening of inflammation. Where anthelmintic drugs are necessary, corticosteroids are used to suppress the inflammatory response. Laser photocoagulation has been used to destroy ocular granulomas.

### *Onchocerca volvulus* infection causes river blindness and is transmitted by *Simulium* flies

*O. volvulus* infection is transmitted by biting *Simulium* flies, which take up microfilariae (larvae) from the skin of infected hosts. These larvae develop further in the *Simulium* fly to become infective and infect a new host at a future feed. Adult worms live in subcutaneous nodules and are comparatively harmless. The microfilariae, released by the females in enormous numbers, induce intense inflammatory reactions in the skin (see Ch. 27). The larvae migrate through the subcutaneous tissue, and invasion of the eye (resulting in river blindness) is particularly common in regions of Africa, Yemen and Central America. Onchocercal eye disease is associated with lengthy exposure to infection.

Inflammatory responses in the eye cause a number of pathologic changes, which may affect both the anterior and posterior chambers (Fig. 26.11). These include:

- punctate and sclerosing keratitis
- corneal scarring
- iridocyclitis
- chorioretinitis
- optic atrophy.

The disease is called *river blindness* because the *Simulium* flies develop in fast-flowing rivers, and people living near these sites are most affected. In the past, blindness rates have reached 50% of the adult population in endemic areas, but vector control and especially ivermectin treatment are important in reducing the incidence of new infections. Unfortunately, once established, the blindness is irreversible.

## KEY FACTS

- The external surfaces of the eye are vulnerable to infection. They are protected by the eyelids and by factors such as lysozyme in tears.

- It can be difficult to make a diagnosis regarding the aetiology of conjunctivitis on clinical signs and symptoms alone.

- The consequences of eye infection are always potentially serious given that sight is dependent upon the presence of an intact transparent cornea.

- Pathogens infecting the conjunctiva have specific attachment mechanisms.

- Inflammatory responses, though designed to limit invasion and repair damage, can irreversibly damage conjunctival and corneal surfaces.

- Relatively few organisms invade the retina, and those that do are potentially sight threatening.

- Some of the most serious infection-related diseases of the eye involve invasion by protozoan or helminth parasites. The diagnosis then often follows rather than precedes the development of visual impairment.

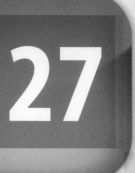

# 27

# Infections of the skin, soft tissue, muscle and associated systems

## Introduction

### Healthy intact skin protects underlying tissues and provides excellent defence against invading pathogens

The microbial load of normal skin is kept in check by various factors (Box 27.1). Alterations in these factors (e.g. prolonged exposure to moisture) upset the ecologic balance of the commensal flora and predispose to infection.

The number of bacteria on the skin varies from a few hundred/cm² on the arid surfaces of the forearm and back to tens of thousands/cm² on the moist areas, such as the axilla and groin. This normal microbiota plays an important role in preventing foreign organisms from colonizing the skin, but it, too, needs to be kept in check.

A small number of pathogens cause diseases of muscle, joints or the haemopoietic system. Invasion of these sites is generally from the blood, but the reason for localization to particular tissues is often obscure. Circulating pathogens tend to localize in growing or damaged bones (acute osteomyelitis) and in damaged joints, but we do not know why coxsackieviruses or *Trichinella spiralis* invade muscle. On the other hand, some viruses infect a given target cell, and plasmodia invade erythrocytes because they have specific attachment sites for these cells.

---

### Box 27.1 — Factors Controlling the Skin's Microbial Load

- The limited amount of moisture present
- Acid pH of normal skin
- Surface temperature less than optimum for many pathogens
- Salty sweat
- Excreted chemicals (sebum, fatty acids, urea)
- Competition between different species of the normal flora

---

## Infections of the skin

In addition to being a structural barrier, the skin is colonized by an array of organisms that forms its normal flora. The relatively arid areas of the forearm and back are colonized with fewer organisms, predominantly gram-positive bacteria and yeasts. In the moister areas, such as the groin and the armpits, the organisms are more numerous and more varied and include gram-negative bacteria. The normal microbiota of the skin and other body sites plays an important role in defending the surface from foreign invaders.

An appreciation of the structure of the skin helps in understanding the different sorts of infection to which the skin and its underlying tissues are prone (Fig. 27.1). If organisms breach the stratum corneum, the host are mobilized, the epidermal Langerhans cells elaborate cytokines, neutrophils are attracted to the site of invasion and complement is activated via the alternative pathway.

### Microbial disease of the skin may result from any of three lines of attack

These lines of attack are:

- breach of intact skin, allowing infection from the outside
- skin manifestations of systemic infections, which may arise as a result of bloodborne spread from the infected focus to the skin or by direct extension (e.g. draining sinuses from actinomycotic lesions, necrotizing anaerobic infection from intraabdominal sepsis)
- toxin-mediated skin damage due to production of a microbial toxin at another site in the body (e.g. scarlet fever, toxic shock syndrome [TSS]).

The sequence of events in the pathogenesis of mucocutaneous lesions caused by bacterial, fungal and viral infections is outlined in Fig. 27.2. Breaches in the skin range from microscopic to major trauma, which may be accidental (e.g. lacerations or burns) or intentional (e.g. surgery). Hospitalized patients are liable to other skin breaches (e.g. pressure sores and intravenous catheter insertions), which may become infected. Infections in compromised individuals such as patients with burns are discussed in Chapter 31. Here we will consider primary infections of the skin and underlying soft tissues, together with mucocutaneous lesions resulting from certain systemic viral infections. Examples of systemic bacterial and fungal infections that cause mucocutaneous lesions are summarized in Table 27.1.

**Fig. 27.1** Infection of the skin and soft tissue can be related to the anatomy of the skin. Pathogens usually enter the lower layers of the epidermis and dermis only after the skin surface has been damaged.

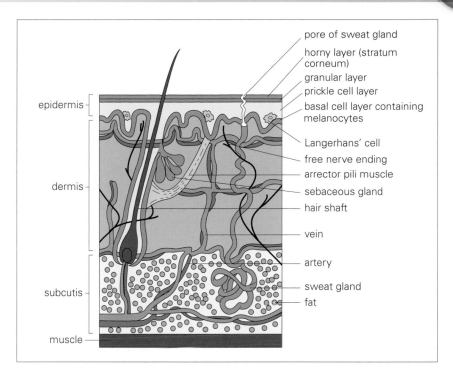

pore of sweat gland
horny layer (stratum corneum)
granular layer
prickle cell layer
basal cell layer containing melanocytes
Langerhans' cell
free nerve ending
arrector pili muscle
sebaceous gland
hair shaft
vein
artery
sweat gland
fat

epidermis
dermis
subcutis
muscle

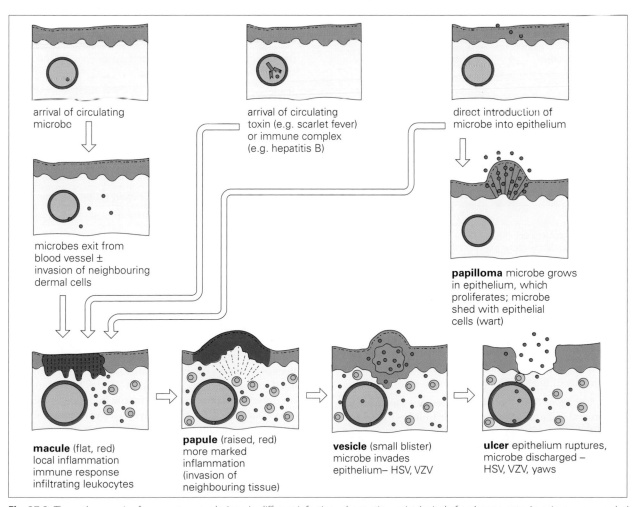

arrival of circulating microbe

arrival of circulating toxin (e.g. scarlet fever) or immune complex (e.g. hepatitis B)

direct introduction of microbe into epithelium

microbes exit from blood vessel ± invasion of neighbouring dermal cells

**papilloma** microbe grows in epithelium, which proliferates; microbe shed with epithelial cells (wart)

**macule** (flat, red) local inflammation immune response infiltrating leukocytes

**papule** (raised, red) more marked inflammation (invasion of neighbouring tissue)

**vesicle** (small blister) microbe invades epithelium– HSV, VZV

**ulcer** epithelium ruptures, microbe discharged – HSV, VZV, yaws

**Fig. 27.2** The pathogenesis of mucocutaneous lesions. In different infections, the starting point (arrival of pathogen or toxin or immune complex) and the final picture (e.g. maculopapular rash, vesicle) will be different. HSV, Herpes simplex virus; VZV, varicella-zoster virus.

**Table 27.1** Skin manifestations of systemic infections caused by bacteria and fungi

| Organisms | Disease | Skin manifestation |
|---|---|---|
| *Salmonella typhi, S. schottmuelleri* | Enteric fever | Rose spots containing bacteria |
| *Neisseria meningitidis* | Septicaemia, meningitis | Petechial or maculopapular lesion containing bacteria |
| *Pseudomonas aeruginosa* | Septicaemia | Ecthyma gangrenosum, skin lesions pathognomonic if infected by this organism |
| *Treponema pallidum* <br> *T. pertenue* | Syphilis <br> Yaws | Disseminated infectious rash seen in secondary stage of disease after infection |
| *Rickettsia prowazekii* <br> *R. typhi* <br> *R. rickettsii* | Typhus <br> Spotted fever | Macular or haemorrhagic rash |
| *Streptococcus pyogenes* | Scarlet fever | Erythematous rash caused by erythrogenic toxin |
| *Staphylococcus aureus* | Toxic shock syndrome | Rash and desquamation due to toxin |
| *Blastomyces dermatitidis* | Blastomycosis | Papule or pustule develops into granuloma lesions containing organisms |
| *Cryptococcus neoformans* | Cryptococcosis | Papule or pustule, usually on face or neck |

Skin lesions are often associated with systemic infection with particular bacteria and fungi. The lesions may provide useful diagnostic aids. Sometimes they are a site from which organisms are shed.

**Table 27.2** Direct entry into skin of bacteria and fungi

| Structure involved | Infection | Common cause |
|---|---|---|
| Keratinized epithelium | Ringworm | Dermatophyte fungi (*Trichophyton, Epidermophyton* and *Microsporum*) |
| Epidermis | Impetigo | *Streptococcus pyogenes* and/or *Staphylococcus aureus* |
| Dermis | Erysipelas | *S. pyogenes* |
| Hair follicles | Folliculitis <br> Boils (furuncles) <br> Carbuncles | *S. aureus* |
| Subcutaneous fat | Cellulitis | *S. pyogenes* |
| Fascia | Necrotizing fasciitis | Anaerobes and microaerophiles, usually mixed infections |
| Muscle | Myonecrosis gangrene | *Clostridium perfringens* (and other clostridia) |

Direct introduction of bacteria or fungi into the skin is the most common route of skin infection. Infections range from mild, often chronic conditions such as ringworm to acute and life-threatening fasciitis and gangrene. Relatively few species are involved in the common infections.

## BACTERIAL INFECTIONS OF SKIN, SOFT TISSUE AND MUSCLE

### These can be classified on an anatomic basis

The classification depends upon the layers of skin and soft tissue involved, although some infections may involve several components of the soft tissues:

- *Abscess formation.* Boils and carbuncles are the result of infection and inflammation of the hair follicles in the skin (folliculitis).
- *Spreading infections.* Impetigo is limited to the epidermis and presents as a bullous, crusted or pustular eruption of the skin. Erysipelas involves the blocking of dermal lymphatics and presents as a well-defined, spreading erythematous inflammation generally on the face, legs or feet and often accompanied by pain and fever. If the focus of infection is in subcutaneous fat, cellulitis (a diffuse form of acute inflammation) is the usual presentation.
- *Necrotizing infections.* Fasciitis describes the inflammatory response to infection of the soft tissue below the dermis. Infection spreads, often with alarming rapidity, along the fascial planes causing disruption of the blood supply. Gangrene or myonecrosis may follow infection associated with ischaemia of the muscle layer. Gas resulting from the fermentative metabolism of anaerobic organisms may be palpable in the tissues (gas gangrene).

The common causative organisms are shown in Table 27.2. Note that the same pathogen (e.g. *Streptococcus pyogenes*) can cause different infections in different layers of the skin and soft tissue.

## Staphylococcal skin infections

### *Staphylococcus aureus* is the most common cause of skin infections and provokes an intense inflammatory response

*S. aureus* causes minor skin infections such as boils or abscesses as well as more serious postoperative wound infection. Infection may be acquired by self-inoculation from a carrier site (e.g. the nose) or acquired by contact with an exogenous source, usually another person. People who are nasal carriers of virulent *S. aureus* may suffer from recurrent boils, but an inoculum of approximately 100,000 organisms is thought to be required in the absence of a wound or foreign body. *S. aureus* can also cause serious skin disease due to toxin production (scalded skin syndrome, TSS; see later). In addition, skin and soft tissue infections caused by community-associated methicillin-resistant *S. aureus* (CA-MRSA) strains are of concern (see Ch. 37).

A boil begins within 2–4 days of inoculation as a superficial infection in and around a hair follicle (folliculitis; Fig. 27.3). In this site the organisms are relatively protected from the host defences, multiply rapidly and spread locally. This provokes an intense inflammatory response with an influx of neutrophils. Fibrin is deposited, and the site is walled off. Abscesses typically contain abundant yellow creamy pus formed by the massive number of organisms and necrotic white cells. They continue to expand slowly, eventually erode the overlying skin, come to a head and drain. Drainage inward can result in seeding of the staphylococci to underlying body sites to cause serious infections such as peritonitis, empyema or meningitis.

### *S. aureus* infections are often diagnosed clinically, and treatment includes drainage and antibiotics

*S. aureus* is the most common cause of boils, and diagnosis is made on clinical grounds. Isolation and further characterization of the infecting staphylococcus in hospital patients and staff are important in the investigation of hospital infections (see Ch. 37).

Treatment involves drainage, and this is usually sufficient for minor lesions, but antibiotics may be given in addition when the infection is severe and the patient has a fever. Most *S. aureus* are beta-lactamase producers, but methicillin-susceptible *S. aureus* (MSSA) can be treated with addition of a beta-lactamase inhibitor (e.g. amoxicillin/clavulanate) or enzyme-stable penicillins such as nafcillin. Isolates resistant to these compounds (i.e. MRSA; see Ch. 34) may be treated with vancomycin, linezolid, quinupristin-dalfoprisin or daptomycin. Treatment with these agents does not necessarily eradicate carriage of the staphylococci.

Recurrent infections may be treated in nasal carriers of *S. aureus* with nasal creams containing antibiotics. For example, mupirocin has been used successfully for carriers of methicillin-resistant staphylococci (see Ch. 37). Good skin care and personal hygiene should be encouraged.

### Staphylococcal scalded skin syndrome is caused by toxin-producing *S. aureus*

This condition, also known as *Ritter disease* in infants and *Lyell disease* or *toxic epidermal necrolysis* in older children, occurs sporadically and in outbreaks. It is caused by strains of *S. aureus* producing a toxin known as *exfoliatin* or *scalded skin syndrome toxin*. The initial skin lesion may be minor, but the toxin causes destruction of the intercellular connections and separation of the top layer of the epidermis. Large blisters are formed, containing clear fluid, and within 1–2 days the overlying areas of skin are lost (Fig. 27.4), leaving normal skin underneath. The baby is irritable and uncomfortable but rarely severely ill. However, treatment should consider the risk of increased loss of fluid from the damaged surface, and fluid replacement may be needed. As mentioned, antimicrobial chemotherapy would employ beta-lactamase stable penicillins (e.g. nafcillin) against MSSA, whereas vancomycin, linezolid, quinupristin-dalfoprisin or daptomycin would be used for MRSA.

### Toxic shock syndrome is caused by TSS toxin–producing *S. aureus*

This systemic infection came to prominence in the 1980s through its association with highly absorbent tampons (since taken off the market) in healthy women, but it is not confined to women and can occur as a result of *S. aureus* infection at nongenital sites (e.g. a wound). TSS involves multiple organ systems and is characterized by fever, hypotension and a diffuse macular erythematous rash followed by desquamation of the skin, particularly on the soles and palms (Fig. 27.5). TSS is caused by exotoxins of *S. aureus*, most commonly TSST1,

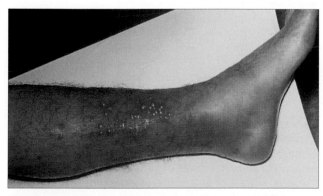

**Fig. 27.3** Folliculitis. A superficial infection is shown here localized in the hair follicles on the leg. The boils contain creamy-yellow pus and masses of bacteria. *Staphylococcus aureus* is the most common cause. (Courtesy A. du Vivier.)

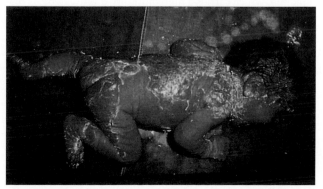

**Fig. 27.4** Scalded skin syndrome results from infection of the skin with strains of *Staphylococcus aureus* producing a specific toxin, which destroys the intercellular connections in the skin, resulting in large areas of desquamation. The appearance may be confused with a burn. (Courtesy A. du Vivier.)

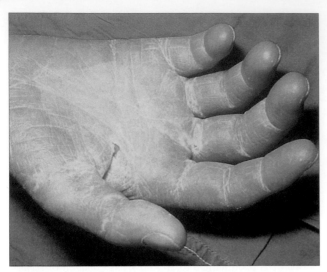

**Fig. 27.5** Toxic shock syndrome results from systemic infection with *Staphylococcus aureus* but has skin manifestations in the form of desquamation, particularly of the palm and soles. (Courtesy M.J. Wood.)

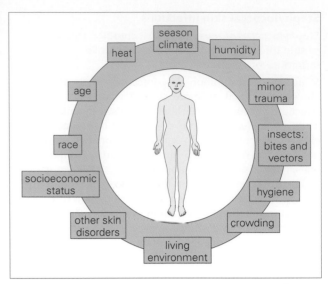

**Fig. 27.6** Various factors are involved in the development of streptococcal skin infections. Particular M types of *Streptococcus pyogenes* have a predilection for skin, but various factors predispose the host (usually a child) to infection. Mixed infections with *Staphylococcus aureus* are also common.

which behaves as a superantigen (stimulating T-cell proliferation and cytokine release; see Ch. 17). While the prevalence of TSS in the United States is low (estimated at <200 cases per year), >90% of adults carry antibodies to TSST1. Treatment of TSS includes steps to open the infected site (e.g. drainage), fluid replacement and antistaphylococcal chemotherapy.

## Streptococcal skin infections

### Streptococcal skin infections are caused by *S. pyogenes* (group A streptococci)

Streptococcal impetigo develops independently of streptococcal upper respiratory tract infection, and, although up to 35% of patients carry the same strain in their nose or throat, colonization may well occur after the skin has become infected. The organisms are acquired through contact with other people with infected skin lesions and may first colonize and multiply on normal skin before invasion through minor breaks in the epithelium and the development of lesions. The various risk factors involved in the development of streptococcal impetigo are shown in Fig. 27.6. *S. pyogenes* may also cause erysipelas, an acute deeper infection in the dermis. About 5% of patients with erysipelas go on to develop bacteraemia, which carries a high mortality if untreated. As discussed previously, impetigo may also be caused by *S. aureus* and occasionally presents in more extreme bullous form (i.e. bullous impetigo) as blisters resembling localized scalded skin syndrome (see earlier).

*S. pyogenes* possesses certain surface proteins (M and T), which are antigenic. In the past, the species has been subdivided (typed) on the basis of these antigens, and it has been recognized that certain M and T types are associated with skin infection (and these differ from the types associated with sore throats). T proteins play no known role in virulence, and their function is unknown. M proteins are important virulence factors because they inhibit opsonization and confer on the bacterium resistance to phagocytosis. A variety of additional factors contribute to the virulence of the organism, such as lipoteichoic acid (a component of the gram-positive cell wall) and F protein, which facilitate binding to epithelial cells.

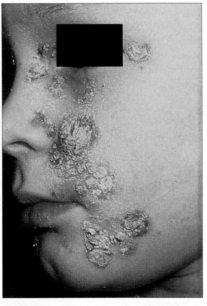

**Fig. 27.7** Impetigo is a condition limited to the epidermis, with typically yellow crusted lesions. It is commonly caused by *Streptococcus pyogenes* either alone or together with *Staphylococcus aureus*. (Courtesy M.J. Wood.)

### Clinical features of streptococcal skin infections are typically acute

They develop within 24–48 h of skin invasion and trigger a marked inflammatory response as the host attempts to localize the infection (Figs. 27.7 and 27.8). *S. pyogenes* elaborates a number of toxic products and enzymes, such as hyaluronidase, which help the organism to spread in tissue. Lymphatic involvement is common, resulting in lymphadenitis and lymphangitis.

Lysogenic strains of *S. pyogenes* produce pyrogenic exotoxins (SPE; formally called *erythrogenic toxins*). As with TSST1 in *S. aureus* (discussed earlier), these toxins are

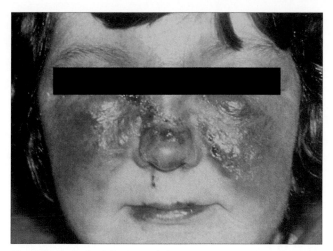

**Fig. 27.8** Erysipelas. Infection with *Streptococcus pyogenes* involves the dermal lymphatics and gives rise to a clearly demarcated area of erythema and induration. When the face is involved, there is often a typical butterfly-wing rash, as shown here. (Courtesy M.J. Wood.)

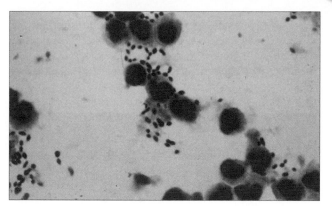

**Fig. 27.9** Gram-positive cocci in pus.

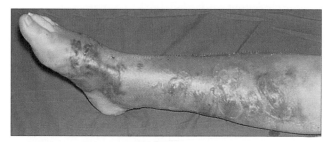

**Fig. 27.10** When the focus of infection is in the subdermal fat, cellulitis—a severe and rapidly progressive infection—is the typical presentation. Large blisters and scabs may also be present on the skin surface. (Courtesy M.J. Wood.)

superantigens with a potent influence on the immune system. The toxins (e.g. SPEA, B, C) also act on skin blood vessels to cause the diffuse erythematous rash of scarlet fever, which may occur with streptococcal pharyngitis. *S. pyogenes* may also cause a form of TSS that has been especially associated with the production of the SPEA.

### M protein is a major virulence factor in *S. pyogenes* with >100 types, some of which (e.g. M49) are specifically associated with diseases such as acute glomerulonephritis

Acute glomerulonephritis (AGN) occurs more often after skin infections than after infections of the throat (see Ch. 19). It is characterized by the deposition of immune complexes on the basement membrane of the glomerulus, but the precise role of the streptococcus in the causation is still unclear (see Ch. 18); 10–15% of individuals infected with a nephritogenic strain will develop AGN about 2–3 weeks after the primary infection. Most people recover completely, and recurrence after a subsequent streptococcal infection is rare. Rheumatic fever (see Ch. 19) very rarely follows skin infections with *S. pyogenes*.

### Streptococcal skin infections are usually diagnosed clinically and treated with penicillin

Gram stains of pus from vesicles in impetigo show gram-positive cocci, and culture reveals *S. pyogenes* sometimes mixed with *S. aureus* (Fig. 27.9). In erysipelas, skin cultures are often negative, although culture of fluid from the advancing edge of the lesion may be successful.

Depending on the cause of infection and antibiotic susceptibility, dicloxacillin is a commonly used drug, although erythromycin, newer macrolides or an oral cephalosporin may be used for penicillin-allergic patients. However, the prevalence of resistance (e.g. to erythromycin) in streptococci is increasing, and these drugs are not effective in mixed infections with *S. aureus*. Severe infections may require hospitalization.

Impetigo is prevented by improving the host factors associated with acquisition of the disease as illustrated in Fig. 27.7. Since AGN rarely recurs on subsequent streptococcal infection, long-term prophylaxis with penicillin is not indicated (in contrast to the long-term prophylaxis following rheumatic fever; see Ch. 19).

## Cellulitis and gangrene

### Cellulitis is an acute spreading infection of the skin that involves subcutaneous tissues

Cellulitis extends deeper than erysipelas and usually originates either from superficial skin lesions such as boils or ulcers or following trauma. It is rarely bloodborne, but conversely it may lead to bacterial invasion of the bloodstream. Infection develops within a few hours or days of trauma and quickly produces a hot red, swollen lesion (Fig. 27.10). Regional lymph nodes are enlarged, and the patient suffers malaise, chills and fever.

The great majority of cases of cellulitis are caused by *S. pyogenes* and *S. aureus*. Occasionally, in patients who have had particular environmental exposure, other organisms may be implicated. For example, *Erysipelothrix rhusiopathiae* is associated with cellulitis in butchers and fishmongers, while *Vibrio vulnificus* and *V. alginolyticus* may complicate traumatic wounds acquired in saltwater environments.

The pathogen causing cellulitis is isolated in only 25–35% of cases, and initial therapy should cover streptococci and staphylococci. Attempts can be made to confirm the clinical diagnosis by culture of:

- aspirates from the advancing edge of the cellulitis
- the site of trauma (if present)
- skin biopsies
- blood.

Treatment should be initiated on the basis of the clinical diagnosis because of the potential for rapid progression of the disease.

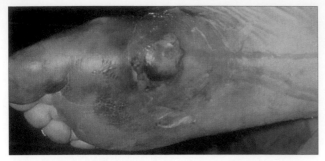

**Fig. 27.11** Severe progressive cellulitis of the foot. Such cellulitis is usually caused by anaerobic bacteria or a mixture of aerobes and anaerobes and is a particular problem in diabetic patients with peripheral vascular and neuropathic damage. (Courtesy J.D. Ward.)

### Anaerobic cellulitis may develop in areas of traumatized or devitalized tissue

Such damaged tissue is associated with surgical or traumatic wounds or is found in ischaemic extremities. Diabetic patients are particularly prone to anaerobic cellulitis of their feet (Fig. 27.11). The causative organisms depend upon the circumstances of the trauma: infections in the lower parts of the body are most often caused by organisms from the faecal flora, whereas wounds from human bites are infected with oral organisms. Foul-smelling discharge, marked swelling and gas in the tissues are characteristic of anaerobic cellulitis, and a mixture of organisms is usually cultured from the wound. Treatment needs to be aggressive to halt the spread of infection, and both antibiotics and surgical debridement are required. Osteomyelitis (see later) is a common sequela.

### Synergistic bacterial gangrene is a relentlessly destructive infection

This rare infection is caused by a mixture of organisms, typically *microaerophilic streptococci* and *S. aureus*. The gangrene most commonly follows surgery in the groin or genital area, starting at the site of a drain or suture. Cellulitis develops in the surrounding skin and extends rapidly (within hours), leaving a black necrotic centre. The condition is often fatal, and treatment requires radical excision of the necrotic area and systemic antibiotic therapy.

## Necrotizing fasciitis, myonecrosis and gangrene

### Necrotizing fasciitis is a frequently fatal mixed infection caused by anaerobes and facultative anaerobes

Although apparently resembling synergistic bacterial gangrene, necrotizing fasciitis is a much more acute and highly toxic infection causing widespread necrosis and undermining of the surrounding tissues such that the underlying destruction is more widespread than the skin lesion (Fig. 27.12). Necrotizing fasciitis has been most prominently linked by the popular media with *S. pyogenes* (e.g. flesh-eating bacteria), and the more recently described invasive group A streptococci are clear etiologic agents. However, the infection may be caused by a variety of other organisms, especially MRSA. Patients with necrotizing fasciitis deteriorate rapidly and frequently die. Radical excision of all necrotic fascia is an essential part of therapy, along with antibiotics given both locally to the wound and systemically.

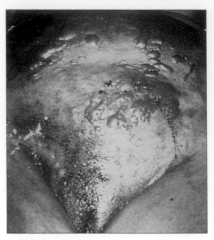

**Fig. 27.12** Necrotizing fasciitis of the abdominal wall. In patients such as this, infection can be seen rapidly spreading from its origin and causing deep and widespread necrosis. Complete debridement and intensive antimicrobial therapy is required, but the condition is often fatal. (Courtesy W.M. Rambo.)

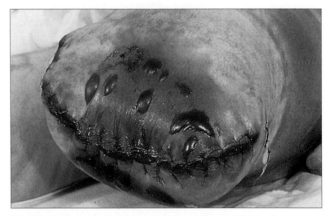

**Fig. 27.13** Gas gangrene caused by *Clostridium perfringens*. Organisms from the fecal flora may contaminate a wound and grow and multiply in poorly perfused (anaerobic) tissue. Infection spreads rapidly, and gas can be felt in the tissue and seen on radiographs. (Courtesy J. Newman.)

### Traumatic or surgical wounds can become infected with *Clostridium* species

*Clostridium tetani* gains access to the tissues through trauma to the skin, but the disease it produces is entirely due to the production of a powerful exotoxin (see Ch. 18).

Gas gangrene, or clostridial myonecrosis, can be caused by several species of Clostridia, but *C. perfringens* is the most common. The organism and its spores are found in the soil and in human and animal faeces and can therefore gain access to traumatized tissues by contamination from these sources. Infection develops in areas of the body with poor blood supply (anaerobic), and the buttocks and perineum are common sites particularly in patients with ischaemic vascular disease or peripheral arteriosclerosis. The organisms multiply in the subcutaneous tissues, producing gas and an anaerobic cellulitis, but a characteristic feature of clostridial infection is that the organisms invade deeper into the muscle where they cause necrosis and produce bubbles of gas, which can be felt in the tissue and sometimes seen in the wound (Fig. 27.13). The infection proceeds very rapidly and causes acute pain. Much of the damage is due to the

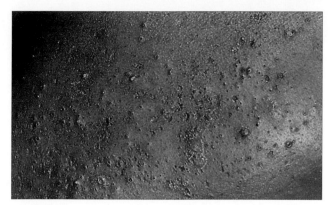

**Fig. 27.14** Typical lesions of acne. Blackheads are seen when plugs of keratin block the pilosebaceous duct. (Courtesy A. du Vivier.)

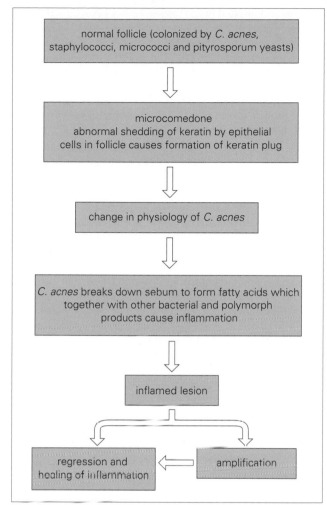

**Fig. 27.15** The proposed mechanism of the pathogenesis of acne. Hormonal changes in the host initiate the formation of comedones from normal follicles and thereby change the environment of *Cutibacterium acnes* and its physiologic properties. *C. acnes* is also known to be an immunostimulator.

production by *C. perfringens* of a lecithinase (also known as *alpha toxin*), which hydrolyses the lipids in cell membranes resulting in cell lysis and death. The presence of dead and dying tissue further compromises the blood supply, and the organisms multiply and produce more toxin and more damage. Other extracellular enzymes may also play a role in helping the clostridia to spread. If the toxin escapes from the affected area and enters the bloodstream, there is massive haemolysis, renal failure and death.

### Amputation may be necessary to prevent further spread of clostridial infection

Because of the rapid progression and fatal outcome of this type of clostridial infection, gangrenous areas require immediate surgery to excise all the affected tissue, and amputation may be necessary. Although some reports suggest that anti-alpha toxin may help if given early enough, antitoxin treatment is not generally viewed as effective, while treatment in a hyperbaric oxygen chamber, where available, may be helpful (i.e. oxygenation of tissue) in some cases.

Antibiotics are adjuncts to, not replacements for, surgical debridement.

Prevention of infection is of foremost importance. Wounds should be cleansed and debrided early to remove dead and poorly perfused tissue, which the anaerobes favour. Prophylactic antibiotics should be given preoperatively to patients having elective surgery of body sites liable to contamination with faecal flora.

### Cutibacterium acnes and acne

*C. acnes* go hand in hand with the hormonal changes of puberty that result in acne

An increased responsiveness to androgenic hormones leads to increased sebum production plus increased keratinization and desquamation in pilosebaceous ducts. Blockage of ducts turns them into sacs in which *C. acnes* and other members of the normal flora (e.g. micrococci, yeasts, staphylococci) multiply. *C. acnes* acts on sebum to form fatty acids and peptides, which, together with enzymes and other substances released from bacteria and polymorphs, cause the inflammation (Fig. 27.14). Comedones (blackheads in popular terminology) are greasy plugs composed of a mixture of keratin, sebum and bacteria and capped by a layer of melanin (Fig. 27.15).

### Treatment of acne includes long-term administration of oral antibiotics

The antibiotics used to treat acne are usually one of the tetracyclines. Other treatments include skin care, keratolytics and, in severe cases, synthetic vitamin A derivatives such as isotretinoin. Orally administered antibiotics reduce the surface numbers of *C. acnes* with a concomitant lowering of the free fatty acids, which act as skin irritants that result from the activity of bacterial enzymes on sebum. Acne can be a problem for teenagers but often disappears in older age-groups as the sebaceous follicles become less active.

Other gram-positive rods related to *C. acnes*, such as corynebacteria and brevibacteria, can also cause skin infections.

## MYCOBACTERIAL DISEASES OF THE SKIN

### Leprosy

**Leprosy is decreasing in incidence but still remains a concern**

Leprosy has been recognized since biblical times, but in the past the word was a generic term applied to several different diseases and implied moral uncleanliness. Leprosy is thought to have spread to Europe in the 6th century, and by the 13th century there were some 200 leper hospitals in England. Over the centuries that followed, leprosy declined in incidence, and by the 15th century it was no longer endemic in England; in contrast, tuberculosis (TB) was on the increase. Now leprosy is rare in the United Kingdom and United States, but the World Health Organization (WHO) estimates that the number of new cases worldwide persists at approximately 200,000 cases per year. The disease remains particularly problematic in Southeast Asia, Africa and the Americas.

### Leprosy is caused by *Mycobacterium leprae*

*M. leprae* was discovered in 1873 by G.A. Hansen, who identified it as the first bacterial agent capable of causing human disease. Leprosy (Hansen disease) appears to be confined to humans. *M. leprae* is found in nine-banded armadillos, chimpanzees and mangabey monkeys; however, epidemiologic studies have not demonstrated a significant link between this carriage and human disease. Transmission of infection is directly related to overcrowding and poor hygiene and occurs by direct contact and aerosol inhalation. Relatively few organisms are shed from skin lesions, but nasal secretions of patients with lepromatous leprosy (LL) are laden with *M. leprae*. Arthropod vectors may play a role in transmission. Leprosy is not highly contagious, and prolonged exposure to an infected source is necessary; it seems that children living under the same roof as an open case of leprosy are most at risk. Ironically, because the lesions of leprosy are more obvious, patients in the past were excluded from the community and gathered in leper colonies, whereas TB is much more contagious, but people with TB were not shunned.

### The clinical features of leprosy depend upon the cell-mediated immune response to *M. leprae*

*M. leprae* cannot be grown in artificial culture media, and little is known about its mechanism of pathogenicity. Two animal models have been used: infection in the armadillo and in the footpads of mice. The organism grows better at temperatures <37°C, hence its concentration in the skin and superficial nerves, and it grows extremely slowly; in the mouse footpad the generation time is 11–13 days. Likewise in humans, the incubation period may be many years.

*M. leprae* grows intracellularly, typically within skin histiocytes and in endothelial cells and the Schwann cells of peripheral nerves. The immune response is all important in deciding the type of disease.

*M. leprae* shares many pathobiologic features with *M. tuberculosis*, but the clinical manifestations of the diseases are quite different. After an incubation period of several years, the onset of leprosy is gradual, and the spectrum of disease activity is very broad depending upon the presence or absence of a cell-mediated immune (CMI) response to *M. leprae* (Fig. 27.16). At one end of the spectrum is tuberculoid leprosy (TT), characterized by blotchy red lesions with anaesthetic areas on the face, trunk and extremities (Fig. 27.17). There is palpable thickening of the peripheral nerves because the organisms multiply in the nerve sheaths. The local anaesthesia renders the patient prone to repeated trauma and secondary bacterial infection. This disease state is equivalent to secondary

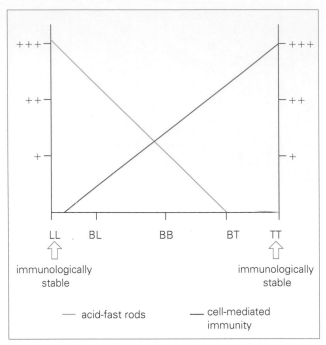

**Fig. 27.16** Immunologic responses in leprosy. In tuberculoid leprosy (TT) the patient is capable of mounting an effective cell-mediated immune (CMI) response, which makes it possible for macrophages to destroy the organisms and contain the infection. At the other extreme, in lepromatous leprosy (LL) the patient is incapable of producing a CMI response and the organisms multiply unhindered. These patients have many acid-fast rods in their skin and nasal secretions and are much more infectious than TT patients. Borderline lepromatous (BL), borderline borderline (BB) and borderline tuberculoid (BT) responses are found between these extremes.

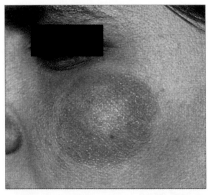

**Fig. 27.17** Tuberculoid leprosy—a characteristic dry blotchy lesion on the face. The diagnosis needs to be confirmed by microscopic examination of skin biopsy (see Fig. 27.20). (Courtesy Institute of Dermatology.)

TB (see Ch. 20), with a vigorous CMI response leading to phagocytic destruction of bacteria and exaggerated allergic responses. TT carries a better prognosis than LL and in some patients is self-limiting, but in others it may progress across the spectrum towards LL.

In LL there is extensive skin involvement with large numbers of bacteria in affected areas. As the disease progresses, there is loss of eyebrows and thickening and enlargement of the nostrils, ears and cheeks, resulting in the typical leonine (lionlike) facial appearance (Fig. 27.18). There is progressive

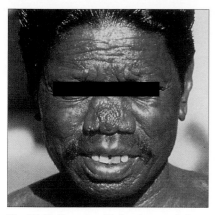

**Fig. 27.18** Extensive skin involvement in lepromatous leprosy results in a characteristic leonine appearance. (Courtesy D.A. Lewis.)

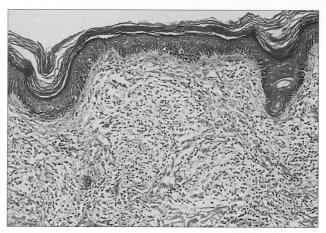

**Fig. 27.20** In tuberculoid leprosy, the organisms are much sparser but characteristic granulomas form in the dermis, as shown in this histologic preparation. (Courtesy C.J. Edwards.)

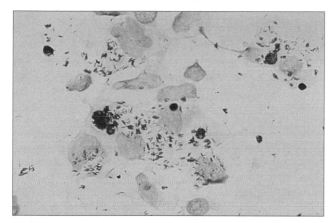

**Fig. 27.19** In lepromatous leprosy, the nasal mucosa is packed with *Mycobacterium leprae*, seen here in an acid-fast stain (Ziehl–Neelsen) of nasal scrapings. (Courtesy I. Farrell.)

destruction of the nasal septum, and the nasal mucosa is loaded with organisms (Fig. 27.19). This form of the disease is equivalent to miliary TB (see Ch. 20), with a weak CMI response and many extracellular organisms visible in the lesions. The gross deformities characteristic of late disease result primarily from infectious destruction of the nasomaxillary facial structures and secondarily from pathologic changes in the peripheral nerves predisposing to repeated trauma of the hands and feet and subsequent superinfection with other organisms.

Whether a patient develops TT or LL may, in part, be genetically determined. Patients with intermediate forms of the disease may progress to either extreme.

### *M. leprae* are seen as acid-fast rods in nasal scrapings and lesion biopsies

Alertness to the possibility of leprosy when confronted with a patient with dermatologic, neurologic or multisystem complaints is of fundamental importance. Although the majority of cases are in people who are not native to Europe or the United States, the diagnosis should also be considered in those who have worked in endemic areas.

Nasal scrapings and biopsies of skin lesions can be stained by Ziehl–Neelsen or auramine stain to demonstrate acid-fast rods. In LL these are numerous, but in TT few if

any organisms are seen, but the appearance of granulomas is sufficiently typical to allow the diagnosis to be made (Fig. 27.20). Remember that, in contrast to *M. tuberculosis*, the organism cannot be grown in vitro.

### Treatment

**Leprosy is treated with dapsone given as part of a multidrug regimen to avoid resistance**

If the disease is diagnosed early and treatment initiated promptly, the patient has a much better prognosis. Dapsone (see Ch. 34) had long been the mainstay of therapy, but multidrug therapy is now used because of dapsone resistance:

- For LL, triple therapy with dapsone, rifampin and clofazimine is commonly given for 1–2 years and may be longer or until all skin scrapings and biopsies are negative for acid-fast rods.
- For TT, a combination of dapsone and rifampin for 6 months is recommended, the rationale being that, in this form of disease, there are many fewer organisms and therefore less chance of emergence of resistant mutants.

As a result of multidrug therapy, which is reasonably cheap, well tolerated and effects a complete cure, steady progress is being made toward the elimination of leprosy as a public health problem.

Destruction of the organisms by effective antimicrobial therapy may result in an inflammatory response, erythema nodosum leprosum, which may be severe and occasionally fatal. Treatment with corticosteroids may be indicated.

Vaccination with bacille Calmette-Guérin has been used in countries with high incidence where potential protection outweighs negative factors such as a positive skin test. Vaccination is not useful for immunocompromised individuals.

### Other mycobacterial skin infections

*Mycobacterium marinum, M. ulcerans* and *M. tuberculosis* also cause skin lesions

*M. marinum* and *M. ulcerans* are two slow-growing mycobacterial species that prefer cooler temperatures and cause skin lesions. As its name suggests, *M. marinum* is associated with water and marine organisms. Human infections

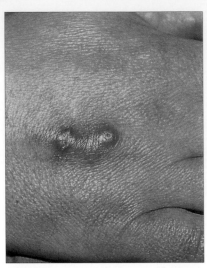

**Fig. 27.21** Fish tank granuloma caused by *Mycobacterium marinum* infection of a lesion acquired while cleaning out a fish tank. (Courtesy M.J. Wood.)

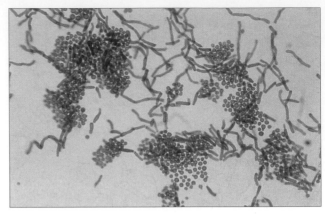

**Fig. 27.22** Infected skin scales stained to show the thick-walled yeast forms of *Malassezia furfur* and the short angular hyphae. (Courtesy Y. Clayton and G. Midgley.)

follow trauma, often minor such as a graze acquired while climbing out of a swimming pool or while cleaning out an aquarium, which becomes contaminated with mycobacteria from the wet environment. After an incubation period of 2–8 weeks, initial lesions appear as small papules, which enlarge, suppurate and may ulcerate. Histologically, the lesions are granulomas, hence the name swimming pool granuloma or fish tank granuloma (Fig. 27.21). Sometimes the nodules follow the course of the draining lymphatic and produce an appearance that may be mistaken for sporotrichosis (see later).

*M. ulcerans* causes chronic, relatively painless cutaneous ulcers known as Buruli ulcers. This disease is seen in Africa and Australia but rarely elsewhere.

TB of the skin is exceedingly uncommon. Infection can occur by direct implantation of *M. tuberculosis* during trauma to the skin (lupus vulgaris) or may extend to the skin from an infected lymph node (scrofuloderma).

## FUNGAL INFECTIONS OF THE SKIN

Fungal infections may be confined to the very outermost layers of the skin and hair shafts or penetrate into the keratinized layers of the epidermis, nails and hair (the superficial and cutaneous mycoses); others develop in the dermal layers (subcutaneous mycoses). In addition, some systemic fungal infections acquired by the airborne route have skin manifestations (see Table 27.1).

### Superficial and cutaneous mycoses

These are some of the most common infections in humans. Superficial infections of the skin and hair (pityriasis versicolor, tinea nigra, black and white piedras) mainly cause cosmetic problems; cutaneous infections (ringworm, tineas) caused by the dermatophyte fungi are more significant. The important causative agents are the superficial basidiomycete yeasts of the genus *Malassezia* and the cutaneous ascomycete dermatophytes *Epidermophyton*, *Trichophyton*, *Nannizzia* and *Microsporum*. Some nondermatophyte molds can also cause skin and nail infections.

### Pityriasis versicolor

#### *Malassezia* is the cause of pityriasis or tinea versicolor

The yeast *Malassezia* (previously known as *Pityrosporum*) is a common skin inhabitant. The change from commensalism to pathogenicity appears to be associated with the phase change from yeast to hyphal forms of the fungus. As part of their adaptation to living in the skin, *Malassezia* secrete acid sphingomyelinases and aspartate proteases, and, as they cannot synthesize fatty acids, they secrete lipases and phospholipases C, which release fatty acids from host lipids. Infections are usually confined to the trunk or proximal parts of the limbs and are associated with hypo- or hyperpigmented macules that coalesce to form scaling plaques. The lesions are not usually itchy, and in some patients they resolve spontaneously.

*Malassezia* yeasts are also involved in the pathogenesis of seborrhoeic dermatitis and dandruff, but the relative roles of the host's immune system, enzymatic activity of *Malassezia* or secondary metabolites in promoting it, have yet to be clearly defined.

#### Diagnosis of pityriasis versicolor can be confirmed by direct microscopy of scrapings

Direct microscopy of scrapings shows characteristic round yeast forms with broad-based budding and short hyphal fragments (Fig. 27.22); appropriate treatment is with a topical azole antifungal (see later) or with selenium sulfide (2.5%) lotion.

### Cutaneous dermatophytes

#### Dermatophyte infections are acquired from many sources and are spread by arthrospores

Species of dermatophytes are described as anthropophilic, zoophilic or geophilic depending upon their primary source (human, animal, soil). The species concerned differ in their geographic distribution, in their predilection for different body sites and in the degree of host response elicited in humans. The source of an infection determines its route of transmission to humans and, to some extent, its distribution in human populations, although population movements (international travel and migration) are changing established patterns. For example, for a time, migration from

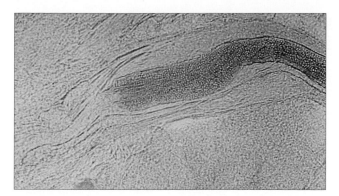

**Fig. 27.23** Arthrospores of *Trichophyton tonsurans* in an infected hair shaft. These thick-walled spores are the form in which infection is spread. They can survive in the environment for weeks or months before infecting a new host. (Courtesy A.E. Prevost.)

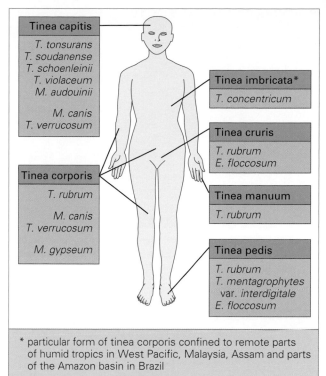

\* particular form of tinea corporis confined to remote parts of humid tropics in West Pacific, Malaysia, Assam and parts of the Amazon basin in Brazil

**Fig. 27.24** Tinea (or ringworm) is the disease of skin, hair and nails caused by dermatophyte fungi. Different species have predilections for different body sites. *E.*, *Epidermophyton*; *M.*, *Microsporum*; *T.*, *Trichophyton*.

Latin America replaced *Microsporum audouinii* by *Trichophyton tonsurans* as the common cause of tinea capitis in the United States, but the latter (which responds poorly to treatment) is now again predominant.

The anthropophilic species are the most common causes of dermatophyte infections. In temperate countries, *T. verrucosum* from cattle, *T. mentagrophytes* from rodents and *Microsporum canis* from cats and dogs are the most common zoophilic causes of human infection. Geophilic species such as *Nannizzia gypsea* (formerly *Microsporum gypseum*) are uncommon causes of human disease but are seen in people who have appropriate exposure, such as gardeners and agricultural workers. Zoophilic and geophilic species tend to cause a greater inflammatory response than anthropophilic species.

Infections are spread by contact with arthrospores, the thick-walled vegetative cells formed by dermatophyte hyphae (Fig. 27.23), which can survive for months. In anthropophilic and zoophilic species, these are shed from the primary host in skin scales and hair.

### Dermatophytes invade skin, hair and nails

The dermatophytes are keratin-loving organisms and invade the keratinized structures of the body (i.e. skin, hair and nails). Dermatophytes have septate hyphae and form arthrospores that adhere to keratinocytes, germinate and invade. In adapting to life in the skin, they produce proteases to break down keratin, Lys M proteins to bind to and mask cell wall components and help evade recognition by the host, and kinases and pseudokinases to modulate host cell metabolism. The Latin word *tinea*, "maggot or grub," or ringworm, is used for these infections because they were originally thought to be caused by a wormlike parasite. Thus tinea capitis affects the hair and skin of the scalp, tinea corporis the body, tinea cruris the crotch, tinea manuum the hands, tinea unguium the nails and tinea pedis the feet (Fig. 27.24).

The typical lesion is an annular or serpentine scaling patch with a raised margin. The main symptom is itching, but this is variable in degree. The skin is often dry and scaly and sometimes cracks (e.g. between the toes in tinea pedis), while infections of hair cause hair loss (Fig. 27.25). The degree of associated inflammation varies with the infecting species. Anthropophilic species usually result in asymptomatic infections or oligosymptomatic chronic infections,

whereas human infection with geophilic or zoophilic species results in a symptomatic inflammatory condition.

Individuals also differ in their susceptibility to infection; tinea capitis is more common in children, whilst tinea unguium is more prevalent in elderly patients in whom the presence of diabetes and peripheral vascular insufficiency may be contributory factors. Human immunodeficiency virus (HIV), immunosuppression, obesity, and smoking are additional predisposing factors for onychomycosis.

### Dermatophyte species differ in their ability to elicit an immune response

Interleukin 17 (IL-17)–based immunity is central to the prevention of uncontrolled growth of superficial dermatophytes and restricting excessive cutaneous inflammation.

In some patients, circulating fungal antigens gives rise to immunologically mediated hypersensitivity phenomena in the skin (e.g. erythema or vesicles) known as *dermatophytid reactions*. When the skin becomes cracked and macerated as a result of infection, it is liable to cause superinfection with other organisms such as gram-negative bacteria in moist sites.

Very rarely, dermatophytes invade the subcutaneous tissues (deep dermatophytosis) via the lymphatics, causing granulomas, lymphoedema and draining sinuses. Further extension to sites such as the liver and brain may be fatal.

### In diagnosis most dermatophyte species fluoresce under ultraviolet light

This feature can be used as a diagnostic aid in the clinic, particularly for tinea capitis. Direct microscopic examination and culture of scrapings or clippings from lesions on Sabouraud dextrose agar or other mycology media, to which

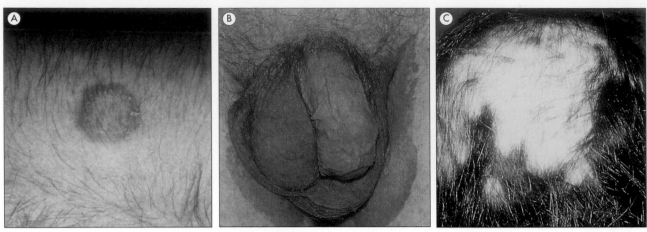

**Fig. 27.25** (A) Classic annular lesion of tinea corporis caused here by infection with a *Microsporum* species. (B) Tinea cruris, or jock itch, is a scaly rash on the thighs; the scrotum is usually spared. (C) Tinea capitis is characterized by scaling on the scalp and hair loss. Some dermatophytes fluoresce under ultraviolet light, and this can be an aid to diagnosis. (A, Courtesy A.E. Prevost; B, courtesy M.J. Wood; C, courtesy M.H. Winterborn.)

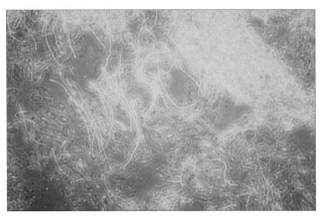

**Fig. 27.26** Dermatophyte infection. Samples of skin, hair and nails need to be cleared by treatment with potassium hydroxide before examining under the microscope for the presence of fungal hyphae. (Courtesy R.Y. Cartwright.)

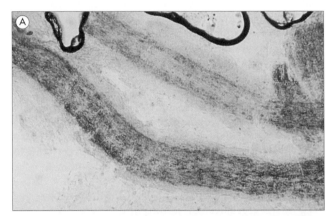

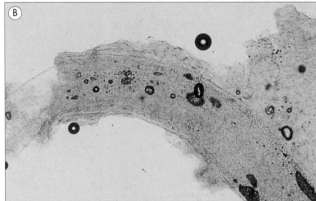

**Fig. 27.27** Dermatophytes may form arthrospores within the hair shafts (endothrix infection) as shown in (A) and less commonly outside the shaft (ectothrix infection) as shown in (B). (Courtesy Y. Clayton and G. Midgley.)

inhibitory agents (antibiotics and cycloheximide) have been added to provide some selectivity, remains important (Fig. 27.26). Dermatophytes infecting hair shows a characteristic distribution, which may be helpful for identification:

- Some, such as most *Microsporum* spp., form arthrospores on the outside of the hair shaft (ectothrix infections).
- The majority of *Trichophyton* infections form arthrospores within the hair shaft (endothrix infection; Fig. 27.27).

Confirmation of identity is useful for determining the source of infection and depends upon the colonial and microscopic characteristics of the fungi cultured on Sabouraud dextrose agar (Fig. 27.28). Growth may take up to 3 weeks, so more rapid molecular-based methods are also deployed (Table 27.3)

### Dermatophyte infections are treated topically if possible

A range of agents is available for topical treatment (see Ch. 34), both antifungals (e.g. miconazole) and keratolytic agents such as Whitfield ointment (a mixture of salicylic and benzoic acids). To prevent relapse, treatment should be continued for 1–2 weeks after resolution of clinical signs.

Systemic therapy with oral antifungal drugs is required for scalp infection and is more effective than topical agents for nail infections. Terbinafine or itraconazole are now used in preference to griseofulvin. These newer agents may give a cure rate of 70–80% for nail infections. The recent emergence and worldwide spread of terbinafine-resistant *Trichophyton indotineae*, causing difficult-to-treat dermatophytosis, is a major clinical concern.

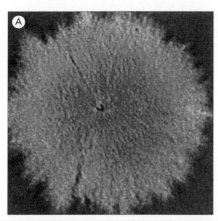

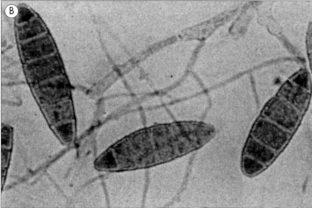

**Fig. 27.28** (A) Macroscopic growth (colony) and (B) microscopic preparation showing the macroconidia of *Microsporum gypseum*.

## *Candida* and the skin

### *Candida* requires moisture for growth

The relative dryness of most areas of skin limits the growth of fungi such as *Candida* that require moisture. *Candida* is found in low numbers on healthy intact skin but rapidly colonizes damaged skin and intertriginous sites (opposed skin sites that are often moist and become chafed; Fig. 27.29). *Candida* also colonizes the oral and vaginal mucosa, and overgrowth may result in disease in these sites (oral or vaginal candidiasis; see Ch. 22). However, a substantial lowering of host resistance (e.g. neutropenia leading to invasion via the gastrointestinal tract) is necessary for *Candida* to invade deeper subcutaneous tissue, and disseminated candidiasis does not often originate from skin infection unless there is disruption to the skin barrier (e.g. presence of a central venous catheter).

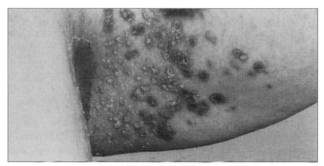

**Fig. 27.29** *Candida* infection of the skin. Here, infection has occurred between two apposing skin surfaces, which provide a suitably moist environment for this yeast to multiply. (Courtesy A du Vivier and St Mary's Hospital.)

**Table 27.3** A summary of the diagnostic methods in use for detecting dermatophytes. (Some are only available in reference laboratories)

| Diagnostic method | Advantages | Disadvantages | Time to results |
|---|---|---|---|
| Direct examination | • Noninvasive<br>• Low cost | • Unable to determine species | Minutes |
| Wood lamp | • Noninvasive<br>• Low cost | • Not all species fluoresce | Minutes |
| Microscopy | • Can detect unique features of species<br>• Low cost | • Unable to distinguish dead and alive fungi | Minutes |
| Culture | • Low cost<br>• Easy to perform<br>• Can distinguish between species | • Requires expertise to determine species<br>• Can be contaminated by saprophytes | Days–weeks |
| PCR | • Highly sensitive<br>• Can distinguish between species | • Unable to distinguish dead and alive fungi | Hours–days |
| ELISA | | • False positives due to past infections | Hours–days |
| MALDI-ToF | • Highly sensitive<br>• Can distinguish between species | • Only detect species in library | Minutes–hours |
| Genetic analysis | • Can distinguish between species<br>• Highly sensitive | • Unable to distinguish dead and alive fungi | Hours–days |

Modified from Moskaluk AE, VandeWoude S. Current topics in dermatophyte classification and clinical diagnosis. *Pathogens*. 2022;11(9):957. doi:10.3390/pathogens11090957.

## Subcutaneous mycoses

### Subcutaneous fungal infections can be caused by a number of different species

Lesions usually develop at sites of trauma (a thorn, a bite) where the fungus becomes implanted. With the exception of sporotrichosis, subcutaneous fungal infections are rare, but similar diseases can be caused by certain bacteria such as *Actinomyces* and atypical mycobacteria and, therefore, it is important to establish the cause to select optimal therapy. In case of eumycetoma, the fungi involved are difficult to eradicate with antifungal agents, and surgical intervention in the form of excision or even amputation is often required.

### Sporotrichosis is a nodular condition caused by *Sporothrix*

*Sporothrix* is a saprophytic dimorphic fungus that is widespread in nature in soil and on rose and berberis bushes, tree bark and sphagnum moss. Sporotrichosis can be caused by certain species of *Sporothrix*, most commonly *S. schenckii* in the United States. Infection is often acquired through trauma (e.g. a thorn) and is an occupational hazard for people such as farmers, gardeners and florists. Clinical presentation depends on host immune status, size and depth of inoculum, pathogenicity and thermal tolerance of the infecting strain. Commonly, a small papule or subcutaneous nodule develops at the site of trauma 1 week to 6 months after inoculation, and infection spreads, producing a series of secondary nodules along the lymphatics that drain the site (Fig. 27.30). By 2018, in Brazil and neighboring countries, the species *S. brasiliensis* emerged as a zoonotic disease that is spread from cats to humans through bites and scratches of infected cats. This species appears to cause more severe disease among humans and animals than other *Sporothrix* species.

Diagnosis is made by culture of drained or aspirated material onto Sabouraud dextrose agar and histopathology of biopsy material. Molecular diagnosis such as polymerase chain reaction (PCR) is more rapid and can be helpful in culture-negative cases. Serologic tests (e.g. IgG enzyme-linked immunosorbent assay [ELISA]) are commercially available but can vary in performance depending on the disease presentation. Azole drugs are highly effective, and itraconazole has replaced treatment with oral potassium iodide.

Disseminated disease can occur following cutaneous or pulmonary infection (acquired by inhalation) with *S. schenckii*. It is more common in compromised patients such as those with underlying carcinoma or sarcoidosis, but many cases occur in people in whom no underlying disease is recognized. Disseminated or severe pulmonary infection is treated with amphotericin B induction therapy followed by itraconazole. Long-term maintenance therapy may be needed when it is not possible to reverse underlying immunosuppression.

Other species causing subcutaneous infections include *Exophiala, Fonsecaea, Rhinocladiella, Cladophialophora* and *Phialophora* (chromoblastomycosis). This infection is mostly reported in Latin America and the Caribbean, Asia, Africa, and Australia. It was added to WHO's list of neglected tropical disease in 2017.

### Mycetoma

Mycetoma is a chronic progressive subcutaneous infection that gives rise to tumourlike swellings complicated by the development of sinuses discharging grains. It most commonly involves the foot (hence Madura foot), but it can affect the hand or other parts of the body. The lesion develops after trauma that introduces the infecting organism into subcutaneous tissue, so it is more common in farmers and the poor who may have no footwear. Its true global distribution and prevalence are not established. Most cases have been reported from Mexico, Sudan and India. As a result of global migration patterns, clinicians in regions considered nonendemic for mycetoma are now seeing imported cases for the first time.

There are two types of mycetoma:

- eumycetoma, caused by fungi, of which *Madurella mycetomatis* is the commonest causative agent
- actinomycetoma, caused by bacteria, usually *Nocardia brasiliensis* and *Streptomyces somaliensis*.

Biopsy for histopathology, bacterial and fungal culture is required to establish the diagnosis and identify the infecting organism. PCR is valuable in identifying the organism responsible, but culture is essential for antimicrobial susceptibility testing.

Actinomycetoma responds well to antibiotic therapy (e.g. co-trimoxazole). Eumycetoma requires surgery in addition to prolonged antifungal therapy with an azole antifungal, often itraconazole, and where possible wide local excision should be performed. Repeat operation may be necessary to deal with recurrent disease, and amputation may be required in advanced cases.

### Systemic fungal infections with skin manifestations include blastomycosis, coccidioidomycosis, talaromycosis (penicilliosis), histoplasmosis and cryptococcosis

Skin lesions occur in 40–80% of cases of blastomycosis, a disease endemic in Central and North America and Africa and caused by the dimorphic fungus *Blastomyces dermatitidis* and *B. gilchristii*. Infection is acquired by aspiration of the fungal spores and spreads from the primary site in the lung. Blastomycosis can be a systemic disease in apparently immunologically normal hosts (Fig. 27.31). It also causes disease in horses and dogs.

Other systemic fungal infections that may have skin manifestations are those caused by *Talaromyces marneffei, Coccidioides immitis, Coccidioides posadasii, Histoplasma* species and *Cryptococcus neoformans*.

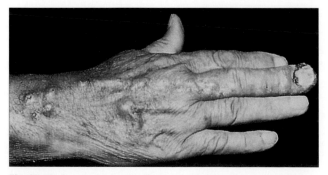

**Fig. 27.30** *Sporotrichosis* spreading up the draining lymphatics of the hand following a primary infection in the nailbed of the third finger. (Courtesy T.F. Sellers, Jr.)

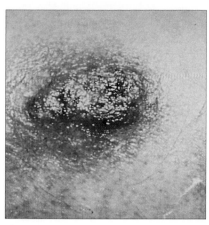

**Fig. 27.31** Typical skin lesion of blastomycosis. Infection is acquired by the respiratory route, and the primary site of infection is the lung. However, in chronic blastomycosis the skin is the most common extrapulmonary site of infection. (Courtesy K.A. Riley.)

## PARASITIC INFECTIONS OF THE SKIN

The skin is a major route of entry for parasites, which may penetrate directly (e.g. schistosomes, hookworm) or be injected by blood-feeding vectors. Many of these parasites leave the skin almost immediately as they progress through their life cycle, but some remain there (e.g. the scabies mite) or remain nearby in subcutaneous tissue and deposit larvae in the skin (e.g. *Onchocerca*), whilst others (e.g. animal parasites unable to complete their life cycle in humans) may become trapped. A few parasites actually exit from the body through the skin (e.g., release of Guinea worm larvae). Pathologic responses to parasites associated with the skin range from mild to disablingly severe. Some species causing severe conditions are described briefly later.

### Leishmaniasis may be cutaneous or mucosal (formerly termed *mucocutaneous*)

Two of the three major disease complexes caused by the protozoan *Leishmania* affect the skin, and both are transmitted by the bite of sandfly vectors:

- The cutaneous leishmaniases, which occur in both the Old World (Asia, Africa, Southern Europe) and New World (Central and South America), include conditions ranging from localized self-healing ulcers to noncuring disseminated lesions similar to leprosy in appearance.
- In the New World, mucosal leishmaniasis occurs when the parasite in the skin invades mucosal surfaces (nose, mouth), giving rise to chronic disfiguring conditions. Leishmaniasis is discussed in detail in Chapter 28.

### Schistosomal infection can cause a dermatitis

Transmission of schistosomal infection to humans is achieved via active skin penetration by larvae (cercariae) released into fresh water by the snail intermediate host (see Ch. 28). This stage of infection can give rise to cercarial dermatitis, commonly known as *swimmer's itch*. However, there are many more species of schistosomes that infect birds or mammals, and it is the cercariae of nonhuman schistosomes that are thought to be the cause of most cases of swimmer's itch. It is relatively common where natural water used for

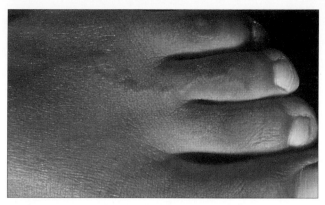

**Fig. 27.32** Cutaneous larval migrans (creeping eruption) showing the raised inflammatory track left by the invading hookworm larvae. (Courtesy A. du Vivier.)

recreation is populated with aquatic birds and a frequent problem in lakes in North America. Topical antiinflammatory treatments are effective therapy. Occasionally, topical 1% hydrocortisone ointment is required for treatment.

### Cutaneous larval migrans is characterized by itchy inflammatory hookworm larvae trails

Human hookworm (the nematodes *Ancylostoma* and *Necator*) invade the body through the skin, the infective larvae burrowing into the dermis then migrating via the blood to eventually reach the intestine. Invasion may cause an itchy popular erythematous rash, usually on the feet (known as *ground itch*), which becomes more severe upon repeated infection. Humans, however, can also be invaded by the larvae of the cat and dog species of *Ancylostoma*. Infection is acquired when exposed skin comes into contact with soil that has been contaminated by animals carrying the adult worms in their intestines. Eggs in the faeces hatch and release rhabditiform larvae, which go on to produce filariform larvae, the infective stage, that remain viable in the soil for some weeks depending on local environmental conditions. As the human host is foreign for these species, the nonhuman hookworm larvae fail to escape from the dermis after invasion and may live for some months in the absence of antiparasitic treatment, migrating parallel to the skin and leaving intensely itchy sinuous inflammatory trails (creeping eruption), which are easily visible at the surface (Fig. 27.32). Treatment is with topical thiabendazole paste where available, topical albendazole, oral albendazole or oral ivermectin.

### Onchocerciasis is characterized by hypersensitivity responses to larval antigens

Onchocerciasis is also known as *river blindness*. The adult-stage worms of *Onchocerca volvulus* live for an average of 10 years in subcutaneous nodules. Each day, female worms release several hundred live microfilariae, which migrate away from the nodules, remaining largely in the dermal layers but also capable of invading the eye, causing river blindness (see Ch. 26). The continuing buildup of parasite numbers and the development of a hypersensitivity response to the antigens released by living and dying larvae and their endosymbiont *Wolbachia* bacteria give rise to inflammatory skin conditions. In the early stages these appear as erythematous maculopapular rashes accompanied by intense itching. Later there are lichenified hyperkeratotic lesions. In long-standing infections, elasticity is lost, resulting in atrophied skin and excessive wrinkling. Depigmentation is also common. The microfilariae can be killed by ivermectin treatment, but the skin changes, once advanced, are irreversible.

Dermal inflammatory conditions and secondary bacterial infection of the skin are not uncommon during infection with lymphatic filarial nematodes.

### Arthropod infections

#### Some flies, mainly in the tropics and subtropics, have larvae that develop within the skin

Myiasis is a condition associated with invasion of the body by the larvae (maggots) of dipteran flies such as *Dermatobia*. Several species of fly have a cycle in which the larvae feed and grow in the skin of a mammal, just below the surface, escaping before or after pupation to continue their life cycle and lead ultimately to the release of adult forms. Female flies lay eggs, or larvae, directly onto the skin or attach eggs to the abdomen of a mosquito, which then delivers the larva, or lays eggs onto soiled clothing, depending on the species of fly. Larvae then penetrate the skin but may also invade wounds or natural orifices. The activities and feeding of the larvae cause intensely painful reactions, and large lesions may develop, consisting of multiple furuncular lesions. A number of dipteran species have been found to infect humans and have been recorded in many countries, although primarily in tropical and subtropical climatic zones. Treatment involves removal of the larvae, ensuring it is complete, alleviation of symptoms and prevention of secondary bacterial infection.

Maggot debridement therapy uses maggots of nonmyiasis species, usually *Lucilia sericata*, to treat troublesome wounds, achieving debridement, disinfection of the wound and possibly stimulation of tissue growth to aid healing.

#### Certain ticks, lice and mites live on blood or tissue fluids from humans

Some feed nonselectively on humans, the normal hosts being animals (e.g. *Ixodes scapularis*, the deer tick); other species are human specific (e.g. *Pthirus pubis*, the pubic louse). The feeding processes and the inevitable release of saliva give rise to skin irritation, which becomes more intense as the body responds immunologically to the proteins present in the saliva. Prolonged feeding, as practised by ticks, may leave painful lesions in the skin, which can become secondarily infected. Species such as lice and scabies mites, which spend the greater part or the whole of their lives on the human body, can cause severe skin conditions when populations accumulate. These conditions arise from:

- the activity of the arthropods themselves
- their production of excreta
- the oozing of blood and tissue fluids from the feeding sites
- the host's inflammatory reaction.

Pediculosis—infection with head and body lice of the genus *Pediculus*—can result in pruritus due to sensitization to louse antigens. Severe infestations can give rise to encrusting inflammatory masses in which fungal infections may establish. Good personal hygiene and reducing social deprivation

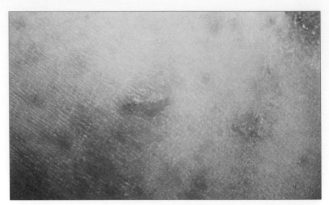

**Fig. 27.33** A characteristic cutaneous burrow in scabies. (Courtesy M.J. Wood.)

prevents infestation with body lice, but head lice can still be transmitted even under good hygienic conditions, close contact being a key factor. Use of insecticidal creams, lotions, shampoos and powders helps to clear the insects directly, but resistance to some insecticides (e.g. permethrin, malathion) is well documented in head lice infection.

The scabies mite has a more intimate contact with the human host than lice, living its whole life in or on the skin. Males remain superficial, but females burrow into the skin and lay eggs there. Burrows often occur in interdigital web spaces on the hands and on the wrists, but the area of infection can spread from the original site to cover large areas of the body (Fig. 27.33; see Ch. 22). Infection causes a characteristic rash with itching, excoriation is commonly seen and secondary infections may follow. Very heavy infections may develop in immunocompromised individuals or in people who are unable to care adequately for themselves. Under these conditions there is extensive thickening and crusting of the skin (Norwegian scabies). Treatment with permethrin or malathion is recommended; benzyl benzoate can also be used on unbroken skin but is less effective. Oral ivermectin is required in addition to topical therapy for Norwegian scabies.

## MUCOCUTANEOUS MANIFESTATIONS OF VIRAL INFECTIONS

Rashes can be divided into vesicular (blistering) eruptions, maculopapular (flat, papules) and erythematous (red) types. In addition, rashes are described according to where the virus is restricted to the body surface at the site of initial infection and where the virus spreads systemically through the body (Table 27.4). The skin rash has a characteristic distribution in many infectious diseases, but, with the exception of zoster, which involves the dermatome of the skin innervated by the affected nerve and dorsal root ganglion, the reason for this is unknown.

Rashes are particular features of human infection and are rare in animals. This is because human skin is naked and is a turbulent, highly reactive tissue in which immune and inflammatory events are clearly visible. Rashes cause discomfort and may be painful, but they may be very helpful for the clinician who needs to make a diagnosis. The veterinarian is less privileged because the skin of most other mammals is largely covered with fur, and skin lesions generally involve hairless areas such as udders,

**Table 27.4** Mucocutaneous manifestations of viruses

| Virus | Lesion | Virus shedding from lesion |
|---|---|---|
| **No systemic spread** | | |
| Papillomavirus (wart) | Common wart; plantar wart; genital wart | + |
| Molluscum contagiosum virus (poxvirus) | Fleshy papule | + |
| Orf (poxvirus from sheep, goats) | Papulovesicular | + |
| **Systemic spread** | | |
| Herpes simplex virus Varicella-zoster virus | Vesicular (neural spread and latency) | + |
| Coxsackievirus A (9, 16, 23) | Vesicular, in mouth (herpangina) | + |
| Coxsackievirus A16 Enterovirus 71 | Vesicular (hand, foot and mouth disease) | + |
| Parvovirus B19 | Facial maculopapular (erythema infectiosum) | − |
| Human herpesvirus 6 | Exanthem subitum (roseola infantum) | − |
| Measles virus | Maculopapular skin rash | − |
| Rubella virus Echoviruses | Maculopapular skin rash not distinguishable clinically | − |
| Dengue and other arthropod transmitted viruses | Maculopapular skin rash | − |

The pathogenesis of these diseases is illustrated in Fig. 27.2. Papillomas and vesicular lesions are generally sites of virus shedding. The distribution as well as the nature of the lesion can be important in diagnosis (e.g. varicella), but many maculopapular rashes are clinically indistinguishable.

scrotums, ears, prepuces, teats, noses or paws, all of which have the human properties of thickness, sensitivity and vascular reactivity.

## Papillomavirus infection

### Over 200 different types of papillomavirus can infect humans and are species specific

Papillomaviruses are 55 nm in diameter, icosahedral, double-stranded (ds), unenveloped DNA viruses that infect epithelial cells in skin and both oral and genital mucosa. Over 650 distinct animal and human papillomavirus (HPV) types have been identified, of which are species specific and distinct from animal papillomaviruses. They are highly adapted to human skin and mucosa and are ancient associates of our species; therefore, for most of the time, they cause little or no disease. Papillomas, also called *warts*, are often benign skin infections, but HPV infection can lead to neoplastic transformation of cells. The squamous epithelial cell in the skin and mucosal lesions can undergo low- and high-grade dysplasia (abnormal cells). High-grade dysplasia is a premalignant state. There are low- and high-risk HPV types, and the latter cause anogenital and some head and neck cancers. HPV shows some adaptation to definite sites on the body; some examples are as follows:

- At least 40 types, including HPV 6, 11, 16 and 18, can infect the anogenital tract and other mucosal areas and are sexually transmitted.
- HPV 1, 4, 27 and 57 tend to cause plantar warts (on the underside of the foot), and other cutaneous HPV types include 2, 3, 7 and 10.

Papillomaviruses are generally transmitted by direct contact, but they are stable and can spread indirectly. For instance, plantar warts can be acquired from contaminated floors or from the nonslip surfaces at the edges of swimming pools,

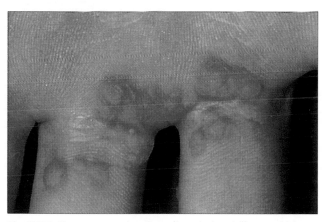

**Fig. 27.34** Common warts (papillomas) on the hand. (Courtesy M.J. Wood.)

and, in a given individual, warts can be spread from one site to another by shaving as they are autoinoculated.

### Papillomavirus infects cells in the basal layers of skin or mucosa and are tissue tropic

After entering the body via surface abrasions, the virus infects cells in the basal layers of the skin or mucosa (see Fig. 27.2). There is no spread to deeper tissues. Virus replication is slow and is critically dependent on the differentiation of host cells. Viral DNA is present in basal cells, but viral antigen and infectious virus are produced only when the cells begin to become squamified and keratinized as they approach the surface. The infected cells are stimulated to divide, and, finally 1–6 months after initial infection, the mass of infected cells protrudes from the body surface to form a visible papilloma or wart (Fig. 27.34). There is marked proliferation of prickle cells, and vacuolated cells are present in the more superficial layers. Warts can be:

- filiform with fingerlike projections
- flat topped
- flat because they grow inwards due to external pressure (plantar warts)
- a cauliflower-like protuberance (e.g. genital warts)
- a flat area of dysplasia on the cervix.

Immune responses eventually bring virus replication under control and, several months after infection, the wart regresses. Antibodies are demonstrable, but CMI responses are more important in recovery. Viral DNA remains in a latent state in the basal cell layer, infecting an occasional stem cell, and is, therefore, retained within the layer as epidermal cells differentiate and are shed from the surface. When patients are subsequently immunocompromised (e.g. posttransplant), crops of warts may result from reactivation of latent virus in the skin.

### Papillomavirus infections are associated with cancer of the cervix, vulva, penis, rectum, head and neck

Globally, HPV infection is associated with approximately 700,000 newly diagnosed cancers, constituting 5% of all cancers. It is second to *Helicobacter pylori* in infections that can cause cancer.

Of the HPV-associated cancers, 83% are cervical cancer, of which 72% are due to HR-HPV types 16 and 18 (these cause almost all male HPV-associated cancers) and 17% to HPV types 31, 33, 45, 52 and 58.

The association between genital warts and cancer of the cervix, vulva, penis and rectum is referred to in Chapter 18. Infection with specific genital HPVs causes invasive cervical cancer. There is a rare autosomal recessive disease, epidermodysplasia verruciformis, characterized by multiple warts containing many different HPV types normally seen causing skin warts and immunologic defects. Warts may undergo malignant change (squamous cell carcinomas) in approximately 30% of these patients, usually in sun-exposed sites.

### Diagnosis of cutaneous papillomavirus infection is clinical, and there are a variety of treatment options

Wart viruses cannot be cultivated in the laboratory, and serologic tests are mainly of epidemiologic rather than diagnostic use. HPV DNA detection methods can be used to examine samples not only for the HPV type but also to quantify the viral load.

Many treatments have been used for warts, some of them doubtless, seeming effective because skin warts eventually disappear without treatment. Treatments of skin warts include the application of karyolytic agents such as salicylic acid and destruction of wart tissue by cryotherapy and freezing with dry ice (solid carbon dioxide) or with liquid nitrogen. The latter is the most commonly used and most effective treatment. Genital intraepithelial lesions, especially cervical lesions, can lead to malignant disease, and treatment to eliminate the infection may involve laser therapy, loop excision and surgery. Immunotherapeutic drugs include Toll-like receptor agonists, such as imiquimod, that activate innate immunity and stimulate proinflammatory cytokines and type 1 interferons. Therapeutic HPV vaccines targeting the E6 and E7 proteins that can enhance T-cell responses have shown promise, as have immune checkpoint inhibitors such

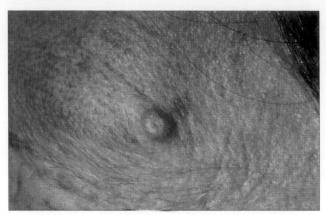

**Fig. 27.35** Single umbilicated lesion in *Molluscum contagiosum*. (Courtesy M.J. Wood.)

as nivolumab and pembrolizumab that block programmed cell death protein 1 and have been used in clinical trials but may need to be combined with other treatments.

### Molluscum contagiosum is an umbilicated lesion caused by a poxvirus

This DNA poxvirus infects epidermal keratinocytes to form a fleshy lesion, often with an umbilicated centre (Fig. 27.35). It only infects humans, is one of the five most common skin infections globally and is mainly seen in children, sexually active adults and immunocompromised individuals. Molluscum contagiosum (MC) is spread by contact or, in the case of genital lesions, by sexual intercourse; the incubation period is thought to be 2–8 weeks. There are four antigenically distinct types, and molluscum contagiosum virus (MCV)-1 and -2 are the most prevalent. Poxvirus particles can be seen by electron microscopy (see Ch. 3), but the characteristic lesions lead to a clinical diagnosis that can be augmented by using reflectance confocal microscopy. MC is self-limiting but may take months to resolve. MC may cause discomfort and can be severe in immunocompromised individuals, and treatments are available. These are similar to cutaneous HPV, cryotherapy, curettage, immunomodulatory, chemical (with potassium hydroxide) and antiviral. However, promising results have been reported with topical cantharidin, a terpenoid compound that weakens and degrades keratinocytes. In addition, a nitric oxide–releasing gel has an antiviral effect and immune modulation, possibly by protein nitrosylation and modulating the transcription factor NF-κB that regulates aspects of the innate and adaptive immune system.

### Orf is a papulovesicular lesion caused by a poxvirus

Orf (contagious pustular dermatitis) is an uncommon infection of the epidermis and is acquired by direct contact with infected sheep or goats. There is a papulovesicular lesion, generally on the hands, that may ulcerate. It is a clinical diagnosis and can be confirmed by electron microscopy or by molecular methods.

### Smallpox virus infection

Smallpox (variola) was a major scourge of humankind for at least 3000 years. It was caused by a poxvirus and spread from person to person by contact with skin lesions and via the respiratory tract. The disease was severe, with a

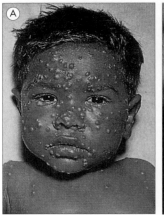
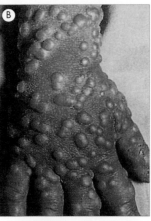
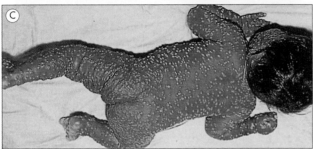

**Fig. 27.36** Smallpox. (A–C) These pictures were used as smallpox recognition cards by the World Health Organization during its smallpox eradication campaign. After upper respiratory tract infection, the virus reached the skin, where it replicated to cause a widespread vesiculopustular rash, with later scarring, especially on the face. The fatality rate was up to 40%, depending on the age of the host and the strain of the virus. (Courtesy the World Health Organization.)

generalized rash (Fig. 27.36), and was fatal in up to 40% of cases depending upon the strain of virus.

### Global smallpox eradication was officially certified in December 1979

During the first part of the 20th century, smallpox was largely eradicated from Oceania, North America and Europe by widespread vaccination, as originally developed by Edward Jenner (see Ch. 35) using a live attenuated strain of virus (vaccinia virus) with strict controls at frontiers. In 1967 WHO started a campaign to eradicate smallpox from the world, focusing on South America, Africa, India and Indonesia, making use of vaccination, surveillance and containment of cases. Despite such daunting difficulties as cultural barriers, warfare and transport to remote areas, the campaign was successful. Occasional cases had continued to occur in the United States until the 1940s, and in 1974 there were 218,000 cases worldwide, mostly in Asia, but the last case was recorded in Somalia in October 1977. The total cost to WHO was about US$150 million.

### Global eradication of smallpox was possible for a variety of reasons

The reasons are as follows:

- There were no subclinical infections, so cases could be readily identified.
- The virus was eliminated from the body on recovery, with no carriers.

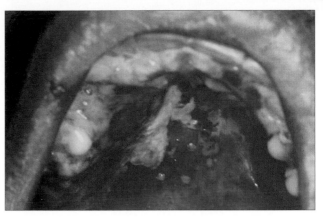

**Fig. 27.37** Primary herpes simplex virus infection. There are shallow ulcers with white exudate on the palate and gums. (Courtesy J.A. Innes.)

- Humans were the only host (no animal reservoir).
- An effective vaccine was available.

For a few years there were concerns about monkeypox (mpox), a simian disease caused by a similar virus and acquired by contact with infected monkeys in Africa. It was, however, thought to be poorly transmitted from human to human until the multicountry outbreak of mpox in 2022 (see Ch. 22). Concerns about the use of smallpox by bioterrorists have resulted in countries making contingency plans for the potential threat, which include the stockpiling of smallpox vaccine.

### Monkeypox caused a multicountry outbreak in 2022

Mpox is an orthpoxvirus in the Poxviridae family and became another emerging virus infection in 2022 resulting in WHO declaring the outbreak a global health emergency. The incubation period is 5–21 days, and symptoms include fever, headache, myalgia with clinical signs of maxillary, cervical or inguinal lymphadenopathy and rashes on the face and oral cavity before becoming generalized. The rash goes from being macular, to papular, vesicular and then pustular. The 2022 outbreak mostly involved the men who have sex with men (MSM) group, and anogenital vesicular lesions were mostly seen, with inguinal lymphadenopathy (see Ch. 22).

## Herpes simplex virus infection

### Herpes simplex virus infections are ubiquitous

Herpes simplex virus (HSV) is a medium-sized (120-nm in diameter) dsDNA virus of the herpesvirus group. Two types, HSV-1 and HSV-2, are distinguishable antigenically. It is a ubiquitous infection in early childhood. They cause a wide variety of clinical syndromes, the basic lesion being an intraepithelial vesicle from which the virus is shed.

Infection is usually transmitted from the saliva or cold sores of other individuals and frequently by kissing and sexual intercourse.

### Clinical features of HSV infection include painful vesicles and a latency state

After infection, the virus replicates in cells in the oral mucosa and forms virus-rich vesicles that ulcerate and become coated with a whitish-grey slough (Fig. 27.37).

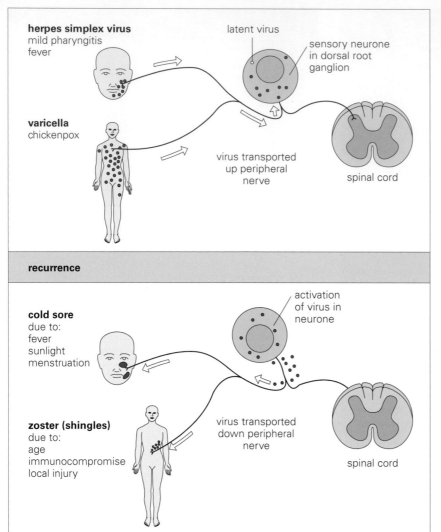

**Fig. 27.38** Pathogenesis of cold sores and zoster. In both herpes simplex virus and varicella-zoster virus infections, the virus in mucocutaneous nerve endings travels up the axon to reach the dorsal root ganglion where it becomes latent. Recurrences are due to reactivation of the virus within the dorsal root ganglion to become infectious followed by passage of virus down the axon to mucocutaneous site(s) and local spread and replication to form clinical lesion(s).

During the primary infection, virus particles enter sensory nerve endings, supplying the affected, area of the skin, and are transported to the dorsal root ganglion where they initiate a latent infection (see Ch. 17). The lesion resolves as antibody, and CMI responses develop. The latent virus remains in the sensory ganglion for life, and, under certain circumstances such as local trauma, can reactivate and spread down sensory nerves to cause cold sores at the site of the original infection (Fig. 27.38).

Primary infection can occur in various sites of the body and may be a result of inadvertent autoinoculation and include:

- in and around the mouth, lips and nose, causing painful, recurrent ulcers
- the eye, to cause conjunctivitis and keratitis, often with vesicles on the eyelids (see Ch. 26)
- the finger, to cause herpetic whitlow
- other skin sites following direct contact with infected individuals where there is rubbing or trauma, for instance in rugby football (scrum pox) or in wrestlers (herpes gladiatorum)
- the genital tract (see Ch. 22). Although HSV-2 arose as a sexually transmitted variant of HSV-1, the sites infected by the two types are less clearly distinct.

Serious complications associated with HSV infection include:

- herpetic infection of eczematous skin areas leading to severe disease in young children, eczema herpeticum (Fig. 27.39)
- acute necrotizing encephalitis following either primary infection or reactivation (see Ch. 25)
- neonatal infection acquired from the genital tract of the mother (see Ch. 24)
- primary or reactivating HSV infection in immunocompromised individuals, causing very severe disease (see Ch. 31).

### HSV reactivation is provoked by a variety of factors

In healthy individuals, HSV reactivation is provoked by:

- certain febrile illnesses (e.g. common cold, pneumonia)
- direct sunlight
- stress
- trauma
- menstruation
- immunocompromise.

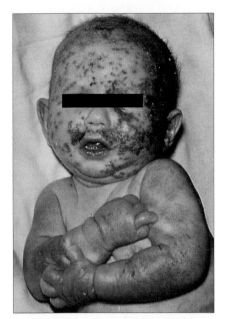

**Fig. 27.39** Eczema herpeticum due to herpes simplex virus infection in an infant. (Courtesy M.J. Wood.)

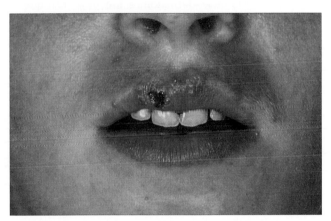

**Fig. 27.40** Recurrent herpes simplex virus vesicles on the mucocutaneous margin of the lip. (Courtesy A. du Vivier.)

Reactivation may be very severe in immunocompromised patients (see Ch. 31).

A sensory prodrome in the affected area may include feeling pins and needles, pain, burning and itching, which precedes the appearance of the lesion and is due to virus activity in sensory neurones. The lesion, a so-called cold sore, generally occurs around the mucocutaneous junctions in the nose or mouth (Fig. 27.40). Less commonly, when the ophthalmic branch of the trigeminal ganglion is involved, the lesion is a dendritic ulcer of the cornea. Large amounts of virus are shed in the cold sore, which scabs over and heals over the course of approximately 1 week. Occasionally the sensory prodrome occurs without proceeding to a cold sore (see also varicella-zoster virus recurrence, later).

### HSV DNA can be detected in vesicle fluid, and infection is treated with aciclovir

HSV DNA may be detected by PCR in vesicular fluid collected from lesions at affected sites. The majority of samples sent to laboratories are from genital lesions, but as HSV can infect various sites; cerebrospinal fluid, skin, eye and mucous membrane swab samples are part of the routine diagnostic laboratory workload. HSV causes a distinct cytopathic effect when grown in cell culture lines such as human embryo lung. However, highly sensitive and specific molecular-based techniques have improved the diagnosis of HSV infection by detecting HSV types 1 and 2 DNA in a variety of samples and replaced virus culture in many laboratories around the world.

Aciclovir revolutionized the treatment of HSV infection (see Ch. 34) and can be used either systemically or topically, although the antiviral drug penetration is better when given systemically. It is relatively nontoxic and acts specifically in virus-infected cells (see Ch. 34). Recurrent HSV can be very disabling, and aciclovir prophylaxis may be successful using a lower dose of aciclovir given twice daily for 6–12 months, at which time treatment can be stopped and the frequency of recurrent infection reassessed.

Other antiviral treatment options include valaciclovir and famciclovir. Aciclovir must be given intravenously when treating severe HSV infections such as herpes simplex encephalitis or disseminated HSV infection in immunocompromised individuals. Alternative antivirals such as ganciclovir, foscarnet or cidofovir may be used when antiviral resistance is being considered.

## Varicella-zoster virus infection

### Varicella-zoster virus infections are highly infectious and cause chickenpox (varicella) and zoster (shingles)

Varicella-zoster virus (VZV) is a medium-sized (100- to 200-nm in diameter) dsDNA virus of the herpesvirus group and is morphologically indistinguishable from HSV. There is only one serologic type. The virus grows more slowly than HSV and is not released from the infected cell. Infection is by inhalation of droplets from respiratory secretions and saliva or by direct contact from skin lesions. Primary infection with VZV causes varicella (chickenpox). Immunity develops and prevents reinfection (a second attack of varicella), but the virus persists in the body and later in life, after reactivation, causes zoster (shingles). Nearly all individuals in resource-rich countries are infected during childhood, but there are many areas of the world where the incidence of chickenpox in children is low (e.g. Africa and the Caribbean islands).

### Varicella is characterized by crops of vesicles that develop into pustules and then scab over

After primary infection, the virus passes across surface epithelium in the respiratory tract to infect mononuclear cells and is then carried to lymphoid tissues. There are no symptoms and no detectable lesions at the site of entry into the body. The virus slowly replicates in lymphoreticular tissues for approximately 1 week and then enters the blood in association with mononuclear cells and is seeded out to epithelial sites. These are mainly the respiratory tract and the skin but also include the mouth, often the conjunctiva and probably the alimentary and urogenital tracts. In the skin, for unknown reasons, the trunk, face and scalp are especially involved. At these epithelial sites, the virus exits from small blood vessels, infecting subepithelial and finally epithelial cells. Multinucleated giant cells with intranuclear inclusions are present in the lesions. In the oropharynx and respiratory tract, the virus reaches the surface and is shed to the exterior to infect other individuals approximately 2 weeks after initial infection. In the skin it takes 1–2 days longer, and it is at this stage when the characteristic varicella vesicles appear in a centripetal distribution that a clinical diagnosis can be made (Fig. 27.41). The mean incubation period is 14 days (range 10–23 days).

The individual remains well until 1–2 days before the rash, when there may be slight fever and malaise, but the illness is usually mild and often unnoticed. The vesicles appear first on the trunk, then on the face and scalp and less commonly on the arms and legs. They often come in crops over the course of several days, and all stages of lesions occur simultaneously then develop into pustules, break down, and scab over. The lesions are deeper than with HSV, and scarring is more common. Lesions in the mouth may be painful.

### Varicella is usually more severe and more likely to cause complications in adults

The skin lesions of varicella can become infected with staphylococci or streptococci to produce secondary impetigo, but varicella in a child is characteristically a mild illness. The main complications are:

- interstitial pneumonia, especially in adults who smoke; secondary bacterial pneumonia can also occur
- central nervous system (CNS) involvement, which may consist of a lymphocytic meningitis or an encephalomyelitis (see Ch. 25).

Thrombocytopenia can occur, but it is usually symptomless. Varicella can be a life-threatening disease in any immunocompromised patient.

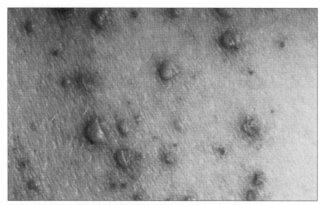

**Fig. 27.41** Early rash in varicella (chickenpox), with macules, papules and vesicles. (Courtesy M.J. Wood.)

After a primary infection during pregnancy, the virus may infect the fetus (see Ch. 24). Congenital varicella syndrome is seen in up to 1–2% if maternal infection occurs in the first or second trimester. Clinical features include skin scarring and hypoplastic limbs; other stigmata involve the eyes and brain. When the mother is infected a few days before or after delivery, the infant is exposed without the protection of maternal antibody and can suffer a serious disease. Prophylaxis to prevent or attenuate the potential infection in the infant can include passive immunization with varicella-zoster immune globulin (VZIG) or antiviral prophylaxis. In 2022 in the United Kingdom, aciclovir was recommended for postexposure prophylaxis for all at-risk groups apart from susceptible babies exposed within 1 week of delivery. VZIG was recommended if oral antivirals were contraindicated.

### Zoster results from reactivation of latent VZV

During primary infection, VZV in mucocutaneous lesions enters sensory nerve endings and establishes latent infection in the dorsal root ganglia (see Fig. 27.38). Later in life, reactivation can occur to cause zoster in the dermatome, the area of skin supplied by that nerve, at the site of the reactivation. Thoracic dermatomes are most commonly affected because these are the most common sites for the original varicella lesions. Zoster is usually unilateral, unless the individual is immunocompromised, because the reactivation is a localized event in a single dorsal root ganglion. Zoster therefore originates from inside the body and is not directly acquired from either varicella or zoster in other individuals. During reactivation in sensory neurones (see Fig. 27.38) there is paraesthesia and pain. Pain may be severe and precedes the development of the erythematous rash in which virus-rich vesicles appear (Fig. 27.42) by several days. It takes a few days for the virus to travel down peripheral nerves and multiply in the skin. Fever and malaise may accompany the rash. Sometimes the immune response controls the reactivating virus before skin lesions have had time to form, and, in this case, the sensory phenomena occur without the skin eruption. This is referred to as *zoster sine herpete*, for the classical scholars amongst the readers.

Conditions that predispose to zoster include:

- increasing age, although zoster is very occasionally seen in childhood, its incidence increases with increasing age, rising from 3/1000/yr in 50- to 59-year-olds to 10/1000/yr in 80- to 89-year-olds

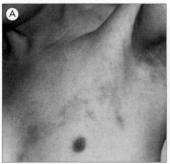 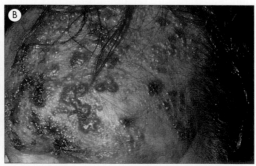

**Fig. 27.42** Zoster rash. (A) A band of faint erythema, an early sign of shingles, along an intercostal nerve. (B) Rash affecting the ophthalmic division of the trigeminal nerve. (Courtesy M.J. Wood.)

- immunocompromise due to leukaemia, lymphoma, acquired immunodeficiency syndrome (AIDS), solid organ transplantation and drug-induced immunosuppression
- trauma or tumours affecting the brain or spinal cord.

The skin areas affected by zoster reflect the distribution of the original varicella rash, as might be expected from its pathogenesis (see Fig. 27.38). Hence the trunk is most commonly involved. Ophthalmic zoster involving the upper eyelid, forehead and scalp is a particularly unpleasant manifestation, which can be sight threatening and is highly infectious as there is an opportunity for a lot of VZV to be shed into the air.

### Postherpetic neuralgia is a common complication of zoster

In the healthy host, postherpetic neuralgia (also known as *zoster-associated pain [ZAP]*) is common especially in the elderly. The pain, which can be severe early in the illness, continues for up to several months after the lesions have resolved. It is difficult to treat, although antiviral agents reduce the incidence, duration and severity of ZAP if started as soon as possible after zoster occurs.

Zoster may be severe in immunocompromised patients. A few days after the localized eruption, the virus, with inadequate control by cell-mediated immunity, spreads via the blood to produce skin and visceral lesions throughout the body. Haemorrhagic complications and pneumonia may occur.

### Laboratory diagnosis of VZV

It is a clinical diagnosis that can be assisted by carrying out molecular tests to detect VZV DNA in swabs from the vesicles. Alternative tests less widely used include immunofluorescence tests on skin lesion scrapings using VZV-specific monoclonal antibodies or by isolating VZV in cell culture, although the cytopathic effect may take a couple of weeks. Herpesvirus particles can be seen by electron microscopy in vesicle fluid but are indistinguishable from other herpesviruses—in particular HSV, which also causes vesicular lesions. Past infection is determined by detecting VZV immunoglobulin G (IgG) by ELISA or other methods. A VZV IgM result may be helpful if the skin lesions have healed and the diagnosis needs to be made for clinical reasons.

### Treatment of varicella and zoster infection

Higher dose aciclovir is given to treat VZV infections, compared with HSV infections, but this drug or the more readily bioavailable valaciclovir or famciclovir can be used orally to treat varicella and zoster. Treating chickenpox is often not considered as it is thought of as a mild infection that causes little discomfort, mostly by those who cannot remember having had chickenpox. However, varicella can cause complications in adolescents and adults, and antiviral treatment should be offered especially as new lesion formation, viral shedding and symptoms will be reduced. Severe infections must be treated with intravenous aciclovir especially in high-risk groups.

VZIG contains a high titre of VZV IgG, pooled from blood donors with a past history of chickenpox. VZIG is used to prevent or attenuate varicella in susceptible individuals at risk of complications such as immunocompromised individuals after exposure to someone with chickenpox or shingles (the latter may be dependent on the site and whether it is covered or not), but it must be given within 7–10 days of exposure to the source. In the United Kingdom, aciclovir prophylaxis had replaced VZIG in this setting; in the United States, varicella vaccine was another recommendation for prophylaxis if there were no contraindications, the contact was VZV IgG negative and it was within 5 days of the exposure. Varicella skin lesions may be treated with calamine lotion to relieve itching and to prevent scratching and secondary infection.

A live attenuated chickenpox vaccine is licensed in a number of countries, and universal childhood immunization was started in the United States in 1995. In addition, a live attenuated shingles (herpes zoster) vaccine called Zostavax was first used in 2006 in the United States that was replaced in 2020 by a recombinant subunit vaccine (Shingrix) that reduces the risk in the target age group (those age ≥70 years) of both developing shingles and ZAP by just over 91% and 89%, respectively. In the United Kingdom, the routine shingles vaccination programme was introduced in 2013 and still includes Zostavax with Shingrix being offered to immunocompromised individuals. Other countries have different age ranges for those eligible in their national shingles vaccination programmes.

## Rashes caused by enteroviruses

### Coxsackieviruses and echoviruses cause a variety of exanthems (skin rashes)

Enteroviruses are positive sense, single-stranded (ss) RNA viruses in the Picornaviridae family. There are 106 human enterovirus types, and the genus has four species, enterovirus A–D within which are the coxsackieviruses, echoviruses, enteroviruses and polioviruses. Sometimes such infections are accompanied by an enanthem (lesions on internal epithelial surfaces such as the oral cavity). These infections are generally seen in young children, are not usually distinguishable on clinical examination and are not severe. These viruses are also responsible for illnesses affecting the CNS (see Ch. 25), the upper respiratory tract (see Ch. 19) and striated and heart muscle (see later). In addition, enterovirus infections have been increasingly associated with the development of type 1 diabetes mellitus.

The lesions are usually vesicular and occur mostly on the buccal mucosa and the tongue. Most children complain of a sore mouth or tongue, and there is slight fever. When vesicular lesions are also seen on the skin, principally on the hands and feet, the condition is called hand, foot and mouth disease (Fig. 27.43). The virus is present in the lesions, and coxsackievirus A16 and enterovirus 71 are the most common causes.

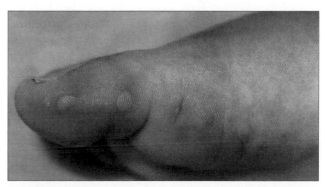

**Fig. 27.43** Vesicular lesions on the foot in hand, foot and mouth disease. (Courtesy M.J. Wood.)

Maculopapular rashes resembling rubella and often occurring in the summer are common manifestations of some coxsackie A and echovirus infections.

### Rashes caused by human parvovirus B19

#### Parvovirus B19 causes slapped cheek syndrome

Viruses are small anyway(!), but parvoviruses, as Latin scholars might know, are very small (22 nm in diameter) ssDNA viruses. Parvovirus B19 was identified by chance in 1974 when serum sample number 19 in panel B gave some odd results when tested in hepatitis B surface antigen assays. At that time, electron microscopy was the catch-all method for detecting viruses, and particles that looked like animal parvoviruses were seen. Parvovirus B19 is the only member of the Parvoviridae family known to cause human disease and is tropic to erythroid progenitor cells and binds to the P antigen cellular receptor. It causes a febrile illness in children with a characteristic maculopapular rash on the face (hence slapped cheek syndrome). The condition is referred to as erythema infectiosum and sometimes fifth disease, it being the fifth of the six common exanthematous infections recognized by 19th-century physicians. Rash, myalgia (muscle pain) and arthralgia (joint pain) may be seen in adults.

#### Symptomless parvovirus B19 infection is common and spreads by respiratory droplets

Nearly 50% of the population has had parvovirus B19 in the past. The virus grows in haemopoietic cells in the bone marrow, and, although this normally causes no more than a temporary and barely detectable fall in haemoglobin levels, it can lead to serious consequences in those with chronic anaemia. In children with sickle cell anaemia, for instance, the effect on erythropoiesis may cause an aplastic crisis. In pregnancy, if the fetus is infected and affected after maternal P19 infection, anaemia can lead to heart failure and hydrops fetalis.

Laboratory diagnosis is made by testing sera for parvovirus B19–specific IgM. Molecular tests may be used to detect B19 DNA in fetal blood when hydrops fetalis is suspected, after the mother has had either a parvovirus infection or an ultrasound examination of the baby showing hydrops. Parvovirus B19 cannot be isolated in cell culture.

### Rashes caused by human herpesviruses-6 and -7

#### Human herpesvirus-6 is present in the saliva of >85% of adults and causes roseola infantum

Human herpesviruses-6 (HHV-6) and HHV-7 were discovered in 1986 and 1990, respectively, the preceding five HHVs being HSV-1, HSV-2, VZV, cytomegalovirus (CMV) and Epstein-Barr virus (EBV). Both infections are ubiquitous globally and occur in most of the population in the first 2 years of life. HHV-6 replicates in T and B cells and in the oropharynx from where it is shed into saliva. The virus persists in the body after initial infection. There are two HHV-6 variants, namely HHV-6A and -6B. Their tissue distribution differs in that HHV-6B can be detected in blood, saliva and brain tissue; 6A occurs more often in the lungs and skin.

HHV-6B is the cause of exanthem subitum (also called roseola infantum), a very common acute febrile illness in infants and young children. After an incubation period of approximately 2 weeks, children develop a high fever that

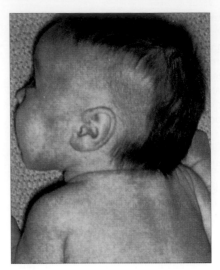

**Fig. 27.44** Maculopapular rash in roseola infantum. (Courtesy M.J. Wood.)

lasts 3–5 days. The disease is mild, and within 2 days of the fever subsiding a maculopapular rash is seen (Fig. 27.44). HHV-6B is also associated with approximately 30% of febrile fits in children, and HHV-6 encephalitis has been reported in bone marrow transplant recipients.

The diagnosis is difficult as HHV-6 DNA may be integrated into human cell chromosomes, so detecting HHV-6 DNA may not be diagnostic of an active infection. This means that the HHV-6 DNA load needs to be quantified in the peripheral blood as well as the sample from the body compartment affected to make a diagnosis of HHV-6 infection.

#### HHV-7 is acquired slightly later in early childhood

HHV-7 has been isolated from CD4-positive T cells. Infection occurs later than HHV-6 during infancy and early childhood. Persistence in the saliva and exanthem subitum has been reported with HHV-7.

#### HHV-8 causes Kaposi sarcoma skin lesions and a number of lymphoproliferative disorders

After a number of epidemiologic reports, it had been thought that a transmissible agent was involved in the development of Kaposi sarcoma (KS), a skin malignancy more common in some Mediterranean areas and in parts of Africa in addition to AIDS-associated KS. A number of molecular technology developments allowed the identification of KS-associated herpesvirus, also known as *HHV-8*, in 1994 in the endothelial cells of KS lesions. It is not a ubiquitous infection and has been associated with two other rare malignancies, primary effusion lymphoma and multicentric Castleman disease.

There are four main subtypes of KS:

- classic (sporadic)
- endemic (sub-Saharan Africa)
- epidemic (AIDS-related)
- iatrogenic (transplant-related).

Patients may present with multifocal skin lesions mucosal lesions or lymph node or organ involvement.

Transmission is mostly via saliva and sexual intercourse, and interactions between defective cellular immune responses, the endothelial system and HHV-8 result in the pathogenesis of KS.

The clinical diagnosis is confirmed in the laboratory by finding HHV-8 DNA in biopsy tissue with the characteristic spindle cell appearance of endothelial cells. In addition, qualitative and quantitative HHV-8 DNA load tests can be carried out by PCR. The incidence of AIDS-associated KS has dropped since the advent of combined antiretroviral therapy. In addition, retrospective studies reported that ganciclovir and foscarnet treatment resulted in a reduction of KS lesions. Treatment differs depending on the KS subtype and may involve surgical excision, cryotherapy, laser therapy for local lesions or immunomodulators, cytotoxic chemotherapy and monoclonal antibody treatment for widespread involvement.

## MEASLES VIRUS INFECTION

Measles has several special features, as follows:

- Nearly all infected individuals become unwell and develop disease. This is in contrast to most other viral infections in which a significant proportion of individuals undergo an asymptomatic or subclinical infection.
- The disease is so characteristic that a clinical diagnosis can nearly always be made without the need for laboratory help. We can recognize measles as described 1000 years ago by Arabian physician Rhazes.
- There is only one antigenic type of measles virus, and humans are the only natural hosts.
- Measles is highly infectious, and nearly all susceptible children contract the disease on exposure. Measles was regarded as a routine inescapable part of childhood, and >99% of individuals were infected until immunisation programmes were developed.
- There is a striking contrast between measles in well-nourished children with good access to medical care in resource-rich countries and measles under conditions of malnutrition or starvation or with less access to medical services in resource-poor countries (Table 27.5).

### Aetiology and transmission

**Measles outbreaks can occur every few years in unvaccinated populations**

Measles virus is a member of the Paramyxoviridae family, is an enveloped, negative sense and nonsegmented ssRNA virus and is transmitted by respiratory droplets. Although the virus is soon inactivated as it dries on surfaces, it is more stable in droplets suspended in the air. In unvaccinated populations, outbreaks tend to occur every few years when the number of susceptible children reaches a high enough level. There were a number of measles outbreaks in Europe in 2011, some of which were large, including >7000 infections in France that resulted in further immunisation campaigns in a number of countries.

It is highly infectious with an $R_0$ value between 12 and 18; in other words, one individual with measles can infect 12–18 contacts. The incubation period is 10–14 days, but the upper range can be 23 days. Although the number of infections globally fell since the turn of the 21st century, they increased between 2016 and 2019 to approximately 870,000, as did the mortality rate.

**Clinical features of measles include respiratory symptoms, Koplik spots and a rash**

The inhaled virus enters the body in the upper or lower respiratory tract or conjunctiva and spreads to subepithelial and local lymphatic tissues, without causing detectable lesions or symptoms. Measles virus infects cells using two receptors, CD150 (also called the signalling lymphocyte activation molecule 1) on lymphocytes, macrophages and dendritic cells, and nectin-4, on respiratory tract epithelial cells. During the next few days there is a primary viraemia, and the virus, which is highly lymphotropic, slowly spreads and multiplies in lymphoid tissues elsewhere in the body, including the spleen and the respiratory tract. There is then a secondary viraemia approximately 5 days after the initial infection, and the virus disseminates to a variety of epithelial sites, including the skin, kidney and bladder. Clinical signs soon appear in the respiratory tract where there are only one or two layers of epithelial cells to traverse. The patient is well until 9–10 days after infection and then develops an acute respiratory illness with a runny nose, fever and cough. Conjunctivitis is also a feature, and as a result of the large amounts of virus being shed in respiratory secretions the patient is highly infectious. The diagnosis may be suspected during this prodromal illness, especially after known exposure to measles. It takes 1–2 days longer for the foci of infection at mucosal and skin surfaces to cause lesions. Koplik spots, pathognomonic of measles, appear inside the cheek (Fig. 27.45), and shortly afterwards at approximately 12 days after infection the maculopapular

**Table 27.5** The clinical impact of measles depends on the condition of the host

| Site | Well-nourished child<br>Good medical care | Malnourished child<br>Poor access to medical care |
|---|---|---|
| Lung | Mild respiratory illness | Life-threatening pneumonia |
| Ear | Otitis media quite common | Otitis media more common, more severe |
| Oral mucosa | Koplik spots | Severe ulcerating lesions |
| Conjunctiva | Conjunctivitis | Severe corneal lesions, secondary bacterial infection, blindness may result |
| Skin | Maculopapular rash | Haemorrhagic rashes may occur (black measles) |
| Intestinal tract | No lesions | Diarrhoea—exacerbates malnutrition, halts growth, impairs recovery |
| Overall impact | Serious disease in a small proportion of those infected | Major cause of death in childhood (estimated 1 million deaths per year worldwide) |

Measles is a much more serious disease in malnourished children with poor access to medical care. The same epithelial surfaces are infected more extensively and with more serious sequelae.

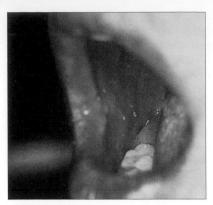

**Fig. 27.45** Koplik spots seen as minute white dots on the inflamed buccal mucosa of a patient with measles. (Courtesy M.J. Wood.)

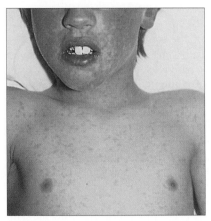

**Fig. 27.46** Maculopapular rash on the face and trunk of a patient with measles. (Courtesy M.J. Wood.)

rash (Fig. 27.46) is seen first on the face, then spreading down the body to the extremities. Individuals are infectious 4 days before until 4 days after rash onset.

### Measles rash results from a cell-mediated immune response

Antibodies are formed, but a CMI response is needed to control the virus in the lungs and elsewhere. Without it, the virus continues to multiply and gives rise to giant cell pneumonia (see Ch. 20). The CMI response is also responsible for the skin lesions, which are not seen in patients with serious defects in this type of immunity. Children with agammaglobulinaemia, on the other hand, have a normal course of disease, develop normal immunity and can be protected by vaccination. In uncomplicated cases, recovery is rapid.

During measles, as in a variety of other acute infections, there are temporary defects in immune responses to unrelated antigens. For instance, at about the time the rash appears, individuals who are known to be tuberculin positive give negative skin test responses to tuberculin. This returns to normal in approximately 1 month. During the virgin-soil epidemic in 1953, when measles reappeared after a long absence in South Greenland and adults as well as children were infected, there was increased mortality in those previously infected with TB. Since then, it has been shown that measles virus can induce T and B memory cell apoptosis and affect the innate immune system causing immune amnesia.

Previous immunologic memory is lost. Furthermore, the virus can block interferon production and signalling.

### Complications of measles are particularly likely among children in resource-poor countries

Complications of measles, due to the loss of memory B and T cells and a resulting generalized immune suppression, include:

- opportunistic bacterial superinfections, which are quite common, especially otitis media and pneumonia, as a result of virus damage to respiratory surfaces
- a primary measles virus pneumonia (giant cell pneumonia), which is seen in patients with serious CMI response defects
- postinfectious encephalitis known as *acute disseminated encephalomyelitis*, which occurs in approximately 1/1000 patients approximately 2 weeks after infection. Measles inclusion body encephalitis can rarely occur in immuno-compromised individuals (see Ch. 25)
- very rarely, subacute sclerosing panencephalitis in 6.5–11/100,000 infections. This develops 1–10 years after apparent recovery from acute infection.

Children in countries where access to medical care is poor and they are malnourished develop a more serious disease (see Table 27.5) especially during famine. This is attributable to:

- poor local mucosal defences, which can be improved by vitamin A administration
- impaired immune defences due to protein–calorie malnutrition, with the added impact of measles virus-induced immunosuppression
- poor medical services, with less ready availability of antibiotics to control secondary infection
- high levels of bacterial contamination of the environment
- exposure to a larger virus dose—a possible factor if others with severe measles shed larger amounts of virus from the respiratory tract.

### Diagnosis, treatment and prevention

#### Measles is usually diagnosed clinically; ribavirin can be used as antiviral treatment if clinically indicated and there is a safe and effective vaccine

Although the clinical diagnosis should be clear, the rash is similar to a number of other viral exanthems that affect the same age group. In addition, immunized individuals may have a milder infection. Koplik spots and conjunctivitis help with the definitive diagnosis, although they may not be seen in immunocompromised individuals with a blunted immune response. Therefore samples should be collected to confirm the diagnosis. In addition, with the success of the vaccine, the incidence of measles infection fell, and it was less likely that health care workers would see children with measles in resource-rich countries. However, after the controversial publication of a study in 1998 in which the measles, mumps and rubella (MMR) vaccine was linked with autism, which was never confirmed and all the subsequent epidemiologic investigations showed there was no link, there was both a reduction in immunisation rates and an increase in measles and mumps infections around the world. Since then, MMR vaccine rates have risen with a corresponding reduction in infection.

Detecting measles virus RNA by PCR in oral fluid or throat swab samples and collecting blood and testing for measles-specific IgM is helpful in confirming the diagnosis. Virus isolation in cell culture is rarely necessary. Complicated measles infection can be treated with ribavirin.

A live attenuated vaccine has been available since 1963. It is effective, safe and long lasting and is combined with MMR vaccine (see Ch. 35). Before a vaccine became available, measles killed 7–8 million children each year worldwide. By 1996 this was reduced to 1 million, and the WHO/UNICEF initiatives included applying the mass immunisation programmes used in the Americas and Europe to resource-poor countries.

## RUBELLA VIRUS INFECTION

**Rubella virus infection causes a multisystem infection, but its main impact is on the fetus**

There is only one serotype of this ssRNA togavirus, and humans are the only known host, its principal impact being on the fetus (see Ch. 24). It is transmitted by droplet infection and is less contagious than measles but more so than mumps.

After entering the body via the upper respiratory tract, the virus replicates for a period in local lymphoid tissues, followed by spread to the spleen and to lymph nodes elsewhere in the body. One week after infection, further multiplication in these tissues leads to viraemia and localization of virus in the respiratory tract and skin, and sometimes the placenta, joints and kidney. The clinical consequences of infection in various tissues of the body are shown in Table 27.6.

After an incubation period of 14–21 days, there is a mild disease with fever, malaise and an irregular maculopapular rash lasting 3 days. Enlarged lymph nodes are often evident behind the ear (posterior auricular or may be suboccipital), but the infection is commonly subclinical.

**Rubella is diagnosed in the laboratory; there is no treatment, but there is a vaccine**

Clinical diagnosis of rubella is sometimes possible but must be confirmed in the laboratory. Laboratory diagnosis is made by demonstrating rubella-specific IgM in a serum sample or detecting rubella virus RNA in oral fluid or throat swab samples (see Ch. 33). Virus isolation from the throat is rarely indicated — virus isolation requires specialized cell lines, and indirect methods are needed to demonstrate its growth. Viral RNA can be detected in samples from different sites.

There is no antiviral treatment. A live attenuated rubella vaccine that is safe and effective is given by injection, generally in combination with MMR vaccine. Prevention of congenital rubella is referred to in Chapter 24.

## OTHER MACULOPAPULAR RASHES ASSOCIATED WITH VIRAL INFECTIONS

The maculopapular rashes seen in certain arthropod-borne virus infections (e.g. dengue) and in zoonotic virus infections (e.g. Marburg disease) are referred to in Chapters 28 and 29. A maculopapular rash may be rarely seen in acute hepatitis B virus (HBV) infection and is immune complex mediated.

## OTHER INFECTIONS PRODUCING SKIN LESIONS

**Other bacterial, fungal and rickettsial infections produce a variety of rashes or other skin lesions**

Most of these are referred to elsewhere in this book, and they are listed in Table 27.1. Rashes in rickettsial infections are often striking, as in the case of Rocky Mountain spotted fever or typhus (see Ch. 28). Most rickettsia invade vascular endothelial cells and are shed into the blood to infect blood-sucking arthropod vectors. Invasion of vascular endothelial cells in the skin provides the basis for the skin rash but is not a source of direct shedding to the exterior.

## KAWASAKI DISEASE

**Kawasaki disease is an acute vasculitis and is probably caused by superantigen toxins**

Kawasaki disease (KD) is a childhood illness that occurs in genetically susceptible hosts with dysregulated T-cell activation after exposure to infectious triggers. Patients, who are generally <4 years of age, develop fever, conjunctivitis and a rash. There is dryness and redness of the lips and red palms and soles with some oedema, desquamation of fingertips, often arthralgia and myocarditis, which gives a case mortality of approximately 2%. The basic pathology is an acute multisystemic vasculitis, and 20% of untreated patients develop coronary artery aneurysms. The disease is more common in those of Asian ethnicity but occurs worldwide. There is no clear evidence for person-to-person transmission, and the disease is endemic with seasonal fluctuations and outbreaks. It is thought to be of infectious origin, and the mechanism of immune activation may be due to either an antigen or superantigen such as the toxins (see Ch. 17) of *S. aureus* or *S. pyogenes*. A superantigen is a group of proteins that can stimulate many T cells by attaching to part of the T-cell receptor in association with the major histocompatibility complex (MHC) class II molecules without needing antigen processing.

Treatment with intravenous immunoglobulin and aspirin reduces the incidence of coronary artery damage and prevents the aneurysms if given early enough. Serum levels of tumor necrosis factor alpha (TNFα), a proinflammatory cytokine, are high in KD and can lead to inflammatory signalling cascades

**Table 27.6** Clinical consequences of rubella virus invasion of different body tissues

| Site | Result | Comment |
|------|--------|---------|
| Respiratory tract | Virus shedding but symptoms minimal (mild sore throat, coryza, cough) | Patient infectious 5 days before to 3 days after symptoms |
| Skin | Rash | Often fleeting, atypical; immunopathology involved (Ag-Ab complexes) |
| Lymph nodes | Lymphadenopathy | More common in posterior triangle of neck or behind ear |
| Joints | Mild arthralgia, arthritis | Immunopathology involved (circulating immune complexes) |
| Placenta/fetus | Placentitis, fetal damage | Congenital rubella |

and further activation of the immune response. Infliximab is a TNFα inhibitor and expands regulatory T cells and has been shown to be beneficial as combination treatment for acute KD.

## VIRAL INFECTIONS OF MUSCLE

### Viral myositis, myocarditis and pericarditis

**Some viruses, particularly coxsackievirus B, cause myocarditis and myalgia**

Patients with cardiomyopathy will present with chest pain, breathlessness and tiredness and there may be other associated symptoms, including myalgia and diarrhoea. The pathogenesis of inflammatory cardiomyopathy, myocarditis together with cardiac dysfunction and heart ventricle remodelling, mostly due to viral infections, is unclear. It looks like it is multifactorial involving viruses, the host immune system and genetic background, plus environmental factors. The outcome may be poor if the cardiac dysfunction involves the left venricle, cardiac failure and/or arrhythmias.

The viruses can be divided into:

- cardiotropic: enteroviruses
- indirectly triggering myocarditis (autoimmune molecular mimicry or cytokine-related cardiotoxicity: influenza A and B viruses, HIV, HCV, SARS-CoV-2, SARS-CoV, MERS CoV)
- ACE2 tropic and mediate direct cardiac injury: SARS-CoV-2, SARS-CoV, MERS CoV and rarely due to COVID-19 messenger RNA (mRNA) vaccines (see Ch. 20)
- vasculotropic: parvovirus B19
- lymphotropic and indirect action: HHV-6, EBV, CMV.

Group B, and to a lesser extent group A, coxsackieviruses and certain enteroviruses were the main viral causes of acute myocarditis and pericarditis. A cytotoxic effect is seen in animal models after viral attachment to the cellular receptors found in cardiac myocytes and macrophages. Adenoviruses and enteroviruses infect cardiomyocytes by binding to a transmembrane receptor leading to direct myocardial injury and a dysregulated immune response. Around 50% of patients recover, but the remainder have poor outcomes as the adenoviruses and enteroviruses persist in the myocardium. However, cardiac dysfunction related to SARS-CoV-2 and COVID-19 is probably underreported. There is a slight male predominance in myocarditis, and both myocarditis and pericarditis can be mistaken for myocardial infarction, yet the prognosis is good and complete recovery is the rule. There is also evidence for persistent infection linked with chronic myocarditis and chronic dilated cardiomyopathy. The most common cause of viral myocarditis in infants is the coxsackievirus B group, and it may be rapid in onset and fatal. These infections are transmitted by the faecal–oral route and occasionally from pharyngeal secretions. Ingested coxsackieviruses spread from the pharynx or gastrointestinal mucosa to the lymphatics and then to the blood. Invasion of striated muscles, heart or pericardium takes place across small blood vessels and results in acute inflammation. Group B coxsackieviruses also cause pleurodynia or epidemic myalgia. This condition is sometimes called Bornholm disease, after the Danish island where there was an extensive outbreak in 1930. There is pain and inflammation involving intercostal or abdominal muscles.

Influenza (especially influenza B in children) can cause pain and tenderness in muscles, but it is not known whether this is associated with viral invasion of muscle. Myalgias are also seen in dengue and in rickettsial and other febrile infections and are probably caused by circulating cytokines.

**Enterovirus RNA detection methods and then typing positive samples and in situ hybridization on endomyocardial biopsy tissue (if available) are key diagnostic tests**

Laboratory diagnosis can be difficult, as molecular-based methods, serology and virus isolation can give only circumstantial evidence for association between that virus infection and a specific organ. Enterovirus serologic tests are mostly insensitive and nonspecific and are being replaced. Many clinicians remember coxsackie IgM testing in individuals with cardiomyopathy from their training days and request the test.

Molecular detection methods have replaced virus isolation from throat swabs, faecal specimens or occasionally pericardial fluid. Endomyocardial biopsy material sent for histopathologic examination is the gold standard diagnostic method but may not be collected as it is very invasive.

The antiviral drug pleconaril has been used to treat enterovirus infections; however, it is no longer in production. Immunomodulators such as interferon β have been used in clinical trials and show promise in clearing the viral infection. Intravenous immunoglobulin may be used. There are no specific vaccines for enterovirus infections. The other causes of myocarditis can be treated with the appropriate antiviral drugs as they may be viral associated rather than virus induced and therefore have more a bystander effect (i.e. antiretroviral drugs for HIV, specific treatment for COVID-19 and influenza virus infections). The mainstay of treatment involves medical management of acute heart failure. This can involve mechanical circulatory support, cardiac drug treatments and extracorporeal membrane oxygenation in some clinical situations.

## POSTVIRAL FATIGUE SYNDROME

**It has been difficult to establish postviral fatigue syndrome as a clinical entity**

The postviral fatigue syndrome or chronic fatigue syndrome (CFS) is sometimes referred to as myalgic encephalomyelitis, but this is inappropriate because there is no evidence for CNS pathology.

The term unexplained postacute infection syndromes is likely to encompass this as the chronic sequelae of specific acute infectious diseases in a proportion of infected individuals for whom a diagnosis cannot be made is well recognized. In particular, 75% of individuals with CFS report a recent episode of infection. Long COVID is the latest example and has been reported in individuals after mild or moderate COVID-19. It has been estimated that 65 million people may have long COVID globally.

CFS consists of:

- chronic and severe muscle weakness, lasting at least 6 months, often as a sequel to an acute febrile illness
- severe tiredness
- less regularly associated symptoms such as depression, headache and anxiety.

It is more reliably identified when the first two symptoms appear in a previously healthy individual with no history of psychosomatic illness. Several viruses have been suggested as causes. Claims have been made for the role of coxsackie

B viruses, based on antibody tests and on the detection of a virus-specific protein in the serum of patients, but the picture remains unclear. A small proportion of cases appear to be due to chronic infection with EBV. Occasional reports have associated the condition with HHV-6 as well as other viruses. It has also been suggested that it is due to allergic reactions triggered by virus infections.

In 2009 a gammaretrovirus called *xenotropic murine leukaemia virus* was detected in peripheral blood mononuclear cells from approximately 67% of people with CFS compared with 4% of healthy controls. However, the association was not confirmed in other studies, and it was a salutary lesson about sensitive methods of detection as well as good laboratory practice as it was shown that the genomic sequences detected were part of the enzymes used in the PCR process.

Long COVID and CFS may well be part of the postacute infection syndromes that have no specific and objective biomarkers and so cannot be given a definitive diagnosis with a clear pathogenesis and management plan for the affected individual. It is interesting that after the SARS epidemic, approximately 10–20% of individuals had post-SARS sequelae after 2 months to 12 years follow-up. The most common symptom was fatigue in approximately 19%.

Longitudinal studies involving specific criteria for CFS and some for the acute infection reported approximately 40% of young adults had persisting symptoms for several weeks after onset of illness, and the number fell to 8–14% at 6 months and 7–9% at 12 months. Depending on whether a diagnosis of the acute infection had been made, the disability may still have been present after ≥2 years.

To help people manage their symptoms, understanding the pathogenesis is key and may include one, some or all of the following:

- Persistent infection that may not be detectable, resulting in chronic stimulation of the immune system (i.e. Ebola virus in sanctuary sites such as the eye and seminal fluid).
- Targeting self-antigens via infection-triggered impairment of regulatory T-cell function and/or molecular mimicry.
- Dysregulation of the microbiota–gut–brain axis.
- Permanent organ damage.

Once again, the theme of this book, the conflict between pathogen and host response, underpins understanding infectious diseases and how to treat the infections.

## PARASITIC INFECTIONS OF MUSCLE

Relatively few protozoan or helminth parasites invade muscle tissues and cause serious disease. Three of the more common are described here to illustrate the variety of organisms and the range of pathology.

### *Trypanosoma cruzi* infection

#### *Trypanosoma cruzi* is a protozoan and causes Chagas disease

Chagas disease is also known as American trypanosomiasis (see Ch. 28). The disease is endemic to Mexico, Central and South America, where WHO estimates 6–7 million people are infected. It is a zoonosis, and *T. cruzi* has been isolated from >150 species of mammal. The parasite is carried by blood-sucking reduviid bugs, which deposit infective trypomastigote stages on to the skin as they defecate while feeding. If these are rubbed into mucous membranes or wounds,

the parasites penetrate cells, transform into amastigotes and multiply. The infected cells then burst, liberating trypomastigotes, and a local superficial lesion is formed in up to 75% of cases. The parasite then disperses around the body to reinvade other cells. It is able to infect any nucleated cell, but its major sites of infection are cardiac muscle, smooth muscle, the intestinal myenteric plexus and nervous tissue, including the peripheral nervous system in some cases.

#### Chagas disease is complicated by cardiac conduction disorders, ventricular aneurysm formation or heart failure many years later

Chagas disease may be asymptomatic from the outset, but 5–10% occur as an acute febrile phase, with intense inflammatory changes, followed by a chronic phase that may produce no apparent damage (indeterminate phase), or progress to cause damage 20–30 years later. In the chronic phase there is gradual tissue destruction with autoimmune damage playing a part. Of those with clinical features of chronic Chagas disease, 95% have cardiac manifestations and 5% have either megaoesophagus or megacolon. The parasite invades the myofibrils of the heart (see Fig. 28.15). *T. cruzi* is capable of immune evasion, and the host's proinflammatory immune response leads to myocarditis. Autoimmune activity leads to fibrosis such that muscle fibrils and Purkinje fibres may be replaced by fibrous tissue. As a result of muscle weakness and conduction defects, the heart enlarges, there are cardiac arrhythmias and heart failure can occur.

Benznidazole or nifurtimox are used to treat the acute phase and in some cases they are used in the indeterminate, or chronic, phase. These drugs are available from WHO. At the time of writing, no vaccine is available, and prevention of infection is the most important measure.

### *Taenia solium* infection

#### The larval stages of *Taenia solium* invade body tissues

Tapeworms are intestinal parasites, but the larval stages of several species may invade deeper tissues. The most important of these are *Echinococcus granulosus*, which causes cystic echinococcosis (previously termed cystic hydatid disease; see Chs. 25 and 29), and the pork tapeworm *T. solium.* Humans acquire adult *T. solium* intestinal tapeworm infection by eating undercooked infected pig meat in which the cysticercus larvae are found as small, bladderlike structures in the muscle tissue. These larvae are digested out in the intestine and mature into the adult tapeworm, which may reach a length of several metres. *T. solium* eggs released in human faeces and ingested by a pig hatch in the pig intestine and release larvae, which cross the intestinal wall and are carried via the bloodstream to muscle. *T. solium* is unusual in that its eggs can hatch directly in the human intestine and behave in the same way as they would in a pig. In areas of poor sanitation this may result from accidental swallowing of water or food contaminated with eggs. Thus it is possible to acquire cysticercosis without ever eating pork. If hatching occurs, larvae can invade and form cysticerci in human muscle or, much more seriously, in the CNS. Forming cysticerci in human tissue is of no advantage to the parasite as it is essentially trapped there and unable to complete its life cycle by becoming an adult worm. Cysts in muscle eventually become calcified and can be seen on radiography

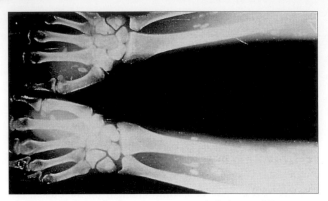

**Fig. 27.47** Radiograph showing numerous calcified cysts of *Taenia solium* in the forearms. (Courtesy R. Muller and J.R. Baker.)

(Fig. 27.47). Muscle infection is not serious, being largely asymptomatic. Infections are common in many parts of the world, particularly South and Central America and Asia. Avoidance of undercooked pork products is the safest precaution against developing adult pork tapeworm infection, whereas good sanitation and good personal hygiene practice are required to avoid ingesting eggs and thus developing cysticercosis.

### *Trichinella* infection

#### The larvae of *Trichinella* invade striated muscle

This nematode has many unique features. It is able to infect almost any warm-blooded animal and has a life cycle in which a complete generation (infective stage to infective stage) develops within the body of a single host. Humans can be infected by a variety of *Trichinella* species, *T. spiralis* being the most common. Transmission depends upon the ingestion of muscle tissue containing viable infective larvae. As far as humans are concerned, the commonest route of transmission is through infected pig meat, but many other meat sources have been known to transmit infection (e.g. bear, boar, horse). Infections occur worldwide. When infected undercooked meat is eaten, the larvae are digested out in the small intestine, invade the small bowel columnar epithelium and develop within 30 h into the adult worms. They mate in the mucosa, each female releasing between 500 and 1500 newborn larvae directly into the intestinal tissues, from where they are carried in blood or lymph around the body. Eventually the larvae penetrate striated muscles and mature into the infective stage, transforming muscle cells into parasite-sustaining nurse cells in approximately 20 days (see Fig. 29.11).

Light infections are asymptomatic, but the migration and penetration of the larvae are associated with inflammatory reactions, which can be severe and life-threatening when a person is heavily infected. Various symptoms are associated with this phase of which fever, muscle pains, weakness and eosinophilia are characteristic. Eosinophilic myocarditis may also occur, although the parasite does not develop in the heart.

Diagnosis on clinical criteria is usually made after the parasites have invaded the muscles, and treatment then is difficult. Albendazole or mebendazole is used to kill adult females in the intestine and prevent production of more larvae. Adjunctive corticosteroids are given in severely symptomatic cases to treat myositis.

### *Sarcocystis*

#### *Sarcocystis* is a rare muscle parasite

*Sarcocystis* is a protozoan related to *Toxoplasma*. Humans are the definitive hosts for *S. hominis* and *S. suihominis*, with cattle or pigs as intermediate hosts. Ingestion of raw or undercooked beef or pork containing sarcocysts in skeletal muscle results in a diarrhoeal illness. Humans can also act as aberrant intermediate hosts for *Sarcocystis* (e.g. *S. nesbitti*). The parasite develops initially in vascular endothelium, followed by sarcocyst formation in muscle. Outbreaks of myalgia and myositis due to *S. nesbitti* occurred in 2011–2012 in visitors to Southeast Asia.

## JOINT AND BONE INFECTIONS

Joints and bones will be considered separately for convenience, but joint lesions often spread to involve neighbouring bone, and vice versa (e.g. in TB).

### Reactive arthritis, arthralgia and septic arthritis

#### Arthralgia and arthritis occur in a variety of infections and are often immunologically mediated

Examples of such infections are outlined in Table 27.7. Joints can become infected by the haematogenous route or directly following trauma or surgery, but in many cases the condition is immunologically mediated rather than due to microbial invasion of the joint. The pathogen responsible is at a distant site in the body and causes a reactive arthritis. Reactive arthritis and arthralgia occur after certain enteric bacterial infections, and the arthralgia in rubella and HBV infections is of similar origin. In this type of arthritis, more than one joint is usually affected.

Ankylosing spondylitis is associated with *Klebsiella* infection, and it has been suggested that the antigenic similarity between *Klebsiella* antigen and human leukocyte antigen (HLA) B27 provokes a cross-reactive immune response that causes the disease. So far, there is no evidence that rheumatoid arthritis is caused by either viruses or other microbes.

#### Circulating bacteria sometimes localize in joints, especially following trauma

Such bacterial localization can then cause a suppurative (septic) arthritis. Generally, a single joint is involved. Joints are very susceptible, particularly if they are already damaged, for instance by rheumatoid arthritis, or if a prosthesis has been inserted. Knees are most commonly affected, followed by hips, ankles (see Fig. 22.5B) and elbows. Signs include a fever, joint pain, limitation of movement and swelling, and usually a joint effusion. Bacteria can be isolated from the joint fluid or seen in the centrifuged deposit, and the commonest organism is *S. aureus*. Sometimes the source of the circulating bacteria is obvious (e.g. a septic skin lesion), but often no source is apparent.

### Osteomyelitis

#### Bone can become infected by adjacent infection or haematogenously

As with joints, infection of bones can be by the direct route (e.g. from a nearby focus of infection, after fractures, after orthopaedic surgery) or from circulating pathogens. The commonest cause of haematogenous osteomyelitis is *S. aureus*, but when

**Table 27.7** Arthralgia and arthritis in infectious diseases

| Infectious agent | Comments |
|---|---|
| **Viral arthritis** | |
| Hepatitis B | Occurs in prodromal period; due to circulating immune complexes |
| Rubella | May occur in up to 70% of adult women with rubella |
| Mumps | Unusual; mostly in men |
| Ross River and other togaviruses | Mosquito-transmitted infections in Australia (Ross River) and Africa |
| Parvovirus | More common in adults, especially women |
| **Reactive arthritis** | |
| *Campylobacter*, *Yersinia*, salmonellae, shigellae, *Chlamydia trachomatis* (Reiter syndrome[a]) | Postinfectious arthritis, human leukocyte antigen (HLA) B27 associated, no bacterial invasion of joint, immune mediated |
| **Septic arthritis** | |
| *Staphylococcus aureus* | Commonest cause of suppurative arthritis |
| Streptococci (group A and B) | Common in adults and children |
| *Haemophilus influenzae* | Occurrence in children has decreased with *H. influenzae* vaccine |
| *Neisseria gonorrhoeae* | May affect multiple joints |
| *Mycobacterium tuberculosis* | Often with bone lesions, especially weight-bearing joints and bones |
| *Borrelia burgdorferi* | Arthritis a late feature of Lyme disease |
| Gram-negative bacilli | Neonates, the elderly, patients with immune deficiency disorders |
| *Sporothrix schenckii* | Fungal infection of joints; increased risk with human immunodeficiency virus infection |

[a]Urethritis, arthritis, uveitis, mucocutaneous lesions; complicates a small percentage of cases of chlamydial urethritis.

infection is from a neighbouring site it is generally mixed, with gram-negative rods and occasionally anaerobes also present. There seems to be no equivalent to reactive arthritis, in which inflammation is due to infection at a distant site.

Acute osteomyelitis typically involves the growing end of a long bone where sprouting capillary loops adjacent to epiphyseal growth plates promote the localization of circulating bacteria. It therefore tends to be a disease of children and adolescents and may follow nonpenetrating injury to the bone.

Osteomyelitis results in a painful tender bone lesion and a general febrile illness.

### Osteomyelitis is treated with antibiotics and sometimes surgery

The infection is diagnosed from blood cultures taken before the start of antimicrobial therapy or, if there is an open lesion, from a bone biopsy. Periosteal reaction and bone loss may be visible radiologically (Fig. 27.48). Treatment is begun on a most likely basis (e.g. nafcillin for MSSA; see earlier) as soon as microbiologic samples have been taken.

Osteomyelitis can become chronic, especially when there are necrotic bone fragments to act as a continued source of infection. Surgical intervention for debridement and drainage, as well as prolonged courses of antibiotics, may be necessary.

TB may affect the spine, hip, knee and bones of the hands and feet, and in resource-rich countries TB is particularly seen in immigrants from the Indian subcontinent. Constitutional disturbances are often absent, but the site is generally painful, and pressure from a tuberculous abscess in the spine can cause paraplegia.

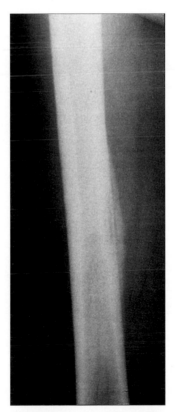

**Fig. 27.48** Acute staphylococcal osteomyelitis in the femur of a 24-year-old woman. There is a well-defined periosteal reaction in relation to the midshaft of the femur and an underlying lucency. (Courtesy A.M. Davies.)

## INFECTIONS OF THE HAEMOPOIETIC SYSTEM

### Many infectious agents cause changes in circulating blood cells

Examples of such agents include:

- *Bordetella pertussis*, which causes lymphocytosis
- EBV and CMV infections, which cause mononucleosis
- *Plasmodium* spp., which cause anaemia and thrombocytopenia.

A smaller number of infectious agents act directly on cells in the bone marrow (human parvovirus) or cause malignant transformation of lymphocytes (e.g. human T-cell lymphotropic virus type 1 [HTLV-1]). The range of possibilities is summarized in Table 27.8. HTLV-1 and HTLV-2 are mentioned earlier (see Ch. 24) but are described more fully later.

## HTLV-1 infection

### HTLV-1 is mainly transmitted by maternal milk

HTLV-1 was first isolated in 1980 from a patient with adult T-cell leukaemia and lymphoma (ATLL). However, it has been present in humans for >20,000 years and may have infected approximately 10 million people globally. Infection is widespread, especially in certain islands in the West Indies and Japan, where 5–15% of the population are infected, and in South America and parts of Africa. Transmission is primarily via maternal milk and sexual intercourse, and by blood-contaminated equipment in injecting drug users.

### HTLV-1 infects T cells, and up to 5% of those infected develop T-cell leukaemia

HTLV-1 infects T cells and persists, integrated, in the host genome. The tax gene product, a transcriptional activator protein, stimulates transcription of host genes controlling production of IL-2, IL-2 receptor and other molecules, thus affecting cell replication. Infected T cells proliferate, and, if in addition there are certain chromosomal abnormalities, malignant transformation takes place.

Clinically, the patient develops a mild febrile disease with lymphadenopathy. The skin is often involved, with nodule and plaque formation, and pleural effusion or aseptic meningitis can occur. There is also increased susceptibility to opportunist infections such as *Pneumocystis jirovecii* and *Strongyloides stercoralis*. Depressed delayed hypersensitivity responses to tuberculin are associated. Polymyositis has been described. Up to 5% of infected individuals eventually develop T-cell leukaemia, which has a high and rapid mortality rate, and a similar proportion progress to tropical spastic paraparesis (TSP), also known as HTLV-associated myelopathy, in which there is primary demyelination (see Ch. 25) depending on the endemic region. Neural cells do not appear to be infected, and it is not known how the virus causes a neurologic disease.

Detection of HTLV-1– and HTLV-2–specific antibody is based on serologic methods with type differentiation by immunoblot. Antiretroviral agents other than protease inhibitors have been shown to inhibit viral replication and may be used as part of the management of individuals with ATLL or TSP. In particular,

**Table 27.8** Examples of pathogens affecting blood cells or haemopoiesis

| Pathogen | Disease | Effect | Mechanism |
|---|---|---|---|
| *Plasmodium* spp. | Malaria | Anaemia | Replication in erythrocytes |
| *Babesia* spp. | Babesiosis (tickborne) | Anaemia | Replication in erythrocytes |
| *Bartonella bacilliformis* | Oroya fever[a] (rare, sandfly transmitted, occurs in Peru) | Anaemia | Replication in erythrocytes |
| *Ehrlichia* spp. (Rickettsiae) | Human ehrlichiosis (tick transmitted in southern United States and Japan) | Leukopenia, thrombocytopenia | Replication in leukocytes |
| Human parvovirus B19 | Erythema infectiosum | Temporary fall in haemoglobin levels<br>Aplastic crisis (individual with chronic anaemia) | Replication in erythroid progenitor cells of the bone marrow |
| Colorado tick fever virus | Colorado tick fever | No effect on survival of infected erythrocytes | Replication in erythropoietic cells |
| Human T-cell lymphotropic virus | T-cell leukaemia/lymphoma | Malignant transformation of infected T cells | Replication in T cells |
| Human immunodeficiency virus | Acquired immunodeficiency syndrome | Immunosuppression | Infection of CD4-positive T cells |
| Epstein-Barr virus | Infectious mononucleosis | Atypical lymphocytosis<br>Thrombocytopenia<br>Haemolytic anaemia | Autoantibody to platelets and erythrocytes |
| Cytomegalovirus (CMV) | Congenital CMV complication of adult infection | Atypical lymphocytosis<br>Thrombocytopenia<br>Haemolytic anaemia | Unknown but may be autoantibody to erythrocytes and platelets in some patients |

[a]A cutaneous form (Verrugas) also occurs; in 1885 a Peruvian medical student, Daniel Carrion, demonstrated the common bacterial origin by inoculating himself with infected blood from the cutaneous form of the disease and developing Oroya fever.

zidovudine, a nucleoside reverse transcriptase inhibitor and type 1 interferon slowed the progress of adult T-cell leukemia (ATL). Treatment with an anti-CCR4 (a chemokine receptor on the cell surface) monoclonal antibody called mogamulizumab, together with cytotoxic chemotherapy, improved survival rates by lysing the CCR4 expressing ATL T cell and reducing the number of immunosuppressive T regulatory cells. The result was that a stronger anti-ATL cell-mediated response was made. Allogeneic bone marrow transplantation has been carried out with some success, with some survivors in those with a graft versus ATLL effect 3 years posttransplant. HTLV infection can be transmitted by HTLV antibody-positive individuals, and they should not donate blood or organs. HTLV antibody screening of blood donors is now included in many countries.

### HTLV-2 infection

HTLV-2 was first isolated in 1982 from a patient with T-cell hairy leukaemia, although it is not the usual cause of this condition. HTLV-2 is closely related to HTLV-1, is transmitted by similar routes and has been reported in injecting drug users and native Amerindian tribes in North, Central and South America. It has been associated with a number of neurologic conditions, including occasional reports of myelopathy.

## KEY FACTS

- The intact skin is an invaluable barrier that defends the body against invasion.

- A wide range of organisms is associated with skin infection and disease.

- Bacteria, fungi and viruses usually gain access through breaches of the barrier caused by trauma.

- Some parasites initiate their own penetration into the skin (hookworm, schistosomes).

- Other pathogens are introduced into the skin by arthropod vectors.

- Once in the skin, pathogens cause local infections or disseminate through the body to distant sites.

- Pathogens may be acquired by other routes, disseminate in the body and then localize in the skin or cause toxic or immunopathologic manifestations in the skin.

- Superficial infections of the skin are among the commonest human infections (boils, impetigo, warts, acne, ringworm).

- Invasion of pathogens deeper into dermal and subdermal tissues may produce severe infections that can be rapidly fatal, as in gangrene, or slow but progressive deformation and destruction, as in leprosy.

- Infections of muscle usually arise from invasion from the outside, whereas infections of joints are more often bloodborne.

- Bone infections may arise either by local spread from an infected joint or as a result of haematogenous seeding.

- Bone marrow cells or leukocytes may be invaded by viruses that interfere with haemopoiesis (parvovirus), cause malignant transformation (HTLV-1) or interfere with the immune system (EBV, HIV).

# 28

# Vector-borne infections

## Introduction

A number of important human diseases caused by organisms ranging from viruses to worms are transmitted by blood-feeding arthropods. These vectors inject the organisms into humans as they take a blood meal. Two classes of arthropods make the major contribution to disease transmission: the six-legged insects and the eight-legged ticks and mites. Arthropod-transmitted infections are commonest in warmer countries but occur worldwide. Of these, malaria is undoubtedly the most important. This chapter will also cover schistosomiasis, a major tropical disease that is often described as vector transmitted, but the aquatic snail vectors are more accurately referred to as *intermediate hosts*.

## Transmission of disease by vectors

### In sparsely populated areas, transmission by insects is an effective means of spread

Disease transmission by insects has major implications for the host, the vector and the parasite. To consider the parasite first, it requires the organism to be present in the right place (in the blood) and at the right time (some insects, for example, bite only at night). Blood is an inhospitable environment, and this may require quite subtle evasion mechanisms for parasite survival. In addition, the conditions found in the vector are likely to be very different from those in the human host, and the parasite may have to make a remarkably complex transition in a short time. With the larger protozoal and helminth parasites, this transition often involves clearly visible changes in appearance and is responsible for much of the complicated nomenclature of parasite life cycles. As some insect vectors have life spans hardly longer than those of their parasites, there is considerable wastage due to death of the vector before the parasite has matured to the infective stage for humans. A difference of a few days in a mosquito's life span can make an enormous difference to the effectiveness of malaria transmission, and indeed this simple factor is believed to underlie much of the difference between the African pattern of endemic infection and the Indian pattern of sporadic epidemics. However, what may be lost from wastage is more than compensated for by the increased distances over which spread of the parasite can occur.

Vector transmission of disease means that the disease may be controlled by controlling the vector, which is, for instance, a major reason why malaria is not endemic in many European countries where it used to be common.

A potential advantage of this type of transmission for the host is that it is sometimes possible to immunize specifically against the stages infective to humans or those responsible for infecting the vector of the parasite. Again, malaria can serve as an example—vaccines against the sporozoites, gametocytes and gametes having been clearly shown to block transmission

in animal models. Once transmission is blocked, there is a mathematically calculable possibility that the disease will die out. The RTS,S in ASO1 vaccine is based on the *Plasmodium falciparum* circumsporozoite protein. In 2021 the WHO recommended that four doses of RTS,S be given to children from 5 months of age if they live in sub-Saharan Africa or another area with moderate to high malaria transmission.

## ARBOVIRUS INFECTIONS

### Arboviruses are arthropod-borne viruses

A wide range of about 500 different viruses is transmitted by arthropods such as ticks, mosquitoes and sandflies. These arboviruses are single-stranded, enveloped, positive sense RNA viruses that multiply in the arthropod vector, and for each virus there is a natural cycle involving vertebrates (various birds or mammals) and arthropods. The virus enters the arthropod when the latter takes a blood meal from the infected vertebrate and passes through the gut wall to reach the salivary gland where replication takes place. Once this has occurred, 1–2 weeks after ingesting the virus, the arthropod becomes infectious and can transmit the virus to another vertebrate during a blood meal. Certain arboviruses that infect ticks are also transmitted directly from adult tick to egg (transovarial transmission) so that future generations of ticks are infected without the need for a vertebrate host.

### World Health Organization 2022 Global Arbovirus Initiative

The arthropod-borne viruses, including dengue, yellow fever, chikungunya and Zika viruses, have epidemic and pandemic potential, and the vectors have a human population of ~4 billion to attack. Global climate change and deforestation have changed environments so that *Aedes* mosquitoes, for example, feel more at home in destinations that were previously inhospitable. The Global Arbovirus Initiative will monitor risk and lead to a level of preparedness that would control outbreaks and avert a potential pandemic.

**Table 28.1** Arboviruses causing fevers and haemorrhagic disease

| Viruses | Disease reservoir | Geographic distribution | Vector | Animal |
|---|---|---|---|---|
| Yellow fever (alphavirus) | Fever, hepatitis | Africa, Central and South America | Mosquito *Aedes* spp. | Nil (monkeys for jungle type) |
| Dengue (four serotypes) (flavivirus) | Fever, rash (haemorrhagic shock syndrome) | India, Southeast Asia, Pacific, South America, Caribbean | Mosquito | Nil |
| Kyasanur Forest (flavivirus) | Haemorrhagic fever | India | Tick | Monkeys, rodents |
| Ross River (alphavirus) | Fever, arthralgia, arthritis | Australia, Pacific Islands | Mosquito | Birds |
| Rift Valley fever (bunyavirus) | Fever, sometimes haemorrhage | Africa | Mosquito | Sheep, cattle, camels |
| Sandfly fever (bunyavirus) | Fever (mild disease) | Asia, South America, Mediterranean | Sandfly | Gerbils |
| Congo-Crimean haemorrhagic fever (bunyavirus) | Fever, haemorrhage | Asia, Africa | Tick | Rodents |
| Colorado tick fever (reovirus) | Fever, myalgia | United States (Rocky Mountains) | Tick | Rodents |
| La Crosse (bunyavirus) | Fever | United States | Mosquito | Rodents |

There are many other less important arboviruses. For example, there are ~200 in the *Bunyavirus* family, most of which are arthropod borne, with ~40 occasionally causing human disease.

## A number of arboviruses are important causes of human disease

Most arboviruses belong to the *Togaviridae* (*Alphavirus* genus) and *Flaviviridae* family (*Flavivirus* genus).

Alphaviruses include chikungunya virus (CHIKV), eastern and western equine encephalitis virus (EEV), Venezuelan equine encephalitis (VEE) virus, Ross River virus, Barmah Forest virus and O'nyong'nyong virus.

Flaviviruses include dengue virus, West Nile virus (WNV), yellow fever virus, Zika virus, Japanese encephalitis virus (JEV), Kyansur Forest disease virus, louping ill virus, Murray Valley encephalitis virus, Omsk haemorrhagic fever virus, St. Louis encephalitis virus, tickborne encephalitis (TBE) virus and Usutu virus (USUV).

In addition, other arboviruses include some bunyaviruses, namely Crimean-Congo haemorrhagic fever (CCHF), La Crosse encephalitis virus, Rift Valley fever virus and Toscana virus (TOSV).

These are listed to give a flavour of the wide geographic distribution associated with the different vectors.

Arboviruses tend to replicate in vascular endothelium, the central nervous system (CNS), skin and muscle and are therefore multisystem infections. They are generally named after the clinical disease (e.g. yellow fever) or the place where they were first discovered (e.g. Rift Valley fever, Japanese encephalitis). A few (e.g. Ross River virus in Australia and the Pacific virus and CHIKV in Africa and Asia) cause arthritis.

The human stage of the virus cycle may be essential (e.g. urban yellow fever, dengue), there being no other vertebrate host, or it may be accidental from the virus's point of view, with humans acting as dead-end hosts who do not form a necessary part of the natural cycle (e.g. equine encephalitides, WNV).

## Arboviruses and haemorrhagic fevers

### Arboviruses are major causes of fever in endemic areas of the world

Arbovirus infections are often subclinical or mild, but occasionally there is a severe haemorrhagic illness. Some of the best known of these infections are listed in Table 28.1. Laboratory diagnosis detection of viral genome, demonstration of a rise in antibody and virus isolation are possible in special centres.

### CCHF fever, a tickborne virus infection

CCHF, a severe haemorrhagic fever with shock and disseminated intravascular coagulation, was described clinically during a large outbreak in the Crimea, part of the former Soviet Union, in 1944. The CCHF virus of the *Bunyaviridae* family, *Nairovirus* genus, was identified in 1967 and has a wide geographic range, including Africa, Asia, Central and Eastern Europe and the Middle East.

It is transmitted by the bite of ixodid ticks (both reservoir and vector), by contact with infected animals or person to person by exposure to infected body fluids, including blood.

CCHF has been reported in Iraq since 1979, and numbers started increasing in 2021 when 33 confirmed infections with 49% mortality were reported. Between January and May 2022, 212 probable infections were reported with 27 deaths. Most of those with confirmed infections had direct contact with animals and were livestock breeders or butchers.

A number of nosocomial outbreaks have been reported around the world. Although mortality rates of up to 80% have been reported, supportive management and ribavirin treatment have been shown to be effective.

## Yellow fever

### Yellow fever virus is transmitted by mosquitoes and is restricted to Africa, Central and South America and the Caribbean

Yellow fever virus is an RNA virus of the family *Flaviviridae*. It was taken by the early slave traders to the Americas where the first recorded case was in Yucatan in 1640. The virus is transmitted by three different cycles:

- from human to human by the mosquito *Aedes aegypti*, which is well adapted to breeding around human habitations; the infection can be maintained in this way as urban yellow fever

- from infected monkeys to humans by mosquitoes such as *Haemagogus*; this is sylvatic or jungle yellow fever and is seen in Africa and South America
- mosquitoes that breed in the wild and around households infect monkeys and humans with increased contact between infected mosquitoes and humans; this is intermediate yellow fever and is more common in Africa.

Yellow fever is not transmitted directly from human to human by day-to-day contact, but transmission from ill patients to healthcare workers has been reported notably after needlestick injury.

Yellow fever outbreaks have been seen in 2020 in West and Central Africa, as well as Uganda, Ethiopia, South Sudan and Venezuela in 2021. A concern is that yellow fever virus epidemiology has changed since the start of the 21st century. Countries previously thought to be low risk have reported outbreaks involving urban vector transmission in 2016 in Brazil, Angola and the Democratic Republic of Congo.

### Clinical features of yellow fever may be mild, but in 10–20% of cases, classic yellow fever with liver damage occurs, which can prove fatal

The virus enters dermal tissues or blood vessels at the site of a mosquito bite and spreads through the body. The liver is the most affected organ, but the kidneys, spleen, lymph nodes and heart are also damaged. Studies in Africa estimated that the ratio of inapparent to apparent infection was 7–12:1. When symptoms occur, after an incubation period of 3–6 days, there is a sudden onset of fever, nausea, vomiting, headache and muscular aches. Although mild cases occur, severe infection results in hepatocellular jaundice and renal failure, including acute tubular necrosis and shock. Coagulation defects are due to reduced synthesis and increased consumption of clotting factors and cause haemorrhage into the gastrointestinal tract (manifesting as haematemesis and melena) and elsewhere. The case fatality rate is ~20% in Africa and 40–60% in South America. Yellow fever is endemic in ~34 African countries and in 13 South American countries. It was estimated in 2013 that there were between 84,000 and 170,000 severe infections and between 29,000 and 60,000 deaths in those regions.

### Clinical diagnosis is unreliable; there is no specific treatment, but there is a vaccine

Yellow fever RNA can be detected by reverse transcriptase polymerase chain reaction (PCR) from blood during the acute stage. A postmortem histopathologic diagnosis can be made from the severe midzonal changes and acidophilic inclusion bodies (Councilman bodies) seen in the liver. Virus-specific immunoglobulin M (IgM) is detectable after a week, but there is cross-reactivity with other flaviviruses, a particular problem in endemic areas. No specific antiviral treatment is available.

The best prevention is to give the live attenuated 17D yellow fever vaccine to those who may be exposed. Vaccination is necessary for entry into and for travel through endemic areas. Protection is long lasting, and in 2016 the International Health Regulations (IHR) stipulated that the period of protection provided by the vaccine changed from 10 years to the lifetime of the person vaccinated. Boosters are given to immunocompromised individuals. The IHR permit a state to require a valid certificate of vaccination from a traveller from an endemic area to another country where the right mosquitoes are present but the disease does not occur. Vaccines based on recombinant DNA technology have been developed. As with all arthropod-borne infections, control of arthropod vectors (insecticides, attention to breeding sites) and reduced exposure (insect repellents, mosquito nets) are also important.

## Dengue fever

### Dengue virus is transmitted by mosquitoes and occurs in Southeast Asia, the Pacific area, India and South and Central America

Dengue virus is one of the most rapidly reemerging arbovirus diseases, with infections reported to the World Health Organization (WHO) having increased from ~500,000 in the year 2000 to 5.2 million in 2019. It has been estimated that there may be ~400 million infections annually with 96 million symptomatic people. Dengue virus is a flavivirus with four antigenic subtypes, all of which circulate in Asia, Africa and the Americas. It is endemic in ~130 countries with ~70% of infections seen in Asia. Dengue fever (DF) has spread to the Eastern Mediterranean, and outbreaks in other parts of Europe have been seen. Local transmission was reported in France and Croatia. The mosquito *A. aegypti* is the principal human vector. The virus also circulates in monkeys and can be transmitted by mosquitoes to cause jungle dengue in humans, a disease analogous to jungle yellow fever.

### DF may be complicated by dengue haemorrhagic fever/dengue shock syndrome

Dengue virus replicates in dendritic cells, peripheral blood monocytes, liver parenchymal cells and macrophages in lymph nodes, liver and spleen. After an incubation period of 4–8 days, there is malaise, fever, headache, arthralgia, nausea, vomiting and sometimes a maculopapular or erythematous rash. Recovery may be followed by prolonged fatigue and/or depression.

DF ranges from a mild febrile illness to severe dengue haemorrhagic fever (DHF) and dengue shock syndrome (DSS). In 2009 WHO classified DF disease into uncomplicated and severe DF.

In the past, mortality rates were high, but with prompt access to expert hospital care, a fatality rate of <1% can be achieved. The pathogenesis of this syndrome is shown in Fig. 28.1. After an earlier attack of dengue, antibodies are formed that are specific for that serotype. On subsequent infection with a different serotype, the antibodies bind to the virus and not only fail to neutralize it (as might be expected for a different subtype), but also enhance its ability to infect monocytes. The Fc portion of the virus-bound immunoglobulin molecule attaches to Fc receptors on monocytes, and entry into the cell by this route increases the efficiency of infection. Infection of increased numbers of monocytes results in an increased release of cytokines into the circulation (see Ch. 18), and this leads to vascular damage, shock and haemorrhage especially into the gastrointestinal tract and skin. Similar enhancing antibodies are formed in many other virus infections, but it is only in DHF that they are known to play a pathogenic role. A number of other factors can influence the course of dengue infection, including

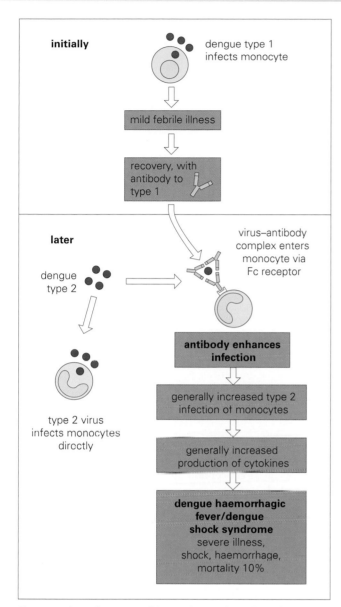

**Fig. 28.1** The pathogenesis of dengue haemorrhagic fever/dengue shock syndrome. There are four serotypes of dengue virus. Types 1 and 2 are illustrated as examples. Antibody to type 1 binds to type 2 without preventing infection with type 2.

age, female gender, several human leukocyte antigen (HLA) class I alleles and dengue virus strain virulence. It has been reported that a higher dengue viremia during the initial fever phase was associated with vascular leakage, severe dengue and admission to hospital irrespective of infection serotype or host immune status. Other studies concluded that dengue serotype 2 was associated with more severe outcomes. There are still questions about pathogenesis of DHF and DSS, and these are key to developing treatment strategies in the future.

There is no antiviral therapy for DF. Treatment is supportive. It has taken many years to develop a dengue vaccine. It was essential that it be tetravalent to avoid the danger that a vaccine could induce the type of antibody associated with DHF/DSS. Three live attenuated vaccines have shown promise. The Dengvaxia vaccine, the only one licensed so

far, is based on the yellow fever virus 17D live attenuated vaccine strain in which specific genes were replaced by homologous genes from each of the four dengue virus serotypes. It generated a strong neutralizing antibody response to all four serotypes and, in a challenge study, protected 92% of immunized monkeys against wild-type dengue virus 1–4.

## Chikungunya virus infection

ChikV is an arbovirus of the family *Togaviridae* transmitted mainly by *A. aegypti* or *A. albopictus*. The disease is present mostly in Africa, Asia and the Americas, but sporadic outbreaks have occurred elsewhere, including in Italy in 2007 and 2017 (~300 probable and confirmed infections in both outbreaks) and in France in 2010, 2014 and 2017. These were autochthonous infections (i.e. indigenous spread having originated from travellers from Asia and Africa). *A. aegypti* has not been seen in mainland Europe yet, but *A. albopictus* is established in southern and central Europe and is spreading. In March 2023 there were >110,000 infections and 43 deaths globally.

The incubation period is 3–7 days with a range of 1–12 days. ChikV infection presents with fever, severe joint pain and swelling (the name comes from the African Makonde language and translates as "bent over in pain"), rash, myalgia and headache. The illness is similar to dengue and Zika virus infections, but sudden-onset high fever and severe joint pain is very common, and retro-orbital pain is rare in CHIKV.

The diagnosis is confirmed by detecting CHIKV RNA by PCR, and serology tests are available.

Treatment is supportive and there is no vaccine.

## Zika virus infection

**Zika virus infection was declared a public health emergency of international concern in February 2016, but infections dramatically fell by the following year**

Zika virus, a single-stranded, positive sense, nonsegmented enveloped RNA virus of the *Flaviviridae* family, was discovered in 1947 in a rhesus macaque in the Zika Forest of Uganda and was recognized as a cause of human disease in 1953. It remained an uncommon cause of human illness but rose to prominence in 2013 in the Pacific and from 2015 in the Americas, Africa, Asia and the Pacific. Thus a little-known arbovirus long thought to result in only mild illness has become a major threat to humans. Possible reasons for its spread through Latin America include changes in climate and in land use, poverty and movement of people. In February 2016, WHO declared that the spread of the Zika virus was a public health emergency of international concern that was ended by November 2016. There was a lot of anxiety about travel to Brazil at the time of the Olympic games in 2016 as Zika virus infection was reported in the international news with pictures of babies with microcephaly (small heads). The reduction in infections was quite dramatic, and by 2017 to date, low-level transmission has occurred in endemic areas, especially the Americas. Indigenous mosquito-transmitted Zika virus disease was reported in France, Madeira, Turkey, Georgia and Russian Federation by 2022, and there was a Zika virus outbreak in India in 2021. Around 89 countries and territories have reported Zika virus infections.

**Table 28.2** Arboviruses causing encephalitis

| Virus and disease | Geographic distribution | Vector for human infection | Vertebrate reservoir | Severity of infection |
|---|---|---|---|---|
| Eastern equine encephalitis (alphavirus) | United States (Atlantic Gulf states) | *Aedes* spp. mosquitoes | Wild birds, horses (dead-end hosts) | 50% case fatality |
| Western equine encephalitis (alphavirus) | United States (west of Mississippi River) | *Culex* spp. mosquitoes | Wild birds, horses (dead-end hosts) | Up to 2% case fatality |
| West Nile encephalitis (flavivirus) | Africa, Europe, Central Asia, North America | *Culex* spp. mosquitoes | Birds | Up to 5% case fatality |
| St. Louis encephalitis (flavivirus) | United States (southern, central and western states) | *Culex* spp. mosquitoes | Wild birds | 10% case fatality |
| California encephalitis (bunyavirus) | United States (northern and central states) | *Aedes* spp. mosquitoes | Small mammals | Fatalities rare |
| Japanese encephalitis (flavivirus) | Far East, Southeast Asia | *Culex* spp. mosquitoes | Birds, pigs | >10% case fatality |
| Murray Valley encephalitis (flavivirus) | Australia | *Culex* spp. mosquitoes | Birds | Up to 70% case fatality |
| Tickborne encephalitis (flavivirus) | Eastern Europe | Tick | Mammals, birds | Up to 10% case fatality (variable) |
| Venezuelan encephalitis (alphavirus) | Southern United States, Central and South America | Mosquito | Rodents | 70% case fatality (cases rare) |
| Powassan (flavivirus) | United States, Canada | Tick | Rodents | Cases rare |

The great majority of infections are either subclinical or associated with nonspecific febrile illness (e.g. 70% case fatality in encephalitis due to Venezuelan encephalitis virus, but only 3% develop encephalitis).

The virus is transmitted by the mosquito vectors *A. aegypti* or *A. albopictus*. The incubation period is 3–14 days. Infection acquired during pregnancy can lead to vertical infection of the fetus with resulting microcephaly or other congenital abnormality. Infection can also be transmitted by sexual intercourse or via blood transfusion. Sexual transmission just before onset of infection or shortly after symptoms had resolved, between any sexual partners and to women from asymptomatic men has been recognized. Viral RNA is present in blood (up to 83 days), vaginal secretions (up to 6 months), semen (69 days by virus isolation, therefore replication competent; 370 days in an immunocompetent and >900 days in an immunocompromised male) and urine.

Zika virus is neurotropic and infects neural progenitor cells, causing cellular apoptosis. Placental cells can be infected too, both targets leading to the characteristic congenital abnormalities reported.

Symptoms and signs of Zika virus infection include mild fever, a maculopapular rash, arthralgia, myalgia and conjunctivitis. Guillain-Barré syndrome, neuropathy and myelopathy can ensue. Congenital Zika syndrome includes microcephaly, a variety of ocular abnormalities, craniofacial disproportion, spasticity and seizures.

Zika virus RNA can be detected by reverse transcription PCR on serum, saliva, semen and urine collected and by antibody detection (IgM and IgG) after the first week of symptoms. Flavivirus antibodies show significant cross-reactivity, and care is required in test interpretation to differentiate Zika virus infection from dengue.

Prevention involves controlling the mosquito population and avoiding being bitten. As can be seen from viral RNA detection at different sites, especially in vaginal secretions and semen, guidance for couples considering pregnancy both in and when visiting endemic areas to avoid sexual transmission at conception and during pregnancy is quite complicated.

There is no vaccine currently available for Zika virus, but Zika virus strains are strongly conserved at the nucleotide level, raising the possibility of a vaccine to protect against all strains.

## Arbovirus encephalitis

Of the 10 encephalitis arboviruses listed in Table 28.2, 6 cause disease in the United States; although most infections are subclinical or mild, fatal encephalitis can occur. The viruses replicate in the CNS, but a cell-mediated immune response to infection makes a major contribution to the encephalitis.

Many arboviruses can cause meningoencephalitis by direct invasion of the CNS and postinfectious immune-mediated conditions, including autoimmune encephalitis and acute demyelinating encephalomyelitis seen with some Japanese encephalitis, WNV and CHIKV.

After the vector has attached to the skin, viral replication occurs in the Langerhans dendritic cells and then to the regional lymph nodes. There is a transient viremia allowing the virus to travel to the reticuloendothelial system and invade the CNS.

### WNV swept across North America since first appearing in 1999

Prior to the mid-1990s WNV, a flavivirus transmitted from infected wild birds by *Culex* spp. mosquitoes and for which humans are considered to be dead-end hosts, was not considered a major public health problem, but viral changes then resulted in individuals presenting with severe neurologic disease. The virus, which had not previously been reported from the Western Hemisphere, was recorded in New York in 1999 and since then has spread widely in the United States, Canada, Mexico and the Caribbean. In 2006 the Centers for Disease Control and Prevention (CDC) reported >1500 human infections in the United States that included >150 blood donors. By 2021, ~3000 human infections were reported, ~70% of which had neuroinvasive disease. Just over 2000 human infections were reported in Europe in 2018 with a 9% mortality rate. How the virus crossed the Atlantic is unknown, although it has been suggested that it may have been a viable mosquito that managed to get on a plane that may have infected a wild bird in New York.

Most infections are asymptomatic, and ~20% will develop headache, fever, myalgia, muscle weakness and arthralgia; <1% will develop neuroinvasive disease presenting with fever, headache, photophobia, seizures, confusion and muscle weakness, especially those >60 years of age and immunocompromised individuals. There may be a transient maculopapular rash in one-third of patients, mostly in those with West Nile fever, lymphadenopathy and splenomegaly.

The incubation period is 3–5 days with the upper range of 2 weeks. West Nile neuroinvasive disease can be divided into three different syndromes: meningitis, encephalitis and acute flaccid paralysis. Cerebrospinal fluid (CSF) cell count and protein are elevated.

Specific diagnosis can be made by detecting of WNV RNA in blood, urine and CSF and WNV IgM detection in serum (and CSF where appropriate). Viral culture can be carried out in reference laboratories and plaque reduction neutralization tests used.

Management is supportive, and no antiviral treatment is available. A WNV vaccine is available for horses; clinical trials are underway for humans.

### JEV causes at least 70,000 infections annually in Southeast Asia and Western Pacific regions

JEV is another mosquito-borne flavivirus that has an enzootic transmission cycle involving *Culex* spp. mosquitoes, herons, egrets and bittern wading birds. Pigs are amplifying hosts and involved in animal outbreaks that can lead to human infections.

The incubation period is 4–14 days. Most infections are mild, but more severe symptoms include fever, myalgia and confusion; children, who are mostly affected, may also have gastrointestinal symptoms and seizures. Humans and horses can develop fatal encephalitis and are dead-end hosts. There are ~70,000 infections annually in Asia, and the fatality rate can be up to 30%.

In February 2022 JEV caused an increased number of stillbirths and piglets with neurologic disease at commercial pig farms in three eastern Australian states. By May 2022, 70 piggeries across four states had been affected. The first human JEV infections were reported in early March 2022, and by May 2022 there were 30 confirmed JEV infections causing encephalitis and 5 deaths.

The diagnosis is made by testing for JEV-specific IgM in CSF and serum, detectable 3–8 days after illness onset. Treatment is supportive, and there are three inactivated and one live attenuated vaccine available to prevent infection.

### TBE is one of the most common tickborne diseases reported in 24 European countries

TBE virus is a Flavivirus and causes neurologic disease around Europe and is being seen in Western Europe and in Northern China, Mongolia, and the Russian Federation.

There have been three cases of probable or confirmed TBE in England since 2019, including the first confirmed infection in the Yorkshire area in 2022. The tick species carrying the virus is widespread in the United Kingdom and has been detected in various counties. Nearly 4000 TBE infections were reported in 24 European countries in 2020, 95% of which occurred from May to November, peaking in July.

TBE virus is mainly transmitted by *Ixodes* spp. tick bites, and, rarely, infection is due to ingesting unpasteurized milk from infected goats, sheep or cows. People come in contact with the ticks during outdoor activities in forested areas.

Most infections are asymptomatic. The incubation period is 2–28 days (most commonly 7–14 days). Around 30% of people present with fever, tiredness and headache; then in ~10% of infections there is a second phase of the disease with fever, meningitis, encephalitis and/or myelitis. There is a 1% mortality rate. In the first phase, the diagnosis is made by TBE virus RNA detection by reverse-transcriptase PCR; by the second phase, the virus has been cleared in the CSF and blood, so detecting virus-specific IgM and IgG in CSF and blood is more helpful.

There is no specific treatment. Prevention includes covering as much of the body as possible when hiking or camping in endemic areas and looking for ticks attached to the skin and removing them. There are four whole inactivated virus vaccines that are safe and effective.

### TOSV is neurotropic and is a common cause of aseptic meningitis in southwest Europe

TOSV is an enveloped, tri–single-stranded, segmented RNA virus that is part of the *Phlebovirus* genus in the *Phenuiviridae* family. It is transmitted to humans by infected female sandfly bites. The geographic distribution of TOSV is highly dependent on this vector abundance. It is endemic in the Mediterranean area; most infections occur in the warm season and are asymptomatic or mildly symptomatic. The incubation period is 3–7 days, and range is up to 14 days. TOSV is neurotropic, causing meningitis and encephalitis. In France, Italy and Tunisia it is a common cause of aseptic meningitis. Diagnosis is made by detecting TOSV RNA in CSF and blood, IgM tests and virus isolation in reference centres. There is no specific treatment.

### USUV is an emerging arbovirus that can cause encephalitis, and blood donor screening may be needed in endemic areas

USUV is another neurotropic member of the *Flaviviridae* family transmitted mainly by *Culex* spp. mosquitoes. They are the vectors that feed on birds, especially sparrows, magpies, blackbirds and owls, and that act as hosts and reservoirs. USUV was first seen in 1959 near the Usutu River in South Africa, but it was in 2016 that dead infected birds were found in several parts of Europe with sporadic infections in humans, horses and bats. The incubation period is 3–12 days. Again, many human infections are asymptomatic, but fever, rash and jaundice may be seen. After two immunocompromised individuals in Italy were diagnosed with USUV meningoencephalitis in 2009, then 12 individuals were found to have USUV RNA in CSF and blood samples, and national surveillance was started in 2017. By 2018, 38 Italian blood donors were found to have Usutu viraemias, and other European countries reported a USUV antibody prevalence between 0.02 and 3%. By 2022, >100 human infections have been reported, 30 of whom had neurologic symptoms.

Diagnosis is made by detecting USUV RNA by reverse-transcriptase PCR in blood and CSF samples, serology (although there is cross-reactivity with WNV antibody) and virus isolation. There is no specific treatment.

### The equine encephalitis viruses: eastern equine encephalitis is rare, western equine encephalitis even more so, but Venezuelan equine encephalitis virus has caused large outbreaks in humans and horses in the past

Eastern equine encephalitis (EEE) caused by the mosquito-borne eastern EEV (EEEV) is a single-stranded positive sense RNA virus in the *Alphavirus* genus of the *Togaviridae* family. EEEV affects horses, humans and other vertebrate hosts with a mortality rate up to 40% and neurologic sequelae in 50% of survivors. The enzootic cycle between *Culiseta melanura* and passerine birds maintains EEEV, and other vectors, including *A. albopictus*, transmit to the dead-end hosts, horses and humans.

There are intermittent outbreaks of EEE in eastern and midwestern United States, with around six to eight infections annually. There has been a rise in virus activity, with outbreaks in both human and horses. There were 110 infections in different US states between 2011 and 2020.

Western equine encephalitis (WEE) is also seen in horses and humans and is contracted via the bite of infected *Culex tarsalis* mosquitoes having fed on infected birds. WEE is found mostly in western and central United States, and 639 infections were reported between 1964 and 2012.

VEE resulting from VEE virus infection is reported in Central and South America. One of the largest outbreaks in horses recorded was in 1995 and led to up to 100,000 human infections in Colombia and Venezuela, with ~3000 neurologic sequelae and 300 deaths reported.

Laboratory diagnosis is carried out in special centres using PCR tests to detect viral RNA, serology may be helpful and occasionally virus isolation. Management is supportive with no antiviral treatment available.

Equine vaccines are available against WEE, EEE and VEE; they are not licensed for humans but could be considered in an emergency, having been used in studies in laboratory workers. However, an inactivated JEV vaccine is also available for at-risk travellers.

## INFECTIONS CAUSED BY RICKETTSIAE

The rickettsiae are a group of intracellular, arthropod-transmitted gram-negative aerobic rods (see Pathogen parade). Previously the group included, among others, the genera *Rickettsia*, *Bartonella*, *Coxiella*, *Ehrlichia* and *Orientia*. Genomic-based analysis has resulted in a complete reclassification of the group, and only the genera *Rickettsia* and *Orientia* remain in the family *Rickettsiaceae*. *Bartonella*, *Coxiella* and *Ehrlichia* have been transferred to other families

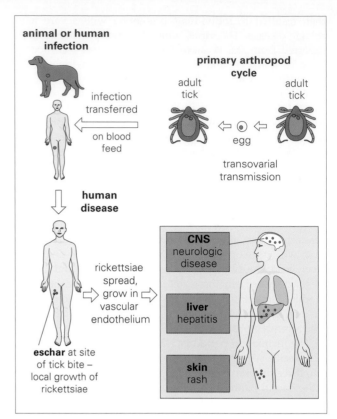

**Fig. 28.2** Typical events in rickettsial infection. There is no direct person-to-person spread. Typhus is unusual because the infected arthropod transmits from person to person, eventually dies and there is no eschar. CNS, Central nervous system.

and are not discussed further in this chapter. The rickettsiae are obligate intracellular parasites carried in arthropod or animal reservoirs (Fig. 28.2). Person-to-person transmission does not occur.

### The rickettsiae are small bacteria, and infections tend to be persistent or become latent

Howard T. Ricketts identified Rocky Mountain spotted fever in 1906 and showed that the infection was transmitted transovarially in ticks. Rickettsiae probably arose as parasites of blood-sucking or other arthropods in which they were maintained by vertical transmission transfer to the arthropod's vertebrate host being initially accidental and not necessary for rickettsial survival. The infected arthropod does not appear to be adversely affected. *Rickettsia prowazekii* is perhaps a more recent parasite of the human body louse because the louse dies 1–3 weeks after infection. As with most arthropod-borne infections, transmission from person to person does not occur.

### Typical clinical symptoms of rickettsial infection are fever, headache and rash

Rickettsiae multiply in the vascular endothelium to cause vasculitis in skin, CNS and liver and hence are multisystem infections (Table 28.3). In spite of immune responses there is a tendency for rickettsial infections to persist in the body for long periods or become latent.

The typical clinical features are fever, headache and rash. A history suggesting contact with rickettsial vectors or reservoir

**Table 28.3** The principal rickettsial diseases in humans

| Organism | Disease | Arthropod vector | Vertebrate reservoir | Clinical severity | Geographic distribution |
|---|---|---|---|---|---|
| **Spotted fevers**[a] | | | | | |
| *Rickettsia rickettsii* | Rocky Mountain spotted fever | Tick[b] | Dogs, rodents | ++ | Rocky Mountain states, eastern United States |
| *R. akari* | Rickettsial pox | Mite[b] | Mice | – | Asia, Far East, Africa, United States |
| *R. conorii* | Mediterranean spotted fever | Tick | Dogs | + | Mediterranean |
| **Typhus** | | | | | |
| *R. prowazekii* | Epidemic typhus | Louse | Human[c] | + + | Africa, South America |
| *R. typhi* | Endemic typhus | Flea | Rodents | – | Worldwide |
| *Orientia tsutsugamushi* | Scrub typhus | Mite[b] | Rodents | + + | Far East |

[a]Other rickettsiae cause similar tickborne fevers in Africa, India and Australia.
[b]Vertically transmitted in arthropod.
[c]Nonhuman vertebrates are possibly also involved.

animals may suggest a diagnosis (e.g. camping, working and engaging in military activities in endemic areas).

## Laboratory diagnosis is based on serologic tests

Microimmunofluorescence methods are the most common serologic approach, and demonstration of a fourfold or greater rise in titre is considered to be a positive result. Western blot analysis is used in reference laboratories. Seroconversion occurs 7–15 days after the onset of illness but can take as long as 28 days. Infected patients also make antibody to the rickettsiae that cross-react with the O antigen polysaccharide of various strains of *Proteus vulgaris*, as detected by agglutination in the Weil-Felix test. Although the phenomenon is of interest, the Weil-Felix test is not of great value, however, because of false-positive and false-negative results. Earlier diagnosis can often be made by fluorescent antibody staining of skin biopsy material. PCR tests are deployed on skin biopsies or swabs from eschars, but a negative PCR does not exclude rickettsial infection. Isolation of rickettsiae is difficult and dangerous, and laboratory infections have occurred.

## All rickettsiae are susceptible to tetracyclines

Prevention is based on reducing exposure to the vector (e.g. ticks). A killed *R. prowazekii* vaccine has been used in the past by the military, but at present there is no commercially available anti-*Rickettsia* vaccine.

## Rocky Mountain spotted fever

### Rocky Mountain spotted fever is transmitted by dog ticks and has a mortality of ≥10%

The rickettsiae causing this disease are carried by the dog tick (*Dermacentor variabilis*) or by wood ticks (*D. andersoni*) and are transmitted vertically from adult tick to egg. Human infection occurs in the warm months of the year as ticks become active. Children are most commonly infected, but their disease is milder.

The rickettsiae multiply in the skin at the site of the tick bite, then spread to blood and infect vascular endothelium in the lung, spleen, brain and skin. After an incubation period

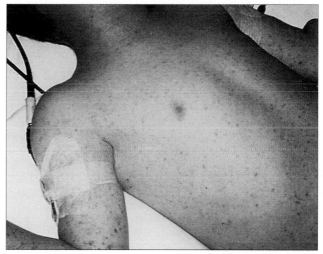

**Fig. 28.3** Generalized maculopapular rash with petechiae in Rocky Mountain spotted fever. (Courtesy T.F. Sellers, Jr.)

of ~1 week, there is onset of fever, severe headache, myalgia and often respiratory symptoms. A generalized maculopapular rash develops 2–4 days after the onset of fever, becoming petechial or purpuric in 50–60% of cases (Fig. 28.3). Splenomegaly may occur, and neurologic involvement is frequent, with later onset of clotting defects (disseminated intravascular coagulation), shock and death. Fatal cases are usually those with a delayed diagnosis. Peak mortality is seen in 40–60-year-olds.

## Mediterranean spotted fever

### Mediterranean spotted fever is transmitted by dog ticks

Mediterranean spotted fever is caused by *Rickettsia conorii*, which is carried by the dog tick *Rhipicephalus sanguineus*. Human infection, which occurs mainly in the summer, is known in all Mediterranean countries and can occur in urban as well as rural areas. After an incubation period of ~1 week, 50% of cases develop fever, headache and myalgia, then 2–4 days later a maculopapular rash, especially on the palms and soles, may develop. Approximately 50–75% of cases show an eschar.

## African tick-bite fever

Eight pathogenic rickettsial species are currently recognized in Africa. *R. africae* is found mainly in urban areas, and *R. conorii* is found in semirural and rural areas. African tick-bite fever is regularly seen in travellers returning from Africa to the temperate zone.

## Rickettsialpox

### Rickettsialpox is a mild infection

About 5 days after the bite of a rodent-associated mite (*Liponyssoides sanguineus*) infected with *R. akari*, a local eschar develops with fever and headache occurring ~1 week later. After a few more days, a generalized papulovesicular rash appears. The disease is, however, self-limiting and usually settles in 14–21 days.

## Epidemic typhus

### Epidemic typhus is transmitted by the human body louse

Epidemic typhus is transmitted from person to person by *Pediculus humanus*. The rickettsiae (*R. prowazekii*) multiply in the gut epithelium of the louse and are excreted in faeces during the act of biting. The rickettsiae enter the skin when the bite is scratched. The disease cannot maintain itself unless enough people are infested with lice. Epidemic typhus is therefore classically associated with poverty and war, when clothes and bodies are washed less frequently. There were 30 million cases in Eastern Europe and the Soviet Union from 1918 to 1922. The disease is seen in Africa, Central and South America and sporadically (as a sylvatic form) in the United States. As there is no direct person-to-person spread, outbreaks can be terminated by delousing campaigns.

### Untreated epidemic typhus has a mortality as high as 60%

Rickettsiae proliferate at the site of the bite and then spread in the blood to infect vascular endothelium in skin, heart, CNS, muscle and kidney. About 10–14 days after the louse bite (there is no eschar), the infected person develops fever, headache and flulike symptoms. A generalized maculopapular rash appears 5–9 days later in 20–40% of cases. Neurologic involvement occurs in 80%, and sometimes there is severe meningoencephalitis with delirium and coma. In untreated cases mortality can range from 20% in healthy individuals to as high as 60% in elderly or compromised patients, owing to peripheral vascular collapse or secondary bacterial pneumonia. Well-treated cases have a mortality rate of ~4%.

Convalescence may take months. In some individuals the rickettsiae are not eliminated from the body on clinical recovery and remain in the lymph nodes. As much as 50 years later the infection can reactivate to cause Brill-Zinsser disease, and the patient once again acts as a source of infection for any lice that may be present.

## Endemic (murine) typhus

Endemic typhus is caused by *R. typhi* and is transmitted to humans by the rat flea. The disease is similar to epidemic typhus but is less severe and can present as a nonspecific febrile illness.

## Scrub typhus

Scrub typhus is a severe illness caused by *Orientia tsutsugamushi* and is transmitted to humans by larval trombiculid mites. It occurs throughout Asia where it is a common cause of fever in rural areas. The rickettsiae are maintained in the mites by transovarial transfer and are transmitted to humans or rodents during feeding. There is fever, headache and an eschar, then a macular rash appears after 5–8 days of illness. Pneumonitis, meningitis, disseminated intravascular coagulation and circulatory collapse may ensue. Immunochromatographic rapid diagnostic tests are available and should improve diagnosis in the field. Treatment is with doxycycline or azithromycin and must be given early. The human immune response to *O. tsutsugamushi* is unable to produce sterile, long-lasting, cross-protective immunity. As a result, attempts to develop a vaccine have so far proven unsuccessful, but work is underway to identify candidate antigens recognized by T cells.

# BORRELIA INFECTIONS

## Relapsing fever

### The epidemic form of relapsing fever is caused by *Borrelia recurrentis*, which is transmitted by human body lice

*B. recurrentis* is a gram-negative spirochete consisting of an irregular spiral 10–30 μm long and is highly flexible, moving by rotation and twisting.

Epidemics of relapsing fever (Fig. 28.4) are due to transmission of infection by the human body louse. Bacteria multiply in the louse, and when louse bites are rubbed, the lice are crushed and the bacteria are introduced into the bite wound. *B. recurrentis* can also penetrate intact mucosa and skin. Lice are essential for person-to-person transmission of louseborne relapsing fever. As with other louseborne infections (e.g. typhus), spread of the disease in humans is favoured when people rarely wash and when clothes are not

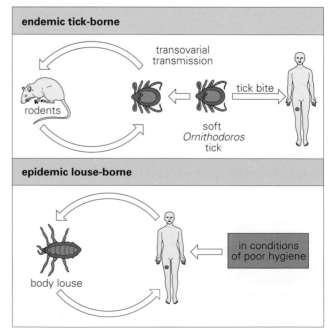

**Fig. 28.4** Transmission in relapsing fever.

**Fig. 28.5** Course of events in relapsing fever.

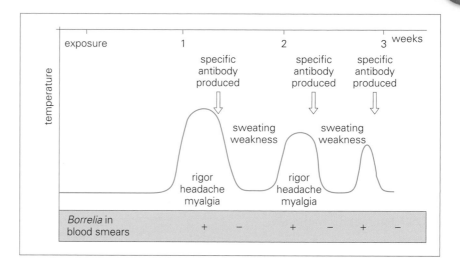

changed (e.g. in wars, natural disasters). The last great epidemic in North Africa and Europe during the Second World War caused 50,000 deaths, and it remains an infection of public health concern in North and East Africa.

### The endemic form of relapsing fever in humans is transmitted by tick bites

Infections with other species of *Borrelia* are endemic in rodents in many parts of the world, including western United States, and are primarily transmitted by soft ticks of the genus *Ornithodoros*. *Borrelia miyamotoi* is the cause of hard tick relapsing fever and is transmitted by the deer tick *Ixodes scapularis*. Within *Ornithodoros* ticks, the bacteria are transmitted transovarially from generation to generation, which, together with their ability to survive for up to 10 years, helps maintain the endemic cycle of this form of relapsing fever.

### Relapsing fever is characterized by repeated febrile episodes due to antigenic variation in the spirochetes

The bacteria multiply locally and enter the blood. After an incubation period of 3–10 days, there is a sudden onset of illness with chills and fever lasting for 3–5 days (Fig. 28.5). The afebrile period lasts about a week before there is a second attack of fever, which is followed by another afebrile period. Generally, there are 3–10 such episodes of diminishing severity. More serious illness can occur if there is extensive growth of the bacteria in the spleen, liver and kidneys.

Agglutinating and lytic antibodies are formed against the infecting bacteria, which are cleared from the blood. Under the pressure of this immune response, a new antigenic type emerges and is free to multiply and cause a fresh febrile episode.

Antigenic variation involves switching of variable proteins on the bacterial surface. The *Borrelia* spp. have arrays of genes (variable large proteins and variable small proteins) that are altered and activated by gene conversion involving plasmids carrying collections of these genes. The result is that a single cloned bacterium can give rise spontaneously to ~30 serotypes, and switching occurs at a rate of 1:1000–1:10,000/cell generation. Similar phenomena are seen in trypanosomes. Direct person-to-person transmission does not occur. Mortality with endemic (tickborne) relapsing

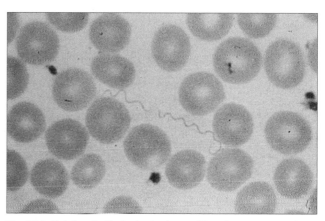

**Fig. 28.6** Tightly coiled helical spirochetes of *Borrelia recurrentis* in the blood of a patient with relapsing fever. (Courtesy T.F. Sellers.)

fever is <5% but may be up to 40% in untreated epidemic (louseborne) relapsing fever (4% if treated).

### Relapsing fever is diagnosed in the laboratory and treated with tetracycline

The bacteria can be cultivated in the laboratory and in ~70% of cases can be seen in Giemsa-stained smears of blood taken during the febrile period (Fig. 28.6). Enzyme-linked immunosorbent assay (ELISA) or immunofluorescence assays can detect specific antibody after 1 week of infection. PCR and molecular typing are available in reference laboratories.

Tetracycline is used in treatment and to prevent relapses. A Jarisch-Herxheimer reaction with worsening of symptoms, high fever, rigors and hypotension occurs in the first few hours after the start of treatment in 50–75% of cases. The best preventative measure against louse-borne relapsing fever is good personal hygiene, good sanitation and good control of the louse vector. For tickborne relapsing fever, a key measure is avoidance of the vector.

## Lyme disease

### Lyme disease is caused by *Borrelia* spp. and is transmitted by *Ixodes* ticks

Lyme disease (or Lyme borreliosis) occurs in Europe, the United States and most continents of the world and is named

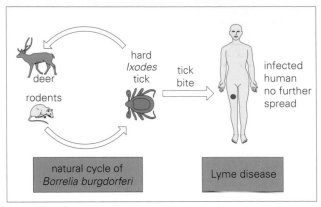

**Fig. 28.7** Transmission of Lyme disease.

after the town in Connecticut (US state) where the first cases were recognized in 1975. About 30,000 new cases of Lyme disease are reported each year in the United States; however, recent estimates by the CDC suggest 476,000 patients are treated for Lyme disease annually. Lyme disease is primarily caused by *B. burgdorferi* in the United States, with infections by other species including *B. mayonii* and possibly *B. bissettii* occurring less frequently. In Europe infections are caused by *B. garinii* and *B. afzelii*, with *B. burgdorferi* less common. The natural cycle of infection takes place in small mammals in which it is transmitted by hard ticks of the genus *Ixodes* (Fig. 28.7). Human infection follows the bite of an infected tick (most commonly the nymph). In Europe and the United States, infection is commoner in summer months when recreational exposure to infected ticks is more likely. Person-to-person transmission does not occur.

### Erythema migrans is a characteristic feature of Lyme disease

The bacteria multiply locally and, after an incubation period of ~1 week, fever, headache, myalgia, lymphadenopathy and a characteristic lesion at the site of the tick bite develop. The skin lesion is called *erythema migrans* (Fig. 28.8), its name describing its main features. It begins as a macule and enlarges over the next few weeks, remaining red and flat, but with the centre clearing until it is several centimetres in diameter. In 50% of patients, fresh transient lesions appear on the skin elsewhere in the body. Immunologic findings

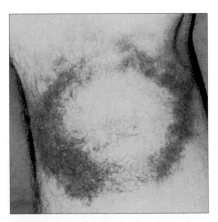

**Fig. 28.8** Rash of erythema chronicum migrans on the leg in Lyme disease. (Courtesy E. Sahn.)

include circulating immune complexes and sometimes elevated serum IgM levels and cryoglobulins that contain IgM. *Borrelia* is capable of evading the human immune response, and mechanisms include antigenic variation and the ability to evade complement-mediated killing.

### Lyme disease commonly causes additional disease 1 week to 2 years after the initial illness

In 75% of untreated patients, in spite of antibody and T-cell responses to the *Borrelia*, there are additional later manifestations of disease. These are seen from 1 week to >2 years after the onset of illness. The initial manifestations to appear are neurologic (meningitis, encephalitis, peripheral neuropathy) and cardiologic (heart block, myocarditis). The subsequent manifestations are arthralgia and arthritis, which may persist for months or years (referred to as *posttreatment Lyme disease syndrome*). Immune complexes are found in affected joints. These late manifestations are immunologic in origin and are probably due to antigenic cross-reactivity between *Borrelia* and host tissues. The *Borrelia* themselves are rarely detectable at this stage.

### Lyme disease is diagnosed serologically and treated with antibiotics

*Borrelia* can be cultured (in BSK or MKP medium) from early-stage cutaneous tissues, but culture has low sensitivity (40–60% in erythema migrans) and may take several weeks. Thus Lyme disease is primarily diagnosed on clinical presentation and known exposure. When indicated, serologic tests such as ELISA are useful, with Western blot confirmation of all positive and equivocal results. Specific IgM antibodies are detected 3–6 weeks after infection and IgG antibodies at a later stage. PCR diagnosis has been disappointing except for Lyme arthritis in which synovial fluid PCR is positive in 70–85% of cases.

Doxycycline or amoxicillin is effective in treatment of early disease. Late disease, especially with neurologic complications, may require more aggressive therapy (e.g. with intravenous ceftriaxone for up to 28 days).

Prevention of Lyme disease is by avoidance of tick bites. A vaccine is available for use in dogs (which can become naturally infected), but there is no Lyme vaccine currently licensed for humans. A Lyme vaccine based on recombinant outer surface protein A (Osp A) was marketed in North America for human use from 1998–2002, but concerns were expressed that it might induce arthritis and uptake was poor, so it was voluntarily withdrawn from the market. Current Lyme research is exploring the option of a vaccine to block both tick feeding and *Borrelia* transmission.

## PROTOZOAL INFECTIONS

### Malaria

#### Malaria is initiated by the bite of an infected female anopheline mosquito

Between 2000 and 2019 the global malaria case incidence is estimated to have decreased by 30%, but in association with service disruption due to COVID-19, it then rose in 2020, resulting in an additional 13.4 million cases of malaria worldwide. Malaria is a formidable opponent, with ~247 million cases per year worldwide. Its geographic distribution is restricted to areas where the anopheline mosquitoes can

**Table 28.4** Human malaria parasites

| Species | Plasmodium falciparum | P. vivax | P. malariae | P. ovale (P. o. curtisi and P. o. wallikeri) | P. knowlesi |
|---|---|---|---|---|---|
| Major distribution | West, East and Central Africa; Middle East; Far East; South America | India, North and East Africa, South America, Far East | Tropical Africa, India, Far East | Tropical Africa | Asia-Pacific region |
| Common name | Malignant tertian | Benign tertian | Quartan | Ovale tertian | |
| Duration of liver stage (incubation period) | 6–14 days | 12–17 days (with relapses up to 3 yr) | 13–40 days (with recrudescence up to 50 yr) | 9–18 days (with rare relapses) | 9–12 days |
| Duration of asexual blood cycle (fever cycle) | 48 h | 48 h | 72 h | 50 h | 24 h |
| Major complications | Cerebral malaria, anaemia, hypoglycaemia, jaundice, pulmonary oedema, shock | | Nephrotic syndrome | | Respiratory distress; renal failure |

The most important and life-threatening complications occur with *P. falciparum*, hence its old name malignant tertian malaria.

breed (i.e. latitudes between 60°N and 40°S except areas >2000 m). Ninety-five percent of malaria cases occur in the WHO African region. Drug and insecticide resistance present major challenges to malaria elimination, and there are ~619,000 malaria deaths globally each year. International travel, now rebounding after a fall during the COVID-19 pandemic, means malaria is regularly seen as an imported disease in non-malarious countries and, unless the possibility of malaria is constantly borne in mind, the diagnosis may be delayed or missed altogether with fatal results. Malaria can also be transmitted by blood transfusion, needlestick accidents or from mother to fetus or neonate.

### The life cycle of the malaria parasite comprises three stages

Five species of *Plasmodium* cause malaria in humans, of which *P. falciparum* and *P. knowlesi* are the most virulent (Table 28.4). All have similar life cycles, which are the most complex of any human infection, comprising three quite distinct stages and characterized by alternating extracellular and intracellular forms (Figs. 28.9 and 28.10).

Invasion of red cells requires at least two separate receptor–ligand interactions; the lack of one red cell surface receptor, the Duffy blood group antigen (Duffy antigen-chemokine receptor), explains the absence of *P. vivax* from most West Africans as there is a high prevalence of Duffy-negative people in the region. However, *P. vivax* infection of Duffy-negative individuals has now been confirmed, indicating that this malaria parasite is capable of using other receptors to invade erythrocytes and suggesting it is evolving rapidly. Nevertheless, the Duffy binding protein of *P. vivax* merozoites is a key target antigen for vaccine development. Other genetic traits that contribute to partial protection from malaria include haemoglobin S (sickle cell), haemoglobin C, alpha-thalassaemia and glucose-6-phosphate dehydrogenase (G6PD) deficiency.

### Clinical features of malaria include a fluctuating fever and drenching sweats

Symptoms range from fever to fatal cerebral disease or multiorgan failure and are associated exclusively with the asexual blood stage (see Fig. 28.9). The clinical picture depends upon the age and immune status of the patient and the species of parasite. The most characteristic feature is fever, which follows rupture of erythrocytic schizonts and is mainly due to the induction of cytokines such as interleukin 1 (IL-1) and tumour necrosis factor (TNF). The synchronous cycle in red cells means that the different species of malaria give characteristic patterns of fever, with either a 48-h (tertian: days 1 and 3), 72-h (quartan: days 1 and 4) or, rarely, 24-h (quotidian: daily) periodicity (Fig. 28.11). However, this classical pattern of fever is seldom seen in clinical practice in which a chaotic fever pattern is common. Furthermore, it is possible to be afebrile yet obviously very unwell with malaria. A typical paroxysm starts with a feeling of intense cold with shivering, followed by a hot, dry stage and finally a period of drenching sweats. Headache, muscle pains and vomiting are common. The symptoms of malaria closely resemble those of influenza, which is a common misdiagnosis. Jaundice may be present and may lead to an erroneous diagnosis of viral hepatitis. Fever may be the only physical sign in early malaria, but later enlargement of the spleen and liver is common, and anaemia is almost invariable.

*P. vivax* produces a chronic debilitating febrile illness resulting in significant morbidity and mortality in endemic areas. Indeed, there are proven cases of *P. vivax* infection that fulfill the case definition for severe malaria, manifesting as severe anaemia and respiratory distress. In the absence of reinfection, *P. ovale* and *P. malariae* malarias are normally self-limiting, although debilitating, infections. *P. malariae* may persist in the blood at a low level for decades and recrudesce to cause symptoms from time to time. Relapses (defined as hypnozoite-induced) may occur with *P. vivax* and *P. ovale* months or even 1–2 years after the initial malarial illness.

*P. falciparum* malaria is frequently fatal during the first 2 weeks because of a variety of complications (see Table 28.4). In hyperendemic areas, complicated falciparum malaria is most common in children aged between 6 months and 5 years and in pregnant, particularly primigravid, women. However, it can occur at any age in nonimmune individuals (e.g. tourists). The most dangerous complication is cerebral malaria, with convulsions and diminished level of

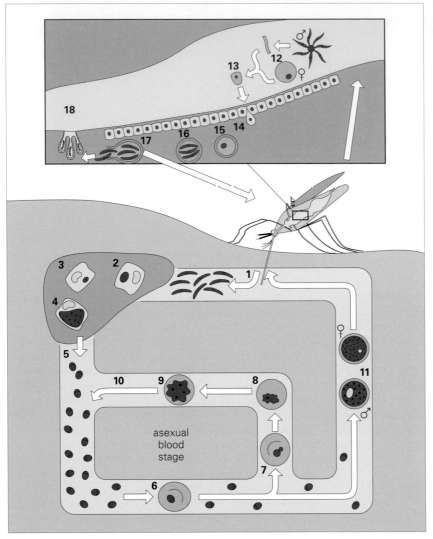

**Fig. 28.9** The life cycle of malaria in human and mosquito. In the symptomless preerythrocytic stage, sporozoites from the saliva of an infected *Anopheles* mosquito are injected into the human bloodstream when the mosquito bites (*1*). They then enter the parenchymal cells of the liver (*2*), where they mature in ~2 weeks into preerythrocytic (tissue) schizonts (*4*), finally rupturing to produce 10,000–40,000 merozoites (*5*). These circulate in the blood for a few minutes before entering the red blood cells (*6*) to initiate the asexual blood stage. For *Plasmodium vivax* and *P. ovale* only, some parasites, however, remain within the liver to lie dormant as hypnozoites (*3*), which are the cause of relapses. Once in the red blood cells the merozoites mature into the ring form (*7*), trophozoite (*8*) and schizont (*9*), thus multiplying and completing the cycle by maturing to release merozoites back into the circulation (*10*). This cycle may last for months or even years. Some merozoites, however, go on to initiate the sexual stage, maturing within the red blood cells to form male and female gametocytes (*11*), which can be taken up by the *Anopheles* mosquito on feeding. On entering the gut of the insect, the male gametocyte exflagellates (*12*) to form male microgametes, which fertilize the female gamete to form the zygote (*13*). This then invades the mosquito gut mucosa (*14*), where it develops into an oocyst (*15*). This matures to produce thousands of sporozoites (*16*), which are released (*17*) and migrate to the salivary glands of the insect (*18*), whence the cycle begins again.

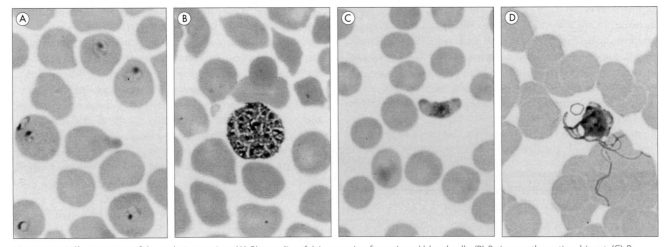

**Fig. 28.10** Different stages of the malaria parasites. (A) *Plasmodium falciparum* ring forms in red blood cells. (B) *P. vivax* erythrocytic schizont. (C) *P. falciparum* female gametocyte. (D) *P. vivax* male gametocyte exflagellating to form microgametes 20–25 μm long.

consciousness progressing to coma. Parasitized erythrocytes adhere to the walls of capillaries, a processs known as *sequestration*. This leads to vascular congestion, hypoperfusion, and localized hypoxia. Additional factors include endothelial dysfunction, increased permeability of the blood-brain barrier, dysregulation of coagulation pathways and a cytokine storm with excessive induction of proinflammatory cytokines such as TNF. Cerebral malaria is an important cause of mortality in African children; even if successfully treated, almost a quarter of children who recover from

**Fig. 28.11** Malaria fever charts showing cyclic fluctuations in temperature. The peaks coincide with the maturation and rupture of the intraerythrocytic schizonts, occurring every 48 h (*Plasmodium falciparum, P. vivax* and *P. ovale*) or every 72 h (*P. malariae*), when the cycles are synchronized. Classically synchronized fever charts are seldom seen in clinical practice.

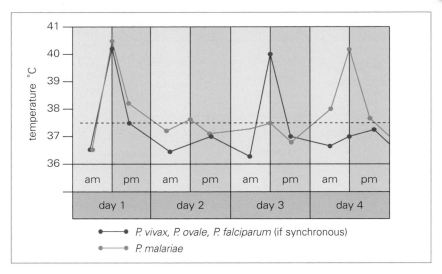

cerebral malaria plus malarial retinopathy have persistent neurologic symptoms such as seizures, cerebral palsy and cognitive impairment.

Also common is severe anaemia, which is due partly to haemolysis of infected and uninfected red cells and partly to dyserythropoiesis in the bone marrow. Of the other complications, hypoglycaemia in children is associated with increased malaria mortality especially if lactic acidosis is also present. Acute kidney injury (AKI) is an important complication of falciparum malaria. Several mechanisms contribute to malarial AKI: hypovolaemia and hypoperfusion (especially in children), endogenous nephrotoxins, sequestration, haemolysis, endothelial activation and disruption of the microcirculation. Prolonged renal hypoperfusion can lead to acute tubular necrosis. *P. malariae* may result in immune complex-mediated diffuse proliferative or focal glomerulonephritis, leading to the nephrotic syndrome (quartan malarial nephropathy).

In children, the main components of severe malaria are cerebral malaria, severe malarial anaemia and metabolic acidosis. In adults, multiorgan failure is seen, with metabolic acidosis, acute renal failure, jaundice and acute respiratory distress syndrome, with or without cerebral malaria.

### Malaria has an immunosuppressive effect and interacts with human immunodeficiency virus infection

The strong epidemiologic correlation between malaria and endemic Burkitt lymphoma probably reflects reduced T-cell cytotoxicity against Epstein-Barr virus–infected cells. It develops in germinal centre B lymphocytes with chromosomal translocations that result in upregulated expression of the *MYC* gene and activation-induced activity of cytidine deaminase, which promotes hypermutation in B cells. Malaria may also interfere with the immune response to vaccines against common viral or bacterial infections.

Malaria and human immunodeficiency virus (HIV) coinfection increases the severity and mortality for both diseases. In pregnant females, HIV-1 infection is associated with more peripheral blood parasitaemia, more placental malaria, higher parasite densities, more fever and increased risk of adverse birth outcomes. The odds ratio for developing severe malaria is higher in coinfected children than in coinfected adults, and coinfected children with cerebral malaria have lower CD4 T-cell, B-cell, and natural killer–cell counts. In semi-immune nonpregnant adults, HIV-1 infection is associated with higher rates of malaria infection, higher parasitaemia, and a significantly increased odds ratio of developing severe malaria. In nonimmune, nonpregnant adults, HIV-1 infection is associated with higher rates of severe malaria and death. HIV-infected patients have a higher rate of malaria treatment failure.

### Immunity to malaria develops gradually and seems to need repeated boosting

Immunity to malaria develops in stages, and in endemic areas, children who survive early attacks become resistant to severe disease by about 5 years of age. Parasite levels fall progressively until adulthood. In areas of hyperendemic malaria transmission, asymptomatic malaria parasitaemia may be found in as many as 75% of individuals. Repeated boosting is needed to maintain it, however, and 1 year spent away from exposure is sufficient for much of this semi-immunity to wane, albeit incompletely. The actual mechanisms are still being worked out but involve both antibody- and cell-mediated immunity (Fig. 28.12).

### Malaria is diagnosed by finding parasitized red cells in thin and thick blood films

Malaria microscopy in routine practice can detect 10–90 parasites per microlitre and remains the method of choice in most diagnostic laboratories. Lateral-flow devices (dipsticks) to detect malarial antigen are also widely used and can be performed without the need for a laboratory, but they are best deployed alongside microscopy where facilities and resources exist. Molecular assays to detect malarial DNA or RNA are much more sensitive. Initially performed only in reference laboratories, they are becoming more widely available in kit form.

In the case of *P. falciparum* infection, later (schizont) stages may be sequestered in deep tissues, so parasites may be deceptively scarce in or even absent from the peripheral blood, resulting in a negative blood film. Nonfalciparum malarias generally have lower parasitaemias. Therefore

| stage | mechanism |
|---|---|
| 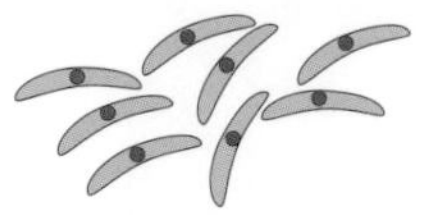 sporozoites | antibody (IgG1, IgG3, IgM) complement CD4 T cells |
| 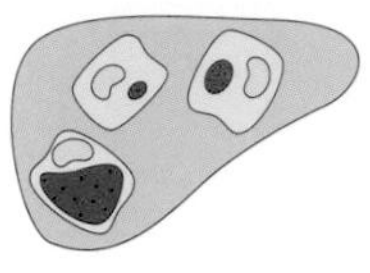 liver stage | cytotoxic T cells TNF IFN-α IL-1 |
| 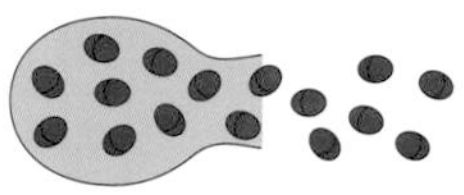 merozoites | antibody (IgG1, IgG3, IgM) complement antibody-dependent cellular mechanisms |
| 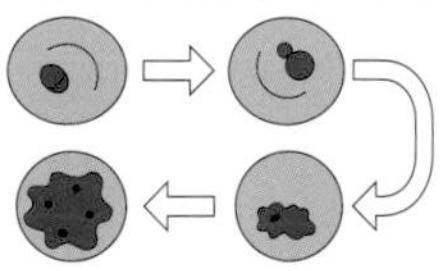 asexual erythrocyte stage | antibody opsonization and phagocytosis ROI RNI ECP TNF |
| 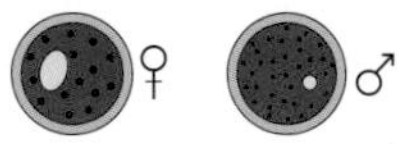 gametocytes | antibody complement |
| 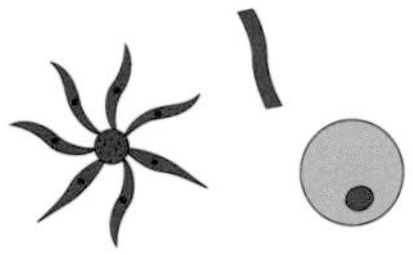 gametes | antibody complement |

**Fig. 28.12** Immunity to malaria. The principal mechanisms thought to be responsible for immunity at each stage of the cycle. CD, Cluster of differentiation; ECP, eosinophil cationic proteins; IFN, interferon; Ig, immunoglobulin; IL, interleukin; RNI, reactive nitrogen intermediates; ROI, reactive oxygen intermediates; TNF, tumour necrosis factor.

a single negative blood film does not exclude malaria of any species, and additional blood samples should be taken 12–24 h and 48 h later. A severe febrile illness, especially with anaemia, splenomegaly or cerebral signs with a negative blood film in a patient who conceivably could have malaria may therefore need to be treated as malaria while healthcare workers continue to look for other diagnoses and seek expert help. However, the presence of parasites in the blood of an ill patient from an endemic area does not mean that malaria is the only contributing factor to the illness, so additional causes of fever should still be borne in mind while they receive treatment for malaria. For example, they might have lobar pneumonia and coincidental malarial parasitaemia, as low-grade parasitaemia may be asymptomatic in those with partial malarial immunity.

Where available, intravenous artesunate (in combination with other antimalarials to avoid the development of drug resistance) is the drug of choice for severe malaria. Intravenous quinine is used if artesunate cannot be obtained without delay.

Uncomplicated falciparum malaria is treated with oral artemisinin combination therapy (ACT). Malaria due to *P. vivax*, *P. ovale*, *P. knowlesi* or *P. malariae* is treated with oral ACT or oral chloroquine (for *P. ovale*, *P. knowlesi* or *P. malariae* and for *P. vivax* from most geographic areas). Severe or complicated malaria due to any of these species is treated as for severe falciparum malaria. Primaquine (contraindicated in G6PD deficiency and in pregnancy) is used to kill hypnozoites of *P. vivax* or *P. ovale* in the liver and thus prevent relapses of these infections. Tafenoquine (also contraindicated in G6PD deficiency and in pregnancy) is available as an alternative to primaquine in some countries.

In endemic areas the most important method of prevention is the use of long-lasting insectide-impregnated bed nets. Indoor residual spraying with insecticides has an important effect in rapidly reducing malaria transmission when at least 80% of houses in a given area are sprayed. Other measures include seasonal malaria chemoprevention, intermittent preventive treatment of malaria in pregnancy, intermittent preventive treatment in infants and intermittent preventive treatment of malaria in school-aged children. Development of malaria vaccines is discussed in Chapter 35.

## Trypanosomiasis

### Three species of the protozoan *Trypanosoma* cause human disease

*Trypanosoma brucei gambiense* and *T. b. rhodesiense* cause human African trypanosomiasis (HAT) or sleeping sickness, and *T. cruzi* causes American trypanosomiasis or Chagas disease. The diseases differ markedly in the insect vector and the localization of the parasite. Their pathologic features are therefore considered separately in this chapter.

## Human African trypanosomiasis

### HAT is transmitted by the tsetse fly and restricted to equatorial Africa

The vector of HAT is the tsetse fly *Glossina*.

Humans are the main reservoir for *T. b. gambiense*. *T. b. rhodesiense* has a reservoir in domestic livestock and wild animals. In humans, *T. brucei* remains extracellular, first in the tissues near the insect bite and then in the lymphatics and blood, where it continues to divide. Trypanosomes are also found in the skin and in significant numbers in adipose tissue.

### Clinical features of HAT include lymphadenopathy and sleeping sickness

A few days after an infected bite, a swollen chancre develops at the site (*T. b. rhodesiense* mainly, rarely with *T. b. gambiense*) with related lymph node enlargement. Posterior cervical lymphadenopathy (Winterbottom's sign; Fig. 28.13A) is typical of *T. b. gambiense*. The parasite establishes in the blood and multiplies rapidly, with fever, splenomegaly and often signs of myocardial involvement. The CNS may become involved (earlier in the course of the illness in the East African *T. b. rhodesiense* than the West African *T. b. gambiense*), with the gradual development of headache, psychological changes, weight loss and finally coma (sleeping sickness; see Fig. 28.13B) and death. Parasitologically cured HAT can leave the patient with severe residual neurologic and mental disability.

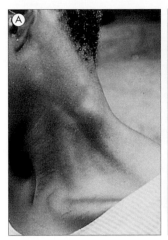
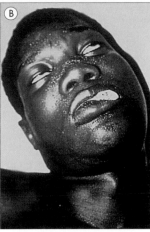

**Fig. 28.13** African trypanosomiasis. (A) Enlargement of the lymph nodes in the neck (Winterbottom's sign). (B) Coma (sleeping sickness) due to generalized encephalitis. (A, Courtesy P.G. Janssens; B, courtesy M.E. Krampitz and P. de Raadt.)

### *T. brucei* evades host by varying the antigens in its glycoprotein coat

*T. brucei* survives freely in the blood because of its remarkable degree of antigenic variation based on switching between some 900 different genes for its variant surface glycoprotein coat (VSG). Initially thought to express only one VSG at a time, *T. brucei* has now been shown to express several distinct VSGs in each wave of parasitaemia. This strategy is advantageous to the parasite, not only to facilitate chronic infection in an already infected individual, but also to counter herd immunity when infecting a new host. A high concentration of immunoglobulins, especially IgM, directed mainly at VSG is found in the blood and later in the CSF, and this is manufactured by morular-shaped plasma cells (Mott's cells), a feature of the predominantly lymphocytic infiltrate seen as perivascular cuffing around blood vessels in the brain (Fig. 28.14) and in white matter infiltration.

HAT is diagnosed by demonstrating parasites microscopically in blood, lymph nodes (by puncture) or in late cases in the CSF. Molecular diagnostics (PCR or loop-mediated isothermal amplification assays) are available in reference laboratories. Detection of antitrypanosomal antibody is used to screen populations for *T. b. gambiense*, with further parasitologic examination of those who are seropositive.

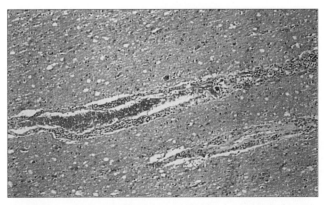

**Fig. 28.14** Lymphocytic infiltration around a blood vessel in the brain in *Trypanosoma brucei* infection (H&E stain). (Courtesy R. Muller and J.R. Baker.)

Immunochromatographic antibody detection tests have been developed for field use.

Treatment of HAT is determined by which trypanosome is involved and the disease stage present. Drugs available include fexinidazole, pentamidine, suramin, eflornithine, nifurtimox and melarsoprol.

### Control of HAT

Some 85–95% of HAT cases are due to *T. b. gambiense*. Its control is based on case finding and treatment and supported by vector control and bite avoidance. Bed nets are ineffective, as the flies feed during daylight hours. Due to its long half-life, prophylaxis with pentamidine was used in HAT control programmes >50 years ago, but its use for that purpose has long been discontinued.

## Chagas disease

### *T. cruzi* is transmitted by the reduviid (kissing) bug

*T. cruzi* is transmitted by reduviid (kissing) bugs, which readily inhabit poor housing. Almost all species of mammal can act as reservoirs of infection. Vectorial transmission occurs in parts of North, Central and South America. Oral transmission via food or drink contaminated by reduviid bugs also occurs in endemic areas. Vertical transmission from mother to fetus and transmission by blood or organ donation also take place and can occur in nonendemic areas.

Chagas disease has traditionally been characterized as a disease of the rural poor, but increasing urbanization has been followed by significant vectorial transmission of *T. cruzi* in cities (e.g. in Peru and Bolivia).

Due to such migration from rural to urban settings, many people with Chagas disease now live in the large cities of Latin America and, as a result of international migration, in the United States and parts of Europe. More than 300,000 people in the United States are estimated to have *T. cruzi* infection, but only ~1% have been diagnosed. Similarly, in Europe, ~96% of infected people are undiagnosed.

### Chagas disease has serious long-term effects, which include fatal heart disease

The parasite invades mammalian host cells, with a tropism for adipose, reticuloendothelial, myocardial and neuroglial tissues. Most infections are asymptomatic or oligosymptomatic, but ~10% produce more specific symptoms. A nodular lesion (chagoma) or oedematous swelling of the eyelid (Romaña's sign) may develop at the site of infection, with a transient febrile illness, regional lymphadenopathy and hepatosplenomegaly. Acute myocarditis due to myocyte invasion and necrosis may lead to cardiac failure and death. Meningoencephalitis can also occur and is life threatening in the immunocompromised host. After the acute phase, the disease pursues an extremely slow and chronic course. Approximately 70% of infected individuals remain in the indeterminate phase of chronic asymptomatic infection and do not develop complications. In cases where the disease does progress, the major complications, which can take years to appear, involve the heart (20–30% of infections), gastrointestinal tract (15–20%) and the peripheral nervous system (<5%, manifest as sensory polyneuropathy). The major cause of death is cardiomyopathy, with progressive weakening and dilatation of the ventricles due to destruction of cardiac muscle as a result

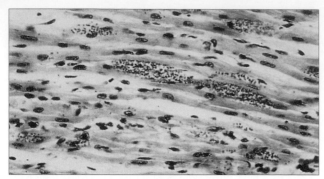

**Fig. 28.15** Amastigote forms of *Trypanosoma cruzi* in cardiac muscle in Chagas disease (H&E stain). (Courtesy H. Tubbs.)

**Table 28.5** *Leishmania* species—their distribution and clinical syndromes

| Species | Distribution | Diseases |
|---|---|---|
| *L. donovani* *L. infantum* | Africa, India Mediterranean | Visceral leishmaniasis |
| *L. chagasi* | South America | |
| *L. major* *L. tropica* | Africa, India Mediterranean | Cutaneous leishmaniasis |
| *L. aethiopica* | Africa | |
| *L. Mexicana* | Mexico and Central America | |
| *L. braziliensis* | South America | |

of parasite persistence and the host's inflammatory response (Fig. 28.15). Cardiac ventricular aneurysm and heart block are particularly serious features. Dilatation of the intestinal tract is due to similar processes in nerve cells, such that the organs become incapable of proper peristalsis; megaoesophagus and megacolon are the two commonest manifestations.

### Chronic Chagas disease is usually diagnosed serologically

In the acute phase, parasites may be seen in a blood film, but the chronic disease is usually diagnosed by serology for IgG antibody using two different types of assay (e.g. ELISA and indirect fluorescent antibody technique and, if available, PCR on peripheral blood). *T. cruzi* parasites can also be detected by xenodiagnosis. Clean reduviid bugs are fed on the patient and their rectal contents examined 1–2 months later or they are homogenized and injected into mice in which even a single trypanosome will produce a patent infection. The use of PCR on bug faeces instead of microscopy increases the sensitivity of xenodiagnosis. Performance of xenodiagnosis requires maintenance of a colony of clean, uninfected reduviid bugs to feed on the patient, which limits its availability.

Antiparasitic therapy of Chagas disease is with oral benznidazole or oral nifurtimox. Children respond better to antitrypanosomal drugs than do adults. Treatment is recommended in infants and children with congenital infection, girls and nonpregnant women of childbearing age (to prevent vertical transmission) and individuals with acute *T. cruzi* infection. Despite the low certainty of evidence, antiparasitic treatment is also now recommended for patients with indeterminate disease and may be of particular benefit to those at highest risk of Chagas disease reactivation (transplantation, people living with HIV, and immunosuppressive therapy). Both benznidazole and nifurtimox commonly produce significant side effects, so patients need to be followed carefully during treatment.

Prevention is achieved by improved housing and living standards, vector control, plus active case finding and treatment. However, vector control by insecticides is difficult, as some triatomine bugs can adapt to different habitats and reinvade houses after spraying. *T. cruzi* is adept at evading the immune response—a major challenge to vaccine development. However, therapeutic vaccines as immunotherapy for those with chronic or indeterminate Chagas disease are now in preclinical studies. Of particular interest is the possibility of deploying a therapeutic vaccine for pregnant women to prevent congenital transmission of *T. cruzi*.

## Leishmaniasis

### *Leishmania* parasites are transmitted by sandflies and cause New World and Old World leishmaniasis

Several species of *Leishmania* parasites cause disease in both the New World and the Old World (Table 28.5) and resulting in between 700,000 and 1 million new cases each year. Dogs can act as an important reservoir of infection for *L. donovani infantum* in the Mediterranean, whilst rodents such as gerbils are reservoirs for *L. major*. All are transmitted by sandflies.

### *Leishmania* is an intracellular parasite and inhabits macrophages

*Leishmania* evades the killing mechanisms of macrophages (Fig. 28.16) by way of a series of virulence factors that enable it to survive in the hostile environment of the macrophage's parasitophorous vacuole. Examples are superoxide dismutase and trypanothione reductase, both of which protect the parasite from oxidative stress, and cysteine proteinases which can degrade lysosomal proteases. The two principal sites of parasite growth are the spleen, liver and bone marrow (visceral leishmaniasis [VL]) and the skin (cutaneous leishmaniasis [CL]).

### Untreated VL (kala-azar) is fatal in 95% of cases

VL, or kala-azar, usually develops slowly, with fever and weight loss, anaemia, hepatomegaly and especially

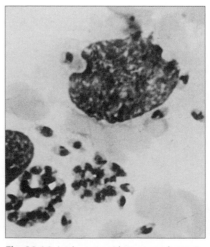

**Fig. 28.16** *Leishmania* within macrophages in aspirate from a lesion of New World leishmaniasis. (Courtesy M.J. Wood.)

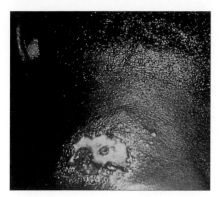

**Fig. 28.17** Cutaneous lesion on the neck in *Leishmania braziliensis* infection. (Courtesy P.J. Cooper.)

splenomegaly. With appropriate treatment, only those who are very ill at diagnosis die. Skin lesions known as post–kala-azar dermal leishmaniasis (PKDL) may appear following treatment. They can take the form of hypopigmented patches, erythematous papules or plaques and nodular lesions. PKDL lesions contain *Leishmania* amastigotes and constitute a reservoir of infection that can infect biting sandflies.

### CL is characterized by plaques, nodules or ulcers

Classic CL progresses insidiously from a small papule at the site of infection to a large ulcer. This may eventually heal with considerable scarring (Fig. 28.17), leaving the patient relatively immune to reinfection. Old World leishmanial lesions are known by various colloquial terms such as Oriental sore or Baghdad boil. New World leishmaniasis causing localized cutaneous lesions due to *L. mexicana* infection of the pinna is referred to as Chiclero's ulcer. Espundia refers to mucosal leishmaniasis, a disfiguring and potentially fatal disease of the mucosa of the upper respiratory tract beginning in the nasal septum and progressing in some cases to involve the pharynx, palate and larynx. Espundia is usually caused by *L. (Viannia) braziliensis*.

### Immunodeficient patients may suffer more severe leishmaniasis

In individuals lacking delayed type hypersensitivity, widespread chronic skin lesions can occur—diffuse CL—analogous to lepromatous leprosy. VL is a major complication of HIV infection not only in the tropics but also around the Mediterranean, although it is now easier to manage with antileishmanial drugs since the advent of highly active antiretroviral therapy. VL is also found in other patients severely immunocompromised by transplantation, leukaemia, lymphoma, systemic lupus erythematous, corticosteroid or other immunosuppressive therapy. A newly emerging risk factor for more severe leishmaniasis is monoclonal antibody therapy directed against TNFα. More cases are therefore likely to be seen, as such biologics are increasingly being used to treat a variety of medical conditions. Immunocompromised patients with VL have lower cure rates and higher relapse rates.

### Leishmaniasis is diagnosed by demonstrating the organism microscopically and treament is determined by the infecting species

Demonstration of the organism by microscopy of splenic aspirate or biopsies of bone marrow or skin lesions (depending upon the clinical picture) is definitive proof of leishmaniasis. PCR is more sensitive than microscopy and culture and has the advantage of determining the infecting species. Where available, PCR is now the method of choice for the detection and species identification of *Leishmania* in skin biopsies. Detection of antileishmanial antibody by the *Leishmania* direct agglutination test and the rK39 rapid test is valuable in the diagnosis of VL.

The precise choice of antiparasitic agent depends on the infecting species, hence the importance of diagnosis by PCR, but in principle, CL is treated by local injection of the edge of the ulcer with meglumine antimoniate (an antimonial). Intravenous meglumine antimoniate is used to treat multiple or potentially disfiguring lesions. Oral miltefosine is an alternative. The agent of choice for the treatment of VL is intravenous liposomal amphotericin B. Intravenous meglumine antimoniate is an alternative, though there is now significant antimony-resistant VL in parts of India. Oral miltefosine is an alternative.

Prevention depends on the use of insect repellent, bed nets and insecticides. Sandflies are smaller than mosquitoes and can pass through smaller holes in bed nets, so insecticide-impregnated bed nets should be used to protect against the sandfly vector.

*L. infantum* vaccines are available for use in dogs, with reported efficacy rates of 70–80%.

Currently there are no anti-*Leishmania* vaccines licensed for use in humans, but the ChAd63-KH vaccine, based on a simian adenovirus encoding a synthetic gene for expression of *Leishmania* antigens, has entered phase II clinical trials as a therapeutic vaccine against PKDL. Candidate antigens for expression in mRNA vaccines are under consideration.

## HELMINTH INFECTIONS

### Schistosomiasis

More than 230 million cases of schistosomiasis occur each year. Of these cases, 95% occur in sub-Saharan Africa; about two-thirds of them are caused by *Schistosoma haematobium*.

### Schistosomiasis is transmitted through snail vectors (intermediate hosts)

All digenean flukes must pass through a mollusc intermediate host to complete their larval development. However, schistosomes are the only group in which larvae released by the snails penetrate directly into the final host.

The life cycle of schistosomes is illustrated in Fig. 28.18. Infected freshwater snails, which are always aquatic, release fork-tailed larvae into the surrounding water. These penetrate the host's skin, enter the dermis and pass via the bloodstream through the lungs to the liver, where they mature and form male and female pairs before relocating to their final site:

- the veins surrounding the bladder for *S. haematobium*
- the mesenteric veins around the colon for *S. japonicum* and *S. mansoni*.

Worm pairings are now known not to be permanent; male–male competition and mate choice of females both occur such that schistosomes can change mates. The life cycle is completed when eggs laid by the female worms move across the walls of the bladder or bowel and leave the body in urine or faeces.

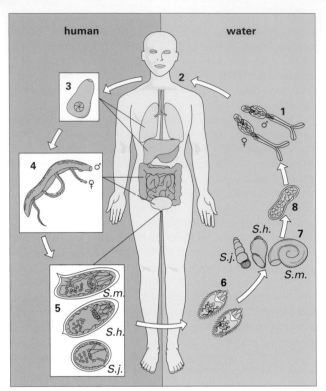

**Fig. 28.18** Life cycle of schistosomes. Free-swimming cercariae in water (*1*) penetrate unprotected skin. (*2*) During penetration, they lose their tails to become schistosomulae. (*3*) These migrate through the bloodstream via the lungs and liver to the veins of the bladder (*Schistosoma haematobium, S.h.*) or bowel (*S. mansoni, S.m.; S. japonicum, S.j.*), where they mature (*4*) to produce characteristic eggs (*5*) within 6–12 weeks. The eggs then penetrate the bladder or colon to be passed in the urine or the faeces (*6*). Eggs passed into fresh water release miracidia, which penetrate snail intermediate hosts (*7*) where they mature into sporocysts (*8*). These release cercariae (*1*) into the water to complete the cycle.

### Clinical features of schistosomiasis result from allergic responses to the different life cycle stages

The stages of skin penetration, migration and egg production are each associated with pathologic changes, collectively affecting many body systems. Penetration can cause a dermatitis, which becomes more severe on repeated reinfection. The developmental stages are associated with the onset of allergic symptoms (e.g. fever, eosinophilia, lymphadenopathy, spleno- and hepatomegaly, diarrhoea), but the most severe pathology arises following the onset of egg laying. The body becomes hypersensitive to antigens released by the eggs as they pass through tissues to the outside world or become trapped in other organs after being swept away in the bloodstream.

- In urinary schistosomiasis caused by *S. haematobium*, movement of eggs through the bladder wall causes haemorrhage. With time, the bladder wall becomes inflamed. Infiltrated polyps develop, and malignant changes may follow; nephrosis may also occur (see Ch. 21). In recent years it has increasingly been recognized that *S. haematobium* does not simply result in urinary pathology but causes genitourinary schistosomiasis. In males it can result in pelvic and ejaculatory pain, abnormal ejaculates, haematospermia and infertility. Female genital schistosomiasis (FGS) can result in vaginal bleeding or itching,

dyspareunia, and formation of sandy patches on the cervix and uterus. Left untreated it can result in infertility, miscarriage, ectopic pregnancy and spontaneous abortion. FGS is associated with increased susceptibility to HIV infection in those affected.

- Release of the eggs of *S. japonicum* and *S. mansoni* similarly causes intestinal haemorrhage and inflammation.

A more serious consequence of these infections results from the inflammatory responses to eggs that become trapped in other organs of the body, primarily the liver but also the lung and CNS. There is a CD4 Th2-driven granulomatous response directed against schistosome eggs and the antigens they secrete. Reactions around eggs in the presinusoidal capillaries interfere with blood flow and, together with extensive periportal fibrosis (Symmers' pipestem fibrosis), which occurs in ~10% of those infected with *S. mansoni*, lead to portal hypertension. As a consequence, there is hepatosplenomegaly, collateral connections form between the hepatic vessels and oesophageal varices develop. The collateral circulation can lead to eggs being washed into the capillary bed of the lungs.

Ectopic adult worm pairs laying eggs in the paravertebral venous plexus can result in spinal schistosomiasis, leading to paraplegia.

### Schistosomiasis is diagnosed by microscopy and treated with praziquantel

Diagnosis of schistosomiasis is made by visualization of eggs on microscopy of stool or urine samples. Serum antibody detection, commonly with an IgG ELISA to soluble egg antigen, is helpful in nonendemic areas, especially in travellers. Antigen detection assays and molecular diagnostics are in use in some centres.

Treatment of individuals with praziquantel destroys the adult worms but does not kill the eggs, which die naturally in ~2 months. In advanced cases the pathology is irreversible. There are currently no schistosomal vaccines licensed for human use. Candidate vaccines directed against *S. mansoni* fatty acid–binding protein, *S. mansoni* tetraspanin, *S. mansoni* large-subunit calpain and *S. haematobium* glutathione S-transferase are in preclinical or clinical studies.

Control of infection at a population level is achieved by breaking the transmission cycle through avoidance of infected water and improvement in sanitation, supported by health education campaigns. Control of snail intermediate hosts is practised in some regions. In the case of *S. japonicum* for which bovines are major intermediate hosts, transmission-blocking vaccines for veterinary use are under evaluation. Mass drug administration (MDA) programmes aim to reduce morbidity but can also reduce transmission. On the way to eradication it is hoped to move from MDA to selective treatment, but that will require more sensitive diagnostics suitable for field use.

### Filariasis

#### Filarial nematodes depend upon blood-feeding arthropod vectors for transmission

The filarial nematodes parasitize the deeper tissues of the body (see Ch. 6). The most important species can be divided into those located in the lymphatics (*Brugia, Wuchereria*) and those in subcutaneous tissues (*Onchocerca*). A number of less harmful species also occur. In all species, the female worms release live larvae (microfilariae), which are picked up by the vector from the blood (lymphatic species) or skin (*Onchocerca*). Both groups can cause severe inflammatory responses, reflected in a variety of pathologic responses in the skin and lymph nodes, but each is associated with additional and characteristic pathology. (Descriptions of the diseases caused by *Onchocerca* are given in Chs. 26 and 27.)

### Lymphatic filariasis caused by *Brugia* and *Wuchereria* is transmitted by mosquitoes

Mosquitoes introduce infective larvae into the skin as they feed. These larvae migrate to the lymphatics and develop slowly into long, thin adult worms (females 80–100 mm × 0.25 mm) found in the lymph nodes and lymphatics of the limbs (usually lower) and groin. Adult females live for ~7 years. Infections become patent after ~8–12 months when sheathed microfilariae appear in the blood. Approximately two-thirds of infections are asymptomatic but produce subclinical lymphangiectasia; other infected individuals may show few clinical signs or have acute manifestations such as fever, rashes, eosinophilia, lymphangitis, lymphadenitis (Fig. 28.19) and, in men, funiculitis, epididymitis and orchitis. Initial damage to the lymphatics is vessel dilatation in response to mediators released by the adult worms. In addition, *Wolbachia*, an endosymbiont bacterium present in *Wuchereria bancrofti* and in *Brugia* spp. needed for survival and reproduction of adult worms, plays a part in stimulating the proinflammatory response to the adult worms themselves.

Gradual impairment of lymphatic contractility follows. The lymphatic valves become incompetent, resulting in lymphatic stasis. Collateral lymph vessels form. Later, chronic obstructive changes caused by repeated episodes of lymphangitis may block lymphatics, leading to hydrocoele and to the gross enlargement of breasts, scrotum and limbs—the latter condition being known as *elephantiasis*, in which there is significant tissue fibrosis (Fig. 28.20). Chyluria (milky white urine) may also occur. Most episodes of local inflammation are due to secondary bacterial (e.g. with streptococci) or fungal infection of

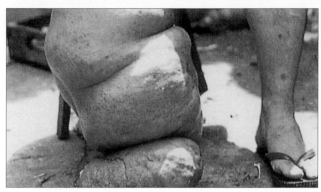

**Fig. 28.20** Elephantiasis of the leg caused by *Brugia malayi*. (Courtesy A.E. Bianco.)

the skin and are of major importance in the development and progression of filarial adenolymphangitis.

A feature of filarial infections in endemic regions is that not everyone exposed develops symptomatic infections. Many, although microfilaraemic and thus contributing to disease transmission, remain asymptomatic, and relatively few show gross pathology (Fig. 28.21). Some individuals develop pulmonary symptoms known as *tropical pulmonary eosinophilia* (see Ch. 20). Various factors influence susceptibility to lymphatic filariasis, including socioeconomic status, day-to-day activities, age, gender and host genetics. Polymorphisms of host defence pathway genes mannose-binding lectin, vascular endothelial growth factor, HLA, Toll-like receptor, programmed cell death-1, IL 10 and chitotriosidase increase susceptibility to bancroftian filariasis. However, variability of genetic polymorphisms and the associations they have with disease susceptibility are found in different ethnic groups.

### Few drugs are really satisfactory for treating filariasis

Diethylcarbamazine (DEC), which primarily kills microfilariae, is no longer used for the treatment of onchocerciasis as it produces a violent allergic response when microfilariae are killed. A single low dose of DEC is, however, used in the Mazzotti test to diagnose onchocerciasis in patients whose skin snips are negative for microfilariae. Onchocerciasis is treated with ivermectin plus doxycycline.

DEC is still used to treat lymphatic filariasis in combination with doxycycline, which kills the *Wohlbachia* bacterial symbionts in the adult worm. Albendazole plus either DEC or ivermectin, or ivermectin plus DEC and albendazole in countries without onchocerciasis, is used in MDA programmes.

Elimination of lymphatic filariasis is possible using preventive chemotherapy with MDA supplemented by vector control and prevention of biting. Factors affecting the success of programmes to eliminate lymphatic filariasis include the initial level of disease endemicity, the effectiveness of the local vector mosquitoes, the regimen used for MDA and acceptance of the proposed intervention by the local population. Since the Global Programme to Eliminate Lymphatic Filariasis was launched by WHO in 2000, 17 countries/ territories have eliminated lymphatic filariasis as a public health problem.

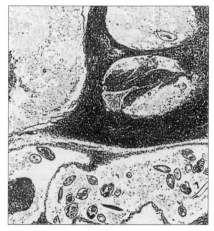

**Fig. 28.19** Lymph node containing adult *Wuchereria*, showing dilated lymphatics and tissue reaction in the vessel walls. (Courtesy R. Muller and J.R. Baker.)

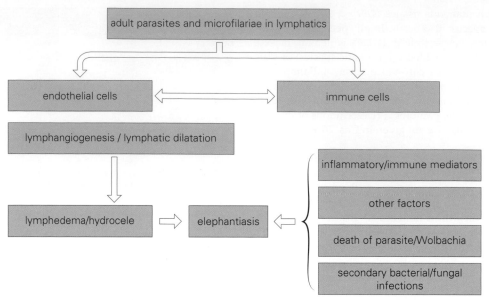

**Fig. 28.21** Pathogenesis of lymphatic filarial disease (lymphedema, hydrocele, elephantiasis). Live filarial parasites and/or their products directly affect lymphatic endothelial cells and the cells of the innate and adaptive immune system, thus contributing to disease development. (Modified from Gavins FNE, Stokes GK. Ch. 16. In: Vascular Response to Pathogens. Academic Press; 2016.)

## KEY FACTS

- Many important infections (arboviruses, rickettsiae, *Borrelia*, protozoa, helminths) are transmitted by vectors such as insects, ticks or snails.

- Some infections are chronic (Lyme disease, leishmaniasis, schistosomiasis) or can be lethal (malaria, HAT, viral encephalitis).

- Often they are restricted to tropical countries because of the distribution of the vector. Climate change may alter this distribution and therefore the pattern of diseases transmitted.

- Strong immune responses are mounted, often leading to immunopathologic complications. Treatment is usually by chemotherapy.

- Vector control is difficult but can lead to disease eradication.

- With very few exceptions (yellow fever), vaccines are not available for this group of diseases.

# Multisystem zoonoses

29

## Introduction

### Some multisystem infections in humans are animal diseases (i.e. zoonoses)

In these infections a nonhuman vertebrate host is the reservoir of infection, and humans are involved only incidentally. The human infection follows contact with or ingestion of infective material passed by an infected host, but infection of a human is not essential for the pathogen's life cycle or for its maintenance in nature. One striking feature of zoonotic infections, and of the arthropod-borne infections described in Chapter 28, is that few are transmitted effectively between humans, who thus represent dead-end hosts for the infecting organism. However, the largest Ebola virus disease (EVD) outbreak to date, between 2013 and 2016, demonstrated that there is the potential to do so and how important it is to control and prevent these infections.

Sometimes the zoonotic origin of these infections is less clear. For example, tularaemia can be acquired either by direct contact with the reservoir host or from an arthropod vector and is included in this chapter. Plague is included because it is transmitted from infected rats via the rat flea, although it is also transmissible directly from human to human.

Other zoonoses are dealt with in their relevant chapters (e.g. toxoplasmosis in Chs. 24–26, rabies in Ch. 25, salmonellosis in Ch. 23).

## VIRAL HAEMORRHAGIC FEVER IS A MULTISYSTEM SYNDROME TRIGGERED BY A GROUP OF VIRUSES THAT CAUSE SEVERE DAMAGE TO THE VASCULAR SYSTEM

Viruses from the following families can cause viral haemorrhagic fever and are zoonoses:

- Arenaviridae (i.e. Lassa fever virus)
- Hantaviridae (i.e. Hantaan, Seoul and Puumala viruses)
- Filoviridae (i.e. Ebola and Marburg viruses)

Nairoviridae (Crimean-Congo haemorrhagic fever virus), Phenuiviridae (Rift Valley fever virus) and Flaviviridae (dengue, yellow fever, Omak haemorrhagic fever and Kyansur Forest disease viruses) are all borne by arthropod vectors (see Ch. 28). The intermediate hosts, mode of transmission and illness severity differ between virus species.

### ARENAVIRUS INFECTIONS

#### Arenaviruses are transmitted to humans in rodent excreta

Many zoonoses are caused by enveloped single-stranded RNA viruses with a genome consisting of two RNA segments called arenaviruses. On electron microscopy (Fig. 29.1) these pleomorphic virus particles with a diameter of 50–300 nm can be seen to contain ribosomes that have a sandlike granular appearance, giving rise to the name arena (Latin: *arena*, "sand"). Arenaviruses are carried by various species of rodent in which they cause a harmless lifelong infection with continuous excretion of virus in urine and faeces of apparently healthy infected animals. Humans may become infected via direct contact with infected rodents, inhalation

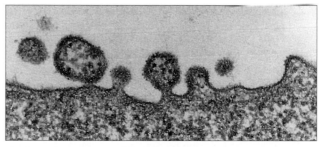

**Fig. 29.1** Electron micrograph of lymphocytic choriomeningitis virus budding from the surface of an infected cell. The sandlike granules in the virus particles are characteristic of arenaviruses. (Courtesy K. Mannweiler and F. Lehmann-Grübe.)

of infectious excreta, working in agricultural environments or trekking in areas where the rodents exist and may develop severe and often lethal disease involving extensive haemorrhaging and multiorgan involvement. A selection of arenaviruses and the diseases they cause are included in Table 29.1. Since 2007 nine new arenaviruses have been identified, some as a result of recombination events within one segment. They are divided into the Old World (Eastern Hemisphere) and New World (Western Hemisphere) groups based on geography and genomic differences. Old World viruses are found in Africa, Europe and Asia of which Lassa fever and lymphocytic choriomeningitis virus (LCMV) are associated with the most common human infections involving this family. New World viruses are found in North and South America.

The distribution of the host is concordant with the distribution of the virus. LCMV is the only arenavirus with a worldwide distribution, the rest being seen in Africa or the

**Table 29.1** Viral fevers and haemorrhagic diseases acquired from vertebrates or from unknown sources

| Virus | Virus group | Disease | Animal of origin | Lethality | Geographic distribution |
|---|---|---|---|---|---|
| Lymphocytic choriomeningitis (LCM) | Arenavirus | LCM | Mouse, hamster | - | Worldwide |
| Lassa fever | Arenavirus | Lassa fever | African bush rat (*Mastomys natalensis*) | + | West Africa |
| Machupo | Arenavirus | Bolivian haemorrhagic fever | Bush mouse (*Calomys callosus*) | + | Northeast Bolivia |
| Junin | Arenavirus | Argentinian haemorrhagic fever | *Calomys* spp., mice | + | Argentina |
| Hantaan | Hantavirus | Haemorrhagic fever Fever with renal syndrome (Korean haemorrhagic fever severe pulmonary syndrome) | } Mice, rats | + | Far East, Scandinavia, Eastern Europe, US Southwest |
| Marburg | Filovirus | Marburg disease | Fruit bats | ++ | Africa (lab, infections in Marbug, Germany) |
| Ebola | Filovirus | Ebola disease | Fruit bats | ++ | Africa (Sudan, Zaire, Sierra Leone, Guinea, Liberia) |

New World. As with most zoonoses, infection is not transmitted, or is transmitted with low efficiency, from human to human. However, health care workers have been infected by direct contact with blood or secretions from patients infected with Lassa fever virus, but this can be prevented by using barrier nursing techniques. Of the New World Tacaribe serocomplex viruses, serious illness is associated with the Junin and Machupo viruses that cause Argentine and Bolivian haemorrhagic fevers, respectively. LCMV can cause acute central nervous system (CNS) disease.

## Arenavirus infection is diagnosed by viral genome detection, serology or virus isolation

Diagnosis by testing for viral genome or specific antibodies or by isolating viruses can be carried out in reference centres.

Prevention of infection by reducing exposure to the virus concerned was dramatically illustrated when rodent trapping terminated outbreaks of Bolivian haemorrhagic fever (Box 29.1 and Fig. 29.2). Treatment with the antiviral agent ribavirin has been successful if used early in Lassa fever infection. Postexposure prophylaxis with oral ribavirin has been used. There are no World Health Organization (WHO)–approved vaccines against arenaviruses. However, a live attenuated Junin virus vaccine was licensed in 2006 for use only in Argentina.

## Lassa fever virus is an arenavirus that occurs naturally in bush rats in parts of West Africa

Lassa fever, one of the viral haemorrhagic viruses, is endemic in various West African countries but especially in Nigeria and Sierra Leone. It is a single-stranded enveloped RNA virus that may have originated in Nigeria >1000 years ago. Viral entry into host cells is directed by a fusion glycoprotein sited in the viral outer lipid envelope. The cellular receptor for Lassa fever virus is matriglycan, an oligosaccharide found on a peripheral membrane protein called α-*dystroglycan*. Once bound, the virions are endocytosed after which conformational changes allow release of virus into the cytosol.

The first person with Lassa fever was reported in 1969. She was a missionary nurse working in a rural clinic near Lassa, Nigeria. Sadly she died, as did two of three nurses looking after her, then one of two researchers working on the virus isolate also died. Infection arising from human exposure to infected rats (*Mastomys natalensis*) by eating them or being exposed to their urine results in a febrile disease that is generally not very severe.

There are ~300,000 infections with 5000 deaths annually in West Africa. In 2022, 929 confirmed and 6769 suspected infections were recorded with 71% reported from three states in Nigeria, part of an ongoing outbreak. The mortality rate varies but is ~20–30%. There is a seasonal distribution, and, although infections can occur around the year, January to March are peak times.

Lassa fever is a travel-related infection, and human-to-human transmission occurred in February 2022 in the United Kingdom when two family members (one of whom died) were infected by another family member who returned from Mali and was subsequently symptomatic and diagnosed with Lassa fever.

## Laboratory diagnosis is important as the initial symptom may be a febrile illness

Lassa fever virus RNA testing by polymerase chain reaction (PCR) is key, and serology tests include Lassa fever virus antigen-capture and immunoglobulin M (IgM; but IgM can persist for months after infection) and IgG enzyme-linked immunosorbent assays (ELISAs).

It is thought that the majority of Lassa fever virus infections are asymptomatic or mild and so the different infections could be related to strain differences and the amount of virus people have been exposed to as well as their genetic susceptibility. The incubation period is 5–10 days, and people present with a few days of fever, sore throat, vomiting and coughing. Around 20% will have a viral haemorrhagic fever with bleeding from various body sites, including the mucosa. Haemorrhage, capillary damage, haemoconcentration and collapse with multiorgan failure result in death ~2 weeks after the onset of symptoms.

## Box 29.1 ▪ Lessons in Microbiology

### Bolivian haemorrhagic fever: a lesson in ecology

In 1962 there was an outbreak of a severe and often lethal infectious disease in the small town of San Joachim, Bolivia. Patients developed fever, myalgia and an enanthem (internal rash), followed by capillary leakage, haemorrhage, shock and a neurologic illness. This disease was termed *Bolivian haemorrhagic fever* and had a mortality rate of 15%. Extensive investigations failed to incriminate an arthropod vector, but the evidence pointed to a role for mice in the epidemic. Acting on this possibility, hundreds of mousetraps were airlifted to the beleaguered town, and it was soon shown that trapping mice had a dramatic effect on the incidence of the disease. The epidemic was completely halted. Quite separately, a virus was isolated from the tissues of a trapped local bush mouse (*Calomys callosus*). The virus was shown to cause a harmless lifelong infection in this animal with continued excretion of virus in urine and faeces. The virus (given the name Machupo) was an arenavirus, a group that includes lymphocytic choriomeningitis virus (LCMV; infecting mice and hamsters) and Lassa fever virus (infecting an African bush rat). These viruses cause a harmless, persistent infection in the natural rodent host but an often severe disease in humans exposed to infected animals.

This outbreak of Bolivian haemorrhagic fever provided an important lesson in ecology. Because of the high incidence of malaria in the San Joachim area, extensive dichlorodiphenyltrichloroethane (DDT) spraying had been carried out to control mosquitoes. As a result, geckos (small lizards that eat insects) accumulated DDT in their tissues, and the local cats that preyed on geckos began to die with lethal concentrations of DDT in their livers. The shortage of cats, in turn, allowed the bush mice to invade human dwellings. The close vicinity of infected mice to humans and human food led to the epidemic (see Fig. 29.2).

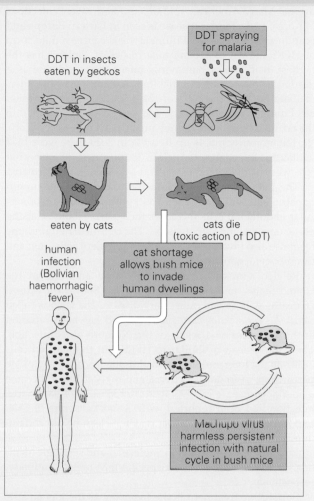

**Fig. 29.2** Bolivian haemorrhagic fever—a lesson in ecology. DDT, Dichlorodiphenyltrichloroethane. (Courtesy the late Dr. Davis Ellis, London School of Hygiene & Tropical Medicine.)

Prognosis is determined by measuring various parameters, including Lassa fever virus RNA viraemia, liver enzymes and renal function. If these are high and there is a cytopaenia, low red and white blood cells and platelets, the prognosis is poor.

Supportive therapy is the mainstay of treatment together with the early addition of the antiviral drug ribavirin.

### LCMV occurs worldwide

LCMV is an enveloped single-stranded virus discovered after studies investigating the outbreak of the encephalitis epidemic in 1933 in St. Louis, Missouri. The common house mouse (*Mus musculus*) is the host. It has caused sporadic infection in people living in mouse-infested dwellings and has been reported in children possessing apparently healthy but infected hamsters. There is generally a nonspecific febrile illness, but occasionally aseptic lymphocytic meningitis occurs with recovery as was reported in 2021 in Australia when a mouse plague occurred in New South Wales and spread to adjoining regions. A farmer developed photophobia, neck stiffness, headache and had an abdominal rash having had contact with mice carcasses and droppings. A rare diagnosis was made having collected a careful history and excluding other causes. LCMV can be a rare cause of congenital infection as women have acquired the infection in pregnancy, and it has a fetal mortality rate of ~30% and can lead to severe neurologic sequelae. Hantavirus infections can cause haemorrhagic fever with renal syndrome (HFRS) and hantavirus pulmonary syndrome (HPS).

Hantaviruses belong to the *Hantaviridae* family and are single-stranded enveloped negative sense RNA viruses. They cause two zoonotic diseases, HFRS in Europe and Asia due to species including Puumala, Seoul, Dobrava Belgrade and Hantaan viruses (Old World) and HPS in the Americas due to Sin Nombre and Andes viruses (New World).

Each particular species of hantavirus has a particular rodent as its intermediate host. Humans get infected by inhaling aerosolized urine and saliva from infected rodents. They differ from other bunyaviruses that are transmitted by arthropod vectors. The incubation period is 9–33 days (median 14–17 days).

Hantaan virus was isolated from infected field rodents near the Hantan River in South Korea in 1978. After exposure to the urine of infected animals, there is a febrile illness, myalgia, fatigue, headache, nausea, vomiting and diarrhoea that can lead to hypotension, haemorrhage and a renal syndrome. Many American soldiers suffered severe infections in Korea, and a milder disease is seen in Eastern Europe and Scandinavia. In Europe, Puumala virus causes a mild form of HFRS known as *nephropathia epidemica*. Finland has the highest incidence of hantavirus infections worldwide as it has large areas of forest inhabited by bank voles, the intermediate host. Nearly 13% of the adult Finnish population has Puumala virus antibody, and ~6% of those admitted to the hospital with acute kidney injury need temporary dialysis; the mortality rate is up to 0.4%. In 2020 there were 1647 hantavirus infections reported in 28 countries in Europe, but 85% were from Finland (71%) and 14% were from Germany.

The pathogenesis is multifactorial and includes immunopathologic and host genetic background. Infection of vascular endothelial cells increases their permeability, causing tissue oedema and hypotension. The cell-mediated immune response also involves increased complement activation and thrombocytopaenia.

Related viruses are present in mice and rats in the United States, and outbreaks in the US Southwest caused 26 deaths with severe pulmonary disease. The latter is called *hantavirus cardiopulmonary syndrome* and has been reported in the Americas as a result of Sin Nombre virus infection. The pathogenesis is similar to HFRS, but the infected cells infiltrate the lung and myocardial tissue leading to cytokine production, pulmonary oedema and myocarditis. It became a notifiable disease in 1995; in 2020, 833 cases of hantavirus infection had been reported, with a mortality rate of 35%. Exposure to hantaviruses occurs when cleaning out rodent-infested outdoor buildings.

Laboratory diagnosis is by molecular and serologic methods, detecting viral RNA or specific IgM or IgG antibody, respectively.

Supportive treatment is the mainstay as there is no specific antiviral therapy, together with intensive care support, dialysis and extracorporeal membrane oxygenation for the different diseases.

## EBOLA AND MARBURG HAEMORRHAGIC FEVERS

### Fruit bats are the reservoir for Ebola and Marburg viruses

Ebola and Marburg haemorrhagic fevers occur in central and east Africa, are infections caused by Ebola virus (EBOV) and Marburg virus, are members of the family *Filoviridae* and are long filamentous single-stranded RNA viruses (Fig. 29.3). There are six EBOV species in the *Ebolavirus* genus, of which Zaire (EBOV), Sudan, Tai Forest and Bundibugyo viruses

can infect humans and primates. Reston EBOV is also a member but does not cause disease in humans, and Bombali EBOV was found in 2018 in bats in Sierra Leone.

The incubation period for EBOV and Marburg virus infection is 2–21 days, with a mean of 8–10 days. Ebola and Marburg virus–infected individuals can develop fever, headache, myalgia, rash and then haemorrhage, disseminated intravascular coagulation (see Ch. 18) and multiorgan failure.

The reservoir of origin and natural cycle of maintenance for Marburg virus was not known until Marburg virus RNA was detected in cave-dwelling fruit bats after a small outbreak of Marburg haemorrhagic fever was seen in some miners in Uganda in 2007. EBOV is also thought to have a fruit bat reservoir.

Marburg virus infection was first recognized in 1967 in Marburg, Germany, after exposure of laboratory workers to infected African green monkeys from Uganda. However, these monkeys are not the natural hosts. Mortality was ~20%, and, as with EBOV infection, it was noted that the virus could be detected in semen for months after clinical recovery; one patient transmitted the infection to his wife by this route.

### EVD—gradual evolution of outbreaks to an unprecedented epidemic in West Africa from 2013–2016

Outbreaks of a similar disease to Marburg virus infections occurred in 1976 in southern Sudan and in the region of the Ebola River in Zaire (now Democratic Republic of the Congo [DRC]). Overall, there were 602 people with EVD and 397 deaths. Person-to-person transmission took place in local hospitals via contaminated syringes and needles, burial preparations and sexual contact.

The virus enters through mucous membranes or abraded skin. Infection does not occur through aerosol transmission. In 1989 monkeys infected with EBOV were inadvertently imported into the United States from the Philippines. A number of the monkeys died, but although at least four people were infected, none developed disease.

A large epidemic was seen in Kikwit, Zaire, in 1995, with 315 cases and 244 deaths. Gabon had three epidemics between 1994 and 1997. EVD appeared in northern Uganda in 2000 and caused large outbreaks with high mortality rates in Congo-Brazzaville in 2003, also killing many gorillas and chimpanzees, and then again in Angola between 2004 and 2005.

The largest and longest epidemic of EVD occurred between December 2013 and April 2016 in West Africa in Guinea, Liberia and Sierra Leone. Overall, 28,616 people had

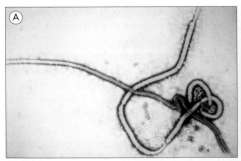
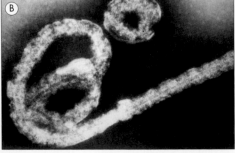

**Fig. 29.3** (A, B) Electron micrographs of Ebola Zaire virus. (Courtesy the late Dr. David Ellis, London School of Hygiene and Tropical Medicine.)

been seen with suspected, probable and confirmed EVD, with 11,310 deaths, although the true figures were likely to have been greater. Due to local travel and EBOV-infected health care workers returning home, there were 36 people with EVD reported in Nigeria, Senegal and Mali and the United States, Great Britain, Spain and Italy, respectively.

It was thought to have started in Guinea, where a 2-year-old boy had died within 2 days of falling ill with the Zaire EBOV strain (see Fig. 29.3B), possibly having been in contact with a bat. Subsequently, direct contact with blood or body fluids of EBOV-infected symptomatic individuals was the main route of transmission. The outbreaks in West African countries varied in size owing to the time period of the growth rate of the epidemic and the population size. In addition, a proportion of EBOV-infected individuals were super-spreaders who infected the majority of people who made up the next generation of infected individuals.

The 2018–2020 outbreak in the DRC led to ~3500 confirmed infections and >2000 deaths. In January 2023 Uganda declared the most recent outbreak over with ~164 infections and 77 deaths.

### Interventions that reduced the transmission rate

The effective control measures included finding symptomatic people, contact tracing, isolation of patients and contacts, admission of patients to specific Ebola treatment centres where clinical supportive care could be given, ensuring good infection control practices and providing safe burials. In the absence of antiviral treatments, components of the management of symptomatic people that were critical involved relatively simple measures such as carrying out blood tests to measure electrolyte imbalances and intravenous rehydration. The development of a vaccine and rapid diagnostic tests in biocontainment field laboratories helped, too, in terms of protection and faster EVD detection, respectively.

The epidemic peaked in September 2014 after 10 months, and further EBOV infections were seen for another 18 months, with the end determined by the passing of two incubation periods, 42 days, from the last reported EBOV-infected person. It was known that transmission could occur in the absence of a viraemia as viral RNA could be detected in semen, breast milk, eye fluid and cerebro spinal fluid (CSF).

### Complications after the acute Ebola virus infection and viral persistence in sanctuary sites

Reactivation from sanctuary sites could also result in a viraemia leading to transmission. Little had been known about potential clinical sequelae whilst recovering from EVD, but a clinic in Sierra Leone reported that 76% of survivors had arthralgia, 18% had uveitis and 24% had hearing loss.

Since then, recognized complications reported include arthralgia, eye pain and redness, dryness, photophobia and blurred vision, hearing loss and tinnitus, abdominal pain, headache, impaired memory, peripheral neuropathy and tremors as well as mental and sexual health issues. In addition, new-onset fever and relapse can occur.

EBOV may persist in sanctuary or immune privileged sites. These include the inner eye, brain and spinal cord, testes and mammary glands. The virus can be detected in these sites as well as in semen and breast milk for >9 months.

This means specialist support and care is needed; it is advised that safe sexual practices are practiced for 1 year after acute infection or until the semen has twice tested as negative.

### Rapid development of diagnostic tests, antiviral agents and vaccines

A major global effort by the international community led to ~40 field laboratories being built in West Africa, with biocontainment facilities and the equipment to carry out extraction of nucleic acid from various sample types and real-time reverse transcriptase PCR (RT-PCR) assays to detect EBOV RNA.

In those 27 people who were medically evacuated for care in their countries of origin in Europe and in the United States, including those diagnosed with EVD in those countries having been infected with EBOV in West Africa, careful monitoring, intravenous rehydration, correcting electrolyte imbalances and critical care management were all critical in the ~82% survival figure.

Experimental treatments were also used, including immunotherapies such as convalescent plasma, monoclonal antibodies (ZMapp, ZMab or MIL77) and antiviral agents such as brincidofovir and favipravir. It was impossible to determine whether they had an effect as there were small numbers of patients and no controls (Box 29.2).

Since then, Inmazeb (REGN-EB3)—a combination of three humanized monoclonal (antibodies atoltivimab, maftivimab, and odesivimab)—and Ebanga (mAb114 or ansuvimab) that targets the EBOV glycoprotein have been developed and were approved for treating Zaire EBOV infection in adults and children in 2020. The glycoprotein is the only viral protein expressed on the virus surface and is key for host cell attachment, endosomal entry and membrane fusion.

In August 2022 WHO published the first EBOV treatment guidelines based on REGN-EB3 and mAb114 separately, reducing mortality compared with ZMapp, remdesivir, or standard care in individuals with EBOV.

### Infection control strategies to manage travellers from EBOV-affected countries

From an infection control perspective, screening algorithms were prepared across the world for managing people travelling from the countries in West Africa where there were EBOV outbreaks. The key questions involved whether the traveller had had a fever in the previous 24 h and had developed symptoms within 21 days of leaving an EBOV-affected country. Screening at airports and other ports of entry into countries involved measuring the person's temperature and asking about symptoms, preparing isolation rooms in emergency departments in hospitals for travellers or contacts with symptoms and making arrangements in laboratories to both test samples and send samples for EBOV RNA as well as malaria, the latter being the most common diagnosis. In addition, ambulance and hospital staff were trained on what protective equipment to wear when in contact with people with potential EBOV infection and to know which infectious disease containment facilities they were to be admitted to for management if found to have EVD.

### Immunogenicity and safety data from various clinical trials demonstrated vaccine efficacy for Zaire Ebola vaccine regimens

A number of vaccines were rapidly developed, starting with virus inactivation and moving on rapidly to DNA

## Box 29.2 ■ Lessons in Microbiology

Although there have been a number of Ebola virus disease (EVD) outbreaks in Africa, complications in survivors had not been recognized. A number of health care workers were repatriated to their countries having volunteered to assist in managing patients with EVD in the epidemic in West Africa and subsequently developed symptoms associated with Ebola virus (EBOV) infection. One nurse became symptomatic having returned to Great Britain. She was transferred to a specialist infectious disease high containment unit and received intravenous fluid and electrolyte replacement, an antiviral agent called *brincidofovir* and convalescent plasma that had been collected from another survivor. However, she developed respiratory failure and needed mechanical ventilation, high-volume diarrhoea, erythroderma and mucositis. The initial high plasma EBOV RNA load, with a reverse transcriptase PCR (RT-PCR) crossing threshold (CT) value of 25, had become raised at a value of 13 by day 6 of admission. This fell after two doses of ZMAb, an experimental monoclonal antibody raised against an EBOV glycoprotein, had been given; plasma EBOV RNA was not detectable by day 25.

She was then discharged from the hospital, but 3 weeks later developed thyrotoxicosis, an overactive thyroid gland, due to thyroiditis. Plasma EBOV RNA was not detected in blood, a test carried out after she had developed joint pains and some ankle joint effusions. However, 9 months after discharge, she had a fever, severe headache and meningism. A diagnosis of EBOV relapse was made when a lumbar puncture was carried out and EBOV RNA was detected at a CT of 24 in the cerebrospinal fluid (CSF) and 31 in the plasma. No other pathogens were detected in the CSF sample. She subsequently developed meningoencephalitis, had two tonic–clonic seizures and was given another monoclonal antibody drug, MIL 77, that had to be discontinued. An experimental nucleoside analogue, GS-5734, that had successfully treated EBOV-infected nonhuman primates was then given, together with a steroid, dexamethasone, and she improved slowly and was again discharged after ~2 months.

The central nervous system was the most likely site of EBOV relapse, probably after viral dissemination during the acute infection and persistence in this immunologically privileged sanctuary site. EBOV sequence analysis showed that the virus had not changed since the initial infection.

Careful monitoring of EVD survivors is critical, together with continuing research and development of effective antiviral therapies.

## Box 29.3 ■ Lessons in Microbiology

Molecular epidemiology, phylogenetic analyses, high-throughput sequencing and bioinformatics have revolutionized the approach to investigating outbreaks of infections, determining the origin, evolution and spread.

High-throughput sequencing of Ebola virus (EBOV) genomes in the 2013–2016 Ebola virus epidemic in West Africa allowed rapid real-time molecular epidemiologic investigation of transmission chains that resulted in improved outbreak responses.

Analysis of the genome sequences answered the key question as to whether one cross-species transmission event involving humans occurred or a number of zoonotic events from a widespread animal EBOV reservoir occurred, leading to the epidemic. It was likely the former as the EBOV genomes sequenced at the start of the epidemic were genetically similar. Molecular clock analyses showed that all recorded human Ebola virus disease (EVD) outbreaks shared a common ancestor around 1975, close to the first described outbreak in southern Sudan and in the region of the Ebola River in 1976.

Genomic data were used to assist with infection control and public health policies during the epidemic. Phylogeographic approaches were used to determine how EBOV spread through the communities, allowing direct intervention to be employed in transmission hotspots. Phylogenetic analyses shed light on individual transmission events, showing that sexual transmission had occurred and that multiple reoccurrences happened during the epidemic and how they were related to transmission events involving survivors, together with the human superspreaders.

**Ecologic niche modelling has been used to predict where to find these filovirus infections**

Interestingly, Ebola mapped to the broadleaf tropical rainforest and humid areas in equatorial Central Africa and parts of West Africa (although Angola did not fit this model). Marburg, however, mapped to the opposite, drier, more open areas away from the equator. In these models, bats were thought to be the potential reservoir hosts. Subsequently, tropical rainforest fruit bats were identified as the Ebola virus reservoir. Developments in high-throughput next-generation sequencing and large-scale sequence data sets and bioinformatics analyses allowed molecular epidemiologic investigations of EBOV transmission chains that could assist outbreak management (Box 29.3).

**In 2023 Marburg virus outbreaks were reported in Tanzania and Equatorial Guinea**

Having been notified on February 13, the outbreak in Equatorial Guinea was declared over on June 8, 2023, with 17 confirmed (12 deaths) and 23 probable infections reported.

There is no treatment, postexposure prophylaxis or vaccine prevention option for Marburg virus infections.

**Rabies is a zoonotic viral disease affecting the CNS**

Rabies virus infection (see Ch. 25) can affect wild and domestic animals, including dogs, bats, cats, foxes, raccoons

vaccines, recombinant viral vector vaccines and recombinant and subunit proteins. All involved expressing the EBOV glycoprotein, which is involved in attachment and virus–cell membrane fusion and is a target for neutralizing antibodies. Two vaccines that underwent clinical investigation were a replication-competent vesicular stomatitis virus-based vaccine, expressing the glycoprotein of the Zaire strain of EBOV (ZEBOV), and a monovalent, replication-deficient chimpanzee adenovirus type 3 vector-based ZEBOV vaccine.

The ERVEBO(R) (ZEBOV) vaccine protected people from the species Zaire EBOV and was given to ~350,000 people in Guinea and in the 2018–2020 outbreak in the DRC; it was approved in 2020.

and skunks. Transmission from animals to humans is via saliva, usually through bites, scratches or direct contact with mucosal surfaces, including eyes, mouth or open wounds. After developing discomfort at the site of the bite and a sore throat, headache and fever, the patient becomes excited, with muscle spasms and convulsions. Once rabies has developed, it is fatal, death occurring following cardiac or respiratory arrest. Paralysis is often a major feature of the disease.

Rabies is present on all continents except Antarctica, and prophylaxis can be given preexposure by immunizing individuals at risk or postexposure with rabies-specific immunoglobulin and immunization, depending on the rabies risk assessment in the country where the exposure incident occurred.

## Q FEVER

### *Coxiella burnetii* is the rickettsial cause of Q fever

The disease Q fever was first recognized in Australia in 1935, but the cause was unknown for several years—hence Q (query) fever. The causative rickettsia, *C. burnetii*, differs from other rickettsiae (see Ch. 28) in the following ways:

- It is not transmitted to humans by arthropods.
- It is relatively resistant to desiccation, heat and sunlight and is therefore stable enough to be acquired from infected material by inhalation.
- Its main site of action is the lung rather than vascular endothelium elsewhere in the body, so there is usually no rash.

### *C. burnetii* is transmitted to humans by inhalation

*C. burnetii* can infect many species of wild and domestic animals. In many countries (e.g. United States) infection of livestock is quite common, but there are few human cases (178 acute and 34 chronic cases reported in 2019 in the United States). The largest known Q fever outbreak occurred in the Netherlands between 2007 and 2009. Infected dairy goat farms were the source of infection. More than 3500 human infections were notified over that time period. The southern part of the Netherlands was most affected, with >12% of the population found to have *C. burnetii* antibodies. People who come into contact with infected animals, especially their placentas (e.g. veterinarians, farmers, abattoir workers) are at risk from aerosolized organisms. Unpasteurized milk, tissue fluids and dust from infected stock can also transmit the disease.

After inhalation, the microbe multiplies in the terminal airways of the lung, and ~3 weeks later the patient develops fever, severe headache, often respiratory symptoms and an atypical pneumonia. The rickettsia can also spread to the liver, commonly causing hepatitis. Recovery is usually complete in 2 weeks, but the disease can become chronic. The heart is then sometimes involved (endocarditis), with thrombocytopenia and purpura in some patients, and this condition is fatal if untreated.

### Q fever is diagnosed serologically and treated with antibiotics

PCR can be used to determine whether a patient has Q fever; however, the sensitivity of this approach decreases after the first week of illness. *C. burnetti* cannot be detected in blood cultures and cannot be isolated by culture except in specialized laboratories. Thus serologic diagnosis is important. There are two antigenic forms of the rickettsial lipopolysaccharide: phase 1 and phase 2. Increased antibody to phase 2 compared with phase 1 is seen in acute Q fever, while the reverse (higher antibody titres in phase 1 than in phase 2) is seen in chronic disease. Definitive serologic confirmation of acute Q fever is demonstrated by increased (≥1:1024) phase 1 IgG antibody. The Weil-Felix test (see Ch. 28) is not used.

Acute infection is treated with oral tetracyclines; chronic infections may require drug combinations such as rifampin and doxycycline or trimethoprim-sulphamethoxazole. A killed vaccine is available (although not in the United States) for those at risk. The rickettsiae are destroyed when milk is pasteurized.

## ANTHRAX

### Anthrax is caused by *Bacillus anthracis* and is primarily a disease of herbivores

Most members of the genus *Bacillus* are harmless saprophytes, present in soil, water, air and vegetation. *Bacillus cereus* is a cause of food poisoning, but *B. anthracis* is the principal pathogen. It is a large, aerobic and nonmotile gram-positive rod and is unique in having an antiphagocytic capsule made of D-glutamic acid. It forms spores that survive for years in soil.

Anthrax is a disease of herbivores such as sheep, goats, cattle and horses, and bacilli are excreted in faeces, urine and saliva. Humans are relatively resistant, infection occurring following direct contact with infected animals or by contact with spores present in animal products. The spores can enter the body via the skin and mucous membranes or less commonly via the respiratory tract. In resource-rich countries where animal infection is now uncommon, human infection is rare and, when present, has been due to exposure to contaminated imported goods such as hides, skin, wool, goat hair and bristles, bones and bonemeal in fertilizers. Spores have also been used in bioterrorism.

### Anthrax is characterized by a black eschar, and the disease can be fatal if untreated

*B. anthracis* spores germinate in tissues at the site of entry. The bacteria then multiply and produce the anthrax toxin, which consists of a protective antigen, an oedema factor (an adenylate cyclase) and a lethal factor; all of them are plasmid coded. Toxic activity requires the protective antigen and at least one of the other two. Host defences are inhibited by the antiphagocytic capsule surrounding the bacillus (see Ch. 15).

The skin is the usual site of entry. As the toxic material accumulates, there is oedema and congestion, and a papule develops within 12–36 h. The papule ulcerates, the centre becoming black and necrotic to form an eschar or malignant pustule (although there is no pus), which is painless and is often surrounded by a ring of vesicles (Fig. 29.4). The bacilli spread to the lymphatics and, in ~10% of cases, reach the blood to cause septicaemia. Continued multiplication and production of the toxin causes generalized toxic effects, oedema and death.

When the spores are inhaled and enter alveolar macrophages, bacterial growth in the lung leads to pulmonary oedema and mediastinal haemorrhage, with spread to the blood and subsequent death. Pulmonary anthrax is now very rare in most resource-rich countries, where it was referred to as *woolsorter's disease*.

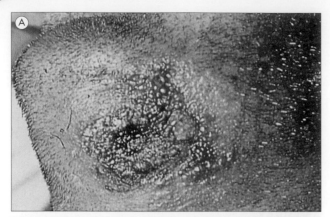

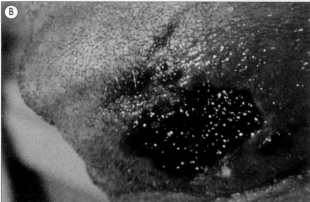

**Fig. 29.4** Anthrax. (A) Characteristic black eschar surrounded by a ring of vesiculation. (B) Some 8 days later the eschar has enlarged to cover the previously vesicular area, and the surrounding oedema has diminished. (Courtesy F.J. Nye.)

### Cutaneous anthrax is diagnosed by culture and treated with ciprofloxacin

Films from skin lesions show gram-positive bacilli, but diagnosis can be confirmed and the organism distinguished from nonpathogenic bacilli by culture on blood agar or by PCR assay. Antibodies to toxin antigens indicate presence of the bacillus.

Cutaneous anthrax is successfully treated by ciprofloxacin. Cutaneous anthrax is fatal in 20% of cases when untreated. Systemic anthrax is treated with combination antimicrobial therapy plus antitoxin.

### Anthrax, as a natural infection, is now mainly confined to resource-poor countries. Vaccines are available. Bioterrorism is an important threat

The disease is largely confined to resource-poor countries (parts of Asia, Africa and Middle East).

Animals can be protected by vaccination with live avirulent bacteria. Infected animals are isolated, killed and buried or cremated without autopsy. A vaccine consisting of purified protective antigen is available for humans at high risk. Human infection is reduced by rigidly controlled disinfection of imported animal products such as hides, hair and wool.

Anthrax is one of six etiologic agents categorized by the US Centers for Disease Control and Prevention as a high-priority (Category A) bioterrorism threat. Although decades ago (i.e. 2001), 22 people in the United States infected by spores sent by mail are still remembered for generating

renewed interest in anthrax as an agent of bioterrorism and antimicrobial postexposure control (e.g. a fluoroquinolone or doxycycline).

## PLAGUE

### The plague is caused by *Yersinia pestis*, which infects rodents and is spread from them by fleas to humans

*Y. pestis* is a small gram-negative rod with a surrounding antiphagocytic capsule that is associated with virulence. The sylvatic reservoirs are rodents such as rats, squirrels, gerbils and field mice in which the infection is generally mild, the bacteria being spread between animals and to humans by fleas (Fig. 29.5). Infections in urban rats have been the most important sources of plague in humans, and the disease has at times decimated populations and influenced the course of history. In the 14th century, ~25% of the population of Europe died in plague epidemics (Box 29.4). Early in the 20th century the disease arrived in North America and is at present endemic in wild rodents in the western United States. Plague in humans is now extremely rare in Europe and uncommon in the United States.

The rat flea (*Xenopsylla cheopis*) carries infection from rat to rat and from rat to human. *Y. pestis* causes blood to clot in the gut of the flea, multiplies profusely in the clot and eventually blocks the gut lumen so that the flea regurgitates infected material as it attempts to feed. As infected rats sicken, their fleas leave and may bite humans, thus transmitting bubonic plague. This disease is not generally transmitted from person to person. However, when there is extensive replication of bacteria in the lung with bronchopneumonia and large numbers of bacteria in the sputum, the infection can spread from person to person by droplets, causing pneumonic plague with extremely rapid onset.

Rodent infection is endemic in India, Southeast Asia, central and southern Africa, South America, Mexico and the western United States. Sporadic plague continues with between 1000 and 2000 cases occurring each year worldwide.

### Clinical features of plague include buboes, pneumonia and a high death rate

The infecting bacteria multiply at the site of entry in the skin and spread via the lymphatics to local and regional lymph nodes. They produce a number of virulence factors, including an antiphagocytic capsular antigen (fraction 1, coded by a plasmid), endotoxin and various other protein toxins. Lymph nodes in the axilla or groin become very tender and enlarge to form buboes with haemorrhagic inflammation 2–6 days after the flea bite. The patient develops fever. In mild forms, the infection is arrested at this stage, but spread to the blood often occurs, with septicaemia, haemorrhagic illness and multisystem involvement (spleen, liver, lungs, CNS).

Common complications are disseminated intravascular coagulation, pneumonia and meningitis. The death rate is ~50% in untreated bubonic plague and ~100% in pneumonic plague. On recovery there is solid immunity, and bacteria are eliminated from the body.

### Plague is diagnosed microscopically and treated with antibiotics

Organisms can be recovered in fluid aspirated from lymph nodes or from sputum in pneumonic plague and stained

**Fig. 29.5** The epidemiology of plague.

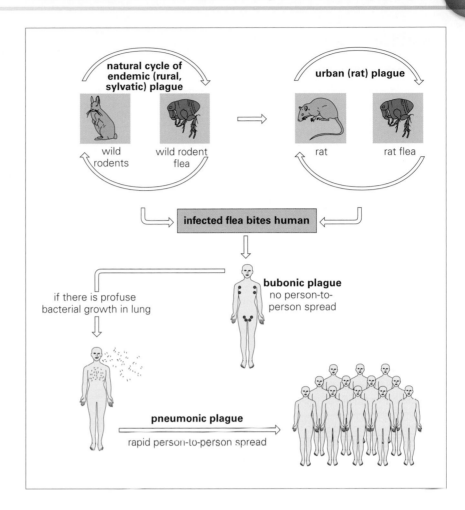

with Giemsa, Gram or fluorescent antibody (the staining is bipolar); they can also be cultivated. Gentamicin, doxycycline or ciprofloxacin, and streptomycin (less available in the United States) are commonly used in treatment.

Plague has been prevented by the following measures:

- classically, by quarantine measures in ports and on ships
- by rodent control, especially of rats at the site of entry of ships and aircraft into plague-free countries
- by strict isolation of patients with plague
- by chemoprophylaxis during an epidemic or visit to an affected area
- by vaccination of military personnel and of certain workers in endemic areas.

An older vaccine formulation consisting of formalin-killed bacteria has been replaced by a more effective (recombinant) formulation.

### *YERSINIA ENTEROCOLITICA* INFECTION

*Y. enterocolitica* is a cause of diarrhoeal disease (see Ch. 23) and is mentioned here because it has a reservoir in rodents, rabbits, pigs and other livestock.

### TULARAEMIA

**Tularaemia is caused by *Francisella tularensis* and is spread by arthropods from infected animals**

Tularaemia is caused by the small gram-negative rod, *F. tularensis*, first isolated from rodents in Tulare County,

California, in 1912 and later shown by Edward Francis to cause human disease. It is present in rodents and in a wide variety of other wild animals in many countries in the Northern Hemisphere, including the United States (especially Arkansas and Missouri), Russia, Scandinavia and Spain and can occur in contaminated water. The variety found in North America causes a more severe disease than that found in Europe and Asia. In the infected animal it causes a plaguelike disease and is spread via ticks, mites, lice and biting flies. In *Dermacentor* ticks, the bacteria are transmitted vertically by infected female ticks to her offspring via the ovum. Human infection is sporadic, the normal means of infection being contact with the carcass of an infected animal (e.g. skinning of hares, rabbits, muskrats) or the bite of an arthropod vector. There is no spread from person to person.

**Clinical features of tularaemia include painful swollen lymph nodes**

*F. tularensis* parasitizes the reticuloendothelial system and lives intracellularly in macrophages, inhibiting phagosome–lysosome fusion. It spreads at the site of entry, aided by an antiphagocytic capsule, and after 3–5 days forms a skin ulcer. There is a febrile illness, and lymphatic spread results in swollen painful regional lymph nodes. Blood invasion and involvement of lungs, gastrointestinal tract and liver is not uncommon, with the formation of granulomatous nodules around infected reticuloendothelial cells. There may be a rash. Mortality in untreated patients is 5–15%. The

## Box 29.4 ■ Lessons in Microbiology

### The Black Death in 14th-century England

For thousands of years, *Yersinia pestis* has been endemic in rodents in the Far East, with occasional epidemic spread into Europe and elsewhere. In January 1348, three galleys laden with spices from the East brought the plague to the port of Genoa, Italy. The disease, for reasons that are not clear, became known as the *Black Death* and soon spread to the rest of Europe, arriving in London in December 1348. To the medieval mind, the speed and violence with which the illness passed from person to person (in the pneumonic form in the winter) was its most terrifying feature. The bubonic form was also important especially in the warmer summer months, with there being at least one family of black rats per household and three fleas to a rat.

The disease was attributed to earthquakes, to the movement of the planets, to a Jewish or Arab plot (350 massacres of Jews took place during the Black Death in Europe) and most commonly to God's punishment for human wickedness. One could become infected without touching a plague victim, and to many it seemed that there was something—a miasma or a poison—in the air. Physicians wore strange masks, and infected houses were labelled and boarded up, together with the inhabitants. But it was impossible to isolate all those who were sick. Rich and poor perished.

The population of England was ~4 million, and over a period of 2.5 years, ~35% (>1 million) died. The clergy, for unknown reasons, suffered an even greater mortality of ~50%. Altogether in Europe, at least 25 million people died. The Black Death was a major human disaster, with lasting effects on economic and social structure. There were five less severe outbreaks in England in the 14th century. The epidemic in 1665, the year before the Great Fire of London, was graphically described by Daniel Defoe (who was only 5 years old at the time) in his *Journal of a Plague Year in London*. The last pandemic arose in China and reached Hong Kong in 1894, where Yersin and (independently) Kitasato described the causative bacillus.

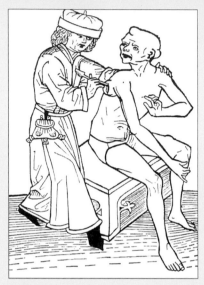

**Fig. 29.6** Fifteenth-century German woodcut showing incision of a bubo. (Courtesy the World Health Organization.)

conjunctiva or oral mucosa can be infected via contaminated fingers, resulting in ocular or oral manifestations. Infection by inhalation is less common and gives a febrile illness with respiratory symptoms.

**Tularaemia is diagnosed clinically and serologically; streptomycin is the drug of choice, although other antimicrobials have been used (doxycycline and gentamicin)**

Infected tissues can be examined by fluorescent antibody staining, but isolation of bacteria is not often attempted because of the high risk of laboratory infection. Antibody tests are more commonly used in diagnosis.

Streptomycin gentamicin, doxycycline and ciprofloxacin are commonly used in treatment. A live attenuated bacterial vaccine has been available for people with an occupational risk (e.g. fur trappers) but has issues of toxicity and incomplete protection. However, the vaccine is not available in the United States, and efforts are now underway to develop a more effective preparation. Handling animals with gloves, particularly when skinning or eviscerating, gives protection, and contact with ticks should be avoided.

### *PASTEURELLA MULTOCIDA* INFECTION

**P. multocida is part of the normal flora of cats and dogs and is transmitted to humans by an animal bite or scratch**

*P. multocida* is an encapsulated gram-negative rod and is distributed worldwide. A number of capsular types exist. It is part of the normal oral flora in cats, dogs and other domestic and wild animals in which it can also cause pneumonia and septicaemia. It is transmitted to humans by animal bites (especially cat bites) or scratches.

**P. multocida infection causes cellulitis, is diagnosed by microscopy and is treated with amoxicillin/clavulanate**

Local multiplication of bacteria leads within 1–2 days to cellulitis and lymphadenitis; other types of bacteria, including anaerobes, are often present in the lesion. Infection can become systemic in patients with compromised immune systems. Virulence factors include endotoxin and the capsule.

*P. multocida* can be cultivated and identified in material from the wound.

Amoxicillin/clavulanate is an effective treatment and has been used in prophylaxis after cat or dog bites. Bite wounds should be cleansed and debrided.

### LEPTOSPIROSIS

**Leptospirosis is caused by the spirochete *Leptospira interrogans*, which infects mammals such as rats**

Leptospires are tightly coiled spirochetes 5–15 μm long. They show active rotational movement and have two flagella originating at each end but located within the cell as in *Borrelia*. Their delicate outline is best seen by dark field microscopy because they are not well stained by dyes. There are many species, each with several serotypes.

**Table 29.2** Disease caused by the three main serogroups of the *Leptospira interrogans* complex

| Leptospiral serogroups | Animal host | Geographic distribution | Clinical features |
|---|---|---|---|
| Canicola | Dog | Worldwide | Influenza-like illness (canicola fever, 7-day fever) is the commonest; can progress to aseptic meningitis, liver and kidney damage (Weil disease) |
| Icterohaemorrhagiae | Rat | Worldwide | |
| Hebdomadis | Mice, voles, rats, cattle | Japan, Europe | |

There are 19 different serogroups of this organism. Other serogroups include Seroja (pigs) and Pomona (swine and cattle in United States and Europe). Among the serogroups there are 172 different serotypes.

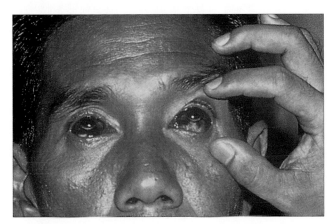

**Fig. 29.7** Conjunctival haemorrhages in a jaundiced patient with leptospirosis. (Courtesy D. Lewis.)

The *biflexa* complex is free living; the *interrogans* complex is pathogenic. The ends of *L. interrogans* are bent into a question-mark shape, hence the specific name. This species infects many domestic and wild mammals in various parts of the world (Table 29.2), dogs and rats being important sources of infection. Infected animals develop a chronic kidney infection with excretion of large numbers of bacteria in urine. The spirochetes are soon killed on drying, heating and exposure to detergents or disinfectants, but they remain viable for several weeks in stagnant alkaline water or wet soil. Humans are infected by ingestion of, or exposure to, contaminated water or food. The bacteria, aided by their motility, enter through breaks in skin or mucosae, so infection can be acquired by swimming, working or playing in contaminated water. Therefore miners, farmers, sewage workers, and water sports enthusiasts are especially at risk. There are ~50 cases per year in England and Wales and ~100 cases per year in the United States. Bacteria are excreted in human urine, but person-to-person transmission is rare. Immunity is serotype specific.

### Clinical features of leptospirosis include kidney and liver failure

The bacteria reach the blood and, after an incubation period of 1–2 weeks, cause a febrile, influenza-like illness. In ~90% of cases this resolves uneventfully, but multiplication can cause:

- hepatitis, jaundice and haemorrhage in the liver
- uraemia and bacteriuria in the kidney
- aseptic meningitis and conjunctival or scleral haemorrhage in the CSF and the aqueous humor (Fig. 29.7).

The main clinical signs result from damage to the endothelia of blood vessels, the clinical picture depending to some extent upon the particular type of leptospire involved. Weil disease, the severe form with haemorrhagic complications and kidney and liver failure, occurs in only 5–10% of patients with leptospirosis.

### Leptospirosis is diagnosed mainly by serologic tests and treated with antibiotics

There is often a history of exposure. Bacteria can be isolated from blood, CSF and urine, and a rise in agglutinating serotype-specific antibody can be demonstrated.

Penicillin and doxycycline have been valuable in treatment when given within 1–2 days of onset of illness, and doxycycline will prevent disease in those exposed to infection.

Measures for prevention include rodent control, protective clothing and prophylactic doxycycline after cuts and abrasions in those at risk.

## RAT-BITE FEVER

### Rat-bite fever is caused by bacteria transmitted to humans by a rodent bite

This uncommon but worldwide condition is caused by one of two species: *Spirillum minus*, a gram-negative spiral-shaped organism (spirillar fever), or *Streptobacillus moniliformis*, a gram-negative filamentous bacillus (streptobacillary fever). These bacteria are found in the oropharyngeal flora of 50% of healthy wild and laboratory rats and in other rodents. Transmission to humans is by biting.

### Clinical features of rat-bite fever can include endocarditis and pneumonia

After an incubation period of 7–10 days there is an onset of fever, headache and myalgia. Bacteria multiply at the site of the bite, and, in the case of *S. moniliformis*, cause an inflamed local lesion. Spread of infection to lymph nodes and the blood leads to lymphadenopathy, rash and arthralgia. Fever may be recurrent if untreated.

Complications include endocarditis and pneumonia, and there is a mortality of up to 10% in untreated patients.

### Rat-bite fever is diagnosed by microscopy or culture and is treated with antibiotics

*S. moniliformis* can be cultured from the wound site, lymph nodes and blood, but *S. minus* cannot be cultivated and must be demonstrated in tissues by dark field microscopy.

Penicillin and tetracyclines are effective treatments.

Measures for prevention include rodent control and prevention of rat bites in laboratory workers.

## BRUCELLOSIS

### Brucellosis occurs worldwide and is caused by *Brucella* species

Brucellae are small gram-negative nonmotile coccobacilli adapted to intracellular replication. Four species cause disease in humans: *Brucella abortus*, *Brucella melitensis*, *Brucella suis*, *Brucella canis*, but based on DNA homology, these are all variants of *B. melitensis*. The first three share common A and M antigens (*B. abortus* primarily A and *B. melitensis* primarily M); *B. canis* is distinct.

Brucellae are primarily animal pathogens, infecting humans after contact with infected animals or their products (Fig. 29.8):

- *B. abortus* infects cows worldwide but has been eliminated from several resource-rich countries. It causes mild disease in humans.
- *B. melitensis* infects goats and sheep and is common in Malta and other Mediterranean countries, Mexico and South America. It causes more severe disease in humans.
- *B. suis* infects pigs in the United States, South America and Southeast Asia. It causes severe disease with destructive lesions in humans.
- *B. canis* infects dogs and is an uncommon cause of mild disease in humans.
- In cows and goats, brucellae localize in the placenta, causing contagious abortion, and in mammary glands from where they are shed for long periods in milk. They are present in uterine discharges, faeces and urine.

Human brucellosis (undulant fever, Malta fever) occurs when the bacteria enter the body via abrasions in the skin, via the alimentary tract or most commonly via the respiratory tract. Infection is therefore more common in farmers, veterinarians and abattoir workers. Unpasteurized cows' milk (United Kingdom, United States), goats' milk or cheese (Mediterranean countries) are less frequent sources of infection. There is no spread from person to person. Infection is common worldwide, but incidence is low in the resource-rich world.

### Clinical features of brucellosis are immune mediated and include an undulant fever and chronicity

The infecting bacteria pass from the site of entry into local and regional lymph nodes, the thoracic duct and thus the blood (septicaemic phase). Reticuloendothelial cells are infected (liver, spleen, bone marrow, lymphoid tissues), and here the bacteria can survive for prolonged periods. The result is an inflammatory (granulomatous) reaction with epithelioid and giant cells, central necrosis and peripheral fibrosis.

Quite commonly, the infection is subclinical. The symptoms of acute brucellosis begin after an incubation period of 2–6 weeks with a gradual onset of malaise, fever, drenching sweats, aching and weakness. A rising and falling (undulant) fever is seen in a minority of patients. Enlarged lymph nodes and spleen may be detected, and hepatitis can occur (Fig. 29.9). The bone marrow lesions may progress to osteomyelitis, and cholecystitis, endocarditis and meningitis are occasionally seen. Abortion occurs in infected cows, sows and goats but not in humans who lack the sugar compound, erythritol, which stimulates bacterial growth in the placenta.

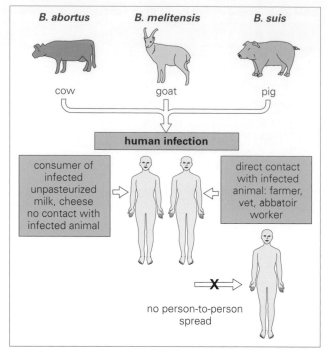

**Fig. 29.8** Transmission of brucellosis. Human infection follows contact with infected animals or consumption of infected animal products.

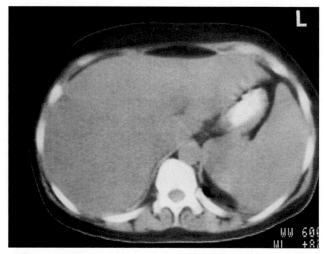

**Fig. 29.9** Computed tomography scan showing hepatosplenomegaly in *Brucella melitensis* infection. (Courtesy H. Tubbs.)

The patient generally recovers after a few weeks or months, but a chronic stage (>1 year) can develop with tiredness, aches and pains, anxiety, depression and occasional fever. Relapses and remissions may occur. Brucellae cannot be isolated at this stage, and chronic brucellosis is often a difficult diagnosis. Agglutinin titres are generally high, but antibodies are less relevant than cell-mediated immunity for this intracellular parasite.

### Brucellosis is diagnosed by culture and by serologic tests and treated with antibiotics

Brucellae can be isolated in some cases from blood cultures (or from bone marrow or lymph nodes), and urine culture may be successful. This takes up to 4 weeks. IgM antibodies are present in acute brucellosis, and IgG and IgA are present in chronic brucellosis. A rising titre suggests a current infection.

Brucellosis is typically susceptible to tetracycline and streptomycin; co-trimoxazole is also used. Because of the intracellular location of the bacteria, brucellosis is typically treated with combination therapy (e.g. doxycycline plus rifampicin or an aminoglycoside) for a minimum of 6 weeks.

Brucellae in milk are destroyed by pasteurization. In the United States and United Kingdom, brucellosis has gradually declined (~100 cases per year now reported in the United States) following eradication and control programmes. Protective clothing and goggles may be used by those in close contact with infected animals (farmers, veterinarians, abattoir workers). There is no satisfactory vaccine available for humans. Indeed, veterinarians may develop illness when accidentally infected with the live RB51 animal vaccine.

## HELMINTH INFECTIONS

### Few helminth infections are true multisystem diseases

It is a somewhat arbitrary decision to include a particular helminth (worm) infection in a chapter on multisystem zoonotic infections. Many of the helminth parasites that can be acquired from animals have stages that are capable of invading a number of the body systems. Others are primarily located in a particular organ but cause pathologic changes that can be widespread in their effects. Conversely, although stages of certain helminths may be widely distributed in the body, their pathologic effects are commonly associated with a particular organ. For example:

- The larvae of the pork tapeworm *Taenia solium*, which cause the disease cysticercosis, develop in a variety of tissues, especially muscle. However, the most serious pathology is caused by larvae found in the CNS or the eye. Accordingly, this infection is discussed in Chapter 25.
- After infection with eggs of the dog nematode *Toxocara canis*, larvae migrate through the body, causing visceral larval migrans or ocular larva migrans. Again, the most serious effects are associated with larvae in the CNS (see Ch. 25) and the eye (see Ch. 26).

However, three helminths can be considered as genuinely multisystem in their effects. These are the tapeworm *Echinococcus granulosus*, the nematode *Trichinella spiralis* and the nematode *Strongyloides stercoralis*.

### Echinococcus

*Echinococcus* adults are tiny tapeworms in the small intestine of dogs or foxes, and their larvae cause echinococcosis (hydatid disease) in humans. They cause two major types of echinococcosis, both of which result in significant human morbidity.

#### E. granulosus (cystic echinococcosis; cystic hydatid disease)

The adults of this species live as tiny (3- to 5-mm long) tapeworms in the intestine of the dog. Eggs laid by the worm are passed in faeces, surviving for long periods outside the host. If swallowed (by sheep or accidentally by humans), the eggs hatch, releasing larvae that then penetrate the small intestinal mucosa to enter a blood vessel. Larvae then spread to and lodge in the tissues, most commonly of the liver, with

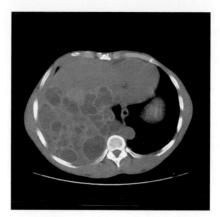

**Fig. 29.10** Computed tomography scan showing extensive cystic echinococcosis of the liver. (Courtesy P.L. Chiodini.)

the lung next most common, but any organ can potentially be affected. They then grow slowly into large, thick-walled, fluid-filled echinococcal cysts. The resulting symptoms and signs are largely due to the mechanical pressure exerted by the cysts (Fig. 29.10), but patients may also present with fever due to cyst leakage or to secondary bacterial infection of the cyst itself. Rupture of a liver cyst can result in disseminated disease with numerous cysts present throughout the peritoneum.

Cystic echinococcosis is diagnosed by ultrasonography, computed tomography or magnetic resonance imaging scans. Serologic tests assist diagnosis, but the sensitivity and specificity of serology are variable and are influenced by the site and stage of the cyst. Initial testing for antibody by ELISA is followed by confirmation with a species-specific Western blot. Finding hooks and protoscoleces in aspirated cyst fluid provides confirmation, but suspected echinococcal cysts in the lung must never be aspirated. Treatment is according to the WHO CE (Cystic Echinococcosis) ultrasound classification (see Bibliography). Depending on cyst type, therapy is with albendazole plus praziquantel in some cases, and with or without PAIR (puncture, aspiration, injection and reaspiration) or open surgery. Dead echinococcal cysts do not require treatment. Special care must be taken during aspiration or surgical removal to prevent leakage of fluid from the cysts. Not only may this trigger anaphylactic responses in sensitized individuals, but also the numerous protoscoleces present in the fluid (produced by asexual division) can cause local recurrence or metastatic infection in other sites.

#### *Echinococcus multilocularis* (alveolar echinococcosis; alveolar hydatid disease)

*E. multilocularis* results in the formation of a multilocular mass lesion consisting of hundreds of small vesicles. The parasite generally occurs as a fox–rodent cycle in China, Northern Europe, Siberia and parts of North America, and human infections occur via ingestion of eggs spread by contamination of the environment with fox faeces. Its pathogenesis and clinical features are significantly different from those of cystic echinococcosis, and the macroscopic appearance of alveolar echinococcosis (AE) is similar to that of a hepatic carcinoma. Almost all cases occur in the liver, where the parasite leads to obstructive jaundice, abdominal pain and weight loss. Metastasis to the lung and brain may occur. At clinical presentation, no more than 40% of AE liver lesions are resectable. Before effective antiparasitic therapy was available, the 10-year survival rate for such patients was <10%, but it is now 80%. Treatment of hepatic disease is with radical excision plus albendazole. Inoperable cases of AE require lifelong albendazole therapy. Liver transplantation is sometimes needed.

## Trichinella

### *Trichinella spiralis* is transmitted in undercooked pork and causes the disease trichinosis

The genus *Trichinella* consists of eight different species, and the genus is capable of infecting almost any warm-blooded animal. Its natural cycle involves predators (e.g. bears, seals) and their prey, or scavengers, and the carrion on which they feed, but a domestic cycle has become established in pigs and rats.

Humans are infected by eating raw or undercooked meat (pork, horse or wild game animal [e.g. wild boar]) containing the encysted infective larval stages. These larvae mature rapidly into adults in the small intestine, their invasion of the mucosa causing acute enteritis.

### The clinical features of trichinosis are mainly immunopathologic in origin

Female worms release live larvae, which invade the blood vessels and become distributed around the body, into the mucosa. The larvae attempt to invade the cells of many organs (including the heart and CNS), although they can mature and encyst only in striated muscles (Fig. 29.11). Severity depends on the number of larvae originally ingested by the patient, and there is a wide spectrum of pathologic features such as fever, joint and muscle pains, eosinophilia, periorbital oedema, myositis and petechial haemorrhage. Encephalitis and myocarditis may also occur. These signs are mainly caused by hypersensitivity and inflammatory responses.

### Trichinosis is diagnosed by microscopy and serology and treated with anthelmintics and antiinflammatories

Diagnosis of trichinosis is by demonstration of specific antibody by ELISA or indirect fluorescent antibody test, but these tests are negative in the first 3 weeks of infection. Muscle biopsy is sometimes required. Molecular methods are required for species identification. Treatment is with benzimidazoles, which kill the adult worms and thus prevent further release of larvae. Benzimidazoles do not kill larvae encysted in the muscles, so they need to be given as early as possible in the course of the infection. Systemic corticosteroid therapy is administered in moderate to severe cases, and nonsteroidal antiinflammatory agents are given in mild cases.

## Strongyloides

### *Strongyloides* infections are generally passed between humans but can develop in animal hosts, including dogs

*Strongyloides* infection is acquired by the penetration of infective larvae through the skin. The larvae migrate to the lung, enter the alveoli, pass up the bronchi and trachea and are then swallowed. Only females develop in the human host. They reproduce parthenogenetically and lay eggs into the intestinal mucosa (Fig. 29.12). The eggs hatch within the intestine to release larvae that pass out with the faeces

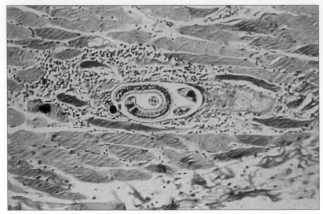

**Fig. 29.11** Inflammatory reaction around a nurse cell containing a coiled larva of *Trichinella spiralis*. Trichrome stain. (Courtesy I.G. Kagan.)

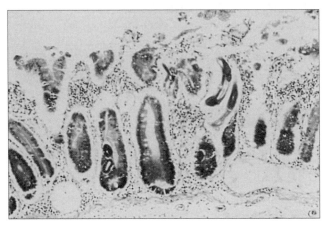

**Fig. 29.12** *Strongyloides stercoralis*. Adults and larvae in the mucosa of small intestine, showing disruption of the villous surface.

and require warm, moist soil to become infective. The geographic distribution of strongyloidiasis is similar to that of hookworm (in tropical and subtropical areas and in rural southern United States).

Infections are most often passed between humans, but two species can also develop in animal hosts, including dogs (*Strongloides stercoralis*) and African primates (*Strongloides fuelleborni*). Faecal larval stages may develop directly into the infective stage whilst still in the intestine and penetrate the mucosa or perianal skin to reinfect the host in the process of autoinfection. This capability represents a major survival advantage for the parasite.

### *Strongyloides* infections are usually asymptomatic but can cause disseminated disease in patients with immunodeficiency states or malnutrition

Many infected individuals are asymptomatic, although abdominal pain, vomiting or diarrhoea may occur. However, in immunodeficiency due to corticosteroid therapy, immunosuppression for transplantation, advanced malignancy, human T-cell lymphotropic virus (HTLV) infection and malnutrition, autoinfection can lead to hyperinfection or disseminated strongyloidiasis, the larvae invading almost all organs and causing severe and sometimes fatal pathology. Infected patients may show vomiting, abdominal pain, diarrhoea with malabsorption and dehydration, paralytic ileus and pneumonitis. Eosinophilia is often absent in *Strongyloides* hyperinfection. Disseminated strongyloidiasis can arise long after initial infection. It has been firmly established that infections can persist for many years (>30), being maintained by low-level autoinfection, then disseminate once the patient's immune defences are reduced. HTLV-1 antibody testing should be advised in patients found to have strongyloidiasis as antiparasitic treatment is less efficacious in patients coinfected with *Strongyloides* and HTLV-1. Furthermore, HTLV-1 coinfection is a major risk factor for disseminated strongyloidiasis. In addition, any patients for whom immunosuppression is planned should be asked about their residence and travel history. If they have been potentially exposed to *Strongyloides*, they should be screened for it ideally before immunosuppression is commenced.

*Strongyloides* infection is diagnosed by microscopy and *Strongyloides* culture of faeces to detect larvae. They are often scarce in asymptomatic infections but are very readily seen in hyperinfection as the parasite load is so high in that condition. Faecal PCR is used in some centres, but is not yet widely deployed. Serology for IgG antibody to *Strongyloides* is helpful in migrants from endemic areas but less sensitive in travellers. It may be negative in hyperinfection.

Treatment of *Strongyloides* infection is with ivermectin. Thiabendazole is also effective, but it is much less well tolerated by the patients. Albendazole is inferior to both.

## KEY FACTS

- The multisystem infections described in this chapter are zoonoses, being maintained naturally in a reservoir of nonhuman vertebrates.

- Humans are infected incidentally, generally from rodents (arenaviruses, hantaviruses, plague, tularaemia, leptospirosis), bats (filoviruses, rabies virus) or domestic animals (brucellosis, leptospirosis, trichinosis).

- There is generally no transmission from person to person except for plague and Ebola virus infections.

- The nature and the extent of human–animal contact are determining factors.

- Some of these infections are highly virulent.

- When the reservoir host is common in crowded human communities (e.g. plague), disease epidemics have been major events in history.

- Most of these infections are now less frequent in resource-rich countries (e.g. anthrax, brucellosis, echinococcosis), but they remain as frequent causes of disease in other parts of the world and thus may present in migrants from those regions.

- Anthrax is seen as a major bioterrorism threat.

- There are satisfactory antimicrobial agents for most nonviral infections, but effective vaccines are generally not available.

- The Ebola virus epidemic between 2013 and 2016 demonstrated the potential for transmission worldwide and how planning and preparedness is critical in terms of prevention, infection control and management.

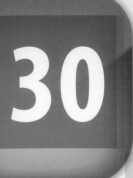

# 30 Fever of unknown origin

## Introduction

**Fever is an abnormal increase in body temperature and may be continuous or intermittent**

The homeostatic mechanisms of the body maintain a constant body temperature with daily fluctuations (circadian temperature rhythm) not exceeding ±1–1.5°C (1.8–2.7°F). Although 37°C (98.6°F) is considered a normal temperature, individuals vary in their body temperature; in some it may be as low as 36°C (96.8°F) and in others as high as 38°C (100.4°F). Fever is defined as an abnormal increase in body temperature—an oral temperature >37.6°C (100.4°F) or a rectal temperature >38°C (101°F)—and may be continuous or intermittent:

- In continuous fever the body temperature is elevated over a 24-h period and swings <1°C (1.8°F); this is characteristic of, for example, typhoid and typhus fever.
- In an intermittent fever the temperature is above normal throughout a 24-h period but swings >1°C (1.8°F) during that time. A swinging fever is typical of pyogenic infections, abscesses and tuberculosis.

Fever may be produced in response to:

- exogenous pyrogen such as endotoxin in gram-negative cell walls
- endogenous pyrogen such as interleukin 1 released from phagocytic cells.

It is thought that fever may be a protective response by the host (Fig. 30.1).

## DEFINITIONS OF FEVER OF UNKNOWN ORIGIN

Fever is a common complaint of patients presenting to a doctor. The cause is usually immediately apparent or is discovered within a few days, or the temperature settles spontaneously. However, if the patient's fever is >38.3°C (101°F) on several occasions and continues for >3 weeks despite 1 week of intensive evaluation, a provisional diagnosis of fever of unknown origin (FUO) is made based on the classic definition of FUO. However, increased awareness of FUO causes and an increasing number of patients with serious underlying diseases successfully kept alive by modern medicine has led to additional categorization of FUO with regard to particular patient risk groups (Table 30.1).

## CAUSES OF FUO

### Infection is the most common cause of FUO

For centuries, fever has been recognized as a characteristic sign of infection, and historically infection has been the most common cause of FUO, especially in children. However, there are important noninfectious causes of fever, most notably malignancies and collagen vascular diseases. These noninfectious causes need to be differentiated from infections during the investigation of a patient with FUO. Despite intense and prolonged investigations, the cause of fever may remain undiagnosed in a significant number of patients. However, in the absence of significant weight loss or indication of severe underlying disease, the outcome, although potentially long term, is generally positive. The reported incidence of different FUO aetiologies has varied over time, owing in part to patient demographics and advances in medical diagnostics. One must also consider that patients may have a factitious fever (produced artificially by the patient [e.g. in Munchausen syndrome]).

### Infective causes of classical FUO

The most common infective causes of classic FUO are shown in Table 30.2. These can be divided into two main groups:

- infections such as tuberculosis and typhoid fever caused by specific pathogens
- infections such as biliary tract infections and abscesses, which can be caused by a variety of different pathogens.

Most of these infections are described in detail elsewhere in this book. Bacterial endocarditis, which was long associated with FUO but now more easily diagnosed, is discussed later.

Significant infection may be present in the absence of fever in some groups of patients, notably:

- seriously ill neonates
- the elderly
- patients with uraemia
- patients receiving corticosteroids
- those taking antipyretic drugs continuously.

In these people, other signs and symptoms of infection have to be sought. This chapter deals only with patients whose presenting complaint is fever.

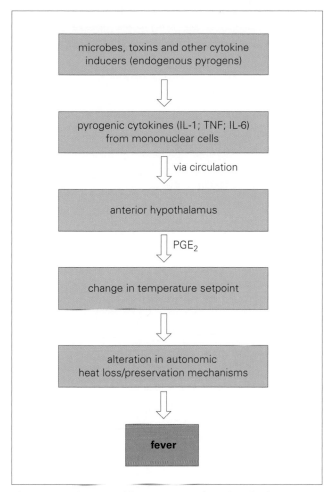

**Fig. 30.1** Mechanisms of fever. Fever may be induced either by exogenous pyrogens such as pathogens or their toxins or by endogenous pyrogens released in the host, and may have a protective effect. IL, Interleukin; PG, prostaglandin; TNF, tumour necrosis factor.

## INVESTIGATION OF CLASSIC FUO

### Steps in the investigative procedure

Because of the many possible infectious and noninfectious causes of FUO, it is clearly not practical to attempt specific investigations for each at the outset. However, guidelines for the minimum diagnostic evaluation necessary to categorize a presenting case as FUO have remained consistent over the years, an example of which is shown in Box 30.1. In addition, the diagnostic pathway can be divided into a series of stages, each stage attempting to focus the investigation on the likely (e.g. infective) causes (see Table 30.2).

Stage 1 comprises careful history taking, physical examination and screening tests

Careful history taking is essential and should include questions about travel, occupation, hobbies, exposure to animals and known infectious hazards, antibiotic therapy within the previous 2 months, substance misuse and other habits. Some of the infections listed in Table 30.2 are zoonoses (e.g. leptospirosis, spotted fevers), whereas others are vectorborne (e.g. malaria, trypanosomiasis) and/or of more limited geographic distribution (e.g. histoplasmosis), hence the importance of a travel history.

In light of the history and the differential diagnosis, a complete physical examination of the patient with FUO is essential, in particular:

- the skin, eyes, lymph nodes and abdomen should be examined
- the heart should be auscultated.

It is also important to confirm that the patient does have a fever. In some series, as many as 25% of patients whose presenting complaint was FUO may not have a fever but rather a naturally exaggerated circadian temperature rhythm. The possibility of a factitious fever must also be considered.

Routine investigations such as chest radiography and blood tests should be performed at this stage.

**Table 30.1** Definitions of fever of unknown origin (FUO)

| Definition | Symptoms | Diagnosis |
|---|---|---|
| Classical FUO | Fever (>38.3°C) on several occasions and >3-wk duration | Uncertain despite appropriate investigations after at least three outpatient visits or 3 days in hospital, including at least 2 days of incubation of microbiologic cultures |
| Nosocomial (health care–associated) FUO | Fever (>38.3°C) on several occasions in a health care setting; infection not present or incubating on admission | Uncertain after 3 days despite appropriate investigations, including at least 2 days of incubation of microbiologic cultures |
| Neutropenic FUO | Fever (>38.3°C) on several occasions; neutrophil count <500/mm³ in peripheral blood, or expected to fall below that number within 1–2 days | Uncertain after 3 days despite appropriate investigations, including at least 2 days of incubation of microbiologic cultures |
| HIV-associated FUO | Fever (>38.3°C) on several occasions; fever of >4-wk duration as an outpatient or >3-day duration as an inpatient; confirmed positive HIV serology | Uncertain after 3 days despite appropriate investigations, including at least 2 days of incubation of microbiologic cultures |

The classic definition of FUO requires that the fever is of >3-week duration, but infections in compromised patients frequently progress rapidly because of inadequate host defences. Consequently, the pace of the investigations needs to be rapid if appropriate therapy is to be initiated. HIV, Human immunodeficiency virus.

**Table 30.2** Representative infective causes of fever of unknown origin (FUO)

| Infection | Usual cause |
|---|---|
| **Bacterial** | |
| Tuberculosis | *Mycobacterium tuberculosis* |
| Enteric fevers | *Salmonella typhi* |
| Osteomyelitic | *Staphylococcus aureus* (also *Haemophilus influenzae* in young children, *Salmonella* in patients with sickle cell disease) |
| Endocarditis | Oral streptococci, *S. aureus*, coagulase-negative staphylococci |
| Brucellosis | *Brucella abortus*, *B. melitensis*, and *B. suis* |
| Abscesses (esp. intraabdominal) | Mixed anaerobes and facultative anaerobes from gut microbiota |
| Biliary system infections | Gram-negative facultative anaerobes (e.g. *Escherichia coli*) |
| Urinary tract infections | Gram-negative facultative anaerobes (e.g. *E. coli*) |
| Lyme disease | *Borrelia burgdorferi* |
| Relapsing fever | *Borrelia recurrentis* |
| Leptospirosis | *Leptospira interrogans* serovar icterohaemorrhagiae |
| Rat bite fever | *Streptobacillus moniliformis*, *Spirillum minus* |
| Typhus | *Rickettsia prowazekii* |
| Spotted fever | *Rickettsia rickettsii*, *R. conorii* |
| Psittacosis | *Chlamydophila psittaci* |
| Q fever | *Coxiella burnetii* |
| **Parasitic** | |
| Malaria | *Plasmodium* spp. |
| Trypanosomiasis | *Trypanosoma brucei gambiense* |
| Amoebic abscesses | *Entamoeba histolytica* |
| Toxoplasmosis | *Toxoplasma gondii* |
| Fungal | |
| Candidiasis | *Candida albicans* |
| Cryptococcosis | *Cryptococcus neoformans* |
| Histoplasmosis | *Histoplasma capsulatum* |
| **Viral** | |
| Acquired immunodeficiency syndrome | Human immunodeficiency virus |
| Infectious mononucleosis | Epstein-Barr virus, cytomegalovirus |
| Hepatitis | Hepatitis viruses |

A wide range of infections can present as FUO. Some, such as brucellosis, are zoonoses, and many are vectorborne. Therefore the patient must have had appropriate exposure to contract these infections. For example, there are ~2000 cases of malaria annually in both the United Kingdom and the United States, the overwhelming majority of which are contracted outside the country. A travel history is therefore very important.

**Stage 2 involves reviewing the history, repeating the physical examination and performing specific diagnostic tests and noninvasive investigations**

A review of the patient's history, particularly after discussion with colleagues and perhaps carried out by a second physician, is valuable to check for omissions such as exposure to particular risk factors in the recent or more distant past. The physical examination should also be repeated because rashes and other signs of infection can be transient.

Clues to the diagnosis elicited by careful history taking should direct specific investigations. As the most common cause of unexplained fever is infection, collection and careful

examination of appropriate specimens are essential. Skin tests may also be appropriate at this stage. The most important specimens include:

- blood for culture
- blood for examination of antibodies. A sample of serum collected when the patient presents should also be stored for comparison with later samples to detect rising antibody titres even if the patient is some weeks into the infection. Serologic tests are helpful, particularly in the diagnosis of cytomegalovirus and Epstein-Barr virus infection, toxoplasmosis, psittacosis and rickettsial infections. Positive results in syphilis serology should be

## Box 30.1     Example of Minimum Diagnostic Evaluation Necessary to Categorize a Case as Classical Fever of Unknown Origin

- Comprehensive history (including travel history, risk for venereal diseases, hobbies, contact with pet animals and birds, etc.)
- Comprehensive physical examination (including temporal arteries, rectal digital examination, etc.)
- Routine blood tests (complete blood count, including differential, ESR or CRP, electrolytes, renal and hepatic tests, creatine phosphokinase, lactate dehydrogenase)
- Microscopic urinalysis
- Cultures of blood, urine (and other normally sterile compartments if clinically indicated [e.g. joints, pleura, cerebrospinal fluid])
- Chest radiograph

- Abdominal (including pelvic) ultrasonography
- Antinuclear and antineutrophilic cytoplasmic antibodies, rheumatoid factor
- Tuberculin skin test
- Serologic tests directed by local epidemiologic data
- Further evaluation directed by abnormalities detected by above test (e.g. HIV antibodies depending on detailed history)
- CMV-IgM and EBV serology in case of abnormal differential WBC count
- Abdominal or chest helical CT scan (also consider FDG-PET)
- Echocardiography in case of cardiac murmur

CMV, Cytomegalovirus; CRP, C-reactive protein; CT, computed tomography; EBV, Epstein-Barr virus; ESR, erythrocyte sedimentation rate; FDG-PET, fluorodeosyglucose-positron emission tomography; HIV, human immunodeficiency virus; Ig, immunoglobulin; WBC, white blood cell.

viewed with caution as other infections can cause biologic false positives (see Ch. 22)
- direct examination of blood to diagnose malaria, trypanosomiasis and relapsing fever.

Repeated sampling of blood, urine and other body fluids may be required, and the laboratory should be alerted to search for unusual and fastidious organisms (e.g. nutritionally variant streptococci as a cause of endocarditis; see later). If possible, serial cultures should be collected before antimicrobial therapy is commenced.

Technical advances in diagnostic imaging techniques have provided the physician with a wide range of noninvasive investigative methods such as $^{18}$F-fluorodeoxyglucose-positron emission tomography, diffusion-weighted magnetic resonance imaging and computed tomography scans (Fig. 30.2).

### Stage 3 comprises invasive tests

Biopsy of liver and bone marrow should always be considered in the investigation of classic cases of FUO, but other tissues such as skin, lymph nodes and kidney may also be sampled. It is undesirable or impossible to repeat biopsies; therefore it is important to organize the laboratory examination of material carefully to maximize the information obtained.

### Stage 4 involves therapeutic trials

Trials of corticosteroids (e.g. prednisone, dexamethasone) or prostaglandin inhibitors (e.g. aspirin, indometacin) may be indicated if a noninfectious cause has been essentially eliminated. There are few indications for empiric antimicrobial or cytotoxic chemotherapy in the management of classic FUO. However, a trial of antituberculosis drugs may be advocated in patients with a history of tuberculosis in the absence of supporting microbiologic evidence. Infections can progress very rapidly in people who are neutropenic or have acquired immunodeficiency syndrome (AIDS), and blind therapy is warranted (see later).

## TREATMENT OF FUO

The investigation and management of a patient with FUO requires persistence and an informed and open mind to reach the correct diagnosis. As the range of infective causes of FUO is enormous, the correct diagnosis is an essential prelude to the choice of appropriate treatment. As soon as the cause has been identified, specific therapy, if available, should be given.

## FUO IN SPECIFIC PATIENT GROUPS

### The main difference between FUO in these groups and classic FUO is the time course

As mentioned earlier, an increasing number of people are surviving with severe underlying disease that predisposes them to infection or are receiving treatment, such as cytotoxic drugs, that compromises their defences against infection. These groups of patients are discussed in more detail in Chapter 31, but they are included here because, in addition to classic FUO, other classifications of FUO (see Table 30.1) define:

- nosocomial FUO
- neutropenic FUO
- human immunodeficiency virus (HIV)–associated FUO.

Classically, an FUO may exist for weeks or months before a diagnosis is made, whereas for health care–associated (nosocomial) FUO and in neutropenic patients, the time course is hours to days. The more common infective causes of FUO in these groups are shown in Table 30.3.

Investigation should proceed as noted earlier but with the particular emphasis depending upon the patient. In hospital patients, the emphasis will depend upon:

- the type of operative procedures performed; fever is a common complaint that may indicate graft-versus-host disease in patients who have received transplants

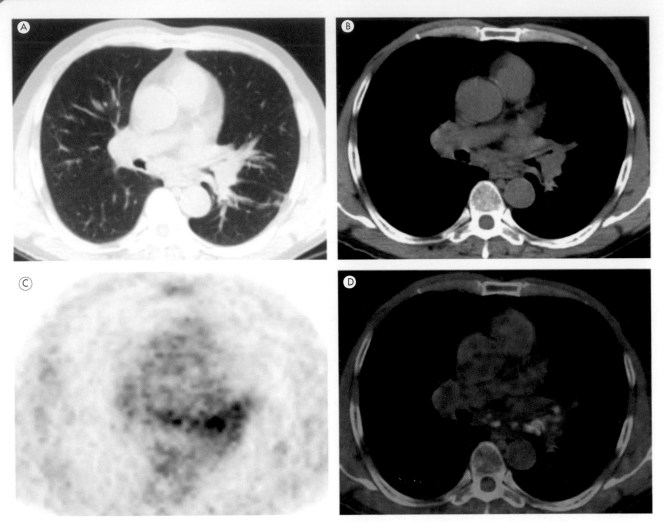

**Fig. 30.2** Bilateral endobronchial metastasis in a patient with prostate cancer visualized by $^{18}$F-fluorodeosyglucose–positron emission tomography (FDG–PET)/computed tomography (CT). Transverse CT (A,B), PET (C), and fusion (D) reveal multiple nodules with FDG uptake. (From Jin C, et al. Bilateral endobronchial metastases from prostate cancer: a case report with literature review. *Resp Med Case Rep*. 2022;30:fig. 3.)

- the presence of foreign bodies, especially intravascular devices
- drug therapy, as drug fevers are a common noninfective cause of FUO
- the underlying disease and stage of chemotherapy in neutropenic patients
- the presence of known risk factors such as intravenous drug misuse, travel and contact with infected individuals in patients with HIV. Although the major opportunist infections in people with AIDS are well described (see Ch. 31), common infections can present atypically and new infections continue to emerge.

## INFECTIVE ENDOCARDITIS

Infective endocarditis often presents as an FUO that is fatal if untreated. The infection involves the endothelial lining of the heart, usually including the heart valves. It may occur as an acute, rapidly progressive disease or as a subacute form. The majority of these patients have a preexisting heart defect, either congenital or acquired (e.g. as a result of rheumatic fever), or a prosthetic heart valve in situ. However, the patient may be unaware of any defect before the infection.

### Almost any organism can cause endocarditis, but native valves are usually infected by oral streptococci and staphylococci

Infection of native valves is most commonly caused by species of oral streptococci viridans group (e.g. *Streptococcus mutans, S. mitis, S. salivarius, S. anginosis, S. bovis*), *Staphylococcus aureus* and coagulase-negative staphylococci (Table 30.4). Intravenous drug misusers have the added complication of infection due to organisms they inject into themselves. Coagulase-negative staphylococci are common causes of early prosthetic valve endocarditis and are probably acquired at the time of surgery. The species causing late infections (>3 months after cardiac surgery) are somewhat more like those causing native valve endocarditis (Fig. 30.3).

Endocarditis is an endogenous infection acquired when organisms entering the bloodstream establish themselves on the heart valves. Therefore any bacteraemia can potentially result in endocarditis. Most commonly, streptococci from the oral flora enter the bloodstream (e.g. during dental procedures or vigorous teeth cleaning or flossing) and adhere to damaged heart valves. It is thought that fibrin-platelet vegetations are present on damaged valves before the organisms

**Table 30.3** Representative infective causes of fever of unknown origin (FUO) in specific patient groups

| Category of FUO | Infection | Usual cause |
|---|---|---|
| Nosocomial | Vascular line related | Staphylococci |
| | Other device related | Staphylococci, *Candida* |
| | Transfusion related | Cytomegalovirus |
| | Cholecystitis and pancreatitis | Gram-negative rods |
| | Pneumonia (related to assisted ventilation) | Gram-negative rods, including *Pseudomonas* |
| | Postoperative abscesses (e.g. intraabdominal) | Gram-negative rods and anaerobes |
| | Postgastric surgery | Systemic candidiasis |
| Neutropenic | Vascular line related | Staphylococci |
| | Oral infection | *Candida*, herpes simplex virus |
| | Pneumonia | Gram-negative rods, *Candida*, *Aspergillus*, cytomegalovirus (CMV) |
| | Soft tissue (e.g. perianal abscesses) | Mixed aerobes and anaerobes |
| Human immunodeficiency virus associated | Respiratory tract | CMV, *Pneumocystis*, *Mycobacterium tuberculosis*, *M. avium-intracellulare* |
| | Central nervous system | *Toxoplasma* |
| | Gastrointestinal tract | *Salmonella*, *Campylobacter*, *Shigella* |
| | Genital tract or disseminated | *Treponema pallidum*, *Neisseria gonorrhoeae* |

Patients with health care–associated FUO are most likely to be infected with health care–associated pathogens, either from their own microbiota or from the health care environment. This also applies to neutropenic patients if they are inpatients, but some are treated as outpatients and may therefore be exposed to a wider range of pathogens. People with acquired immunodeficiency syndrome commonly become infected with opportunistic pathogens, though an increasing range of organisms is now implicated. It is important to take a detailed history, as latent infections can become florid as the patient's immune status deteriorates.

**Table 30.4** Causative agents of endocarditis in different groups of patients (in general order of decreasing importance)

| Patient group | Major aetiologic agents of infective endocarditis |
|---|---|
| Native valve | Oral streptococci and enterococci<br>*Staphylococcus aureus*<br>Coagulase-negative staphylococci<br>Gram-negative (enteric) rods<br>Fungi (mainly *Candida*) |
| Intravenous drug misuser | *S. aureus*<br>Oral streptococci and enterococci<br>Gram-negative (enteric) rods<br>Fungi (mainly *Candida*)<br>Coagulase-negative staphylococci |
| Prosthetic valve (early) | Coagulase-negative staphylococci<br>*S. aureus*<br>Gram-negative (enteric) rods<br>Oral streptococci and enterococci<br>Fungi (mainly *Candida*) |
| Prosthetic valve (late) | Oral streptococci and enterococci<br>Coagulase-negative staphylococci<br>*S. aureus*<br>Gram-negative (enteric) rods<br>Fungi (mainly *Candida*) |

Although almost any organism can cause endocarditis, the majority of cases are caused by a relatively small range of species. The relative importance of these species varies depending upon whether patients have their own heart valves or prosthetic valves.

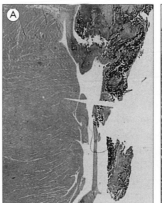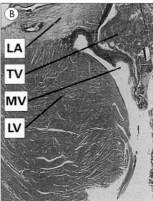

**Fig. 30.3** Bacteria circulating in the bloodstream adhere to, and establish themselves on, the heart valves. Multiplication of the pathogens is associated with destruction of valve tissue and the formation of vegetations, which interfere with, and may severely compromise, the normal function of the valve. These histologic sections show the virtual destruction of the leaflet at the mitral valve by staphylococci. (A) Gram stain. (B) Eosin–Van Gieson stain. LA, Left atrium; LV, left ventricle; MV, remnant of mitral valve; TV, thrombotic vegetation. (Courtesy R.H. Anderson.)

further fibrin and platelet deposition. In this position, they are protected from the host defences, and vegetations can grow to several centimetres. This is probably quite a slow process, and correspondingly the time period between the initial bacteraemia and the onset of symptoms averages ~5 weeks.

### A patient with infective endocarditis almost always has a fever and a heart murmur

The signs and symptoms of infective endocarditis are quite varied but relate essentially to four ongoing processes:

implant and that adherence is probably associated with the ability of the organisms to produce dextran as well as adhesins and fibronectin-binding proteins. Having attached themselves to the heart valve, the organisms multiply and attract

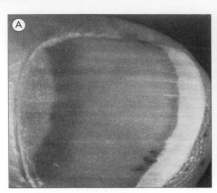
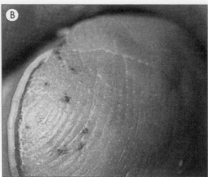
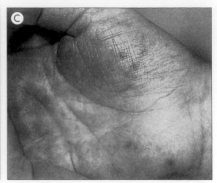

**Fig. 30.4** Outward signs of endocarditis may be helpful in suggesting the diagnosis. These result from the host's response to infection in the form of immune complex–mediated vasculitis, focal platelet aggregation and vascular permeability. (A and B, different views.) Splinter haemorrhages in the nailbed and petechial lesions in the skin. (C) Osler nodes. These are tender nodular lesions that tend to affect the palms and fingertips. (Courtesy H. Tubbs.)

- the infectious process on the valve and local intracardiac complications
- septic embolization to virtually any organ
- bacteraemia, often with metastatic foci of infection
- circulating immune complexes and other factors.

The patient almost always has a fever and a heart murmur and may complain of nonspecific symptoms such as anorexia, weight loss, malaise, chills, nausea, vomiting and night sweats—symptoms that are common to many of the causes of FUO listed in Table 30.2. Peripheral manifestations may also be evident in the form of splinter haemorrhages and Osler nodes (Fig. 30.4). Microscopic haematuria resulting from immune complex deposition in the kidney is characteristic (see Ch. 18).

### Blood culture is the most important test for diagnosing infective endocarditis

Microbiologic and cardiologic investigations are of critical importance. The blood culture is the single most important laboratory test. Ideally, three separate samples of blood should be collected within a 24-h period and before antimicrobial therapy is administered. Isolation of the causative organism is essential so that antibiotic susceptibility tests can be performed and optimum therapy prescribed. Nutritionally variant strains of oral streptococci are known to cause infective endocarditis. These may fail to grow in blood culture media but grow as satellite colonies around *S. aureus* colonies on blood agar.

### The mortality of infective endocarditis is ~20–40% despite treatment with antibiotics

In the past, most organisms causing infective endocarditis have been susceptible to a range of antimicrobials. However, antibiotic resistance has become an increasing issue (see Ch. 34). Even with appropriate treatment, complete eradication takes weeks to achieve, and relapse is common. This is probably due to factors such as:

- relative inaccessibility of the organisms within the vegetations both to antibiotics and to host defences
- the organism's high population density and relatively slow rate of multiplication.

Before the advent of antibiotics, infective endocarditis had a mortality of 100%. Even today, despite appropriate antimicrobial chemotherapy and depending on individual circumstances, the mortality remains at ~20–40%.

### The antibiotic treatment regimen for infective endocarditis depends upon the susceptibility of the infecting organism

For example, with prosthetic valve endocarditis due to penicillin-susceptible streptococci, high-dose penicillin is the treatment of choice. Patients with a good history of penicillin allergy may be treated with ceftriaxone or vancomycin. Minimum inhibitory concentration (MIC) and minimum bactericidal concentration (MBC) tests (see Ch. 34) should be performed to detect organisms that are less susceptible or tolerant to penicillin (inhibited, but not killed; e.g. MBC = 32 × MIC). Organisms less susceptible to penicillin and enterococci, which are always more resistant to penicillin, are treated with a combination of a beta-lactam antibiotic and an aminoglycoside. Combinations such as this act synergistically against streptococci and enterococci (see Ch. 34). However, vancomycin-resistant enterococci (usually *Enterococcus faecium*) pose a therapeutic challenge and require drugs such as linezolid or daptomycin.

Staphylococcal endocarditis, particularly in prosthetic valve endocarditis when the organisms may be health care associated and, consequently, often resistant to many antibiotics, often presents a more difficult therapeutic challenge. The increasing incidence of methicillin-resistant staphylococci requires a combination approach (e.g. vancomycin plus rifampin and gentamicin). A number of sources exist for detailed treatment regimens, including the American Heart Association and the British Society for Antimicrobial Chemotherapy.

### In some cases, prophylactic antibiotics may be indicated before or during invasive procedures

Guidelines for the use of prophylactic antibiotics to reduce the risk of bacteraemia has become a topic of major discussion, and many guidelines have reduced the indications. However, certain risk groups (e.g. people with known heart defects or prosthetic heart valves) remain candidates for prophylactic antibiotics to protect them during dental surgery and any other invasive procedure that is likely to cause a transient bacteraemia.

### Most people with an FUO have a treatable disease presenting in an unusual manner

The clinical investigation needs to be individualized, but this chapter outlines the essential stages in the investigation of patients and draws attention to the important infective causes of FUO.

Although classically a patient with FUO presents with a long history (weeks or months of fever), patients also present with fevers that are not immediately diagnosed by routine laboratory investigations. Definitions of FUO have also been proposed for these groups (nosocomial, neutropenic, HIV associated). The list of pathogens causing fever in these patients is growing.

The clinician's aim in the investigation of every patient with FUO should be to discover the cause (i.e. to change an FUO to a fever of known origin) and to initiate appropriate treatment.

## KEY FACTS

- Fever is the body's response to exogenous and endogenous pyrogens. It is a common symptom and may have a protective effect.

- The term *fever of unknown origin (FUO)* is used when the cause of fever is not obvious, has classically exceeded a 3-week duration, and is not revealed by routine clinical and laboratory investigations.

- Increased numbers of immunocompromised patients have prompted the definition of FUO groups other than classical (i.e. nosocomial, neutropenic, HIV-associated FUO).

- Among the causes of FUO, infection is the most common, but neoplasms and autoimmune diseases are also significant. Cases of FUO often remain undiagnosed.

- The list of infective causes is long; therefore the first stage of investigation (i.e. the patient's history and results of physical examination and screening tests) is a critical pointer to subsequent specific diagnostic tests.

- Therapeutic trials may be indicated if a diagnosis has not been achieved, but they may confuse the results of further tests.

- The correct diagnosis is paramount to direct appropriate and specific therapy.

- Infective endocarditis is a classic example of FUO. It is usually caused by gram-positive cocci, the species depending upon the patient's underlying predisposition, and is fatal unless treated.

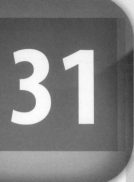

# 31

# Infections in the compromised host

## Introduction

The human body has a complex system of protective mechanisms to prevent infection. This involves both the adaptive (cellular and humoral) immune system and the innate defence system (e.g. skin, mucous membranes). (These have been described in detail in Chs. 10–12.) So far we have concentrated on the common and serious infections occurring in people whose protective mechanisms are largely intact. In these circumstances, the interactions between host and microorganism are such that the microorganism has to use all its guile to survive and invade the host, and the healthy host is usually able to combat such an invasion. The focus of this chapter involves the infections that arise when the host defences are compromised by disease or treatment, resulting in the host–microorganism equation being weighted heavily in favour of the microorganism.

## THE COMPROMISED HOST

Compromised hosts are individuals with one or more defects in their body's natural defences against microbial invaders. Consequently, they are much more liable to suffer from severe and life-threatening infections. Modern medicine has effective methods for treating many types of cancers, is improving organ transplantation techniques and has developed technology that enables people with otherwise fatal diseases to lead prolonged and productive lives. A consequence of these achievements, however, is an increasing number of compromised people prone to infection. In addition, viral infections (including human immunodeficiency virus [HIV] and human T-cell lymphotropic virus [HTLV]) result in a compromised immune system referred to as *acquired immunodeficiency syndrome (AIDS)* (see Ch. 22) and *adult T-cell leukaemia/lymphoma,* respectively.

### The host can be compromised in many different ways

Compromise can take a variety of forms, falling into two main groups:

- defects, accidental or intentional, in the body's innate defence mechanisms
- deficiencies in the adaptive immune response.

These disorders of the immune system can be further subclassified as primary or secondary (Table 31.1):

- Primary immunodeficiency is inherited or occurs by exposure in utero to environmental factors or by other unknown mechanisms. It is rare and varies in severity depending upon the type of defect.
- Secondary or acquired immunodeficiency is due to an underlying disease state (Table 31.2) or occurs as a result of treatment for a disease.

### Primary defects of innate immunity include congenital defects in phagocytic cells or complement synthesis

Congenital defects in phagocytic cells confer susceptibility to infection, and, of these, perhaps the best known is chronic granulomatous disease (Fig. 31.1) in which an inherited failure to synthesize cytochrome b-245 leads to a failure to produce reactive oxygen intermediates during phagocytosis. As a result, the neutrophils cannot kill invading pathogens.

The central role of complement in the innate defence mechanisms is undisputed, and inability to generate classical C3 convertase (see Ch. 10) through congenital defects in the synthesis of the early components, particularly C4 and C2, is associated with a high frequency of extracellular infections.

### Secondary defects of innate defences include disruption of the body's mechanical barriers

A variety of factors can disrupt the mechanical nonspecific barriers to infection. For example, burns, traumatic injury, and major surgery destroy the continuity of the skin and may leave poorly vascularized tissue near the body surface, providing a relatively defenceless site for pathogens to colonize and invade. In health, the mucosal barriers of the respiratory and alimentary tract are vital to prevent infection. Damage sustained through endoscopy, surgery or radiotherapy, for example, provides easy access for infecting organisms. Devices such as intravascular and urinary catheters or procedures such as lumbar puncture or bone marrow aspiration allow organisms to bypass the normal defences and enter normally sterile parts of the body. Foreign bodies such as prostheses (e.g. hip joints or heart valves) and cerebrospinal fluid (CSF) shunts alter the local nonspecific host responses and provide surfaces that pathogens can colonize more readily than the natural equivalents.

The adage "obstruction leads to infection" is a valuable reminder that the defences of many body systems work partly through the clearance of undesirable materials (e.g. by urine flow, ciliary action in the respiratory tract, peristalsis in the gut). Interference with these mechanisms as a result of pathologic obstruction, central nervous system (CNS) dysfunction or surgical intervention tends to result in infection.

**Table 31.1** Factors that make a host compromised

| Factors affecting innate systems | |
|---|---|
| Primary | Complement deficiencies, phagocyte cell deficiencies |
| Secondary | Burns, trauma, major surgery, catheterization, foreign bodies (e.g. shunts, prostheses), obstruction |
| **Factors affecting adaptive systems** | |
| Primary | T-cell defects, B-cell deficiencies, severe combined immunodeficiency |
| Secondary | Malnutrition, infectious diseases, neoplasia, irradiation, chemotherapy, splenectomy |

### Primary adaptive immunodeficiency results from defects in the primary differentiation environment or in cell differentiation

The major congenital abnormalities arising in the adaptive immune system are depicted in Fig. 31.2. A defect in the stromal microenvironment in which lymphocytes differentiate may lead to failure to produce B cells (Bruton-type agammaglobulinaemia) or T cells (DiGeorge syndrome).

Differentiation pathways themselves may also be affected. For example, a nonfunctional recombinase enzyme will prevent the recombination of gene fragments that form the B-cell antibody or the T-cell receptor variable regions for antigen recognition, with a resulting severe combined immunodeficiency.

The most common form of congenital antibody deficiency—common variable immunodeficiency—is characterized by recurrent pyogenic infections and is heterogeneous in mechanism. A number of single gene defects have been reported in the tumour necrosis factor (TNF) receptor superfamily molecules, including the transmembrane activator and calcium modulator and cyclophilin ligand interactor, encoded by *TNFRSF13B* that is found in 8–10% of patients although also in healthy individuals. Other genes identified in these patients include those in the CD19 complex and costimulatory molecules like CD20, as well as epigenetic changes, cytosolic and nuclear factors.

**Table 31.2** Infections that cause immune deficiency states

| Microorganism | Affected immunocyte | Immune dysregulation |
|---|---|---|
| HIV-1 and -2 | T cells (CD4 positive) <br>• Macrophages | CD4-positive cell depletion |
| HTLV-1 | T cells <br>• NK cells | Induces cytotoxic T cells to kill virus-infected cells <br>• Alter CD4-positive T-cell function and cytokine production <br>• Decreases NK cell activation |
| CMV | T cells | Lower frequency of naïve T cells and accumulation of memory T cells <br>• Immune senescence |
| EBV | B cells | Depletion of B cells <br>• Mono/polyclonal gammopathy <br>• Autoimmunity <br>• Cancer |
| SARS-CoV-2 MERS | T cells | CD4-positive T-cell depletion |
| Influenza A viruses | Neutrophils | Deactivation of chemotaxis, respiratory burst, degranulation, bacterial killing <br>• Interferon gamma, alpha, beta triggered and depresses macrophage function |
| Measles virus | T cells <br>• Dendritic cells | Reduced lymphocyte proliferation <br>• Reduced antibody production <br>• Increased susceptibility to range of infections |
| Leishmania | Macrophages | Decreased MHC class II expression <br>• Decreased IL-1 production |
| Malaria | T cells <br>• Dendritic cells | Impaired dendritic cell maturation and activation <br>• Increased susceptibility to coinfections <br>• Decreased vaccine efficacy <br>• Reactivation of EBV infection with increased susceptibility to develop lymphoma |
| *Mycobacterium tuberculosis* | Macrophages | Inhibits macrophage activation |
| *Mycobacterium leprae* | Macrophages | Inhibits macrophage activation |
| *Bordetella pertussis* | Airway macrophages <br>• Neutrophils | Delayed neutrophil recruitment and influx into airways <br>• Depletion of airway neutrophils |

CMV, Cytomegalovirus; EBV, Epstein-Barr virus; HIV, human immunodeficiency virus; HTLV, human T-cell lymphotropic virus; IL, interleukin; MHC, major histocompatibility complex; NK, natural killer; MERS, Middle Eastern respiratory syndrome; SARS-CoV-2, severe acute respiratory syndrome coronavirus 2.
Adapted from Sullivan KE, Stiehm ER, editors. *Stiehm's Immune Deficiencies*, Elsevier; 2020:1035–1058.

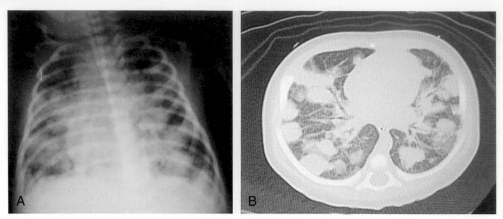

**Fig. 31.1** Neonate with chronic granulomatous disease and invasive pulmonary aspergillosis: (A) chest X-ray and (B) CT scan of the chest. (From Saito S, et al. A neonatal case of chronic granulomatous disease, initially presented with invasive pulmonary aspergillosis. *J Infect Chemother.* 2014;20(3):220–223.)

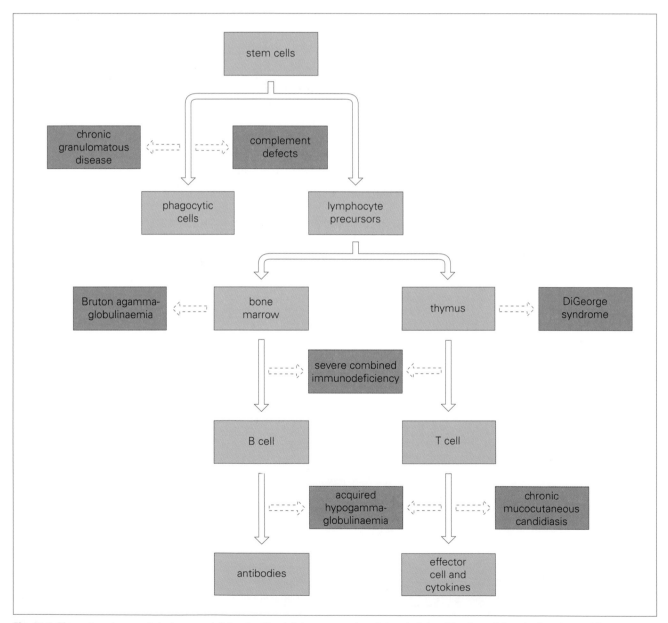

**Fig. 31.2** The major primary cellular immunodeficiencies. The deficiency states (*purple boxes*) derive either from defects in the primary differentiation environment (bone marrow or thymus) or during cell differentiation (*dashed arrows* derived from the differentiation state indicated).

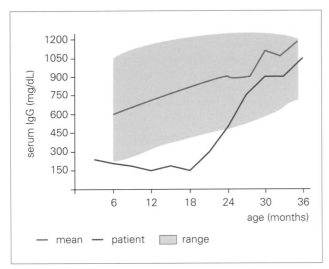

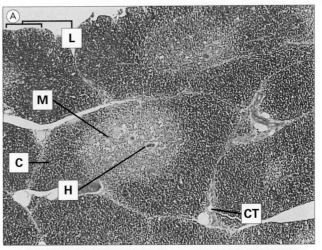

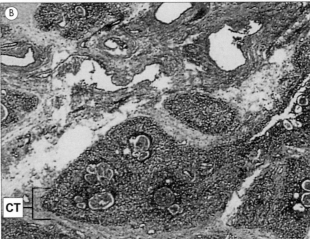

**Fig. 31.3** Serum immunoglobulin concentrations in a boy with transient hypogammaglobulinaemia compared with the range of normal controls. The patient developed mild paralytic polio when immunized at 4 months of age with live attenuated (Sabin) vaccine.

Although the number of immature B cells in the marrow tends to be normal, the peripheral B cells are either low in number or in some cases absent. Where present, they are unable to differentiate into plasma cells in some cases or to secrete antibody in others.

Transient hypogammaglobulinaemia of infancy, characterized by recurrent respiratory infections, is associated with a low serum immunoglobulin G (IgG) concentration, which often normalizes abruptly by 3–4 years of age (Fig. 31.3).

Immunoglobulin deficiency occurs naturally in human infants as the maternal serum IgG concentration decays. It is a serious problem in very premature babies as, depending on the gestational age, maternal IgG may not have crossed the placental barrier.

**Fig. 31.4** Thymic histology in normal children and children with protein–energy malnutrition (PEM). (A) Normal thymus showing a cortex and medullary zones. (B) Acute involution in PEM characterized by lobular atrophy, loss of distinction between cortex and medulla, depletion of lymphocytes, and enlarged Hassall corpuscles. C, Cortex; CT, connective tissue; H, Hassall corpuscle; L, lobule; M, medulla. (Courtesy R.K. Chandra.)

## Causes of secondary adaptive immunodeficiency include malnutrition, infections, neoplasia, splenectomy and certain medical treatments

Worldwide, malnutrition is common and is the most important cause of acquired immunodeficiency. The major form, protein–energy malnutrition, presents as a wide range of disorders, with kwashiorkor and marasmus at the two poles. It results in:

- drastic effects on the structure of the lymphoid organs (Fig. 31.4)
- gross reductions in the synthesis of complement components
- sluggish chemotactic responses of phagocytes
- lowered concentrations of secretory and mucosal IgA
- reduced affinity of IgG
- in particular, a serious deficit in circulating T-cell numbers (Fig. 31.5), leading to inadequate cell-mediated responses.

Infections themselves are often immunosuppressive (see Table 31.2), and none is more so than HIV infection, which gives rise to AIDS (see Ch. 22). Neoplasia of the lymphoid system frequently induces a state of reduced immuno-reactivity, and splenectomy results in impaired humoral responses.

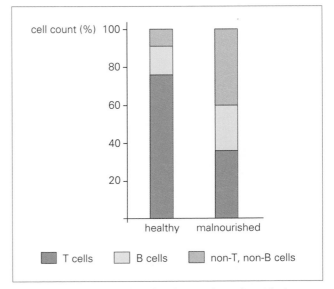

**Fig. 31.5** The proportion of T cells is decreased in malnourished patients compared with healthy controls. B-cell counts are usually unaltered, and lymphocytes lacking T- and B-cell markers are increased.

Treatment of disease can also cause immunosuppression. For example:

- Cytotoxic agents such as cyclophosphamide and azathioprine cause leukopenia or deranged T- and B-cell function.
- Monoclonal antibody immunotherapy such as rituximab binds to CD20, a glycosylated transmembrane protein on the surface of developing B cells.
- Immunomodulatory drugs such as lenalidomide alter cytokine production, regulate T-cell costimulation and augment natural killer cell cytotoxicity.
- Chimeric antigen receptor (CAR) T-cell therapy reprogrammes the T cells of the patient to target cancer cells by genetically modifying them to express a T-cell receptor targeting a tumour-specific antigen. Fourth-generation CAR T-cells have an extra effect as they induce a proinflammatory environment around the cancer cells. So, although this is an exciting new form of immunotherapy, CAR T-cell treatment can cause immunosuppression.
- Corticosteroids reduce the number of circulating lymphocytes, monocytes and eosinophils and suppress leukocyte accumulation at sites of inflammation.
- Radiotherapy adversely affects the proliferation of lymphoid cells.

Therefore a patient receiving treatment for neoplastic disease will be immunocompromised as a result of both the disease and the treatment.

It is important to recognize immunodeficiencies and to understand which procedures are likely to compromise the natural defences of a patient. Due to improvements in medical technology, many immune defects, particularly immunosuppression resulting from radiotherapy or cytotoxic drugs, are transient, and patients who survive the period of immunosuppression have a good chance of a complete recovery.

### Pathogens that infect the compromised host

Immunocompromised people can become infected with any pathogen able to infect immunocompetent individuals as

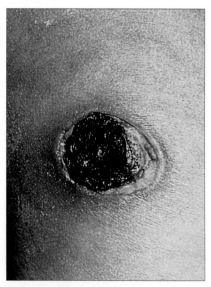

**Fig. 31.6** Ecthyma gangrenosum in a child with *Pseudomonas* septicaemia associated with immunodeficiency. (Courtesy H. Tubbs.)

well as those opportunist pathogens that do not cause disease in a healthy person. They may be lethal when the host defences are lowered. Different types of defect predispose to infection with different pathogens depending on the critical mechanisms operating in the defence against each microorganism (Fig. 31.6). Here, we will concentrate mainly on the opportunistic infections and refer to other chapters for information about other pathogens.

## INFECTIONS OF THE HOST WITH DEFICIENT INNATE IMMUNITY DUE TO PHYSICAL FACTORS

### Burn wound infections

#### Burns damage the body's mechanical barriers, neutrophil function and immune responses

Burn wounds are sterile immediately after the burn is inflicted, but they inevitably become colonized within hours with a mixed bacterial flora. Burn injuries cause direct damage to the mechanical barriers of the body, abnormalities in neutrophil function and immune responses. In addition, there is a major physiologic derangement with loss of fluids and electrolytes. The burn provides a highly nutritious surface for organisms to colonize, and the incidence of serious infection varies with the size and depth of the burn and the age of the patient. Topical antimicrobial therapy should prevent infection of burns of <30% of the total body area, but larger burns are always colonized. Noninvasive infection is confined to the eschar, which is the nonviable skin debris on the surface of deep burns. It is characterized by rapid separation of the eschar from the underlying tissue and a heavy exudate of purulent material from the burn wound. The systemic symptoms are usually relatively mild. However, organisms can invade from heavily colonized burn eschars into viable tissue beneath and rapidly destroy the tissue, converting partial-thickness burns into full-thickness skin destruction. From here, it is a small step to invasion of the lymphatics and thence to the bloodstream or direct invasion of blood vessels, and to septicaemia. Septicaemia in patients with burns is often polymicrobial.

#### The major pathogens in burns are aerobic and facultatively anaerobic bacteria and fungi

The most important pathogens in burn wounds are:

- *Pseudomonas aeruginosa* and other gram-negative rods
- *Staphylococcus aureus*
- *Streptococcus pyogenes*
- other streptococci
- enterococci.

*Candida* spp. and *Aspergillus* together account for ~5% of infections. Anaerobes are rare in burn wound infections. Herpesvirus infections have been reported and are most likely due to reactivation at a damaged skin site.

#### *P. aeruginosa* is a devastating gram-negative pathogen of patients with burns

*P. aeruginosa* is an opportunist gram-negative rod that has a long and infamous association with burn infections. It grows well in the moist environment of a burn wound, producing a foul, green-pigmented discharge and necrosis. Invasion is common, and the characteristic skin lesions (ecthyma gangrenosum) that are pathognomonic of *P. aeruginosa* septicaemia may appear on unburned areas (see Fig. 31.5). Host factors predisposing to infection include:

- abnormalities in the antibacterial activities of neutrophils
- deficiencies in serum opsonins.

Added to these are the virulence factors of the organism, which include the production of elastase, protease and exotoxin. This combination makes *P. aeruginosa* the most devastating gram-negative pathogen of burned patients. Treatment is difficult because of the organism's innate resistance to many antibacterial agents. A combination of aminoglycoside, usually gentamicin or tobramycin, with one of the beta-lactams such as ceftazidime or imipenem is usually favoured, but several units have reported strains resistant to these agents.

It is virtually impossible to prevent colonization. Prevention of infection depends largely on inhibiting the multiplication of organisms colonizing the burn by applying topical agents such as silver nitrate.

### *Staphylococcus aureus* is the foremost pathogen of burn wounds

The most important predisposing factor to *S. aureus* infection in burn patients appears to be an abnormality of the antibacterial function of neutrophils. Infections follow a more insidious course than streptococcal infections (see later), and it may be several days before the full-blown infection is apparent. The organism is capable of destroying granulation tissue, invading and causing septicaemia. *S. aureus* infections of skin are discussed in detail in Chapter 27. Treatment with antistaphylococcal agents such as flucloxacillin or a glycopeptide if methicillin-resistant *S. aureus* is isolated should be administered if there is evidence of invasive infection. Every effort should be made to prevent the spread of staphylococci from patient to patient. Although transmissible by both airborne and contact routes, the contact route is by far more important.

### The high transmissibility of *Streptococcus pyogenes* makes it the scourge of burns units

*S. pyogenes* (group A strep) infections of skin and soft tissue are discussed in some detail in Chapter 27. *S. pyogenes* was the most common cause of burn wound infection in the preantibiotic era and is still to be feared in burns wards. The infection usually occurs within the first few days of injury and is characterized by a rapid deterioration in the state of the burn wound and invasion of neighbouring healthy tissue. The patient may become severely toxic and will die within hours unless treated appropriately. *S. pyogenes* rarely infects healthy granulation tissue, but freshly grafted wounds may become infected, resulting in destruction of the graft. Every effort should be made to prevent spread. Penicillin is the drug of choice for treatment, and erythromycin or vancomycin can be used for penicillin-allergic patients.

Beta-haemolytic streptococci of other Lancefield groups (notably groups C and G) and enterococci are also important pathogens of burn wounds.

## Traumatic injury and surgical wound infections

Both accidental and intentional trauma destroy the integrity of the body surface and leave it liable to infection. Accidental injury may result in pathogens being introduced deep into the wound. The species involved will depend upon the nature of the wound, as discussed in Chapter 27.

### *Staphylococcus aureus* is the most important cause of surgical wound infection

*S. aureus* surgical wound infection (see Ch. 37) may be acquired during surgery or postoperatively and may originate from the patient or from another patient or staff member. The wound is less well defended than normal tissue; it may have a damaged blood supply, and there may be foreign bodies such as sutures. Classical studies of wound infections have shown that far fewer staphylococci are needed to initiate infection around a suture than in normal healthy skin. Wound infections can be severe, and the organisms can invade the bloodstream, with consequent seeding of other sites such as the heart valves, causing endocarditis (see Ch. 30), or bones, causing osteomyelitis (see Ch. 27), thereby further compromising the patient.

### Catheter-associated infection of the urinary tract is common

Urinary catheters disrupt the normal host defences of the urinary tract and allow organisms easy access to the bladder. Such catheter-associated infection of the urinary tract is especially common if catheters are left in place for >48 h (see Ch. 21). The organisms involved are usually gram-negative rods from the patient's own faecal or periurethral flora, but cross-infection also occurs (see Ch. 37).

### Staphylococci are the most common cause of intravenous and peritoneal dialysis catheter infections

Intravenous and peritoneal dialysis catheters breach the integrity of the skin barrier and allow organisms from the skin flora of the patient or hands of the carer easy access to deeper sites. Staphylococci are the most common cause of infection, but coryneforms, gram-negative rods and *Candida* are also implicated.

Coagulase-negative staphylococci, particularly *S. epidermidis*, account for >50% of the infections. These opportunists are members of the normal skin flora and for many years were considered to be harmless. However, they have a particular propensity for colonizing plastic and can therefore seed sites adjacent to plastic devices and cause invasive infections. Their ability to produce an adhesive slime material and grow as biofilms on plastic surfaces is important. They are sticky bacterial clusters attached to the surface and embedded in an extracellular matrix. Protection is provided against antibiotics and host defence by the mechanical barrier, slowing cell processes such as protein synthesis and replication as well as being made up of cells that are less susceptible to antibiotics. There are a number of virulence factors that promote biofilm production, and these include proteins, adhesins and polysaccharides. Infections are characteristically more insidious in onset than those caused by the more virulent *S. aureus*, and recognition is hampered by the difficulty in distinguishing the infecting strain from the normal flora. Treatment is also difficult because many *S. epidermidis* strains carry multiple antibiotic resistances, and agents such as a glycopeptide (vancomycin or teicoplanin) and rifampicin may be required (see Ch. 34). Whenever possible, the plastic device should be removed.

## Infections of plastic devices in situ

The technical developments in plastics and other synthetic materials have enabled many advances in medicine and surgery but in the process have produced further ways of introducing infectious agents. *S. epidermidis* is an important cause of infection of cardiac pacemakers, vascular grafts and CSF shunts.

### *Staphylococcus epidermidis* is the most common cause of prosthetic valve and joint infections

Patients with prosthetic heart valves or prosthetic joints are compromised by:

- the surgery to implant the prosthesis
- the continued presence of a foreign body.

*S. epidermidis* is again the most common pathogen, gaining access either during surgery or from a subsequent bacteraemia originating from, for example, an intravascular line infection. Endocarditis associated with prosthetic heart valves is discussed in Chapter 30.

The most common complication of joint replacement is loosening of the prosthesis, while infection is the second most common complication and is much more likely to lead to permanent failure of the procedure. The difficulties of treatment have been outlined earlier, but there is understandably great reluctance to remove a prosthetic device even though it is sometimes the only way to eradicate an infection.

## Infections due to compromised clearance mechanisms

Stasis predisposes to infection, and in health, the body functions to prevent stasis. In the respiratory tract, damage to the ciliary escalator predisposes the lungs to invasion, particularly in patients with cystic fibrosis who are infected with *S. aureus* and *Haemophilus influenzae* and later with *P. aeruginosa* (see Ch. 20). *Aspergillus fumigatus* is the most common fungal pathogen that is frequently recovered from the airway of patients with cystic fibrosis.

Obstruction and interruption of normal urine flow allows gram-negative organisms from the periurethral flora to ascend the urethra and to establish themselves in the bladder. Septicaemia is an important complication of urinary tract infection superimposed on obstruction.

## INFECTIONS ASSOCIATED WITH SECONDARY ADAPTIVE IMMUNODEFICIENCY

The underlying immunodeficiency state determines the nature and severity of any associated infection, and in some cases infection is the presenting clinical feature in a patient with an immunologic deficit. However, septicaemia and related infectious complications of immunodeficiency are most encountered in patients hospitalized for chemotherapy for malignant diseases or organ transplantation. In these patients, infection continues to be a major cause of morbidity and mortality (Table 31.3). Increasingly, these infections are iatrogenic and caused by opportunist pathogens acquired in hospital.

## Haematologic malignancy and bone marrow transplant infections

### A lack of circulating neutrophils following bone marrow failure predisposes to infection

Susceptibility to infection of patients with haematologic malignancies is primarily due to the lack of circulating neutrophils that inevitably follows bone marrow dysfunction that is either due to the disease or the treatment. Septicaemia may be the presenting feature, but it is much more common when the patient has received cytotoxic chemotherapy to induce a remission of the disease. Neutropenia, defined as a neutrophil count of $0.5 \times 10^9/\text{L}$, may persist for a few days to several weeks. Similarly, prolonged periods of neutropenia occur after bone marrow transplantation until engraftment has taken place.

The length of time over which the patient is neutropenic influences the nature of any associated infection and the frequency with which it occurs. For example, fungal infections are much more common in patients who are neutropenic for >21 days. Although gram-negative rods such as *Escherichia coli* and *P. aeruginosa* from the bowel flora have, in the past, been the most common cause of septicaemia in neutropenic patients, gram-positive organisms such as staphylococci, streptococci and enterococci are also important. *S. epidermidis* septicaemia associated with intravascular catheters (see earlier) is common. Infections caused by fungi are also increasing partly because more patients are surviving the early neutropenic period with the aid of modern antibacterial agents and granulocyte transfusions. Cytomegalovirus (CMV) infections may reactivate in the more intensive type of bone marrow transplantation known as allogeneic transplants in which the recipient receives bone marrow from a matched donor, compared with autologous transplants in which the patient receives their own stem cells, having received cytotoxic chemotherapy, for example. CMV reactivation is often associated with the development of graft-versus-host disease. The antiviral drug letermovir is effective as CMV prophylaxis when given to CMV IgG-positive recipients in the first 100 days postallogeneic transplant. In addition, adenovirus, Epstein-Barr virus (EBV), and BK virus (BKV) infections may be seen, especially in allogeneic bone marrow transplant recipients. Aciclovir prophylaxis is effective at preventing other latent herpesvirus infections such as herpes simplex virus (HSV) and varicella-zoster virus (VZV) from reactivating.

## Solid organ transplant infections

### Most infections occur within 3–4 months of transplantation

Suppression of a patient's cell-mediated immunity is necessary to prevent rejection of an engrafted organ, and the immunomodulatory regimens used will suppress humoral immunity to some extent as well. In addition, high doses of corticosteroids to suppress inflammatory responses are required. The combination of these factors results in a severely compromised host, and those that have an effect on infection in recipients of solid organ transplants include:

- the underlying medical condition of the patient
- the patient's previous immune status
- the type of organ transplant

**Table 31.3** Examples of opportunist pathogens in immunocompromised hosts

| Bacteria |
| --- |
| **Gram positive** |
| Staphylococcus aureus |
| Coagulase-negative staphylococci |
| Streptococci |
| Listeria spp. |
| Nocardia asteroides |
| Mycobacterium tuberculosis |
| Mycobacterium avium-intracellulare |
| **Gram negative** |
| Enterobacteriaceae |
| Pseudomonas aeruginosa |
| Legionella spp. |
| Bacteroides spp. |
| **Fungi** |
| Candida spp. |
| Aspergillus spp. |
| Cryptococcus neoformans |
| Histoplasma capsulatum |
| Pneumocystis jiroveci[a] |
| **Parasites** |
| Toxoplasma gondii |
| Strongyloides stercoralis |
| **Viruses** |
| Herpesviruses (e.g. HSV, CMV, VZV, EBV, HHV-6, HHV-7, HHV-8) |
| Hepatitis B |
| Hepatitis C |
| Polyomaviruses (e.g. BKV, JCV) |
| Adenoviruses |
| HIV |

[a]Formerly *P. carinii*.
BKV, BK virus; CMV, cytomegalovirus; EBV, Epstein-Barr virus; HIV, human immunodeficiency virus; HHV, human herpesvirus; HSV, herpes simplex virus; JCV, JC virus; VZV, varicella-zoster virus.

• the immunosuppressive regimen
• the exposure of the patient to pathogens.
The organisms that cause the most common and most severe infections are shown in Table 31.3. Some of the viral infections are latent and reactivate when cell-mediated surveillance is suppressed.

From 3 to 4 months after transplantation, the risk of infection is reduced but remains for as long as the patient is immunosuppressed.

### HIV infection leading to AIDS

**The clinical definition of AIDS includes the presence of one or more opportunistic infections**

Individuals with AIDS are often infected concomitantly with multiple pathogens, which they fail to eradicate despite prolonged, appropriate and aggressive antimicrobial chemotherapy. Most of the pathogens involved are intracellular pathogens that require an intact cell-mediated immune response for effective defence. As the HIV-infected individual progresses to AIDS (see Ch. 22), organisms that are usually controlled by cell-mediated immunity are able to reactivate to cause disseminated infections not seen in the immunologically intact individual. Improved immune surveillance as a result of combined antiretroviral therapy (cART) has reduced the incidence of infections that are the hallmark of AIDS, including *Candida*, Kaposi sarcoma (KS) and other opportunist pathogens described in more detail later.

Many of the pathogens that cause infections in the immunocompromised host (see Table 31.3) are described elsewhere in this book.

## OTHER IMPORTANT OPPORTUNIST PATHOGENS

### Fungi

The yeast *Candida* is an opportunist pathogen in a variety of patients and in various body sites. It is the cause of:

• vaginal and oral candidiasis (thrush) (see Ch. 22)
• skin infections (see Ch. 27)
• endocarditis, particularly in injecting drug users (see Ch. 30).
   *Candida* manifests itself in different ways depending on the nature of the underlying compromise:

• **Chronic mucocutaneous candidiasis.** This is rare and is a persistent but noninvasive infection of mucous membranes, hair, skin and nails in patients, often children, with a specific T-cell defect rendering them anergic to *Candida* (Fig. 31.7). The condition is associated with autoimmune endocrinopathies. Treatment is with azole drugs; repeated or long-term treatment may be required. Diminished sensitivity to these agents may occur after repeated use.
• **Oropharyngeal and oesophageal candidiasis.** This is seen in a variety of patients who are compromised, including HIV-infected individuals (Fig. 31.8) and those with haematologic malignancies; transplant recipients; people with ill-fitting dentures or diabetes mellitus or those on prolonged antibiotics or high-dose treatment with corticosteroids. Oropharyngeal candidiasis generally responds to treatment with antifungal mouthwashes (nystatin or an azole compound). Those individuals who do not respond

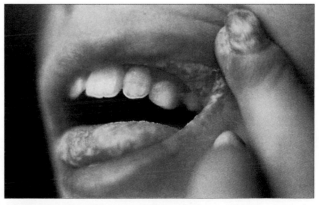

**Fig. 31.7** Chronic mucocutaneous candidiasis in a child with impaired T-cell response to antigens. (Courtesy M.J. Wood.)

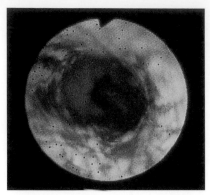

**Fig. 31.8** *Candida* oesophagitis. Endoscopic view showing extensive areas of whitish exudate. (Courtesy I. Chesner.)

can be treated with fluconazole. Oesophageal candidiasis requires systemic therapy, usually with fluconazole.

- **Gastrointestinal candidiasis.** This is seen in patients who have undergone major gastric or abdominal surgery and in those with neoplastic disease. The organism can pass through the intestinal wall and spread from a gastrointestinal focus. Antemortem diagnosis is difficult, and as many as 25% of patients do not have any symptoms in the early stages of disease. If there is dissemination from the gut, blood cultures may become positive, and *Candida* mannan antigens and anti-mannan antibody may be detectable in the serum. In addition, tests for beta-D-glucan are in common use, although this antigen occurs in many other fungi, so it is not specific for *Candida*. A high index of suspicion is required to initiate antifungal therapy early in these patients, but disseminated disease is often fatal.

- **Disseminated candidiasis.** This is probably acquired via the gastrointestinal tract but also arises from intravascular catheter-related infections. Patients with lymphoma and leukaemia, transplant recipients, and those on intensive care units are most at risk. Bloodborne spread to almost any organ can occur. Infections of the eye (endophthalmitis; Fig. 31.9) and the skin (nodular skin lesions) are important because they provide diagnostic clues, and without these the nonspecific symptoms of fever and septic shock make early diagnosis difficult. Immunocompromised patients are often given antifungal therapy blindly if they have a fever and fail to respond to broad-spectrum antibacterial agents. *Candida*

bloodstream infections are diagnosed by detection of yeast cells in blood cultures.

**Cryptococcus neoformans infection is most common in people with impaired cell-mediated immunity**

*C. neoformans* is an opportunistic yeast with a worldwide distribution. It can cause infection in the immunocompetent host, but infection is seen more frequently in people with impaired cell-mediated immunity. The onset of disease may be slow and usually results in lung infection or meningoencephalitis; occasionally other sites such as skin, bone and joints are involved.

*C. neoformans* can be demonstrated in the CSF and is characterized by its large polysaccharide capsule (see Fig. 25.6). Rapid identification can be made by antigen detection in a latex agglutination test using specific antibody-coated latex particles or with a lateral flow assay. Treatment involves a combination of fluconazole, amphotericin B and flucytosine (see Ch. 34). The prognosis depends largely upon the patient's underlying disease; in the severely immunocompromised, mortality is ~50% but may be >70% in low-income countries. Fluconazole can be given as posttreatment prophylaxis.

**Disseminated *Histoplasma capsulatum* infection may occur years after exposure in immunocompromised patients**

This is a highly infectious fungus that causes an acute but benign pulmonary infection in healthy people, but it can produce chronic progressive disseminated disease in the compromised host. The organism is distributed throughout the world and notably in the so-called histoplasmosis belt of the central United States, particularly in the Ohio and Mississippi river valleys. The fungus also lives in parts of Central and South America, Africa, Asia and Australia. The natural habitat of the organism is the soil. It is transmitted by the airborne route, and the fungal spores are deposited in the alveoli, from where the fungus spreads via the lymphatics to the regional lymph nodes. As disseminated disease may occur many years after the initial exposure in immunocompromised patients, it may present in patients who have long since left endemic areas. The infection may occur in HIV-positive individuals who have visited such regions.

Cultures of blood, bone marrow, sputum and CSF may yield *Histoplasma*, but culture can take an average of 2 weeks, or as long as 6–8 weeks, and sensitivity is low. Therefore biopsy and histologic examination of bone marrow, liver or lymph nodes is often required to make the diagnosis (Fig. 31.10). Serology

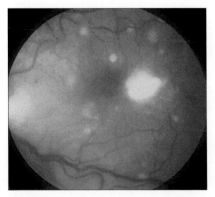

**Fig. 31.9** *Candida* endophthalmitis. Fundal photograph showing areas of white exudate. (Courtesy A.M. Geddes.)

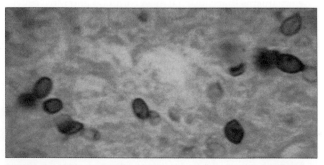

**Fig. 31.10** Histologic section of the lung showing yeast forms of *Histoplasma capsulatum* (methenamine silver stain). (Courtesy T.F. Sellers Jr.)

is of limited value in immunosuppressed patients. Antigen detection (e.g. *Histoplasma* galactomannan) is valuable in cases of disseminated histoplasmosis. Approximately 50% of cases of progressive disease in the immunocompromised are successfully treated with amphotericin followed by itraconazole.

African histoplasmosis, caused by *H. duboisii,* is found in Equatorial Africa. Patients may present with localized cutaneous or disseminated disease.

### Invasive aspergillosis has a very high mortality rate in the compromised patient

The role of *Aspergillus* spp. in diseases of the lung has been outlined in Chapter 20, but this fungus is also recognized as a cause of invasive disease in compromised patients, usually in profoundly neutropenic patients, those receiving high-dose corticosteroids and, increasingly, in recipients of allogeneic haematopoietic stem cell transplants and solid organ transplant recipients (Fig. 31.11). Like *Histoplasma,* aspergilli are found in soil and have a worldwide distribution. Infection is spread by the airborne route, and the lung is the site of invasion in almost every case. Dissemination to other sites, particularly the CNS (Fig. 31.12) and heart, occurs in ~25% of compromised individuals with lung infection. Serology is unhelpful in invasive aspergillosis. Diagnosis involves microscopy, culture, antigen detection and polymerase chain reaction (PCR) on bronchoalveolar lavage specimens. Galactomannan antigen detection is widely deployed. Lung biopsy may be required to make a tissue diagnosis as respiratory cultures for *Aspergillus* have low sensitivity.

Invasive aspergillosis has a high fatality rate in the compromised patient. Prophylactic antifungal agents, early diagnosis and institution of treatment (see Ch. 34), together with a reduction in corticosteroid and cytotoxic therapy wherever possible, appear to improve the prognosis. Antifungal therapy for invasive aspergillosis is with voriconazole, isavuconazole or posaconazole. Liposomal amphotericin B is an alternative. Outbreaks of hospital-acquired infection have been reported (see Ch. 37), especially in relation to recent building work.

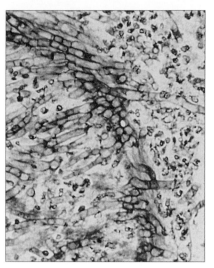

**Fig. 31.12** Numerous septate hyphae invading a blood vessel wall in cerebral aspergillosis (periodic acid-Schiff stain). (Courtesy W.E. Farrar.)

### *Pneumocystis jiroveci* (formerly *P. carinii*) causes symptomatic disease only in people with deficient cellular immunity

*P. jiroveci* is an atypical fungus, which appears to be widespread; a large proportion of the population has antibodies to the organism, but it only causes symptomatic disease in people whose cellular immune mechanisms are deficient. There is therefore a high incidence of *P. jiroveci* pneumonia in patients receiving immunosuppressive therapy to prevent transplant rejection and in individuals with HIV/AIDS. It is very rare to find *Pneumocystis* infection in any other site in the body, but the reason for this is unknown.

Diagnosis is not easy and requires a high index of suspicion. The symptoms are nonspecific and can mimic a variety of other infectious and noninfectious respiratory diseases. In addition, unlike the other fungi described earlier, the organism cannot be isolated in expectorated sputum using conventional culture methods. Induced sputum is tested initially, but it is often necessary to perform invasive techniques such as bronchoalveolar lavage. In samples obtained by these techniques, the organism can be demonstrated by silver or immunofluorescent stains (Fig. 31.13). DNA amplification by PCR in respiratory

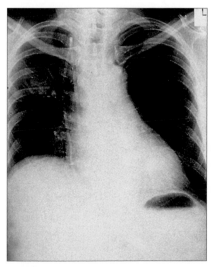

**Fig. 31.11** Chest radiograph showing invasive aspergillosis in the right lung of a patient with acute myeloblastic leukaemia. (Courtesy C. Kibbler.)

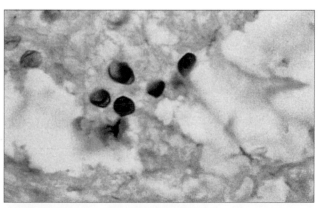

**Fig. 31.13** Darkly staining cysts of *Pneumocystis jiroveci* in an open lung biopsy from an AIDS patient with pneumonia (Grocott silver stain). (Courtesy M. Turner-Warwick.)

samples together with detection of β-D-glucan antigen in serum improves the sensitivity of the diagnostic tests.

Treatment is with high-dose co-trimoxazole (trimethoprim-sulfamethoxazole). Pentamidine is an alternative (see Ch. 34). Adjunctive corticosteroid therapy is given in moderate to severe infections in HIV-coinfected individuals. Co-trimoxazole is used prophylactically.

## Microsporidia

Infections with microsporidia cause diarrhoea in people with AIDS and in other immunosuppressed patients, especially in those whose CD4 count is <100. *Enterocytozoon bieneusi* is the most common cause, although *Encephalitozoon intestinalis* also occurs. Albendazole treatment is effective against *E. intestinalis* but has disappointing activity against *E. bieneusi*. When feasible, immune reconstitution is the mainstay of treatment.

## Bacteria

### *Nocardia asteroides* is an uncommon opportunist pathogen with a worldwide distribution

The family Actinomycetes, relatives of the mycobacteria but resembling fungi in that they form branching filaments, contains two pathogenic genera: *Actinomyces* and *Nocardia*. *N. asteroides* infections have been reported in immunocompromised, especially in renal transplant, patients. The lung is usually the primary site (Fig. 31.14), but infection can spread to the skin, kidney or CNS. As with *Aspergillus*, hospital outbreaks of nocardiosis have been described.

*Nocardia* can be isolated on routine laboratory media but is often slow to grow and is consequently easily overgrown by commensal flora. Therefore, the laboratory staff should be informed if nocardiosis is suspected clinically so that appropriate media are inoculated. The organism is a gram-negative branching rod and weakly acid fast (Fig. 31.15).

Sulphonamides or co-trimoxazole is the drug of choice, but treatment can be difficult, and various other regimens involving aminoglycosides or imipenem have been described.

### *Mycobacterium avium-intracellulare* consists of two mycobacterium species, *M. avium* and *M. intracellulare*

Although mycobacterial infections are well documented in immunosuppressed patients, the association between AIDS and mycobacteria includes disseminated infection not only with *M. tuberculosis* but also with *M. avium-intracellulare*

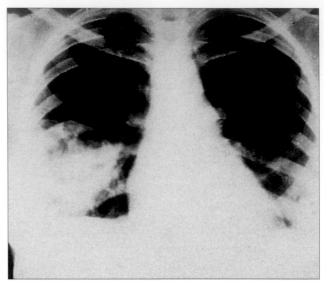

**Fig. 31.14** Pulmonary nocardiosis. Chest radiograph showing a large rounded lesion in the right lower zone with multiple cavities. (Courtesy T.F. Sellers Jr.)

(*M. avium* complex [MAC]). These organisms can be isolated from blood cultures from patients with AIDS. *M. tuberculosis* has been described in detail in Chapter 20. *M. avium-intracellulare* belongs to the so-called atypical mycobacteria or mycobacteria other than tuberculosis found in the environment (soil and water) and in animals. It resembles *M. tuberculosis* in that it is slow growing, but it is resistant to the conventional antituberculosis drugs. MAC causes lung disease, cervical lymphadenitis and disseminated disease. Inhalation is likely to lead to lung disease, and entry via the gastrointestinal tract is thought to be the main route in immunocompromised patients, especially with HIV infection. MAC invades and multiplies in macrophages and will disseminate in immuncompromised individuals. In those whose immune system is intact, there is cytokine release, including of interleukin-8 as well as further macrophage activation that will lead to intracellular killing of both MAC and granulomas.

Patients may present with fever, lymphadenopathy, tiredness and weight loss in general with breathlessness and chronic productive cough in pulmonary MAC (often with underlying lung disease) or abdominal pain and diarrhoea in

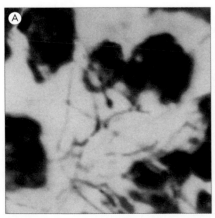
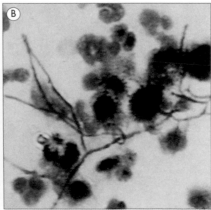

**Fig. 31.15** *Nocardia asteroides* in sputum. (A) Acid-fast stain. (B) Gram stain. (A, Courtesy T.F. Sellers Jr; B, courtesy H.P. Holley.)

disseminated disease (in the immunocompromised). Imaging, sputum and blood culture investigations are key; depending on the results, bone marrow aspirate for culture and bronchoscopy may be needed. Recommended multidrug therapy is to give in pulmonary disease with macrolides such as azithromycin or clarithromycin plus ethambutol and rifampicin or rifabutin. In severe disease and cavitating disease, streptomycin or amikacin is added. Treatment continues until a year after sputum conversion with two consecutive sputa tests. For disseminated MAC, azithromycin or clarithromycin and ethambutol treatment is advised initially, but if the patient is severely immunosuppressed, some of the other drugs mentioned earlier may be added. Some patients may require surgery, too, involving a lobectomy or pneumonectomy.

## Protozoa and helminths

### *Cryptosporidium* and *Cystoisospora belli* infections cause severe diarrhoea in AIDS

*Cryptosporidium* (Fig. 31.16) is a protozoan parasite that causes human disease and is well known to veterinarians as an animal pathogen. It causes significant but self-limiting diarrhoea in healthy people with an intact immune system (see Ch. 23) but leads to severe and chronic diarrhoea, with stool volumes as high as 17 L/day, in severely immunocompromised people (e.g. immunosuppressed transplant recipients or those living with advanced HIV infection). Combined active antiretroviral therapy (cART) in individuals with AIDS infected with *Cryptosporidium* has been reported to improve the diarrhoea symptoms. Paromomycin reduces oocyst output but does not clear infection. Nitazoxanide is effective in HIV-negative patients but is only partially active in those coinfected with HIV. *Cystoisospora belli* (Fig. 31.17) is another protozoan parasite very similar to *Cryptosporidium* and also produces severe diarrhoea in people with advanced HIV infection. Unlike *Cryptosporidium*, however, it responds to co-trimoxazole.

*Cyclospora cayetanensis*, also related to *Cryptosporidium*, likewise produces prolonged and severe diarrhoea in immunosuppressed individuals. Co-trimoxazole treatment is effective, whilst ciprofloxacin is partially effective.

### Immunosuppression may lead to reactivation of dormant *Strongyloides stercoralis*

*S. stercoralis* is a parasitic roundworm that remains dormant for years, probably for the life of the host, following initial

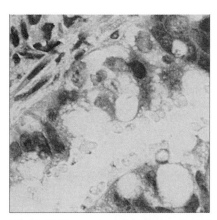

**Fig. 31.16** Numerous organisms in the brush border of the intestine in cryptosporidiosis. (Courtesy J. Newman.)

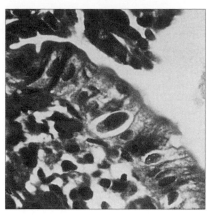

**Fig. 31.17** Human coccidiosis with a single *Cystoisospora belli* organism within an epithelial cell and a chronic inflammatory reaction in the lamina propria. (Courtesy G.N. Griffin.)

infection, but it may be reactivated by immunosuppression (e.g. with steroid therapy) to produce massive autoinfection, known as the *Strongyloides hyperinfection syndrome (SHS)*. HTLV type 1 infection is associated with disseminated strongyloidiasis due to the modified immune response to this enteric helminth. Considerable multiplication occurs, and the parasites disseminate widely beyond the intestine and lungs to involve the liver, brain, heart and urinary tract. Gram-negative bacteraemia is a recognized complication of SHS, and mortality is high. Although rare in the United Kingdom and most of the United States, *Strongyloides* should be borne in mind in patients who have lived in endemic areas such as the tropics and southern United States, even if this was many years before their immunosuppression.

## Viruses

### Certain virus infections are both more common and more severe in compromised patients, and regular surveillance is critical

The virus infections that are more common or more severe in the compromised patient (see Table 31.3) have been described in detail elsewhere in this book. Many of these represent reactivation of latent infections. Pretransplantation baseline serology is carried out to determine both the donor and recipient status for a number of virus infections, including HIV, HTLV, hepatitis B and C, CMV, EBV and HSV.

Suppression of specific virus infections using antiviral agents is part of the management of the recipient in conjunction with regular virologic surveillance posttransplantation using viral genome detection methods that have superseded antigen detection.

As part of a preemptive treatment strategy, blood samples are collected for early detection of viraemia or antigenaemia, which precedes disease. For example, transplant donors and recipients are screened for CMV IgG. CMV causes a broad spectrum of clinical disease in this setting, including pneumonitis, oesophagitis, colitis, hepatitis and encephalitis. If there is a transplant mismatch (i.e. the donor is CMV IgG positive and the recipient CMV IgG negative), the infection may be acquired from the donor organ or bone marrow. If possible, transplant centres try to avoid this situation, as the risk of a primary CMV infection in the first month posttransplantation is extremely high as is the morbidity and mortality. In this case, CMV DNA monitoring is carried out on blood samples on a regular basis posttransplantation to detect early infection and start antiviral therapy as soon as possible. A primary CMV infection is usually detected at 4 weeks posttransplantation compared with reactivation at 6–8 weeks. Some centres involved in solid organ transplantation offer antiviral therapy in the immediate posttransplant period in this clinical setting to delay the onset of infection to a time when the recipient is less immunosuppressed.

CMV IgG-positive recipients are at risk of reactivation and need to be monitored regularly posttransplantation. Letermovir, a nonnucleoside antiviral drug that targets the later stage of CMV replication by inhibiting the viral terminase complex, was licensed in 2017 to prevent CMV reactivation in CMV IgG-positive allogeneic bone marrow transplant recipients.

Antiviral prophylaxis for HSV reactivation that may occur in the immediate posttransplantation period is often given to bone marrow transplant recipients for prolonged periods posttransplantation. Aciclovir is given at a low dose and is effective in preventing HSV and VZV reactivation. Virus surveillance is therefore not carried out, but if a breakthrough infection occurs, it is important to collect material from the lesions for virus isolation or genome sequence analysis to determine the antiviral susceptibility. Herpetic lesions can be persistent and involve the lips, oesophagus and other parts of the gastrointestinal tract and may cause a pneumonitis, hepatitis or encephalitis.

Herpes zoster, a reactivation of VZV infection, may occur within a few months posttransplantation, affecting the skin dermatome supplied by the involved nerve. Sometimes the distribution may be multidermatomal, and dissemination can occur to other sites.

Human herpesvirus 6 (HHV-6) and HHV-7 infection, reinfection, or reactivation has been reported in transplant recipients, in particular with neurologic conditions, including encephalitis. HHV-8 has been associated with the development of KS in individuals with AIDS as well as classic and endemic KS in HIV-negative individuals. If a recipient or donor has had a hepatitis B virus (HBV) infection previously, antiviral prophylaxis with lamivudine, tenofovir or entecavir is also given to prevent reactivation. HBsAg and HBV DNA monitoring is also carried out on blood samples.

### EBV infection can lead to tumour development

EBV infection has been associated with the development of Hodgkin disease, non-Hodgkin lymphomas in HIV-positive individuals, posttransplantation lymphoproliferative disease and smooth muscle tumours in immunosuppressed children. EBV has a broad spectrum of clinical syndromes ranging from infectious mononucleosis to malignancies, which include EBV-associated posttransplant lymphoproliferative disorder (PTLD), containing clonal chromosomal abnormalities with a high mortality rate, especially with the monoclonal tumours. The risk factors recognized for PTLD development in solid organ transplant recipients include posttransplantation primary EBV infection, mismatched donor and recipient CMV status, CMV disease and intensity and type of immunosuppressive therapy. With respect to EBV infection, EBV-susceptible recipients have a tenfold to seventy-six fold higher risk of PTLD compared with recipients with previous EBV exposure.

As the two peaks of primary EBV infection are in children and adolescents, the incidence of PTLD is higher in paediatric transplant recipients. In addition, without an effective cytotoxic T-cell response owing to posttransplant immunosuppression to prevent graft rejection, the EBV-infected B lymphocytes may proliferate in an uncontrolled fashion. This results in B-cell hyperplasia with CD20-positive lymphocytes that ranges from polyclonal and benign to development of a monoclonal or oligoclonal B-cell lymphoma. The prevalence of PTLD in paediatric liver transplant recipients ranges from 4 to 14%, depending on the immunosuppressive regimen. Retrospective studies have shown that up to 50% of paediatric transplant recipients with primary EBV infections are at risk of developing PTLD. The infection may be acquired in the community or in the transplant setting from the donor organ or blood products. The natural history of EBV infection and pathophysiology of posttransplant EBV-driven lymphoproliferation is not well understood.

Diagnostic criteria for EBV-associated PTLD have been developed. However, in the absence of randomized, placebo-controlled trials, there is little information on the efficacy of specific treatment protocols. The treatment of PTLD includes reducing immunosuppression to allow a better host response to control the infection, although there is a risk of rejecting the graft, using rituximab, an anti-CD20 monoclonal antibody that targets the B cells with the EBV receptor, and chemotherapy. Treatment of posttransplant lymphomas by adoptive transfer of EBV-specific cytotoxic T lymphocytes has been reported.

### Respiratory virus infections

Immunocompromised patients, especially transplant recipients, are at increased risk of pneumonia and death if they develop respiratory tract infections with viruses such as SARS-CoV-2, influenza, respiratory syncytial virus (RSV), parainfluenza and adenoviruses. Preventive measures include influenza and SARS-CoV-2 (COVID) immunisation, prophylaxis with palivizumab, an RSV-specific monoclonal antibody that is used in specific clinical settings, and early diagnosis of an upper respiratory tract infection using sensitive tests such as viral genome detection. There are some specific antiviral treatments that include oseltamivir for influenza and ribavirin for RSV infections.

### Adenovirus infection has a high mortality rate

Primary and reactivated adenovirus infections can result in disseminated disease in immunocompromised hosts, in particular paediatric and adult bone marrow transplant recipients. Hepatitis and pneumonia are most frequently reported. Again, adenovirus surveillance is often carried out in centres by collecting blood samples posttransplantation, which are tested for adenovirus DNA to detect early viraemia. Where adenovirus viraemia is detected, management options include reducing immunosuppression and treating with an antiviral agent such as cidofovir (or ribavirin if cidofovir is contraindicated). However, there are few reports of successful outcomes in patients with disseminated infections.

### Hepatitis B and C infection in transplant recipients

HBV infection has an immunopathologic pathogenesis, with jaundice occurring after cytotoxic T cells have lysed the hepatitis B surface antigen–bearing hepatocytes. The virus is integrated in the hepatocytes after acute hepatitis B. Bone marrow transplant recipients with evidence of previous, not current, hepatitis B infection are likely to suffer a hepatitis B reactivation posttransplantation. They will be asymptomatic as they are immunosuppressed and will not mount a cytotoxic T-cell response until they have engrafted. It is at that stage they will become symptomatic, develop jaundice, and the morbidity and mortality can be high. Antiviral prophylaxis with antiviral agents such as lamivudine, tenofovir or entecavir is given to prevent reactivation, together with HBV DNA monitoring. Antiviral treatment will be given pre- and posttransplant if a transplant recipient has a current HBV infection (i.e. is hepatitis B surface antigen positive).

Hepatitis C overtook hepatitis B as the main viral cause of cirrhosis leading to liver transplantation when antiviral treatment options for hepatitis B became available. HCV-infected individuals with advanced liver disease can be treated with direct-acting antivirals and may not need a liver transplant.

HCV infection is also associated with venoocclusive disease in bone marrow transplant recipients. Venous congestion occurs in the liver, owing to a nonspecific vasculitis, and results in liver necrosis. Multiorgan failure can be precipitated because of increased capillary permeability throughout the body.

### Polyomaviruses can cause haemorrhagic cystitis and progressive multifocal leukoencephalopathy

BK or JC viruses are polyomaviruses acquired via the respiratory tract that lie latent in the kidney and may be detected in the urine of bone marrow transplant recipients (see Ch. 21). BK viraemia and viruria are associated with haemorrhagic cystitis. Reduction of immunosuppression, supportive care with bladder washouts when clots form and, in rare occasions, intravesical cidofovir may be indicated. Cidofovir treatment has been shown to be ineffective in a number of controlled studies.

JC virus can reactivate and disseminate to cause CNS infections such as progressive multifocal leukoencephalopathy (PML) in individuals with AIDS. However, since the advent of cART, resulting in higher CD4 counts and suppressed HIV load, PML is seen less often.

## KEY FACTS

- A compromised person is one whose normal defences against infection are defective. Immunodeficiencies may involve the innate or adaptive immune systems and may be primary or secondary.

- Compromised patients can be infected with any of the pathogens capable of infecting immunocompetent individuals. In addition, they suffer many infections caused by opportunist pathogens. The type of infection is related to the nature of the compromise.

- Effective antimicrobial therapy is often difficult to achieve in the absence of a functional immune response, even when the pathogen is susceptible to the drug in vitro.

- Important bacterial opportunists include *P. aeruginosa*, especially in neutropenic patients and those with major

burns, and *S. epidermidis* in patients with plastic devices in situ. In AIDS, the predominant bacterial opportunists are intracellular pathogens benefiting from the lack of cell-mediated immunity.

- Neutropenia following cytotoxic therapy and in advanced HIV infection (AIDS) predisposes to fungal infections (e.g. *Candida*, *Aspergillus* and *Cryptococcus*), especially when the patient has received previous antibacterial therapy.

- Viral infections are more common and severe in immunodeficient patients than in immunocompetent patients, particularly reactivation of latent infections (e.g. HSV, CMV, BKV).

# Diagnosis and Control

**32.** Diagnosis of infection and assessment of host defence mechanisms     468

**33.** Epidemiology and control of infectious diseases     485

**34.** Attacking the enemy: antimicrobial agents and chemotherapy     495

**35.** Protecting the host: vaccination     540

**36.** Specific and nonspecific immunotherapy     559

**37.** Infection control     567

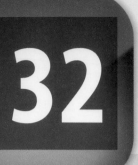

# Diagnosis of infection and assessment of host defence mechanisms

## Introduction

### Good-quality specimens are needed for reliable microbiologic diagnoses

The precise identification of the causative organism in infection has become increasingly important now that therapeutic intervention is possible. The ability to achieve this depends upon a positive interaction between the clinician and the microbiologist; the clinician must be aware of the complexity of the tests and the time required to achieve a result. In turn, the microbiologist must appreciate the nature of the patient's condition and be able to assist the clinician in interpreting the laboratory report. A fundamental step in any diagnosis is the choice of an appropriate specimen, which ultimately depends upon an understanding of the pathogenesis of infections.

Microbiology differs from other clinical laboratory disciplines in the amount of interpretative input required. When a specimen is received, decisions are made regarding the appropriate processing pathway, and when the result is received, it must be interpreted in relation to the specimen and the patient.

## AIMS OF THE CLINICAL MICROBIOLOGY LABORATORY

The aims of the microbiology laboratory are:

- to provide accurate information about the presence or absence of microorganisms in a specimen that may be involved in a patient's disease process
- to provide accurate information about the presence or absence of antibodies in a serum sample to help in the diagnosis of an acute or past infection
- to assess the response to treatment by measuring, for example, the viral load in the relevant sample
- to provide information on the antimicrobial susceptibility of the microorganisms isolated or detected by polymerase chain reaction (PCR) and sequence analysis where relevant.

### Identification is achieved by detecting the microorganism or its products or the patient's immune response

Laboratory tests are performed to detect (1) microorganisms or their products in specimens collected from the patient and (2) evidence of the patient's immune response (production of antibodies or T cell response) to infection. Although there are different protocols for different specimens (urine, faeces, genital tract, blood, etc.), the tests fall into three main categories:

1. *Identification of microorganisms by isolation and culture.* Microorganisms may grow in artificial media or, in the case of viruses, in cell cultures. In some instances, quantification is important (e.g. $>10^5$ bacteria/mL of urine is indicative of infection whereas lower numbers are not; see Ch. 21). Once an organism has been isolated in culture, its susceptibility to antimicrobial agents can be determined.

2. *Identification of a specific microbial gene or product.* Nonculture techniques that do not depend upon the growth and multiplication of microorganisms to detect them have the potential to yield more rapid results. These techniques include the detection of structural components of the cell (e.g. cell wall antigens) and extracellular products (e.g. toxins). Alternatively, molecular approaches are available such as the detection of specific gene sequences in clinical specimens using DNA probes or the polymerase chain reaction (PCR; see later). They are potentially applicable to all microorganisms, but actual antimicrobial susceptibilities cannot be determined without culture, although the presence of resistance genes may be detectable using molecular methods.

3. *Detection of specific antibodies to a pathogen.* This is especially important when the pathogen cannot be cultivated in laboratory media (e.g. *Treponema pallidum*, many viruses and many parasites) or when culture would be particularly hazardous to laboratory staff (e.g. culture of *Francisella tularensis*, the cause of tularaemia, or the fungus *Coccidioides immitis*). Detection of IgM and/or IgG antibodies in a single serum collected during the acute phase of illness can be helpful in diagnosis of, for example, rubella by specific IgM, hepatitis A by IgM and hepatitis B by hepatitis B surface antigen or in rare diseases such as Lassa fever. The classic diagnostic method is by detection of a rise (fourfold or greater) in antibody titre between paired sera, collected in the acute phase of an infection (5–7 days after onset of symptoms) and in convalescence (e.g. after 3–4 weeks). Such tests therefore tend to result in a delayed or retrospective diagnosis and are therefore of limited help for clinical management.

## SPECIMEN PROCESSING

### Specimen handling and interpretation of results is based upon a knowledge of normal microbiota and contaminants

Specimens intended for cultivation of microorganisms can be divided into two types:

- those from sites that are normally sterile
- those from sites that usually have commensal microorganisms (Box 32.1; see also Ch. 9).

A thorough knowledge of the microorganisms normally isolated from specimens from nonsterile sites and the common contaminants of specimens collected from sterile sites is important to ensure that specimens are properly handled and the results are correctly interpreted. Some specimens from sites that are normally considered sterile (e.g. bladder urine, sputum from the lower respiratory tract) are usually collected after passage through orifices that have a normal flora, which may contaminate the specimens. This needs to be considered when interpreting the culture results of these specimens.

In an ideal world, each specimen arriving in the laboratory would be considered, in turn, together with the information provided about the patient on the request form so that the microbiologist could assess the pathogens likely to be present and devise an individualized processing plan. In reality, however, this approach is not practical because of constraints on time and money. Thus specimens tend to be processed by type (e.g. urine, blood, faeces), and the microbiologist looks for easily cultivated pathogens known to be associated with each sample type. However, if the laboratory is provided with suitable information, such as a history of international travel and a statement of possible aetiology, more fastidious or unusual pathogens can be sought and relevant antibiotic susceptibilities assessed. To obtain a test result that correctly identifies the infection, it is important to collect an appropriate specimen, to use the appropriate transport conditions and to deliver specimens rapidly to the laboratory. These conditions all affect the accuracy of the laboratory report and therefore its value to the clinician and ultimately to the patient. Key points to remember about specimen collection are summarized in Box 32.2.

### Routine culture takes at least 18 h to produce a result

Time is a key factor because the conventional methods of microbiologic diagnosis depend upon growth and identification of the pathogen. Reliable results of routine bacterial culture cannot be achieved in <18 h and may take much longer (e.g. several weeks) for a minority of pathogens such as the mycobacteria, which grow very slowly. Antibiotic susceptibility tests involve a further incubation period. Thus specimen processing can be categorized according to the time required to achieve a result and the method—cultural or noncultural. An alternative, more immediate route to the diagnosis of an infection is an immunologic one, relying on the detection of an antibody response to the putative pathogen in the patient's blood, or a molecular one such as PCR and nucleic acid probes (see later).

---

**Box 32.1    Sampling Sites, the Normal Microbiota and Interpretation of Results**

**Body sites that are normally sterile**

- Blood and bone marrow
- Cerebrospinal fluid
- Serous fluids
- Tissues
- Lower respiratory tract
- Bladder

**Body sites that have normal commensal organisms**

- Mouth, nose and upper respiratory tract
- Skin
- Gastrointestinal tract
- Female genital tract
- Urethra

Some sites in the body are sterile in health so that growth of any organism is indicative of infection provided that the specimen has been properly collected, transported and examined in the laboratory without delay. The significance of isolates from sites that have a commensal flora depends upon the identity of the isolate and the quantity as well as the immune status of the patient.

---

**Box 32.2    Important Steps in Specimen Collection and Delivery to the Laboratory**

- Take the appropriate specimen (e.g. blood and cerebrospinal fluid in suspected meningitis).
- Collect the specimen at the appropriate time during the acute phase of the disease (e.g. virus isolation, viral genome detection, IgM detection).
- If possible, collect the specimen before the patient receives anti-microbial treatment.
- Collect enough material and an adequate number of samples (e.g. enough blood/serum for more than one set of blood cultures).
- Avoid contamination: from normal flora (e.g. midstream urine from nonsterile equipment).
- Use the correct containers and appropriate transport media.
- Label specimens properly.
- Complete request form with enough clinical information, including a history of recent travel and a statement of possible aetiology.
- Inform the laboratory if special tests are required.
- Transport specimens rapidly to the laboratory.

Responsibility does not end with collection of the specimen and requesting tests. Good communication with the microbiologist is essential.

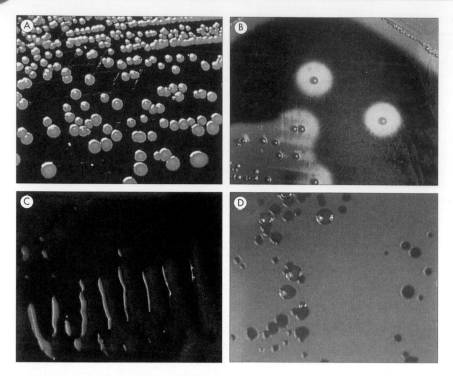

**Fig. 32.1** Bacterial colonies. A bacterial cell implanted on a solid nutrient medium will multiply to produce a colony containing millions of cells. Different species produce characteristically different colonies, and this feature can be used as a preliminary clue to the identity of the organism. (A) Golden colonies of *Staphylococcus aureus*. (B) Additional features such as the ability to lyse red blood cells can be demonstrated by culturing bacteria on blood-containing media. Here, beta haemolysis (complete haemolysis) is produced by *Streptococcus pyogenes* on blood agar. (C) Culture media can be made selective by including agents that are inhibitory to some species. For example, MacConkey agar contains bile salts so only those organisms tolerant to bile will grow. In addition, it contains lactose and a pH indicator. Species that ferment lactose change the indicator to bright pink. (D) Nonlactose-fermenting species, such as *Salmonella* and *Shigella*, form yellowish colonies.

## CULTIVATION (CULTURE) OF MICROORGANISMS

### Bacteria and fungi can be cultured on solid nutrient or liquid media

While cultures can be made in liquid media (broth), it is not possible to tell whether there is more than one species present. Therefore solid media are more useful in diagnostic microbiology. Bacteria and fungi grow on the surface of solid nutrient media (agar-based) to produce colonies composed of thousands of cells derived from a single cell implanted on the surface. Colonies of different species often have characteristic appearances, which can give a clue to their likely identity (Fig. 32.1).

### Different species of bacteria and fungi have different growth requirements

It is possible to grow the majority of species of bacteria and fungi of medical importance in artificial media in the laboratory, but there is no single culture medium that will support the growth of them all, and there are still some species that can be grown only in experimental animals (e.g. *Mycobacterium leprae* and *Treponema pallidum*). Some bacteria that cannot be cultivated on artificial media (e.g. *Chlamydia* and *Rickettsia*) can be grown in cell cultures (see later).

Many culture media are designed not only to support the growth of the desired organisms but also to inhibit the growth of others (i.e. they are selective media).

Specimens collected from body sites that have a normal commensal microbiota will contain a mixture of organisms from which the pathogen has to be recognized. Specimens are plated out on a carefully chosen range of nutrient and selective media to produce single colonies to ensure a pure culture. These are subcultured to fresh media for identification and antibiotic susceptibility tests (see later), a procedure that can take ≥48 h by conventional (nonmolecular) approaches.

Parasites such as *Leishmania* and *Trichomonas* can be cultivated in liquid media to allow small numbers present in the original specimen (e.g. bone marrow or vaginal secretions) to multiply and thus become easier to detect by microscopic examination. *Strongyloides* can be grown from faeces applied to a nutrient agar plate, but parasites do not form colonies on solid media in the same way as bacteria and fungi.

### Growth of viruses *Chlamydia* and *Rickettsia* requires cell or tissue cultures

This is because these organisms are incapable of a free-living existence. Cell cultures used are human or animal cells adapted to growth in vitro that can be stored at −80°C until required. The specimen is introduced into the cell culture medium where growth/replication ultimately allows detection. Cell culture techniques are specialized and labour intensive and take time to produce an observed result (>1 week for cytomegalovirus). Therefore alternative methods such as antigen and antibody detection (see later) and PCR-based approaches are important for diagnosis.

## IDENTIFICATION OF MICROORGANISMS GROWN IN CULTURE

### Bacteria are identified by simple characteristics and biochemical properties

A preliminary identification of many of the bacteria of medical importance has traditionally been made on the basis of the following few simple characteristics of the cells (Fig. 32.2):

- Gram reaction
- cell morphology (e.g. rod or coccus) and arrangement (e.g. pairs or chains)
- ability to grow under aerobic or anaerobic conditions
- growth requirements (simple or fastidious).

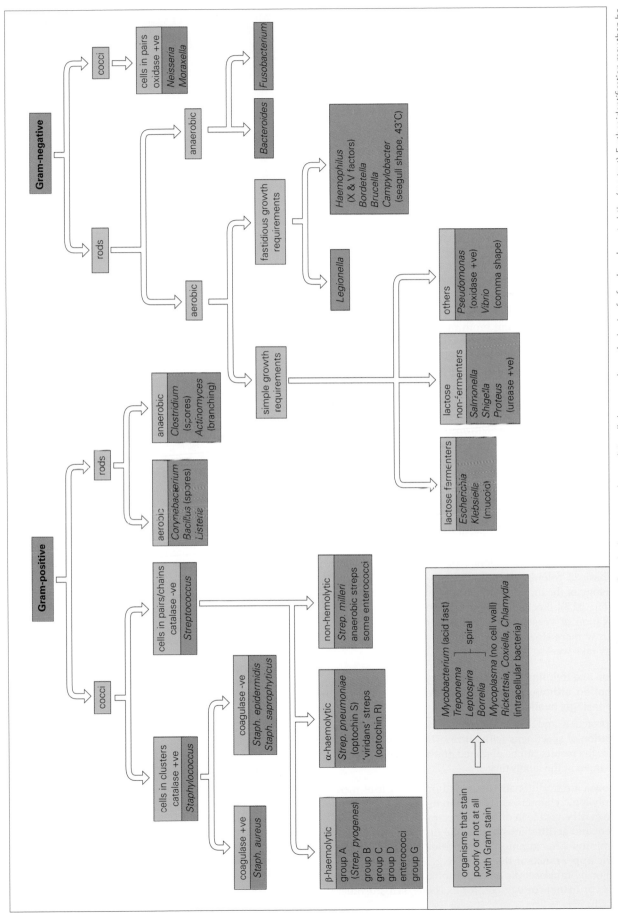

**Fig. 32.2** Identifying bacteria. The preliminary investigation of the bacteria of medical importance has traditionally been made on the basis of a few key characteristics (see text). Further identification may then be made on the basis of biochemical and serologic tests.

Further identification is made on the basis of biochemical properties such as:

- the ability to produce enzymes that can be detected by simple tests
- the ability to metabolize sugars via an oxidative pathway or by fermentation (aerobically or anaerobically)
- the ability to use a range of substrates for growth (e.g. glucose, lactose, sucrose).

While these tests were historically done individually (e.g. in broth media containing the specifically required reagents), they are now commonly performed using commercial kits or automated systems that have the potential to give a rapid (e.g. 2–4 h) indication of pathogen identity based on biochemical profiles.

Some species are identified on the basis of their antigens by reacting cell suspensions with specific antisera.

### Antibiotic susceptibility can be accurately determined only after the bacteria have been isolated in a pure culture

A variety of methods are available for antimicrobial susceptibility testing, including broth microdilution and automated instrument approaches. However, the most widely used method assesses antibiotic susceptibility by applying filter paper disks that contain different antibiotics onto a lawn of the test organism that has been seeded onto an agar plate (i.e. disk diffusion). During overnight incubation, the organisms grow and multiply, and the antibiotics diffuse out from the disks and inhibit growth around the disk. Therefore after isolation of bacteria from a specimen, a further incubation period (overnight for disk diffusion testing) is required before antibiotic susceptibility results are available. Methods for antibiotic susceptibility tests are described in more detail in Chapter 34.

### Fungi are identified by their colonial characteristics and cell morphology

Fungi are identified from colonies or pure cultures largely on the basis of colonial characteristics (e.g. colour) and the morphology of the individual cells viewed under the microscope (Fig. 32.3). Biochemical tests can be used for detailed identification of yeasts of medical importance. In general, fungi grow more slowly than bacteria, and final identification may take weeks.

### Protozoa and helminths are identified by direct examination, although newer molecular methods are increasingly available

Many protozoa and parasites can be identified by direct examination of specimens without resorting to culture, and therefore the results can be obtained on the day of receipt of the specimen in the laboratory.

- Protozoa are traditionally identified on the basis of their morphologic characteristics—different stages of the life cycle may be visible in different specimens from the same patient and at different stages in the disease (Fig. 32.4).
- Helminths are commonly identified by the macroscopic appearance of the worm (e.g. *Ascaris* or *Enterobius*) or by microscopic examination of specimens (e.g. faeces or urine) for eggs of, for example, schistosomes (see Ch. 23).

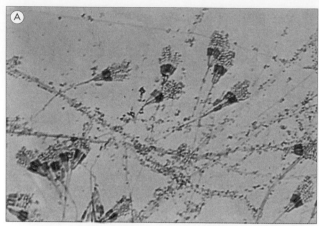

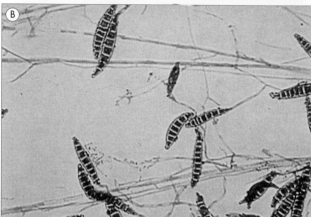

**Fig. 32.3** Fungi under the microscope. Fungi can be grown on agar culture media in the same way as bacteria, but most species grow much more slowly than bacteria and it may take weeks for a colony to form. Colonial characteristics (such as colour) are helpful in the identification of fungi, but confirmation depends upon microscopic examination of the hyphae and sporing structures. (A) *Penicillium* in a wet preparation showing the conidiophores and free conidia. (B) Macroconidia of *Microsporum canis* stained with lactophenol cotton blue.

However, microscopy may miss low numbers of cysts, ova and larvae in clinical specimens, is labour intensive and requires significant technical expertise. The introduction of molecular approaches has improved diagnosis over traditional methods, especially for malaria, leishmaniasis and giardiasis.

### Viruses are usually identified using serologic and nucleic acid–based tests

A number of viruses are identified by nucleic-acid-based tests (e.g. PCR; see below), as well as detection of viral antigens and the presence of specific antibodies in the patient's serum (see below).

### Mass spectrometry heralds a novel diagnostic era

One of the most promising approaches to the identification of bacteria and fungi involves the use of mass spectrometry or, more specifically, matrix-assisted laser desorption–ionization time-of-flight mass spectrometry (MALDI-TOF). MALDI-TOF is being increasingly used for the identification of microbial pathogens through analysis of their predominant mass spectral protein fingerprints, which can then be compared with established databases of known organisms.

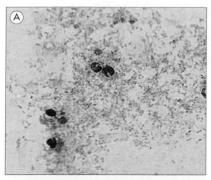

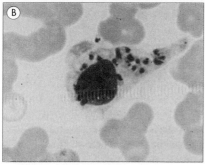

**Fig. 32.4** Although some parasites can be cultivated in the laboratory, identification is usually based on microscopic appearances in the specimen. (A) Acid-fast stain of *Cryptosporidium* in faeces. Like mycobacteria, this organism is able to retain the pink carbol fuchsin stain when challenged with acid alcohol. (B) *Leishmania donovani* (Leishman-Donovan bodies) in a stained preparation from a specimen of bone marrow.

## NONCULTURAL TECHNIQUES FOR THE LABORATORY DIAGNOSIS OF INFECTION

### Noncultural techniques do not require microorganism multiplication before detection

Although medical microbiology has long been synonymous with the cultivation of microorganisms from patient specimens, these techniques are labour intensive and slow to produce results (days rather than hours) because replication of organisms is a necessary but rate-limiting step. In addition, some microorganisms cannot be cultured in artificial media, and viable organisms may be difficult to recover from specimens of patients who have received antimicrobial therapy. Noncultural techniques do not require multiplication of the microorganism before its detection. Techniques such as microscopy, detection of microbial antigens in specimens (especially DNA probes) and amplification of DNA by PCR provide a rapid answer (e.g. minutes to hours).

### Microscopy

#### Microscopy is an important first step in the examination of specimens

Microscopy plays a fundamental role in microbiology. Although microorganisms show a wide range in size (see Ch. 1), they are too small to be seen individually by the naked eye, and therefore a microscope is an essential tool in microbiology. The light microscope magnifies objects and therefore improves the resolving power of the naked eye from about 100,000 nm (0.1 mm) to 200 nm; although not routinely used in the clinical microbiology laboratory, the electron microscope can improve this to 0.1–1.0 nm.

### Light microscopy

#### Bright field microscopy is used to examine specimens and cultures as wet or dry (stained) preparations

Bright field microscopy is used to demonstrate:

- blood cells and pathogens in fluid specimens (wet preparations) such as urine, faeces or cerebrospinal fluid (CSF)
- cysts, ova, larvae and parasites in faeces (wet and stained preparations)
- fungi in skin (wet and stained preparations)
- blood and tissue protozoa and helminths (wet and stained preparations).

Living organisms can be examined to detect motility.

Dyes are used to stain cells so that they can be seen more easily. Stains are usually applied to dried material that has been fixed (by heat or alcohol) onto the microscope slide. Samples from specimens themselves, or pure cultures, can be stained. The slide can then be viewed in the light microscope with an oil immersion lens, which improves the resolving power of the microscope. Correct configuration of the microscope (e.g. for Köhler illumination, a specific way of ensuring correct illumination and optimal image resolution) is essential, especially when observing the internal structure of suspected protozoal cysts.

#### The most important differential staining technique in bacteriology is the Gram stain

Differential staining procedures exploit the fact that cells with different properties stain differently and thus can be distinguished. Based on their reaction to Gram stain (Fig. 32.5), bacteria are divided into two broad groups:

- gram positive (stain purple)
- gram negative (stain pink).

This difference is related to differences in the structure of the cell walls of the two groups (see Ch. 2).

#### Acid-fast stains are used to detect mycobacteria

Some organisms, particularly mycobacteria, which have waxy cell walls, do not readily take up the Gram stain. To demonstrate their presence, special staining techniques are used that rely on the ability of such organisms to retain the stain in the presence of decolourizing agents such as acid and alcohol. The Ziehl–Neelsen stain (see Fig. 20.30) is a classic differential staining procedure that uses heat to drive the fuchsin stain into the cells; mycobacteria stained with fuchsin withstand decolourization with acid and alcohol and are therefore known as acid and alcohol fast (typically abbreviated AFB: acid-fast bacteria), whereas other bacteria lose the stain after acid and alcohol treatment. Alternatively, many laboratories use a fluorescent auramine-rhodamine stain, which has a strong affinity for the waxy cell wall of mycobacteria, to demonstrate these organisms by fluorescence microscopy (Fig. 32.6).

#### Other staining techniques can be used to demonstrate particular features of cells

Examples of such features to aid identification include stains to detect bacterial spores, polymetaphosphate storage (volutin) granules in *Corynebacterium* spp. (dark spots in blue-green cells using Albert stain) and lipid storage granules in *Bacillus* spp. stained with Sudan black (black lipid against red cells).

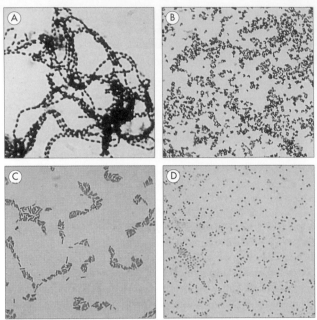

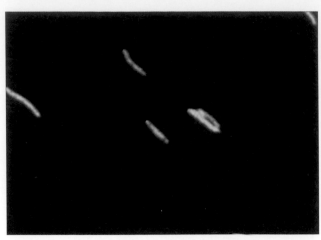

**Fig. 32.6** Fluorochrome stain of *Mycobacterium tuberculosis* with a mixture of auramine O and rhodamine B. Mycobacteria appear fluorescent under ultraviolet light. (Courtesy D.K. Banerjee.)

**Fig. 32.5** The Gram stain is the most important stain for studying bacteria. The combination of the violet dye (crystal violet) and iodine (acting as a mordant) binds to the cell wall. Gram-positive cells retain the stain when challenged with acetone and remain purple. Gram-negative cells lose the purple stain and appear colourless until stained with a pink counterstain (neutral red or safranin). Examination of Gram-stained films also allows the shape of the cells to be noted. Some examples are shown: (A) gram-positive cocci in chains (*Streptococci*); (B) gram-positive rods (*Listeria*); (C) gram-negative rods (*Escherichia coli*); (D) gram-negative cocci (*Neisseria*).

### Dark field (dark ground) microscopy is useful for observing motility and thin cells such as spirochetes

The light microscope may be adapted by modifying the condenser so that the object appears brightly lit against a dark background. Living organisms can be examined by dark field microscopy and thus motility can be observed. The method is also used for visualizing very thin cells such as spirochetes because the light reflected from the surface of the cells makes them appear larger and therefore more easily visible than when examined by bright field microscopy (Fig. 32.7).

### Phase contrast microscopy increases the contrast of an image

This technique enhances the very small differences in refractive index and density between living cells and the fluid in which they are suspended and therefore produces an image with a higher degree of contrast than that achieved by bright field microscopy.

### Fluorescence microscopy is used for substances that are either naturally fluorescent or have been stained with fluorescent dyes

If light of one wavelength shines on a fluorescent object, it emits light of a different wavelength. Some biologic substances are naturally fluorescent; others can be stained with fluorescent dyes and viewed in a microscope with an ultraviolet light source instead of white light (see Fig. 32.6).

Fluorescence microscopy is widely used in microbiology and immunology and has been developed to detect microbial antigens in specimens and tissues by staining with specific antibodies tagged with fluorescent dyes

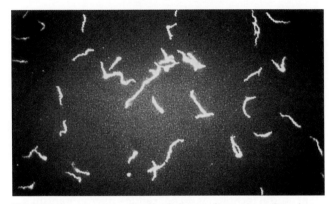

**Fig. 32.7** Spirochetes visualized by dark ground microscopy. Spirochetes and leptospires are much thinner than most bacterial cells (~0.1 μm in diameter compared with 1 μm for *Escherichia coli*), but they appear larger when viewed by dark ground illumination.

(immunofluorescence). The method can be made more sensitive or can be adapted to the detection of antibody by labelling a second antibody in an indirect test (Fig. 32.8).

## Electron microscopy

### Although not routinely used in the clinical laboratory, electron microscopy provides the ultimate in microbe visualization, which can aid in microbe identification

The electron microscope uses a beam of electrons instead of light, and magnets are used to focus the beam instead of the lenses used in a light microscope. The whole system is operated under a high vacuum. Electron beams penetrate poorly, and a single microbial cell is too thick to be viewed directly. To overcome this, the specimen is fixed and mounted in plastic and cut into thin sections that are examined individually. Electron-dense stains such as osmium tetroxide, or uranyl acetate, are applied to the specimen to improve contrast. The electrons pass through the section and produce an image on a fluorescent screen. Alternatively, electrons interact with the specimen at an angle to produce a view in three dimensions (scanning electron microscopy). In either case, images are photographed and enlarged so that the original specimen is magnified many thousand-fold.

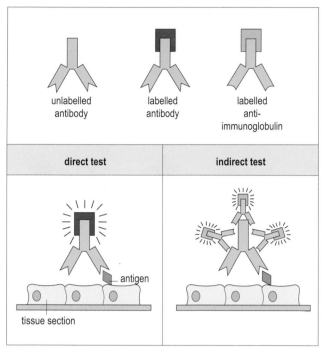

**Fig. 32.8** The fluorescent antibody test for detection and identification of microbial (or tissue) antigens or antibodies directed against them. In the direct test, antibody labelled with a fluorescent dye is applied to a tissue section bearing the antigen, unbound antibody is washed away, and the bound antibody showing the presence and location of the antigen is visualized by fluorescence microscopy. In the indirect test, antigen is revealed by successive treatments with unlabelled antigen-specific antibody and then fluorescent-labelled anti-immunoglobulin, which amplifies the signal (thus if the first antibody is human, the labelled antibody will be an anti-human Ig).

It is a catch-all method as, for example, any virus structure can be seen as long as there are at least 1 million particles per mL of fluid and an experienced electron microscopist is viewing the grid containing the sample.

## Detection of microbial antigens in specimens

Detection of specific microbial antigens can be a more rapid method for detecting the presence of an organism than attempting to grow and identify the microbe. The methods include:

- those that detect antigens by their interaction with specific antibodies
- those that detect microbial toxins.

They are summarized in Box 32.3. Detection of microbial genes using DNA probes and PCR is discussed later in this chapter.

### Specific antibody coated onto latex particles will react with the organism or its product, resulting in visible clumping

For example, common causative agents of bacterial meningitis (e.g. *Streptococcus pneumoniae* and *H. influenzae*) can be detected in CSF by mixing the specimen with specific antibody coated onto latex particles. If the antigen (i.e. the organism or its product) is present, the particles will clump together (Fig. 32.9). These tests give results within minutes of receipt of the specimen and are especially useful when the

---

**Box 32.3** **Nonculture Techniques for Detection of Microbial Products**

**Nonspecific techniques for detection of microbial products**

Fatty acid end products of metabolism of anaerobes can be detected in fluid specimens (e.g. pus, blood) by gas liquid chromatography.

**Antigen detection**

Soluble carbohydrate antigens can be detected by agglutination of antibody-coated latex particles or red blood cells (see Fig. 32.9); for example:

- *Streptococcus pneumoniae* capsule in CSF and urine
- *Haemophilus influenzae* type b capsule in CSF and urine
- *Cryptococcus neoformans* capsule in CSF and urine
- *S. pyogenes* group antigen in throat swabs.

Detection of particular antigens by binding to antibodies labelled with:

- enzymes (see Fig. 32.10; e.g. ELISA for hepatitis B, rotavirus)
- fluorescent molecules (see Fig. 32.8).

**Toxin detection**

Detection of exotoxins has historically involved tissue culture or injection into animals. Endotoxin from cell walls of gram-negative bacteria has been historically detected by clotting of amoebocyte extracts *Limulus*, the horseshoe crab (*Limulus* lysate assay), and by colorimetric and turbidimetric assays.

Identification of specific microbial products can be a more rapid method for detecting microorganisms than isolation and culture. The available techniques vary in their specificity. Toxins may be detected either by virtue of their antigenic properties or by demonstrating their action. Molecular methods such as the polymerase chain reaction (PCR) are used to assess the potential of microorganisms to produce specific microbial products (e.g. toxins) by detecting the presence of their respective genes.

---

patient has received antibiotics and organisms may appear morphologically unidentifiable in the CSF and fail to grow in culture.

### Immunoassays can be used to measure antigen concentration

Usually an antibody is adsorbed for convenience to a solid phase, and the amount of bound antigen is assessed using a second antibody labelled with an enzyme that acts on a substance to produce a colour or luminescence (Fig. 32.10) or is labelled with a fluorescent probe.

- The test employing an enzyme label is referred to as an *enzyme-linked immunosorbent assay (ELISA)*.
- The use of chemiluminescent or time-resolved fluorescent labels gives assays of very high sensitivity.

With modern techniques, multiple assays can be performed on single samples (see later).

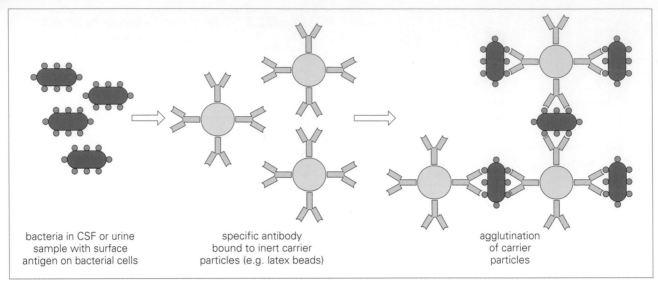

**Fig. 32.9** When a specimen of cerebrospinal fluid (CSF) containing bacteria (e.g. *Haemophilus influenzae*) is mixed with a suspension of latex particles coated with specific antibody (e.g. *H. influenzae* anticapsular antibodies), the interaction between antigen and antibody causes an immediate agglutination of particles, which is visible to the naked eye.

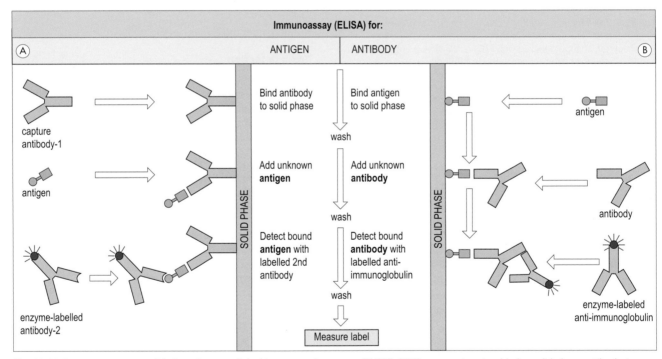

**Fig. 32.10** Immunoassay on a solid phase (enzyme-linked immunosorbent assay [ELISA]). (A) The test antigen is added to solid phase antibody-1 and the occupancy measured by adding an enzyme-labelled second antibody and then quantitating bound enzyme (e.g. peroxidase or alkaline phosphatase) through a colorimetric or luminometric reaction. In some cases, particularly with small antigens, unoccupied sites can be detected by adding a standard amount of labelled antigen. (B) Antibody to be tested is added to solid phase antigen and is detected by addition of an enzyme-labelled anti-immunoglobulin. (Compare with the indirect test in Fig. 32.8, which uses a fluorescent anti-immunoglobulin to detect bound antibody. Similarly, the label in the above assays can be a fluorescent probe rather than an enzyme.)

## Monoclonal antibodies can distinguish between species and between strains of the same species on the basis of antigenic differences

Hybridomas produced by the fusion of immortal B-cell tumours and individual normal antibody-producing cells provide a copious source of monoclonal antibodies, all with identical specificities for their relevant antigen (see Ch. 12). These monoclonal antibodies can be used as diagnostic tools.

In direct ELISA (see earlier), enzyme-conjugated monoclonal antibodies can be used to detect antigens in specimens from patients. Rotavirus antigen in faeces and hepatitis B surface antigen in sera can be detected directly with monoclonal antibodies in ELISAs. *Chlamydia trachomatis* infection can be diagnosed within a few hours by a direct fluorescent antibody test using a monoclonal antibody labelled with fluorescein (see Fig. 32.8; Ch. 22).

## Detection of microbes by probing for their genes

### Organisms can be identified using nucleic acid probes that match specific gene sequences

A gene probe is a nucleic acid molecule which, when in a single-stranded state and labelled, can be used to detect a complementary sequence by hybridizing to it. Historically this was accomplished by hybridizing a fluorescently labelled nucleic acid probe to the extracted microbial nucleic acid that has been denatured (to make single stranded) and immobilized onto a nitrocellulose membrane. The labelled probe can be visualized by chemiluminescent methods, depending on the label used. However, such blotting techniques are time consuming and prone to contamination in routine use and are now only used in a more automated (e.g. kit) form for a few organisms (e.g. *Mycobacterium tuberculosis* and *M. avium* complex, *M. kansasii* and *M. gordonae*, *Gardnerella vaginalis*, *Trichomonas vaginalis*, *Candida* spp.). However, probe use is increasingly being superseded by PCR methods.

### PCR can be used to amplify a specific DNA sequence to produce millions of copies within a few hours

PCR has the capability to rapidly detect a single gene target—that is, a single organism in the sample being analysed (Fig. 32.11)—within 1–3 hours, depending on the type of technology used. It is particularly useful for diagnostic work with pathogens (e.g. viruses and protozoa) that are difficult to culture. Earlier methods required the PCR products to be analysed on agarose gels and, for diagnostic certainty, some form of nucleic acid probe technique to unequivocally identify the target. This added a considerable amount of time to the analysis.

### For diagnostic purposes, traditional PCR has largely been replaced by real-time PCR

Real-time PCR uses the same basic reagents and techniques as the original PCR method but with the addition of fluorescently labelled sequence-specific probes. The TaqMan is one of the most widely used types of probes because it is relatively easy to design and it demonstrates inherently low levels of background fluorescence (Fig. 32.12A). The nucleotide probe sequence has two fluorescent molecules attached: at the 5′ end a reporter dye, and at the 3′ end a quencher molecule. When the probe is intact, no signal is detected, owing to reporter–quencher proximity; any fluorescence given off by the reporter is immediately absorbed, a feature contributing to the low background of the reaction. During the PCR the polymerase removes the 5′ nucleotides to which the reporter dye is attached. The reporter is now free to move away from the quencher, and its fluorescence can be detected. This 5′–3′ exonuclease activity is an inherent proof-reading ability of the enzyme, removing unexpected double-stranded regions of DNA and restricting the probe to register fluorescence only when the PCR is working. The result is the ability to monitor the amplification process in real time (hence the name). The amount of fluorescence detected during the reaction is directly proportional to the amount of amplicon produced (see Fig. 32.12B). By including a set of prequantified DNA standards, coamplified during the reaction, the copy number of nucleic acid in the original sample can be estimated. Because

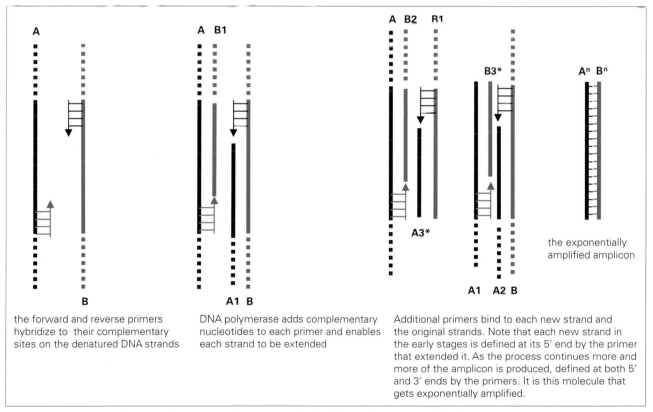

the forward and reverse primers hybridize to their complementary sites on the denatured DNA strands

DNA polymerase adds complementary nucleotides to each primer and enables each strand to be extended

Additional primers bind to each new strand and the original strands. Note that each new strand in the early stages is defined at its 5′ end by the primer that extended it. As the process continues more and more of the amplicon is produced, defined at both 5′ and 3′ ends by the primers. It is this molecule that gets exponentially amplified.

**Fig. 32.11** Conventional polymerase chain reaction. Short oligonucleotides (about 20 bases of DNA) hybridize to complementary sequences on each DNA strand to be amplified. The strands are separated by denaturation, enabling the primers to bind, which are extended by the thermostable polymerase adding complementary nucleotides by repeating the thermal cycling rounds of denaturation, annealing and extension 30–60 times. The original strands to be amplified are shown in the figure as A and B with subsequent amplified copies numbered (e.g. A2, A3) After rounds of amplification, the desired fragment of DNA (amplicon) is copied exponentially.

Ⓐ

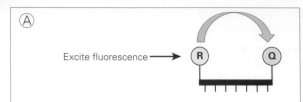

Excite fluorescence ⟶ Ⓡ Ⓠ

Step1: The intact TaqMan probe consists of approximately 20 bases of DNA complementary to a specific region of the target gene. A reporter (R) fluorophore and a quencher fluorophore (Q) are attached to the 5' and 3' ends respectively. When fluorescence is excited by the thermal cycler's LED, the quencher, due to its close proximity, absorbs fluorescence from the reporter and no signal is detected.

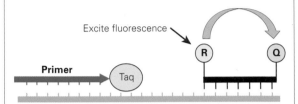

Step 2: The probe binds to its complementary region on the target strand, together with one of the primers. Now that the primer is bound, the Taq polymerase begins to extend it, moving towards the probe, which is still intact and so no signal is detected.

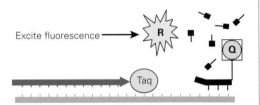

Step 3: As the Taq encounters the probe, the inherent 5'-3' nuclease activity of the polymerase cleaves nucleotides and releases the reporter fluorophore. The reporter is now free from quenching and able to fluoresce and its signal detected

Ⓑ

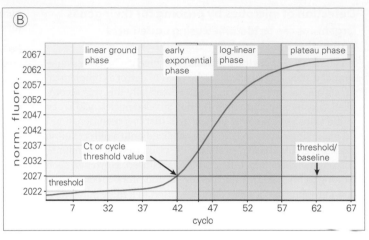

**Fig. 32.12** Real-time polymerase chain reaction (PCR). (A) The steps involved in real-time detection of PCR products by TaqMan probes. (B) A typical S-shaped real-time PCR amplification curve. The number of cycles in the reaction is shown on the X-axis; the levels of fluorescence, derived from the TaqMan probe and representing the accumulating amplicon, is shown on the Y-axis. The threshold or baseline value can be set by the user. The Ct value represents the PCR cycle number at which the exponential phase of amplification begins. Ct, cycle threshold.

there is no need for post-PCR analysis, the reaction tubes do not need to be opened, which reduces the potential for contamination and provides results in as little as 1 h. If the pathogen's nucleic acid is in the form of RNA, it must first be converted into complementary DNA (cDNA) before it can be amplified. This is achieved in an enzymatic step using a reverse transcriptase prior to the PCR (RT-PCR). RT-PCR tests for the severe acute respiratory syndrome coronavirus 2 (SARS-CoV-2) Spike protein were shown to have high specificities and were much more sensitive than the antigen detection lateral flow tests (see later).

### More than one pathogen can be detected in a single reaction—multiplexing

The PCR can be multiplexed by adding primers and probes for more than one pathogen, further reducing costs and time to diagnosis. Multiplexing is an extremely useful approach to diagnostic PCR, which apart from its economic benefits allows tests to be grouped into disease syndromes such as respiratory or sexually acquired infections, making the requesting

and diagnostic procedure much more efficient. This syndromic approach can also provide a diagnosis for multiple infections and pathogens not originally requested by the clinician. For example, analysis of a swab from the buttock region of a patient attending a sexual health clinic whose likely diagnosis is herpes simplex virus could reveal herpes zoster (shingles), not considered as part of the original differential diagnosis.

### Advances in molecular diagnoses for infectious diseases: sequencing-based techniques

#### Dideoxy chain terminator sequencing

This method was developed in the 1970s by Fredrick Sanger and colleagues (Sanger sequencing), and, although newer techniques continue to be developed, it is still the cornerstone of sequencing technology. The reaction is similar to PCR; a DNA polymerase is used to make copies of the nucleic acid to be sequenced. However, in addition to the four standard deoxynucleotide triphosphate bases (dNTPs), four dideoxynucleotide (ddNTPs) base analogues are used (Fig. 32.13).

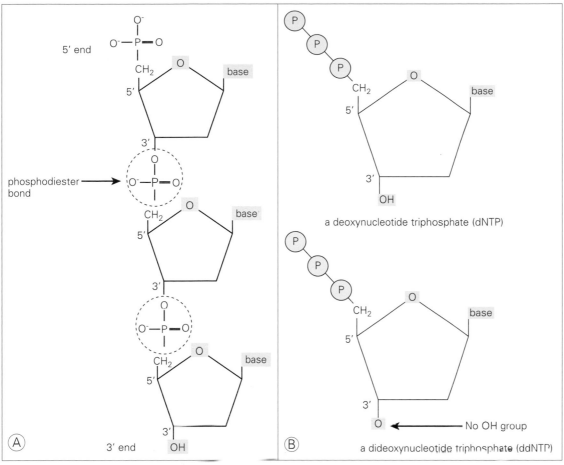

**Fig. 32.13** Dideoxy chain terminator sequencing. (A) Polymerization occurs in a 5'–3' direction via the formation of phosphodiester bonds. (B) Dideoxynucleotides lack reactive –OH on 3' carbon. The 5'–C can form a phosphodiester bond with the previous nucleotide in the chain, but the 3'–C cannot form a bond with the incoming dNTP (no OH group). Addition of a ddNTP during DNA replication stops chain elongation.

The ddNTPs lack the 3'–OH group on ribose of the dNTPs necessary for extending the DNA molecule. When one of these molecules is incorporated into the growing chain, extension is terminated (hence the name). The four ddNTPs are each labelled with different fluorescent dyes emitting light at different wavelengths. The fragments are separated according to their lengths by electrophoresis. A laser excites the different fluorescent dyes, the resulting different wavelengths emitted are detected and the sequence of the original nucleic acid is read as a series of fluorescent peaks.

### Second-generation sequencing by synthesis

The need for greater speed in generating data and reducing costs has led to significant improvements in sequencing methods. One of the most widely used (the so-called *next or second generation*) is sequencing by synthesis. The basic methodology is similar to dideoxy sequencing, but there are differences in how the reactions are carried out. The method uses a flow cell, which simplifies the addition of new reagents and the removal of previous reactants at each cycle of the process. A library of the microbe's DNA is created by randomly cutting the genome into short (50–80 bases) fragments either enzymatically or mechanically and attaching (ligating) adapters of known DNA sequence to both ends of the fragments. The adapters are complementary to primers already attached to the surfaces of the flow cell channels. As

illustrated in Fig. 32.14, the fragments are denatured, and the single-stranded products are bound to the complementary primers. The library is amplified for sequencing, resulting in the formation of double-stranded bridge structures, which are denatured to form templates for further amplification, eventually producing millions of cluster copies in the flow cell channels. The design of the fluorescence detection allows sequences to be read from each cluster in each of the channels simultaneously in such a way that a whole bacterial genome can be read in a single run in <24 h. Subsequent computer analysis assembles the generated sequence fragments as they overlap to produce the final contiguous sequence, often by comparison with a known reference sequence (see Ch. 37).

### Single-molecule sequencing—the third generation

Further developments promise even more rapid and cost-effective data acquisition. These methods focus on sequencing a single molecule and do not need PCR amplification of the pathogen's genome. One of the most promising of these techniques is based on the movement of the molecule to be sequenced through a protein nanopore. Each base has its own individual electronic signature and disturbs the current flowing across the pore in a specific manner, allowing each base to be uniquely identified as it passes through the pore. This approach is capable of producing longer stretches of sequence more amenable to assembly and analysis.

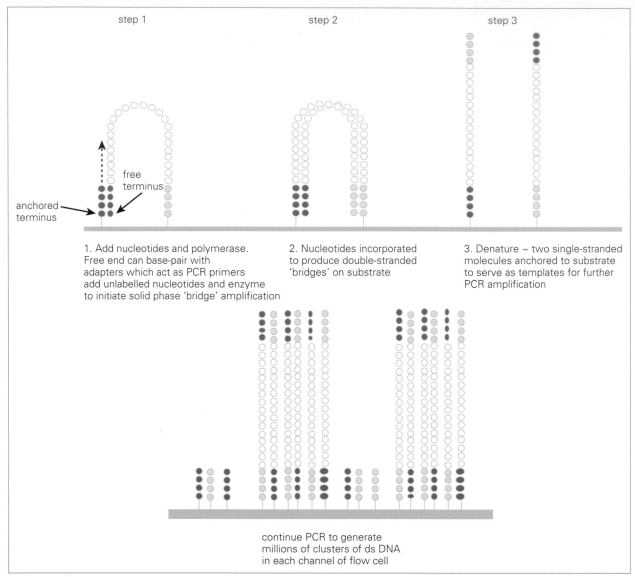

**step 1**

**step 2**

**step 3**

free
terminus

anchored
terminus

1. Add nucleotides and polymerase.
Free end can base-pair with
adapters which act as PCR primers
add unlabelled nucleotides and enzyme
to initiate solid phase 'bridge' amplification

2. Nucleotides incorporated
to produce double-stranded
'bridges' on substrate

3. Denature ~ two single-stranded
molecules anchored to substrate
to serve as templates for further
PCR amplification

continue PCR to generate
millions of clusters of ds DNA
in each channel of flow cell

**Fig. 32.14** The steps involved in second-generation sequencing by synthesis. PCR, Polymerase chain reaction.

### Amplification-based techniques and point-of-care tests

By definition, a point-of-care (POC) test requires a specimen to be tested at or near the patient with the results available instantly or within a very short time to provide an immediate diagnosis and enable rapid and appropriate treatment. As noted earlier, traditional culture-based microbiologic methods can take at least 24 h for a result. In a molecular laboratory, the test itself can be completed in 1–2 h, allowing rapid decisions about the management of the patient, with many of the bottlenecks removed because the patient is next to the testing device. This dictates that the equipment used should be small and portable such that it could be used conveniently in a consulting room or at the bedside. This is particularly important in infectious disease management in which empiric treatment can lead to inappropriate antibiotic use and the development of microbial resistance. In addition, infection control issues involving isolating infectious patients can be made quickly. Despite considerable interest in POC testing, there are difficulties related to the need for extracting the sample's nucleic acid and POC analysis by PCR, which have been addressed by some manufacturers using cassette-based or microfluidic

approaches. However, such instrumentation commonly tests only one sample at a time compared with the multiplex capabilities of current real-time applications. In some instances, the size of the equipment may require it to be sited in laboratories, and these have been termed *near-patient tests* (e.g. a near-POC respiratory panel with 17 viral targets plus *Bordetella pertussis, Chlamydophila pneumoniae, Mycoplasma pneumoniae* and *Legionella pneumophila*). More advanced systems are in development to reduce both equipment size and reaction times using microfluidics and nanotechnology analytes, in very small volumes, interact rapidly to changes in temperatures, speeding up the PCR. For example, newly developed approaches to single-molecule sequencing use highly portable devices that may be as small as the size of a USB flash drive.

The SARS-CoV-2 pandemic enabled the general public to use a POC test—the lateral flow antigen detection tests had antibodies to the spike protein captured on the strip that detected the presence of the spike protein (Fig. 32.15). The tests became widely available and proved to be remarkably specific; although they were less sensitive than PCR, they could be carried out without a laboratory or hospital

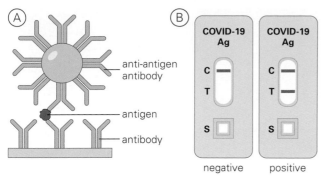

Ⓑ

| COVID-19 Ag | COVID-19 Ag |
|---|---|
| C | C |
| T | T |
| S | S |
| negative | positive |

**Fig. 32.15** Lateral flow test for severe acute respiratory syncrome caronavirus 2 (SARS-CoV-2). A nasal or throat swab is collected, placed into sample buffer and added to the cartridge where it resuspends gold or latex nanoparticles coated with anti-spike antibodies. Any spike antigen is captured by the nanoparticles. These flow up the strip by capillary action, and, if the SARS-CoV-2 spike protein antigen is present, the coated nanoparticles are captured by additional anti-spike antibodies, and a coloured test line develops within about 15 min (T). A control line (C) proves the test is working properly. Lateral flow tests can be modified to detect specific antibodies (e.g. IgM and IgG) by replacing the capture antibodies on the nanoparticles with the spike protein itself and using anti-IgM or anti-IgG as the capture reagents on the test line. (Modified from Budd J, Miller BS, Weckman NE, et al. Lateral flow test engineering and lessons learned from COVID-19. *Nat Rev Bioeng*. 2023;1:13–31.)

(Table 32.1). Home testing for human immunodeficiency virus (HIV) is now also possible.

### Personalized molecular medicine and infectious disease

Personalized medicine is not new; in fact, clinicians have been attempting to tailor treatment to individual patients' needs for centuries. The difference now is the amount of data made available by dramatic technologic advances that are providing clearer insights into the molecular basis of disease. The original concept of personalized medicine relied on interrogating the patient's genetic information to determine the effectiveness of a particular therapeutic regimen. This typically involved the management of genetic disease or chronic disorders such as the use of molecular cancer biomarkers in disease screening to predict treatment efficacy or toxicity in an individual. Use of a combination of molecular techniques and infectious disease diagnosis to achieve personalized medicine is an increasing reality, owing to improvements in PCR, sequencing and the range of clinically useful biomarkers (e.g. immune response, host susceptibility to infection, hypersensitivity to antimicrobial drug treatment). Personalized medicine, although often not considered as such, has been a key driver for the management of HIV/acquired immunodeficiency syndrome (AIDS) since the early 2000s. Sequencing data have been used to guide antiviral treatment based on viral subtype and sequence comparison with known antiretroviral resistance mutations. In the absence of genotyping, inappropriate therapy may be initiated, viral suppression is unlikely and antiretroviral resistance may develop. The development of diagnostic tests in parallel with targeted therapeutics has led to the concept of theranostics. Linking a drug identified through personalized medicine with a companion diagnostic test helps to ensure that the patient will benefit from the drug and determines its long-term usefulness by monitoring the therapy in real time. Other benefits from this approach potentially relate to drug development and comprehensive genomic data applied in selecting candidates

**Table 32.1** Performance of SARS-CoV-2 antigen detection tests

| Patient features and sampling times | Average sensitivity (95% CI) |
|---|---|
| Symptomatic | 72% (63.7–79.0%) |
| Asymptomatic | 58.1% (40.2–74.1%) |
| First week after symptom onset | 78.3% (71.1–84.1%) |
| Second week after symptom onset | 51.0% (40.8–61.0%) |
| High PCR Ct values (≤25) | 94.5% (91.0–96.7%) |
| Low PCR Ct values (>25) | 40.7% (31.8–50.3%) |

The overall specificity of the antigen tests was 99.6% (95% CI 99.0–99.8%). CI, Confidence interval; Ct, cycle threshold; PCR, polymerase chain reaction; SARS-CoV-2, severe acute respiratory syndrome coronavirus 2. (Data from Dinnes J, Deeks JJ, Berhane S, et al. Rapid, point-of-care antigen and molecular-based tests for diagnosis of SARS-CoV-2 infection. *Cochrane Database Syst Rev*. 2021;3(3):CD013705.)

for clinical trials, which will hopefully reduce the outcomes of potentially harmful side effects and the time taken to demonstrate safety and efficacy.

## ANTIBODY DETECTION METHODS FOR THE DIAGNOSIS OF INFECTION

Serologic tests (the study of antigen–antibody interactions) are used to:

- diagnose infections
- identify microorganisms (see earlier)
- type blood for blood banks and tissues for transplantation.

### Diagnoses based on detecting antibodies in patient sera

To detect an active or acute infection, assays detect IgM antibodies present early in infection (7–10 days). IgG antibodies develop after 2–4 weeks and can be detected for a long period afterward, so they may indicate a previous infection. It may also help to show that the patient has seroconverted by demonstrating a fourfold or greater rise in antibody titre between sera collected in the acute and the convalescent phases of the disease.

### Common serologic tests used in the laboratory to diagnose infection

#### Solid-phase immunoassays can be used to estimate antibody in a given sample

These ELISA assays have been described previously (see Fig. 32.10). The amount of antibody binding to the solid-phase antigen is a measure of the antibody content of the original sample and can be detected by adding a second antibody conjugated with a fluorochrome or an enzyme (e.g. phosphatase or peroxidase) that produces a colour or luminescent reaction with a given substrate.

Modern techniques permit the simultaneous assay of several analytes in the same sample. For example, multiplexed arrays of beads core labelled with different fluorochromes and coated with antibodies to cytokines are being increasingly used.

Antibodies to a specific antigen can also be detected using lateral flow tests, as described earlier for the detection of pathogen antigens, but by putting the antigen onto the strip and then using detection systems that will identify IgM antibodies indicating a recent/ongoing infection or IgG antibodies showing that antibody production switched to IgG, which may also indicate a previous infection.

## ASSESSMENT OF HOST DEFENCE SYSTEMS

### Blood samples may be checked for complement components

The complement system is a complex set of blood proteins that work to respond to infection (e.g. inflammation and immune response). Tests for specific complement proteins in the blood provide an indication of the robustness of host immune defence systems.

### Phagocytic activity is a key element of proper immune function

The ability of neutrophils to become phagocytic and concurrently release reactive oxygen (i.e. oxygen burst) has traditionally been assayed by the nitroblue tetrazolium (NBT) test. When yellow NBT dye is added to blood, it forms complexes with heparin or fibrinogen in the sample. These complexes are then phagocytosed by neutrophils that have been activated by the addition of exogenous endotoxin. The dye complex is taken into the stimulated neutrophils and substitutes for oxygen by acting as a substrate for the reduction process, forming blue, insoluble formazan (Fig. 32.16). More recently, flow cytometry (see later) has been used to assess oxidative burst using the dye dihydrorhodamine 123 (i.e. the DHR test).

### T cells

The development of effector T cells to an antigen can often be revealed by intradermal challenge with that antigen. Such an intradermal challenge usually gives rise to erythema and induration, peaking at ~48 h (Fig. 32.17). This time course has led to the reaction being described as delayed-type hypersensitivity and is the basis of the Mantoux skin test for tuberculosis (see Ch. 20).

Overall responsiveness of the T-cell population can be probed with flow cytometry by identifying dividing cells that have incorporated specific modified nucleosides such as bromodeoxyuridine or that express a cell division–associated nuclear protein such as Ki-67. By adding specific antibodies, flow cytometry can also detect the phenotype of the responsive T-cell populations by their fluorescent signal. The technique can also provide information regarding overall T-cell health (e.g. apoptosis). The fluorescence-activated cell sorter separates subpopulations delineated by their cytofluorimetric parameters measuring multiple fluorescent labels simultaneously, allowing both the surface phenotype of the cells and its function to be assessed (Fig. 32.18). The potential of flow

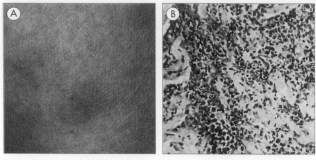

**Fig. 32.17** Tuberculin-type delayed sensitivity. The dermal response to antigens of leprosy bacillus in a sensitive subject (the Fernandez reaction) is characterized by (A) red induration maximal at 48–72 h and (B) dense infiltration of the injection site with lymphocytes and macrophages. (H&E, × 80.)

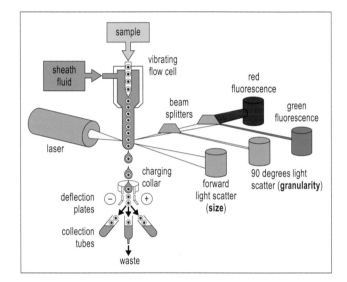

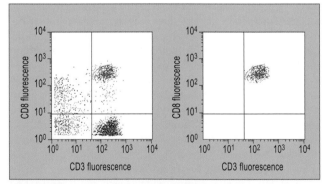

**Fig. 32.18** Flow cytofluorimetry. Cells in the sample are stained with specific fluorescent reagents to detect surface molecules and then stream one at a time past a laser. Each cell is measured for size (forward light scatter) and granularity (90 degrees light scatter), as well as for red and green fluorescence, to detect two different peripheral blood surface markers—in this instance, CD8 and CD3, respectively (but modern instruments can detect many more different fluorophores). In a cell sorter, the flow chamber vibrates the cell stream, causing it to break into droplets, which are then charged according to an arbitrary cutoff gate and can then be steered by deflection plates under computer control to collect different cell populations according to the parameters measured. In the example shown in the left panel, four populations can be seen; after appropriate gating, the CD8 population in the right upper quadrant can be selected; reanalysis gives the plot seen in the right hand panel. (From Male D, Brostoff J, Roth DB, et al. *Immunology*, ed 7, Mosby Elsevier; 2006.)

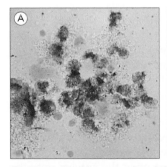 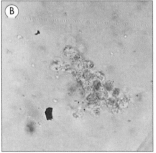

**Fig. 32.16** Nitroblue tetrazolium (NBT) test. In normal neutrophils and monocytes, reactive oxygen intermediates (ROIs) are activated by phagocytosis, and yellow NBT is converted to purple-blue formazan (A). Patients with chronic granulomatous disease (CGD) cannot form ROIs and so the dye stays yellow (B). (Courtesy A.R. Hayward.)

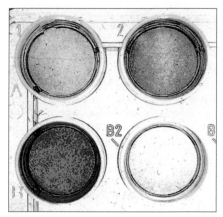

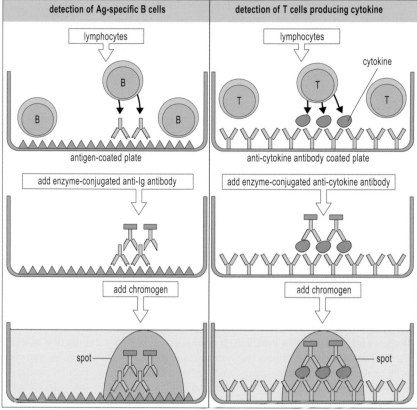

**Fig. 32.19** The ELISPOT assay for counting lymphocytes secreting antibodies or cytokines. The secreted products (antibodies from B cells and cytokines from T cells) are bound by the solid phase capture molecules immediately beneath the cell and revealed by a colour reagent as a spot corresponding with the secreting cell. Wells with different numbers of ELISPOTs are shown *top left*. (From Male D, Brostoff J, Roth DB, et al. *Immunology*, ed 7, Mosby Elsevier; 2006.)

cytometry is limited by the number of distinct channels (and thus cells that have bound different dye-labelled specific antibodies) that can be detected and has increased from ~3–4 in the earliest machines to ≥20. Antibodies can also be labelled with heavy metals enabling their exact molecular weights to be measured: Cytometry by time-of-flight (CyTOF) can detect 30–60 distinct markers, while spectral cytometry, which detects fluorophore-tagged antibodies using a complex process called *spectral unmixing*, can detect 40–60 markers. This means that cell subsets can be identified using not only expression of surface markers and intracellular cytokines or nuclear factors but also their antigen-specificity using multimers.

### Individual cells secreting antibodies or cytokines can be counted by the ELISPOT technique or by cytometry

The lymphocytes are incubated on a membrane impregnated with antigen for antibody detection or for anticytokine monoclonal antibody to detect cytokines (Fig. 32.19). The secreted product is identified by conventional ELISA-type readout. The presence of antigen-specific T cells secreting IFNγ can also be detected by measuring the secreted cytokine in an interferon gamma release assay (IGRA), as used for detecting *M. tuberculosis* infection (see Ch. 20).

An alternative approach utilizes inhibitors of cytokine export (e.g. metabolic poisons such as brefeldin A that trap cytokines within the endoplasmic reticulum) to block cytokine secretion so that these molecules can be immunostained after cellular permeabilization. Cells can then be stained for intracellular cytokines (intracellular cytokine staining) using

specific antibodies followed by flow cytometric analysis as described earlier. Alternatively, the cytokines can be identified with specific antibodies tagged with heavy metals using mass spectrometry or oligonucleotides (see later).

### The ability of cytotoxic T cells to attack targets can also be assayed by flow cytometry

The ability of cytotoxic T cells to attack targets such as virally infected cells was historically accomplished by prelabelling the target with a radioisotope such as $^{51}$Cr and then looking for isotope release into the supernatant from damaged cells. More recently, a variety of more sensitive assays have been developed for use with flow cytometry and immunofluorescent dyes.

### Molecular signatures can provide diagnostic tools as well as identify the pathogen

A specific PCR test can identify a pathogen (e.g. the GeneXpert assay will identify *M. tuberculosis* within 1.5 h). Small host gene signatures may also provide useful diagnostic tests in cartridge-based automated assays.

### Single-cell analysis and complex data analysis are the future

Single cells were previously sorted using a cell sorter, but newer molecular methods for tagging or barcoding individual cells, coupled with staining with oligonucleotide-labelled antibodies, now mean that the phenotype and function of an individual cell can be identified. Such methodologies are showing that our divisions of the immune cells into CD4 and CD8 T-cell subsets or type 1 or 2 cytokine producers are simplistic and there are many more subpopulations of cells. Will the key to immune protection for a particular infection be a particular cell subset or subpopulation, perhaps? Such detailed knowledge will hopefully help identify correlates of protection and biosignatures that could be exploited in vaccine trials, for example. But here microbiologists and immunologists need the help of bioinformaticians and artificial intelligence techniques to enable us to work with what are enormous data sets.

## PUTTING IT ALL TOGETHER: DETECTION, DIAGNOSIS AND EPIDEMIOLOGY

As seen more fully in Chapter 33, understanding the epidemiology of an infection can help to define the correct strategies for control at the population level. However, this understanding and decisions about control depend heavily upon the ability to recognize outbreaks of disease, to follow their progress and to identify the causative organism concerned. Detection and diagnosis are therefore key activities here, as they are for treatment of infection at the level of the individual.

Descriptive epidemiology involves asking questions about an outbreak of disease that will help to identify the pathogen and the source of infection. It is important to have a case definition, which includes the symptoms of the disease as well as details of the individuals involved and the timing of events. Analysis of these data should make it possible to say where and how the outbreak has arisen, who is at risk and what treatment is necessary to control further infection (Box 32.4). Measures used may involve antibiotic treatment of those immediately affected or vaccination if a large number are at risk (e.g. meningitis outbreaks in university students). For sexually transmitted disease (see earlier), an important element of detection is to establish contact patterns, or mixing matrices, so that individuals who may acquire an infection can be treated and further transmission prevented.

This approach to outbreaks of known or new disease follows their chance discovery as a result of clinical

**Box 32.4    Lessons in Microbiology**

**Importance of DNA sequencing in understanding the Ebola virus outbreak**

Nanopore sequencing was used in the 2015–2016 Ebola outbreak in West Africa. By combining data with those of a second group working in Sierra Leone, evidence of frequent transmissions across the border with Guinea was demonstrated. Importantly, data were released regularly throughout the investigation and enabled complicated clinical diagnoses to be discussed with other workers in the study based in different areas of the epidemic. Although the epidemic was officially declared over on 14 January 2016, hours later a new case was confirmed in Sierra Leone. Genomic surveillance is crucial in understanding the sources of new outbreaks by determining links to previously infected individuals and eliminating any zoonotic connections (also see Ch. 37).

observations, exemplified by the discovery of AIDS in 1981 through the increased occurrence of *Pneumocystis jiroveci* infection and of Kaposi sarcoma in men who have sex with men. A more systematic approach to detection relies on a regular notification system — a surveillance system that routinely records episodes of a number of legally notifiable diseases. Such systems operate nationally through government or federal health organizations as well as internationally through the World Health Organization. Regular monitoring of this kind makes it easier to identify outbreaks because it provides the baseline against which the occurrence of cases in excess of expectancy (the definition of an epidemic) can be measured.

Once outbreaks of infectious disease have been detected, the pathogen concerned can be identified by conventional diagnostic procedures to ensure that the appropriate antibiotic or vaccination is given.

## KEY FACTS

- Microbiologic confirmation of a clinical diagnosis of infection depends upon the collection of high-quality specimens and their rapid dispatch to the laboratory with all the necessary supporting information.

- Laboratory tests detect microorganisms or their products or evidence of a patient's immune response to infection.

- Although coming from different perspectives, culture and serologic methods are both important as cooperative approaches to the identification of clinically important pathogens.

- Molecular techniques involving PCR and other methods such as mass spectroscopy are increasingly used to detect pathogens rapidly; however, antimicrobial susceptibility is most accurately determined and

- appropriate treatment information provided by isolating organisms in pure culture.

- Growth of bacteria requires at least 18 h (isolation of viruses and of fungi may take much longer); therefore standard culture results cannot be expected in <24 h, although newer diagnostic tests are more rapid.

- Interpretation of culture results depends upon the source of the specimen. From sites that are normally sterile, any isolated organism is significant. From sites colonized by commensal flora, isolating and identifying the pathogen can be more difficult.

- Good communication between the clinician and the microbiologist is extremely important.

# Epidemiology and control of infectious diseases

# 33

Epidemiology is the study of the distribution or determinants of health-related states or events in specified populations and its application to the control of health problems.

The coronavirus 2019 (COVID-19) pandemic gave the global population a first-hand, real-time, practical understanding of epidemiology. Everyone became involved with infectious disease concepts, including time of infection, reproductive rate, transmission; diagnostic testing with tracking and tracing; and protection and prevention involving isolation, herd immunity, immunization and antiviral agents.

In epidemiology, we are concerned with populations rather than individuals. What we want to know of a disease in a population is who, where, when and why.

The field of epidemiology is divided into observational and interventional epidemiology. Interventional or experimental epidemiologic studies are designed to test a hypothesis by allocating an exposure or intervention to one group of people but not the other and measuring the disease outcome.

Epidemiologists talk about outcomes and exposures. The outcome is usually a disease or event such as death, infection or onset of new symptoms. Sometimes outcomes are laboratory markers. These outcomes are sometimes called intermediate outcomes because they may not represent a definite clinically important end point. Exposures are either risk factors or interventions.

## WHAT IS EPIDEMIOLOGY?

Epidemiology can provide the clinician or microbiologist with the evidence on which to base the treatment or control of infectious diseases. Disease surveillance describing the number of notifiable disease cases such as measles, meningitis or cholera is an example of observational descriptive epidemiology. Studies showing an association between human papillomavirus infection and cervical cancer are examples of analytical epidemiologic studies. Examples of intervention studies are randomized controlled trials investigating efficacy of a new vaccine. Examples of outcomes might be the laboratory marker C-reactive protein, or human immunodeficiency virus [HIV] viral load. Risk factors might include a specific behaviour (or use of a harmful substance) or interventions such as drugs, vaccines, or health education.

An example of the investigation of "who, where, when and why" is provided by Hepatitis A outbreaks which are often associated with institutions, restaurants and specific food. It is therefore important to determine who – which individuals ate the frozen organic strawberries, where – at home but purchased from particular supermarkets, when – between which dates in 2023 – they developed hepatitis A, and why fresh imported berries in particular batches supplied to various supermarkets were contaminated with a genetically identical strain of hepatitis A to that which has previously caused an outbreak in 2022 in the US.

## OUTCOME MEASUREMENTS

It is important to clearly define health-related outcomes. A definition should include the methods used to identify a case, the definition of a case and the unit of analysis. For example, eye disease secondary to *Chlamydia trachomatis* (see Ch. 26) is an important public health issue globally. The trachomatous inflammation is graded clinically into whether it involves follicular inflammation of the eyelid, abnormally positioned eyelashes or corneal scarring. When defining a case of trachomatous inflammation, it is important to describe (1) the methods and procedures used to determine a case (clinical examination vs. direct immunofluorescence microscopy of conjunctival smear), (2) the definition of a case (e.g. follicular inflammation only compared with including all three clinical grades) and (3) the unit of analysis (in this case, one or two eyes).

Disease prevalence and incidence are the two main types of measures of occurrence (disease frequency) used in epidemiology. Prevalence ($P$) is the number of existing cases in a population at a given point in time. Incidence ($I$) is the number of new cases occurring in a population during a specified period of time. $P$ is influenced by occurrence of new cases ($I$) and the duration ($D$) of each case (i.e. $P = I * D$). Thus prevalence of diseases with short durations such as viral gastroenteritis is mainly influenced by incidence, whereas prevalence of chronic diseases with relatively low mortality is likely to be high even if incidence is low. An example of the interaction between prevalence, incidence and mortality is shown in Box 33.1.

**The interaction between prevalence, incidence, mortality and treatment**

When HIV is introduced into an HIV-negative population, HIV prevalence and incidence grow exponentially (see Fig. 33.1). As more people become infected, the proportion of individuals not infected decreases. With fewer individuals susceptible to infection, the likelihood that an infectious HIV-positive individual will be in contact with an HIV-uninfected individual is reduced. This in turn reduces incidence, but prevalence continues to rise. The median time of survival in the natural course of HIV disease (without antiretroviral treatment) is 6–8 years. Thus after a time lag, HIV mortality grows, which reduces HIV prevalence. However, if HIV treatment becomes available, survival is prolonged and prevalence grows.

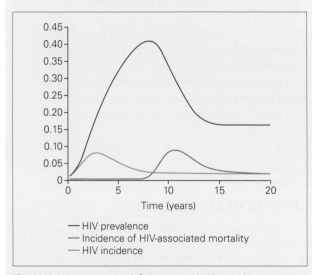

**Fig. 33.1** Human immunodeficiency virus (HIV) prevalence, incidence and mortality in a hypothetical population. (Modified from Trends in HIV incidence and prevalence: natural course of the epidemic or results of behavioural change? UNAIDS Best Practice Collection in collaboration with Wellcome Trust Centre for the Epidemiology of Infectious Disease; 1999.)

## TYPES OF EPIDEMIOLOGIC STUDIES

### Cross-sectional studies

Cross-sectional studies measure the frequency of an outcome and/or exposure(s) in a defined population at a particular point in time (Fig. 33.2A). These studies can be either descriptive, measuring the burden of disease, or analytical, comparing the frequency of disease in people exposed and unexposed to a risk factor.

Examples of study questions addressed by cross-sectional studies are:

- What proportion of the population has evidence of a past infection with Lyme disease?
- Is hepatitis B associated with hepatocellular carcinoma?

Cross-sectional studies are relatively inexpensive and quick. They are useful to determine the scale of a problem (prevalence of disease or prevalence of a risk factor in the population),

to assess hypotheses for possible causal associations and to evaluate diagnostic tests (Box 33.2). As cross-sectional studies can only measure disease prevalence, it is therefore difficult to differentiate between exposures causing the disease or improving the survival. With cross-sectional studies, outcome and exposure are determined at the same time, so there remains uncertainty whether the exposure preceded the outcome, which is a crucial requirement for causality. Sometimes it is difficult to exclude reverse causality (i.e. the outcome caused the exposure).

### Case control studies

Case control studies identify people with the outcome (cases) and a representative group of people in the population from which cases arose but without the outcome (controls). Cases and controls are then compared with regard to differences in their past exposure (see Fig. 33.2B). These studies are always analytical studies, as they ask the question, "Does exposure A cause disease B?"

Examples of study questions addressed by case control studies are:

- Are women with cervical cancer more likely to be infected with human papillomavirus than women without cervical cancer?
- Is injecting drug use associated with hepatitis C?

Case control studies are usually less expensive and time consuming than cohort or intervention studies. Rare diseases and diseases with long duration between exposure and outcome are most efficiently investigated using a case control design, as case control studies start with diseased and nondiseased individuals. However, when the exposure is rare, case control studies are impractical. Unbiased ascertainment of exposure is often difficult, especially when it relies on the participant to self-report. Neither disease prevalence nor incidence is measured in a case control study; only the increased risk of disease if individuals are exposed compared with if they are unexposed is measurable. Exposure is determined when the outcome has occurred, and thus reverse causality might be the reason for an association between an exposure and disease.

### Cohort studies

Cohort studies follow a group of people who do not initially have the outcome of interest and determine whether they develop the disease (descriptive cohort study). Analytic cohort studies classify people at the start of the study as exposed or unexposed to a certain risk factor. Both groups are followed over time, and the occurrence of disease is compared between the exposed and unexposed group (see Fig. 33.2C).

Examples of study questions addressed by cohort studies are:

- How high is the mortality among patients with methicillin-resistant *Staphylococcus aureus* septicaemia?
- Does infection with human herpesvirus 8 cause Kaposi sarcoma in human immunodeficiency virus–infected individuals?

Cohort studies measure disease incidence and ascertain risk factors before the outcome occurred. Thus they provide more robust evidence that an association between disease and exposure is likely to be causal. As cohort studies select disease-free exposed and unexposed individuals, they are particularly useful to investigate associations between rare exposures and disease, but they are inefficient when investigating rare diseases. Minimizing loss to follow-up is sometimes challenging but important to ensure comparability between exposure groups and validity of the study results. Cohort studies are often expensive in terms of the costs and manpower needed, as well as time consuming unless historical information (e.g. electronic health records of both exposures and subsequent outcomes) is available.

### Intervention studies

In an intervention study, disease-free and exposure-free individuals are actively allocated to an exposure (intervention) or no exposure (no intervention) group. The two

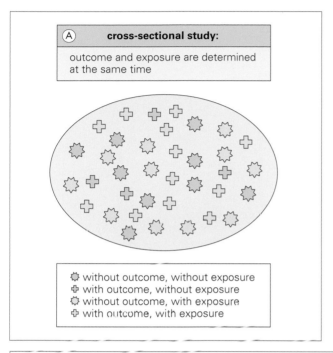

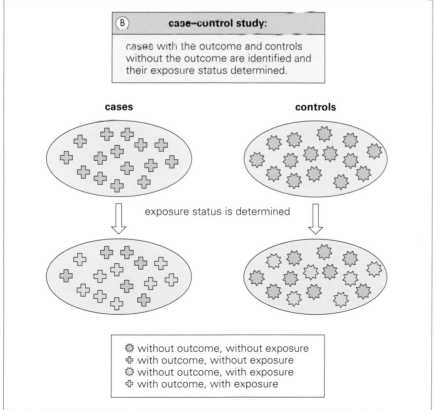

**Fig. 33.2** (A) Cross-sectional study: Outcome and exposure are determined at the same time. (B) Case control study: Cases with the outcome and controls without the outcome are identified and their exposure status determined. *(Continued)*

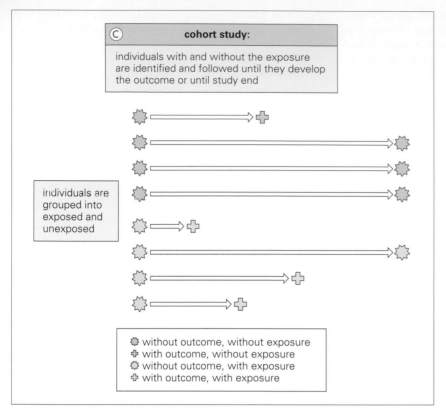

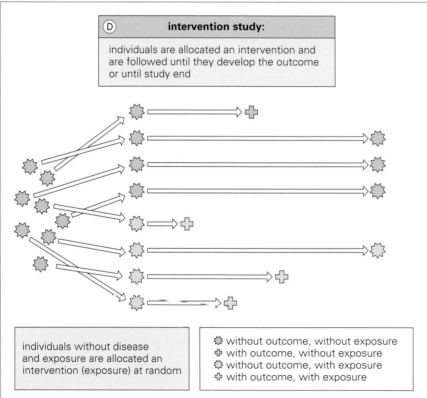

**Fig. 33.2 cont'd.** (C) Cohort study: Individuals with and without the exposure are identified and followed until they develop the outcome or until study end. (D) Intervention study: Individuals are allocated an intervention (exposure) and are followed until they develop the outcome or until study end.

## Box 33.2   Lessons in Microbiology

### Sensitivity, specificity and positive and negative predictive value

New diagnostic tests are usually evaluated using a cross-sectional study design. The new test is compared against a gold standard test and sensitivity and specificity are determined.

Sensitivity is the proportion of true positives correctly identified by the new test, and specificity is the proportion of true negatives correctly identified by the new test. Both sensitivity and specificity are intrinsic to the test and do not vary according to disease prevalence. However, they can be influenced by operators and environmental conditions.

From the patient's and physician's point of view, the more interesting question is, "What are the chances of me having the disease if I have a positive test result?" This question is answered by the positive predictive value (PPV), which is the proportion of individuals with a positive test result who actually have the disease. The negative predictive value (NPV) is the proportion of individuals with a negative test result who are free of disease. Both PPV and NPV are related not

only to the sensitivity and specificity of a test, but also to the prevalence of disease in a population.

The Xpert MTB-RIF is an automated molecular test for diagnosis of *Mycobacterium tuberculosis* (see Ch. 20). Diagnosis of tuberculosis (TB) previously relied on smear microscopy in most resource-limited settings and liquid culture in resource-rich settings. Smear microscopy has a low sensitivity and detects only patients with relatively advanced disease. Liquid culture is the gold standard of TB diagnosis, but it takes days to weeks to become positive.

A hypothetical evaluation study in 7000 TB suspects in a high-TB–prevalence setting revealed a sensitivity of the Xpert MTB-RIF of 92% and a specificity of 98% (Table 33.1A). The prevalence of TB among these 7000 TB suspects was 10%. PPV was 93% and NPV 99%.

The evaluation study was repeated in a population survey with 10,000 participants, among whom TB prevalence was 1%, sensitivity and specificity remained the same, but PPV was 53% and NPV was 100% (Table 33.1B).

**Table 33.1A** Results of the Xpert MTB-RIF evaluation among tuberculosis suspects

| | | Liquid culture (gold standard) | | |
| --- | --- | --- | --- | --- |
| | | Positive | Negative | Total |
| Xpert MTB-RIF | Positive | 645 | 50 | 695 |
| | Negative | 55 | 6250 | 6305 |
| | Total | 700 | 6300 | 7000 |

Sensitivity = 645/700 = 92%.
Specificity = 6250/6300 = 98%.
Positive predictive value = 645/695 = 93%.
Negative predictive value = 6250/6305 = 99%.

**Table 33.1B** Results of the Xpert MTB-RIF evaluation in a population survey

| | | Liquid culture (gold standard) | | |
| --- | --- | --- | --- | --- |
| | | Positive | Negative | Total |
| Xpert MTB-RIF | Positive | 92 | 80 | 172 |
| | Negative | 8 | 9820 | 9828 |
| | Total | 100 | 9900 | 10,000 |

Sensitivity = 92/100 = 92%.
Specificity = 9820/9900 = 98%.
Positive predictive value = 92/172 = 53%.
Negative predictive value = 9820/9828 = 100%.

groups are then followed over a period of time, and the frequency of the outcome is compared between the two groups (see Fig. 33.2D). Randomized controlled studies are a subtype of intervention studies and are considered the gold standard type of study because, when rigorously designed and conducted, they provide very strong evidence of causal associations. The intervention is allocated at random, which means that the only reason a participant receives the intervention is by chance alone. This ensures that the group receiving the intervention and the group not receiving the

intervention are equally balanced and comparable. The control group often receives a placebo, such as a tablet or injection containing no active compounds. Some intervention studies are double blinded, which means that neither investigator nor participant knows who receives the active intervention and who receives the placebo.

Examples of study questions addressed by intervention studies are:

• Is a new vaccine effective in preventing pneumococcal disease in children?

• Do steroids improve the outcome in children with meningococcal disease?

Randomized, placebo-controlled, double-blinded studies potentially deal with most problems experienced in observational studies: confounding, recall and observer bias. Confounding occurs when there is unequal distribution of a risk factor between exposed and unexposed individuals, and thus the observed association between exposure and disease is due to this other factor. Recall bias is a systematic error, which occurs when the way a participant answers a question is affected by either the disease status (in case control or cross-sectional studies) or the exposure status (in cohort studies). Observer bias arises when the accuracy of exposure (in case control or cross-sectional studies) or outcome (cohort studies) data recorded by the investigator differs systematically between subjects in different outcome or exposure groups. Outcome data are determined prospectively in intervention studies, and thus standard case definitions can be applied. Intervention studies may be expensive and time consuming, and loss to follow-up can be challenging. Large sample sizes or long follow-up may be needed if disease incidence is low or duration between exposure and disease is long. Allocation of a harmful exposure or withholding of a beneficial intervention is unethical. Intervention studies cannot be conducted under these circumstances.

## TRANSMISSION OF INFECTIOUS DISEASE

An infectious disease is transmitted from one person to another either directly or indirectly. Indirect transmission occurs when the infectious agent is transferred from one person to another via an intermediary (e.g. vector or vehicle). The occurrence of a case depends on the occurrence of at least one previous case (source), and each case can itself lead to another case. Disease events in infectious diseases are dependent. Therefore we investigate the spread of infectious diseases through a population over time to determine ways to control it (Fig. 33.3).

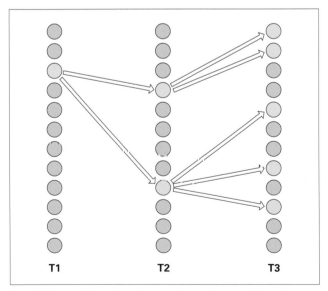

**Fig. 33.3** Transmission of an infectious disease in a population. One case of disease (source) at T1 transmits the disease to two cases (secondary cases) at T2; those cases transmit the disease to five cases at T3. Note that individuals who had the disease at T1 and T2 do not have the disease at T3 due to immunity.

### Infectiousness (Box 33.3)

The infectiousness of a disease in a population depends on several factors:

• the infectious agent: time between infection of a person and becoming infectious
• duration of infectiousness
• the probability of transmission given a contact between an infectious person and a susceptible person
• the environment:
  • the type of contacts between infectious and susceptible individuals
  • the number of contacts
  • whether it is well ventilated in the case of respiratory infections
  • use of mass transport: buses, trains, aeroplanes, boats
• the characteristics of the individuals in the population:
  • susceptibility of the population (number of susceptible individuals and degree of susceptibility)
  • infectiousness of the infected person.

### Time periods of infections

When infected, a susceptible individual enters the latent period (Fig. 33.4, Box 33.4). The latent period is the period

---

### Box 33.3    Lessons in Microbiology

#### Infectiousness—example syphilis

An individual infected with syphilis develops a painless but very infectious sore (chancre) at the site of infection on average 3 weeks following infection. The lesion may persist for 3–6 weeks. The individual cannot transmit the infection before the chancre lesion develops. Once the lesion is present, the likelihood of transmitting the infection is increased the more frequently the individual has sexual intercourse and the longer the lesion persists (if the frequency of intercourse remains constant). Therefore the duration of infectiousness and the number of contacts influence transmission. The probability of transmission is reduced if the individual uses condoms.

---

### Box 33.4    Lessons in Microbiology

#### Terminology: latency

In epidemiologic terms, the latent period is the time from infection until the infected individual is able to transmit the disease. A child infected with measles becomes infectious before symptoms occur. Thus the latent period is shorter than the incubation period. In contrast, an individual infected with *P. falciparum* malaria will experience symptoms 7–14 days following infection when parasites are multiplying in and destroying erythrocytes but will be infectious to mosquitoes only after about 24 days when gametocytes appear in the host's peripheral blood. Sometimes disease stages are called latent, such as latent tuberculosis or syphilis. Latent disease in that context describes periods of inactivity of the disease with regard to signs and symptoms.

**Table 33.2** Latent, infectious and incubation periods for a variety of viral and bacterial infections

| Infectious disease | Latent period[a] (days) | Infectious period (days) | Incubation period (days) |
|---|---|---|---|
| Measles | 6–9 | 6–7 | 8–13 |
| Mumps | 12–18 | 4–8 | 12–26 |
| Whooping cough (pertussis) | 21–23 | 7–10 | 6–10 |
| Rubella | 7–14 | 11–12 | 14–21 |
| Diphtheria | 14–21 | 2–5 | 2–5 |
| Varicella | 8–12 | 10–11 | 13–17 |
| Poliomyelitis | 1–3 | 2–3 | 7–12 |
| Influenza | 1–3 | 2–3 | 1–3 |

[a]Here the latent period is the preinfectious period, which is then followed by the infectious period.

between infection and becoming infectious (able to transmit the infection) and is often called the *preinfectious period* to avoid confusion with the other uses of the term *latent* (when the infection is quiescent in the body). Knowing this preinfectious period is important for understanding disease transmission, and it is followed by the infectious period during which the infected individual is able to transmit the infectious agent. This is followed by the noninfectious period due to death or recovery. If surviving, the individual might be immune or remain susceptible to reinfection.

The sum of the average latent and infectious periods is called the *average generation interval* of the infection. Latent and infectious periods are different for different diseases (Table 33.2). For measles the latent period is 6–9 days followed by an infectious period of 6–7 days.

### Time periods of infectious disease

Not all infected individuals will develop the disease. Disease and infection differ with regard to symptoms and clinical signs. Infected individuals without symptoms and signs have asymptomatic infections. For some infectious agents such as cytomegalovirus, the majority of infections will be asymptomatic.

The incubation period starts with the time of infection and ends when the individual develops symptoms. The time interval between onset of symptoms of the index case and that of the contact, who becomes the secondary case, is called the *serial interval*. The time interval between the time of infection/exposure in the index individual and the time of infection/exposure in the secondary case is the generation interval. When you can identify the index case and contact who developed the infection (the secondary case), this is a pairwise transmission chain (see Fig. 33.4). The time of infection of the index case will not be known, but the time of infection of the contact/secondary case can be determined by the contact tracing history.

Knowing the incubation period means it is possible to prevent or attenuate the symptoms in the contact by giving prophylaxis that can be either an antimicrobial drug or active or passive immunization. The incubation period is then followed by the symptomatic period. The symptomatic period ends with death or recovery.

The incubation period for measles is 8–13 days and much longer for hepatitis B (6 weeks–6 months, median 2.5 months), although the longer range is rare and seen more often in immunocompromised individuals due to the

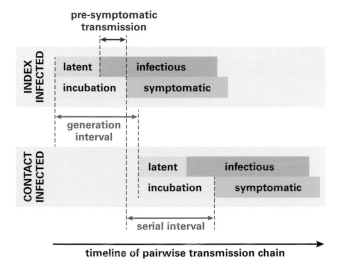

**Fig. 33.4** Time periods of infections and infectious diseases. Time lines of transmission between the index case and a contact case are shown. The time periods of infections (latent period + infectious period) and of infectious diseases (incubation period and symptomatic period) are shown. (Modified from Zhao S, Tang B, Musa SS, et al.: Estimating the generation interval and inferring the latent period of COVID-19 from the contact tracing data. *Epidemics* 2021;36:100482.)

immunopathogenesis involving T cells. With a blunted T cell response, that part of the hepatocyte injury is delayed, although infection has occurred and the jaundice appears when the T cells have returned to the fray. Thus an individual infected with measles is infectious before developing symptoms, as persons become infectious after 6–9 days. Therefore, importantly, isolation at the time of symptoms will not prevent transmission.

### Basic and net reproduction number

The basic reproduction number ($R_0$) is the average number of secondary infections produced by one infected individual in a totally susceptible population.

Disease incidence:

- is static if each case leads to one new case ($R_0 = 1$)
- increases if each case leads to more than one infective secondary case ($R_0 > 1$)
- decreases if each case leads to less than one infective secondary case ($R_0 < 1$), which will result in disease control and eradication.

The basic reproduction number is key in predicting the spread of an infection in a population and depends on the duration of infectiousness of the case ($d$), the number of contacts per unit time ($c$) and the transmission probability ($p$): $R_0 = c * p * d$. This formula shows that the basic reproduction number is not specific to an infectious agent only in terms of infectivity and how it is transmitted, but also to the characteristics of the host population at a particular point in time. If $R_0 > 1$, an outbreak will increase, with every case infecting more than one other person. The $R_0$ for HIV is different for women, men and commercial sex workers. Table 33.3 shows basic reproduction number for different diseases. Measles has a very high basic reproduction number of 15–17, whereas influenza has a basic reproductive rate of 2–3.

$R_0$ is an estimated number based on the incidence of infection and the diagnostic test used. The sensitivity and specificity of the test, sample type and testing strategy are all part of the calculation. The testing strategy could be based on testing only those with symptoms, contacts of those with symptoms or a group without symptoms. Together with mutations in key virulence determinants that are specific to the infection, all these factors can affect the $R_0$.

During the first wave of the COVID-19 pandemic, international surveillance included whole genome sequence analysis of new severe acute respiratory syndrome coronavirus 2 (SARS-CoV-2) infections identifying variants of concern (VOCs), variants of interest (VOIs) or variants under monitoring (VUMs) (Table 33.4) and subvariants, too. There was the original wild-type virus, Wuhan-Hu-1, that was first detected in Wuhan, China and then variants with names as Alpha, followed by Beta, Gamma and Delta. The more easily transmissible Omicron variant then appeared. The key factors with regard to the effects on the population of the waves of variants included transmissibility, illness severity and potential protection by previous infection, immunization or ability to evade the immune system (Box 33.5).

Mutations in the spike protein, part of the virus receptor binding domain (RBD), drove viral diversity. The RBD is an important viral binding site to the cellular ACE-2 receptor and is a target of neutralizing antibodies, part of the host defence. T-cell responses induced by either infection or immunization also act to clear infection quickly and reduce disease severity. The Omicron variant $R_0$ was ~8.2, compared with an $R_0$ of 2.3–3.8 in Wuhan-Hu-1, showing the increased rate of transmissibility with the Omicron variant infecting around two to four times more people over a certain period.

**Table 33.3** Basic reproductive rate for a variety of infectious diseases

| Infectious disease | Basic reproductive rate ($R_0$) |
| --- | --- |
| Measles | 15–17 |
| Mumps | 10–12 |
| Whooping cough (pertussis) | 15–17 |
| Rubella | 7–8 |
| Diphtheria | 5–6 |
| Poliomyelitis | 5–6 |
| Influenza | 2–3 |

**Table 33.4** Examples of types of severe acute respiratory syndrome coronavirus 2 (SARS-CoV-2) variants

| VOC | Lineage | Country first detected and date detected | Number of key spike mutations | Impact on transmissibility | Impact on immunity |
| --- | --- | --- | --- | --- | --- |
| Omicron | BA.2 | South Africa November 2021 | 28 | Increased | Increased |
| Omicron | BA.4 | South Africa January 2022 | 3 | No evidence | Increased |
| Omicron | BA.5 | South Africa February 2022 | 3 | Increased | Increased |
| **VOI** | **Lineage** | **Country first detected and date detected** | **Number of key spike mutations** | **Impact on transmissibility** | **Impact on immunity** |
| Omicron | BA.2.75 and sublineages | India May 2022 | 8 | No evidence | Increased |
| Omicron | BQ.1 | Unknown | 2 | No evidence | Increased |
| Omicron | XBB and sublineages | Unknown | 2 | No evidence | Increased |
| Omicron | XB.1.5 | USA | 3 | No evidence | Increased |
| **VUM examples** | **Lineage** | **Country first detected and date detected** | **Number of key spike mutations** | **Impact on transmissibility** | **Impact on immunity** |
| Omicron | BA.2.3.20 | Unknown | 3 | No evidence | No evidence |
| Omicron | BF.7 | Unknown | 2 | No evidence | No evidence |

The different SARS-CoV-2 variants had variants of concern (VOCs) that showed a significant impact on transmissibility, severity and/or immunity. Variants of interest (VOIs) had preliminary or uncertain evidence on genomic properties, epidemiologic evidence or in vitro evidence that could imply a significant impact on transmissibility, severity and/or immunity. Variants under monitoring (VUMs) were detected through epidemic intelligence, rules-based genomic variant screening or preliminary scientific evidence present in at least one outbreak, detected in a community or evidence that there is community transmission.
Modified from European Centre for Disease Prevention and Control: SARS-CoV-2 variants of concern as of 29 June 2023. Author; 2023.

| Box 33.5 | Lessons in Microbiology |

**Household transmission of the SARS-CoV-2 Omicron variant in Denmark: interplay between transmission and the effect of immunization**

A 2022 report by Lyngse and colleagues in *Nature Communications* is a classic example. The Delta variant of concern (VOC) was the dominant variant in Denmark in December 2021. On 8 December 2021, Danish authorities stopped tracing close contacts for those with Omicron VOC infections.

This household study period was from 9–15 December 2021, when those infected with either variant were treated approximately equally as active case finding had stopped.

Danish register data were used as all individuals had a unique identification number, and complete data on all COVID-19 tests from the Danish Microbiology Database were available, together with vaccination records from the Danish Vaccination Register. Households with two to six members were included, and a primary case was the first individual to test as severe acute respiratory syndrome coronavirus 2 (SARS-CoV-2) positive within the study period. A secondary case was defined by having a positive test, and the VOC was determined in all samples and households classified as Omicron or Delta.

The three groups were those (1) unimmunized, (2) fully immunized (2 doses of vaccine) or (3) booster immunized (3 doses of vaccine); 8568 primary infections with the Omicron VOC and 18,107 with the Delta VOC were included. Overall, the secondary attack rate (SAR) was 29% in Omicron households and 21% in Delta households. Unimmunized contacts had similar attack rates in Omicron (28%) and Delta households (27%), while fully immunized individuals had an SAR of 30% in Omicron and 19% in Delta households, respectively. For booster-immunized individuals, Omicron had a SAR of 23% and for Delta it was 11%.

The probability of contacts testing positive increased from 3% and 5% on day 1 to 21% and 29% on day 7, when the primary case was infected with the Delta and Omicron VOC, respectively.

For households infected with the Delta VOC, the odds ratio (OR) of infection was estimated as 2.4 for unimmunized contacts compared to fully immunized contacts and an OR of 0.4 for booster-immunized contacts compared to fully immunized contacts. The OR is a way to look at how strongly associated risk factors/exposures and outcomes are; if the OR is <1, the odds are reduced for an outcome, and with an OR >1, the odds are increased for that outcome.

The corresponding OR estimates for households infected with the Omicron VOC was 1.1 for unimmunized contacts and 0.6 for booster-immunized contacts, both compared to fully immunized contacts.

Unimmunized primary cases were associated with an OR of infection of 1.4 compared to fully immunized primary cases, while booster-immunized primary cases were associated with an OR of infection of 0.8.

The OR was estimated as 1.1 when comparing unimmunized contacts living in households infected with the Omicron VOC relative to unimmunized contacts living in households infected with the Delta VOC.

The OR was 2.4 when comparing fully immunized contacts between variants, and the OR was 3.2 when comparing booster-immunized contacts between variants.

There was an increased susceptibility with age of the household contact, an increased infectiousness with increasing age of adult primary cases and a decreased infectiousness with increasing age for children.

---

As mentioned earlier, $R_0$ values can vary at different times in different countries, and the minimum and maximum range can be quite wide. Percentage estimates of transmissibility are probably easier to understand. A general review of published data estimated that, initially, the Alpha variant was ~50% more transmissible than Wuhan-Hu-1; Beta was also ~50% more transmissible, and Delta was ~40–60% more transmissible than Alpha. The number of spike mutations increased, reaching ~28 in Omicron BA.2 in 2023—a much higher number compared with previous VOCs. However, although more transmissible, the illness severity fell. When Omicron was the predominant VOC in the United States, the rate of admissions to hospital per week per 100,000 adults peaked at 38.4 compared with 15.5 during the Delta peak. The Omicron variant wave involved high infection rates globally and reached a higher peak than previous waves.

A completely susceptible population is unusual. More commonly, a population consists of susceptible and immune individuals. The net reproduction number ($R$) is the average number of secondary cases in a population in which not all individuals are susceptible. The net reproduction number depends on the basic reproduction number ($R_0$) and the proportion of susceptible individuals ($x$): $R = R_0 * x$.

The lower the proportion of susceptible individuals in a population, the lower is the probability that an infectious individual will be in contact with a susceptible individual. Thus if the proportion of susceptibles ($x$) is small enough, $R$ will be <1 and the disease can be eradicated. The proportion of the population immune to an infection is called *herd immunity* (*HI*): $HI = 1 - x$. The herd immunity threshold (HIT) is the proportion of the population that needs to be immune for a disease to eventually die out ($R < 1$): $HIT = R_0 - 1 / R_0$. Susceptible individuals become immune once they are vaccinated with a highly effective vaccine. The basic reproduction number allows us to estimate the vaccination coverage, which needs to be achieved to control an infectious disease. The critical vaccination coverage needs to be very high (92–95%) for measles due to the high reproductive rate (15–17). Rubella has a lower reproductive number (7–8), and thus for disease control vaccination, coverage needs to be only 85–87%.

## VACCINE EFFICACY

Vaccines protect individuals directly by making them less susceptible (more immune) to the disease. They also protect individuals indirectly (even individuals who did not receive the vaccine) through increased herd immunity.

Vaccine efficacy is the most commonly used measure of effect when evaluating vaccines in randomized controlled trials. Vaccine efficacy is the reduction in the incidence of disease in vaccinated individuals compared with unvaccinated individuals:

Vaccine efficacy = Incidence of disease in unvaccinated individuals − Incidence of disease in vaccinated individuals/ Incidence of disease in unvaccinated individuals.

Thus vaccine efficacy measures only the direct effect of the vaccine. Measurement of the indirect effect of vaccines requires more complex study designs.

## KEY FACTS

- Epidemiologic studies can be observational or interventional.

- Prevalence is the number of existing cases in a population at a given point in time. Incidence is the number of new cases occurring in a population during a specified period of time.

- Infectiousness depends on the infectious agent itself, the environment and the characteristics of the individuals in the population, such as whether they are immune or susceptible.

- Infections can also be characterized by the latent or preinfectious period, the infectious period, the incubation period until symptoms develop and the symptomatic period: individuals can become infectious before they develop symptoms.

- Vaccine efficacy is the reduction in the incidence of disease in vaccinated individuals compared with unvaccinated individuals. When a significant proportion of the community is protected by vaccination, unvaccinated individuals are also less likely to acquire disease; this is called *herd immunity*.

# Attacking the enemy: antimicrobial agents and chemotherapy

# 34

## Introduction

The interactions between host, microbial pathogen and antimicrobial agent can be considered as a triangle, and any alteration in one side will inevitably affect the other two sides (Fig. 34.1). In this chapter, two sides of the triangle will be examined in greater detail:

• the interactions between antimicrobial agents and microorganisms
• the interactions between antimicrobial agents and the human host.

Laboratory aspects of antimicrobial susceptibility tests and assays will also be outlined. The third side of the triangle, the interactions between microorganisms and the human host, has been considered in detail in other chapters. The concluding part of the present chapter will draw together the three sides of the triangle.

## SELECTIVE TOXICITY

The term *selective toxicity* was proposed by the immunochemist Paul Ehrlich (Box 34.1). Selective toxicity is achieved by exploiting differences in the structure and metabolism of microorganisms and host cells; ideally, the antimicrobial agent should act at a target site present in the infecting organism but absent from host cells. This is more likely to be achievable in microorganisms that are prokaryotes than in those that are eukaryotes, as the former are structurally more distinct from the host cells. (A comparison of the cellular organization of prokaryotic and eukaryotic cells is given in Ch. 1.) At the other end of the spectrum, viruses are difficult to attack because of their obligate intracellular lifestyle. A successful antiviral agent must be able to enter the host cell but inhibit and damage a virus-specific target. The desirable features of ideal antimicrobial agents are summarized in Box 34.2.

## DISCOVERY AND DESIGN OF ANTIMICROBIAL AGENTS

The term *antibiotic* has traditionally referred to natural metabolic products of fungi, actinomycetes and bacteria that kill or inhibit the growth of microorganisms. Antibiotic production has been historically associated with soil microorganisms, and in the natural environment it is thought to provide a selective advantage for organisms in their competition for space and nutrients. Antibacterial agents derived from natural sources (e.g. penicillins, aminoglycosides) are usually chemically modified (i.e. semisynthetic) to improve their antibacterial or pharmacologic properties. However, some agents are totally synthetic (e.g. sulphonamides, quinolones). Therefore the term *antibacterial* or *antimicrobial agent* is often used in preference to antibiotic. Agents used against fungi, parasites and viruses can also be included under antimicrobial agents, but the terms *antifungals, antiprotozoans, anthelmintics* and *antivirals* are more often used.

The discovery of new antimicrobial agents was once entirely a matter of chance. Pharmaceutical companies undertook massive screening programmes searching for new soil microorganisms that produced antibiotic activity. In the light of our greater understanding of the mechanisms of action of existing antimicrobial agents, the processes have become rationalized, searching either for new natural products by target site–directed screening or synthesizing molecules predicted to interact with a microbial target. Genomic approaches to the identification of novel targets have revolutionized this approach. In addition, knowledge of the crystal structure of the key enzymes involved in viral replication such as protease, reverse transcriptase and helicase leads to the design of new drugs. At the start of the COVID-19 pandemic these types of approaches were accelerated in an open, global collaboration named COVID Moonshot, involving a collaboration between academics, biotechnologists and pharmaceutical companies, to develop antiviral treatments. The steps in a rational design programme are summarized in Box 34.3.

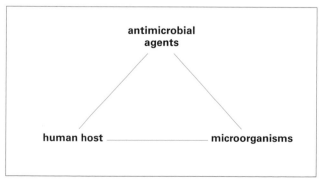

**Fig. 34.1** The interactions between antimicrobial agents, microorganisms and the human host can be viewed as a triangle. Any effect on one side of the triangle will have effects on the other two sides.

## Box 34.1 ▪ Lessons in Microbiology

### Paul Ehrlich (1854–1915)

Just as Pasteur towers over immunomicrobiology, Ehrlich (Fig. 34.2) is the father figure of immunochemistry. His contributions to the science of medicine at all levels are quite extraordinary. He was the first to propose that foreign antigens were recognized by side chains on cells (1890), a brilliant insight that took 70 years to confirm. He also discovered the mast cell, invented the acid-fast stain for the tubercle bacillus and devised a method to manufacture and commercialize a strong diphtheria antitoxin. He pioneered the development of antibiotics with his work on 606 (or Salvarsan), a treatment for syphilis, for which he was denounced by the church for interfering with God's punishment for sin.

While working on the treatment of infections caused by trypanosomes, Ehrlich set forth the concept of selective toxicity, as illustrated by the following quote:

*But, gentlemen, it should be made clear that in general this task is much more complicated than that using serum therapy. These chemical agents, in contrast to the antibodies, may be harmful to the body. When such an agent is given to a sick organism, a difference must exist between the toxicity of this agent to the parasite and its toxicity to the host. We must always be aware of the fact that these agents are able to act on other parts of the body as well as on the parasites.*

Like Pasteur, he had a grasp of the continuum from the whole body to the cell and the three-dimensional structure of molecules, and throughout his life he stressed the importance of molecular interaction as the basis of all biologic function; this is summed up in his famous maxim *corpora non agunt nisi fixata* or "things do not interact unless they make contact." A Nobel Prize winner in 1908, his name was systematically eliminated from the records by the Nazi regime on account of his Jewish birth, but he was restored to honour by a reconstruction of his laboratory at the Seventh International Congress of Immunology in Berlin in 1989.

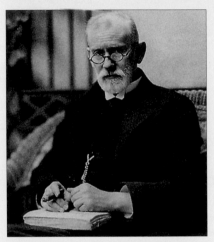

**Fig. 34.2** Paul Ehrlich (1854–1915).

## Box 34.2 ▪ Desired Properties of a New Antimicrobial Agent

In the design of new antimicrobial agents, both antimicrobial activity and pharmacologic properties of the antibiotic for the host have to be considered.

### Antimicrobial properties

- Selectivity for microbial rather than mammalian targets
- Cidal activity (antibacterial and antifungal agents)
- Slow emergence of resistance
- Narrow spectrum of activity[a]

### Pharmacologic activities

- Nontoxic to the host
- Long plasma half-life (once-a-day dosing)
- Good tissue distribution, including CSF
- Low plasma-protein binding
- Oral and parenteral dosing forms
- No interference with other drugs

## Box 34.3 ▪ Rational Design of an Antimicrobial Agent

The discovery process of new antimicrobial agents has moved away from historical random screening of soil microorganisms toward a rational design programme informed by computer modelling and genomics. From discovery to development and marketing can take over 10 years and cost at least US$1 billion. This list identifies different steps in this programme.

- Select an appropriate target.
- Identify a chemical lead (i.e. a new molecule with inhibitory activity on the target).
- Modify the lead compound to enhance potency.
- Evaluate in vitro activity.
- Evaluate in vivo activity and toxicity.
- Test in clinical trials and develop.

[a]The desired attribute depends on drug usage. Narrow-spectrum drugs cause less disturbance to the microbiota and may contribute less to emergence of antibiotic resistance, whereas broad-spectrum compounds are more useful for empiric therapy and treatment of polymicrobial infections. CSF, Cerebrospinal fluid.

# CLASSIFICATION OF ANTIBACTERIAL AGENTS

There are three ways of classifying antibacterial agents:

1. according to whether they are bactericidal or bacteriostatic
2. by target site
3. by chemical structure.

### Some antibacterial agents are bactericidal, others are bacteriostatic

Some antibacterial agents kill bacteria (bactericidal), while others only inhibit their growth (bacteriostatic). Thus the bactericidal process is irreversible, and bacteriostasis is reversible. Nevertheless, bacteriostatic agents are successful in the treatment of some infections because they prevent the bacterial population from increasing, and host defence mechanisms can consequently cope with the static population. However, in immunocompromised patients, bacteriostatic drugs may be less efficacious, and certain infections (e.g. endocarditis) require a bactericidal drug even in an immunocompetent patient.

As a means of classification, the distinction between bactericidal and bacteriostatic agents can be somewhat blurred (e.g. some bacteriostatic agents may tend toward bactericidal activity at higher concentrations).

### There are five main target sites for antibacterial action

A convenient way of classifying antibacterial agents is on the basis of their site of action. This classification does not allow an accurate prediction of which antibacterial agents will be active against which bacterial species, but it does help in understanding the molecular basis of antibacterial action and, conversely, in the elucidation of many of the synthetic processes in bacterial cells. The five main target sites for antibacterial action are:

- cell wall synthesis
- protein synthesis
- nucleic acid synthesis
- metabolic pathways
- cell membrane function.

These targets differ to a greater or lesser degree from those in the host (human) cells and so allow inhibition of the bacterial cell without concomitant inhibition of the equivalent mammalian cell targets (selective toxicity).

Each target site encompasses a multitude of synthetic reactions (enzymes and substrates), each of which may be specifically inhibited by an antibacterial agent. A range of chemically diverse molecules may inhibit different reactions at the same target site (e.g. protein synthesis inhibitors).

### Antibacterial agents have diverse chemical structures

Classification based on chemical structure alone is not of practical use because there is such diversity. However, a combination of target site and chemical structure provides a useful working classification to organize antibacterial agents into specific families (see later).

## RESISTANCE TO ANTIBACTERIAL AGENTS

Resistance to antibacterial agents is a matter of degree. In the medical setting we define a resistant organism as one that will not be inhibited or killed by an antibacterial agent at concentrations of the drug achievable in the body after normal dosage. "Some men are born great, some achieve greatness, and some have greatness thrust upon them" (William Shakespeare, *Twelfth Night*). Likewise, some bacteria are born resistant, and others have resistance thrust upon them. In other words, some species are innately resistant to some families of antibiotics because they lack a susceptible target and are impermeable to or enzymatically inactivate the antibacterial agent. The gram-negative rods with their outer membrane layer exterior to the cell wall peptidoglycan are less permeable to large molecules than gram-positive cells. However, within species that are innately susceptible, there are also strains that develop or acquire resistance.

### The genetics of resistance

In parallel with the rapid development of a wide range of antibacterial agents since the 1940s, bacteria have proved extremely adept at developing resistance to each new agent that comes along. This is illustrated for *Staphylococcus aureus* by the timeline shown in Fig. 34.3. The rapidly increasing incidence of resistance associated with slowing down in the

**Fig. 34.3** Time line illustrating the chronologic emergence of antibiotic resistance in gram-positive cocci. *S. aureus, Staphylococcus aureus.*

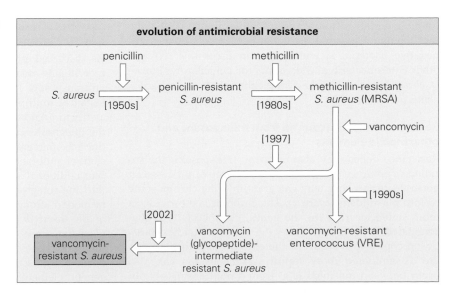

discovery of novel antibacterial agents to combat resistant strains is now recognized worldwide as a serious threat to the treatment of life-threatening infections.

## Chromosomal mutation may result in resistance to a class of antimicrobial agents (cross-resistance)

Resistance may arise from:

- a single chromosomal mutation in one bacterial cell resulting in the synthesis of an altered protein (e.g. streptomycin resistance via alteration in a ribosomal protein or the single amino acid change in the enzyme dihydropteroate synthetase resulting in a lowered affinity for sulphonamides); a mutational event could also alter (i.e. increase or decrease) the production of a protein resulting in increased resistance
- a series of mutations (e.g. changes in penicillin-binding proteins [PBPs] in penicillin-resistant pneumococci).

In the presence of antibiotics, these spontaneous mutants have a selective advantage to survive and outgrow the susceptible population (Fig. 34.4A). They can also spread to other sites in the same patient or by cross-infection to other patients and therefore become disseminated. Chromosomal mutations are relatively rare events (i.e. usually found once in a population of $10^6$–$10^8$ organisms) and generally provide resistance to a single class of antimicrobials (i.e. cross-resistance to structurally related compounds).

## Genes on transmissible plasmids may result in resistance to different classes of antimicrobial agents (multiple resistance)

Not content with surviving the antibacterial onslaught by relying on random chromosomal mutation, bacteria are also able to acquire resistance genes on transmissible plasmids (see Fig. 34.4B; see also Ch. 2). Such plasmids often code for resistance determinants to several unrelated families of antibacterial agents. Therefore a cell may acquire multiple resistance to many different drugs (i.e. in different classes) at once, a process much more efficient than chromosomal mutation. This so-called infectious resistance was first described by Japanese workers studying enteric bacteria but is now recognized to be widespread throughout the bacterial world. Some plasmids are promiscuous, crossing species barriers, and the same resistance gene is therefore found in widely different species. For example, TEM-1, the most common plasmid-mediated beta-lactamase in gram-negative bacteria, is widespread in *Escherichia coli* and other enterobacteria and accounts for penicillin resistance in *Neisseria gonorrhoeae* and ampicillin resistance in *Haemophilus influenzae*.

## Resistance may be acquired from transposons and other mobile elements

Resistance genes may also occur on transposons, the so-called *jumping genes*, which by a replicative process can generate copies that may integrate into the chromosome or into plasmids (see Ch. 2). The chromosome provides a more stable location for the genes, but they will be disseminated only as rapidly as the bacteria divide. Transposon copies moving from the chromosome to plasmids are disseminated more rapidly. Transposition can also occur between plasmids (e.g. from a nontransmissible to

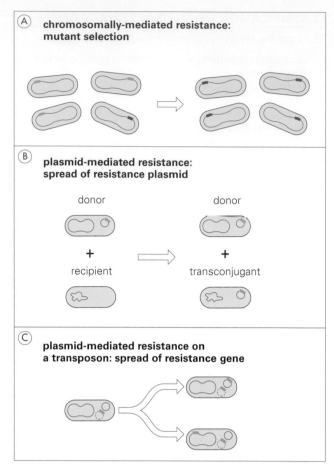

**Fig. 34.4** A chromosomal mutation (A) can produce a drug-resistant target, which confers resistance on the bacterial cell and allows it to multiply in the presence of antibiotic. Resistance genes carried on plasmids (B) can spread from one cell to another more rapidly than cells themselves divide and spread. Resistance genes on transposable elements (C) move between plasmids and the chromosome and from one plasmid to another, thereby allowing greater stability or greater dissemination of the resistance gene.

a transmissible plasmid), again accelerating dissemination (see Fig. 34.4C).

## Cassettes of resistance genes may be organized into genetic elements called integrons

As discussed previously, antibiotic-resistance genes may individually reside on plasmids, on the chromosome or on transposons found in both locations. However, in some instances multiple resistance genes may come together in a structure known as an *integron*. As shown in Fig. 34.5A, the integron encodes a site-specific recombination enzyme (int gene; integrase), which allows insertion (and also excision) of antibiotic-resistance gene cassettes (resistance gene plus additional sequences, including an attachment region) into the integron attachment site (att). In classic operon fashion, a strong integron promoter controls transcription of the inserted genes. Based on their integration mechanism (integrase, etc.), integrons have been organized into different classes found in both gram-negative and gram-positive organisms. Whether acting as independent mobile genetic elements or inserted into transposons, integrons

**Fig. 34.5** (A) Basic integron structure and (B) overall interrelationship between integrons and other DNA elements. att, Integron attachment site; int, integrase.

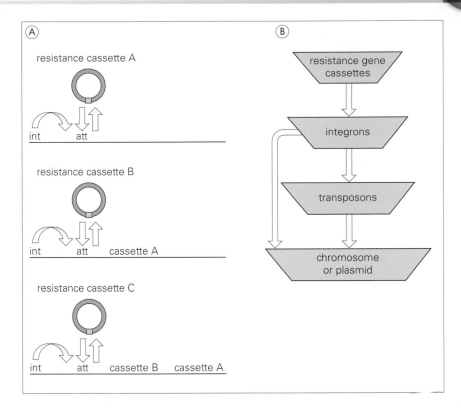

are capable of moving into a variety of DNA molecules, the overall hierarchy of which is depicted in Fig. 34.5B. With their ability to capture, organize and rearrange different antibiotic-resistance genes, integrons represent an important mechanism for the spread of multiple antibiotic resistance in clinically important microorganisms.

### Staphylococcal genes for methicillin resistance are organized into a unique cassette structure

Staphylococcal genes responsible for resistance to the antibiotic methicillin (discussed later) are found in a specialized cassette arrangement termed staphylococcal chromosomal cassette *mec* (SCC*mec*). SCC*mec* inserts into a unique target site on the staphylococcal chromosome. The cassette represents a highly recombinogenic region, which may not only rearrange internally but may also serve as a target for the insertion of other resistance elements (e.g. transposons and plasmids).

### Mechanisms of resistance

Resistance mechanisms can be broadly classified into three main types. These are summarized in Table 34.1 and described in more detail where relevant for each antibiotic in later parts of this chapter. Where bacterial mechanisms of antimicrobial resistance have been elucidated, they appear to involve the synthesis of new or altered proteins. As mentioned, the genes encoding these proteins may be found on plasmids or on the chromosome.

### The target site may be altered

The target may be altered so that it has a lowered affinity for the antibacterial agent, but it still functions adequately for normal metabolism to proceed. Alternatively, an additional (more resistant) target (e.g. enzyme) may be synthesized.

### Access to the target site may be altered (altered uptake or increased exit)

This mechanism involves decreasing the amount of drug that reaches the target by either altering entry (e.g. by decreasing the permeability of the cell wall) or pumping the drug out of the cell (known as an *efflux mechanism*).

### Enzymes that modify or destroy the antibacterial agent may be produced (drug inactivation)

There are many examples of such enzymes especially including:

- beta-lactamases
- aminoglycoside-modifying enzymes
- chloramphenicol acetyl transferases.

These will be described in the relevant parts on these antibiotics.

## CLASSES OF ANTIBACTERIAL AGENTS

The following parts of this chapter deal with groups of antibacterial agents based on their target site and chemical structure. In each case, the discussion attempts to summarize the answers to the questions set out in Table 34.2, reviewing the interactions between the antibacterial agent and the bacteria and between the antibacterial agent and the host (i.e. two sides of the triangle in Fig. 34.1).

## INHIBITORS OF CELL WALL SYNTHESIS

Peptidoglycan, a vital component of the bacterial cell wall (see Ch. 2), is a compound unique to bacteria and therefore provides an optimum target for selective toxicity. Synthesis of peptidoglycan precursors starts in the cytoplasm; wall subunits are then transported across the cytoplasmic membrane and finally inserted into the growing peptidoglycan

**Table 34.1** Mechanisms of resistance can be classified into three main types

| Antibacterial | Mechanism of resistance | | |
|---|---|---|---|
| | Altered target | Altered uptake | Drug inactivation |
| Beta-lactams | + | + | + |
| Glycopeptides | + | | |
| Aminoglycosides | + | + | + |
| Tetracyclines | + | + | |
| Chloramphenicol | | + | + |
| Macrolides/ketolides | + | + | + |
| Lincosamides | + | | |
| Streptogramins | + | | |
| Oxazolidinones | + | | |
| Fusidic acid | + | | |
| Sulphonamides/trimethoprim | + | + | |
| Quinolones | + | + | |
| Rifampicin | + | | |
| Cyclic lipopeptide | + | | |

For antibiotics where more than one mode of resistance exists, drugs vary as to which is more frequently encountered.

**Table 34.2** To understand the nature and optimum use of an antibacterial agent, the questions listed here must be answered

| | |
|---|---|
| What is it? | Chemical structure: natural or synthetic product |
| What does it do? | Target site, mechanism of action |
| Where does it go? (and therefore preferred route of administration) | Absorption, distribution, metabolism and excretion of the drug in the body of the host |
| When is it used? | Spectrum of activity and important clinical uses |
| What are the limitations to its use? | Toxicity to the human host; lack of toxicity (i.e. resistance of the bacteria) |
| How much does it cost? | Great variation between agents but cost is a serious limitation on availability of some agents in resource-poor countries |

molecule. Several different stages are therefore potential targets for inhibition (Fig. 34.6). The antibacterials agents that inhibit cell wall synthesis are varied in chemical structure. The most important of these agents are the beta-lactams, the largest group, and the glycopeptides, which are active only against gram-positive organisms. Bacitracin (primarily used topically) and cycloserine (mainly used as a second-line medication for treatment of tuberculosis [TB]; see later) have many fewer clinical applications.

## Beta-lactams

### Beta-lactams contain a beta-lactam ring and inhibit cell wall synthesis by binding to PBPs

Beta-lactams comprise a very large family of different groups of bactericidal compounds, all containing the beta-lactam ring. The different groups within the family are distinguished by the structure of the ring attached to the beta-lactam ring—in penicillins, this is a five-membered ring; in cephalosporins, a six-membered ring—and by the side chains attached to these rings (Fig. 34.7).

PBPs are membrane proteins (e.g. carboxypeptidases, transglycosylases, transpeptidases) capable of binding to penicillin (hence the name PBP) and are responsible for the final stages of cross-linking of the bacterial cell wall structure. Inhibition of one or more of these essential enzymes results in an accumulation of precursor cell wall units, leading to activation of the cell's autolytic system and cell lysis (Fig. 34.8).

### Most beta-lactams have to be administered parenterally

Different beta-lactams are administered intramuscularly, intravenously, or orally. Most achieve clinically useful concentrations in the cerebrospinal fluid (CSF) when the meninges are inflamed (as in meningitis) and the blood-brain barrier becomes more permeable. In general, they are not effective against intracellular organisms.

A few of the cephalosporins, notably cefotaxime, are metabolized to compounds with less microbiologic activity. Beta-lactams are excreted in the urine, and for some, such as benzylpenicillin, this is very rapid; hence the need for frequent doses. Probenecid can be administered concurrently to slow excretion and maintain higher blood and tissue concentrations for a longer time.

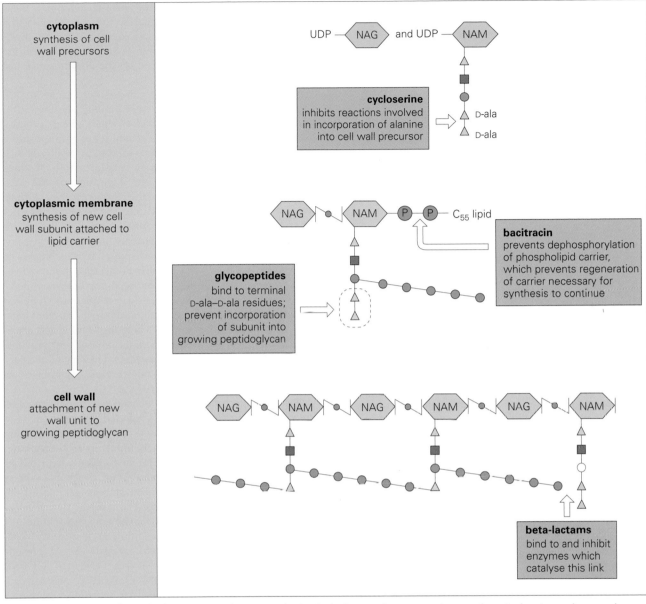

**Fig. 34.6** The synthesis of peptidoglycan is a complex process that begins in the cytoplasm, proceeds across the cytoplasmic membrane and leads to the attachment of new wall units to the growing peptidoglycan chain. This synthetic pathway can be inhibited at a variety of points by antibacterial agents. NAG, *N*-acetyl glucosamine; NAM, *N*-acetyl muramic acid; UDP, uridine diphosphate.

## Different beta-lactams have different clinical uses but are not active against species that lack a cell wall

A vast array of beta-lactam antibiotics are currently registered for clinical use. Some, such as penicillin, are active mainly against gram-positive organisms, whereas others (e.g. semisynthetic penicillins; carboxypenems; monobactams; second-, third-, fourth- and fifth-generation cephalosporins) have been developed for their activity against gram-negative rods. The more recent beta-lactams are also active against innately more resistant organisms such as *Pseudomonas aeruginosa* (Table 34.3).

It is important to remember that beta-lactams are not active against species that lack a cell wall (e.g. *Mycoplasma*), those with very impenetrable walls such as mycobacteria or intracellular pathogens such as *Brucella*, *Legionella* and *Chlamydia*.

## Resistance to beta-lactams may involve one or more of the three possible mechanisms

*Resistance by alteration in target site.* Methicillin-resistant staphylococci (e.g. *S. aureus* [MRSA], *S. epidermidis* [MRSE]) synthesize an additional PBP (PBP2a), which has a much lower affinity for beta-lactams than the normal PBPs and is therefore able to continue cell wall synthesis when the other PBPs are inhibited. Although the *mecA* gene, which codes for PBP2a, is present on the chromosome in all cells of a resistant population, in many instances it may only be transcribed in a proportion of the cells resulting in a phenomenon known as heterogeneous resistance. In the laboratory, special cultural conditions are used to enhance expression and demonstrate resistance. Methicillin-resistant staphylococci commonly produce beta-lactamase (see later) and are resistant to all

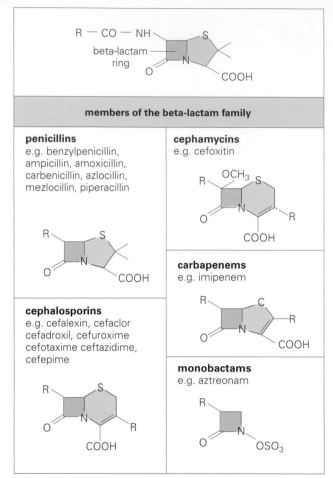

**Fig. 34.7** The beta-lactam family. The ring structure is common to all beta-lactams and must be intact for antibacterial action. Enzymes (beta-lactamases) that catalyse the hydrolysis of the beta-lactam bond render the agents inactive. The penicillins and cephalosporins are the major classes of beta-lactam antibiotics, but other members of the family and new beta-lactam beta-lactamase inhibitor combinations are the focus of new developments.

other beta-lactams with the exception of ceftaroline, a fifth-generation cephalosporin and the first approved by the US Food and Drug Administration for activity against MRSA. This cephalosporin binds to PBP2a with an affinity 2000-fold better than other beta-lactams and is thus effective in treating infections caused by MRSA. Another fifth-generation cephalosporin, ceftobiprole, has a similar spectrum of activity and is available in a number of countries.

Other organisms such as *Streptococcus pneumoniae, N. gonorrhoeae* and *H. influenzae* may also utilize PBP changes to achieve beta-lactam resistance, which may vary depending on the compound employed.

***Resistance by alteration in access to the target site.*** This mechanism is found in gram-negative cells where beta-lactams gain access to their target PBPs by diffusion through protein channels (porins) in the outer membrane. Mutations in porin genes result in a decrease in permeability of the outer membrane and hence resistance. Strains resistant by this mechanism may exhibit cross-resistance to unrelated antibiotics that use the same porins.

***Resistance by production of beta-lactamases.*** Beta-lactamases are enzymes that catalyse the hydrolysis of the beta-lactam ring to yield microbiologically inactive products. Genes encoding these enzymes are widespread in the bacterial kingdom and are found on the chromosome and on plasmids.

The beta-lactamases of gram-positive bacteria are released into the extracellular environment (see Fig. 34.8), and resistance will only be manifest when a large population of cells is present. The beta-lactamases of gram-negative cells, however, remain within the periplasm (see Fig. 34.8).

To date, thousands of different beta-lactamase enzymes have been described. All have the same function but with differing amino acid sequences that influence their affinity for different beta-lactam substrates. Some enzymes specifically target penicillins or cephalosporins, while others are especially troublesome in broadly attacking most beta-lactam compounds (e.g., extended-spectrum beta-lactamases [ESBLs], carbapenemases). Some beta-lactam antibiotics (e.g. carbapenems) are hydrolysed by very few enzymes (beta-lactamase stable), whereas others (e.g. ampicillin) are much more labile. Beta-lactamase inhibitors such as clavulanic acid are molecules that contain a beta-lactam ring and act as suicide inhibitors, binding to beta-lactamases and preventing them from destroying beta-lactams. They have little bactericidal activity of their own and are used in combination with beta-lactam antibiotics (Fig. 34.9).

***Extended-spectrum beta-lactamases and carbapenemases are especially problematic.*** The extended spectrum of new beta-lactam antibiotics has represented a survival challenge for the affected pathogens, which, unfortunately, they have been fully prepared to meet. Similar to events depicted in Fig. 34.3, new iterations of beta-lactam drugs have been met with mutations in genes encoding beta-lactamases (i.e. ESBLs) in gram-negative bacteria. The carriage of such genes on plasmids has allowed their movement both within and between pathogenic species resulting in widespread dissemination of the associated drug resistance. At present there is a myriad of such enzymes (e.g. TEM, SHV, CTX-M, OXA beta-lactamases; IMP, VIM, OXA, KPC, NDM-1 carbapenemases). An extended spectrum of activity coupled in some instances with resistance to beta-lactam beta-lactamase inhibitor combinations has produced organisms with few if any remaining therapeutic options. For this reason, as noted in the book introduction, carbapenem-resistant and ESBL-producing Enterobacteriaceae are now categorized by the World Health Organization (WHO) as critical and third on the list of 12 pathogens identified as priority for the research and development of new antibiotics.

## Side effects

***Toxic effects of beta-lactam drugs include mild rashes and immediate hypersensitivity reactions.*** Statistics regarding allergy to beta-lactam drugs are complicated by the fact that the problem historically involves self-reporting by patients who are often mistaken in their diagnosis. Nevertheless, serious allergy to beta-lactam drugs in the form of an immediate (type 1) hypersensitivity reaction may occur in ca. 0.5–4% of patients, although anaphylaxis occurs much less frequently (c. 0.004–0.04% of penicillin treatment courses). Mild idiopathic reactions, usually in the form of a rash, are

**Fig. 34.8** Penicillin-binding proteins (PBPs) play a key role in the final stages of peptidoglycan synthesis. They catalyse the cross-linkage of wall subunits, which are then incorporated into the cell wall. Beta-lactams are able to enter the cell (e.g. through pores in the outer membrane of gram-negatives) and bind to the PBP. This prevents it from catalysing the cross-linkage of subunits, leading to their accumulation in the cell and the release of autolytic enzymes, which causes cell lysis. Within the periplasmic space of gram-negatives (b1) beta-lactamases can inactivate beta-lactams before they reach their target PBPs, thereby protecting the cell from antibiotic action. Alternatively, mutant PBPs fail to bind with beta-lactams, thus allowing peptidoglycan synthesis to occur. In gram-positive bacteria (b2) beta-lactams may be extracellularly destroyed by beta-lactamases or rendered ineffective, as in gram-negatives, by mutant PBPs.

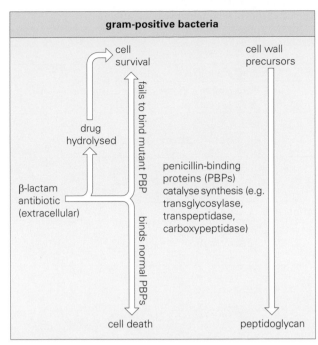

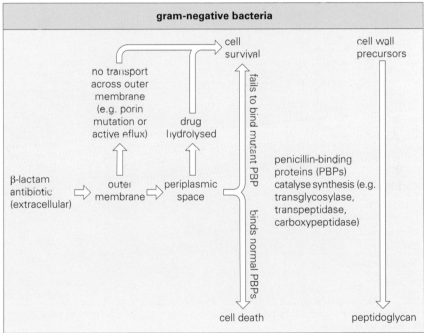

more common (>1% of treatment courses) especially with ampicillin. Patients who are allergic to penicillin can be allergic to cephalosporins (less with newer-generation compounds), but aztreonam, a monobactam, shows negligible cross-reactivity.

Neurotoxicity and seizures can occur with all the beta-lactams if improperly dosed for body weight and kidney function, especially in patients with renal impairment. This toxicity is manifest as fits, unconsciousness, myoclonic spasms and hallucinations. Carbenicillin can cause platelet dysfunction and sodium overload (because it is given as a sodium salt) especially in patients with liver failure, renal failure and congestive heart failure.

## Glycopeptides

### Glycopeptides are large molecules and act at an earlier stage than beta-lactams

Glycopeptides include vancomycin (with structurally related oritavancin, telavancin and dalbavancin) and teicoplanin. Both vancomycin and teicoplanin are very large molecules and therefore have difficulty penetrating into gram-negative cells. Teicoplanin is a natural complex of five different but closely related molecules.

Glycopeptides are bactericidal and interfere with cell wall synthesis by binding to terminal D-alanine-D-alanine at the end of pentapeptide chains that are part of the growing

**Table 34.3** Characteristics of representative beta-lactams

| Drug class | Category | General spectrum of activity |
|---|---|---|
| **Pencillins** | | |
| Pencillin G, V[a] | Natural penicillin | Gram-positive bacteria |
| Nafcillin[a]<br>Oxacillin[a] | Semisynthetic (beta-lactamase resistant) pencillin | Gram-positive bacteria, including beta-lactamase producers |
| Amoxicillin[a,b]<br>Ampxicillin[a,b] | Semisynthetic (amino) penicillin | Gram-positive bacteria<br>Gram-negative bacteria, including spirochetes, *Listeria monocytogenes*, *Proteus mirabilis* and some *Escherichia coli* |
| Carbenicillin[a]<br>Mezlocillin<br>Piperacillin[b] | Semisynthetic (carboxy) penicillin<br>Semisynthetic (ureido) penicillin | Gram-positive bacteria<br>Enhanced coverage of gram-negatives, including *Pseudomonas* and *Klebsiella* |
| **Cephalosporins** | | |
| Cefadroxil[a]<br>Cefazolin<br>Cephalexin[a] | First generation | Gram-positive bacteria |
| Cefaclor[a]<br>Cefprozil[a]<br>Cefuroxime[a] | Second generation | |
| Cefdinir[a]<br>Cefditoren[a]<br>Cefpodoxime[a]<br>Cefotaxime<br>Ceftazidime<br>Ceftibuten[a]<br>Ceftriaxone | Third generation | |
| Cefepime | Fourth generation | Improved activity against gram-negative bacteria |
| Ceftolozane[b]<br>Ceftabiprole<br>Ceftaroline | Fifth generation | Improved activity against gram-negative bacteria<br>Improved activity, especially against methicillin-resistant *Staphylococcus aureus* |
| **Cephamycin[c]** | | |
| Cefotetan<br>Cefoxitin | | Gram-positive bacteria<br>Improved activity against *Bacillus fragilis* |
| **Carbapenems** | | |
| Ertapenem<br>Imipenem<br>Meropenem<br>Doripenem | | Gram-positive and gram-negative bacteria |
| **Monobactams** | | |
| Aztreonam | | Gram-negative bacteria, including *Haemophilus influenza* and *Pseudomonas aeruginosa* |

Although there are many beta-lactam agents available, the most commonly used ones are listed, together with their main indications.
[a]Oral formulation available.
[b]Can be formulated in combination with beta-lactamase inhibitors (see Fig. 34.9).
[c]Often classified with second-generation cephalosporins.

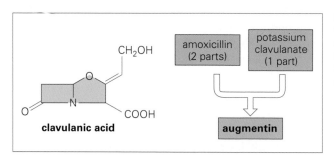

**Fig. 34.9** Clavulanic acid, a product of *Streptomyces clavuligerus*, inhibits the most common beta-lactamases (e.g. TEM enzymes) and allows amoxicillin to inhibit cells producing these enzymes. Augmentin is the most widely used of these combination drugs. Other combinations include ampicillin and sulbactam, piperacillin and tazobactam, ceftolozane and tazobactam, and ceftazidime and avibactam.

bacterial cell wall structure (see Fig. 34.6). This binding inhibits the transglycosylation reaction and prevents incorporation of new subunits into the growing cell wall. As glycopeptides act at an earlier stage than beta-lactams, it is not useful to combine glycopeptides and beta-lactams in the treatment of infections.

### Vancomycin and teicoplanin must be given by injection for systemic infections

Vancomycin and teicoplanin are not absorbed from the gastrointestinal tract and do not penetrate the CSF in patients without meningitis. However, bactericidal concentrations are achieved in most patients with meningitis because of the increased permeability of the blood-brain barrier. Excretion is via the kidney.

### Both vancomycin and teicoplanin are active only against gram-positive organisms

Vancomycin and teicoplanin are used mainly for:

- the treatment of infections caused by gram-positive cocci and gram-positive rods that are resistant to beta-lactam drugs, particularly MRSA and MRSE
- for patients allergic to beta-lactams
- the treatment of *Clostridioides difficile* in antibiotic-associated colitis, although concerns that this may promote emergence of glycopeptide-resistant enterococci in the gut flora have led to the increasing use of alternative compounds.

### Resistance

*Some organisms are intrinsically resistant to glycopeptides.* As mentioned, gram-negative bacteria are naturally resistant to the glycopeptides because these compounds are too large to efficiently move through the outer membrane to the peptidoglycan. Other organisms have an altered glycopeptide target, such as pentapeptides, terminating in D-alanine-D-lactate (e.g. *Erysiplothrix, Leuconostoc, Lactobacillus, Pediococcus*) or D-alanine-D-serine (e.g. *Enterococcus gallinarum, E. casseliflavus*).

*Organisms may acquire resistance to glycopeptides.* Historically, the most clinically relevant acquired glycopeptide resistance has been observed in *E. faecium* and *E. faecalis* (vancomycin-resistant enterococci [VRE]), first reported by UK investigators in 1986. Since that time, a variety of resistance phenotypes have been described that can be differentiated by transferability (e.g. plasmid association), inducibility and extent of resistance (Table 34.4). The genes associated with the highest levels of glycopeptide resistance are *vanA*, *vanB*, and *vanD*, which encode ligase-producing pentapeptides terminating in D-alanine-D-lactate.

**VanA** *is the best understood mechanism of acquired glycopeptide resistance.* *VanA*-type glycopeptide resistance has been the most extensively studied and is characterized by inducible high-level resistance to both vancomycin and teicoplanin. *VanA* is associated with the transposable element *Tn1546* (ca. 11 kb in size), which may be carried either chromosomally or on a plasmid, the latter being transferable in nature.

*VanB* is associated with inducible high-level resistance to vancomycin but not teicoplanin (although teicoplanin resistance can be induced by prior exposure to vancomycin). *VanB* resistance may be chromosomal or plasmid linked and is associated with very large transposable elements such as *Tn1549* (34 kb).

*VanD* is chromosomal in nature and thus nontransferable, resulting in constitutive resistance to high levels of vancomycin but low levels of teicoplanin.

*Glycopeptide resistance in the staphylococci occurs by mutation or by acquisition from the enterococci.* Within the coagulase-negative staphylococci (central nervous system [CNS]), *S. epidermidis* and *S. haemolyticus* are especially prone to development of glycopeptide resistance by mechanisms that remain incompletely understood but likely include cell wall thickening. Resistant clinical and laboratory-generated isolates have been shown to differ from their susceptible counterparts in a variety of ways, including changes in glycopeptide-binding capacity, membrane proteins and cell wall synthesis and composition.

Coagulase-positive staphylococci (i.e. *S. aureus*) showing decreased susceptibility to glycopeptides (but not fully resistant) were first described by Japanese investigators in 1996. The reduced susceptibility of these vancomycin-intermediate or glycopeptide-intermediate isolates may be either homogeneously or heterogeneously expressed. In either case, resistance is not associated with *vanA*, B, or D but, instead, involves other mechanisms affecting cell wall composition (leading to increased thickness, etc.).

Unfortunately, high-level glycopeptide resistance has also been observed in *S. aureus* (vancomycin-resistant *S. aureus*) because of plasmid-associated movement of the *vanA* gene from VRE. Although highly troubling, this event has fortunately been rare (<20 isolates worldwide).

### Side effects

*The glycopeptides are potentially ototoxic and nephrotoxic.* Vancomycin is usually given by intravenous infusion, administered slowly to avoid red-man syndrome caused by histamine release. Particular care must be taken to prevent toxic concentrations accumulating in patients with renal impairment. Oral vancomycin is used for treatment of antibiotic-associated pseudomembranous colitis caused by *C. difficile*. Teicoplanin is less toxic than vancomycin and can be given by intravenous bolus and by intramuscular injection.

**Table 34.4** Characteristics of glycopeptide resistance in enterococci

| Type | Resistance | Expression | Transmissible |
|------|-----------|------------|:---:|
| VanA | Vancomycin Teicoplanin | Inducible | + |
| VanB | Vancomycin | Inducible | + |
| VanD | Vancomycin (variable) Teicoplanin (variable) | Constitutive | − |

## INHIBITORS OF PROTEIN SYNTHESIS

Although protein synthesis proceeds in an essentially similar manner in prokaryotic and eukaryotic cells, it is possible to exploit the differences (e.g. 70 S vs 80 S ribosome) to achieve selective toxicity. The process of translation of the messenger RNA (mRNA) chain into its corresponding peptide chain is complex, and a range of antibacterial agents act as inhibitors (Fig. 34.10).

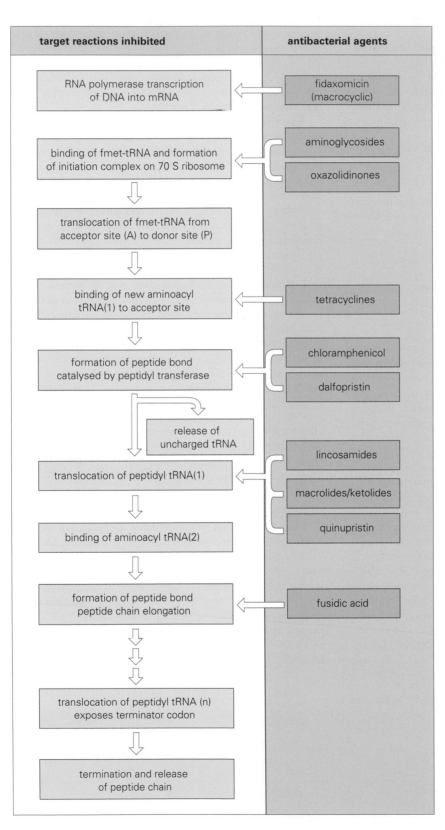

| target reactions inhibited | antibacterial agents |
| --- | --- |
| RNA polymerase transcription of DNA into mRNA | fidaxomicin (macrocyclic) |
| binding of fmet-tRNA and formation of initiation complex on 70 S ribosome | aminoglycosides / oxazolidinones |
| translocation of fmet-tRNA from acceptor site (A) to donor site (P) | |
| binding of new aminoacyl tRNA(1) to acceptor site | tetracyclines |
| formation of peptide bond catalysed by peptidyl transferase | chloramphenicol / dalfopristin |
| release of uncharged tRNA | |
| translocation of peptidyl tRNA(1) | lincosamides / macrolides/ketolides / quinupristin |
| binding of aminoacyl tRNA(2) | |
| formation of peptide bond peptide chain elongation | fusidic acid |
| translocation of peptidyl tRNA (n) exposes terminator codon | |
| termination and release of peptide chain | |

**Fig. 34.10** The synthetic pathway leading to the production of new protein in bacterial cells is extremely complex. A number of different groups of antibacterial agents act by inhibiting proteins with specific reactions in this synthetic pathway. The macrocyclic drug fidaxomycin inhibits the earliest step (mRNA transcription), while the others can be grouped into those that act on the 30 S subunit of the ribosome (e.g. aminoglycosides and tetracyclines) and those that act on the 50 S subunit (e.g. chloramphenicol, lincosamides, macrolides and fusidic acid). fmet-tRNA, Formylmethionyl-transfer RNA; mRNA, messenger RNA.

## Aminoglycosides

### The aminoglycosides are a family of related molecules with bactericidal activity

The aminoglycosides contain either streptidine (streptomycin) or 2-deoxystreptamine (e.g. gentamicin; Table 34.5). The original structures have been modified chemically by changing the side chains to produce molecules such as amikacin and netilmicin that are active against organisms that have developed resistance to earlier aminoglycosides.

Aminoglycosides act by binding to specific proteins in the 30 S ribosomal subunit, where they interfere with the binding of formylmethionyl-transfer RNA (fmet-tRNA) to the ribosome (see Fig. 34.10), thereby preventing the formation of initiation complexes from which protein synthesis proceeds. In addition, aminoglycosides cause misreading of mRNA codons and tend to break apart functional polysomes (protein synthesis by multiple ribosomes tandemly attached to a single mRNA molecule) into nonfunctional monosomes.

### Aminoglycosides must be given intravenously or intramuscularly for systemic treatment

Aminoglycosides are not absorbed well from the gut, do not penetrate well into tissues and bone and do not cross the blood-brain barrier. Thus they are usually administered as an intravenous infusion. Intrathecal administration of streptomycin is used in the treatment of tuberculous meningitis, while gentamicin and amikacin may be administered by this route in the treatment of gram-negative meningitis in neonates. Aminoglycosides are excreted via the kidney.

### Gentamicin and the newer aminoglycosides are used to treat serious gram-negative infections

Gentamicin, tobramycin and amikacin are important for the treatment of serious gram-negative infections, including those caused by *P. aeruginosa* (Box 34.4). They are not active against streptococci or anaerobes but are active against staphylococci. Against *P. aeruginosa,* amikacin is most active. Amikacin may be active against strains resistant to gentamicin and tobramycin (see later). Streptomycin is now reserved almost entirely for the treatment of mycobacterial infections. Neomycin is not used for systemic treatment but can be used orally in gut decontamination regimens in neutropenic patients.

### Production of aminoglycoside-modifying enzymes is the principal cause of resistance to aminoglycosides

Although relatively uncommon, resistance to aminoglycoside antibiotics may occur by alteration of the 30 S ribosomal target protein (e.g. a single amino acid change in the P12 protein prevents streptomycin binding). In addition, methylation of 16 S ribosomal RNA (rRNA) can prevent aminoglycoside binding to the ribosomal aminoacyl site. Resistance may also arise through alterations in cell wall permeability or in the energy-dependent transport across the cytoplasmic membrane.

Production of aminoglycoside-modifying enzymes is the most important mechanism of acquired resistance (Fig. 34.11). The genes for these enzymes are often plasmid mediated, located on transposons and transferable from one bacterial species to another. The enzymes alter the structure of the aminoglycoside molecule, thus inactivating the drug. The type of enzyme determines the spectrum of resistance of the organism containing it.

### The aminoglycosides are potentially nephrotoxic and ototoxic

The therapeutic window between the serum concentration of aminoglycoside required for successful treatment and that which is toxic is small. Blood concentrations should be monitored regularly, particularly in patients with renal impairment.

## Tetracyclines

### Tetracyclines are bacteriostatic compounds that differ mainly in their pharmacologic properties rather than in their antibacterial spectra

Tetracyclines are a family of large cyclic structures that have several sites for possible chemical substitutions (Fig. 34.12).

Tetracyclines inhibit protein synthesis by binding to the small ribosomal subunit in a manner that prevents aminoacyl tRNA from entering the acceptor sites on the ribosome (see Fig. 34.10). While this process may occur with both prokaryotic and eukaryotic ribosomes, the selective action of tetracyclines is due to their much greater uptake by prokaryotic cells.

Tetracyclines are usually administered orally. Doxycycline and minocycline are more completely absorbed than tetracycline and so result in higher serum concentrations and less gastrointestinal upset because there is less inhibition of normal gut flora. Tetracyclines are well distributed and penetrate host cells to inhibit intracellular bacteria. They are excreted primarily in bile and urine.

### Tetracyclines are active against a wide variety of bacteria, but their use is restricted due to widespread resistance

Tetracyclines are used in the treatment of infections caused by mycoplasmas, chlamydiae and rickettsiae. Resistance in other genera is common partly due to the widespread use of these drugs in humans and to their use as growth promoters in animal feed. The resistance genes are carried on a transposon, thus facilitating their spread, and new cytoplasmic membrane proteins are synthesized in the presence of tetracycline. As a result, tetracycline is positively pumped out of resistant cells (efflux mechanism). Although included with the tetracyclines (see Fig. 34.12), tigecycline is a member of a related class of compounds (glycylcyclines) derived from minocycline, with activity against bacteria resistant to tetracyclines.

### Tetracyclines should be avoided in pregnancy and in children <8 years of age

Tetracyclines suppress normal gut flora, resulting in gastrointestinal upset and diarrhoea and encouraging overgrowth by resistant and undesirable bacteria (e.g. *S. aureus*) and fungi (e.g. *Candida*).

Interference with bone development and brown staining of teeth occurs in the fetus and in children. Systemic administration may cause liver damage. The potential for photosensitization is another caveat associated with the use of tetracyclines in all patients.

## Chloramphenicol

### Chloramphenicol contains a nitrobenzene nucleus and prevents peptide bond synthesis with a bacteriostatic result

Chloramphenicol is a relatively simple molecule containing a nitrobenzene nucleus, which is responsible for some of the toxic

**Table 34.5** Aminoglycoside-aminocyclitol antibiotics classified according to their chemical structure

| 4,6-Distributed 2-deoxystreptamines | |
|---|---|
| Gentamicin[a] | Complex of three closely related structures; first aminoglycoside with broad spectrum |
| Tobramycin[b] | Activity very similar to gentamicin but slightly better against *Pseudomonas aeruginosa* |
| Amikacin | Semisynthetic derivative of kanamycin; active against many gentamicin-resistant gram-negative rods |
| **4,5-Disubstituted 2-deoxystreptamines** | |
| Neomycin[b] | Too toxic for parenteral use but has topical uses in decontaminating mucosal surfaces |
| **Streptidine-containing** | |
| Streptomycin[b] | Oldest aminoglycoside; now use restricted to treatment of tuberculosis |

They are also differentiated by the genus of microorganisms that produces them, and this is reflected in the spelling of the names.
[a]Micins from *Micromonospora* species.
[b]Mycins from *Streptomyces* species.

## Box 34.4 ■ Indications for Aminoglycoside Therapy

Aminoglycosides are valuable additions to the clinician's armamentarium despite their potential toxicity. They are important agents active against gram-negative facultative bacteria and are often used in combination with beta-lactams to broaden the spectrum to include streptococci and some anaerobes, which are not susceptible to aminoglycosides alone. Resistance to aminoglycosides, particularly among enterobacteria and staphylococci, is mediated by the production of aminoglycoside-modifying enzymes, which react with groups on the aminoglycoside molecule to yield an altered aminoglycoside product. This competes with the unmodified aminoglycoside for uptake into the cell and binding to the ribosome.

### Basic rule: use only in severe, life-threatening infections

- Gram-negative septicaemia (including *Pseudomonas*) usually in combination with beta-lactam
- Septicaemia of unknown aetiology arising from:
  - healthcare-associated respiratory infections
  - major trauma, major surgery or major burns
  - intravenous catheter
  - complicated urinary catheter-associated infections
- Bacterial endocarditis for synergy with beta-lactam
- *Streptococcus aureus* septicaemia in combination with beta-lactam
- Pyelonephritis for difficult cases
- Postsurgical abdominal sepsis in combination with antianaerobe therapy

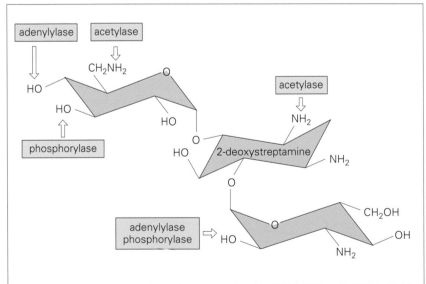

| aminoglycoside-modifying enzyme | reactive group on aminoglycoside | co-factor | modiﬁed aminoglycoside product |
|---|---|---|---|
| acetylase | –NH$_2$ | acetyl CoA | –NHAc |
| adenylylase (nucleotidyl transferase) | –OH | ATP | –O–AMP |
| phosphorylase | –OH | ATP | –O–PO$_2$–OH |

**Fig. 34.11** Prototype structure of aminoglycoside consisting of aminohexoses linked via glycosidic linkage to a central 2-deoxystreptamine nucleus. Hydroxyl and amino groups are sites at which these compounds can be inactivated by phosphorylation, adenylation or acetylation catalysed by enzymes produced by resistant strains.

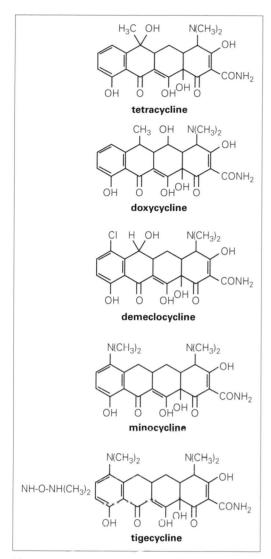

**Fig. 34.12** Tetracyclines are four-ring molecules with different sites around the rings for substitution, thereby giving rise to a family of molecules with different substituents at different sites. Members of the family differ more in their pharmacologic properties than in their spectrum of activity.

problems associated with the drug (see later). Other derivatives have been produced, but none is in widespread clinical use.

Chloramphenicol has affinity for the large (50 S) ribosomal subunit where it blocks the action of peptidyl transferase, thereby preventing peptide bond synthesis (see Fig. 34.10). The drug has some inhibitory activity on human mitochondrial ribosomes (which are also 70 S), which may account for some of the dose-dependent toxicity to bone marrow (see later).

Chloramphenicol is well absorbed when given orally, but it can be given intravenously if the patient cannot take drugs by mouth. Topical preparations are also available. It is well distributed in the body and penetrates host cells. Chloramphenicol is metabolized in the liver by conjugation with glucuronic acid to yield a microbiologically inactive form that is excreted by the kidneys.

### Resistance and toxicity have limited the use of chloramphenicol

Chloramphenicol has been used in the treatment of bacterial meningitis (particularly *H. influenzae*) since the drug achieves satisfactory concentrations in the CSF. Chloramphenicol is active against a wide variety of bacterial species, both gram-positive and gram-negative, aerobes and anaerobes, including intracellular organisms. However, its potential serious toxic effects (see later) and issues of resistance have all but eliminated the systemic use of chloramphenicol in countries where alternative agents are readily available.

The most common mechanism of chloramphenicol resistance involves the inactivation of the drug by a plasmid-mediated enzymatic mechanism, which is easily transferred within gram-negative bacterial populations. Chloramphenicol acetyl transferases produced by resistant bacteria are intracellular but capable of converting chloramphenicol in the immediate environment of the cell to an inactive form that fails to bind to the ribosomal target.

### The most important toxic effects of chloramphenicol are in the bone marrow

Nitrobenzene is a bone marrow suppressant, and the structurally similar chloramphenicol molecule has similar effects. This toxicity takes two forms:

- dose-dependent bone marrow suppression, which occurs if the drug is given for long periods and is reversible when treatment is stopped
- an idiosyncratic reaction causing aplastic anaemia, which is not dose dependent and is irreversible. It can occur after treatment has stopped but fortunately is rare.

Chloramphenicol is also toxic to neonates, particularly premature babies whose liver enzyme systems are incompletely developed. This can result in grey baby syndrome. Thus chloramphenicol serum concentrations should be monitored in neonates.

### Macrolides, lincosamides and streptogramins

These three groups of antibacterial agents share overlapping binding sites on ribosomes, and resistance to macrolides confers resistance to the other two groups.

#### Macrolides

*Erythromycin is a widely used macrolide preventing the release of tRNA after peptide bond formation.* The macrolides are a family of large cyclic molecules all containing a macrocyclic lactone ring (Fig. 34.13A) and bacteriostatic in activity. Erythromycin is the best known, but the newer agents (azithromycin, clarithromycin) have fewer side effects and improved activity and pharmacology.

Macrolides bind to the 23 S rRNA in the 50 S subunit of the ribosome and block the translocation step in protein synthesis, thereby preventing the release of tRNA after peptide bond formation (see Fig. 34.10).

Macrolides are usually administered by the oral route but can also be given intravenously. They are well distributed in the body and penetrate to reach intracellular organisms. The drugs are concentrated in the liver and excreted in the bile. A small proportion of the dose is recoverable in the urine.

*Macrolides are an alternative to penicillin for streptococcal infections, but resistant strains of streptococci are common.* Macrolides are active against gram-positive cocci and an important alternative treatment of infections caused by streptococci in patients allergic to penicillin. They are active against *Legionella pneumophila* and *Campylobacter jejuni*. They are also active against *Mycoplasma* and *Chlamydia* spp. and are therefore important drugs in the treatment of atypical pneumonia and chlamydial infections of the urogenital tract.

Resistance is primarily due to either plasmid-encoded *mef* or *erm* genes for efflux or alteration in the 23 S rRNA target by methylation of two adenine nucleotides in the RNA, respectively. The methylase enzyme may be either inducible or constitutively expressed. Macrolides are better inducers of resistance than the lincosamides, but strains resistant to macrolides will also be resistant to lincomycin and clindamycin, so-called *macrolide-lincosamide-streptogramin (MLS)* resistance. Induction also varies between bacterial species, and resistant strains of gram-positive cocci such as staphylococci and streptococci are common. In contrast to methylation, efflux, while active against macrolide and streptogramin B antibiotics, does not affect streptogramin A and lincosamide drugs.

## Newer macrolide-related (macrocycle) drugs show promise for targeted therapy

The term *macrocycle* generally refers to compounds with a ring structure containing at least eight atoms. This includes not only the macrolides but also a newer class of compounds termed *macrocyclic antibiotics*. Fidaxomicin is a newly approved member of this group. This orally administered bactericidal compound is interesting in its specific targeting of the problem pathogen *C. difficile* (see Ch. 23) without major disturbance of the intestinal microbiota. The drug acts by interfering with mRNA transcription inhibiting bacterial RNA polymerase (see Fig. 34.10).

## Ketolides are semisynthetic derivatives of erythromycin with improved activity against respiratory pathogens

Modification of the macrolide ring structure (see Fig. 34.13B) provides ketolides with increased activity against a variety of gram-positive (and some gram-negative) bacteria, especially those associated with respiratory infections. Ketolides are administered orally and act in a manner similar to erythromycin. However, their higher affinity for the 50 S ribosomal subunit allows them to bind to ribosomes, which are resistant to erythromycin. While active against methicillin-susceptible *S. aureus* that are either susceptible or inducibly

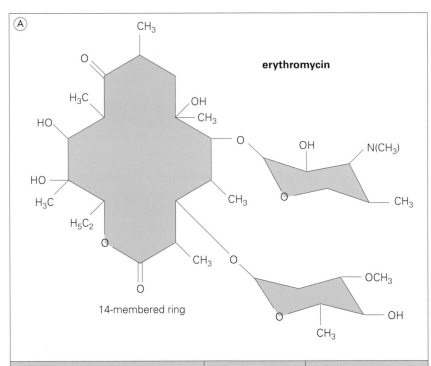

erythromycin

14-membered ring

**Fig. 34.13** (A) The macrolides are antibacterial agents composed of large structures that may be 14-, 15- or 16-membered rings. Erythromycin is the oldest of these, and newer agents with improved activity and fewer side effects are available.

| newer macrolides | in vitro activity compared with erthyromycin | human pharmacokinetics |
|---|---|---|
| azithromycin (15-membered ring) | improved against Gram-negative bacteria | high tissue concentrations, once-daily administration |
| clarithromycin (14-membered ring) | improved against Gram-positive bacteria and *Legionella* spp. | improved peak serum concentration compared with erythromycin |
| **new macrocyclic** | | |
| fidaxomicin | specifically targets *Clostridium difficile* | minimal systemic adsorption |

**Fig. 34.13—cont'd** (B) Major differences in ketolide chemical structure compared with erythromycin (i.e. positions of 3-keto and carbamate on the backbone ring structure).

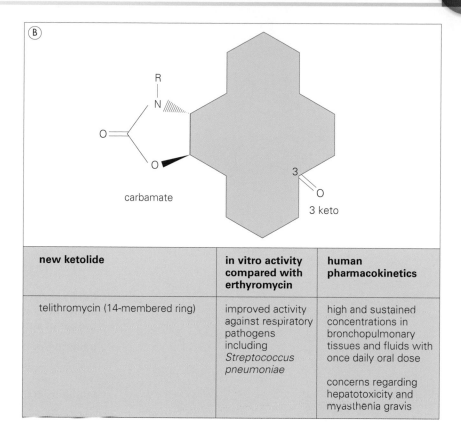

carbamate

3 keto

| new ketolide | in vitro activity compared with erythromycin | human pharmacokinetics |
|---|---|---|
| telithromycin (14-membered ring) | improved activity against respiratory pathogens including *Streptococcus pneumoniae* | high and sustained concentrations in bronchopulmonary tissues and fluids with once daily oral dose<br><br>concerns regarding hepatotoxicity and myasthenia gravis |

resistant to erythromycin, ketolide activity is poor against erythromycin-resistant MRSA. In addition, telithromycin has had major issues related to hepatotoxicity and exacerbations of myasthenia gravis.

## Lincosamides

*Clindamycin inhibits peptide bond formation.* Clindamycin is a chlorinated more active derivative of the lincosamide lincomycin and represents the most important and most clinically used drug in this class.

Lincosamides bind to the 50 S ribosomal subunit and inhibit protein synthesis in a manner similar to macrolides (see Fig. 34.10), hence the MLS resistance combination noted earlier. The selectively toxic action results from a failure to bind to the equivalent mammalian ribosomal subunit.

Clindamycin is usually given orally but can be administered intramuscularly or intravenously. It penetrates well into bone but not into CSF, even when the meninges are inflamed. Clindamycin is actively transported into polymorphonuclear leukocytes and macrophages. It is metabolized in the liver to several products with variable antibacterial activity, and clindamycin activity persists in faeces for up to 5 days after a dose.

*Clindamycin has a spectrum of activity similar to that of erythromycin.* Clindamycin is much more active than macrolides against anaerobes, both gram-positive (e.g. *Clostridium* spp.) and gram-negative (e.g. *Bacteroides*). However, *C. difficile* is often resistant and may be selected in the gut, causing pseudomembranous colitis (see later). The activity of clindamycin against *S. aureus* and its penetration into bone make it an option for the treatment of osteomyelitis. Clindamycin is not active against aerobic gram-negative bacteria because of poor penetration of the outer membrane.

As clindamycin is a less potent inducer of 23 S rRNA methylase (see MLS resistance, earlier), erythromycin-resistant strains may appear susceptible to clindamycin in vitro. However, resistance will be manifest in vivo.

*Pseudomembranous colitis caused by* C. difficile *was first noted following clindamycin treatment.* Pseudomembranous colitis caused by *C. difficile* follows treatment with many antibiotics. The pathogenesis of this complication is described in Chapter 23, and it should be treated with drugs such as metronidazole, oral vancomycin or fidaxomicin.

## Streptogramins

The streptogramin formulation currently available is a mixture of streptogramin B and A compounds—quinupristin and dalfopristin, respectively (Fig. 34.14)—that are bacteriostatic individually but synergistically bactericidal in combination. Both compounds bind to 23 S RNA in the large (50 S) ribosomal subunit (dalfopristin facilitates binding of quinupristin). Dalfopristin inhibits protein synthesis at an earlier stage than quinupristin (see Fig. 34.10), and they, together, interfere with elongation and extension of peptide chains.

Resistance may develop by altering the quinupristin binding site (MLS resistance; see earlier), enzymatic inactivation or efflux.

The quinupristin-dalfopristin combination is active against gram-positive cocci, including multidrug-resistant isolates. Activity is good against *E. faecium* but not *E. faecalis* (most probably due to an intrinsic efflux mechanism). However, there has been concern that commercial use of streptogramin compounds (e.g. virginiamycin) to prevent disease

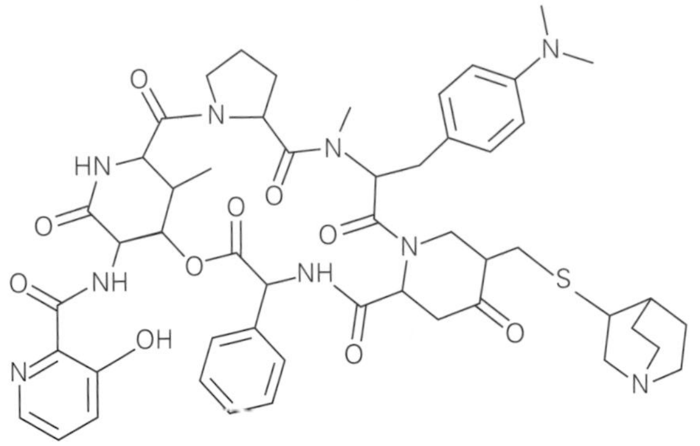

**quinupristin**
(streptogramin B)

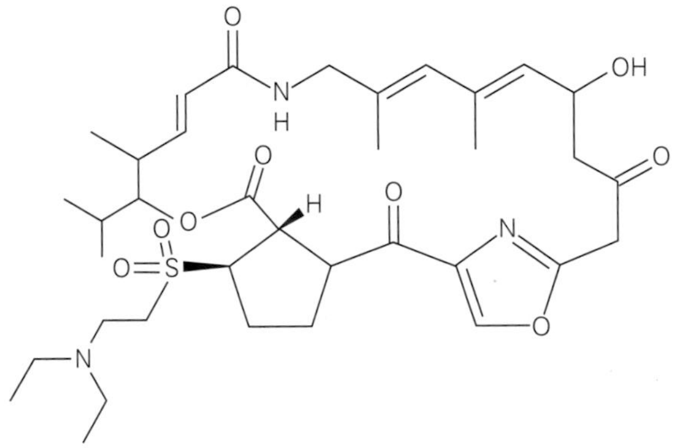

**dalfopristin**
(streptogramin A)

Fig. 34.14 Chemical structure of the streptogramins.

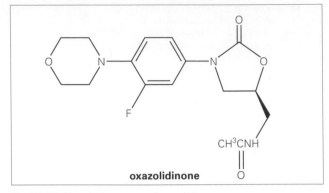

**oxazolidinone**

Fig. 34.15 Chemical structure of oxazolidinones.

## Box 34.5     Inhibitors of Nucleic Acid

**Inhibition of nucleic acid takes place at different stages in its synthesis and function, and different groups of antimicrobial agents are involved**

**Inhibitors of DNA replication**

• Quinolones

**Inhibitors of RNA polymerase**

• Rifampicin

**Antimetabolites inhibiting precursor synthesis**

• Sulphonamides, trimethoprim

and promote growth in poultry could contribute to quinupristin-dalfopristin resistance among gram-positive pathogens in humans.

Quinupristin-dalfopristin is administered intravenously and primarily metabolized in the liver.

## Oxazolidinones

Oxazolidinones are a newer class of synthetic bacteriostatic antimicrobial agents (Fig. 34.15). Linezolid is active against a wide range of gram-positive bacteria, including multiresistant strains. Linezolid inhibits initiation of protein synthesis (see Fig. 34.10) by targeting 23 S rRNA in the 50 S subunit in a manner that prevents formation of a functional 70 S complex. Linezolid is administered orally or intravenously and is metabolized in the liver. A newer oxazolidinone tedizolid is administered and acts similarly to linezolid but appears to have lower haematologic toxicity. Due to the unique oxazolidinone mechanism of action, emergence of resistance is low.

## Fusidic acid

### Fusidic acid is a steroidlike compound that inhibits protein synthesis

Fusidic acid is a bacteriostatic agent that inhibits protein synthesis by forming a stable complex with elongation factor

EF-G (the bacterial equivalent of the human EF-2), guanosine diphosphate and the ribosome.

Fusidic acid can be administered orally or intravenously. It is well absorbed and penetrates well into tissues and bone but not into the CSF. Topical preparations are also available, but their use should not be encouraged because of the rapid emergence of resistance (see later). Fusidic acid is metabolized in the liver and excreted in the bile.

### Fusidic acid is a treatment for staphylococcal infections but should be used with other antistaphylococcal drugs to prevent emergence of resistance

Fusidic acid is active against gram-positive cocci, and its most important use is in the treatment of staphylococcal infections resistant to beta-lactams or in patients who are allergic to alternative staphylococcal agents. Fusidic acid should be given in combination with another antistaphylococcal agent to prevent the emergence of resistant mutants with altered EF-G, which can emerge rapidly in staphylococcal populations exposed to the drug.

### Fusidic acid has few side effects

Occasionally, fusidic acid causes jaundice and gastrointestinal upset.

## INHIBITORS OF NUCLEIC ACID SYNTHESIS

Antibacterial agents that act as inhibitors of nucleic acid synthesis do so in one of three main ways, as listed in Box 34.5.

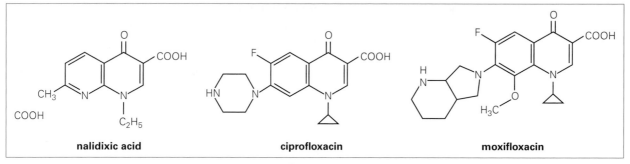

**Fig. 34.16** The quinolones form a large group of synthetic antibacterial agents.

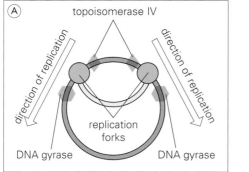
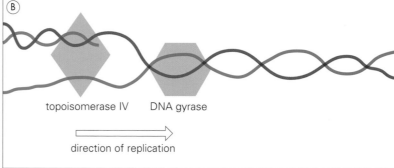

**Fig. 34.17** (A) An overview and (B) an enlarged view of the role played by bacterial gyrase and topoisomerase enzymes in replication of the bacterial chromosome.

## Quinolones

### Quinolones are synthetic agents that interfere with replication of the bacterial chromosome

Quinolones represent a large family of bactericidal synthetic agents which, in a manner similar to the cephalosporins, are sometimes discussed in terms of generations based on their spectrum of activity. However, these categories are less clear than for the cephalosporins. Nalidixic acid was the first-generation prototype, but the addition of fluorine at position 6 of the main quinolone ring (i.e. fluoroquinolones [e.g. ciprofloxacin, moxifloxacin]) (Fig. 34.16) has improved antibacterial activity, leading to the synthesis of many additional, more commonly used compounds.

The antibacterial activity of quinolones is due to their ability to inhibit the activity of bacterial DNA gyrase and topoisomerases. During replication of the bacterial chromosome, DNA gyrase produces and removes supercoils in DNA ahead of the replication fork to maintain the proper tension required for efficient DNA duplication. Topoisomerase IV similarly acts to remove supercoils and to separate newly formed DNA daughter strands after replication (Fig. 34.17). These enzymes thus act in concert to ensure that the DNA molecule has the proper conformation for efficient replication and packaging within the cell. Quinolones are able to interfere with these essential enzymes in bacteria while not affecting their counterparts in mammalian cells.

### Resistance to quinolones is usually chromosomally mediated

Chromosomally mediated resistance is exhibited in two forms:

- mutations, which change the target enzymes in a manner that affects quinolone binding
- changes in cell wall permeability, resulting in decreased uptake, or by efflux. These mechanisms may also lead to cross-resistance to other unrelated agents affected by the same process.

Plasmid-encoded quinolone resistance involves production of a protein (termed *qnr*) that protects the target DNA from quinolone binding.

### Quinolones are used as alternatives to beta-lactam antibiotics for treating a variety of infections

Quinolones are primarily administered orally since they are readily absorbed from the gastrointestinal tract, achieving significant serum concentrations and good distribution throughout the body compartments.

Ciprofloxacin, gemifloxacin, levofloxacin, moxifloxacin and ofloxacin are the drugs most commonly used. Excretion is mostly in the urine; however, drugs such as moxifloxacin are excreted to a significant amount in faeces.

The newer quinolones have improved activity against gram-negative rods, including *P. aeruginosa*. In addition to the treatment of urinary tract infections, the newer quinolones are useful for systemic gram-negative infections and in the treatment of chlamydial and rickettsial infections. They are also useful in infections caused by other intracellular organisms, such as *L. pneumophila* and *Salmonella typhi*, and in combination with other agents for atypical mycobacteria. They have activity against staphylococci, but many strains of MRSA now exhibit high-level resistance, and there is limited use against streptococci and enterococci.

## Fluoroquinolones are not recommended for children or pregnant or lactating women because of possible toxic effects on cartilage development

Gastrointestinal disturbances are the most common side effect of quinolones. Neurotoxicity and photosensitivity reactions are less common. All fluoroquinolones have the potential to cause tendon ruptures in active patients who may tend to push their workout regimens. This risk is increased when quinolones and corticosteroids are simultaneously administered.

## Rifamycins

### Rifampicin is clinically the most important rifamycin and blocks the synthesis of mRNA

Rifampicin is the most important member of the rifamycin family in clinical use. It is a large molecule with a complex structure. Other family members such as rifabutin and rifapentine are also available. All are bactericidal in activity.

Rifampicin binds to DNA-dependent RNA polymerase and blocks the synthesis of mRNA. Selective toxicity is based on the far greater affinity for bacterial polymerases than for the equivalent human enzymes.

Rifampicin is administered orally, is well absorbed and is very well distributed in the body. It crosses the blood-brain barrier and reaches high concentrations in saliva. It also appears to have an affinity for plastics, which can be valuable in the treatment of infections involving prostheses.

Rifampicin is metabolized in the liver and excreted in bile. The compound is red, and the urine, sweat and saliva of treated patients turn orange. This is harmless, although disturbing for the patient, but it is good evidence of patient compliance.

The newer rifamycins, rifabutin and rifapentine are excreted more slowly than rifampicin, thereby allowing less frequent administration—a feature particularly attractive in the treatment of TB.

### The primary use for rifampicin is in the treatment of mycobacterial infections, but resistance is a concern

While used primarily against mycobacteria, rifampicin may also be used for the prophylaxis of close contacts of meningococcal and *Haemophilus meningitis*. However, highly resistant meningococcal strains may emerge; thus short courses only (maximum 48 h) should be given.

While staphylococci rapidly develop resistance to rifampicin, the drug can be efficacious if used in combination with another agent, particularly in the treatment of prosthetic valve endocarditis.

Resistance is provided by chromosomal mutations that alter the RNA polymerase target, which then has lowered affinity for rifampicin and escapes inhibition. The prevalence of rifampicin-resistant *Mycobacterium tuberculosis* is increasing, which is problematic for anti-TB therapy.

### Rashes and jaundice are side effects of rifampicin treatment

Intermittent rifampicin can lead to hypersensitivity reactions.

## ANTIMETABOLITES AFFECTING NUCLEIC ACID SYNTHESIS

Several commonly used antimicrobial agents inhibit bacterial metabolic pathways, including those that produce precursors for nucleic acid synthesis.

## Sulphonamides

### Sulphonamides are structural analogues of and act in competition with *para*-aminobenzoic acid

This group of molecules is produced entirely by chemical synthesis (i.e. they are not natural products). In 1935 the parent compound sulphanilamide became the first clinically effective antibacterial agent. The *p*-amino group is essential for activity, but modifications to the sulphonic acid side chain have produced many related agents (Fig. 34.18).

Sulphonamides are bacteriostatic compounds that act in competition with *para*-aminobenzoic acid (PABA) for the active site of dihydropteroate synthetase, an enzyme that catalyses an essential reaction in the synthetic pathway of tetrahydrofolic acid (THFA), which is required for the synthesis of purines and pyrimidines and therefore for nucleic acid synthesis (Fig. 34.19). Selective toxicity depends on the fact that many bacteria synthesize THFA, whereas human cells lack this capacity and depend on an exogenous supply

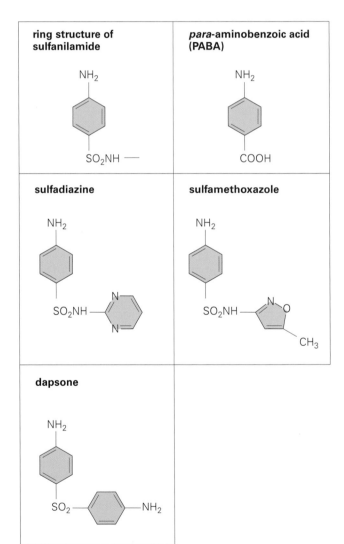

**Fig. 34.18** The ring structure of the sulphonamides is very similar to the structure of the normal substrate (PABA) of the dihydropteroate synthetase enzyme, which the sulphonamides inhibit. The sulphonamides differ in their pharmacologic properties more than in their spectrum of activity. Dapsone is important in the treatment of *Mycobacterium leprae*.

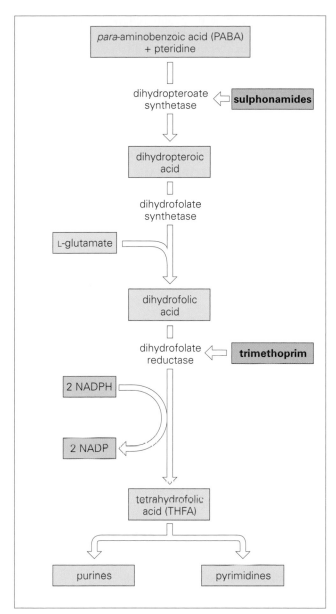

**Fig. 34.19** Sulphonamides and trimethoprim inhibit in series the steps in the synthesis of tetrahydrofolic acid by interacting with key enzymes in the pathway. NADP, Nicotinamide adenine dinucleotide phosphate; NADPH, nicotinamide adenine dinucleotide phosphate reduced form.

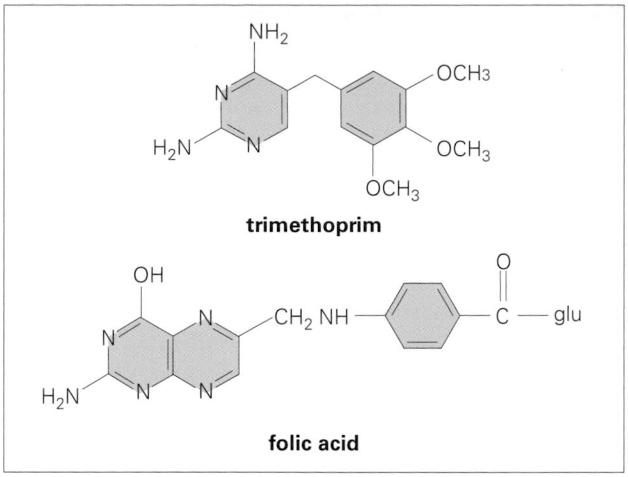

**Fig. 34.20** Trimethoprim resembles the aminohydroxypyrimidine moiety of folic acid and, in this way, antagonizes the enzyme dihydrofolate reductase.

of folic acid. Bacteria that can use preformed folic acid are similarly unaffected by sulphonamides.

Sulphonamides are usually administered orally, often in combination with trimethoprim as co-trimoxazole (see later). Different molecules within the family differ in their solubility and penetrability. Metabolism occurs in the liver, and free and metabolized drug is excreted by the kidneys.

### Sulphonamides are useful in the treatment of urinary tract infection, but resistance is widespread

The sulphonamides have a spectrum of activity primarily against gram-negative organisms (except *Pseudomonas*). Therefore they are useful in the treatment of urinary tract infections (see Ch. 21). However, susceptibility cannot be assumed, as resistance is widespread with plasmid-mediated genes coding for an altered dihydropteroate

synthetase. This is essentially unchanged in its affinity for PABA but has a greatly decreased affinity for the sulphonamide. Therefore a possesses two distinct enzymes: a sensitive chromosome-encoded enzyme and a resistant plasmid-encoded enzyme.

### Rarely, sulphonamides cause Stevens-Johnson syndrome

Sulphonamides are relatively free of toxic side effects, but rashes and bone marrow suppression can occur.

### Trimethoprim (and co-trimoxazole)

#### Trimethoprim is a structural analogue of the aminohydroxypyrimidine moiety of folic acid and prevents the synthesis of THFA

Trimethoprim is one of a group of pyrimidine-like molecules analogous in structure to the aminohydroxypyrimidine moiety of the folic acid molecule (Fig. 34.20). Other agents with a similar structure and mechanism of action include the antimalarial pyrimethamine and the anticancer drug methotrexate.

Trimethoprim, like sulphonamides, prevents THFA synthesis, but at a later stage by inhibiting dihydrofolate reductase (see Fig. 34.19). This enzyme is present in mammalian cells as well as bacterial and protozoan cells, and selective toxicity depends upon the far greater affinity of trimethoprim for the bacterial enzyme.

Trimethoprim is often given in combination with sulphamethoxazole as co-trimoxazole. The advantages of this combination over either drug alone are as follows:

- Mutant bacteria resistant to one agent are less likely to be resistant to the other (i.e. double mutation).
- The two agents act synergistically against some bacteria (i.e. the combined action of the two bacteriostatic agents has a bactericidal effect that is greater than the action of either agent alone).

Trimethoprim can be given orally (either alone or as co-trimoxazole) or by intravenous infusion (alone or accompanied by sulphonamide). Trimethoprim is excreted in urine, and in patients with severe renal failure it is excreted more rapidly than sulphonamide so that the synergistic ratio of the combination may be lost.

## Trimethoprim is often given with sulphamethoxazole as co-trimoxazole for urinary tract infections

Trimethoprim alone is active against gram-negative rods, with the exception of *Pseudomonas* spp., and its main use is in the treatment (and long-term prophylaxis) of urinary tract infection (see Ch. 21); however, the development of resistance is a concern.

Co-trimoxazole is active against a wide range of urinary tract pathogens and against *S. typhi*. This combination is also valuable for the treatment of pneumonia caused by the fungus *Pneumocystis jirovecii* (formerly *P. carinii*), although pentamidine, another pyrimidine derivative, is probably the preferred alternative. Co-trimoxazole is also useful for the treatment of nocardiosis.

## Resistance to trimethoprim is provided by plasmid-encoded dihydrofolate reductases

Plasmid-encoded dihydrofolate reductases with altered affinity for trimethoprim allow the synthesis of THFA to proceed unhindered by the presence of trimethoprim. The replacement enzymes are ~20,000-fold less susceptible to trimethoprim while retaining their affinity for the normal substrate. Bacteria that are resistant to sulphonamide and trimethoprim are also resistant to co-trimoxazole.

## Trimethoprim and co-trimoxazole

Trimethoprim alone and in combination with sulphamethoxazole can cause neutropenia. Nausea and vomiting may occur.

## OTHER AGENTS THAT AFFECT DNA

### Nitroimidazoles

#### While nitroimidazoles are generally known for their antiparasitic activity, metronidazole also exhibits antibacterial properties

After entry into the microbial cell, the molecule is activated by reduction, and the reduced intermediate products are responsible for antimicrobial activity probably through interaction with, and breakage of, the cell's DNA. The reactive intermediates are short lived and decompose to nontoxic inactive end products. Metronidazole is active only against anaerobic organisms because only these can produce the low redox potential necessary to reduce the parent drug.

Metronidazole has also been used as a hypoxic cell sensitizer in radiotherapy.

Metronidazole is usually given orally or rectally. It is well absorbed and well distributed in tissues and CSF. The drug is metabolized, and most of the parent compound and metabolites are excreted in the urine.

#### Metronidazole was originally introduced for the treatment of the flagellate parasite *Trichomonas vaginalis*

Metronidazole is also effective against other protozoan parasites such as *Giardia duodenalis* and *Entamoeba histolytica*. It is an important agent for the treatment of infections caused by anaerobic bacteria.

Metronidazole resistance is of increasing concern in *T. vaginalis*, *G. duodenalis* and several anaerobic and microaerophilic bacteria and commonly involves either an alteration in uptake or a decrease in cellular reductase activity, thereby slowing the activation of the intracellular drug. *Helicobacter pylori*, a microaerophilic bacterium causing ulcers and gastritis, has been frequently treated with metronidazole. However, resistance can rapidly develop.

#### Rarely, metronidazole causes CNS side effects

The most serious side effects of metronidazole involve the CNS and include peripheral neuropathy, however, these are relatively uncommon and are usually only seen in patients on large doses or prolonged treatment.

## INHIBITORS OF CYTOPLASMIC MEMBRANE FUNCTION

The cytoplasmic membranes that encompass all kinds of living cells perform a variety of vital functions. The structure of these membranes in bacterial cells differs from that in mammalian cells and allows the application of some selectively toxic molecules, but these are few in number compared with those acting at other target sites.

### Lipopeptides

#### Lipopeptides are a newer class of membrane-active antibiotics

Daptomycin is a lipopeptide antibiotic with bactericidal activity against a wide variety of gram-positive bacteria, including vancomycin-resistant *E. faecalis* and *E. faecium* and methicillin-resistant *S. aureus* and *S. epidermidis* (Fig. 34.21). The drug has been especially useful in treating complicated skin and skin structure infections and bactaeremia. The compound acts in a calcium-dependent matter to insert and depolarize the bacterial cytoplasmic membrane, leading to a number of consequences, including the inability to synthesize ATP and interference with uptake of nutrients. At present, resistance to daptomycin has been relatively rare and seems to occur in a stepwise fashion over time.

### Polymyxins

#### Polymyxins act on the membranes of gram-negative bacteria

In addition to the polymyxins, the polyene antifungal agents (e.g. amphotericin B, nystatin) also act by inhibiting membrane function (see later). Polymyxins are bactericidal cyclic polypeptides that disrupt the structure of cell membranes.

The free amino groups of polymyxins act as cationic detergents, disrupting the phospholipid structure of the cell membrane. Polymyxin B is the most common member of the family still in clinical use.

In the past, polymyxins have been used systemically, but due to poor distribution in tissues, neurotoxicity and nephrotoxicity, their general use has been superseded by less toxic agents.

#### There is renewed interest in polymyxins as a last-effort option for treating multiresistant gram-negative infections

Polymyxins are active against most gram-negative organisms except *Proteus* spp. They have been especially used topically in ointments. After oral administration, polymyxins are not absorbed from the gut, and polymyxin E (colistin)

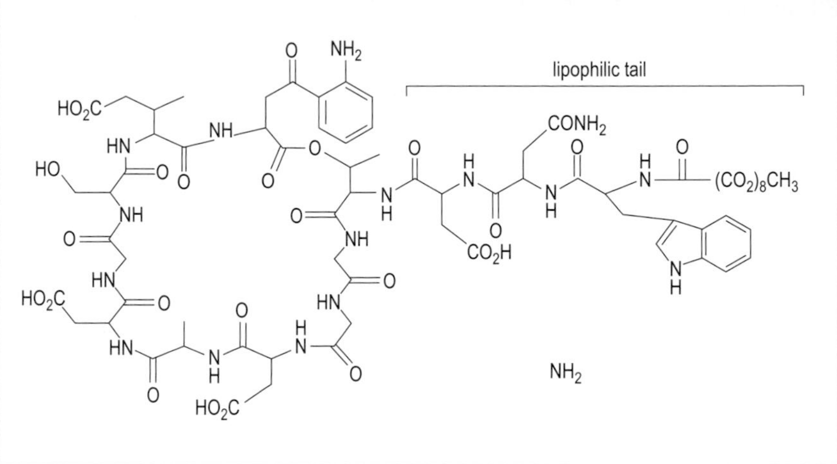

**Fig. 34.21** Chemical structure of the cyclic lipopeptide, daptomycin, consisting of a 13-member amino acid cyclic lipopeptide with a lipophilic tail, which attacks the bacterial cell membrane, causing depolarization and a potassium iron efflux.

has been used in some gut decontamination regimens for neutropenic patients, although with caution owing to concerns regarding renal toxicity. Concerns regarding the lack of effective antibiotics for treating multidrug resistant gram-negative bacteria (especially *Pseudomonas* and *Acinetobacter* spp.) have led to renewed interest in polymixin/colistin combination therapy.

Resistance is due to both chromosomal and plasmid encoded (e.g., mcr) mechanisms, which alter membrane structure or antibiotic uptake.

## URINARY TRACT ANTISEPTICS

### Nitrofurantoin and methenamine inhibit urinary pathogens

Nitrofurantoin and methenamine are both synthetic compounds that, when taken orally, are absorbed and excreted in the urine in concentrations high enough to inhibit urinary pathogens. Nitrofurantoin has activity only in acid urine. Methenamine is hydrolysed at acid pH to produce ammonia and formaldehyde; it is the formaldehyde that has the antibacterial activity. Nitrofurantoin is used to treat uncomplicated urinary tract infection, and both agents are used to prevent recurrent urinary tract infections, although there are concerns with adverse reactions in the young and elderly. While resistance rarely develops in susceptible bacterial populations, resistance to nitrofurantoin prior to treatment is a concern.

## ANTITUBERCULOSIS AGENTS

### *M. tuberculosis* and other mycobacterial infections need prolonged treatment

The treatment of infections caused by *M. tuberculosis* and other mycobacteria presents an enormous challenge to medicine and the pharmaceutical industry because these organisms:

- have a waxy outer layer that makes them naturally very impermeable and difficult to penetrate with antibiotics
- have an intracellular location, often in cells surrounded by a mass of caseous material, that also makes it difficult for antibiotics to get to them

- grow and multiply extremely slowly, and effective inhibition (and therefore cure) takes weeks or months to achieve. Long-term therapy is therefore a challenge for drug delivery, and orally administrable drugs are consequently highly desirable. It also follows that the emergence of resistance among the mycobacteria and toxicity in the patient are more likely than with the short sharp shock treatment more often administered for bacterial infections
- are common and increasing in the wake of the acquired immunodeficiency syndrome (AIDS) epidemic in resource-poor countries, where the cost of drug treatment can be prohibitive.

### The drugs for first-line therapy of TB are isoniazid, ethambutol, rifampicin and pyrazinamide

Treatment regimens vary between countries and the susceptibility of the infecting strain, but where susceptibility is uncertain, an initial course of isoniazid, ethambutol, rifampicin and pyrazinamide is typically followed for 2 months followed by a two-drug (e.g. isoniazid and rifampicin) continuation phase for an additional 18 weeks. If the strain is susceptible to both isoniazid and rifampicin, ethambutol is then discontinued. The structure and mechanism of action of rifampicin have been described earlier this chapter.

### Isoniazid

#### Isoniazid inhibits mycobacteria and is given with pyridoxine to prevent neurologic side effects

Isoniazid is isonicotinic acid hydrazide, a compound that inhibits mycobacteria but does not affect other species of bacteria or humans to any great extent. Its bactericidal activity results from inhibition of mycolic acid synthesis, which also accounts for its specificity. It is well absorbed after oral administration, and a single daily dose is usually prescribed except in more difficult cases such as meningitis or miliary TB. The main toxic effects in humans are neurologic complications (which can be prevented by the concurrent administration of pyridoxine) and hepatitis.

## Ethambutol

### Ethambutol inhibits mycobacteria but can cause optic neuritis

Ethambutol is a synthetic molecule that inhibits but does not kill mycobacteria. It acts by inhibiting the polymerization of arabinoglycan, a critical constituent of the mycobacteria cell wall. It is well absorbed after oral administration and well distributed in the body, including the CSF. Resistance appears fairly rapidly if the drug is used alone. Thus it is combined with other drugs in anti-TB therapy. An important toxic side effect is optic neuritis, and visual acuity should be monitored during therapy.

## Pyrazinamide

Pyrazinamide is a synthetic analogue of nicotinamide, which appears to target mycolic acid synthesis. After oral administration, the drug is readily absorbed from the gastrointestinal tract and well distributed in body tissues and fluids. It is primarily metabolized in the liver and excreted by the kidney. As with ethambutol, resistance during monotherapy requires that the drug be used in combination with other first-line agents. The most important toxic side effect of pyrazinamide is hepatotoxicity.

## Mycobacterial resistance

### Drug resistance and immunocompromised patients complicate TB therapy

Despite the use of antibiotics in combination, the incidence of resistance among mycobacteria is a persistent and increasing problem. Infections with mycobacteria other than *M. tuberculosis* are on the increase as opportunist infections in people with AIDS and these organisms tend to be innately more resistant than *M. tuberculosis*.

## Treatment of leprosy

### The development of resistance during dapsone monotherapy for leprosy has led to its use in combination with rifampicin

Infection caused by *M. leprae* is characterized by persistence of the organism in the tissues for years and necessitates very prolonged treatment to prevent relapse. For many years dapsone, related to the sulphonamides (see Fig. 34.18), has been used. This drug has the advantages that it is given orally and that it is cheap and effective. However, monotherapy has resulted in the emergence of resistance, and a combination of dapsone, rifampicin and clofazimine, a phenazine compound (mechanism of action not well understood), is now commonly used as multidrug therapy.

## ANTIBACTERIAL AGENTS IN PRACTICE

It is clear from the preceding sections of this chapter that although there are certain rules of thumb about the resistance of bacteria to an antibiotic, it is often impossible to do more than guess in the absence of laboratory tests. Susceptibility tests performed in the laboratory examine the interaction between antibiotics and bacteria in an isolated and rather artificial fashion. At best, the results are a helpful guide to the likely outcome of therapy; at worst, they are misleading. Patient factors such as age, underlying disease, site and type of infection, renal and liver impairment and drug pharmacodynamics must be taken into account in the antibiotic management of an infection.

## Susceptibility tests

Laboratory tests for antibiotic susceptibility fall into two main categories: disk diffusion tests and dilution tests.

### Diffusion tests involve seeding the organism on an agar plate and applying filter paper disks containing antibiotics

The isolate to be tested is seeded over the entire surface of an agar plate, and filter paper disks containing the antibiotics are applied. After overnight incubation the plate is observed for zones of inhibition around each antibiotic disk (Fig. 34.22). The amount of antibiotic in the disk is related to, among other things, the achievable serum concentration and therefore differs for different antibiotics. In addition, antibiotics differ in their ability to diffuse in agar, so the size of the inhibition zone (and not simply its presence) is an indicator of susceptibility of the isolate. The zone sizes are compared with those for reference organisms (either tested in parallel or established previously and published in reference tables) and the result recorded as S (susceptible), I (intermediate) or R (resistant). An I result indicates that the isolate is less susceptible than the norm but may respond to higher doses of antibiotic or in sites where the antibiotic is concentrated (e.g. in urine in the bladder for antibiotics excreted by the kidneys).

### A dilution test provides a quantitative estimate of susceptibility to an antibiotic

A more quantitative estimate of the susceptibility of an organism to an antibiotic can be achieved by performing a minimum inhibitory concentration (MIC) test (i.e. a test to find the lowest concentration that will inhibit visible growth of the bacterial isolate in vitro). Serial dilutions of the test antibiotic are prepared in broth or agar medium and inoculated with a suspension of the test organism. After overnight incubation the MIC is recorded as the highest dilution in which there is no macroscopic growth (Fig. 34.23). These tests can be performed in a microtitre plate format and form

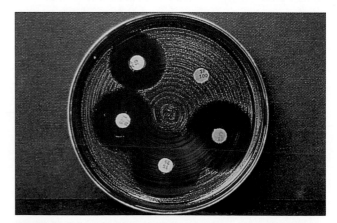

**Fig. 34.22** The antibiotic susceptibility of an organism can be tested by the application of filter paper impregnated with antibiotic onto a lawn of the organisms seeded on an agar plate. After overnight incubation the organism grows and the antibiotics diffuse to produce a zone of inhibition that indicates the degree of susceptibility: disk susceptibility test indicating sulphonamide resistance. SF100 is the sulphonamide disk. (Courtesy D.K. Banerjee.)

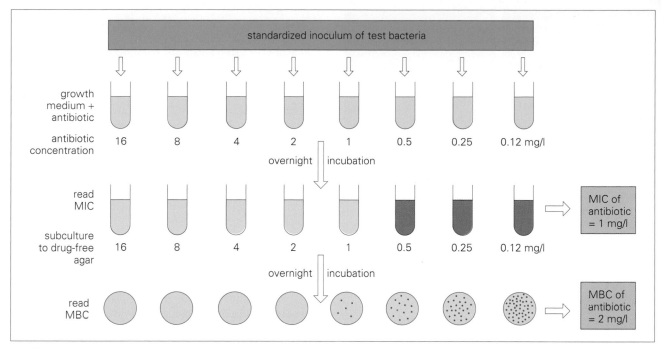

**Fig. 34.23** More precise measures of the amount of antibiotic required to inhibit and kill a bacterial population can be estimated by establishing the minimum inhibitory concentration (MIC) and minimum bactericidal concentration (MBC) of the antibiotic. Using the standard method as outlined in this illustration, the MIC result is available after 24 h and the MBC result after 48 h. A number of variables such as the inoculum size, the growth medium and the interpretation of the results affect the outcome of MIC tests.

the basis of some automated susceptibility test systems. An alternative approach is the E-test in which a filter paper strip impregnated with a gradient of antibiotic is laid on an agar plate seeded with the test isolate. The concentration on the strip at which growth is inhibited indicates the MIC.

MIC tests are clearly more time consuming and costly than disk diffusion tests in terms of time and materials and are not routinely performed in the clinical laboratory; they can, however, yield useful information for the management of difficult infections or for patients who are failing to respond to apparently appropriate therapy.

An advantage of a MIC test is that it can be extended to determine the minimum bactericidal concentration (MBC), which is the lowest concentration of an antibiotic required to kill the organism. To discover whether the agent has actually killed the bacteria rather than simply inhibited their growth, the test dilutions are subcultured onto a fresh drug-free medium and incubated for a further 18–24 h (see Fig. 34.23). The antibacterial agent is considered to be bactericidal if the MBC is equal to or not greater than fourfold higher than the MIC.

### Killing curves provide a dynamic estimate of bacterial susceptibility

One of the disadvantages of MIC and MBC tests is that the result is read at only one point in time. A more dynamic estimate of bacterial susceptibility can be gained by measuring the decrease in viability of the population with time (Fig. 34.24). As with MIC and MBC tests, killing curves are more time consuming and costly than disk diffusion tests and are only typically performed on a research basis. A number of the automated susceptibility test systems use a measure of bacterial viability (e.g. turbidity, electrical impedance) in the presence of an antibacterial agent as their indicator

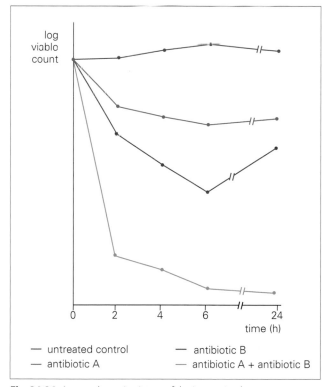

— untreated control  — antibiotic B
— antibiotic A  — antibiotic A + antibiotic B

**Fig. 34.24** A more dynamic picture of the interaction between an antibiotic and a bacterial population can be gained from producing killing curves. In these experiments a culture of $2 \times 10^6$ colony-forming units/mL was treated with antibiotics A and B alone and in combination. Compared with the untreated control, both A and B inhibit the growth of the bacterial culture, but B is more active than A. However, in combination, the activity of A plus B is synergistic (i.e. it is more active than the sum of the activities of the two antibiotics alone). The combination also prevents the regrowth seen after 6–24 h when the antibiotics are used singly.

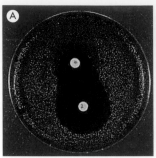
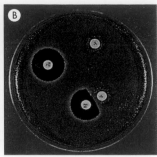

**Fig. 34.25** (A) Synergy of two antibacterial agents. Disks containing sulphonamide and trimethoprim have been placed to demonstrate the synergistic activity of these two agents against *Escherichia coli*. Synergy can be recognized by the fact that the zones of inhibition become continuous between the two disks. (B) Antagonism. Nitrofurantoin is capable of antagonizing the activity of nalidixic acid. When the disks are placed far apart, nalidixic acid inhibits the test organism, but when placed close together, this inhibition is antagonized by the presence of nitrofurantoin as demonstrated by the foreshortening of the zone of inhibition.

system. These machines can produce results more rapidly (e.g. within a few hours) than conventional susceptibility tests. However, fastidious organisms (e.g. *S. pneumoniae*, *N. meningitidis*) or resistance that is characteristically difficult to detect (e.g. borderline oxacillin MICs in *S. aureus*, ESBLs in gram-negative isolates) can be problematic.

## Combining antibacterial agents can lead to synergism or antagonism

Hospital patients frequently receive more than one antibacterial agent, and these agents may interact with each other (and with other drugs such as diuretics).

Antibacterial combinations are described as:

- synergistic if their activity is greater than the sum of the individual activities
- antagonistic if the activity of one drug is compromised in the presence of the other.

Both disk diffusion and dilution tests allow the action of combinations of antibiotics to be studied. Although synergy often can be demonstrated in vitro (Fig. 34.25), it is difficult to confirm in vivo. Co-trimoxazole is an example of a combination that is frequently used (see earlier). Another example is the combination of penicillin (or ceftriaxone) with gentamicin in the treatment of endocarditis caused by a penicillin-susceptible strain, as this combination has been shown to be clearly superior to the effect of the beta-lactam alone (Box 34.6).

Antagonism can be demonstrated between some pairs of antibiotics in vitro but is rarely evident in vivo.

## ANTIBIOTIC ASSAYS

In the preceding parts of this chapter the pharmacokinetic properties (i.e. absorption, distribution, excretion) of antibacterial agents have been summarized. Some antibacterial agents have a narrow therapeutic index (i.e. the concentration required for successful treatment and the concentration toxic to the patient are not very different). The concentrations of such antibiotics should be monitored both to prevent toxicity and to ensure that therapeutic concentrations are achieved. Other less toxic agents should be monitored in some circumstances in some patients (Box 34.7). Serum

---

### Box 34.6    Use of Antibiotic Combinations

**Reasons for using antibiotic combinations**

Ideally, single drugs are used, but antibiotic combinations are justifiable under certain circumstances:

- to obtain a synergistic effect (e.g. co-trimoxazole)
- to prevent or delay emergence of persistent organisms (e.g. isoniazid, rifampicin, ethambutol and pyrazinamide for TB)
- to treat polymicrobial infections (e.g. intraabdominal abscesses in which the different microbes have different susceptibilities)
- to treat serious infection in the stage before the infectious agent is identified.

---

### Box 34.7    Importance of Antibiotic Assays

Assays of antibiotics in clinical practice are particularly important when the antibiotic is potentially toxic, but there are other situations in which assays are important:

- when an antibiotic has a narrow therapeutic index (e.g. aminoglycosides)
- when the normal route of excretion of antibiotic is impaired (e.g. in patients with renal failure for agents excreted via the kidney)
- when the absorption of the antibiotic is uncertain (e.g. after oral administration)
- to ascertain concentrations in sites of infection into which penetration of antibiotics is irregular or unknown (e.g. in cerebrospinal fluid)
- in patients receiving prolonged therapy for serious infections (e.g. endocarditis)
- in neonates with serious infections
- in patients who fail to respond to apparently appropriate therapy
- to check on patient compliance.

---

concentrations are usually measured, but urine, CSF and other body fluids can be assayed if applicable.

Antibiotic assays may be performed by a variety of methods such as high-performance liquid chromatography and direct assays for biologic activity (bioassay). However, the most common approach uses immunologic methods that can be automated. In this method, the antibiotic in the patient specimen is an antigen that competes with a specific level of labelled tracking antibiotic for binding sites on an antidrug antibody. Thus increased antibiotic levels in a patient sample result in decreased binding of tracking antibiotic, etc. Such assays are rapid, require only small volumes of serum and are highly specific. However, they are obviously only applicable in instances in which specific antidrug antibody is available.

## ANTIVIRAL THERAPY

### Antiviral drugs do not kill viruses but stop viral replication

The range of targets and the number of antiviral agents licensed to treat (unlike James Bond, as they cannot kill)

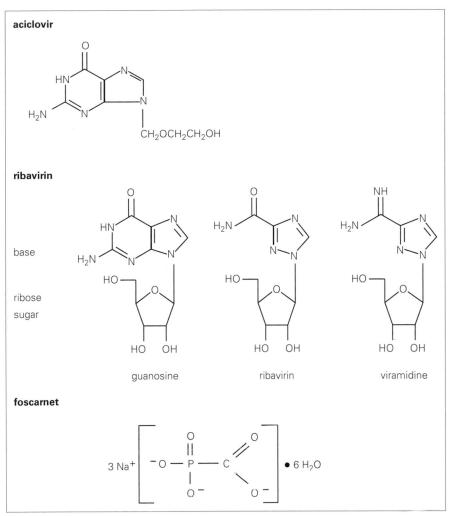

**Fig. 34.26** Examples of the structures of different antiviral drugs that cause chain termination by being guanosine analogues that can be incorporated into viral DNA and inhibit the viral DNA polymerase (aciclovir), use a similar mechanism but with RNA polymerase (ribavirin, which also has an effect intracellularly to ribavirin monophosphate, which competitively inhibits inosine monophosphate dehydrogenase causing depletion of guanosine triphosphate needed for viral RNA synthesis), or bind at the viral polymerase active site (foscarnet).

viral infections have been part of the huge successes in clinical virology. Initially, the first antiviral drug, idoxuridine, was approved in 1963, and the armamentarium increased slowly but surely over the next 50 years. However, by 2023 there were >91 antiviral drugs, not including novel combinations and immunomodulators, that were being used to treat human immunodeficiency virus (HIV), hepatitis B and C viruses (HBV and HCV), herpesviruses (including herpes simplex virus [HSV], varicella-zoster virus [VZV] and cytomegalovirus [CMV]), influenza A and B, respiratory syncytial virus (RSV), human papillomavirus (HPV) and severe acute respiratory syndrome coronavirus 2 (SARS-CoV-2) infections (Fig. 34.26). They are all virustatic rather than virucidal; in other words, they do not kill viruses but suppress their replication. Of the increasing array of antiviral agents licensed for treatment, there has been a revolution in treating the viral infections that cause chronic infection and disease, namely HIV, HBV and HCV infections. The number and range of drugs continue to increase, and compliance and ease of taking these treatments have improved by reducing pill burden by combination therapy and by being able to offer single-tablet oral treatment. Combination antiretroviral therapy (cART)

has made HIV infection a chronic, controllable infection as it has improved survival and reduced hospital admission. It can also be used as pre- and postexposure prophylaxis (PrEP and PEP) to reduce transmission. By 2023 a number of antiretroviral drugs used in the previous 2 decades had been discontinued, with a focus on a more selective list comprising seven different classes of drug (summarized in Table 34.6), including many single-tablet two- to four-drug combination pills as well as a long-acting injectable integrase inhibitor and nonnucleoside reverse transcriptase inhibitor (NNRTI) combination.

In addition, a rapid change in the treatment landscape was seen with HCV infection, with new drugs and combinations becoming past history as others replaced them in short time periods, leading to sustained virologic responses (SVRs) translating into viral clearance after short treatment courses. The problem in developing new antivirals has been mostly due to the difficulty of interfering with viral activity in the cell without adversely affecting the host. This is because viruses are dependent on the host cell's protein synthetic machinery.

Reports have highlighted the importance of making an early diagnosis in short incubation period viral infections, such as influenza, in order for antiviral treatment to be

**Table 34.6** Antiviral drugs

| DNA viruses | |
|---|---|
| CMV | Ganciclovir<br>Valganciclovir<br>Foscarnet<br>Cidofovir<br>Letermovir (prophylaxis in transplant settings) |
| HSV and VZV | Aciclovir<br>Valaciclovir<br>Famciclovir<br>Ganciclovir<br>Foscarnet<br>Cidofovir |
| HBV | Tenofovir<br>Entecavir<br>Emtricitabine<br>Lamividine<br>Interferon-α |
| **RNA viruses** | |
| Influenza A and B viruses | Oseltamivir<br>Zanamavir<br>Peramivir<br>Baloxavir |
| RSV | Ribavirin |
| ***HIV*** | |
| Nucleoside and nucleotide reverse transcriptase inhibitors | Abacavir<br>Emtricitabine<br>Lamivudine<br>Tenofovir disoproxil fumarate<br>Tenofovir alafenamide<br>Zidovudine |
| Fusion inhibitor | Enfuvirtide |
| CCR5 inhibitor | Maraviroc |
| Nonnucleoside reverse transcriptase inhibitors | Doravirine<br>Efavirenz<br>Etravirine<br>Nevirapine<br>Rilpivirine |
| Integrase strand transfer inhibitors | Bictegravir<br>Dolutegravir<br>Elvitegravir<br>Raltegravir<br>Cabotegravir |
| Protease inhibitors | Atazanavir<br>Darunavir<br>Fosamprenavir<br>Lopinavir + ritonavir (Kaletra) |
| Attachment inhibitor<br>Postattachment inhibitor | Fostemsavir<br>Ibalizumab |
| HIV combination drugs:<br>a few examples of single- or two-tablet regimens | Bictegravir/emtricitabine/tenofovir AF<br>Dolutegravir + emtricitabine/tenofovir AF or emtricitabine/tenofovir DX<br>Dolutegravir/lamivudine<br>Dolutegravir/lamivudine/abacavir<br>Darunavir + cobicistat or ritonavir + emtricitabine + tenofovir AF or tenofovir DX<br>Doravirine + emtricitabine or lamivudine + tenofovir AF or tenofovir DX<br>Efavirenz + emtricitabine or lamivudine + abacavir or tenofovir AF or tenofovir DX<br>Raltegravir + emtricitabine + tenofovir AF or tenofovir DX<br>Rilpivirine[a] + emtricitabine/tenofovir DX or AF<br>Rilpivirine[a] + abacavir/lamivudine<br>Elvitegravir/cobicistat + emtricitabine/tenofovir AF |

**Table 34.6** Antiviral drugs—cont'd

| HCV | |
| --- | --- |
| NS5B polymerase inhibitor | Sofosbuvir |
| NS5B polymerase/NS5A inhibitor | Sofosbuvir/velpatasvir |
| NS5B polymerase/NS5A/NS3/4A inhibitor | Sofosbuvir/velpatasvir/voxilaprevir |
| NS3/4A protease/NS5A inhibitor | Glecaprevir/pibrentasvir |
| NS3/4A protease/NS5A inhibitor | Grazoprevir/elbasvir |
| | Ribavirin |
| | Interferon-α |

AF, Alafenamide; CMV, cytomegalovirus; DX, disoproxil fumarate; HBV, hepatitis B virus; HCV, hepatitis C virus; HIV, human immunodeficiency virus; HSV, herpes simplex virus; NS, nonstructural; RSV, respiratory syncytial virus; VZV, varicella-zoster virus.
[a]Or doravirine, nevirapine or efavirenz.

successful. Moreover, virus-specific replication steps can be identified (Fig. 34.27) and interrupted, one of which involves identifying virus-induced enzymes.

Bearing in mind that antivirals can be used to treat acute and chronic viral infections and, in the latter case, may be given for many years or for life, considerations include the length of the treatment course, single versus combination therapy, drug pharmacokinetics and interactions, adverse effects and antiviral resistance. Monitoring viral load as a marker of prognosis and treatment response is important in chronic viral infections such as HIV, HBV and HCV, together with occasional therapeutic drug monitoring and genotypic and phenotypic resistance tests.

Antiviral resistance occurs with varying prevalence in different patient populations (e.g. aciclovir-resistant HSV and ganciclovir-resistant CMV are mostly seen in immunocompromised individuals at a low level). Aciclovir may still be used at a later date, having detected aciclvir-resistant HSV as the virus, and can revert to wild type. Antiretroviral resistance is seen across all the main classes of agents—nucleoside reverse transcriptase inhibitors (NRTIs), nonnucleoside reverse transcriptase inhibitors (NNRTIs), protease inhibitors (PIs) and integrase strand transfer inhibitors (INSTIs)—with increasing frequency in resource-rich countries. Lamivudine-resistant HBV is well recognized and is usually detected after a couple of years of treatment. Drug resistance involving most of the other agents used to treat chronic HBV infection also occurs but much less frequently. One issue with antiviral resistance is that the replication fitness of the drug-resistant variants is often less than the wild-type strain. In addition, in the case of a number of viruses including HBV and HCV, the response varies depending on the viral genotype.

Some viral infections have an immunopathologic basis, such as CMV pneumonitis in which host T cells recognize a virally encoded protein in the lung interstitium in which case an antiviral is given in combination with an immunoglobulin preparation. This may be human normal immunoglobulin or virus-specific immunoglobulin (i.e. CMV hyperimmune globulin).

Palivizumab is an example of a humanized monoclonal antibody produced to prevent infection. It is directed against the RSV fusion protein and has potent neutralizing and fusion inhibitory activity. It is used in specific clinical settings to prevent severe lower respiratory tract infections caused by RSV requiring hospitalization in children born at ≤35 weeks' gestation who are <6 months old at the onset of the RSV season. In addition, it may be used in children <2 years of age with specific respiratory and cardiac conditions such as bronchopulmonary dysplasia.

Finally, in the case of some viral respiratory tract infections, antibiotics are often given to control or act as prophylaxis against a secondary bacterial infection. Influenza infection is an example in which staphylococcal and streptococcal pneumonia may occur after the initial virologic insult.

It is difficult to group the antiviral drugs in the same way as the antibiotics. One can either look at them as, for example, anti-HIV, anti-HBV and anti-HCV drugs or group them under mechanism of action. The following are classified using the latter heading.

## Prodrugs that target the viral DNA polymerase

These include aciclovir, valaciclovir, famciclovir, ganciclovir, valganciclovir and cidofovir.

### Aciclovir (acycloguanosine)

*Aciclovir inhibits HSV and VZV DNA polymerase.* Aciclovir is used in the treatment of HSV and VZV infections. A number of other agents include valaciclovir, the L-valyl ester of aciclovir, and famciclovir. Aciclovir is inactive until phosphorylated and is an example of a prodrug. Aciclovir (Fig. 34.28) is phosphorylated by the herpesvirus thymidine kinase, and the monophosphate is then converted by cellular kinases to the triphosphate, which inhibits the herpesvirus DNA polymerase. As it is taken up and efficiently phosphorylated by HSV-infected cells, the action on cellular DNA polymerase is minimal, and toxic side effects such as neutropenia and thrombocytopenia are rare. The drug is also incorporated into viral DNA, resulting in chain termination. As it is excreted by the kidney, the drug can crystallize in the renal tract in individuals with renal failure, causing acute tubular necrosis. Otherwise, aciclovir has an excellent safety profile. Aciclovir resistance is rare and is most often due to mutations in the thymidine kinase gene but is sometimes due to polymerase gene mutations.

Systemic aciclovir revolutionized the treatment of HSV encephalitis and HSV and VZV infections in immunocompromised patients. It is effective in treating primary and recurrent genital herpes. In shingles (herpes zoster), recovery is accelerated and postzoster pain reduced. As with HSV, the VZV remains latent in ganglia and can reactivate.

As the oral bioavailability is only 15–20%, aciclovir is given intravenously in a number of clinical settings initially. Valaciclovir and famciclovir have improved bioavailability

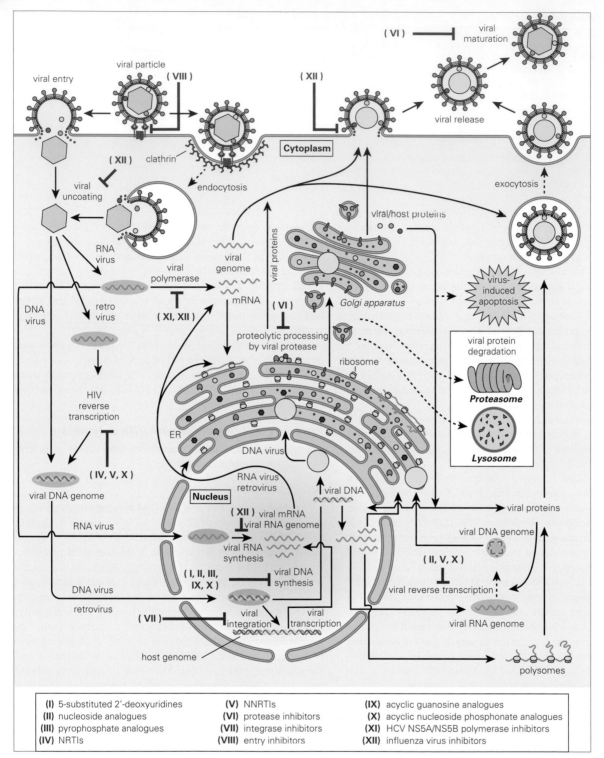

| (I) | 5-substituted 2′-deoxyuridines | (V) | NNRTIs | (IX) | acyclic guanosine analogues |
| (II) | nucleoside analogues | (VI) | protease inhibitors | (X) | acyclic nucleoside phosphonate analogues |
| (III) | pyrophosphate analogues | (VII) | integrase inhibitors | (XI) | HCV NS5A/NS5B polymerase inhibitors |
| (IV) | NRTIs | (VIII) | entry inhibitors | (XII) | influenza virus inhibitors |

**Fig. 34.27** Site of action of antiviral agents during the viral life cycle. Twelve groups of drugs are shown at the bottom (*red roman numerals*). Inhibitory drug action at major stages of the viral life cycle are highlighted (*red arrows*). Solid black arrows indicate direct biologic pathways involving viral replication, and dotted black arrows show biologic pathways with intermediate pathways inside host cells. Major viral stages are illustrated, including endocytosis, exocytosis, virus entry, reverse transcription, virus integration, viral transcription, viral translation, virus budding/release, virus maturation and other pathways associated with cellular compartments (e.g. Golgi apparatus, mitochondria, endoplasmic reticulum [ER], ribosome, proteasome, polysome and endosome). Replication pathways of DNA viruses (HCMV, human cytomegalovirus; HBV, hepatitis B virus; HPV, human papillomavirus; HSV, herpes simplex virus and VZV, varicella-zoster virus), RNA viruses (HCV, RSV, respiratory syncytial virus and influenza virus) and retroviruses (HIV) diverge after entering host cells. The RNA viruses replicate in the cytoplasm, but DNA viruses and retroviruses replicate in the nucleus. Drug group XIII is not displayed since the group acts mainly as immunoregulatory or antimitotic agents not directly targeting viral proteins. Shapes and sizes of proteins and cellular components are not to scale. HCV, Hepatitis C virus; HIV, human immunodeficiency virus; mRNA, messenger RNA; NNRTI, nonnucleoside reverse transcriptase inhibitor; NRTI, nucleoside reverse transcriptase inhibitor. (From De Clercq E, Guangdi L. Approved antiviral drugs over the past 50 years. *Clin Microbiol Rev.* 2016;29[3], fig 4, with permission.)

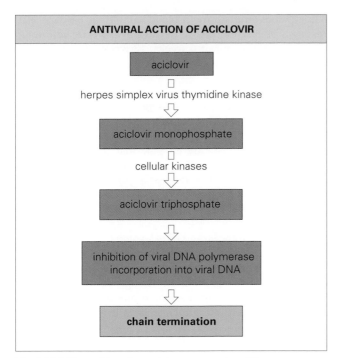

**ANTIVIRAL ACTION OF ACICLOVIR**

aciclovir

herpes simplex virus thymidine kinase

aciclovir monophosphate

cellular kinases

aciclovir triphosphate

inhibition of viral DNA polymerase
incorporation into viral DNA

**chain termination**

**Fig. 34.28** The activity of an antiviral agent against different herpesviruses is correlated with the ability of the viruses to induce a thymidine kinase; hence aciclovir is most active against herpes simplex virus and least active against cytomegalovirus.

profiles in comparison with aciclovir, resulting in less frequent daily dosages.

### Ganciclovir (dihydroxypropoxy-methylguanine)

Ganciclovir is structurally similar to aciclovir but has an extra hydroxyl group. The range of activity is broader than that of aciclovir, and the drug is active against CMV infections. CMV does not encode a thymidine kinase, but rather the drug is monophosphorylated by a virus *UL97* gene–specified kinase and then further phosphorylated by cellular kinases. However, selective toxicity is not seen; it is myelosuppressive, and its main adverse effect is bone marrow toxicity. Ganciclovir triphosphate inhibits CMV DNA polymerase. It is given intravenously because of limited oral bioavailability. However, an oral agent, valganciclovir, has improved the outpatient management of individuals with CMV infections as it has equivalent activity to intravenous ganciclovir.

Ganciclovir is given to treat individuals with CMV viraemia in a variety of clinical settings as well as immunocompromised individuals with end-organ disease such as CMV colitis, pneumonitis and encephalitis. It is also used as preemptive therapy in bone marrow transplant as well as solid organ transplant recipients who are monitored regularly for the presence of CMV in their blood as this may lead to CMV dissemination.

Ganciclovir resistance, most often seen when the drug has been given, stopped and restarted a few times, may be detected in 5–12% of patients and is due to mutations in the *UL97* gene that encodes the viral DNA phosphotransferase or the *UL54* viral polymerase gene.

### Valganciclovir

Valganciclovir is the valine ester of ganciclovir, has similar bioavailability, but has the advantage of being given orally.

### Cidofovir

Cidofovir is another chain terminator that targets the viral DNA polymerase. It is phosphorylated intracellularly to the diphosphate form and is then added to the 3 end of the viral DNA chain. It can be used to treat CMV, but a disadvantage is that it is given infrequently, once weekly initially and then every 2 weeks, so it is unlikely to provide constant suppression. Cidofovir has also been used to treat adenovirus infections. When given topically or intralesionally, it has activity against genital warts and can be used to treat aciclovir-resistant HSV infections. It has to be given intravenously and is nephrotoxic.

### Pyrophosphate analogue that blocks the pyrophosphate-binding site on the viral DNA polymerase

#### Foscarnet

This compound attaches to the pyrophosphate-binding site of the herpesvirus DNA polymerase, preventing nucleotide binding and therefore inhibiting viral replication. It is used in treating CMV infections, is active against HSV and VZV and can be used to treat aciclovir-resistant HSV infections. It is nephrotoxic and can have compliance issues as it has other adverse effects, including nausea and vomiting, electrolyte disturbance and mucosal ulceration and is often used as a second-line agent.

### Antiviral agent with a unique mechanism of action by inhibiting the CMV terminase complex

#### Letermovir

CMV replication involves cleaving viral DNA and packaging each genome into preformed virus capsids mediated by the CMV–terminase complex of three proteins, UL51, UL56, and UL89. Letermovir inhibits CMV replication by binding to the UL51 and/or UL56 components of the terminase complex. In 2017 it was shown that oral letermovir reduced the risk of clinically significant CMV infection when given as prophylaxis in CMV IgG–positive allogeneic bone marrow transplant recipients. It also reduced the risk of all-cause mortality at 6 months post-transplant compared with placebo.

### Antiretroviral drugs

Antiretroviral drugs are divided into seven classes; all are named after their mechanism of action:

- Integrase strand transfer inhibitors (INSTIs)
- Nucleoside reverse transcriptase inhibitors (NRTIs)
- Nonnucleoside reverse transcriptase inhibitors (NNRTIs)
- Protease inhibitors (PIs)
- Fusion inhibitors
- Chemokine CCR5 antagonists
- Postattachment inhibitors.

The aim of antiretroviral therapy is to lower and keep the plasma HIV-1 RNA load below the limit of assay detection and therefore maintain the CD4 count. HIV treatment started in the late 1980s with just NRTI monotherapy, then dual NRTI therapy until NNRTIs and PIs were welcome additions that, in various combinations, resulted in rapid reductions in HIV-1 RNA load. By 2023 the number of drugs had been reduced dramatically to ~30, with at least 20 fixed-drug combinations and at least 7 drugs discontinued due to their side effects.

The uses and combinations of these seven classes of antiretroviral drugs are too complex to summarize, and treatment guidelines are updated regularly. By 2016 cART was recommended for all individuals with an acute HIV infection as well as all those who were viraemic. The reduction in pill burden by combining drugs together with the increased range of antiretroviral agents has increased choice and ease of switching regimens to improve tolerability, compliance, antiretroviral resistance, drug interactions and potential adverse effects such as in pregnancy, chronic viral hepatitis and renal dysfunction.

INSTIs, together with combinations of NRTIs, NNRTIs and/or PIs, constituted recommended treatment regimens in 2023 in resource-rich countries.

## Multiclass antiretroviral drug resistance can be transmitted and acquired and is a global issue

By the early 2020s low- and middle-income countries reported that both transmitted and acquired antiretroviral drug resistance had significantly increased, with 21–91% NRTI and NNRTI resistance in different regions due to significant pretreatment exposure and interrupted access to antiretroviral drugs, HIV load and drug resistance testing. Transmitted drug resistance ranged from 6–11% in resource-rich settings.

## PrEP is part of HIV prevention, adding to the recommended PEP in a number of clinical settings

Daily oral PrEP with a fixed-dose combination of either tenofovir disoproxil fumarate (DX) or tenofovir alafenamide (AF) with emtricitabine was reported to reduce HIV acquisition in a variety of HIV-discordant couples, together with other safer sex practices. Regular HIV testing was also recommended, and breakthrough infections were very rare and attributed to suboptimal PrEP adherence or drug-resistant HIV infection having developed in those who took PrEP but had an undetected acute HIV infection at the time. It is important to be HIV negative when taking PrEP as the latter may induce drug resistance and affect treatment options.

In 2015 WHO recommended offering oral PrEP for HIV prevention; by 2021, 144 countries had adopted that into national guidelines. The United Nations Acquired Immunodeficiency Syndrome program reported that ~1.6 million people globally had received oral PrEP at least once in 2021, ~1 million of whom were in East and South Africa.

In 2022 WHO released guidance for using injectable cabotegravir as long-acting PrEP as two injections 1 month apart and then given every 2 months.

PEP may be used in nonoccupational and occupational settings. In both settings, the risk assessment is key; in nonoccupational settings (sexual exposure, injecting drug use or other), the recipient should have an HIV test when possible. If the transmission risk is assessed as substantial, a 4-week course of a triple-drug regimen such as tenofovir plus emtricitabine plus raltegravir or dolutegravir, should be offered. Alternative regimens can be considered depending on the setting.

The same is true in the occupational setting, although the type of exposure incident will be more varied in a clinical setting, and, after storing a blood sample (or baseline HIV testing in some countries) at the time of exposure, follow-up testing is carried out at 6 weeks, 12 weeks, and 6 months after exposure.

## Integrase inhibitors

*Bictegravir, dolutegravir, elvitegravir, raltegravir, cabotegravir.* INSTIs are HIV integrase strand transfer inhibitors and became more common as first-line treatment. Integrase is a nucleotidyltransferase enzyme that catalyses the integration involving transferring virally encoded DNA into the host chromosome. It is a three-step process, including the formation of a preintegration viral DNA complex, 3' processing and strand transfer. The latter covalently links the viral and host DNA.

INSTIs inhibit the strand transfer step by interacting with two divalent cations at the active site of the integrase and blocking integration of viral DNA into the host genome by preventing the covalent bond forming with the host DNA. INSTIs are also active against HIV strains that are resistant to other classes of antiretroviral agents. Side effects are mostly gastrointestinal.

The second-generation INSTIs dolutegravir, bictegravir and cabotegravir were developed as resistance to the first-generation INSTIs increased. These had a higher genetic barrier to resistance as well as fewer side effects and were highly active, leading to them becoming a key backbone with other drug classes for future antiretroviral management.

Examples of cART that may be given to individuals with newly diagnosed HIV infection include fixed-dose combination tablets such as bictegravir plus emtricitabine plus tenofovir AF, dolutegravir plus emtricitabine plus tenofovir AF or dolutegravir plus lamivudine.

## Nucleoside and nucleotide reverse transcriptase inhibitors

*Abacavir, emtricitabine, lamivudine, tenofovir DX and tenofovir AF.* This class of drugs (see Table 34.6) has similar modes of action and is combined and given with other drug classes as cART.

Zidovudine (AZT) was an anticancer drug originally; it was subsequently found to inhibit HIV replication, and by the mid-1980s was given as the first antiretroviral drug. It is an analogue of the nucleoside thymidine in which the hydroxyl group on the ribose is replaced by an azido group. After conversion to the triphosphate by cellular enzymes (Fig. 34.29), it acts as an inhibitor of, and substrate for, the viral reverse transcriptase. The azido group prevents the formation of phosphodiester linkages. Proviral DNA formation is blocked because AZT triphosphate is incorporated into the DNA, with resulting chain termination.

AZT was given orally. Toxicity was a problem, with bone marrow suppression (macrocytic anaemia, neutropenia, leukopenia) and less commonly nausea, vomiting, headache, myalgia and malaise. This was more often seen in the early days of HIV treatment when the drug was given at a high dose. Other adverse events included lactic acidosis, hyperlipidaemia, lipoatrophy and insulin resistance or diabetes mellitus.

Other nucleoside analogues were synthesized that were converted to triphosphates and inhibited the HIV reverse

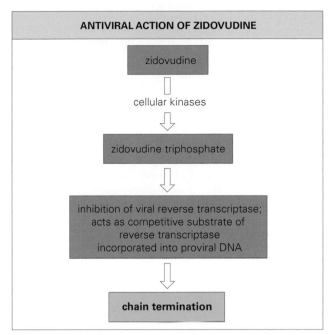

**ANTIVIRAL ACTION OF ZIDOVUDINE**

zidovudine

↓ cellular kinases

zidovudine triphosphate

↓

inhibition of viral reverse transcriptase; acts as competitive substrate of reverse transcriptase incorporated into proviral DNA

↓

**chain termination**

**Fig. 34.29** Human immunodeficiency virus reverse transcriptase is 100 times more sensitive than host cell DNA polymerase to zidovudine triphosphate, but toxic effects are not uncommon.

transcriptase. Many have been discontinued due to side effect profiles, including pancreatitis associated with didanosine and lipodystrophy (fatty tissue redistribution from subcutaneous areas such as the face and limbs, to the neck and abdominal viscera) and peripheral neuropathy associated with stavudine. Mitochondrial toxicity due to inhibition of the mitochondrial DNA polymerase and lactic acidosis was also reported. By 2023 using NRTI monotherapy was part of history, and the number of NRTI drugs had been reduced to mainly abacavir, emtricitabine, lamivudine and tenofovir DX and tenofovir AF. Combinations as fixed-dose treatments included emtricitabine plus tenofovir and lamivudine plus abacavir given with another class of antiretroviral drug such as bictegravir (i.e. bictegravir and emtricitabine plus tenofovir).

Tenofovir is a nucleotide reverse transcriptase inhibitor and is phosphorylated to the diphosphate form that acts as chain terminator.

An INSTI plus two NRTIs is the recommended initial treatment for those with HIV-2. Alternatively, a boosted PI such as darunavir or lopinavir against HIV-2 plus two NRTIs can be used. The nonnucleoside RTIs cannot be used, and the fusion inhibitor, enfuvirtide, has reduced HIV-2 activity.

### Nonnucleoside reverse transcriptase inhibitors

*Doravirine, efavirenz, etravirine, nevirapine, and rilpivirine.* These act as noncompetitive inhibitors of HIV-1 reverse transcriptase by binding to a hydrophobic pocket proximal to the enzyme catalytic site. They are inactive against HIV-2. The NNRTIs are inducers of cytochrome P450, and it is important to consider potential drug interactions. The most common adverse effect with nevirapine is a skin rash. Efavirenz may cause vivid dreams and sleep disturbance initially and should not be used in the first trimester of pregnancy.

A single mutation in the reverse transcriptase leads to resistance to these drugs, effectively removing this class of drug from the treatment regimen. They are given in combination with other drug classes, and examples are doravirine and emtricitabine/tenofovir or lamivudine plus abacavir.

### Protease inhibitors

*Atazanavir, darunavir, fosamprenavir and lopinavir are all boosted by either ritonavir or cobicistat.* The protease enzyme acts in the post-translational cleavage of the gag and gag-pol polyproteins into the structural proteins and enzymes critical for viral replication. The result of protease inhibition is the production of immature, defective viral particles. PIs were introduced to HIV treatment combinations in 1996 and had a great effect on the control of HIV infection. Their use led to the term *highly active antiretroviral therapy,* which was replaced by *cART.* They are peptidomimetic inhibitors of the viral protease and prevent the cleavage of the gag and gag-pol polyproteins into functional structural proteins and enzymes. They are very potent drugs that lead to a rapid fall in the plasma HIV RNA load, especially in those individuals with very high HIV loads. Side effects include gastrointestinal disturbances, lipodystrophy syndrome (body fat redistribution), increased triglycerides and insulin resistance leading to diabetes.

Drug resistance is well recognized, and a number of protease mutations result in cross-resistance. Boosting atazanavir and darunavir with low-dose ritonavir or cobicistat (an inhibitor of cytochrome P450 3A enzyme) leads to greater virologic activity, owing to improved pharmacodynamics. However, higher rates of side effects are seen.

### Fusion inhibitor

*Enfurvitide.* Enfuvirtide, also known as T-20, is a peptide that blocks HIV before it enters the host cell by competitively binding to gp41, the transmembrane glycoprotein, and blocking the postfusion structure from forming. It therefore should not cross-react with the other classes of antiretroviral drugs. It is given twice daily as a subcutaneous injection and may be used in specific circumstances as salvage therapy in those treatment-experienced individuals with resistance mutations to the other drug classes. Adverse events include pain at the injection site and rare hypersensitivity reactions.

### Chemokine receptor antagonists

*Maraviroc.* HIV-1 entry into host cells involves the viral envelope protein binding to the CD4 receptor and subsequently to a chemokine coreceptor. Two coreceptors identified are CCR5 and CXCR4. Tests that identify the viral phenotype have been used to determine the populations of virus in someone with HIV, and these are referred to as R5-tropic, X4-tropic or dual/mixed. Diagnostic laboratories use genotypic tests to predict viral coreceptor tropism, R5 or X4, based on the sequence of the viral envelope on the basis of algorithms.

Maraviroc is a CCR5 chemokine coreceptor antagonist and was approved for adults who had been given cART and had R5 HIV-1 infection.

### Attachment and postattachment inhibitors

*Fostemsavir (attachment) and ibalizumab (postattachment).* Fostemsavir is a first in its class attachment inhibitor that is an oral prodrug of temsavir and is active after hydrolysis in the gastrointestinal tract. Temsavir attaches directly to part of the gp120 envelope glycoprotein. Once bound, it locks gp120 into a conformational state that stops binding to the CD4 receptor.

Fostemsavir has no cross-resistance to other entry inhibitors, including maraviroc, enfuvirtide and ibalizumab. It is active against HIV with both CXCR and CCR5 tropism and may be offered to those with heavy treatment experience and limited treatment options.

Ibalizumab is a recombinant humanized monoclonal antibody that binds to the extracellular domain 2 of CD4 cells and was approved for treating multidrug-resistant HIV-1 infection. It is given intravenously fortnightly. Drug resistance has been reported due to a fall in expression or loss of potential N-linked glycosylation sites in the gp120 V5 loop.

## Inosine monophosphate dehydrogenase inhibitor

### Ribavirin

This guanosine analogue is triphosphorylated by cellular enzymes. It has various actions, including inhibition of production of guanosine triphosphate pools needed for viral nucleic acid synthesis. Ribavirin can target both RNA and DNA viruses. Once triphosphorylated, it can also interfere with the viral RNA polymerase. It can be used clinically as an aerosol for treating severe RSV infection in infants. Ribavirin can be used to treat arenavirus infections such as Lassa fever. Oral ribavirin could be used as PEP for Lassa fever in the case of high-risk exposure incidents. It is also active against measles virus and hepatitis E virus infections (see later). There is controversy about treating individuals with Crimean-Congo haemorrhagic fever with ribavirin. It has in vitro activity, and there are some case reports of successful treatment.

## Antivirals targeting influenza viruses

Oseltamivir, zanamivir, peramivir and baloxavir (and amantadine and rimantadine) have selective activity against influenza viruses and so have been grouped together with this header rather than by their mode of action. Amantadine and rimantadine have activity only against influenza A and are used rarely, if ever. The neuraminidase inhibitors (NAIs) zanamivir, oseltamivir, peramivir and baloxavir, a cap-dependent endonuclease inhibitor, have increased the range of activity by inhibiting both influenza A and B viruses.

### M2 ion-channel inhibitors

*Amantadine and rimantadine.* These are mentioned here only because they are classic drugs that specifically inhibit the replication of influenza A viruses with an interesting mode of action but have no effect on influenza B and other respiratory viruses. They act by inhibiting the penetration of virus into the cell or its uncoating. Fusion of the viral envelope with a cell membrane, which normally occurs at a low pH, is prevented. Amantadine acts on the viral matrix protein (M2) ion channel, thus stopping hydrogen ion passage, raising the pH in intracellular vacuoles and therefore blocking infection. The standard dose can cause minor neurologic side effects such as insomnia, dizziness and headache especially in elderly patients, and this has discouraged its widespread use. Amantadine can be given prophylactically during community outbreaks of influenza A. It can also be used for treatment, and, if taken within 48 h of symptoms, there is a reduction in disease severity. However, rapid emergence of drug-resistant variants can occur, and, due to the inactivity against influenza B and CNS side effects and the development of the NAIs, this class of drugs is of less importance in the influenza armamentarium.

### Neuraminidase inhibitors

*Oseltamivir, zanamavir and peramivir.* Neuraminidase is one of the two surface glycoproteins studded on the influenza virus surface. It cleaves *N*-acetylneuraminic acid, also known as *sialic acid,* residues from the host cell, thus releasing the virus and allowing further spread in the respiratory tract.

The NAIs are *N*-acetylneuraminic acid analogues and act as competitive reversible inhibitors of the neuraminidase enzyme active site. Zanamivir is an inhaled agent and can be given intravenously, oseltamivir is an oral drug and peramivir is an intravenous agent, all of which are cleaved by esterases to the active carboxylate form and act on influenza A and B. The importance of having an increased armamentarium of NAIs was demonstrated during 2007–2008 and 2008–2009 as oseltamivir resistance emerged globally amongst the influenza A H1N1 viruses. In the United States, oseltamivir resistance was seen in ~20% and 90% of influenza A H1N1 viruses tested during both the above seasons, respectively.

These drugs reduce viral shedding, disease severity, duration and symptoms if given early in infection and can be used as prophylaxis. They are effective against the circulating influenza strains, including the avian influenza H5N1 virus.

### Influenza cap-dependent endonuclease inhibitor

*Baloxavir.* The influenza virus polymerase complex is a different target to those mentioned previously and is important when one considers the emergence of antiviral resistance. The polymerase is made up of three protein subunits, one of which, PB2, binds to the cap of host cellular pre-mRNA. The cap-dependent endonuclease is in another part of the polymerase complex, and it cleaves PB2 from the cap, providing an RNA primer for the viral mRNA to be transcribed by the RNA-dependent RNA polymerase, also within the polymerase complex. Given the complexity of this part of viral replication, it is a relief that baloxavir is easy to pronounce and should not be confused with any Old English terminology for making a mess of something.

Oral baloxavir was reported in 2018 to be effective in alleviating influenza symptoms in individuals with uncomplicated influenza A and B virus infections.

### A nucleoside analogue targeting the influenza polymerase

*Favipiravir.* This novel antiviral drug is licensed in Japan and is active against influenza A and B viruses, including strains that are resistant to other antiviral drugs. It seems to act by competing with endogenous guanine and adenine nucleotides, incorporating into viral RNA, and then terminating RNA synthesis. It may also cause genome mutation, resulting in inhibiting viral replication.

### SARS-CoV-2 (COVID-19) treatments

*The world waited while understanding the pathogenesis of COVID-19 led to the identification of potential treatments, the first of which was an adjunct therapy focusing on the host response.* After first being detected in December 2019 in Wuhan, China, SARS-CoV-2 that caused coronavirus disease 2019 (COVID-19) was classified as a pandemic by WHO in March 2020. Immediately there was a worldwide call to identify potential treatments, develop new antiviral drugs and race to develop vaccines.

By 2023 a number of treatment options with an array of mechanisms of action were available starting in 2020 with drugs targeting the host immune response—namely, anti-inflammatory immunodulators and anti-thrombotic drugs. In addition, convalescent antibody treatment was considered early in the pandemic on the basis of previous reports treating individuals with severe influenza. However, convalescent plasma treatment for adults with mild to moderate COVID-19 was not found to have any clinical benefit, although greater viral clearance than standard of care treatment was reported. As new variants emerged, cross-neutralization was unlikely to be seen.

Gradually, antiviral drugs that inhibited viral replication and recombinant neutralizing monoclonal antibodies became available that blocked viral entry into host cells. Randomized clinical trials tested the safety and efficacy of these agents, and the leader was the Randomised Evaluation of COVID-19 Therapy group, known as RECOVERY, that reported the effectiveness of dexamethasone.

The categories of treatment included:

- anti-inflammatory drugs
- antivirals
- anti-thrombotic drugs
- SARS-CoV-2 neutralizing antibody passive immunotherapy.

### Drugs targeting inflammation

Dexamethasone, a synthetic corticosteroid immunomodulator, was shown to reduce mortality in patients with COVID-19 after 28 days of treatment in tandem with invasive mechanical ventilation for oxygen support compared with placebo. This highlighted how effective a national health service could be in an emergency, as 176 UK hospitals participated in the RECOVERY studies involving >11,000 patients, >6000 of whom were randomized to receive dexamethasone or standard care at that time between March and June 2020. The WHO Rapid Evidence Appraisal for COVID-19 (REACT) working group meta-analysis showed the odds ratio for 28-day mortality after treatment was 0.66. In other words, the odds of someone dying were 66% less after treatment compared with placebo.

Tocilizumab is a recombinant humanized monoclonal antibody that binds to the interleukin-6 receptor and therefore blocks proinflammatory cytokine activity. When given around the second day of the disease course, mortality at 28 days was lower than in patients given standard care at the time.

Along similar lines, the Janus tyrosine kinase (JAK) proteins are signalling mediators involved in proinflammatory cytokine activity. Baricitinib is an oral JAK1 and JAK2 inhibitor with antiinflammatory properties. It had also been shown to reduce 28-day mortality. Unsurprisingly, both tocilizumab and baricitinib can be used to treat rheumatoid arthritis.

### Anti-thrombotic drugs

Critically and moderately ill inpatients with COVID-19 were shown to benefit from heparin-based anticoagulation. Anti-platelet treatment (i.e. aspirin) was not found to have any benefit.

### Targeting SARS-CoV-2

*Remdesivir, nirmatrelvir-ritonavir (Paxlovid), and molnupiravir.* Remdesivir is a prodrug that is an intravenously administered nucleoside analogue that inhibits the viral RNA-dependent RNA polymerase. Studies reported an 87% reduction in risk of death or hospital stay compared with placebo as well as a 5-day shorter time to recovery.

Nirmatrelvir-ritonavir (Paxlovid) is an oral combination of a protease inhibitor (nirmatrelvir) and an enhancer or booster (ritonavir) that is a cytochrome P450 inhibitor. Studies reported an 89% reduction in risk of death or hospital stay compared with placebo.

Molnupiravir is an oral cytidine analogue that is incorporated into newly synthesized viral RNA and results in lethal mutagenesis. Studies reported a 33% reduction in risk of death or hospital stay compared with placebo.

*Neutralizing monoclonal antibody passive immunotherapy*
- Sotrovimab
- Casirivimab plus imdevimab
- Bamlanivimab plus etesevimab
- Bebtelovimab
- Tixagevimab plus cilgavimab (Evusheld)

Recombinant neutralizing monoclonal antibodies (mAbs) were made that targeted the viral receptor-binding Spike protein that binds to the host cell angiotensin-converting enzyme 2 (ACE2), mediating viral entry. The ACE2 receptor can be found on cells in the respiratory and gastrointestinal tract and endothelium.

Individuals who were SARS-CoV-2 antibody negative and at high risk of severe infection with mild/moderate COVID-19 and at home were involved in randomized controlled trials that showed early treatment with mAbs reduced the risk of hospital admission or death.

Recombinant mAbs were not as effective at neutralizing SARS-CoV-2 variants that emerged in 2022.

Tixagevimab plus cilgavimab (Evusheld) has a prolonged half-life and was recommended in the United States as PrEP in specific at-risk groups.

### Hepatitis B antiviral treatment

The aim of treating individuals with chronic HBV and HCV infections is to reduce the risk of cirrhosis, liver failure and hepatocellular carcinoma by suppressing HBV DNA and HCV RNA levels, respectively.

Treatment regimens offered to individuals with chronic HBV infection include nucleoside and NRTIs such as lamivudine, adefovir, entecavir, telbivudine, tenofovir and emtricitabine. Entecavir and tenofovir have a higher barrier to resistance and are more potent than the other drugs and are preferred. Antiviral treatment is recommended in all those in the immune active phases of chronic HBV infection and those with cirrhosis and detectable HBV DNA, acute liver failure and exacerbations of chronic HBV. After stopping treatment, the antiviral response may be reversed, and continuing treatment in the long term may lead to the development of antiviral resistance, although the virus will be less fit than the wild type.

Before treatment is started, high alanine aminotransferase levels and low HBV DNA are associated with high rates of hepatitis B early antigen (HBeAg) and hepatitis B surface antigen (HBsAg) responses to both pegylated interferon-α (IFNα) and nucleoside and nucleotide analogues. From an HBV genotyping perspective, response to nucleoside and nucleotide analogues cannot be predicted, but genotype A is associated with the highest rate of HBeAg and HBsAg clearance after pegylated IFNα treatment.

### Pegylated IFNα is used less commonly than nucleoside/nucleotide analogues

Immunomodulation using pegylated IFNα, which has a longer half-life than IFN preparations that do not include polyethylene glycol, enhances the innate immune response by binding to the type 1 IFN receptor. This leads to upregulation of multiple IFN-stimulated genes limiting viral replication. In HBeAg-positive and HBeAg-negative infections, 48 weeks of pegylated IFNα results in HBeAg loss in 30% and HBsAg loss in ~4%, respectively, within 6 months of treatment completion. However, IFNs have a large side effect profile, including flu-like symptoms, depression and neutropenia.

### Only three nucleoside/nucleotide drugs are preferred for treatment

*Entecavir, tenofovir DF or AF, and lamivudine.* Of the nucleoside analogues, lamivudine therapy results in undetectable HBV DNA, improved liver histology and liver enzyme levels in 40–44%, 49–62% and 41–77% of patients, respectively. However, with entecavir, these are 67%, 72% and 68%, respectively. The genetic barrier to resistance is low, as only one mutation is needed to lead to lamivudine resistance compared with entecavir and tenofovir. The lowest rates of drug resistance are therefore seen with entecavir and tenofovir.

Emtricitabine cannot be used as single-agent therapy owing to high rates of resistance. Telbivudine is effective but has a low genetic barrier to resistance.

Adefovir and tenofovir are acyclic nucleoside phosphonates, with tenofovir being more effective than adefovir. They are prodrugs as they need to be phosphorylated to become active and are analogues of adenosine monophosphate. They affect the HBV polymerase by competitively inhibiting deoxyadenosine 5'-triphosphate, resulting in chain termination. The major side effect is nephrotoxicity. Tenofovir is available in two forms, alafenamide and disoproxil fumarate (TDF). There are reports of no TDF resistance after 10 years of treatment and of no tenofovir alafenamide resistance after 3 years of treatment. Both versions are effective in treating HBV that is resistant to the other nucleoside/nucleotide drugs.

Entecavir is a deoxyguanosine analogue that is one of the more effective drugs. It inhibits the HBV DNA polymerase by preventing the following functions: priming of the HBV DNA polymerase, reverse transcription of the negative strand from the pregenomic mRNA and synthesis of positive-strand HBV DNA. Entecavir resistance at 5 years occurs in ~1% of those not treated with lamivudine and 50% of those who previously had been treated with lamivudine, respectively.

These oral antiviral agents have changed the treatment landscape in chronic HBV infection as seen by a 78%

reduction in hepatocellular carcinoma in HBeAg-positive infection in which the HBV DNA load is higher. However, after stopping the oral drug treatment, although viral relapse is the rule, 40–60% of individuals have a clinical relapse within 2 years.

HBsAg is cleared after 10 years of treatment in ~3–5% of patients with chronic HBV infection, so oral treatment is given long term.

### To cure HBV infection, multiple steps are needed, including complete replication suppression, stopping HBsAg production and restoring innate and HBV-specific immune responses

To achieve cure, combinations of drug classes will be needed. There are new therapeutic approaches with direct-acting antivirals (DAAs) targeting other parts of the HBV life cycle. These include entry inhibitors, capsid assembly modulators, translation inhibitors (small interfering RNAs or antisense oligonucleotides) silencing HBV RNA, drugs targeting the covalently closed circular DNA (cccDNA), drug combinations as well as drugs that interfere with the host cell functions that allow viral persistence as assisting the immune response against HBV. In the case of translation inhibitors, HBsAg levels fall, and HBV-specific host immune responses may increase, but sustained clearance is rare. Therapeutic vaccines expressing HB core or polymerase antigens might be effective and may be enhanced by using immune checkpoint inhibitors.

This illustrates, once again, the importance of understanding both the pathogen and the host response.

### Entry inhibitors block HBV entry into hepatocytes and show promise in chronic HDV infection

*Bulevirtide.* Hepatitis delta virus coinfection can exacerbate chronic HBV infection and relies on the presence of HBsAg for infection. Sodium taurocholate cotransporting polypeptide is the cell entry receptor for both HBV and HDV. The entry inhibitor, bulevirtide, a synthetic N-acylated pre-S1 lipopeptide, blocks the binding of HBsAg enveloped particles to the cell entry receptor. Clinical trials of 24/48 weeks bulevirtide monotherapy or combined with pegylated IFNα reported reduced HDV viremia and ALT levels. The combination had a synergistic effect compared with either on their own.

### Hepatitis C antiviral treatment

The days of pegylated IFNα combined with ribavirin as the standard treatment of chronic HCV infection have long gone. However, the aim of antiviral treatment leading to an SVR and long-term clinical benefit is shown by the serum HCV RNA being undetectable 12–24 weeks after the end of treatment. In 2011 everything started moving as fast as the Olympic 100-metre sprint champion, as DAAs were shown to improve the SVR rates in even the more difficult to treat HCV infections. By 2020, 8–12 weeks of oral DAA treatment resulted in HCV RNA clearance in >98% of HCV-infected individuals.

The HCV nonstructural (NS) protein targets included the NS3 protease inhibitor drugs, starting with telaprevir and boceprivir, which were rapidly replaced by simeprevir, asunaprevir and paritaprevir. The NS5 polymerase inhibitors included daclatasvir, elbasvir, ledipasvir, ombitasvir, sofosbuvir and velpatasvir. By 2015 the antiviral action of sofosbuvir, a nucleotide analogue inhibitor, had been elucidated. Its active form is 2′-F′-2′-C-methyluridine monophosphate. This is incorporated into the growing HCV RNA strand affecting the formation of hydrogen bond networks and stopping the conformational changes in the RNA-dependent HCV polymerase, which disrupts the viral RNA chain. Suddenly, 99% of SVRs were being reported across almost all HCV genotypes, the exception being the recalcitrant genotype 3, which includes people previously treated with the older agents as well as those with cirrhosis. If that was not amazing enough, this was achieved with a combination of sofosbuvir and velpatasvir given orally once daily for 3 months. As for genotype 3, the SVR was still ~95% in treatment-naive patients and was improved by adding ribavirin. In 2017 another pan-genotypic regimen was approved, glecaprevir and pibrentasvir, an NS3/4A protease and NS5A inhibitor, respectively. Antiviral combinations recommended in DAA-naive individuals with known genotype and compensated cirrhosis in 2021 were complex. One example is for genotype 1a, 1b, 2, 4, 5, 6 HCV infection previously treated with pegylated IFN and ribavirin: glecaprevir and pibrentasvir for 12 weeks (and 16 weeks if genotype 3).

A 12-week three-drug combination (sofosbuvir-velpatasvir-voxilaprevir) was another recommendation in genotype 3 infection with compensated cirrhosis.

HCV is like a puppeteer, pulling the strings of the intracellular environment, using host factors in a positive or negative way, by replicating in an environment of cholesterol and lipid, protected from host ribonucleases, exonucleases and immune responses. In addition, it has been shown that raised 25-hydroxycholesterol levels are found in HCV infection. This induces a microRNA, which affects the cholesterol and lipid environment and reduces HCV replication—a fascinating discovery throwing light on another example of the complex way host and viral factors affect each other.

### Despite improved HCV surveillance, diagnosis and pan-genotypic DAAs, reaching the target of global HCV elimination will ideally need an effective HCV vaccine

The development of noninvasive markers of liver fibrosis, serologic markers and ultrasound techniques also reduced the need for a liver biopsy as part of the disease staging and management.

However, although there is the potential to reduce the hepatologist's workload by making HCV clinics a thing of the past and curing HCV carriers, the DAAs are expensive. Many of those with diagnosed or undiagnosed HCV infection can have difficulty accessing the DAAs, and there are many with undiagnosed HCV globally. The WHO global strategy for viral hepatitis in 2016 aimed for an 80% and 65% reduction by 2030 for new HCV infections and HCV-associated mortality, respectively, with HCV elimination being the holy grail.

### Interferons—immunomodulatory agents

IFNs (see Ch. 10) are natural glycoproteins produced by the innate immune system in response to infections. They have nonvirus-specific antiviral and immunomodulatory actions and trigger a cascade of intracellular reactions that activate IFN-inducible genes. These genes encode proteins thought to inhibit intracellular virus multiplication by inhibiting translation initiation and assisting RNA degradation. IFNα also binds to immune cells, resulting in class I major histocompatibility complex antigen expression, activation of effector cells and a cytokine cascade. Production of T-helper 1 (Th1) cells is stimulated in contrast to Th2 suppressor cells that are reduced. IFNs are generally given as subcutaneous injections, and the side effects are significant and include tiredness, headache, myalgia and psychiatric symptoms.

IFNs have been used to treat individuals with chronic HBV and HCV infections and have an effect on HPV infections when given by intralesional injection, but they are not used routinely.

When IFNs were given in the past as monotherapy, success was limited, owing to the poor SVR rates for both HBV and HCV infections.

### Other targets

Drugs targeting differing parts of the viral life cycle, post-translational processing, virus entry, RNA translation and virus assembly and release as well as host cell-targeting compounds are always being developed. Nucleic acid–based antiviral agents, including antisense oligonucleotides and RNA interference-based agents, have been synthesized as have immunotherapeutic options using antibody-based preparations and therapeutic vaccines.

### Clinical management of antiviral therapy

#### Viral load and antiviral resistance tests as well as therapeutic drug monitoring assist in clinical management

Qualitative and/or quantitative nucleic acid tests are critical in the diagnosis, treatment decision, assessment of response to treatment and prognosis for a number of viral infections. This is true for HIV load testing, together with the CD4 count and percentage. With HCV it is important to determine the HCV genotype and then monitor the plasma HCV RNA load to look for an SVR. For HBV infection, plasma HBV DNA load and antiviral resistance testing are part of the clinical management strategy. Genotypic analysis is also helpful. Another example is CMV DNA monitoring in post-transplant populations to detect early viraemia so that preemptive treatment may be given.

The main causes of treatment failure in HIV infection are either compliance issues or the development of antiviral resistance.

cART has had an enormous impact on HIV disease progression. The development of drug-resistant virus will lead to treatment failure as seen by an increase in HIV load and reduction in CD4 count. Specific mutations can be detected in the varied drug target sites by nucleic acid sequencing. This is referred to as a *genotypic resistance assay*. Key mutations known as primary resistance mutations at specific codons have been associated with a reduction in susceptibility to the various classes of antiretroviral drugs. Some mutations are unique to certain drugs, but many confer cross-resistance, resulting in an entire class of drugs (such as the NNRTIs) being removed from the treatment regimen. In addition, viral tropism assays are carried out in diagnostic laboratories to identify coreceptor use, which is critical when deciding on use of chemokine receptor antagonists. HIV-1 entry into lymphocytes and monocytes involves binding of the gp120 envelope glycoprotein to the CD4 receptor followed by interaction with one of two main coreceptors, CCR5 or CXCR4. This is referred to as *viral tropism,* and whether the virus is X4 or R5 is mainly determined by the amino acid sequence of the V3 region of gp120. Dually tropic strains can use both receptors. In later-stage HIV-1 infection, the CD4 cell count falls, and the minority population X4 or R5/X4 strain rises within the viral quasispecies and can finally emerge as a majority population. HIV-1 tropism can be determined using phenotypic and genotypic methods. Genotypic tropism testing can be carried out in laboratories, and predictions of coreceptor use are based on the amino acid sequence of the gp120 V3 loop using interpretative algorithms. Antiretroviral drug regimens are based on the results of antiretroviral resistance sequencing assays as well as viral tropism assays.

As HIV drug resistance can be transmitted and the prevalence of resistant viruses is increasing in individuals with a new HIV diagnosis, baseline genotypic resistance testing is very important to tailor cART appropriately. In addition, this is being used to optimize the treatment regimen during drug failure episodes. Details of the key mutations can be found on specialist HIV websites together with guidelines for managing HIV-infected individuals.

It is important in HIV infection to continue the drugs while carrying out resistance tests because, without the driver, there is a reversion to the wild-type strain as the minor viral populations that contain the mutations are deselected. Phenotypic analysis may also be helpful.

The effectiveness of cART is dependent on good drug plasma concentrations. Keeping drug concentrations within a therapeutic range is critical, and drug interactions and compliance issues may result in high or low drug levels, leading to toxicity or virologic failure, respectively. Therapeutic drug monitoring is carried out in specialist laboratories and is helpful in finding and correcting any such problems.

## ANTIFUNGAL AGENTS

Compared with antibacterial agents, the number of suitable antifungal drugs is very limited. Selective toxicity is much more difficult to achieve in the eukaryotic fungal cells than in the prokaryotic bacteria and, although the available antifungals have greater activity against fungal cells than they do against human cells, the difference is not as marked as it is for most antibacterial agents. Treatment of fungal infections is further hampered by problems of solubility, stability and absorption of the existing drugs, and the search for new agents is a high priority. Drug resistance is also increasing.

### Antifungals can be classified on the basis of target site and chemical structure

Like antibacterial agents, antifungal can be classified on the basis of target site and chemical structure. This immediately reveals a major difference between antibacterial and antifungal agents, with the major antifungals acting on the synthesis or function of the intracellular membranes. The exceptions are flucytosine (5-fluorocytosine) and griseofulvin, which interfere with DNA synthesis, and echinocandins (anidulafungin, micafungin, caspofungin, rezafungin), which inhibit cell wall formation. There are currently no inhibitors of fungal protein synthesis that do not also inhibit the equivalent mammalian pathway.

### Azole compounds inhibit cell membrane synthesis

Azole antifungals act by inhibiting lanosterol C14-demethylase, an important enzyme in sterol biosynthesis. Clotrimazole, ketoconazole and miconazole are useful as topical preparations. Itraconazole and fluconazole are used in treatment of a variety of serious fungal infections (Table 34.7), and fluconazole is often used in the treatment of *Candida* infections, subject to species identification. Resistance to the azoles is becoming more widespread in both yeasts and filamentous fungi and threatens to compromise this group of compounds. Newer azole compounds include posaconazole and isavuconazole, which are used in aspergillosis unresponsive to amphotericin B and in the treatment of invasive mucormycosis.

### Echinocandins interfere with cell wall synthesis

The echinocandins caspofungin, micafungin and anidulafungin inhibit the enzyme β-(1,3)-D-glucan synthase, which is required for synthesis of an essential part of the fungal cell wall. This important group of compounds offers new therapeutic options against infections such as invasive *Aspergillus*, candidaemia and invasive candidiasis and *Pneumocystis*. However, they are not active against *Cryptococcus neoformans* or other basidiomycetous yeasts and moulds.

### Polyenes inhibit cell membrane function

Amphotericin B and nystatin act by binding to sterols in cell membranes, resulting in leakage of cellular contents and cell death. Their preferential binding to ergosterol over cholesterol is the basis for selective toxicity. With a few exceptions, amphotericin B remains the drug of choice for the treatment of serious systemic fungal infections despite its serious toxic side effects; lipid formulations have lower toxicity and are increasingly preferred. Nystatin is used only in topical formulations.

*Orotomides inhibit DNA synthesis.* The orotomides inhibit fungal dihydroorotate dehydrogenase in the pyrimidine biosynthesis pathway required for DNA synthesis. Olorofim is a novel antifungal agent in this group and active against filamentous fungi, including *Aspergillus* species, but does not act on yeasts or the Mucorales.

*N-phosphonooxymethylenes interfere with cell wall synthesis.* Fosmanogepix is a prodrug metabolized to manogepix, the active compound. Manogepix inhibits the Gwt1 enzyme in the GP1-anchor biosynthetic pathway, thus affecting cell wall integrity. Manogepix has broad-spectrum activity against yeasts and moulds, including *Candida* and *Aspergillus*.

### Flucytosine and griseofulvin inhibit nucleic acid synthesis

Flucytosine (5-fluorocytosine) is deaminated to 5-fluorouracil, which inhibits DNA synthesis. Selective toxicity is based on the preferential uptake by fungal cells compared with host cells. Flucytosine is active only on yeasts (e.g. *Candida* spp. and *Cryptococcus*). Resistance emerges rapidly to flucytosine given as a single agent, so it should be used in combination with amphotericin B, whereby it is sometimes possible to reduce the dose of amphotericin B and therefore the toxic side effects.

**Table 34.7** The major therapeutic applications of antifungal drugs

| Infection | Antifungal of choice | Route of administration |
|---|---|---|
| **Superficial mycoses** | | |
| Ringworm (dermatophytes) | Topical agents (see text) are used to treat most cases; systemic therapy is required for scalp ringworm | Topical |
| | Griseofulvin | Oral |
| Candidiasis | Clotrimazole | Topical |
| | Miconazole | Topical |
| | Nystatin | Topical |
| | Fluconazole | Oral |
| **Systemic mycoses** | | |
| Histoplasmosis | Liposomal amphotericin B | Intravenous |
| | then itraconazole | Oral |
| Blastomycosis | Liposomal amphotericin B | Intravenous |
| | then fluconazole | Oral |
| Coccidioidomycosis | Fluconazole (liposomal amphotericin B for severe infection) | Oral |
| | | Intravenous |
| Paracoccidioidomycosis | Itraconazole | Oral |
| | If severe: | Intravenous |
| | Liposomal amphotericin B | Oral |
| | then itraconazole | |
| Aspergillosis | Voriconazole | Oral |
| | Isavuconazole | Oral |
| | Liposomal amphotericin B | Intravenous |
| Candidiasis | Caspofungin | Intravenous |
| | Liposomal amphotericin B | Intravenous |
| | For ocular or CNS infection or meningitis: | Intravenous |
| | liposomal amphotericin B + | Oral |
| | Flucytosine | |
| Cryptococcosis | Liposomal amphotericin B + | Intravenous |
| | Flucytosine | Oral |
| | Fluconazole | Intravenous or oral |
| Mucormycosis | Liposomal amphotericin B | Intravenous |
| Pneumocystis pneumonia | Trimethoprim-sulfamethoxazole | Intravenous or oral |
| | Pentamidine isethionate | Intravenous |

CNS, Central nervous system.

Griseofulvin appears to inhibit nucleic acid synthesis and to have antimitotic activity, possibly by inhibiting microtubule assembly. It may also have effects on cell wall synthesis by inhibiting chitin synthesis. In the host, griseofulvin binds specifically to newly formed keratin and is active in vivo only against dermatophyte fungi (see Chs. 4 and 27).

### Other topical antifungal agents include Whitfield ointment, tolnaftate, ciclopirox, haloprogin and naftifine

A variety of agents such as Whitfield ointment (a mixture of benzoic and salicylic acids), tolnaftate, ciclopirox, haloprogin and naftifine are available as creams for the topical treatment of superficial mycoses. These are usually available over the counter, and there is little to choose between them.

### No single antifungal agent is ideal

The main uses and adverse effects of antifungals are summarized in Table 34.7. Although there are several effective preparations available, some conditions such as dermatophyte infection of the nails (onychomycosis) or recurrent vulvovaginal candidiasis may prove intractable to treatment. The number of antifungal agents for systemic fungal infections is limited, and their adverse effects are considerable.

### Fungi develop resistance to antifungal agents

Although much less studied than resistance to antimicrobial agents used against bacteria, there is evidence that many similar mechanisms operate in resistance to antifungals. These include:

- enzyme modification
- target modification
- reduced permeability
- active efflux pumps
- failure to activate antifungal agents.

Resistance involving some or all of these mechanisms has been described in *Aspergillus*, *Candida* and *Cryptococcus*, particularly in the case of the azole compounds.

### There is an urgent need for safer, more efficacious antifungal agents

Invasive fungal infections are a significant cause of morbidity and mortality in patients undergoing chemotherapy, immune suppression and transplantation. The incidence of these infections is increasing in parallel with the increasing numbers of such patients and their improved survival due to effective antibacterial therapy. New agents to control these infections (e.g. *Aspergillus, Fusarium, Scedosporium,* Mucorales and *Candida auris*) are needed.

## ANTIPARASITIC AGENTS

### Parasites pose particular problems

Any consideration of antiparasitic agents must take into account the very large number of different parasites capable of infecting humans, the complexities of their life cycles and the differences between them in their metabolic pathways. Thus drugs acting against protozoa are usually inactive against helminths and vice versa. Additionally, protozoa and helminths are eukaryotes and therefore metabolically more similar to humans than are bacteria. Although some antibacterial agents do have antiprotozoal activity (e.g. metronidazole, tetracycline), in general, antibacterial agents are ineffective against parasites. A major challenge has been to identify targets in which there are sufficient differences between host and parasite to facilitate safe drug activity. Some of these targets include:

- unique drug uptake: chloroquine, mefloquine, primaquine in malaria
- differences in folic acid metabolism: pyrimethamine in malaria, sulphonamides in toxoplasmosis, trimethoprim in cyclosporiasis
- polyamine uptake: pentamidine in leishmaniasis
- unique trypanothione-dependent reduction mechanisms: fluoromethylornithine against trypanosomes
- unique neurotransmitters: piperazine, ivermectin, pyrantel against nematodes
- cytoskeletal proteins (tubulin): benzimidazoles against nematodes
- intracellular calcium levels: praziquantel against flukes and tapeworms
- oxidative phosphorylation: niclosamide against tapeworms.

Despite differences between host and parasite in these targets, it remains true that a number of the more effective antiparasitic drugs still carry the risk of significant toxicity.

The wide array of different antiprotozoal and anthelmintic drugs that have been developed is summarized in Tables 34.8 and 34.9, respectively.

### Drug resistance is an increasing problem

As with the antibacterial agents, drug resistance is a significant problem in the treatment of parasitic infections, particularly with malaria. There are four different indications for antimalarial chemotherapy:

- prophylactic: to prevent infection (e.g. intermittent preventive treatment of malaria during pregnancy in malaria-endemic areas; prevention of malaria in travellers from nonendemic locations visiting malarious areas)
- therapeutic: to treat infection (applies to all human malarias)
- radical cure: to prevent relapse following the treatment of acute infection (applies to *Plasmodium vivax* and *P. ovale* only)

- killing malarial gametocytes: to prevent transmission.

*Plasmodium falciparum* malaria resistant to one or more antimalarial agents is now widespread. Chloroquine-resistant falciparum malaria occurs worldwide, and *P. vivax* shows focal resistance to this agent, notably in the Asia-Pacific region. The usual alternative to chloroquine in the tropics was combined sulphadoxine/pyrimethamine, but there is now significant resistance to the antifolate compounds. Mefloquine-resistant falciparum malaria is found in parts of Southeast Asia and parts of South America. Quinine, the original antimalarial agent, is still used to treat severe malaria if artesunate, the drug of choice, is not available, although quinine requires careful monitoring during treatment to avoid toxicity. Development of antimalarial agents from natural products has provided new compounds, the most important being derivatives of artemisinin (from the Chinese drug *quinghaosu,* produced from the plant *Artemisia annua*). Intravenous artesunate has supplanted quinine as the agent of choice for the treatment of severe falciparum malaria. Drug combinations are now deployed for the treatment of falciparum malaria to reduce the chance of developing drug resistance after monotherapy, as happened with chloroquine, and artemisinin combination therapy (ACT) is the first-line treatment of choice. Of considerable concern is the emergence of *P. falciparum* with reduced sensitivity to artesunate characterized by the *pfk13* gene marker. This was detected initially in Southeast Asia in 2007 and then in Africa in 2020. If ACT fails on a large scale, it will have a devastating effect on malaria morbidity and mortality especially in the African Region, which suffers from 95% of world malaria cases and 96% of malaria deaths.

Drug resistance is less of a problem with other protozoa, although cases of giardiasis failing to respond to treatment with metronidazole are increasingly common, especially if the infection was acquired in India. In the case of helminthic infections, although drug resistance to the benzimidazoles is widespread in animal parasitic nematodes, it has not yet become a serious issue with human infections. Treatment of human schistosomiasis relies almost exclusively on praziquantel, and while there is no definitive evidence for reduced sensitivity in the field, there is evidence to suggest that strains with reduced susceptibility to praziquantel are present, so there is no room for complacency.

Protozoa make use of enzyme and target modification to develop resistance (e.g. against antifolates and sulphonamides), but, in addition, active efflux pumps have been described in resistance of *P. falciparum* to chloroquine and mefloquine. Resistance to benzimidazole anthelmintics involves target modification arising from mutations in cuticular tubulins.

## CONTROL BY CHEMOTHERAPY VERSUS VACCINATION

While vaccination is discussed in detail in Chapter 35, it is important to note here the role both chemotherapy and vaccination play in protecting individuals. An important difference is that chemotherapy is usually given after exposure to infection, whereas vaccination is usually given before exposure. Chemotherapy essentially offers short-term protection, which wanes once the drug is no longer given; vaccination can give long-term protection without repeated treatment. Vaccination is therefore more effective than chemotherapy in protecting populations.

**Table 34.8** Therapeutic applications of the major antiprotozoal drugs

| Disease/site | Agent | Route of administration | Comments |
|---|---|---|---|
| **Amoebiasis** | | | |
| Asymptomatic cyst passers | Paromomycin | Oral | |
| Invasive (dysentery or liver abscess) | Metronidazole or tindazole followed by paromomycin | Oral Oral | |
| Cryptosporidiosis | Nitazoxanide (the agent of choice) Paromomycin (limited activity) | Oral Oral | |
| Cyclosporiasis | Trimethoprim-sulphamethoxazole | Oral | |
| Giardiasis | Metronidazole or tinidazole Nitazoxanide Quinacrine (also known as mepacrine) | Oral Oral Oral | |
| **Leishmaniasis** | | | |
| Cutaneous leishmaniasis | Depending on infecting species, site and number of lesions: Local infiltration with meglumine antimoniate (an antimonial) Intravenous meglumine antimoniate Miltefosine | Local intralesional injection IV Oral | |
| Mucosal leishmaniasis | Liposomal amphotericin B meglumine antimoniate or miltefosine | | |
| Visceral leishmaniasis | Liposomal amphotericin B (agent of choice) Meglumine antimoniate Miltefosine | IV IV Oral | |
| **Malaria** | | | |
| Blood stages | Chloroquine (for *P. vivax, ovale* or *malariae* **only**) | Oral | |
| | Quinine | Oral, IV | Used against drug-resistant *P. falciparum* |
| | Mefloquine | Oral | |
| | Atovaquone/proguanil | Oral | |
| | Artemisinin combination therapy (ACT; e.g. artemether/lumefantrine) | Oral | ACTs are the agents of choice for uncomplicated *P. falciparum* malaria. WHO lists six recommended ACTs |
| | Artesunate | IV | The agent of choice for severe malaria |
| | Tetracycline | Oral | Used with or after quinine against drug-resistant *P. falciparum* |
| Pre-erythrocytic stages | Primaquine | Oral | Used along with chloroquine to kill hypnozoites in the liver and achieve radical cure. Required for *P. vivax* and *P. ovale* **only**. Risk of haemolytic anaemia in G6PD-deficient patients |
| | Tafenoquine | Oral | Used along with chloroquine to kill hypnozoites in the liver and achieve radical cure. Required for *P. vivax* and *P. ovale* **only**. Risk of haemolytic anaemia in G6PD-deficient patients |
| Toxoplasmosis | Pyrimethamine plus sulfadiazine | Oral | |
| Microsporidiosis | Albendazole | Oral | Variable, species-dependent response |
| Trichomoniasis | Metronidazole Tinidazole | Oral Oral | |
| **Trypanosomiasis** | | | |
| East African | Suramin for haemolymphatic stage Followed by melarsoprol if CNS involved | IV IV | |
| West African | Pentamidine for stage 1 disease (haemolymphatic stage) | IV | |
| | Nifurtimox-eflornithine combination if CNS involved (stage 2 disease) | Oral nifurtimox IV eflornithine | |
| | Fexinidazole is effective against stage 1 and stage 2 | Oral | The first entirely oral treatment regimen for this disease |
| American (Chagas disease) | Benznidazole Nifurtimox | Oral Oral | |

Several are potentially toxic and must be given under supervision. Some also have antibacterial activity and have been described in detail earlier in the chapter. Drug resistance is a problem, particularly in the treatment of malaria. CNS, Central nervous system; G6PD, glucose-6-phosphate dehydrogenase; IV, intravenous; WHO, World Health Organization.

**Table 34.9** Therapeutic applications of the major anthelmintic drugs

| Disease | Agent | Comments |
|---|---|---|
| **Cestodes (tapeworms)** | | |
| Adult stage infection | Niclosamide<br>Praziquantel | Avoid praziquantel in intestinal *Taenia solium* infection unless concomitant cerebral cysticercosis has been excluded |
| Cerebral cysticercosis (larval *T. solium*) | Albendazole + praziquantel | Under corticosteroid cover |
| Echinococcosis (hydatid) disease | Albendazole | Regimen depends on cyst type |
| **Trematodes (flukes)** | | |
| Schistosomiasis | Praziquantel | |
| Intestinal flukes | Praziquantel | |
| Lung fluke | Praziquantel | |
| Liver flukes except *Fasciola hepatica* | Praziquantel | |
| *F. hepatica* | Triclabendazole | |
| **Nematodes (roundworms)** | | |
| Ascariasis and pinworm (threadworm) infection | Mebendazole<br>Albendazole<br>Pyrantel pamoate<br>Piperazine | |
| Hookworm infection | Mebendazole<br>Albendazole<br>Pyrantel pamoate | |
| Strongyloidiasis | Ivermectin<br>Albendazole<br>Thiabendazole | Less effective<br>Effective but rarely available. Poorly tolerated due to side effects |
| Trichinosis | Albendazole<br>Mebendazole | |
| Trichuriasis | Albendazole<br>Mebendazole | |
| Cutaneous larva migrans (infection with animal hookworm) | Ivermectin orally<br>Albendazole orally<br>Thiabendazole paste (rarely available) | |
| Toxocariasis (visceral larva migrans) | Albendazole | |
| Lymphatic filariasis | Diethylcarbamazine plus doxycycline | |
| Onchocerciasis | Doxycycline plus Ivermectin or moxidectin | |

All are administered orally except thiabendazole paste for cutaneous larva migrans, which is administered topically. Note that many of these drugs are not safe in pregnancy.

There are, of course, exceptions to these: Passive antibody can be used to treat acute infection just as a drug can, while drugs such as mefloquine or atovaquone-proguanil combination preparation are used for prophylaxis against malaria, almost as if they were short-term vaccines. However, in most cases there is a clear-cut distinction between the one- or two-shot vaccine, conferring protection for years, and the daily or twice-daily drug dose.

### The concept of selectivity, or specificity, is central to both chemotherapy and vaccination

Although they appear so different (Table 34.10), both chemotherapy and vaccination developed together from the intensive study that followed the demonstration in the late 1800s that diseases could be caused by microbes.

Louis Pasteur (Box 34.8) showed that killed or weakened microbes (e.g. anthrax, rabies) could be used to induce immunity that was active against that disease, while Ehrlich's work with histologic dyes led him to the idea that particular chemicals (drugs) might bind specifically to particular microbial structures and damage them, thus being active against several diseases. Both, therefore, established the concept of selectively or specifically targeting infectious organisms within the body as a means of controlling disease.

### The specificity of an antimicrobial drug resides in its ability to damage the microbe and not the host

As noted earlier, antimicrobial drugs should ideally bind to a molecule present only in the microbe to ensure specificity

**Table 34.10** Comparison of chemotherapy and vaccination

| | Chemotherapy | | Vaccination | |
|---|---|---|---|---|
| Specificity | Usually high | | Very high | |
| Toxicity | Potentially high | | Usually low | |
| Duration of effect | Usually short | | Usually long | |
| Duration of treatment | May be prolonged | | Usually short, but may need boosting | |
| Effectiveness | Bacteria<br>Viruses<br>Fungi<br>Parasites | High<br>}Moderate<br>High | Viruses<br>Bacteria<br>Fungi<br>Parasites | High<br>}Low/moderate<br>No vaccine yet marked for parasitic infections of humans, a malaria vaccine will be the first |

---

## Box 34.8 ■ Lessons in Microbiology

### Louis Pasteur (1822–1895)

The science of microbiology was established in the 19th century by the work of many distinguished scientists. However, one such scientist, Louis Pasteur, may legitimately be regarded as a founding father of this discipline (Fig. 34.30). He, along with Robert Koch (see Ch. 13), was able to show that living organisms or microbes were the cause of disease and provided a firm scientific basis for their study and control.

Pasteur began work at a time when spontaneous generation was still an accepted explanation for the appearance of microorganisms in decaying material. His elegant experiments showed that sterile organic infusions would not putrefy or ferment if there were no subsequent contact with airborne contaminants, proving that spontaneous generation did not occur and that all microbes must come from pre-existing microbes. This discovery contributed to many fields of science, both basic and applied. Perhaps most important was the contribution Pasteur made to the work of Lister on antiseptics, which revolutionized approaches to surgery.

Pasteur worked in an amazing variety of microbiologic fields, from fermentation in the brewing of beers and production of wines, to identification of silkworm diseases, bringing to each a penetrating scientific insight and making discoveries that brought him national and international renown. His understanding of the roles of organisms in causing diseases and his acute scientific perception enabled him to grasp from a series of mishaps with experiments on chicken cholera that attenuated microbes could induce not disease, but immunity from it. His ideas generated powerful opposition, but his belief then was strong enough to encourage him in 1881 to take part in a public trial of his vaccine against anthrax in domestic animals. Later, he used his insight into rabies, caused by organisms he could not see or culture, to develop an attenuated vaccine made from the dried spinal cords of infected rabbits. This was proven effective in humans in 1885, when Pasteur inoculated Joseph Meister, a 9-year-old boy who had been badly bitten by a rabid dog. Meister survived, and Pasteur's views on vaccination became universally accepted.

Pasteur ended his life as a national hero in his native France, with a worldwide reputation for his work. His name is immortalized not only in the process of sterilization (pasteurization) that he developed, but also in the Institut Pasteur in Paris, which remains one of the most important international centres of microbiologic work.

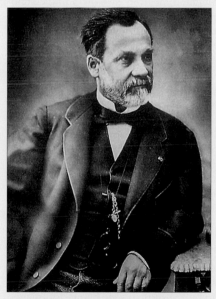

**Fig. 34.30** Louis Pasteur (1822–1895).

---

for the microbe and not the host. The extent to which this can be achieved varies from microbe to microbe. Bacteria, with their prokaryotic cell structure, are much more remote from humans than fungi, protozoa or worms (which are all eukaryotic). It is not surprising therefore that the most effective antibiotics are generally those used against bacteria. As much of the viral life cycle uses host cell components, antiviral chemotherapy has so far been less successful than antibacterial therapy.

Many antimicrobial agents are products of microbes themselves or derivatives of these products. It is presumed that they form part of the self-preservation mechanism by which the microbes prevent overcrowding with their own or other species.

Although it is possible to administer antimicrobial agents in ways that prolong their presence in the body, they are no longer active once concentrations fall below a critical threshold. Continuing antimicrobial activity therefore

**Table 34.11** Strategies for control of infectious diseases

| General features | Water purification (waterborne diseases)<br>Sewage disposal (enteric infections)<br>Improved nutrition (host defence)<br>Improved housing (less crowding, dirt, etc.) |
|---|---|
| Food | Cold storage<br>Pasteurization (milk, etc.)<br>Food inspection (meat, etc.)<br>Adequate cooking |
| Zoonoses and arthropod-transmitted infections | Control of vectors (mosquitoes, ticks, lice, etc.) and bite avoidance<br>Control of reservoir animal (rabies, etc.) |
| Specific disease treatment or prevention | Chemotherapy<br>Vaccines |
| Miscellaneous measures | Changes in personal habits (reduced promiscuity, use of condoms, improved personal hygiene, etc.)<br>Control of intravenous drug abuse<br>Screening of transfused blood and organs |

requires repeated administration as opposed to vaccines, which can provide long-term protection with far less readministration (see Ch. 35).

## CONTROL VERSUS ERADICATION

### Control and eradication are different objectives, although eradication is always an ideal end point

Many infections can be controlled (at least in some parts of the world) by a combination of strategies, including chemotherapy and vaccination (see Ch. 35; Table 34.10) but are certainly not eradicated, even in those countries where control is most effective. Epidemiologic theory (see Ch. 33) predicts that once transmission rates fall below a threshold value, the infection should die out, and this may certainly be true at a local level. However, reservoirs of infection persist where treatment is nonexistent or ineffective, or infection is reintroduced by the movement of peoples, and new epidemics may therefore develop. To date, only one disease (smallpox) has been taken to the point at which the organism has been eliminated. What are the chances that other infectious diseases will follow smallpox into oblivion? Various factors are important in determining the effectiveness of any eradication programme (Table 34.11).

### Realism is required when considering the long-term aims of antimicrobial control strategies

Hopes raised by the early success of antibiotics were soon dashed by the emergence of resistance, and far from the microbial load borne by the human race being diminished in recent years, it has, if anything, increased. Many infections covered in this book (e.g. HIV, Ebola virus, Zika virus, to name but a few) are not featured in older textbooks of microbiology. Infections previously well controlled by antibiotics have become serious problems in hospitals (MRSA, *C. difficile*, carbapenem-resistant, ESBL-producing Enterobacteriaceae). Approaches to the control of infectious diseases are therefore a matter of identifying priorities such as the following:

- Which diseases could, with suitable effort, be eradicated?
- Would the cost of eradication be justified?

- Which diseases need urgent measures to stop them from worsening?
- Which diseases are responsible for the most human suffering and economic loss?
- Inevitably, some diseases will not feature strongly on any such list, and it must be accepted that they may always be with us.

## USE AND MISUSE OF ANTIMICROBIAL AGENTS

Much has been said in this chapter about the interactions between antimicrobial agents and microbes—the mechanisms of selective toxicity and the defences put up by resistant organisms. The distribution, metabolism and excretion of agents by the host have been considered briefly, together with the important toxic side effects of the agents. The choice of antimicrobial agent for treating specific infections is dealt with in the appropriate systems chapter. Dosage regimens have not been included because they vary with the agent, the infection, the age and the underlying condition of the patient and sometimes from one country to another. Practitioners should consult appropriate local pharmacy guidelines.

### Antimicrobial agents should be used only as appropriate for prophylaxis or treatment

In conclusion, we should stand back and ask, "Is antimicrobial therapy necessary for this patient? If so, which agent is appropriate?" Antimicrobial agents can be used to help prevent infection (prophylaxis) and to treat infection. Prophylactic use of antibiotics is appropriate only in a few clearly defined circumstances and is usually of limited duration (e.g. 1–2 days). Specific examples include (1) patients of normal susceptibility who have been exposed to specific pathogens (e.g. bacterial meningitis or TB), (2) individuals with increased susceptibility to infection (e.g. neutropenic patients) and (3) patients undergoing surgery as a perioperative antibiotiv cover.

### Antimicrobial use results in the selection of resistant strains

If antibiotic treatment is necessary, several factors must be considered, and these are summarized in Fig. 34.31.

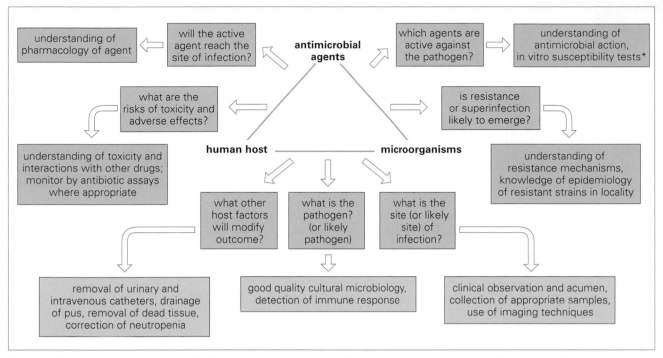

**Fig. 34.31** The interactions between antimicrobial agents, microorganisms and the human host can be summarized by examining the answers to several questions affecting each side of the triangle of interaction. *Other tests include phenotypic and genotypic antiviral susceptibility tests and viral load tests.

It is important to recognize that, during treatment, not only the infecting microbe but also the patient and all the patient's normal microbiota are being exposed to the effects of the antimicrobial agent. Use of antimicrobial agents has been clearly shown to select for resistant strains both in the individual and in the community, and overuse or inappropriate use only increases this risk. History suggests that microbes will never run out of ways of developing resistance, but we may run out of effective antimicrobial agents.

## KEY FACTS

- Infection is unique among the diseases that afflict humans because it involves two distinct biologic systems. Antimicrobial agents are designed to inhibit one system (the microbe) while doing minimal damage to the other (the patient). Antimicrobial agents require selective toxicity.

- Antimicrobial agents are often themselves products of microorganisms (natural products), although most are chemically modified to improve their properties. Other agents are entirely synthetic. Antibacterial agents are the most numerous; designing antiviral, antifungal and antiparasitic drugs that are selectively toxic provides much greater challenge.

- Antibacterial agents are classified by their target site and their chemical family; this helps us to understand better their mode of action and the mechanisms of resistance.

- Antibacterial agents have four possible sites of action in the bacterial cell: cell wall, protein, nucleic acids and cell membrane. Most antibacterial agents act at the cell wall or inhibit protein or nucleic acid synthesis. At each site there are many different molecular targets (enzymes or substrates) that can be specifically inhibited.

- Development of resistance is the major limiting factor of antibacterial agents. It arises through random mutation of bacterial chromosomal genes but more importantly through acquisition, from other bacteria, of resistance genes on integrons, transposons and plasmids.

- Mutated or acquired genes confer resistance by altering the target site of the antibacterial agent, altering the uptake of the drug or producing drug-destroying enzymes.

- The emergence of AIDS and COVID-19, decades later, provided an enormous stimulus to research in developing antivirals, immunomodulators and passive immunotherapies.

- The number of classes of antifungal molecules is very limited. Toxicity (all), difficulty of formulation (polyenes) and emerging resistance (azoles) make effective treatment of fungal infections a serious challenge.

- Although there are many antiparasitic drugs available, a number show toxicity and others are becoming increasingly ineffective because of the development of resistance. This is particularly so in malaria infections in which parasites show resistance to almost all drugs presently available.

- Bacteria can be tested in the laboratory for their susceptibility to antibacterial agents. The results of well-controlled tests provide a valuable guide to appropriate treatment. In vitro tests with antifungals are less reliable and are rarely performed with antivirals in the clinical laboratory setting.

# 35

# Protecting the host: vaccination

## Introduction

Vaccines are one of the most effective public health tools. This chapter reviews how vaccines work and the vaccines in current use. However, although vaccination is a very cost-effective public health measure that saved an estimated 2–3 million deaths each year prior to the severe acute respiratory syndrome coronavirus 2 (SARS-CoV-2) pandemic and perhaps as many as 20 million deaths from SARS-CoV-2 in 2021, a further 1.5 million people still die each year from a vaccine-preventable disease as a result of poor vaccine uptake (Fig. 35.1). Global vaccine coverage fell from 2019–2021 due to the coronavirus disease 2019 (COVID-19) pandemic, and an estimated 25 million children <1 year of age did not receive basic vaccines in 2021. Many others die from infectious diseases such as human immunodeficiency virus (HIV) for which we have no effective vaccine, so new vaccines are also needed (Table 35.1).

Vaccination exploits the ability of the immune system to develop immunologic memory so that it can rapidly mobilize its forces to fight infection when required. Vaccines can be of different types, including live attenuated organisms, killed organisms or subunit vaccines delivered by viral vectors and given as proteins or polysaccharides or injected as messenger RNA (mRNA) in nanoparticles. Depending on the vaccine type, more than one dose may be needed to achieve or maintain optimal protection. Adjuvants are often required to increase immunity particularly with subunit vaccines. Polysaccharide vaccines are a particular challenge as infants do not make a good immune response to polysaccharides unless they are conjugated to a protein. The development of new and more effective vaccines is a major area of research especially with outbreaks of viruses such as SARS-CoV-2, monkeypox, Ebola or Zika virus. Successful vaccination also requires an understanding of the epidemiology of disease transmission to estimate what proportion of the population needs to be vaccinated to produce herd immunity (see Ch. 33). Finally, vaccines need to be safe, as they are given to healthy individuals, and particular care is needed when live attenuated vaccines are used to avoid issues in the immunocompromised person.

## VACCINATION: A 400-YEAR HISTORY

The elimination of smallpox through vaccination has been described as the greatest success story in medicine, and the impact of vaccination on the SARS-CoV-2 pandemic was equally dramatic. Due to the pioneering work of Jenner with vaccinia (Box 35.1, Fig. 35.2), all forms of specific, actively induced immunity are now referred to as *vaccination*.

The principle of vaccination is simple: to prime the adaptive immune system to the antigens of a particular pathogen so that, on first contact with the live organism, a rapid and effective secondary immune response will be induced by memory T and B cells. Vaccination therefore depends upon the ability of the naïve T and B cells to respond to specific antigens and develop into memory T and B cells and represents a form of actively enhanced adaptive immunity. The passive administration of preformed elements such as antibody is considered in Chapter 36.

## AIMS OF VACCINATION

### The aims of vaccination can vary from preventing symptoms to eradicating disease

The most ambitious aim of vaccination is eradication of the disease. This has been achieved for smallpox, the eradication

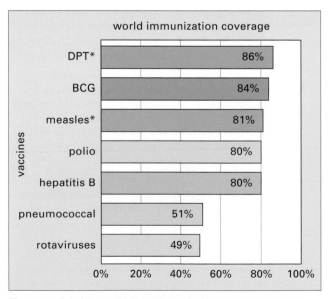

**Fig. 35.1** Global immunization coverage in 2021. Vaccine coverage is good for some vaccines, but many more lives would be saved if available vaccines were more widely used. *, First dose; BCG, bacille Calmette-Guérin; DPT, diphtheria-pertussis-tetanus. (From World Health Organization. *Immunization Data.* WHO; n.d.)

**Table 35.1** Infectious agents that are major killers

| Organism | Disease | Estimated annual deaths (millions) |
|---|---|---|
| Human immunodeficiency virus (HIV) | Acquired immunodeficiency syndrome | 0.65 |
| *Mycobacterium tuberculosis* | Tuberculosis (TB) | 1.60 |
| *Plasmodium* spp. | Malaria | 0.61 |
| Total | | 2.86 |

We currently lack effective vaccines against these organisms, although bacille Calmette–Guérin vaccination can provide protection against disseminated forms of childhood TB and pulmonary TB in some parts of the world, and the RTS,S in ASO1 malaria vaccine provided protection similar to that of seasonal malaria chemoprevention in endemic areas. Most of the deaths from HIV are in Africa, and most of the deaths from malaria are in African children. Deaths from severe acute respiratory syndrome coronavirus 2 (SARS-CoV-2) from 2020–2022 totaled 6.564 million, but a number of protective vaccines have been licensed. From World Health Organization; 2021.

of polio is underway and there was a dramatic downward trend in the incidence of many vaccine-preventable diseases from 1950–1980 (Fig. 35.3).

Most vaccines aim to protect the vaccinated individual against infection. In certain cases the aim of vaccination may be more limited: to protect the individual against symptoms or pathology (e.g. diphtheria and tetanus vaccines induce immunity only against the toxins produced by the bacteria, as it is the effect of these toxins rather than the simple presence of the microbe itself that is harmful).

### The importance of herd immunity

Successful vaccination programmes rely not only on the development and use of vaccines themselves but also on an understanding of the epidemiologic aspects of disease transmission. If enough individuals in a population are immunized or have immunity from a past infection, this will reduce or stop transmission of the infection. This is called *herd immunity*. By having your own child immunized, you therefore help protect the whole community; conversely, when too many parents decide not to vaccinate their children because they think the risk of their child getting the disease is low, this may contribute to the disease becoming more common (see Fig. 35.3). It is therefore important to know how many individuals in a population must be immunized to produce herd immunity and whether immunity should be boosted by revaccination. Giving one dose of pneumococcal vaccine to infants, with a booster dose at 1 year of age, prevents carriage and transmission; giving live attenuated influenza vaccine to school-age children not only protects them but reduces transmission and therefore infection in the more vulnerable elderly population.

## VACCINES CAN BE OF DIFFERENT TYPES

Vaccines can be based on whole organisms, either live or inactivated, or components of the infectious agent that may be delivered by a viral vector or as mRNA that encodes a component of the pathogen such as the SARS-CoV-2 spike protein (Table 35.2). Sometimes two types of vaccine are available for the same disease—and for a good reason.

Live vaccines are designed to induce immunity in a similar way to the actual infection. Live vaccines can use organisms that were attenuated using culture in eggs, animals or in tissue culture (Fig. 35.4); these attenuated organisms replicate to a limited extent in the vaccinated individual but do not cause disease in healthy people. The infectious agent can also be genetically modified to remove genes associated with pathogenicity; however, immunosuppression can produce problems with live vaccines (e.g. infants with HIV infection given bacille Calmette-Guérin [BCG] vaccination can develop disseminated BCGosis). HIV-infected individuals

---

## Box 35.1 ■ Lessons in Microbiology

### Edward Jenner (1749–1823)

English physician Edward Jenner (Fig. 35.2) is regarded as the founder of modern vaccination, but he was by no means the first to try the technique. The ancient practice of variolation dates to 10th-century China and arrived in Europe in the early 18th century via Turkey. The technique involved the inoculation of children with dried material from healed scabs of mild smallpox cases, and it was a striking foretaste of the principles of modern attenuated viral vaccines. This practice was, however, both inconsistent and dangerous, and Jenner's innovation was to show that much safer and more reliable protection could be obtained by deliberate inoculation with cowpox (vaccinia) virus. Milkmaids exposed to cowpox were traditionally known to be resistant to smallpox and so retained their smooth complexions. In 1796 Jenner tested his theory by inoculating 8-year-old James Phipps with liquid from a cowpox pustule on the hand of Sarah Nelmes. Subsequent inoculation of the boy with smallpox produced no disease. Although greeted with skepticism at first, Jenner's ideas soon became accepted, and he went on to inoculate thousands of individuals in a shed in the garden of his house at Berkeley,

Gloucestershire. He ultimately achieved world fame, although his fellowship of the Royal Society was conferred for a quite different piece of work on the nesting habits of the cuckoo!

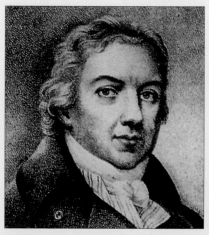

**Fig. 35.2** Edward Jenner (1749–1823).

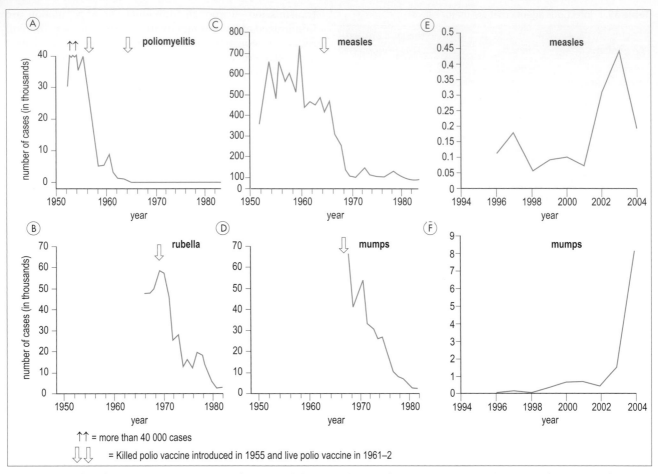

**Fig. 35.3** The effect of vaccination on the incidence of various viral diseases in the United States and United Kingdom. Most infections (A–D) have shown a dramatic downward trend after the introduction of a vaccine (*arrows*), but the right-hand panels (E, F) show the resurgence in disease when vaccine uptake is reduced following vaccine scares. (Modified from Mims and White and the UK Health Security Agency.)

with severe immunosuppression should not be given live vaccines such as those for measles or varicella, but they can be given inactivated vaccines.

Inactivated vaccines are safe to use in the immunocompromised, although they may not be as immunogenic, so a good adjuvant may be needed. Inactivation is usually by fixation (e.g. with formalin). Types of fixatives in use in vaccines are given in Table 35.3. Another difference between live and attenuated vaccines is that immunity induced by inactivated vaccines is not affected by circulating antibody (e.g. maternally derived antibodies in young children). Individual antigens or toxins can also be used as a vaccine with adjuvant. Purified proteins are used in the acellular pertussis vaccine, recombinant surface antigen protein in the vaccines for hepatitis B and the SARS-CoV-2 spike protein in COVID-19 vaccines. A number of protein antigens can be joined together as a fusion protein, as in some candidate tuberculosis (TB) vaccines and the RTS,S malaria vaccine. Polysaccharides form the basis of the pneumococcal vaccine, but as polysaccharide vaccines are not immunogenic in children <2 years of age, who have the highest risk of disease, conjugate vaccines that use a polysaccharide linked to a protein have been developed for pneumococcal and meningococcal disease and for *Haemophilus influenzae* type b (Hib). For some bacteria, it is the toxin that is pathogenic, and this

can be inactivated to make a toxoid, as in the tetanus toxoid vaccine. With individual components of an organism, an adjuvant will be needed to boost immune responses. Multiple doses of protein or polysaccharide are usually needed, as these vaccines are less immunogenic than whole organisms.

One or more vaccine antigens can also be delivered by a viral vector, such as Modified Vaccinia virus Ankara (MVA), which is replication deficient; it was safely used in humans at the end of the smallpox eradication campaign. Delivering the antigen in this way will mimic the natural infection better than giving the proteins in adjuvant. Other viral vectors being tested for new vaccines include adenovirus (Ad26 for respiratory syncytial virus [RSV]) and cytomegalovirus (CMV). This type of technology can be used quickly to make new vaccines and has been exploited to develop vaccines for the Ebola and Zika viruses as well as for SARS-CoV-2.

Rather than using antigen as the vaccine, mRNA encoding the antigen can be used. This enables the antigen to be produced in the body. mRNA vaccines against SARS-CoV-2 proved remarkably effective, and this platform technology is now being explored for other infectious diseases as well as for cancer for which it was originally developed.

Some vaccines are designed to boost immunity using only selected antigens or by using a different delivery route (i.e. prime boost). Some new TB vaccines in development,

**Table 35.2** Types of vaccine

| Types of vaccine | Examples |
| --- | --- |
| **Live attenuated** | |
| Viral[a] | Measles, mumps, rubella, varicella, yellow fever, zoster, oral polio, intranasal influenza, rotavirus |
| Bacterial | Bacille Calmette-Guérin, oral typhoid |
| **Inactivated** | |
| Whole virus | Polio, influenza, hepatitis A, rabies, Japanese encephalitis |
| Whole bacteria | Pertussis, cholera, typhoid |
| **Fractions** | |
| Toxoids | Diphtheria, tetanus |
| Protein subunits[a] | Hepatitis B, influenza, acellular pertussis, papillomavirus, severe acute respiratory syndrome coronavirus 2 (SARS-CoV-2) |
| Polysaccharides | Pneumococcal, meningococcal, *Salmonella typhi* (Vi) |
| Conjugates | *Haemophilus influenzae* type b (tetanus toxoid, nontoxic diphtheria toxoid or *Neisseria meningitidis* outer membrane protein), pneumococcal (diphtheria toxoid), meningococcal (diphtheria toxoid) |

[a]Protein antigens can be delivered by an attenuated viral vector as messenger RNA or with adjuvant. Note that not all types of vaccine are available in all countries. Vaccines are also available for bioterrorism agents such as anthrax and plague and for vaccinia.

**Table 35.3** Fixatives and preservatives used in current vaccines

| **Fixatives** | |
| --- | --- |
| Formalin | DTaP/TdaP, Td, HepA, HepB, Hib,[a] influenza,[a] Japanese encephalitis, meningococcal ACWY,[a] polio, inactivated typhoid, anthrax, IPV |
| Glutaraldehyde | DtaP, Tdap |
| **Preservatives** | |
| EDTA | Influenza,[a] rabies,[a] varicella |
| Phenol | Hib,[a] pneumococcal polysaccharide PPSV23,[a] inactivated typhoid |
| 2-Phenoxyethanol | DtaP, IPV |
| β-Propiolactone | Influenza,[a] rabies |
| Sodium deoxycholate | Influenza[a] |
| Thiomersal[b] | DT/Td,[a] influenza,[a] meningococcal polysaccharide[a] |

[a]Used in some vaccine formulations and in some multidose vials.
[b]Thiomersal (Thimerosal) has now been removed from most vaccines because of concerns about having small traces of mercury in the vaccine. DT/Td, Diphtheria-tetanus; HepA, hepatitis A; HepB, hepatitis B; Hib, *Haemophilus influenzae* type b; IPV, inactivated polio vaccine; PPSV23, pneumococcal polysaccharide vaccine 23; TdaP/DtaP, combined tetanus-diphtheria-pertussis.

for example, would boost the immunity induced by BCG given at birth by using key antigens delivered by a viral vector (Fig. 35.5) or as a fusion protein with adjuvant.

Recipients of haemopoietic stem cell transplants may need to be revaccinated after the infusion of stem cells, as otherwise antibody titres to vaccine-preventable diseases decline.

## Adjuvants

Adjuvants increase the immunity induced by a vaccine in a number of ways. Adjuvants can improve the immune

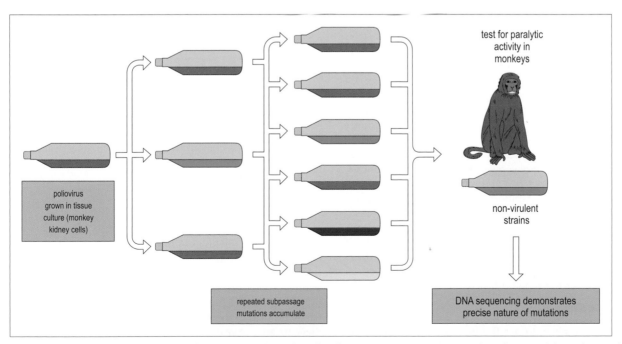

**Fig. 35.4** Live attenuated vaccines (e.g. polio) were originally produced by allowing viruses to grow in unusual conditions and then selecting the randomly occurring mutants that had lost virulence.

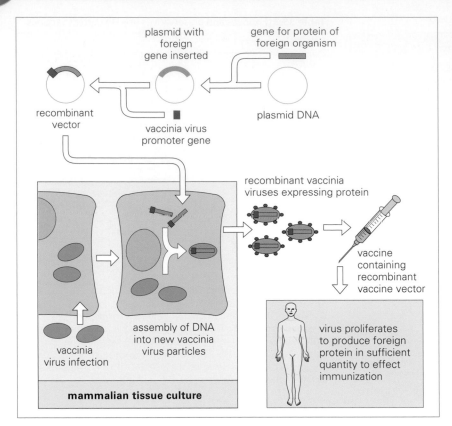

**Fig. 35.5** It is now possible to insert genes coding for antigens of one or more microorganisms into a large virus such as modified Vaccinia virus Ankara or adenovirus so that the virus replicates and antigens are produced in the host. This technology can be exploited to quickly develop new vaccines (e.g. for Ebola or severe acute respiratory syndrome coronavirus 2 [SARS-CoV-2]).

response to the vaccine antigens through inducing activation of Toll-like receptors on dendritic cells to improve antigen presentation or by forming an antigen depot, which allows antigen to persist and to leak out slowly over time. The earliest adjuvants consisted of water-in-oil emulsions: Freund's complete adjuvant, which includes dead mycobacteria in a water-in-oil emulsion, is very effective in animals although not suitable for use in humans. Other adjuvants increase antigen presentation or enhance types of immunity, such as antibodies or T-helper 1 (Th1) immunity. The dramatic effect of adding an adjuvant to a vaccine is shown in Fig. 35.6. Aluminium salts are powerful adjuvants still used in many vaccines (Box 35.2); they induce inflammation when cell products from stressed or dying cells (including heat-shock proteins) interact with damage-associated molecular pattern receptors. Experimentally, cytokines such as interleukin-1 (IL-1), IL-2, interferon-gamma (IFN-γ), IL-12 and IL-18, as well as some chemokines, have been tested as adjuvants. Compounds such as liposomes, lipid-containing vesicles, have also been used (e.g. 3-O-desacyl-4'-monophosphoryl lipid A in the human papillomavirus [HPV] vaccine [Cervarix] as adjuvant). COVID-19 mRNA vaccines do not need an adjuvant, as the lipid nanoparticles in which the mRNA is delivered acts as an adjuvant whereas the mRNA itself induces cytokines such as Type 1 IFNs. Other COVID-19 vaccines based on recombinant spike protein do need an adjuvant, such as the saponin-based adjuvant Matrix-M.

## VACCINE SAFETY

As vaccines are given to healthy individuals, it is critically important that they are safe. In 1926 live *Mycobacterium tuberculosis* was inadvertently given to healthy children instead of

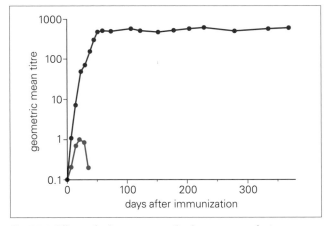

**Fig. 35.6** Effects of adjuvants on antibody responses of mice to egg albumin. Mice were injected subcutaneously with egg albumin in saline or in Freund's incomplete adjuvant. Antibody titres at intervals over time are shown. The blue symbols represent antigen in saline, and the red symbols represent antigen in adjuvant. (Modified from Hunter R. Overview of vaccine adjuvants: present and future. *Vaccine*. 2002;20:S7–S12.)

BCG, leading to the Lubeck disaster; in 1942 US military personnel were vaccinated with yellow fever virus contaminated with hepatitis B virus (HBV). Safety testing is now rigorous, requiring extensive quality controls and animal testing prior to trials or use in humans. Live vaccines will often induce better protection than recombinant or subunit vaccines, but there are an increasing number of people who may be receiving immunosuppressive treatments in whom live vaccines may pose a problem. Some of the more important issues are

## Box 35.2    Examples of Adjuvants in Currently Used Vaccines

Aluminium salts[a]    DTaP, DTaP/IPV/Hib, acellular pertussis, Hib,[b] HepA, HepB, 9vHPV, MenB-4C, PCV13, T-d, Japanese encephalitis

Monophosphoryl lipid A (MPL) (3-O-desacyl-4'-monophosphoryl lipid A)    HPV (Cervarix)

Synthetic oligodeoxynucleotide CpG 1018    HEPLISAV-B (HepB)

AS01 and DOPC[e]    RSV, RTS,S and RZV (ASO1 only)

[a]Aluminium hydroxide/aluminium hydroxysulphate/aluminium phosphate/aluminium potassium sulphate.
[b]Some formulations.
ASO1, Adjuvant system 1 (3-O-desacyl-4'-monophosphoryl lipid A (MPL) and the saponin QS-21; CpG, cytosine and phosphate separated by a phosphate group; DOPC, 1,2-Dioleoyl-sn-glycero-3-phosphocholine; DTaP, diphtheria-tetanus-acellular pertussis; HepA/B, hepatitis A/B; Hib, *Haemophilus influenzae* type b; HPV, human papillomavirus; IPV, inactivated poliovirus vaccine; MenB, meningococcal B vaccine; PCV13, 13-valent pneumococcal conjugate vaccine; RSV, respiratory syncytial virus; RTS,S, Repeat ('R') and T-cell epitope ('T') of the *Plasmodium falciparum* pre-erythrocytic circumsporozoite protein (CSP) together with the hepatitis B virus surface antigen ('S'); RZV, recombinant zoster vaccine, T-d, tetanus-diphtheria.

**Table 35.4** Vaccines may also contain traces of components other than antigens and adjuvant

| Component | Vaccine examples | Comment |
|---|---|---|
| Egg proteins | Influenza, yellow fever | If virus is grown in eggs |
| Yeast proteins | HepA, HepB, 9vHPV | If grown by fermentation of *Saccharomyces cerevisiae* |
| Antibiotics | MMR, MenB-4C, VAR | Such as polymyxin B, neomycin, streptomycin, kanamycin |
| Latex rubber | Diphtheria toxin-containing vaccines, HepA, MenB-4C, RV1 | RV1: oral applicator |
| Gelatin | MMR, VAR | Stabilizes virus; pork derived |

Some vaccines can contain traces of the tissue culture media used to grow the organism or the cell line in which it is grown. Although the concentrations of these compounds may be very low, they could induce allergic responses in some individuals.
HepA, Hepatitis A; HepB, hepatitis B; 9vHPV, 9-valent human papillomavirus; MenB-4C, meningitis B-4 component (proteins); MMR, measles, mumps, rubella; PPSV23, pneumococcal polysaccharide vaccine 23; RV1, rotavirus 1; VAR, varicella.

## Box 35.3    Problems with Vaccine Safety

Both living and nonliving vaccines require rigorous quality and safety control, especially as they are given to healthy individuals. Some of the more important areas of concern are listed.

### Live attenuated vaccines
- Insufficient attenuation
- Reversion to wild type
- Administration to immunodeficient patients
- Persistent infection
- Contamination by other viruses
- Risk of fetal damage

### Nonliving vaccines
- Contamination by toxins or chemicals
- Allergic reactions

### Genetically engineered vaccines
- Possible inclusion of oncogenes

## Box 35.4    Monitoring for Adverse Events

**Local adverse events** (i.e. pain, swelling, redness at injection site)
**Systemic adverse events** (i.e. fever, headache, fatigue [mild/moderate], coagulation disorders or cardiac events, anaphylaxis [severe])

Before licensing a new vaccine, possible adverse events are monitored in safety trials. Following licensure, adverse events are also collected to identify any rare events that might not have occurred in the smaller safety trials. Examples of adverse events as used in trials of severe acute respiratory syndrome coronavirus 2 (SARS-CoV-2) vaccines are given. Both local and systemic adverse events were usually classified as mild or moderate. For new vaccine platforms such as messenger RNA (mRNA) vaccines, adverse events of special interest can be identified related to the specific vaccine platform or the pathogenesis of the disease itself.

and egg proteins may also be present, causing allergic problems for some people (Table 35.4). All vaccines go through rigorous testing for safety before being licensed, and they are monitored for any adverse effects (Box 35.4). It is important to identify whether the adverse event is likely to be causally related to vaccination (e.g. a headache or fever shortly after vaccination) or unrelated (e.g. perhaps death in a road traffic accident). Some adverse events will be very rare and may only be identified once the vaccine is given to large numbers of individuals. Initial clinical trials will involve relatively small numbers of individuals, and rare adverse events such as the myopericarditis and thromboembolism seen with

summarized in Box 35.3. It is vital that vaccines derived from live organisms are completely inactivated to ensure they are safe and that vaccines are preserved appropriately to ensure that vaccine immunogenicity is retained. Examples of fixatives and preservatives used in current vaccines are given in Table 35.3, and some other components such as antibiotics

COVID-19 vaccines were not observed until millions of people were vaccinated.

## NONSPECIFIC BENEFICIAL EFFECTS OF VACCINES

Vaccines can sometimes induce nonspecific effects that are beneficial. Although the prime objective of vaccination is to induce antigen-specific immunity and memory, vaccines can also induce nonspecific protection against irrelevant infections (e.g. BCG vaccination given at birth to protect against TB [see later] can also provide protection against other infections in the neonatal period). This phenomenon is called *innate training* and is associated with epigenetic changes in macrophages and natural killer cells.

## VACCINES IN CURRENT USE

Additional detail to that provided here is available in the Vaccine Parade (*see* eBook).

### Diphtheria, tetanus and pertussis vaccines

The diphtheria vaccine consists of the inactivated toxoid. Toxigenic *Corynebacterium diphtheriae* is grown in liquid culture, and the filtrate is inactivated with formaldehyde to produce the toxoid, with aluminum as the adjuvant. This is a highly effective vaccine, giving >90% protection. Three or four doses are required to give good protection, with a booster every 10 years. It is now given in different formulations in combination with other vaccines.

The inactivated tetanospasmin exotoxin from *Clostridium tetani*, inactivated using formaldehyde, is used to vaccinate against tetanus. Tetanus toxoid was first produced in 1924. Again, this is a very effective vaccine, but boosters are required every 10 years. An initiative to eliminate maternal and neonatal tetanus by vaccinating mothers aims to reduce neonatal tetanus to a level where it is no longer a public health problem. Neonatal tetanus deaths fell from 787,000 in 1988 to 25,000 in 2018; the World Health Organization (WHO) reported that by 2020 only 12 countries had not eliminated neonatal tetanus (<1/1000 live births/district/year).

The first vaccine developed against pertussis was a whole cell vaccine, which was available from the mid-1940s and introduced in the United Kingdom in 1957 (Fig. 35.7). However, although four doses of vaccine induced 70–90% protection against serious whooping cough, concerns over the safety of the vaccine in the United Kingdom and elsewhere in the 1970s led to resurgence of disease and to the development of a safer acellular pertussis vaccine with fewer side effects. Current vaccines contain purified filamentous haemagglutinin, which plays a role in colonization, and pertactin as well as pertussis toxin, with some formulations also including fimbriae types 2 and 4, without preservative. However, cases of pertussis have been increasing since the switch to the acellular vaccine, particularly in infants, so this is an example in which a safer vaccine may not induce as strong immunity.

Global coverage of the combined diphtheria-tetanus-pertussis (DTP) or diphtheria-tetanus–acellular pertussis (DTaP) vaccine is now good, with WHO estimating that 81% of infants worldwide (105 million infants) received three doses of DTP (DTP3) vaccine in 2021. Another formulation for use in adolescents and adults (Tdap) contains tetanus toxoid, with three to five pertussis antigens but less diphtheria toxoid than the paediatric DTaP vaccine.

### Measles, mumps and rubella vaccines

Live attenuated measles vaccine was introduced in the United States in 1963 using the Edmonston B vaccine, which has since been replaced by the more attenuated Edmonston–Enders strain and Schwarz strains, grown in chick embryo fibroblast cells. Children should be given two doses of vaccine, as the first dose fails to induce protective antibodies in 5% of those vaccinated. Vaccination is safe and effective, given either on its own or as part of the measles, mumps and rubella (MMR) vaccine with mumps and rubella or as part of the measles, mumps, rubella and varicella (MMRV) vaccine containing measles, mumps, rubella and varicella. However, maternal antibodies inhibit the induction of immunity, so the first dose is generally given at 12–15 months of age, once maternal-derived antibodies have declined, and the second dose is given at 4–6 years of age. In lower-income countries where the risk of contracting measles is higher, the vaccine may be given earlier, at ~9 months or even at 6 and 12 months to protect children whose levels of maternal antibodies are declining or whose mothers were never exposed to the virus.

Vaccine-induced immunity to measles is long lived, and after two doses, probably lifelong; although reinfections can occur, these are likely to be less symptomatic. Between 2000 and 2015 there was an estimated 79% drop in measles deaths worldwide, with an estimated 20 million deaths from measles prevented by vaccination. The WHO estimated that, at the end of 2021, 81% of children had received one dose of measles-containing vaccine by

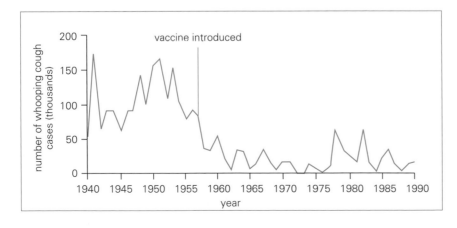

**Fig. 35.7** The number of cases of whooping cough notified fell steadily after the introduction of mass immunization in the United Kingdom in 1958, although epidemics continued to occur at ~4-year intervals. Following the scare about the possible adverse effects of pertussis vaccine, the number of cases rose, and there was a large epidemic in the winter of 1978–1979.

their second birthday and 71% of children had received two doses of measles vaccine. As shown in Fig. 35.3, however, cases of measles increased in the United Kingdom after 2001. The suggestion that the MMR vaccine caused autism, as there was an apparent rise in autism in both California and the United Kingdom that seemed to coincide with the introduction of the vaccine, led to reduced vaccine uptake. However, further studies have failed to show an increased risk of autism after MMR. It is no wonder that parents get worried when bombarded with such scare stories, but they forget that measles infection can kill healthy children. In a measles outbreak in Ireland in 2000, nearly 1500 cases were notified and three children died.

## Mumps vaccine

The current mumps vaccine uses a live attenuated virus (RIT4385 or level B strains) derived from the Jeryl Lynn strain licensed in 1967. Over 97% of those vaccinated make antibodies after a single dose of vaccine, and a study in the United Kingdom showed that 88% of those receiving two doses were protected. The importance of receiving two doses of MMR was illustrated by a mumps outbreak in Northern Ireland where 55.4% of the confirmed cases had received one dose of vaccine, compared with 0.9% of those who had received two doses. After two doses, protection should last >25 years and may be lifelong; as for measles, reinfection can occur but is less likely to be symptomatic. This vaccine is much more effective than an earlier inactivated vaccine, showing how live attenuated viruses induce good immunity.

## Rubella vaccine

The current rubella vaccine is a live attenuated virus (Wistar RA strain 27/3) licensed in 1979. The virus was attenuated by 25–30 cell culture passages in human diploid fibroblasts. A single dose of MMR vaccine is estimated to give 97% protection against rubella. Although rubella itself is a relatively mild infection, it causes real problems if pregnant woman become infected in the first trimester of pregnancy, when congenital rubella syndrome can cause serious damage to the fetus. Thankfully there has been a dramatic reduction in confirmed cases of congenital rubella syndrome due to rubella vaccination: cases fell by 98% in the Americas between 1998 and 2009.

## Polio vaccine

The first polio vaccine licensed in 1955 developed by Salk was a killed vaccine (inactivated polio vaccine [IPV]), which was very effective at reducing the risk of contracting polio. The oral polio vaccine (OPV) developed by Sabin was licensed in 1961. Giving the vaccine on sugar lumps or directly into the mouth was much easier than giving it by injection, and the live vaccine also gives better intestinal immunity. However, the live polio virus used in OPV is not genetically stable and can cause vaccine-associated paralytic polio (VAPP) in approximately one person per million doses administered (Table 35.5). In addition, it has long been recognized that OPV is transmissible from vaccinees to their close contacts, and it can (on rare occasions) persist in the community as circulating vaccine–derived polio viruses (cVDPV) and reacquire virulence. The global polio eradication initiative that began in 1988 emphasized the use of OPV,

**Table 35.5** Inactivated and live attenuated polio vaccines compared

|  | **Inactivated (IPV)** | **Attenuated live (OPV)** |
|---|---|---|
| Virus type | Trivalent types 1–3 | Bivalent types 1 and 3[a] |
| Introduced | Salk 1954 | Sabin 1957 |
| Route | Injection | Oral |
| Adjuvant | Alum | None |
| Advantages | Can be given with other childhood vaccines | Boosts IgA immunity Better immunity in the intestine |
| Disadvantages | More expensive Requires trained staff to vaccinate | Reversion to virulence[b] |

[a]Bivalent oral polio vaccine (OPV) (types 1 and 3) used for routine immunization since April 2016.
[b]Although vaccine-associated paralytic polio only occurs in <1 per million vaccinated, vaccine-derived polio viruses can circulate within the community. IgA, Immunoglobulin A.

but after 2000, most wealthy countries shifted back to IPV to avoid the risk of VAPP. The Global Polio Eradication Initiative has been remarkably successful in reducing the number of polio cases worldwide by >99%, and only one of the three original strains of wild poliovirus (WPV1) is still in circulation (Fig. 35.8). As part of the endgame strategy of the eradication programme, countries are switching to IPV to avoid circulation of VDPV, and trivalent OPV has been replaced by bivalent (1–3) OPV. In 2022–2023, polio was only endemic in two countries, Afghanistan and Pakistan, but there can be outbreaks of cVDPV of all three poliovirus strains (e.g. in London PV2 was detected in sewage in 2022, and wild-type polio that may have derived from Pakistan has spread in Malawi without becoming endemic).

## Pneumococcal vaccines

The challenge in making an effective vaccine against pneumococcal disease is that there are 90 serotypes of *Streptococcus pneumoniae*; luckily, however, a few serotypes cause most infections. The first vaccine was a pneumococcal conjugate vaccine (PCV) with capsular polysaccharide from 14 serotypes. This was replaced in 1983 with a formulation containing 23 capsular polysaccharides from 23 serotypes (PCV23). However, although this vaccine induced antibodies in >80% of adults and is still used in older people, it was not immunogenic in children aged <2 years, who are at highest risk of pneumococcal disease. Conjugate vaccines with 10, 13 or 15 serotypes are now used in children: PCV in which capsular polysaccharides are conjugated to a recombinant non-toxic form of the diphtheria toxin is highly immunogenic in infants and young children and includes the serotypes causing 60% of disease in children <5 years of age. Luckily most of the serotypes causing severe disease are covered by the conjugate vaccines, but their use has resulted in increases in serotypes not included in these vaccines. Further PCV vaccines with additional serotypes are therefore in development. Vaccines are also recommended for adults and older people (e.g. PPV23 only containing polysaccharides from 23 serotypes or PCV conjugates with 15 or 20 serotypes). A further PCV21 adult formulation would include mainly serotypes not present in PCV13.

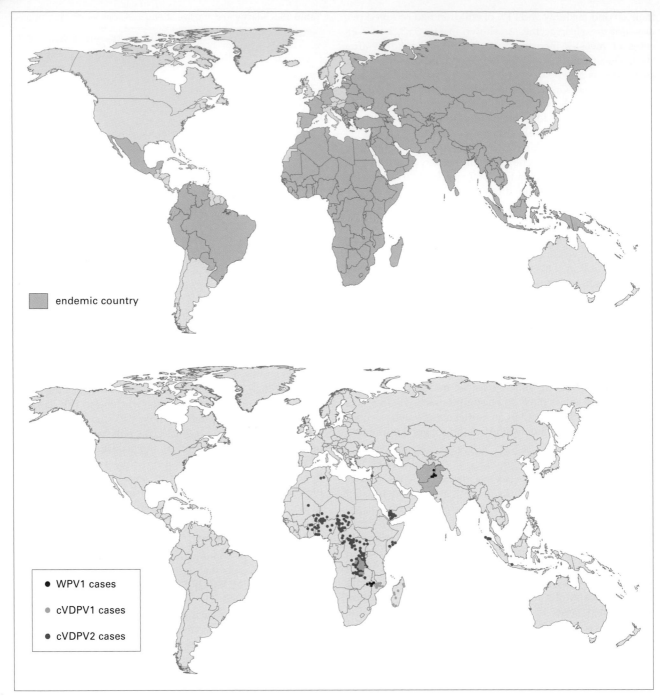

endemic country

WPV1 cases

cVDPV1 cases

cVDPV2 cases

**Fig. 35.8** Progress toward polio eradication. Progress achieved through vaccination is shown by the dramatic decrease in countries endemic for wild poliovirus (*green*) from 1988 (*top map*) to 2022/2023 (*lower map*), where only Afghanistan and Pakistan are still endemic, even though cases of wild poliovirus (*WPV1*) were also detected in Mozambique (*red*). Cases of circulating vaccine–derived poliovirus 1 (*cVDPV*) are shown in yellow and of circulating vaccine–derived poliovirus 2 in *purple*. (Modified from World Health Organization. *Immunization Monitoring*. WHO; 2023; and WHO: *Polio and Global Polio Eradication Initiative*. Geneva: WHO; 2023.)

### Meningococcal vaccines

There are 12 *Neisseria meningitidis* serogroups, 6 of which are responsible for almost all the invasive meningococcal disease: A, B, C, W, X, Y. The first vaccine against meningococcal disease caused by *N. meningitidis* contained polysaccharide alone—first from serogroup C, then a quadrivalent vaccine containing purified capsular polysaccharides for four serotypes: A, C, Y, W-135. Similar to the pneumococcal polysaccharide vaccine, the meningococcal polysaccharide vaccine was not immunogenic in young children, as for other T-independent antigens. Conjugate vaccines containing capsular polysaccharides from the same four serotypes (A, C, W, Y) conjugated to *C. diphtheriae* toxoid (CRM$_{197}$ protein, tetanus toxoid) are now available and induce four times more antibody than the polysaccharide vaccine with better immunologic memory. A new MenACWYX conjugate vaccine is being produced for use in children. The *Neisseria* serotype B strain was not included in these conjugate vaccines,

**Fig. 35.9** Vaccination with a *Haemophilus influenzae* type b (Hib) polysaccharide–tetanus toxoid conjugate vaccine produced a dramatic decrease in the incidence of Hib meningitis in children aged >1 year in Gambia. Dotted lines represent pointwise 90% likelihood-based confidence limits. (From Adegbola R, Secka O, Lahai G, et al. Elimination of *Haemophilus influenzae* type b [Hib] disease from the Gambia after the introduction of routine immunization with a Hib conjugate vaccine: a prospective study. *Lancet*. 2005;366:144–150.)

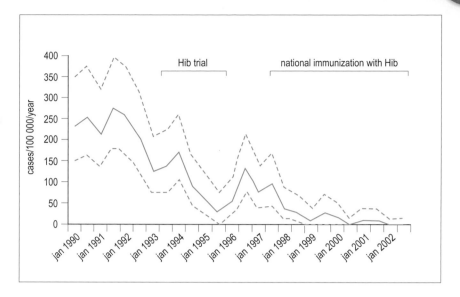

as the B-group polysaccharide is poorly immunogenic and may have some cross-reactivity to the human nervous system; but protein-based vaccines for the B strain are available either containing four components (MenB-4C) with the *Neisseria* heparin-binding antigen, *Neisseria* adhesion A, factor H binding protein (fHbp) or as *N. meningitidis* group B outer membrane vesicles, which is immunogenic in infants and children. For children >10 years of age a bivalent MenB-fHbp is available, combining recombinant fHbp from MenB subfamilies A and B, which may protect against other serogroups as well.

### *Haemophilus influenzae* type b

*H. influenzae* mainly affects children <5 years of age. Although there are six capsular serotypes, one (type b composed of a phosphodiester-linked polymer of ribose and ribitol) causes 95% of disease and so has been the basis of Hib vaccines. The introduction of *H. influenzae* type b (Hib) vaccines has dramatically reduced the incidence of Hib bacterial meningitis (Fig. 35.9). The first polysaccharide vaccine introduced in the United States in 1985 was not immunogenic in children <18 months of age, inducing mostly low-affinity immunoglobulin M (IgM) antibodies similar to other antigens inducing T-cell–independent immune responses. Conjugating the polysaccharide to a T-cell–dependent antigen such as tetanus toxoid or the meningococcal group B outer membrane protein complex overcame this problem. Even so, three or four doses are needed to induce good immunity, as this is another example of how a subunit vaccine is less immunogenic than a live vaccine.

### Influenza

Flu generated great alarm in 2009 when the first flu pandemic since 1968 was caused by a new influenza A (H1N1) virus. The threat from this new virus and from avian influenza (H5N1) highlighted the limited world capacity to produce new flu vaccines quickly in the quantities needed. Three types of vaccine are currently available: trivalent or quadrivalent inactivated vaccines that can be given to anyone aged >6 months by intramuscular or intradermal injection, a live attenuated influenza vaccine given by intranasal spray

to those aged 2–49 years who are healthy and not pregnant that replicates in the mucosa of the nasopharynx and a vaccine with recombinant haemagglutinin.

Flu is a tricky customer, as it changes its haemagglutinin and neuraminidase antigens owing to both point mutations and recombination events, resulting in antigenic drift (Fig. 35.10) and antigenic shift (see Fig. 17.10). Current quadrivalent flu vaccines contain two influenza A subtypes and two influenza B subtypes, with different formulations for the Northern and Southern Hemispheres each year. Links to the recommended compositions of current flu vaccines in the United States (from the Centers for Disease Control and Prevention [CDC]) and globally (from WHO) are referenced in Vaccine Parade (*see* eBook). Flu vaccines can be made as inactivated viruses, as live attenuated viruses delivered intranasally or as recombinant proteins.

Flu vaccination policy varies in different countries. For example, in the United States the inactivated vaccine is offered yearly to everyone aged >6 months, including to pregnant women; children aged 6 months to 6 years being vaccinated for the first time are now given two doses of vaccine. About 80% of the world's flu vaccines are still produced in eggs, although cell-based and recombinant vaccines are also available. In the United Kingdom a live attenuated virus vaccine given intranasally is used for those aged 2–49 years. Cleverly, the live attenuated viruses have been cold adapted so that they only replicate in the nose. For those aged >65 years the inactivated quadrivalent vaccine is given with an adjuvant, or at a higher dose, to improve the immune response generated. Older people may also be protected by herd immunity if more children are vaccinated.

A 2023 report was published about the exciting development of a nucleoside-modified mRNA lipid nanoparticle vaccine encoding haemagglutinin antigens from all 20 known influenza A virus subtypes and B virus lineages. The vaccine response was excellent, and high levels of both cross- and subtype-specific antibodies were detected in mice and ferrets. The response was shown to be effective as the animals were protected when subsequently exposed to a variety of influenza viruses. Such a vaccine would be a real game-changer.

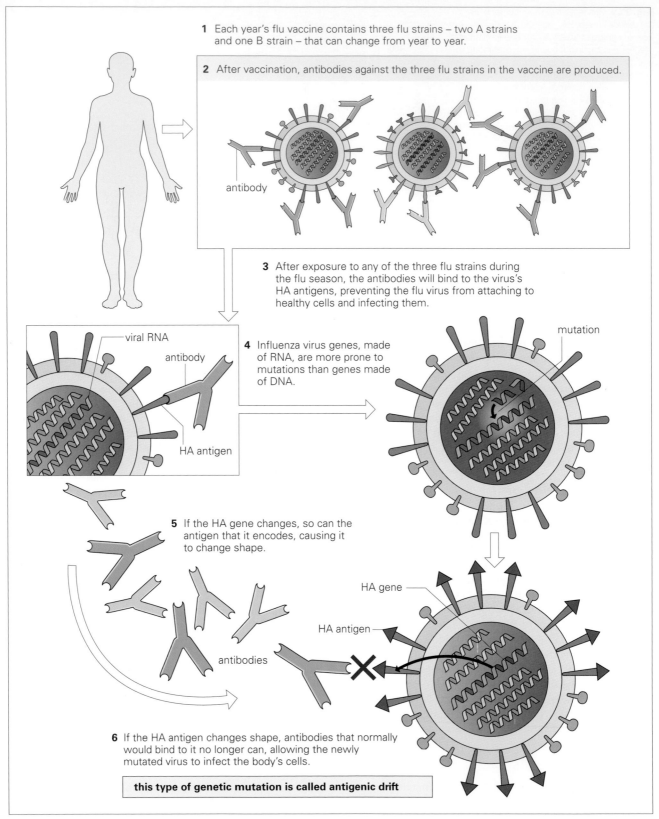

**1** Each year's flu vaccine contains three flu strains – two A strains and one B strain – that can change from year to year.

**2** After vaccination, antibodies against the three flu strains in the vaccine are produced.

antibody

**3** After exposure to any of the three flu strains during the flu season, the antibodies will bind to the virus's HA antigens, preventing the flu virus from attaching to healthy cells and infecting them.

viral RNA

antibody

HA antigen

**4** Influenza virus genes, made of RNA, are more prone to mutations than genes made of DNA.

mutation

**5** If the HA gene changes, so can the antigen that it encodes, causing it to change shape.

antibodies

HA gene

HA antigen

**6** If the HA antigen changes shape, antibodies that normally would bind to it no longer can, allowing the newly mutated virus to infect the body's cells.

**this type of genetic mutation is called antigenic drift**

**Fig. 35.10** Influenza vaccines and antigenic drift. Seasonal influenza vaccines contain three flu strains: two A strains and one B strain. Antibodies to these strains induced by vaccination will protect against infection, but mutations in the influenza genes can cause antigenic drift leading to infection. *HA*, Haemagglutinin. (Modified from National Institute of Allergy and Infectious Diseases. *Flu [influenza]: antigenic drift*. US Department of Health and Human Services; 2011.)

## Box 35.5 ◼ The Race to Deliver the First COVID-19 Vaccine

By April 2020 it was reported that >90 vaccines against severe acute respiratory syndrome coronavirus 2 (SARS-CoV-2) were being developed around the world. Different vaccine types, including a novel messenger RNA (mRNA) vaccine that had been developed as a cancer treatment, were being investigated by research teams in pharmaceutical companies and universities across the world.

Sinovac Biotech in Beijing had started to test an inactivated version of SARS-CoV-2 in humans in July 2020. The vaccines that received most publicity were the Moderna mRNA-1273 and Pfizer/BioNTech BNT162b2 mRNA vaccines, which needed to be refrigerated and frozen (−70°C) before being given. They were in phase 3 clinical trials by July 2020. The Oxford University and AstraZeneca collaboration fridge-stable replication-deficient chimpanzee adenoviral vector ChAdOx1 nCoV-19 vaccine clinical trial results were being reported around the same time. The Janssen/Johnson & Johnson Ad26 recombinant viral vector vaccine had also started trials in July 2020.

On 8 December 2020, a 90-year-old grandmother, Margaret Keenan, became the first person in the world to receive the Pfizer COVID-19 vaccine after it was clinically approved in the United Kingdom. She was immunized at 6.31 am by nurse May Parsons at her local hospital in Coventry, England, a week before her 91st birthday.

It was reported that she said, "I feel so privileged to be the first person vaccinated against COVID-19; it's the best early birthday present I could wish for because it means I can finally look forward to spending time with my family and friends in the New Year after being on my own for most of the year. I can't thank May and the National Health Service (NHS) staff enough who have looked after me tremendously, and my advice to anyone offered the vaccine is to take it—if I can have it at 90 then you can have it, too!"

NHS England Chief Executive Sir Simon Stevens said, "Less than a year after the first case of this new disease was diagnosed, the NHS has now delivered the first clinically approved COVID-19 vaccination—that is a remarkable achievement. A heartfelt thank-you goes to everyone who has made this a reality—the scientists and doctors who worked tirelessly and the volunteers who selflessly took part in the trials. They have achieved in months what normally takes years. Today is just the first step in the largest vaccination programme this country (the UK) has ever seen. It will take some months to complete the work as more vaccine supplies become available, and until then we must not drop our guard. But if we all stay vigilant in the weeks and months ahead, we will be able to look back at this as a decisive turning point in the battle against the virus."

### COVID-19 vaccines

Vaccine development and licensing normally take a decade or longer, with a high risk of failure. Luckily, by using platform technologies developed for cancer, Middle East respiratory syndrome (MERS) and SARS or for TB and malaria, it was possible to develop new vaccines for SARS-CoV-2 within 1 year of the SARS-CoV-2 sequence becoming

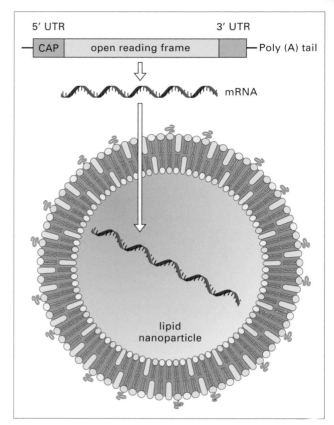

**Fig. 35.11** Use of messenger RNA (mRNA) as a strategy to make vaccines against severe acute respiratory syndrome coronavirus 2 (SARS-CoV-2). The gene of interest, in this case for the SARS-CoV-2 spike protein, is inserted into lipid nanoparticles. Once injected, the mRNA is translated by host cells so that the spike protein is produced. The gene sequence is usually codon optimized.

available (Box 35.5). This accelerated development showed what can be achieved when there is a pandemic and plenty of funding. Because of the urgency, the new vaccines were given emergency or provisional approval, and their use then provided sufficient data for full approval. It has been estimated that ~20 million lives were saved in 2020–2021 by the introduction of new COVID-19 vaccines.

Some of the COVID-19 vaccines used a new mRNA technology (Fig. 35.11). This delivers mRNA into the cell cytosol where it is translated into protein. Such mRNA vaccines may have amino acid substitutions in the protein antigen, in this case the SARS-CoV-2 spike protein, to make them more immunogenic, and they can be codon optimized for mRNA stability and translation efficiency. The mRNA is delivered in lipid nanoparticles; two doses induce ~95% protection against moderate disease or infection. Other COVID-19 vaccines have included viral-vectored vaccines using recombinant human or chimp adenoviruses, the spike protein in adjuvant or inactivated SARS-CoV-2 virus. For SARS-CoV-2 vaccines, the spike protein was an obvious target as antispike antibodies block viral invasion. Luckily the new vaccines induced good virus neutralizing antibody titres as well as some T-cell immunity. Giving a second vaccination markedly boosted the antibody response (Fig. 35.12). Overall, COVID vaccines have proved to give very good protection against severe disease and death. Although the vaccine efficacy against infection was lower, vaccination also

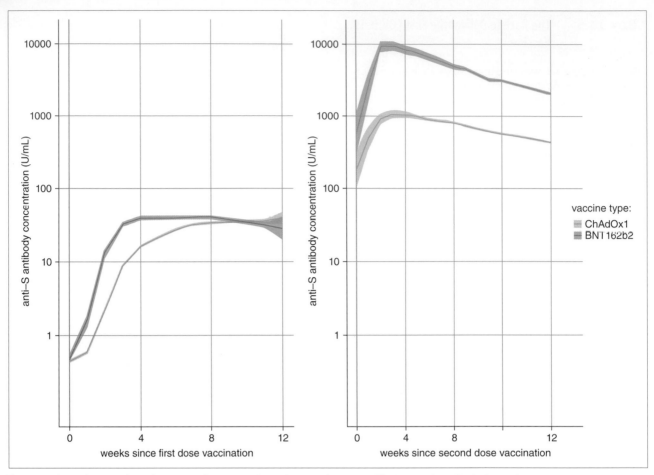

**Fig. 35.12** More than one dose of vaccine is often required to induce good immunity. The increase in antibody titre to the severe acute respiratory syndrome coronavirus 2 (SARS-CoV-2) spike protein in individuals given one or two doses of COVID-19 vaccine is shown. A, Responses after one dose of ChAdOx1 in which the SARS-CoV-2 spike protein was delivered by adenovirus or of BNT162b2 that uses messenger RNA (mRNA) encoding the spike protein. B, Marked improvement in antibody titres after a second dose of the same vaccine. Geometric means and 95% confidence intervals for titres of anti-spike antibodies in units per millilter are shown. Pink indicates those given BNT162b2, and blue indicates those given ChAdOx1. (Modified from Shrotri M, Fragaszy E, Nguyen V, et al. Spike-antibody responses to COVID-19 vaccination by demographic and clinical factors in a prospective community cohort study. *Nat Commun.* 2022;13:5780.)

reduced transmission; however, immunity waned quite rapidly so that at least two further doses were needed, and more were needed in older or more vulnerable people.

### BCG and new vaccines for TB

The oldest vaccine still in use is the BCG vaccine, attenuated following extensive culture of *Mycobacterium bovis* on potato bile medium by Calmette and Guérin. BCG was first used as a vaccine in 1921. Attenuation involved the loss of the RD1 region that encodes the ESAT-6 and CFP-10 antigens used in the currently available commercial diagnostic tests for *M. tuberculosis* infection, the QuantiFERON test (Ch. 20) and the TSPOT-TB ELISPOT assay (Ch. 32).

BCG is usually given to babies shortly after birth and is given to >100 million children annually. Because of concerns that a disseminated BCGosis might occur, the vaccine is not recommended for babies with known HIV infection; in some countries, vaccination is delayed until screening for severe combined immunodeficiency disease is performed.

It provides good (and very cost-effective) prevention of the disseminated forms of childhood TB but variable protection against pulmonary TB in adults (e.g. it induced good protection [>80%] in trials in UK adolescents but no protection in South India or Malawi). The reasons for this may include exposure to environmental mycobacteria that can induce a masking or a blocking effect on the immunity induced by BCG. When BCG is protective, this is associated with induction of a Th1 immune response, although simply measuring IFN-γ induced in response to mycobacterial antigens does not provide a correlate of protection. When induced, protective immunity lasts 10–15 years, and in one study it lasted >50 years. In settings in which BCG is protective, it may protect against infection and disease. A recent trial showed that revaccination with BCG protected against sustained conversion to IFN-γ release assay (IGRA) positivity in South African adolescents; this IGRA test detects an IFN-γ response to *M. tuberculosis* peptides and is positive in those with TB infection.

Because of the variable protection that BCG vaccination gives against TB in adults, the search is on for a new TB vaccine. Candidate vaccines in development include genetically modified BCGs, attenuated *M. tuberculosis*, viral vectors expressing key antigens of *M. tuberculosis* and fusion proteins in adjuvant. An MVA expressing Ag85A, given as

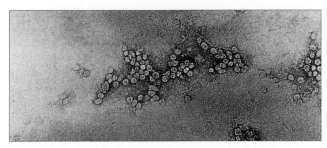

**Fig. 35.13** Electron micrograph of purified 22-nm hepatitis B surface antigens expressed in yeast cells. (Courtesy J.R. Pattison.)

a boosting vaccine following BCG, was the first new vaccine to be tested in children and adults in Africa but was not shown to induce significant protection; new studies are investigating whether giving the vaccine by aerosol might be better. The M72 vaccine containing the Mtb32A and Mtb39A antigens in AS01$_E$ adjuvant induced 54% protection against progression from latent TB infection to TB disease in African adults, and the hunt is on for correlates of protection. Other promising vaccine candidates include a genetically modified BCG that expresses haemolysin (VPM1002), which might enhance activation of CD8 T cells through escape of antigens into the cytoplasm of the infected macrophage, fusion proteins containing various *M. tuberculosis* antigens in adjuvant and an attenuated *M. tuberculosis* vaccine (MTBVAC). Therapeutic vaccines for those with drug-resistant TB are also being developed.

### Vaccines against hepatitis

The first vaccine for HBV consisted of the surface coat antigen of HBV purified from the plasma of virus carriers. This vaccine was protective but required very careful purification and inactivation to ensure it was safe, and it was expensive to produce. The first recombinant hepatitis B surface antigen (HbsAg) vaccine was licensed in the United States in 1986, the first vaccine produced using genetic engineering (Fig. 35.13). Recombinant HBV vaccines produced in yeast containing aluminium salts or synthetic adjuvants have an efficacy of 80–100% against infection or clinical hepatitis B, with immunity lasting >20 years after three vaccine doses.

Inactivated whole cell vaccines are available for hepatitis A. The virus is grown in human cells, purified, inactivated with formaldehyde and adsorbed onto aluminium salts. Again, these vaccines induce excellent immunity when given intramuscularly. Combined vaccines for hepatitis A and B are also available, but, as yet, there is no vaccine available for hepatitis C.

### Human papillomavirus

New HPV vaccines have been introduced in the last decade due to the association between HPV infection and cervical cancer. The first quadrivalent vaccine (Guardasil), which induces immunity against four types of HPV, was licensed in 2006. This contained the L1 capsid protein of HPV from two oncogenic types of virus (HPV16 and HPV18) as well as two non-oncogenic types (HPV6 and HPV11). It was made by recombinant DNA technology and formed viruslike particles. It induced antibody responses in >99.5% of vaccinees. A 9-valent recombinant protein vaccine is now available (with L1 capsid protein from strains 6, 11, 16, 18, 31, 33, 45, 52, 58) and is given to both females and males, as it protects against cervical cancers, some anal/genital cancers and head/neck cancers and genital warts (HPV6 and HPV11 cause ~90% of genital warts).

### Rotavirus vaccine

Rotavirus causes the most serious gastrointestinal disease in infants. The first vaccine was withdrawn when it caused intussusception, a rare cause of bowel obstruction. Two new live oral vaccines are now in use: the RV5 vaccine (RotaTeq) contains five reassortant rotaviruses developed from human and bovine parent strains, and the RV1 vaccine (Rotarix) contains one live attenuated rotavirus strain. These vaccines give 74–87% efficacy against any rotavirus gastroenteritis and 85–98% protection against severe gastroenteritis. Studies from some countries demonstrated marked reductions in hospitalizations and in general practitioner visits for all-cause acute gastroenteritis in children after rotavirus vaccination was introduced.

### Typhoid

Three vaccines are available for typhoid. The live oral vaccine contains a live attenuated mutant strain of *Salmonella typhi*, Ty21a in coated capsules. A second uses the Vi capsular polysaccharide vaccine that is injected intramuscularly but is not immunogenic in young children. These vaccines show a difference in immunogenicity: The oral vaccine needs three to four doses compared with a single injection of the polysaccharide; however, the oral vaccine may be inducing immunity in the right place. To overcome the inability of young children to make good antibody responses to polysaccharide, conjugate vaccines with the Vi polysaccharide conjugated to tetanus toxoid are now also available. An earlier whole *S. typhi* killed cell vaccine was protective but also very reactinogenic, so it is no longer used.

### Varicella

A live attenuated viral vaccine is available against varicella (chickenpox in children). The virus isolated from the vesicular fluid of a child with varicella was attenuated by culturing in three different types of cell lines. The current live attenuated vaccines derived from the Oka strain of the varicella-zoster virus are grown in human diploid cells and can be given to children aged >12 months. Two doses give children 98% protection.

Older individuals are susceptible to developing shingles or postherpetic neuralgia, and a vaccine containing a much higher dose of live attenuated varicella-zoster virus (19,400 plaque-forming units ['s] compared with ≤9772 PFU in the infant vaccines) was initially used for those aged >70 years in the United Kingdom. This was not fully effective but did reduce the risk of shingles by ~50%. A two-dose vaccine with the varicella-zoster glycoprotein E in ASO1$_E$ adjuvant vaccine is now available, which is much more protective and can also be used in those with immunosuppression.

### Respiratory syncytial virus

A new vaccine for RSV to be given to older adults (>60 years) is now approved, containing recombinant glycoprotein F that has been stabilized in the prefusion conformation (RSVPreF3) with ASO1$_E$ adjuvant. Another RSV vaccine containing a bivalent prefusion F protein from subgroups A and B has shown promise when given to pregnant women. The vaccine-induced immunity in the mother then passes to her baby and protects against severe RSV infection in the first 6 months of life (about as long as giving passive immunity with the anti-RSV monoclonal antibody nirsevimab). This would not be the first vaccine to be given to pregnant women to protect their babies, as vaccinating pregnant women against tetanus prevents neonatal tetanus, and currently in the United States pregnant women are also offered vaccination against pertussis and influenza. Other RSV vaccines are in the pipeline, including for older adults.

### Vaccines required for entry into particular countries or regions

The yellow fever vaccine is required for entry into certain countries. A vaccination certificate may be required for all those entering a particular country or for individuals coming from a country where yellow fever is endemic. Luckily this is a very immunogenic vaccine, and a vaccination certificate is now valid for the life of the person vaccinated. Vaccination against meningitis ACWY is compulsory for pilgrims visiting Mecca in Saudi Arabia for the Umrah and Haj pilgrimages, as there was an *N. meningitidis* W-135 outbreak in pilgrims in 2000.

Travellers spending longer periods in areas of rural Asia, where Japanese encephalitis (JE; a mosquito-transmitted flavivirus) is common, can be vaccinated with an inactivated JE virus vaccine. A live attenuated (recombinant) tetravalent dengue vaccine is now licensed in some countries, having shown 79% protection against severe dengue in two phase 3 trials; this contains yellow fever viruses expressing surface membrane and pre-envelope proteins for the four dengue serotypes, with further vaccine candidates in development. However, it is important that the vaccine does not predispose the vaccinees to developing the severe forms of dengue haemorrhagic fever that can occur when someone is reinfected with dengue (see Ch. 18), and so in the United States it is only given to children or adolescents who are seropositive for dengue. Finally, inactivated viral vaccines for tickborne encephalitis have been developed and are available in some countries.

### Vaccines for subgroups at high risk

Rabies vaccination is available for those exposed to rabies or whose work or travel puts them at increased risk. Two types of vaccine are available with inactivated virus from cell cultures of human diploid or chick embryo cells. The cell culture–derived vaccines are considered much safer than earlier brain tissue–based vaccines.

A vaccine has been produced for those working with *Bacillus anthracis*, such as laboratory or animal workers, or some military personnel. Culture filtrate antigens are adsorbed onto an aluminium salt adjuvant. To ensure good protection, three or four doses of vaccine are given with boosters.

Smallpox has been eradicated, but monkeypox (renamed mpox) has still circulated in some countries in West and Central Africa. Normally mpox is a zoonosis, but human-to-human transmission is possible, with an outbreak in 2022–2023 infecting >80,000 people (see Ch. 22). Luckily the original smallpox vaccine and the newer MVA-Bavarian Nordic have proved very effective at protecting against mpox in at-risk groups, including healthcare workers.

In some countries, babies are screened for severe combined immunodeficiency before being given live vaccines such as BCG or rotavirus vaccine.

### Complexity of vaccine schedules

An increasing number of vaccines are being given to infants at a time when their immune system is not fully mature. However, studies have shown that preterm babies can still be vaccinated safely at the right chronologic age for vaccination. Table 35.6 gives an overview of vaccines that were given to infants, children and adolescents in the United Kingdom and the United States in 2022. Links to the current recommended vaccine schedules for the United Kingdom, United States and the rest of the world can be found in Table 35.6.

It is important to ensure that all these vaccines do not interfere with each other and thus reduce vaccine-induced immunity, so testing for noninterference is required before a new vaccine is introduced. It is also generally recommended that an interval of 4 weeks is left between vaccination with different live virus vaccines, as the IFNs produced in response to the first virus can reduce the immune response induced by a second live vaccine.

There may be other factors that affect how well a vaccine works in the real world. Some studies have reported sex differences in vaccine-induced immunity or seasonal effects, and some vaccines do not induce equivalent immunity in all settings. Vaccination is a very powerful public health tool, but not all infants and children will get their vaccines at the right ages or in the recommended order. Vaccines for developing countries therefore need to be tested in the populations most at risk, where other factors and infections such as malaria or intestinal helminths may modulate vaccine-induced immunity.

### Changes in demography mean new vaccine strategies are needed

In many countries the proportion of older individuals is increasing. With age, immunity can be lost; in particular, T-cell immunity is weakened. Hospitalizations for infections such as pneumonia and influenza in older people place a burden on health systems. One strategy is to vaccinate older individuals against flu and pneumococcal disease and in some countries against varicella-zoster (shingles). However, due to the reduced efficiency of the immune system in old age, new vaccine strategies may be needed. If the elderly are vaccinated with the live attenuated varicella-zoster vaccine or the inactivated flu vaccine, they are given 14 times the colony-forming unit of the varicella-zoster virus or 4 times the dose of the haemagglutinin antigen used in the flu vaccine for children to improve immunogenicity.

## NEW VACCINES IN DEVELOPMENT

Improved coverage with available vaccines is reducing child deaths (Fig. 35.14), but if effective vaccines were developed against HIV/acquired immunodeficiency syndrome, malaria and TB, then many more lives could be saved. The development of new vaccines against TB was covered earlier, but what about HIV and malaria?

### HIV vaccines

The first vaccine candidates targeted the HIV-1 envelope glycoprotein Env, which is responsible for viral binding

**Table 35.6** Vaccines used in children and young adults in the United Kingdom (UK) and United States (US)

| Vaccine | UK | US |
|---|---|---|
| Diphtheria, tetanus, acellular pertussis | Given (all) | Given (all) |
| Inactivated polio vaccine | Given (all) | Given (all) |
| *Haemophilus influenzae* type b | Given (all) | Given (all) |
| Pneumococcal conjugate vaccine | Given (all) | Given (all) |
| Meningitis B | Given (all) | Given (not to all) |
| Meningitis AWCY | Given (all) | Given (all)[a] |
| Measles, mumps, rubella | Given (all) | Given (all) |
| Hepatitis A | Given (not to all)[b] | Given (all) |
| Hepatitis B | Given (all) | Given (all) |
| Human papillomavirus | Given (all) | Given (all) |
| Varicella | Special cases[c] | Given (all) |
| Rotavirus | Given (all) | Given (all) |
| BCG[d] | Special cases | Not used |
| Influenza | Given (all) | Given (all) |

Note that the schedules and vaccines given may differ. These indicative schedules are based on recommendations in November 2022; up-to-date schedules can be found at: http://www.nhs.uk/conditions/vaccinations/pages/vaccination-schedule-age-checklist.aspx for the UK, www.cdc.gov/vaccines/schedules/index.html for the US and www.who.int/immunization/policy/immunization_tables/en/ for all other countries.

[a]Given earlier to children with particular health issues such as sickle cell disease.
[b]If required (i.e. travellers).
[c]Offered to those in close contact with someone who is very vulnerable to chickenpox or its complications.
[d]Bacille Calmette-Guérin (BCG) vaccination is given shortly after birth in most countries outside Europe and the United States and can be given to infants considered at greater risk of tuberculosis elsewhere.

**Fig. 35.14** Vaccination has reduced deaths in children. The effect of vaccination on deaths in children aged <5 years from 2000–2015 is shown. However, not all diarrhoeal diseases* or acute respiratory infections* can be prevented by vaccination. (From World Health Organization. *Global Vaccine Action Plan. SAGE/GVAP Assessment Report 2016.* WHO, 2016.)

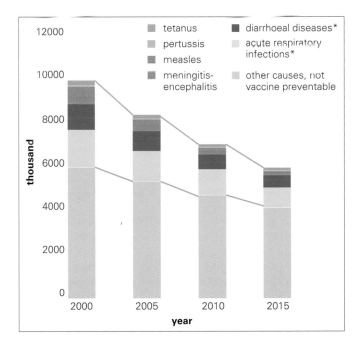

and entry into the host cells and induced antibodies to Env. Further strategies have included using a recombinant adenovirus to deliver the *gag, pol* and *nef* genes. The RV144 trial in Thailand using a priming canary pox vaccine encoding the HIV *gag, pol* and *env* genes and a boosting vaccine with recombinant gp120 showed modest protection of 31.2%, associated with the presence of non-neutralizing antibodies— and no better vaccine has yet been developed. Part of the problem is that mutations in gp120 and viral recombination mean that circulating HIV viruses are highly variable; the

killed virus is not sufficiently immunogenic to use as a vaccine, and the route of infection, mostly through the genital tract, means localized mucosal immunity is needed. This illustrates that, despite huge advances in molecular biology and immunology, it can be difficult to design a protective vaccine. Of course, new mRNA technology is being explored. Some strategies being investigated include novel antigen design strategies to induce non-neutralizing antibodies to the V2 loop of Env, broadly neutralizing antibodies to Env, the use of new vectors such as rhesus CMV to induce

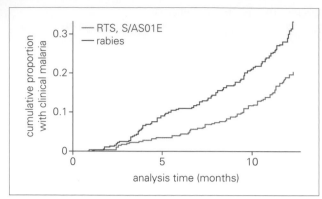

**Fig. 35.15** A new candidate vaccine for malaria that uses parts of the circumsporozoite protein fused to the hepatitis B surface antigen reduces the prevalence of malaria infection in young African children. Children given three doses of the RTS,S vaccine had a longer delay before they developed clinical malaria infection compared with controls given rabies vaccine. If a fourth boosting vaccination was given 18 months after the primary vaccine schedule, efficacy in children aged 5–17 months was 36.3%. (From RTS,S Clinical Trials Partnership. Efficacy and safety of RTS,S/AS01 malaria vaccine with or without a booster dose in infants and children in Africa: final results of a phase 3, individually randomised, controlled trial. *The Lancet*. 2015;386[9988]:31–45.)

**Table 35.7** Serologic correlates of protection

| Vaccine | Assay | Correlate of protection |
|---------|-------|-------------------------|
| Diphtheria | Toxin neutralization | 0.01–0.1 IU/mL |
| Hepatitis A | ELISA | >/= 10 mIU/mL |
| Influenza | Haemagglutinin inhibition | 1/40 dilution |
| Pneumococcus | ELISA Opsonophagocytosis | 0.20–0.35 µg/mL[a] 1/8 dilution |
| Polio | Serum neutralization | 1/4 –1/8 dilution |
| Rubella | Immunoprecipitation | 10–15 mIU/mL |
| Tetanus | Toxin neutralization | 0.1 IU/mL |

Some serologic tests that provide correlates of protection for vaccines in current use are listed. However, sometimes it is secretory antibodies that are more important in protection, and for some vaccines, such as bacille Calmette-Guérin, correlates of protection have not been identified, even though T cells are known to be important.

[a]In children.

ELISA, Enzyme-linked immunosorbent assay.

From Plotkin SA. Vaccines: correlates of vaccine-induced immunity. *Clin Infect Dis*. 2008;47:401.

T-cell memory in the mucosa and using mosaic antigens to generate antibodies to a broad range of HIV epitopes from viruses worldwide.

## Malaria

Malaria has been another challenging disease against which to develop an effective vaccine. The RTS,S in AS01 vaccine is based on the *Plasmodium falciparum* circumsporozoite protein (CSP) and designed to combat the invasive sporozoite stage; the antibodies that are induced immobilize the sporozoites, prevent infection of hepatocytes in the liver and reduce the numbers of clinical cases of malaria (Fig. 35.15). Phase 3 trials have shown that cases halved in the first year after vaccination, and, if given before seasonal transmission, it prevented ~75% of cases, which is similar to seasonal malaria chemo-prevention. In 2021 the WHO recommended that four doses of RTS,S be given to children from 5 months of age if they live in sub-Saharan Africa or another area with moderate to high malaria transmission. Both RTS,S and another vaccine candidate (R21) use the C-terminus and central repeat regions of the circumsporozoite protein (CSP), which is fused to the HBsAg, and both form virus-like particles in yeast. The R21 vaccine, given in MatrixM (a saponin-based adjuvant), achieved 77% efficacy in children age >1 year; it may be more effective because it has a higher ratio of CSP to HBsAg than RTS,S, but yearly boosting, ideally before the rainy season, may be needed for both vaccines. Both vaccines may protect better if given with seasonal malaria chemoprophylaxis. An irradiated attenuated sporozoite vaccine (PfSPZ) looked very promising when given to adults not living in malaria-endemic areas, inducing 100% sterile protection, but it did not protect infants in Kenya in a phase 2 randomized controlled trial; it also needed to be given intravenously, which is not ideal. It would also be difficult to produce sporozoites in sufficiently large quantities, although that may change now that *P. falciparum* sporozoites have been produced in vitro without the need for mosquitoes. Other approaches

include delivering key pre-erythrocytic or blood-stage antigens by viral vectors, as viruslike particles, or trapped within liposomes. For long-term efficacy, a vaccine may need to induce immunity against malaria antigens that are not normally immunogenic and that may be under less immune pressure to evolve. Finally, a vaccine against the sexual forms of malaria that are infectious to mosquitos could help reduce transmission, and candidates are in early trials.

## Vaccines for neglected tropical diseases are also needed

Some infections such as leishmaniasis, leprosy and helminth infections are described as neglected tropical diseases — that is, they are neglected while most emphasis is put on HIV, malaria and TB. Schistosomiasis, onchocerciasis, hookworm, leishmaniasis and trachoma are all examples of neglected tropical diseases for which there is currently no vaccine available, although a glutathione-S-transferase antigen (Sh28GST) in aluminium adjuvant vaccine for *Schistosoma haematobium* has been used in phase II and phase III trials, a vaccine for *Schistosoma mansonii*, with the 14kDa fatty-acid-binding protein in GLA/SE adjuvant is in phase II trials and other candidate vaccines for schistosomiasis, onchocerciasis and hookworm are in early clinical trials. Leprosy also has no vaccine, but luckily the BCG vaccine has been shown to provide partial immunity to leprosy, and hopefully any new TB vaccine will do even better.

## Antibodies provide useful correlates of protection for most of these vaccines

When antibodies provide protection, it is usually possible to determine a quantitative cutoff that is associated with that protection. This can be determined by enzyme-linked immunosorbent assay, by toxin or virus neutralization or in an opsonophagocytosis assay (Table 35.7). It is much easier to have a correlate of protection that can be measured on fingerprick blood or in serum/plasma than one that

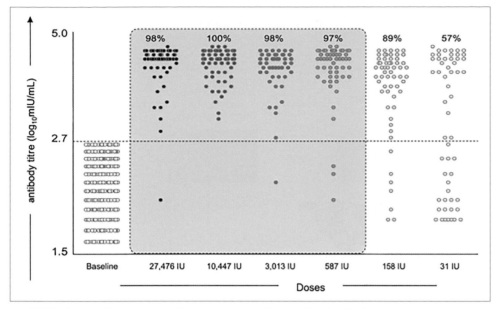

**Fig. 35.16** Use of antibody titres to optimize vaccine dose. The quantity of antibody needed to protect against yellow fever is known, which enabled studies to show that the vaccine could be given at a lower dose without losing protective efficacy, thus dose sparing when vaccine supply was limiting. Similar antibody titres (97% seroconversion) were observed down to 587 IU yellow fever 17DD vaccine dose. The dotted line indicates the cutoff needed for protection. (Modified from Campi-Azevedo AC, de Almedia Estevam P, Coelho-Reia JG, et al. Subdoses of 17DD yellow fever vaccine elicit equivalent virological/immunological kinetics timeline. *BMC Infect Dis.* 2014;14:391.)

requires a T-cell assay (see Ch. 32). Having a correlate of protection can be very useful (e.g. when availability of the yellow fever vaccine was limited, it was possible to show that the vaccine could be given at a lower concentration without losing protection, enabling the available vaccine to be diluted) (Fig. 35.16). For some diseases such as TB it has been surprisingly difficult to identify correlates of protection. This is an area in which new technologies, including multiomics and single cell sequencing, have the potential to characterize what makes one individual a good responder to a vaccine and what makes another person not make a sufficiently robust immune response to give that person protection.

### How quickly can a new vaccine be produced?

The time to make and introduce a new vaccine is critical, as delays mean lives lost. Outbreaks of Ebola in West Africa illustrated how vaccine development can be accelerated. Luckily several potential vaccine candidates were available, existing virus vectors could be used and regulatory processes were accelerated. Within 3 years of the start of the West African Ebola outbreak, results from a phase III trial of a recombinant vesicular stomatitis virus expressing an Ebola glycoprotein (rVSV-ZEBOV) showed the vaccine to be 100% protective. A ring vaccination design was used in which all those exposed to a confirmed Ebola case were vaccinated immediately or 28 days later. ERVEBO is now licensed in the US. Other Ebola vaccines in development include a MVA vaccine (MVA-BNFILO) and adenovirus vectored vaccines (Ad26-ZEBOV, ChAdOx1 biEBOV). As discussed, it was possible to introduce COVID-19 vaccines even more quickly. However, it normally takes decades to develop a vaccine, and accelerating the process only works if a suitable platform technology is already available, such as for viral-vectored vaccines or mRNA vaccines.

Normally vaccine development starts with experiments in the laboratory; the candidate vaccines are first tested in animal models, then move into phase 1 safety and immunogenicity clinical trials before larger phase 2 and 3 trials. This pipeline for TB vaccine development is shown in Fig. 35.17.

### New delivery systems and technologies for future vaccines

Adenoviruses are being tested as vaccine vectors, as they induce good CD8 T-cell responses, but too many individuals already have antibodies to some adenovirus strains, which may reduce the efficacy of the vaccine. For example, although only 20% of individuals in the Netherlands have antibodies to type 5 adenovirus, this rises to 80% in sub-Saharan Africa, so some new vaccine trials are using the Ad35 strain instead, as seroreactivity to Ad35 is lower in Africa. Another strategy used to make a SARS-CoV-2 vaccine was to use a chimpanzee adenovirus rather than a human virus.

Genetic engineering is being used to make more effective vaccines. Viral recombinant vaccines are being developed as new RSV vaccines using parainfluenza virus expressing key RSV proteins. Codon optimization can be used (e.g. for poliovirus) in which reversion to virulence can be reduced by altering the codon usage. For the DEN4CYD dengue vaccine, genes for four dengue strains were inserted into the yellow fever virus genome. Viruslike particles can be made that express key viral proteins yet are replication deficient. The latest papillomavirus vaccines are viruslike particles made from recombinant HPV coat proteins. This approach is also being used for blue-tongue virus vaccine for sheep and for malaria. Genetically modified or transgenic plants can be used to produce immunogens, including glycosylated proteins and even full viruslike particles. Protein glycan coupling technology can also be used in bacteria to produce glycoconjugates.

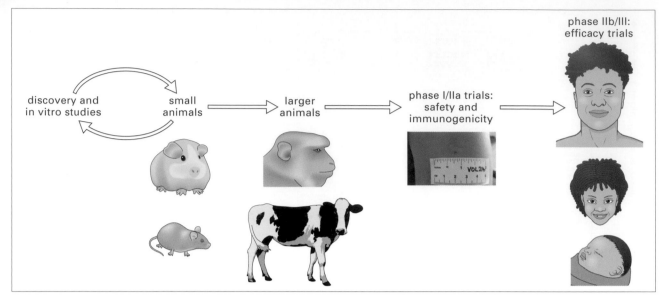

**Fig. 35.17** The vaccine development pipeline. Following initial work to identify the best constituents of a vaccine, the vaccine is usually tested first in small animals such as mice or guinea pigs, then in larger animals such as nonhuman primates (and for bovine tuberculosis [TB] vaccines, cattle), before moving into human trials for safety and immunogenicity (phase I/IIa) and then efficacy (phase IIb/III). The figure illustrates the vaccine development pipeline for TB vaccines. (Redrawn courtesy H. McShane.)

DNA vaccines were thought to hold great promise and have been successfully tested in clinical trials, but so far they have not been licensed for use. However, we now have mRNA vaccine technology, which is already being explored for more than COVID-19 vaccines.

## New routes of vaccination

Some recent studies have shown improved vaccine efficacy if a vaccine is given intravenously rather than intramuscularly, subcutaneously or intradermally (e.g. the irradiated malaria sporozoite vaccine PfSPZ needs to be given intravenously, and the BCG vaccine works better in nonhuman primates if given intravenously rather than intradermally), but this is not an ideal route for administration.

The oral polio vaccine was not the first vaccine to be given orally; the BCG vaccine was originally given by mouth. Dissolvable tablets or wafers may be used under the tongue in the future. If protection is needed in the mucosal-associated lymphoid tissues, then to prime cells in this region is very sensible, and nasal sprays can be used, as in one seasonal flu vaccine formulation. Another approach is to use skin patches. These deliver the vaccine antigens through the transcutaneous route, and for flu this approach can incorporate multiple flu strains and adjuvant as well. Nozzle jet or powder injectors are also being investigated as a means of delivery. Vaccines of the future may be injected using dissolving microneedles, designed to deliver the antigens to cutaneous antigen-presenting cells, which is said to be relatively painless. This is clearly an area where molecular science and technologic developments can make a real impact.

## KEY FACTS

- Vaccination aims to prime the adaptive immune system to the antigens of a particular pathogen so that a first infection induces a faster, more effective secondary immune response.

- Vaccines can use live attenuated organisms, killed whole organisms, subcellular fractions, antigens produced artificially by gene cloning or chemical synthesis that can be delivered by viruses or given with adjuvant, and mRNA-encoding–specific proteins.

- In general, live vaccines are more effective than other types but carry the risk of reverting to virulence or inducing disease in immunocompromised patients.

- The details of vaccine formulation, route, dose and risks have to be considered for each disease individually.

- Overall, vaccination is a very effective public health tool, but many challenges remain, including the effective implementation of existing vaccines worldwide and the design of new vaccines against those infections for which they are not yet available.

# Specific and nonspecific immunotherapy

# 36

## Introduction

Immunotherapy involves any manipulation of the host immune response that results in attenuating or preventing an infection. Vaccines, as described in Chapter 35, protect the host by inducing a protective immune response. Here we will consider other forms of immunotherapy that may be needed particularly in those whose immune system is immunosuppressed, preventing them from making a protective immune response. Moreover, if a person is already infected and antimicrobial agents are either unavailable or ineffective, other forms of immunotherapy are needed. Immunotherapy that acts on the host immune response is now termed *host-directed therapy* and may enhance the immune response or control damaging responses such as excessive inflammation.

The role of immunotherapy is to activate immune effector genes and protective immunity but without enhancing any deleterious side effects they could have, as many events are set in motion when activating innate and adaptive immunity.

**Immunotherapy strategies are divided into:**

1. active or passive approaches, depending on whether the immunotherapy is actively induced in the individual, or just given to them
2. specific or nonspecific approaches, depending on whether the therapy is pathogen specific or not.

## ADOPTIVE IMMUNOTHERAPY WITH T CELLS

T cells recognize and kill target cells, and so adoptive T-cell therapy has been investigated as a way of targeting cells with latent and integrated viral infections. These include herpesvirus and retroviral infections, as well as hepatitis B virus (HBV) infections.

In allogeneic bone marrow transplantation programmes, recipients are at high risk of herpesvirus reactivation, including cytomegalovirus (CMV) and Epstein-Barr virus (EBV) in particular. Other viruses, including herpes simplex virus (HSV) and varicella-zoster virus (VZV), can be suppressed by acyclovir, an antiviral that is relatively free of side effects. Letermovir prophylaxis has been introduced to prevent clinically significant CMV infection in CMV immunoglobulin G (IgG)–positive allogenic bone marrow transplant recipients, and together with monitoring for CMV viraemia has been a further advance in preventing complications of CMV reactivation. An antiviral drug that is effective in reducing EBV replication has yet to be licensed, but a drug called *maribavir* looks promising; only the anti-CD20 monoclonal antibody (MAb), rituximab, is really of use, but it depletes the B-cell population. As a result, producing donor-derived CMV or EBV or adenovirus-specific T cells given as a donor lymphocyte infusion, either prophylactically or as treatment, is another option. If these are not available, donors that have the most common human leukocyte antigen alleles can be used as a source. One concern is that graft-versus-host disease can occur with these infusions.

Chimeric-antigen receptor (CAR)–modified T cells are being used as immunotherapy in haemato-oncology, particularly in aggressive lymphomas, but they were originally investigated as a way of treating individuals with human immunodeficiency virus (HIV) infection. T cells from the patient's blood collected by leukophoresis are genetically modified to recognize an antigen on their tumour, checked for their properties, expanded and then reinfused into the patient (Fig. 36.1). Single chain fragments of antigen-binding domains of antibody heavy and light chains can be used to recognize the antigen, a hinge region linked to a transmembrane domain and an intracellular signalling domain. Other surface receptors can be used, and subsequently costimulatory domains were added. The first approved therapies targeted CD19 or B-cell maturation antigen (BCMA), enabling the CAR T cells to directly recognize the tumour cells, release cytokines and cause lysis of the tumour. Although this is a costly and labour-intensive form of treatment (and currently only given to those with relapsed or refractory disease such as with B-cell acute lymphoblastic leukemia, B-cell non-Hodgkin lymphomas or multiple myeloma), this is an exciting approach. CAR-NK cells and CAR-macrophages may be next. But what about HIV, which is where CAR T cells started? The first-generation CAR T cells for HIV used a CAR with the HIV envelope CD4 receptor protein with the idea that these modified T cells would attack the HIV-infected T cells. It was shown that the CAR T cells found their way to reservoirs of infection in the body, including mucosa, and persisted for years on follow-up.

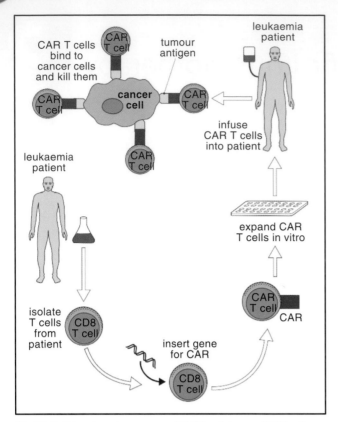

**Fig. 36.1** Chimeric-antigen receptor (CAR) T-cell therapy. CD8 T cells are isolated from a cancer patient's blood, and a gene for a CAR is introduced into the cells. The T cells expressing the new receptor are expanded in vitro and infused back into the patient, to recognize and kill the cancer cells. The extracellular binding domain is linked to a transmembrane region and an intracellular signalling domain (CD3ζ). There have already been several generations of CAR T cells, in which the intracellular domains of the CAR are modified with additional costimulatory domains such as 41BB and CD28 to increase the CAR T-cell function.

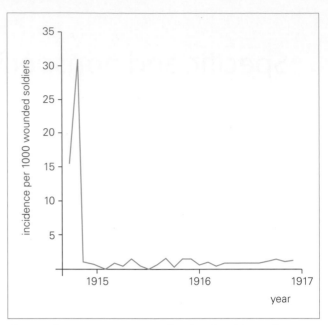

**Fig. 36.2** Passive immunization significantly reduced the incidence of tetanus in the early months of the First World War. The figure shows the incidence of tetanus per 1000 wounded soldiers in British hospitals during 1914–1916. There was a dramatic fall after the introduction of antitetanus serum in October 1914.

However, targeting the limited number of Env-expressing T cells when a person is on antiretroviral therapy (perhaps 1/ million T cells in a person living with HIV) is more challenging than targeting the huge number of malignant cells found in B-cell leukaemias. Even so, HIV-specific CAR T cells are back in the clinic now that the design of CAR T cells has developed further. CMV-CD19 CAR T cells are also being investigated as a treatment for CMV; these could be given to patients with B-cell lymphomas followed by CMV vaccination to expand the CMV-specific CAR T cells.

In 2009 the scientific world was surprised by a report of an HIV-positive person with acute myeloid leukaemia being apparently cured of HIV infection having had an allogeneic bone marrow transplant. A donor who was homozygous for the CCR5 Δ32 mutation, which confers genetic resistance to HIV infection, had been selected.

## PASSIVE IMMUNOTHERAPY WITH ANTIBODIES

### Certain diseases are treated by a passive transfer of immunity, which can be life saving

Once a patient is ill with an acute infectious disease, it can be too late to start inducing an immune response. In the preantibiotic era, such patients were often treated by the injection of preformed antibody in serum. Indeed, the demonstration that immunity to tetanus and diphtheria could be transferred to mice with serum from vaccinated rabbits was a key experiment in the discovery of antibody in the 1890s. Subsequently, the production of antiserum for the passive treatment of diphtheria, tetanus and pneumococcal pneumonia and against the toxic effects of streptococci and staphylococci became an important industry, and generations of horses that had retired from active duty were kept on as the source of immune serum. The introduction of antitetanus serum in the early months of the First World War reduced the incidence of tetanus dramatically by up to thirty-fold (Fig. 36.2). However, giving foreign proteins results in complications, including progressively more rapid elimination and therefore reduced clinical effectiveness as well as serum sickness due to immune complex deposition in, for example, the kidney and skin (see Ch. 18) and even anaphylaxis. Of those receiving horse antibodies, 1 in 20 could develop serum sickness, and skin prick tests were introduced to test for hypersensitivity. These complications can be avoided by using human serum collected during convalescence (normal human immunoglobulin) or following vaccination (disease-specific immunoglobulin) to prevent infection after exposure such as in rabies, HBV and varicella-zoster virus (VZV) infections (Table 36.1). Convalescent human serum from influenza A and Ebola virus disease survivors has been used to treat those with severe infections, especially if antiviral drugs have been ineffective or unavailable. Numerous controlled trials of convalescent plasma use in the coronavirus 2019 (COVID-19) pandemic did not give definitive results in terms of the effectiveness of this treatment. However, a meta-analysis of studies reported that COVID-19 convalescent plasma use was associated with a reduction in mortality when given to immunocompromised individuals with COVID-19.

**Table 36.1** Passive immunotherapy with immunoglobulin for infectious diseases

| Disease-specific immunoglobulin | Normal human immunoglobulin |
|---|---|
| Hepatitis B | Hepatitis A (in addition to hepatitis A vaccine or vaccine alone in some settings) |
| Rabies | Measles |
| Varicella-zoster (being replaced in most situations by acyclovir prophylaxis) | |
| Tetanus | Tetanus (limited availability) |
| SARS-CoV-2[a] | |

SARS-CoV-2, Severe acute respiratory syndrome coronavirus 2.
[a]Effective in immunocompromised patients.

---

## Box 36.1 ■ Indications for Normal Immunoglobulin Therapy

Sufficient antibody to protect immunocompromised patients against common infections can be obtained from pooled human normal plasma.

- X-linked agammaglobulinaemia/hypogammaglobulinaemia
- Common variable deficiency
- Wiskott-Aldrich syndrome
- Ataxia telangiectasia
- Idiopathic thrombocytopenic purpura
- Guillain-Barre syndrome
- Immunoglobulin G (IgG) subclass deficiency with impaired antibody response
- Chronic lymphocytic leukaemia
- Kawasaki disease
- Post–bone marrow transplantation for cytomegalovirus (CMV) pneumonitis in conjunction with an antiviral agent

### Antibody in pooled normal serum can provide protection against infection

With common infections it can be assumed that most immunocompetent people have antibody to the pathogen in their serum. The clearest proof of this is that patients with hypogammaglobulinaemia can be kept free of recurrent infection by regular injections of IgG from pooled normal serum and that immunodeficient children can be protected against measles in the same way (Box 36.1 and Table 36.1). Human normal immunoglobulin (HNIG) is prepared from batches of plasma from at least 1000 healthy donors after screening for a number of infections, including HBV, HCV and HIV. Other infections may be included in the screening tests depending on the prevalence in that country. Intravenous or intramuscular injections may be used. In the United Kingdom, HNIG derived from healthy individuals can be used for treatment of tetanus and given to susceptible contacts to protect them against hepatitis A and measles and to protect pregnant women against rubella. HNIG can also be given to children with symptomatic HIV infection with recurrent bacterial infections.

The immunity conferred by mothers on their newborn infants by placental transfer of IgG and subsequently by colostral IgA (although the latter is not absorbed but remains in the intestine) is further evidence for the protective effect of relatively small amounts of antibody. Thus immunizing a pregnant woman against tetanus will protect her baby from neonatal tetanus.

### An effective therapy is provided by one or more monoclonal antibodies specific for a known target antigen

The first MAb was licensed in 1986, having been generated in mice in 1975 using a hybridoma method (see Ch. 12). MAbs are monovalent antibodies produced by one lymphocyte clone and bind to one epitope. Hybridomas are made by immunizing mice, for example, against a specific epitope on an antigen and then harvesting the B cells from the spleen. These B cells are fused with an immortal cell line creating the hybridoma, which is cultured, and the B-cell clones secrete individual antibodies (MAbs) into the medium. A serious complication with mouse MAbs was that they were highly immunogenic in humans and gave rise to human antimouse antibodies, which accelerated clearance of the MAb from the blood; they also prevent the mouse antibody from reaching its target. To circumvent this, first the variable domains from mouse antibodies were fused to human constant region domains to make chimeric antibodies, and subsequently humanized antibodies containing the mouse sequences for the complementarity determining regions with a human V region were developed.

## Molecular Engineering Has Resulted in Improved Monoclonal Antibodies

### Monoclonal antibodies can be generated by phage display techniques

The next technology developed was based on bacteriophage expression and selection. In essence, messenger RNA (mRNA), preferably from primed human B cells, is converted to complementary, or copy, DNA (cDNA), and the antibody genes or fragments are expanded by the polymerase chain reaction. Single constructs are then made in which the light and heavy chain genes are allowed to combine randomly as *Fab* or single-chain *Fv* (scFv) fragments in tandem with the bacteriophage coat protein gene. This combinatorial library encodes a huge repertoire of antibody fragments expressed as fusion proteins with a filamentous coat protein on the bacteriophage surface. The extremely high number of phages produced by *Escherichia coli* infection can now be panned on solid phase antigen to select those bearing the highest-affinity antibodies attached to their surface (Fig. 36.3). Because the genes that encode these highest-affinity antibodies are already present within the selected phage, they can readily be cloned and the antibody fragment expressed in bulk.

This selection procedure has an enormous advantage over techniques that employ screening because the number of phages that can be examined is several logs higher. To increase the affinities of antibodies produced by these techniques, antigen can be used to select higher affinity mutants produced by random mutagenesis or even more

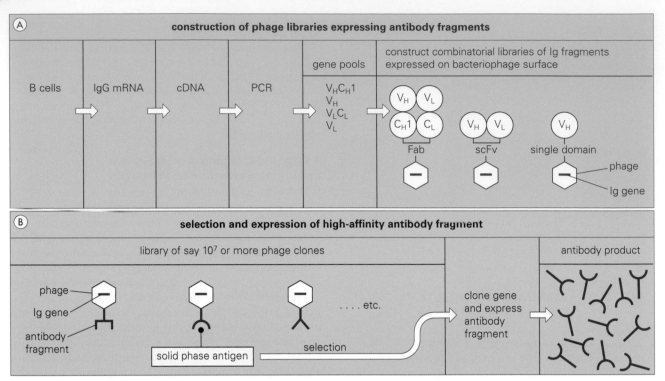

**Fig. 36.3** Pools of genes encoding immunoglobulin (Ig) domains derived from immunoglobulin G messenger RNA (IgG mRNA) are randomly combined and expressed as either *Fab* or single-chain *Fv* (scFv) fragments on the surface of the bacteriophage. Libraries expressing single domains of the heavy chain variable region ($V_H$) (human or sometimes llama) can also be constructed. Phage clones containing genes encoding high-affinity antibody fragments can be selected from these extremely large libraries using solid phase antigen. The appropriate Ig genes can then be cloned and expressed in suitable vectors to produce abundant antibody fragments. cDNA, Complementary, or copy, DNA; $C_H$, constant region of immunoglobulin heavy chain; $C_L$, constant region of immunoglobulin light chain; Fab, fragment (of immunoglobulin) that is antigen binding; IgG, Immunoglobulin G; $V_L$, variable region of immunoglobulin light chain.

effectively by site-directed replacements at mutational hot spots, again mimicking the natural immune response, which involves random mutation and antigen selection. Finally, transgenic mice expressing human antibody genes or immunized humans can now be used to generate fully human antibodies.

### Single-domain variable region fragments (nanobodies) have several advantages

Phage libraries have also been created that express just single heavy or light chain variable region domains ($V_H$ or $V_L$ dAbs). When selected from large naive human phage libraries and fine-tuned by random mutation and further selection, dAbs of surprisingly high affinity, sometimes in the low nanomolar range, can be obtained without the need for prior immunization. Camelids are immunologically curious in that one-half of their antibodies are conventionally composed of heavy and light chains, but the other half are just heavy chains albeit with unusual complementarity-determining regions, which can subserve high-affinity interactions with antigen. Thus a parallel technology was developed in which high-affinity $V_H$ (variable domains from heavy chain antibodies) were selected from immunized llamas.

Both human and llama $V_H$ dAbs have several advantages. They are easy to engineer in bulk cheaply, they can readily be custom tailored by molecular biologic manipulations and they are small and robust in their ability to withstand variations in temperature and acidity, making them relatively insensitive to environmental conditions and the need for

refrigeration and permitting their use for oral therapy and for repeated affinity chromatographic purification of antigens. Another advantage is their low immunogenicity.

Antibody fragments lacking the Fc structures required for secondary activity obviously will not provide protection when complement fixation, phagocytic uptake or extracellular killing is required to eliminate a pathogen. They are effective in blocking cognate enzyme–substrate, hormone or toxin–receptor and microbial addressin–epithelial cell receptor interactions. The latter situation is particularly relevant to mucosal infections in which specific adherence to a cognate epithelial receptor is an essential initial step in the infectious process. Initial studies demonstrated the efficacy of dAbs in preventing experimental rotavirus infection and vaginal candidiasis (Fig. 36.4).

### Monoclonal antibodies can be made more efficacious and are increasingly used in the clinic

Improvements to four-chain MAbs were made by focusing on areas that included pharmacokinetics, immunogenicity, antigen-binding affinity and the effector functions. By pegylating MAbs using polyethylene glycol, the plasma half-life increased. There are also ways to improve effector function, and changing as few as three amino acids in the Fc portion of an antibody can double its half-life in the circulation.

Many human MAbs are now used in the clinic; by 2021, 100 had been licensed by the US Food and Drug Administration. Those licensed include palivizumab for preventing respiratory syncytial virus infections in high-risk infants, raxibacumab for

**Fig. 36.4** Protective activity of an anti-Sap2 (4A7) and an anti-MP65 human variable region single-domain antibody (dAb) against rat vaginal infection by a *Candida albicans* fluconazole-resistant strain (AIDS68). Five rats per group were used. Each animal was administered intravaginally 20 µg of each dAb 30 min before intravaginal challenge with $10^7$ fungal cells. Fluconazole was used as a single intravaginal dose of 50 µg 30 min before challenge. Irrelevant dAbs were not protective. Efficacy in protection against infection paralleled the ability of the dAb to inhibit the adherence of *Candida* to cultures of epithelial cells. CFU, Colony-forming unit. (Courtesy F. de Bernadis and A. Cassone et al.)

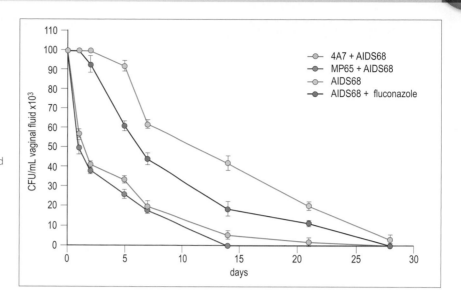

**Table 36.2** Examples of monoclonal antibodies for therapy of infectious diseases

| Licensed | In clinical trials |
|---|---|
| Ebola | Chikungunya |
| Rabies | Malaria |
| Respiratory syncytial virus | *Staphylococcus aureus* |
| Severe acute respiratory syndrome–associated coronavirus | Yellow fever |
| | Zika |

prophylaxis and treatment of anthrax, an antibody cocktail for Ebola and a MAb for postexposure in rabies (Table 36.2). A number of MAbs against other infectious diseases (chikungunya, malaria, *Staphylococcus aureus*, yellow fever, Zika) are also in clinical trials. During the COVID-19 pandemic, an enormous number of neutralizing MAbs were developed, and by March 2023, the Coronavirus Antibody Database listed >10,000 antibodies and nanobodies to severe acute respiratory syndrome coronavirus 2 (SARS-CoV-2). However, they proved to only have clinical efficacy in early or mild COVID-19 disease, which might have been predicted.

Antibodies can also be made in plants; so-called *plantibodies* have been expressed in bananas, potatoes and tobacco plants. The antibodies may also need to be humanized (e.g. plants contain Asn-linked glycans), but promising results have been obtained generating plantibodies to a number of infectious diseases such as HIV, rabies and Ebola (for which a cocktail of three antibodies has been used).

## NONSPECIFIC CELLULAR MODULATION

### Cytokines and other molecular mediators stimulate the immune system

The demonstration by William Coley more than a century ago that crude extracts of bacteria could induce remission and sometimes cure cancers indicated the extent to which the immune system can be nonspecifically overstimulated, with potentially beneficial results. Coley's toxin consisted

of filtered cultures of Streptococci and *Serratia marescens*; it induced a fever and cytokine induction. Many of the compounds used in this way were of microbial origin, but the induction of cytokines and other molecular mediators was probably the basis of action of these older crude materials.

Most of the applications of this type of immunostimulation have been in oncology, and the bacille Calmette-Guérin (BCG) vaccine is still used to treat bladder cancer, instilled directly into the bladder. Some infectious diseases respond to treatment with cytokines. Foremost among these are the interferons (IFNs), notably pegylated IFNα, which has limited antiviral activity but may be used to treat specific individuals with chronic HBV. IFNγ has been found to benefit many cases of chronic granulomatous disease (CGD). However, the unpleasant side effects of high-dose therapy with interleukins (ILs) or IFNs restrict their use and include:

- fever
- malaise leading to fatigue
- muscle pain
- toxicity to the kidney, liver, bone marrow and heart.

### Blocking cytokines can also be useful

Sometimes infectious diseases such as flu, SARS or SARS-CoV-2 and complications such as sepsis involve an excessive release of inflammatory cytokines, termed a *cytokine storm*. This can also be a side effect of CAR T-cell therapy. Steroid treatment can damp down the inflammatory response and can be combined with MAbs such as tocilizumab, a humanized MAb to the IL-6 receptor, or with anakinra, a recombinant human IL-1 receptor antagonist. Anticytokine antibodies such as TNF-blocking antibodies are used to treat disease such as rheumatoid arthritis, ulcerative colitis or Crohn disease, while secukinumab, a MAb to anti-17A, is used to treat psoriasis.

Of course, the use of blocking MAbs can also increase susceptibility to infection; the use of anti-TNF MAbs to treat rheumatoid arthritis resulted in activation of latent tuberculosis (see Fig. 15.9), and anti-IL-17A antibodies used to treat psoriasis can increase the risk of Candidiasis and antibody

## Box 36.2 ■ Host-Directed Therapy

As well as augmenting immunity through antibodies, chimeric-antigen receptor (CAR) T cells and cytokines, damaging host immune responses, can be blocked in a variety of ways by:

- inhibiting components of the innate immune responses (such as complement, neutrophil extracellular traps [NETS])

- using antiinflammatory drugs (such as statins, *N*-acetylcysteine)

- blocking cytokine responses (using antibodies, blocking cytokine signalling, or treatments such as high-dose steroids)

- using immune checkpoint inhibitors, monoclonal antibodies that target molecules such as PD-1, PD-L1 and CTLA-4.

to complement C5 increases susceptibility to *Neisseria menigitidis.*

Another approach used in cancer is to target MAbs to immune checkpoints, key molecules that regulate the immune response, such as PD-1, PD-L1 or CTLA-4. In the future (Box 36.2), this approach could be explored as a way of reducing the T-cell exhaustion seen in some viral infections such as HIV or HBV.

### There is an interesting grey area where immunostimulation and nutrition overlap

A variety of plant products such as saponins, ginseng and Chinese herbal remedies appear to improve resistance to infection and, in some cases, act as adjuvants when combined with vaccines, but the complexity and variability of the extracts makes the active components difficult to track down.

### Gut microbiota to prevent infections in transplant patients

Following transplantation with haemopoietic stem cells or of solid organs, recipients are at risk of developing infections due to immunosuppression. The normal microbiota can also be affected by antibiotic treatment. One possibility is to try to restore the normal gut microbiota, using either transplantation of faecal material or by using probiotics. Probiotics are dietary supplements containing potentially beneficial bacteria or yeast, of which lactic acid bacteria are the most common microorganisms used. They may be given with prebiotics, which are nondigestible fibres that stimulate bacterial growth, a combination known as synbiotics. Probiotic bacterial cultures are intended to assist the body's naturally occurring flora within the digestive tract to reestablish themselves. Many probiotics are present in natural sources such as yoghurt, the commonly used bacteria being *Lactobacillus acidophilus* and *Bifidobacterium bifidum.*

Probiotics have been proposed as treatments for *Clostridium difficile*–associated diarrhoea, irritable bowel disease, and *Helicobacter pylori*; they may also reduce the risk of late-onset neonatal sepsis, of respiratory infections, and of colonization of the gut by harmful microbes. Results in different studies and trials have shown probiotics to be safe, but beneficial effects have been variable. This is another area where more research is necessary!

## CORRECTION OF HOST IMMUNODEFICIENCY

The defects leading to susceptibility to infection are discussed in more detail in Chapter 31, and their correction is an active area of research.

- Antibody defects are the easiest to treat because immunoglobulin can be given as an intravenous infusion and has a reasonably long half-life (~3 weeks for IgG).
- Treatment of T-cell defects is more difficult; thymus or bone marrow grafting has been tried in certain cases with some success.
- Phagocytic defects are the most difficult to correct, and, in practice, antibiotics remain the mainstay of therapy, although the future may lie in gene replacement.
- Gene defects have been identified in certain serious immunodeficiency diseases, including hyper-IgM syndrome, CGD and Bruton agammaglobulinaemia.

Ultimately the correction of gene defects through gene editing may be used in the future. It is now possible to gene edit, for example, using the CRISPR/Cas9 system (Fig. 36.5). CRISPR stands for clustered regularly interspaced short palindromic repeats (found in bacteria such as *E. coli*) that could be used for single RNA-guided cleavage of DNA; the Cas endonuclease was provided by *Streptococcus pyogenes.* Together they enable the precise editing of genes in cells from a patient that can then be reinfused. It is also possible to deliver the endonuclease system directly into patients using a viral or other vector, targeted to a particular tissue. The CRISPR/Cas9 system can be used to delete whole genes if two guide RNAs are used, or can be used to correct or replace a gene using homology-directed repair. Possible future applications include targeting latent or chronic viral infections and even gene editing drug-resistant bacteria so that they revert to become drug sensitive again. Discovering the CRISPR/Cas9 gene editing system won E. Charpeniier and J. Doudna the 2020 Nobel Prize for Chemistry.

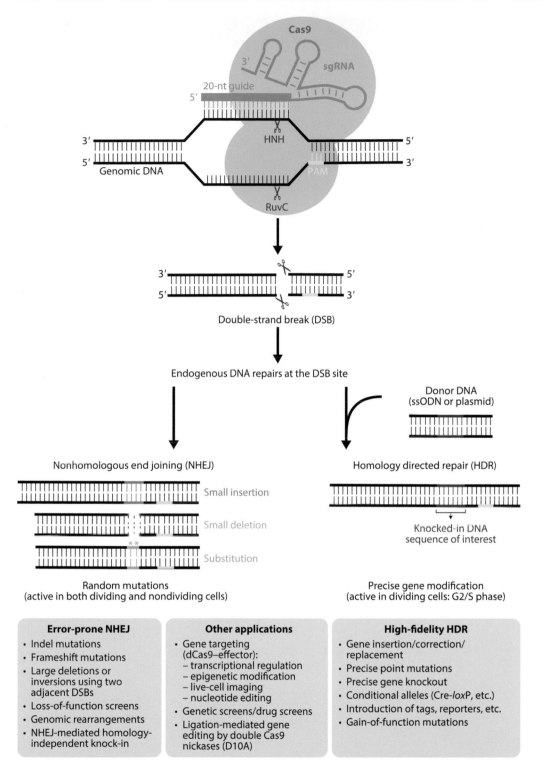

**Error-prone NHEJ**
- Indel mutations
- Frameshift mutations
- Large deletions or inversions using two adjacent DSBs
- Loss-of-function screens
- Genomic rearrangements
- NHEJ-mediated homology-independent knock-in

**Other applications**
- Gene targeting (dCas9–effector):
  – transcriptional regulation
  – epigenetic modification
  – live-cell imaging
  – nucleotide editing
- Genetic screens/drug screens
- Ligation-mediated gene editing by double Cas9 nickases (D10A)

**High-fidelity HDR**
- Gene insertion/correction/replacement
- Precise point mutations
- Precise gene knockout
- Conditional alleles (Cre-*lox*P, etc.)
- Introduction of tags, reporters, etc.
- Gain-of-function mutations

**Fig. 36.5** CRISPR/Cas9 gene editing. Cas9 is an endonuclease enzyme that makes a cut in the DNA. The guide RNA (gRNA) binds to Cas9 and specifies where Cas9 will cut. A single cut will result in the gene being disrupted after the sequence is rejoined. The editing system can also be used to modify or repair genes. The Cas9 endonclease is illustrated in blue. 20-nt guide, 20 Nucleotide guide; HNH and RuvC, two nuclease domains of the Cas9 enzyme; PAM, protospacer adjacent motif; sgRNA, single-guide RNA. (Modified from Jiang F, Doudna JA. CRISPR-Cas9 structures and mechanisms. *Ann Rev Biophys.* 2017;46:505–529, with permission.)

## KEY FACTS

- Transfusion of pooled IgG is the most widely practiced type of passive immunotherapy and is used to treat most forms of antibody deficiency.

- Specific antibodies can be used for certain defined conditions. Such antibodies can be human monoclonal antibodies.

- T cells recognize and kill target cells, and so adoptive T-cell therapy using chimeric-antigen receptor (CAR) T cells with CAR has been investigated as a way of targeting cells with latent and integrated viral infections.

- Fab, single-chain Fv (scFv) or heavy chain variable region domain fragments can be selected by antigen from expression libraries of bacteriophages bearing the antibody fragments as a surface protein.

- These fragments are effective in blocking cognate interactions (such as microbial adherence to mucosal epithelial cells as a precursor to invasion) and are called *nanobodies*.

- Nonspecific stimulation of T-cell–mediated immunity involves cytokines and interferons for viral infections.

- Probiotics may replace the normal microflora affected by antibiotic or immunsuppressive therapy but can give variable results.

- Host-directed therapy may also be increasingly used, including giving licensed drugs such as statins to block unwanted inflammatory immune responses.

- Ultimately gene editing using systems such as CRISPR/Cas9 could be used not only correct gene defects in the immune system, but also to attack latent or chronic viral infections.

# Infection control

## Introduction

**Infections associated with healthcare settings are an increasingly complex issue**

Amassing sick people together under one roof has many advantages but also some disadvantages, notably the easier transmission of infection from one person to another. In the past, the major environment for this interaction has been the hospital, which led to the term *nosocomial infection* (i.e. any infection acquired while in the hospital). Increasing numbers of individuals in skilled nursing and home care settings have prompted the more recent use of the term *healthcare-associated infections (HAIs)*. Nevertheless, hospitals remain the major environment associated with HAI. Hospital infection is generally defined as any infection acquired while in the hospital (e.g. occurring ≥48 h after admission and up to 48 h after discharge). Most of these infections become obvious while the patient is in the hospital, but some (e.g. postoperative wound infections) may not be recognized until after the patient has been discharged. Earlier discharges, encouraged to reduce costs, contribute to these unrecognized infections, although a shorter preoperative stay reduces the chance of acquiring hospital pathogens (see later).

HAI may be acquired from an exogenous source (e.g. from another patient [cross-infection] or from the environment) or an endogenous source (i.e. another site within the patient [self- or autoinfection]). An infection that is incubating in a patient when admitted into hospital is not a hospital infection; however, community-acquired infections brought into hospital by the patient may subsequently become hospital infections for other patients and hospital staff.

### Many HAIs are preventable

In 1850 Semmelweiss demonstrated that many hospital infections are preventable when he made the unpopular suggestion that puerperal fever (an infection in women who have just given birth; see Ch. 24) was carried on the hands of physicians who came directly from attending an autopsy to the delivery ward without washing. The death rate was reduced by introducing the simple measure of hand washing before and after any clinical examination. Recent studies demonstrate that HAIs are significantly less frequent in resource-rich countries compared with those with more limited resources (Fig. 37.1). However, regardless of geographic location, a significant number of these infections can be prevented (e.g. 20–30% in the United States) with success related to the type of infection and available intervention methods. Current US estimates place HAI costs associated with hospital infection at ~2 million infections leading to nearly 100,000 deaths at a cost of US$20 billion annually. On any given day, the US Centers for Disease Control and Prevention (CDC) estimates that 1 in 31 hospital patients has at least one HAI. This number is higher in countries with limited resources.

### COMMON HOSPITAL INFECTIONS

**Hospital infections are frequently associated with indwelling devices**

The infections most commonly acquired in hospitals are:

- surgical wound infection
- respiratory tract infection (pneumonia)

- gastrointestinal infection (e.g. *Clostridioides difficile*; see Ch. 23)
- urinary tract infection (UTI)
- bacteraemia.

A significant number of these infections are associated with medical devices (e.g. catheters, ventilators). Infections may arise from a variety of sources. Bacteraemia, for example, may be:

- primary due to the direct introduction of organisms into the blood (e.g. from contaminated intravenous fluids or via an indwelling device)
- secondary due to a focus of infection already present in the body (e.g. UTI).

Some infections (e.g. gastroenteritis and hepatitis) may contribute to outbreaks in the hospital setting.

### IMPORTANT CAUSES OF HOSPITAL INFECTION

**Staphylococci and *Escherichia coli* have traditionally been the most important gram-positive and -negative causes of infection, respectively; however, the list is expanding**

Almost any microbe can cause a hospital infection, although protozoal infections are rare. The pattern of hospital infection has changed over the years, reflecting advances in medicine and the development of antimicrobial agents. In the preantibiotic era, the majority of infections were caused by gram-positive organisms, particularly *Streptococcus pyogenes* and *Staphylococcus aureus*. With the advent of antibiotics

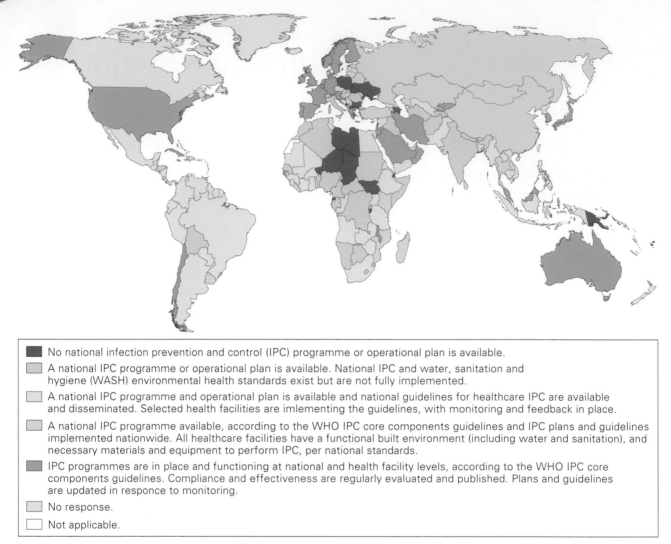

**Fig. 37.1** The prevalence of healthcare-associated infections in resource-rich versus resource-poor countries, 2022. (From *Global Report on Infection Prevention and Control*. World Health Organization, 2022; *Assessment Tool of the Minimum Requirements for Infection Prevention and Control Programmes at the National Level*. World Health Organization; 2021.)

active against staphylococci, gram-negative organisms such as *E. coli* and *Pseudomonas aeruginosa* emerged as important pathogens. More recently, the development of more potent and broad-spectrum antimicrobials and the increase in invasive medical techniques has been accompanied by an increase in the incidence of:

- antibiotic-resistant gram-positive organisms such as coagulase-negative staphylococci, enterococci (especially those resistant to vancomycin [VRE]), methicillin-resistant *S. aureus* (MRSA) and *C. difficile*.
- multidrug-resistant gram-negative organisms, especially including carbapenem-resistant Enterobacteriaceae (e.g. *Klebsiella* spp. and *E. coli*) (see Ch. 34), which in some instances are resistant to the vast majority of (if not, all) available antibiotics
- *Candida*.

Many of these organisms are considered as opportunists—microbes not usually causing disease in healthy people with intact defence mechanisms but able to cause infection in compromised patients or when introduced during invasive procedures. While organisms such as *S. aureus* are a major contributor to healthcare (and hospital) infection, predominant pathogens can vary depending on the specific type of infection (Box 37.1).

## Some infections historically associated with hospitals are now increasingly seen outside of the healthcare setting

Recent reports in numerous countries have documented the emergence of virulent MRSA strains causing infection in individuals outside of the healthcare system. These community-associated MRSA (CA-MRSA) can be transported into the healthcare environment, thus blurring the distinction between community-associated and healthcare-associated infection. This has prompted guidelines for differentiating the increasing number of CA-MRSA infections from those associated with healthcare, summarized in Box 37.2.

## Box 37.1  Order of Pathogen Importance

The general rank order of pathogen importance is listed for the different infection categories. Although a few species are the most important in all kinds of hospital infection, predominant pathogens vary in different infections. *Staphylococcus aureus* is very important in surgical wound infections and bacteraemia but much less important in urinary tract infections. The importance of gram-negative rods has increased since the advent of broad-spectrum antibiotics because these organisms often carry multiple and broad-spectrum antibiotic resistance.

### Urinary tract infections

- *Escherichia coli*
- *Klebsiella pneumoniae*
- *Staphylococcus saprophyticus*
- *Enterococcus* spp.
- Other (e.g. *Pseudomonas aeruginosa*, *Proteus mirabilis*, *S. aureus*, *Candida* spp.)

### Surgical wound infections

- Staphylococci (*S. aureus* and coagulase negative)
- Enterococci
- *E. coli*, *P. aeruginosa* (other gram-negatives to a lesser extent)

### Pneumonia

- *S. aureus*
- *P. aeruginosa* (other gram-negatives to a lesser extent)

### Bloodstream infections

- Staphylococci (*S. aureus* and coagulase negative)
- Enterococci
- *Candida*
- *K. pneumoniae* (other gram-negatives to a lesser extent)

### Gastrointestinal infections

- *Clostridium difficile*

---

## Box 37.2  Criteria for Distinguishing Community-Associated MRSA from Healthcare (Including Hospital)-Associated MRSA

Individuals with methicillin-resistant *Staphylococcus aureus* (MRSA) infections that meet all the following criteria probably have community-associated MRSA (CA-MRSA) infections:

- Diagnosis of MRSA was made in the outpatient setting or by a culture positive for MRSA within 48 h after admission to the hospital
- No medical history of MRSA infection or colonization
- No medical history in the past year of:
  - hospitalization
  - admission to a nursing home, skilled nursing facility or hospice
  - dialysis
  - surgery
- No permanent indwelling catheters or medical devices that pass through the skin

---

### Viral infections probably account for more hospital infections than previously realized

These affect both patients and healthcare workers (HCWs) and include:

- viruses acquired by the respiratory route, especially influenza, as well as respiratory syncytial virus (RSV) and parainfluenza
- viruses acquired by contact with vesicular lesions such as varicella-zoster virus (VZV) and herpes simplex virus
- viruses acquired by contact with contaminated fomites such as noroviruses and rotavirus
- viruses acquired by contact with blood-contaminated fomites, needlestick injury or splash on mucous membranes such as hepatitis B virus (HBV), hepatitis C virus (HCV), human immunodeficiency virus (HIV)

and human T-cell lymphotropic virus. These may also be acquired in countries where blood and blood products are not screened or in the rare instance where the blood donor was in the early incubation (window) period of infection, thereby escaping detection by the screening assay.

The risk of hospital infection is a sum of the transmissibility of the virus and the susceptibility of the patient group. Some viruses, such as VZV, are of low risk in general but very important in paediatric units and particularly in immunocompromised children.

## SOURCES AND ROUTES OF SPREAD OF HOSPITAL INFECTION

### Sources of hospital infection are people and contaminated objects

As stated, the source of infection may be:

- *human* from other patients, hospital staff, and, occasionally, visitors
- *environmental* from contaminated objects (fomites), food, water or air.

The source may become contaminated from an environmental reservoir of organisms (e.g. contaminated antiseptic solution distributed for use into sterile containers) (Fig. 37.2). Eradication of the source will also require eradication of the reservoir.

Human sources may be:

- people who are themselves infected
- people who are incubating an infection
- healthy carriers.

The time period for which a human source is infectious varies with the disease. For example, some infections can be spread during their incubation period, others in the early stages of clinical disease, and others are characterized by a prolonged carrier state even after clinical cure (e.g. typhoid

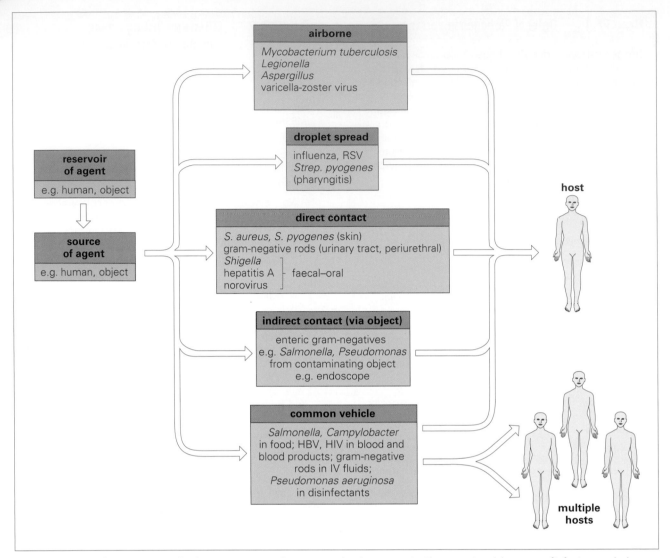

**Fig. 37.2** Hospital infections are spread by the same routes as infections spread in the community. The reservoir and the source of infection may be human or inanimate and may be one and the same (e.g. a nurse with an infected skin lesion). If the reservoir and source are distinct (e.g. contaminated distilled water supply used to prepare a variety of pharmaceuticals), both must be eliminated if the spread of infection is to be halted, otherwise the reservoir may continue to contaminate new sources. HBV, Hepatitis B virus; HIV, human immunodeficiency virus; IV, intravenous; RSV, respiratory syncytial virus.

fever) (Fig. 37.3). Carriers of virulent strains of, for example, *S. aureus* or *S. pyogenes* may act as sources of hospital infection, although they themselves do not develop clinical disease. The carrier state may persist for a long time and go unnoticed unless there is an outbreak or, depending on the significance of the organism, a single case of infection that is traced to the carrier (e.g. HCW with chronic HBV).

**Hospital infections are spread in the air and by contact and common vehicle**

The important routes of spread of infection in hospitals are those common to all infections: airborne, contact and common vehicle. Examples of organisms spread by these routes in hospitals are illustrated in Fig. 37.2. Although theoretically possible, vectorborne spread is very unusual in the healthcare setting, as is sexually transmitted infection. It is important to remember that the same organism may be spread by more than one route. For example, *S. pyogenes* can be spread from patient to patient by the airborne route in droplets or

dust but is also transmitted by contact with infected lesions (e.g. on a nurse's hand). In addition, a patient or HCW with shingles can transmit VZV to a susceptible person having direct contact with rash blisters.

## HOST FACTORS AND HOSPITAL INFECTION

**Underlying disease, certain treatments and invasive procedures reduce host defences**

Host factors play a fundamental role in the infection equation, particularly in hospitals because of the high proportion of hospital patients with compromised natural defences against infection. The spread of an infectious agent to a new host can result in a spectrum of responses: from colonization, through subclinical infection, to clinically apparent disease, which may be fatal. The degree of host response differs in different people depending upon their degree of compromise. The very young are particularly susceptible because of the immaturity of their immune system. Likewise, the elderly suffer a

**Fig. 37.3** Pathogens differ in the time periods for which they can be disseminated from an infected person. For some, it is during the incubation period when infected people may not realize they are ill and infectious. Some people continue to carry organisms such as *Salmonella typhi* and hepatitis B virus long after they have recovered from the clinical disease. Opportunist pathogens are often members of the normal microbiota and may therefore be carried for long periods without the host experiencing any adverse effects.

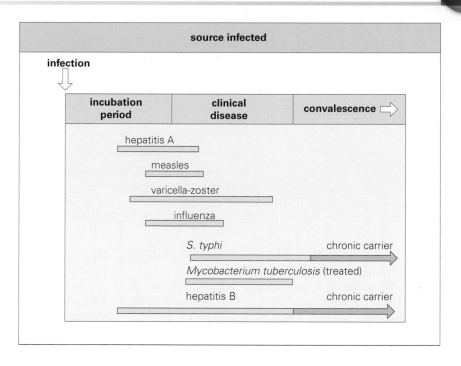

**Table 37.1** Factors that predispose patients to hospital infection

| Age | Patients at extremes of age are particularly susceptible | |
|---|---|---|
| Specific immunity | Patient may lack protective antibodies (e.g. to measles, chickenpox, whooping cough) | |
| Underlying disease | Other (noninfectious) diseases tend to lead to enhanced susceptibility to infection (e.g. hepatic disease, diabetes, cancer, skin disorders, renal failure, neutropenia [either as a result of disease or of treatment]) | |
| Other infections | Human immunodeficiency virus and other immunosuppressing virus infections; patients with influenza prone to secondary bacterial pneumonia; herpes virus lesion may become secondarily infected with staphylococci | |
| Specific medicaments | Cytotoxic drugs (including posttransplant immunosuppression) and steroids lower host defences; antibiotics distrub normal flora and predispose to invasion by resistant hospital pathogens | |
| Trauma<br>  Accidental<br>  Intentional | Burns, stabs or gunshot wounds, road traffic accidents<br>Surgery, intravenous and urinary catheters, peritoneal dialysis | } Disturb natural/host defence<br>} mechanisms |

Hospital patients are not all at equal risk of infection. Some factors that predispose to infection can be influenced by treating underlying disease, improving specific immunity and avoiding inappropriate use of antibiotics, for example. Other factors such as age are unalterable.

greater risk of infection because of predisposing underlying disease, impaired blood supply and immobility, all of which contribute to stasis and therefore to infection in, for example, the lungs. In all age groups, underlying disease and the treatment of that disease (e.g. cytotoxic drugs, steroids) may predispose to infection, while invasive procedures allow organisms easier access to previously protected tissues. The important host factors to be considered in hospital infection are summarized in Table 37.1. Infections in the compromised host are discussed in more detail in Chapter 31.

### A variety of factors predispose to wound infection

Wound infection or wound sepsis is characterized by the presence of inflammation, pus and discharge in addition to the isolation of organisms such as *S. aureus*. Extensive studies of postoperative wound infection have identified a number of predisposing factors:

- Prolonged preoperative stay increases the opportunity for the patient to become colonized with antibiotic-resistant hospital pathogens.

- The nature and length of the operation also have an effect (Table 37.2; see also Ch. 27).
- Wet or open wounds are more liable to secondary infection.

From these studies it has been possible to identify the patients and operations with greatest risk and apply preventive measures such as prophylactic antibiotic regimens and ultraclean air in orthopaedic operating theatres (see later).

### CONSEQUENCES OF HOSPITAL INFECTION

#### Hospital infections affect both the patient and the community

Hospital infection may result in:

- serious illness or death
- prolonged hospital stay, which costs money and results in a loss of earnings and hardship for the patient and family
- a need for additional antimicrobial therapy, which is costly, exposes the patient to additional risks of toxicity

**Table 37.2** Risk factors for postoperative infections

| Length of preoperative stay | Longer stay—more likely to become colonized with virulent and antibiotic-resistant hospital bacteria and fungi |
|---|---|
| Presence of intercurrent infection | Operating on an already infected site more likely to cause disseminated infection |
| Length of operation | Longer—greater risk of tissues becoming seeded with organisms from air, staff, other sites in patient |
| Nature of operation | Any operation that results in faecal soiling of tissues has higher risk of infection (e.g. postoperative gangrene); adventurous surgery tends to carry greater risks |
| Presence of foreign bodies | For example, shunts, prostheses; impair host defences |
| State of tissues | Poor blood supply encourages growth of anaerobes; inadequate drainage or presence of necrotic tissue predisposes to infection |

The risks of infection after surgery have been studied in considerable detail, and surgeons are consequently much more aware of the problems. However, high-tech surgery is often long and difficult, increasing the potential for postoperative infection.

and increases selective pressure for resistance to emerge among hospital pathogens

- the infected patient becoming a source from which others may become infected in the hospital and in the community.

## PREVENTION OF HOSPITAL INFECTION

### There are three main strategies for preventing hospital infection

For reasons outlined earlier, the prevention of hospital infection deserves a very high priority, and the three main strategies are:

- excluding sources of infection from the hospital environment
- interrupting the transmission of infection from source to susceptible host (breaking the chain of infection)
- enhancing the host's ability to resist infection.

### Exclusion of sources of infection

#### Exclusion of inanimate sources of infection is achievable, but it can be difficult to avoid contamination by humans

Exclusion of inanimate sources of infection is both desirable and, to a large extent, achievable. Examples include the provision of sterile instruments and dressings, sterile medicaments and intravenous fluids, clean linen and uncontaminated food and the use of blood and blood products screened for infectious agents. However, many of the sources of infection are human or are objects that become contaminated by humans, in which case exclusion is more difficult. Hospitals must attempt to prevent patient contact with staff who are carriers of pathogens. The problem is the identification of staff who are carriers of pathogens and their relocation to less hazardous positions.

Staff must undergo health screening before employment and should have regular health checks. For example, in the United Kingdom all new HCWs are offered testing for HIV and HCV. HBV immunization is offered, and HCWs must know whether they responded postimmunization and are therefore protected. Any HCW found to have a chronic HBV infection and an HBV load of ≥200 IU/mL (equivalent to the previous limit of 1000 genome equivalents per milliliter) would not be allowed to carry out exposure-prone procedures (EPPs) or carry out clinical work in renal units. It is critical that those carrying out EPPs who either do not know their postimmunization status or have not responded to the

HBV vaccine are checked to ensure that they either do not have a current HBV infection or have a protective level of hepatitis B surface antibody. This is because HBV could be transmitted to the patients if the HCW carrying out EPPs has an active HBV infection and because the unprotected HCW is at risk of infection from a patient with an active HBV infection. There are also guidelines for HCWs with current HIV and HCV infections. Antiviral therapy has revolutionized the guidelines as, for example, those with HCV who are HCV RNA negative for at least 3 months after treatment with directly acting antivirals can return to carrying out EPPs. They are also checked 3 months later. With respect to HIV-infected HCWs, they can perform EPPs if they are on combination antiretroviral therapy (cART) and have a plasma HIV load <200 copies/mL or are an elite controller. The latter is someone not taking ART who has a plasma HIV load <20 copies/mL for at least 1 year and is being monitored every 3 months.

Hospitals have bloodborne virus exposure policies for the management of HCWs and others who may have been exposed to viruses, including HBV, HCV and HIV, having sustained a needlestick injury or mucous membrane splash from a potentially infected source. Prophylaxis includes active and/or passive immunization against HBV and a 4-week course of antiretroviral prophylaxis for HIV exposure (see Ch. 22). The risk of transmission is highest for HBV transmission at ~30–33% in unimmunized recipients, ~0.3% for HIV transmission and 1–3% for HCV but may be higher. However, as reporting of exposure incidents and follow-up of the recipient improves, so too does our understanding of the outcomes of the incident itself. In the United Kingdom it was reported in 2014 that those HCWs who were found to have developed an HCV infection after an exposure incident recovered either spontaneously or after receiving ribavirin and pegylated interferon treatment.

In general, staff should be encouraged to report any incidence of infection (e.g. an infected cut or a bout of diarrhoea). Appropriate immunizations should be offered and in some instances made mandatory. While work restrictions for personnel with infectious diseases are important, healthy carriers of, for example, virulent staphylococci are difficult to identify unless bacteriologic screening is undertaken, which is not feasible on a routine basis. In addition, staff members are sources of opportunist organisms such as coagulase-negative staphylococci or enterobacteria, which are part of their normal microbiota and cannot be excluded.

## Breaking the chain of infection

There are two elements to be considered in breaking the chain of infection: the structure and the human. The structure of the hospital and its equipment can play a role in preventing airborne spread of infection and in facilitating aseptic practises by the staff, but this is of no avail if staff members do not use the facilities correctly and do not themselves act positively to prevent the spread of infection.

### Control of airborne transmission of infection

*Ventilation systems and airflow can play important roles in the dissemination of organisms by the airborne route.* Wards comprising separate rooms have been shown to afford some protection against airborne spread, and rooms with controlled ventilation are even better. However, neither prevents the carriage of organisms into the room on staff members and their clothing, and some studies suggest that this is a more important route of infection than airborne spread. However, *Legionella* infection is acquired by the airborne route, and air-conditioning systems throughout the hospital should be maintained so as to prevent the multiplication of these organisms (see Ch. 20). *Aspergillus* infection in hospitals has been attributed to dissemination of the spores in hospital air, especially when building work is ongoing in the locality.

Ventilation systems in operating theatres must be properly installed and maintained to prevent the ingress of contaminated air and to minimize air currents carrying organisms from the HCWs in the operating room to the operation site. Ultraclean air is air passed through high-efficiency filters to remove bacteria and other particles and has been shown to contribute positively to a reduction in the number of postoperative wound infections developing after long orthopaedic operations.

*Airborne transmission of infection can be reduced significantly by isolating patients.* Patient isolation may be carried out:

- to protect a particularly susceptible patient from exposure to pathogens (i.e. protective isolation)
- to prevent the spread of pathogens from an infected patient to others on the ward (i.e. source isolation).

Isolation also helps to prevent the transmission of infection by other routes by limiting access to the patient and reminding staff of the importance of contact in the spread of infection.

Protective isolation can be provided by a single room on a ward or by enclosing the patient in a plastic isolator. With appropriate positive-pressure ventilation, air should flow from the clean patient area out of the room or isolator. Staff entering the room or in contact with the patient should wear sterile gowns, gloves and masks to prevent organisms they are carrying or have picked up from other patients from coming in contact with the patient.

While source isolation historically involved patient accommodation in an isolation unit in a separate building (e.g. the tuberculosis sanatoria), hospital isolation is typically arranged in a separate ward or in side rooms off the main ward. To prevent airborne transmission of organisms from the patient's room to the ward, air should flow from the ward to the isolation room. In practise, it is difficult to maintain correct airflows without sophisticated designs, including double doors and air locks.

### Facilitation of aseptic behaviour

A general state of cleanliness throughout the hospital is essential, and the design of hospital facilities affects the ease with which the environment can be kept clean and the staff can practise good techniques.

*Bacteriologically, effective hand washing is one of the most important ways of controlling hospital infection.* The hands of staff convey organisms to patients from septic lesions and healthy carrier sites of other patients, from equipment contaminated by these sources and from carrier sites of the staff themselves (Figs. 37.4 and 37.5).

Staff should therefore wash their hands:

- before any procedure for which gloves or forceps are necessary
- after contact with an infected patient or one who is colonized with multiply resistant bacteria
- after touching infective material.

Although soap and water are adequate in many circumstances, emphasis is shifting to the use of fast-drying alcohol-based gels and solutions, which are easier to use and appear to have a greater antibacterial effect. A mandate from the US CDC, for example, has put this approach into practise in US hospitals. Drying hands after any washing procedure is important. A more prolonged and thorough hand decontamination is required before commencing surgery.

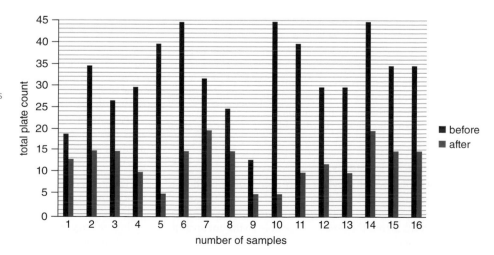

**Fig. 37.4** Bacterial plate counts of demonstrating 60% reduction in plate counts of coagulate-negative staphylococci from the hands of 16 nurses before and after hand washing with soap. (Modified from Nasution TA, Yunita R, Pasaribu AP, et al. Effectiveness hand washing and hand rub method in reducing total bacteria colony from nurses in Medan. *Open Access Maced J Med Sci.* 2019;7(20):3380–3383.)

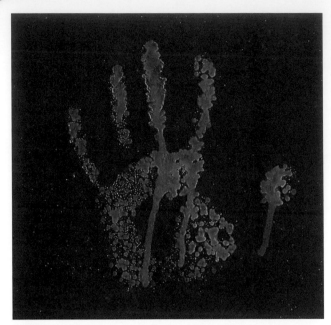

**Fig. 37.5** Gram-negative rods are not usually part of the resident skin flora except in moist environments but are readily carried on hands and can be transferred from a source to a susceptible patient. This impression of a hand shows it was inoculated with ~1000 *Klebsiella* aerogenes.

The design of taps, soap dispensers and other washing facilities, including bedpan washers, has reached a high degree of sophistication. However, human behaviour can be influenced by architectural design to only a limited degree, and there is often a disappointingly low compliance with the simple technique of hand washing. Therefore training and regular reinforcement in appropriate behaviour are essential.

## Enhancing the host's ability to resist infection

### Host resistance can be enhanced by boosting immunity and reducing risk factors

Although attempts can and should be made to control and prevent hospital infection by removing sources of infection and preventing transmission from sources to susceptible hosts, neither of these strategies is fail-safe. In addition, they do not protect the host from endogenous infection. A way of tipping the balance in favour of the host is to enhance the host's ability to resist infection, both by boosting specific immunity and by reducing personal risk factors. The following aspects should be considered:

- boosting specific immunity by active or passive immunization
- appropriate use of prophylactic antibiotics
- care of invasive devices that breach the natural defences (e.g. urinary catheters, intravenous lines)
- attention to the risks predisposing to postoperative infection.

### Boosting specific immunity

*Passive immunization provides short-term protection.* Boosting specific immunity by immunization has been discussed in Chapters 35 and 36. The problem for immunocompromised patients is that they may not be able to mount an antibody response.

## Appropriate use of prophylactic antibiotics

*There are well-documented uses for prophylaxis, but antibiotics tend to be misused.* This is discussed in Chapter 34. There are several well-documented uses for prophylactic antibiotics in so-called dirty surgery and when the consequences of infection would be disastrous (e.g. in cardiac, neurosurgery and transplant surgery). However, there is a tendency to misuse antibiotics:

- first, by using them too often or for too long, thereby increasing the selection pressure for the emergence of resistant organisms
- second, by choosing inappropriate agents.

Treatment (as opposed to prophylaxis) of patients and staff who are carriers of pathogens such as *S. aureus* or *S. pyogenes* has been successful in preventing endogenous infection and to control outbreaks of infection with these organisms. Topical preparations of antibiotics such as pseudomonic acid (mupirocin), a fermentation product of *Pseudomonas fluorescens*, have been shown to be efficacious. However, resistance (both low and high level) to the drug has occurred.

*Gut decontamination regimens and selective bowel contamination aim to reduce the reservoir of potential pathogens in the gut.* Gut decontamination regimens to reduce the aerobic gram-negative flora of neutropenic patients has been practised for some time. With some patients (e.g. patients who have had a liver transplant) in intensive care units, selective bowel decontamination (SBD) has been employed. The aim is to reduce the reservoir of potential pathogens in the gut by oral administration (or via a nasogastric tube) of a high concentration of a mixture of antibiotics. However, at the present time, controversy remains about the efficacy and safety of SBD.

### Care of invasive devices

*Care of invasive devices is essential to reduce the risk of endogenous infection.* It is essential to take care of intravascular devices so as to reduce the risk of endogenous infection from skin organisms and of catheters so as to reduce the risk that the periurethral flora will cause endogenous infection of the bladder in catheterized patients. Guidelines for the care of urinary catheters are discussed in Chapter 21.

*The majority of hospital-associated bacteraemias and candidaemias are infusion related.* These infusion-related bacteraemias and candidaemias derive mainly from vascular catheters. Most bacteraemias associated with invasive devices are caused by the patient's own skin flora, although this may be a more resistant flora acquired during the patient's stay in hospital replacing susceptible resident bacteria. Coagulase-negative staphylococci are the most common aetiologic agents, but enterococci, *Candida* and various gram-negative rods are also implicated. These infections are largely preventable if appropriate steps are taken.

### Reducing the risks of postoperative infection

*Prevention of postoperative infection involves minimizing the risks.* Reducing the risks of postoperative infection involves an understanding of the risks and the ways in which they can be circumvented. For example:

- The preoperative length of stay in hospital should be kept to a minimum.
- Intercurrent infections should be treated appropriately before surgery whenever possible (e.g. treatment of UTI before resection of the prostate).

- Operations should be kept to the minimum duration, consistent with good operating technique.
- Adequate debridement of dead and necrotic tissue is essential, together with adequate drainage and maintenance or reestablishment of a good blood supply to provide the body's natural defences with optimum working conditions.
- Prevention of pressure sores and stasis by good nursing techniques and active physiotherapy minimizes the risks of developing respiratory tract infection or UTI.

## INVESTIGATING HAI

Many of the epidemiologic principles outlined in Chapter 33apply to the investigation of HAI. Outbreaks within hospitals are epidemics; they are detected because the incidence of an infection is seen to be above normal levels for that institution. Investigation, therefore, must determine the extent of the problem, identify the source of infection and the way in which it is spread, identify those at risk and propose effective methods for control. As with infectious diseases in general, the application of statistical techniques (e.g. calculation of risk ratios) and mathematic modelling has helped to provide an analytic and predictive framework for such infections, but day-to-day investigations still require the application of proven microbiologic approaches.

HAI, like community infections, can involve all the major groups of pathogens from viruses to arthropods. However, a particular problem with HAI compared with those commonly occurring in the community is the transmission of antibiotic-resistant bacteria, the emergence of which, and their spread, is favoured by the healthcare environment. The problem with CA-MRSA infections is an unfortunate exception to this trend. Epidemiologic investigations of infections place great importance on molecular (typing) methods to identify and characterize the causative organism. Such molecular epidemiology can make a very important contribution to tracking and controlling infection.

In many hospitals, the responsibility for investigating hospital infection falls on the infection control committee, which includes an infection control officer (who may be a physician or microbiologist) and at least one nurse. The roles of the infection control committee include:

- the surveillance of hospital infection
- the establishment and monitoring of policies and procedures designed to prevent infection (e.g. catheter care policy, antibiotic policy, disinfectant policy, bloodborne virus exposure incidents, including needlesticks and blood splashes)
- the investigation of outbreaks—tracking the source and routes of transmission.

## Surveillance

### Surveillance allows early recognition of any change in the number or type of hospital infections

National and international surveys continue to highlight the prevalence and importance of hospital infection. By maintaining local surveillance, the infection control team can establish the normal trends in their hospital and proactively recognize any change in the number or type of infections. Sources of surveillance data are as follows:

- *Microbiology laboratory reports.* These can be used for general surveillance, for example, monitoring haemodialysis

patients regularly for hepatitis B surface antigen and HCV antibody, as outbreaks of HBV and HCV infection have been reported in renal units around the world, or monitoring for sentinel or alert organisms such as *S. aureus*, VRE and Enterobacteriaceae producing expanded-spectrum beta-lactamases (see Ch. 34).
- *Ward rounds.* New cases of infection can be identified by direct inspection, and previously identified cases of infection can be followed up. Surveys can also be carried out on the wards (e.g. of wound infections after different practices or procedures).
- *Other sources.* These include autopsy reports, staff health records and surveys of patients after discharge from hospital.

## Investigation of outbreaks

When an outbreak (or epidemic) occurs or when routine surveillance highlights an increase in the incidence of infection, the infection control team should initiate an investigation. There is no universally applicable routine for finding the cause of an outbreak, but, in principle, each investigation has an epidemiologic element and a microbiologic element.

### There must be a description of an outbreak in epidemiologic terms

This involves obtaining information about a number of relevant factors:

- How many people are infected?
- When were they admitted?
- When did they develop their infection?
- Are they all on the same ward?
- Are they all treated by the same medical or surgical team?
- Have they all been exposed to the same treatments?

### The causative organism needs to be isolated and/or detected in all patients in the outbreak

It is the role of the microbiology laboratory to attempt to isolate the causative organism and to show that it occurs in all patients in the outbreak (i.e. they are all infected with organisms that are indistinguishable; see later). The identity of the infecting organism can provide clues as to the possible source:

- Respiratory and intestinal viruses implicate the source of infection as a patient or attending medical staff.
- Hepatitis indicates spread via contaminated blood products or hypodermics.
- An outbreak of wound infection with *S. aureus* is likely to be associated with contact spread from staff in theatre or on the ward.
- An outbreak of *Salmonella gastroenteritis* is more likely to originate in the kitchen.
- Infections with *Legionella* or *Pseudomonas* are likely to reflect environmental (e.g. water) contamination.

In addition, the location of the outbreak, whether in a general ward, a surgical ward, a paediatric unit or intensive care unit (once described as the epicentre of hospital infections) may also provide valuable clues.

## Stages in tracking infection

Once the problem has been identified clinically, appropriate specimens should be collected from the patients and, if the indicators are that medical staff are involved, from hospital personnel (see Ch. 32). Likely sources of environmental contamination (surfaces, materials, equipment, water) should also be sampled. This is an important step, as data (using a noninfectious DNA marker as an experimental infectious organism) have shown that after release there is a rapid spread from hands of medical staff to almost all available surfaces (computers, charts, telephones, control knobs, door handles, heater controls, patient monitors). Once samples have been collected, the microbiology laboratory then has the task of identifying and typing the organisms concerned.

While the investigation is proceeding, steps should be taken to contain the outbreak and prevent spread to other patients. Infected patients must be isolated and treated appropriately. Staff who show a similar infection or who are subsequently found to be carriers must be suspended from duty until they have been treated. At the end of the investigation, the relevant procedures must be reviewed to try and prevent the reoccurrence of a similar outbreak.

## Epidemiologic typing techniques

Bacteria are the commonest causes of HAI and of the greatest concern because of the prevalence of antibiotic resistance. For example, in 2018 there were >1.5 million HAIs in the United States resulting in >98,000 deaths. Of the pathogens involved, most were bacteria (see Box 37.1). Tracking infection is therefore disproportionately concerned with bacterial pathogens, although molecular techniques are also applied to monitoring viral infections.

### A variety of phenotypic and genotypic characters are used to fingerprint bacteria for epidemiologic purposes

In epidemiologic studies of the spread of hospital infections, as in the investigation of outbreaks in the community, it is necessary to identify isolates of the infectious organisms to determine whether they are distinct (one commonly does not say that two organisms are the same, only that they are indistinguishable). In the case of bacteria, if the species is a regular member of the normal human flora or is found frequently in the environment, it is necessary to distinguish the outbreak strain from other strains of the same species that are not involved in the outbreak but that may also be isolated during the course of the investigation. Essentially, typing is used to look for evidence of a clonal spread of a particular pathogen.

To be valuable in this context, good typing techniques must:

- be discriminatory (i.e. able to show differences between strains of the same species)
- be reproducible (i.e. the same strain gives the same result when tested on different occasions and in different places)
- have a high degree of typability (i.e. capable of assigning a type to all strains).

## Antibiotic susceptibility patterns

Antibiotic susceptibility testing is readily performed in the diagnostic laboratory (see Chs. 32 and 34) and is useful as a preliminary clue as to whether two isolates are indistinguishable. However, discrimination is poor: Many susceptibility patterns are common, and quite different strains may have the same pattern. Conversely, during an outbreak, strains may gain or lose plasmids carrying antibiotic resistance markers. More specialized typing techniques are commonly performed in reference laboratories. This has the advantage that quality assurance can be optimized, but it also means that there is an inevitable delay in reporting the results and therefore in learning whether an outbreak of hospital infection is caused by a single strain.

## Specialized typing techniques
### Serotyping distinguishes between strains using specific antisera

This classic technique distinguishes between strains by a difference in their antigenic structure, which is recognized by reaction with specific antisera. The O somatic antigens and H flagellar antigens are therefore used to divide salmonellae into types (sometimes referred to as *species*; see Ch. 23). *S. pneumoniae*, *Neisseria meningitidis* and *Klebsiella aerogenes* can be typed on the basis of their capsular (K) antigens and *S. pyogenes* on the basis of its M- and T-cell wall proteins. However, serotyping requires the production and maintenance of appropriate banks of reagents (e.g. antisera), which is both time consuming and costly. Therefore this approach, if still employed, is restricted to reference laboratories.

### Bacteriophage (phage) typing has been used to type *S. aureus*, *S. epidermidis* and *Salmonella typhi*

This technique compares the pattern of lysis obtained when isolates (grown as lawns on agar plates) are exposed to a standard series of phage suspensions. In the past this method has been important for typing *S. aureus*, *S. epidermidis* and *S. typhi* but has also been applied to other species such as *P. aeruginosa*. However, as with serotyping, phage typing requires a reference laboratory for the production, maintenance and testing of the standard phage suspensions and has thus fallen out of favour.

## Molecular typing
### Molecular typing techniques involve characterizing an organism's DNA

The abovementioned methods have been of great use in the epidemiologic analysis of healthcare-associated pathogens but are all variations on the phenotypic characterization of isolates. As the chromosome represents the most fundamental molecule of identity in the cell, genotypic approaches are used for characterization, often referred to as *molecular epidemiology*.

### Plasmid profiles are an example of first-generation molecular epidemiology

Agarose-gel electrophoresis of lysed cell suspensions allows a comparison of plasmid carriage in different isolates. However, the method is useful only for those species that carry a variety of plasmids, and it suffers from the drawback that what is actually being characterized is the plasmid rather than the host organism. However, this method has retained usefulness in mapping the spread of antibiotic-resistant plasmids among healthcare pathogens since gram-negative rods may acquire the same plasmids by conjugation between different species.

## Restriction enzymes and probes represent second-generation molecular epidemiology

Restriction enzyme digestion of total cellular DNA from isolates results in a pattern of different-sized fragments that can be separated and compared by agarose gel electrophoresis–restriction enzyme analysis (REA). All bacterial cells possess chromosomal DNA and can theoretically be analysed by this process. However, the DNA sequences recognized by most restriction enzymes (e.g. *Eco*RI, *Hind*III) are present in hundreds of copies throughout a typical bacterial chromosome. Thus the challenge is to accurately compare electrophoretic patterns comprising hundreds of restriction fragments, which often comigrate in clusters of similar size and may include resident plasmid DNA.

The principle of complementary DNA sequences hybridizing with each other (e.g. Southern hybridization; named after its inventor, Ed Southern) has led to applications in which specific DNA appropriately labelled probes, complementary to target sequences found at various chromosomal locations, are hybridized against isolate REA patterns. Northern blotting is similar in principle but characterizes RNA sequences. Antibiotic resistance genes and a variety of repeated sequences (e.g. transposons) have been especially useful targets in this context. The result is a pattern of hybridization with different restriction fragments commonly termed *restriction fragment length polymorphism (RFLP) analysis*, corresponding to the chromosomal location of the probed sequences, that provides an indication of chromosomal relatedness between different isolates (Fig. 37.6A). For example, copies of the genes for ribosomal RNA (5 S, 16 S and 23 S rRNA) are found at different locations on the chromosome of many medically important bacteria. These highly conserved sequences (i.e. very similar sequences in different species) allow RFLP analysis using a common probe (i.e. ribotyping). However, discrimination between strains of the same species may be less because of the conserved nature of the target sequences. The greatest success with RFLP analysis has primarily involved probes for insertion sequences that provide sufficient coverage (i.e. in number and diversity of chromosomal location) to reflect epidemiologically relevant interrelationships. The use of IS6110 probes in the RFLP analysis of *Mycobacterium tuberculosis* isolates is an example of a successful use of this approach. While superior to REA alone, RFLP analysis remains only moderately discriminatory and is no longer widely used for epidemiologic analysis.

## Pulsed field gel electrophoresis and polymerase chain reaction are third-generation approaches to molecular epidemiology

Instead of using frequently cutting restriction enzymes, chromosomal DNA may be digested using enzymes with rare recognition sites in bacterial chromosomes (e.g. *Not*I, *Sfi*I, *Spe*I and *Xba*I in most gram-negatives; *Asc*I, *Rsr*II, *Sgr*AI and *Sma*I in most gram positives). The extremely large DNA fragments produced are too large to be separated by conventional agarose gel electrophoresis but may be resolved by electrophoretic current pulsed in different directions for different lengths of time-pulsed field gel electrophoresis (PFGE). PFGE has proved to be a powerful epidemiologic tool. The macro restriction patterns produced by PFGE provide a sense of global chromosomal monitoring—genetic events that affect distances between rare restriction site sequences can be inferred from changes in restriction fragment size (see Fig. 37.6B). To date, the major disadvantage to PFGE analysis has been the extra time and effort involved in producing unbroken chromosomal molecules necessary for reproducible macro restriction fragment patterns. For many years the overall success with which PFGE analysis has been employed made it the method of choice (i.e. the gold standard) for the epidemiologic analysis of most pathogens of clinical concern.

Economy, speed and the relatively low level of technical expertise required by the polymerase chain reaction (PCR) (see Ch. 32) have led to a wealth of amplification-based applications for epidemiologic analysis. One of the earliest and most common PCR-based approaches has been randomly amplified polymorphic DNA, also called *arbitrarily primed PCR*. The method is based on the use of relaxing conditions affecting the stringency (i.e. specificity) with which PCR primers bind to DNA templates. PCR primers are allowed to bind randomly to chromosomal sequences of varying homology, resulting in products that can be comparatively analysed by agarose gel electrophoresis. A group of clinical isolates representing interpatient transfer of a single strain would thus be expected to exhibit the same degree of randomness, resulting in identical PCR products (see Fig. 37.6C). However, numerous studies have shown that this method is especially prone to artefactual and inter- and intralaboratory variation. Nevertheless, the overall simplicity and utility of PCR have driven commercialization of this approach, although remaining issues of sensitivity and specificity have hampered its widespread use.

## Fourth-generation molecular epidemiology is based on DNA sequence analysis

Since the chromosome is the most fundamental molecule of identity in the cell, a comparison of actual chromosomal sequences is the most fundamental means of assessing potential interrelationships in healthcare-associated isolates. Thus one could consider sequenced-based analysis fourth-generation molecular epidemiology. While recent years have seen a variety of sequence-based approaches to assessing microbial relatedness, technology now exists to generate and compare the entire chromosomal sequence of isolates via bench-top instrumentation (whole genome sequencing). In the most common approach a library of extracted genomic DNA is sequenced, resulting in multiple copies of short regions (reads) several hundred base pairs in length. Computer algorithms then either de novo assemble the overlapping sequence reads with the goal of reproducing the original sequence or align the sequence reads to a related chromosomal template (reference mapping) (see Fig. 2.22). In either case, bacterial genomes can be divided into core and accessory regions. The core genome represents conserved genes, which are found in all members of a bacterial species, while the presence or absence of other (accessory) genomic regions is variable. Taken together, all the core and variable sequences found in members of a bacterial species are termed the *pan genome*. Bioinformatic analysis of chromosomal sequences then allows a genomic comparison of isolate relatedness either on the basis of single-nucleotide base differences (single-nucleotide polymorphisms) or gene-by-gene differences in the core genome (core-genome multilocus sequence typing).

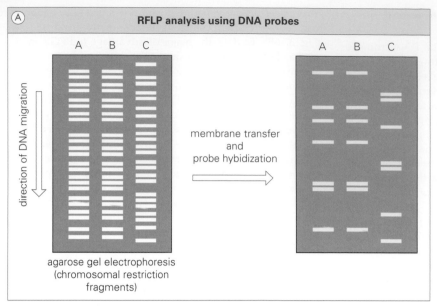

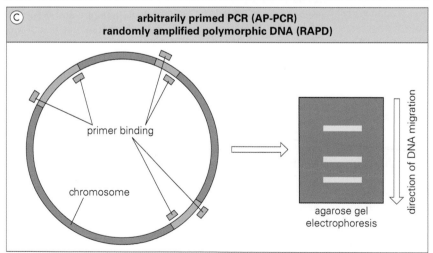

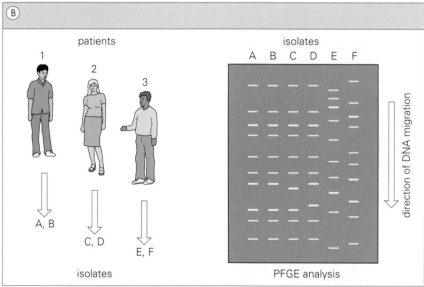

**Fig. 37.6** (A) Restriction fragment length polymorphism (RFLP) analysis using DNA probes. An illustration of three nosocomial isolates (*A* and *B* epidemiologically related; *C* unrelated) analysed by restriction enzyme analysis and subsequently by a specific DNA probe. (B) Pulsed field gel electrophoresis (PFGE) analysis of two bacterial isolates from each of three patients. Isolates in the first two patients are highly related (although slightly different in patient 2). Isolates from patient 3 are epidemiologically unrelated. (C) In the RAPD/AP-PCR approach to epidemiologic analysis, polymerase chain reaction (PCR) products result from the random binding of PCR primers to chromosomal sequences, and the pattern is expected to be similar in epidemiologically related isolates.

## Molecular techniques for epidemiologic fingerprinting have many advantages

Although molecular techniques may require expertise and equipment, they have several advantages. They can be extremely precise, can be performed rapidly, in some instances do not involve handling infectious organisms and provide the potentially most fundamental (i.e. chromosomal) assessment of isolate relatedness. However, it is important to note that available resources may dictate realistic options for epidemiologic fingerprinting, and the use of any of the abovementioned approaches is better than none at all.

## Investigation of viral infections

Nosocomial viral infections usually occur via the airborne route, contaminated fomites or blood-to-blood contact as outlined previously with, for example, RSV, noroviruses or HBV, respectively. These are investigated mostly by detecting virus in samples from symptomatic patients and then, depending on the clinical setting, may rarely involve collecting samples from asymptomatic patients to include in a cohort for broader analysis. In general, only identification of the microbe as a virus is required in outbreaks of viral gastroenteritis, as the management is the same for all the viral causes of gastroenteritis. However, in this setting it is important from an epidemiologic perspective to identify the cause of the outbreak. Surveillance is critical to monitor any changes in the virus as these alterations to parts of its genome may result in the virus evading detection, as the primers used in the molecular diagnostic test may no longer match the complementary sequence of the template. In addition, for those viruses for which we have a vaccine, it is important to know which strains are circulating currently to ensure a good antigenic match with the vaccine strains.

In an outbreak of respiratory infection, identification and typing of the virus are important not only for epidemiologic purposes but also to determine where antiviral treatment and prophylaxis are available.

Molecular detection and typing methodologies such as sequencing may be required, usually for epidemiologic purposes (e.g. severe acute respiratory syndrome coronavirus type 2 [SARS-CoV-2]) rather than for direct management of patients. However, in a setting such as postoperative acute hepatitis B infection, an investigation will be carried out to determine possible routes of transmission. This may include investigating blood products, HCWs who were involved in EPPs, other patients on the operating list, sexual contacts and other risk activities involving potentially blood-contaminated needles. Once the potential sources have been identified, serologic tests may be carried out to seek evidence of current, recent or past hepatitis B infection. Genome detection methods can play an important role in screening blood samples from the individual with acute hepatitis B, as well as the potential source or sources, to help confirm the transmission event or events often by sequence analysis.

## Corrective/preventive measures

### Once tracking is complete, corrective and preventive measures can be introduced

Typing of the aetiologic agent responsible for the outbreak and knowledge of its characteristics and mode of transmission allow preventive measures to be taken. What these include depends to a great extent on the pathogen involved, but all must aim to improve basic hygiene, from more effective hand washing and improved general cleaning to more effectively regulated sterilization of equipment. Hygiene is a crucial factor as agents of HAI can be spread between patients by HCWs. With some organisms that are widely distributed in the environment (e.g. *P. aeruginosa*) or that occur in water supplies (e.g. *Legionella*), corrective measures may involve radical improvements to facilities.

As noted earlier, awareness of the risks of being exposed to bloodborne virus infections in a hospital setting is important to prevent bloodborne virus exposure incidents. Important protective measures include (1) immunization of HCWs, (2) wearing appropriate personal protective equipment (PPE) for procedures that could result in a break in the skin or exposure of mucous membranes and (3) appropriate postexposure steps in the case of an incident.

Transmission of SARS and SARS-CoV-2 (see Ch. 20) has shown how easily airborne infection can be transmitted especially in a hospital or other healthcare setting. The use of PPE (e.g. an N95 respirator, eye protection, mask, gloves, gown) has been critical in reducing the chance of such transmission.

## STERILIZATION AND DISINFECTION

It is clear that the prevention of HAI depends in part on the availability of clean and (where necessary) sterile equipment, instruments and dressings, isolation facilities and the safe disposal of infected material. Sterilization and disinfection are often talked about by microbiologists in relation to the production of sterile culture media and other laboratory activities, but it must be stressed that the concept of sterility is central to almost all areas of medical practice. An understanding of the rationale of sterilization and disinfection will aid intelligent use of the range of sterile equipment (from needles to prostheses) and techniques (from surgery to hand washing) employed in medical practice.

## Definitions

### Sterilization is the process of killing or removing all viable organisms

An item that is sterile is free from all viable organisms — in this sense, viable means capable of reproducing. Sterilization is achieved by physical or chemical means, either by the removal of organisms from an object or by killing the organisms in situ, sometimes leaving toxic breakdown products (pyrogens) in the object.

### Disinfection is a process of removing or killing most, but not all, viable organisms

Disinfection employs either:

- a chemical disinfectant, which kills pathogens but may not kill viruses or spores, or
- a physical process such as boiling water or low-pressure steam, which reduces the bioburden (i.e. the load of viable organisms).

### Antiseptics are used to reduce the number of viable organisms on the skin

Antiseptics are a particular group of disinfectants. Some act differentially, destroying the transient flora but leaving untouched the normal skin flora deep in the skin pores and hair follicles. It is impossible to sterilize the skin, but thorough washing with antiseptic soaps can reduce the numbers of organisms on the surface considerably and therefore reduce contact spread of infection (see earlier). However, the resident bacteria in the hair follicles and ducts of sweat glands can recolonize the skin surface within hours.

### Pasteurization can be used to eliminate pathogens in heat-sensitive products

Pasteurization reduces the total numbers of viable microbes in bulk fluids such as milk and fruit juices without destroying flavour and palatability. It does not affect spores but is effective against intracellular organisms such as *Brucella*, mycobacteria and many viruses.

Since the beginning of recorded history, various other techniques have been used to prevent the multiplication of microorganisms, such as drying and salting of food.

## Deciding whether sterilization or disinfection should be used

Sterilization and disinfection processes are costly, so it is important to choose the appropriate method and the one that causes the least damage to the material involved. A variety of considerations influence the choice of method. The detailed mechanisms of the death process of microorganisms may vary with the sterilizing technique used, but the net effect is similar in that essential cell constituents (nucleic acids or proteins) are inactivated.

### It is easier to sterilize a clean object than a physically dirty one

This is because organic matter protects microbes and hinders penetration of heat or chemicals and may inactivate certain chemicals. In other words, a low bioburden is a prerequisite for cost-effective sterilization.

### The rate of killing of microorganisms depends upon the concentration of the killing agent and time of exposure

The number of organisms surviving sterilization can be expressed by the equation: $N \propto 1/CT$, where $N$ is the number of survivors, $C$ is the concentration of agent and $T$ is time of exposure to the agent. If a population of microbes is exposed to a sterilizing technique and the number of survivors, expressed as a logarithm, is plotted against time, the slope of the graph defines the death rate (Fig. 37.7). These lines may be sigmoid or have shoulders, indicating that individual cells respond slightly differently, some being killed more easily than others. In the case of bacteria, the physiologic state of the organisms influences the shape of the killing curve: Young replicating cells are usually more vulnerable than stationary or decline-phase organisms or those that are sporing. Graphs like those shown in Fig. 37.7 can be used to predict the conditions necessary to achieve sterility. However, these experimental data are usually based on pure cultures in the laboratory (bacterial spores are often used as model systems), whereas in real life the bioburden is mixed. Therefore predictions from such data may be inappropriate for mixed populations.

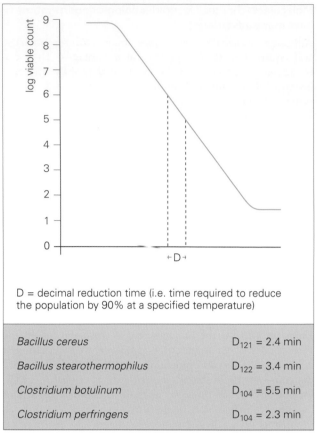

D = decimal reduction time (i.e. time required to reduce the population by 90% at a specified temperature)

| *Bacillus cereus* | $D_{121} = 2.4$ min |
| *Bacillus stearothermophilus* | $D_{122} = 3.4$ min |
| *Clostridium botulinum* | $D_{104} = 5.5$ min |
| *Clostridium perfringens* | $D_{104} = 2.3$ min |

**Fig. 37.7** Theoretically, there is a straight-line relationship between the log viable count of a bacterial population and time when the population is exposed to a lethal temperature. In practice, these lines are usually sigmoid. The *D* value is the time required to reduce the population by 90% at a specified temperature. *Bacillus stearothermophilus* spores are used as biologic indicators of effective heat sterilization by including filter paper strips carrying a standard number of spores into the autoclave cycle. The strips are then incubated to attempt to recover viable organisms. The usual autoclave cycle of 121°C for 15 min is adequate to kill *B. stearothermophilus* with a margin of safety.

## Techniques for sterilization

Sterilization may be achieved by heat, irradiation (gamma or ultraviolet), filtration or chemicals in liquid or gaseous phase. Other techniques of doubtful efficiency include freezing and thawing, lysis, desiccation, ultrasonication and the use of electric discharges, but these are not applied in healthcare practice.

Ultraviolet irradiation is inefficient as a sterilant, and its important uses in the healthcare setting are in inhibiting growth of bacteria in water, in complex apparatus such as autoanalysers and in safety hoods in microbiology laboratories. The potential for damage to the cornea and skin precludes the wider use of ultraviolet irradiation. It should be remembered that the agents of Creutzfeldt-Jakob disease, bovine spongiform encephalopathy and scrapie are highly resistant and are not completely inactivated by formalin, ultraviolet irradiation, ionizing radiation or regular autoclaving. Sterilization can be achieved by boiling in 1 N NaOH for 10 min at atmospheric pressure followed by autoclaving at a higher than normal temperature for a longer period than usual (134°C for 18 min), but obviously this technique cannot be applied to living tissues or materials that are damaged at high temperatures.

## Heat

Heat, as a way of transferring energy, is the preferred choice for sterilization on the grounds of ease of use, controllability, cost and efficiency.

*Dry heat sterilizes by oxidation of the cell components*. Incineration and the use of the laboratory Bunsen burner are examples of sterilization by dry heat. Glassware can be sterilized in a hot air oven at 160–180°C for 1 h.

*The most effective agent for sterilization is saturated steam (moist heat) under pressure*. This can be achieved using an autoclave. Steam under pressure aids penetration of heat into the material to be sterilized (such as dressings), and there is a direct relationship between temperature and steam pressure. Steam under pressure has a temperature in excess of 100°C, which results in increased killing of microbes.

Sterilizing efficiency is improved by evacuating all the air from the autoclave chamber. The subsequently introduced high-pressure steam rapidly penetrates to all parts of the chamber and its load and results in predictable rises in temperature in the centre of articles to be sterilized. The length of an autoclave cycle is determined by the holding time plus a margin of safety and is derived from the thermal death curves for heat-resistant pathogens such as Clostridia. Therefore the usual cycle of 121°C for 15 min is sufficient to kill the spores of *Clostridium botulinum* with an adequate margin of safety. However, the spores of some bacterial species, especially soil organisms, are able to withstand this temperature. The safety margin is reduced in the presence of large numbers of organisms because there is a greater probability of more heat-resistant individuals existing in a large population—hence the importance of cleaning instruments whenever possible, before sterilization.

Moist heat in an autoclave is used to sterilize surgical instruments and dressings and heat-resistant pharmaceuticals. A method for the sterilization of heat-sensitive instruments such as endoscopes uses a solution of 0.55% ortho-phthalaldehyde.

Many of these processes are carried out in a pressure vessel usually available in the hospital central sterile supply department.

*Immersion in boiling water for a few minutes can be used as a rapid emergency measure to disinfect instruments*. Immersion in boiling water for a few minutes will kill vegetative bacteria and many, but not all, spores.

*Pasteurization uses heat at 62.8–65.6°C for 30 min*. This technique was devised by Pasteur to prevent the spoilage of wine by heating it to 50–60°C. It is now used for fluids such as milk to reduce the number of bacteria. This helps to eliminate pathogens present in small numbers and to improve the shelf life of milk. The fluid is held at a temperature of 62.8–65.6°C for 30 min or may be flash pasteurized at 71.7°C for 15 s. After either process, the fluid should be kept at a temperature of <10°C to minimize subsequent bacterial growth.

## Irradiation

*Gamma irradiation energy is used to sterilize large batches of small-volume items*. The use of gamma irradiation energy for sterilization is an industrial process that works well with products such as needles, syringes, intravenous lines, catheters and gloves and even to prevent food spoilage. Although the capital cost of the equipment is high, the process is continuous and 100% efficient. Articles are sterilized while sealed in their original packaging, without any heat gain. The process must be conducted in a suitably constructed building. However, irradiation can cause materials to deteriorate and is thus not suitable for resterilization of equipment. The killing mechanism involves the production of free radicals, which break the bonds in DNA. Irradiation kills spores but at a higher dose than vegetative cells because of the relative lack of water in spores.

Sterilization using ultraviolet irradiation is discussed earlier.

## Filtration

*Filters are used to produce particle- and pyrogen-free fluid*. Solutions that are heat sterilized will contain pyrogens. These heat-stable breakdown products of microbes are capable of inducing fever and are therefore undesirable in products such as intravenous fluids. Filtration or separation of the product from the contamination has a long history in the clarification of water and wine. Modern filters composed of compounds such as nitrocellulose or mixed cellulose ester work by electrostatic attraction and physical pore size to retain organisms or other particles. The resulting fluid should be particle free. Filtration is used in some parts of the world to purify drinking water.

Filtration techniques are also used to recover very small numbers of organisms from very large volumes of fluid (e.g. *Legionella* from cooling tower water) and can be used as a method for quantifying bacteria in fluids.

## Chemical agents

*The gases ethylene oxide and formaldehyde kill by damaging proteins and nucleic acids*. Ethylene oxide and formaldehyde are examples of alkylating gases:

- Ethylene oxide has been widely used to sterilize single-use medical requisites such as heart valves. However, it is toxic and potentially explosive.
- Formaldehyde is not explosive but has an extremely unpleasant odour and is an irritant to mucous membranes. It has been used as a disinfectant to decontaminate rooms (such as isolation rooms) and in the laboratory to disinfect exhaust-protective cabinets. A high relative humidity is essential for effective killing.

*The liquid glutaraldehyde is used to disinfect heat-sensitive articles*. Glutaraldehyde is less toxic than formaldehyde and can be stabilized in solution to remain active for up to several weeks at in-use concentration. It is used for the disinfection of, but does not sterilize, heat-sensitive articles such as endoscopes and for inanimate surfaces.

*Many different antimicrobial chemicals are available, but few are sterilant*. Some, like the derivatives of pine and turpentine, have been known since ancient times, and chloride of lime and coal tar fluids were in use before the germ theory of disease was established. Most fall into the category of disinfectant or antiseptic, but a few are capable of rendering articles sterile. Factors that affect their efficacy include:

- physical environment (e.g. porous or cracked surfaces)
- presence of moisture

**Table 37.3** Examples of disinfectants for use in hospitals

| Group | Examples | Advantages and disadvantages |
|---|---|---|
| Phenolics | Clear-soluble phenolic compounds, white fluids | General-purpose disinfectants used less frequently than in the past; not readily inactivated by organic matter; active against wide range of organisms including *Mycobacterium*; not sporicidal |
| | Chloroxylenols | Inactivated by hard water and organic matter; *Pseudomonas* grows readily in chloroxylenol solutions; limited activity against other gram-negatives |
| Halogens | Hypochlorites (chloramine) | Cheap, effective, act by release of free chlorine; active against viruses and therefore recommended for disinfection of equipment soiled with blood (because of hepatitis and human immunodeficiency virus risk); inactivated by organic material, corrodes metals |
| | Iodine and iodophors | Useful skin disinfectants; sporicidal |
| Quaternary ammonium compounds | Benzalkonium chloride, didecyl dimethyl ammonium bromide | Have detergent properties; low concentrations are bacteriostatic, high concentrations are bacteriocidal |
| Diguanides | Chlorhexidine | Useful disinfectant for skin and mucous membranes, inactivated by many materials and too expensive for environmental use, alcoholic solutions are less easily contaminated, combinations of chlorhexidine and detergent highly effective for disinfection of hands |
| Alcohols | Ethyl alcohol, isopropyl alcohol | Good choice for skin disinfection and for clean surfaces, sometimes used in combination with iodine or chlorhexidine (see above); water must be present for bacterial killing (i.e. 70% ethanol best); isopropyl preferred for skin and articles in contact with patient |
| Aldehydes | Formaldehyde/formalin | Too irritant for use as general disinfectant |
| | Glutaraldehyde | Kills vegetative organisms, including mycobacteria, slowly but effectively; more active, less toxic than formaldehyde; sporicidal (within 6 h when fresh); slightly irritant; used in alkaline solution, which is stable for 1–2 weeks; expensive, limited use (e.g. disinfection of endoscopes) |
| Chlorinated bisphenols | Triclosan | A polychloro phenoxy phenol used in bacteriostatic concentrations in personal products |

Note that no one group of disinfectant has all the properties desirable for use both on skin and on inanimate surfaces.

- temperature and pH
- concentration of the agent
- hardness of water
- the bioburden on the object to be disinfected
- the nature and state of the microbes in the bioburden
- the ability of the microbes to inactivate the chemical agent.

It is obvious that these factors are difficult to control in every circumstance. The main groups of chemical agents are shown in Table 37.3. They act by causing chemical damage to proteins, nucleic acids or cell membrane lipids. The activity of a given disinfectant may result from more than one pathway of damage.

## Controlling sterilization and disinfection

### In general, it is preferable to control the process rather than the product

This means that it is better to run checks on the technique while it is in operation rather than attempting to recognize process failure by isolating microorganisms from the product. Trying to discover whether one or a few viable organisms remain is analogous to trying to find a needle in a haystack. It is known that damaged bacteria can recover, given time and special nutrient recovery media, but it may not

be feasible to hold back a batch of product for such tests. In addition, how many samples of the product should be tested? If too few are examined, the likelihood of missing a failed sample is high; if too many are examined, too much of the batch is used up in quality control to be economically sensible.

The usual process controls are either physical or chemical checks on the technique (e.g. tests showing that the autoclave reached the desired temperature for the desired time). They do not show that there are no viable organisms remaining after the process, but this is assumed if the process satisfies the controls. However, the stringency of the controls can be altered intentionally or accidentally to give either an undersensitive or an oversensitive test.

### Disinfectants can be monitored by microbiologic in-use tests

These tests involve challenging the solution with a bacterial suspension and withdrawing samples, which are then treated to prevent carryover of the disinfectant and cultured. However, these tests are rarely performed in the hospital setting, where the use of disinfectants is guided largely by the manufacturer's recommendations.

## KEY FACTS

- Realization that infection can be associated with a variety of institutional settings has resulted in a preference for the term *healthcare-associated infection* rather than *hospital-acquired infection*.

- Nosocomial infection refers to infection acquired in the hospital.

- Healthcare-associated infections often have serious consequences for the individual, for the healthcare community and for the general community at large. They may be caused by almost any organism, but a few species cause the vast majority of infections.

- The healthcare environment favours the survival of resistant strains, and therefore infections are often caused by organisms with limited antibiotic susceptibility.

- MRSA, traditionally viewed as a problem in hospital infection, is increasingly seen in community-acquired infections in the absence of healthcare contact.

- Most common hospital infections are UTIs, respiratory tract infections, surgical wound infections and bacteraemia (septicaemia).

- The most important bacterial causes are gram-positive cocci (*staphylococci* and *streptococci*) and gram-negative rods (e.g. *E. coli, Pseudomonas*). Multiple antibiotic-resistant organisms are common. *Candida* is the significant fungal cause, and viruses probably cause more hospital infections than has been previously recognized.

- Infecting organisms originate from the patient's own flora (endogenous infection) or from other human or inanimate sources (exogenous or cross-infection). Airborne spread and contact spread are the most important routes of transmission.

- Host factors are of critical importance in determining susceptibility to infection.

- Surveillance should be an ongoing activity to facilitate early recognition of outbreaks of infection. Investigation of outbreaks involves both epidemiologic and microbiologic expertise. Molecular techniques to fingerprint the causative organism are becoming increasingly sophisticated.

- Prevention of healthcare-associated infections by excluding sources, interrupting transmission and enhancing the patient's resistance is fundamental to improving patient care and reducing costs.

- Sterilization and disinfection are key processes in the control and prevention of healthcare-associated infections as well as being central to many areas of medical practice.

# Index

Page numbers followed by "*f*" indicate figures, "*t*" indicate tables, "*b*" indicate boxes, and "*e*" indicate online content.

## A

A subunit, of toxins, 179–180
Abscess
  brain, 364, 365*t*
  in fever of unknown origin, 444
  liver, 324
    amoebic, 324, 325*f*
  lung, 219, 220*f*, 254, 255*f*
  peritonsillar, as complication of *Streptococcus pyogenes*, 208
*Acanthamoeba* spp., 354, 370
Acellular pertussis vaccines, for whooping cough, 217
Acetylcholine release, *Clostridium botulinum*, 365
Aciclovir, 395, 521*f*, 523, 525*f*
Acid-fast stains, for laboratory diagnosis of infection, 473
Acidosis, lactic, malaria and, 421
Acids, mechanisms to counteract, 121
Acne, 381, 381*f*
Acquired immune deficiency syndrome (AIDS), 279
  clinical definition of, 459
  HIV infection leading to, 280, 282*f*, 459
  opportunistic infections and tumours in, 287*t*
  progression to, 284, 287*f*
  treatment of, 286
Acquired immunodeficiency, 452
*Actinobacillus* spp., periodontal disease by, 212
Actinomyces, 388
  peritonitis and, 325
*Actinomyces viscosus*, periodontal disease by, 212
Active immunization, for whooping cough, 217
Acute bacterial prostatitis, in UTIs, 262
Acute bronchitis, 217
Acute epiglottitis, 211
Acute glomerulonephritis (AGN), 186, 187*f*, 379
  as complications of *Streptococcus pyogenes*, 209
Acute otitis media, 211, 211*f*

Acute phase proteins, 81, 81*f*, 82*t*, 137
Acute sinusitis, 211
Acute sore throat, 201
Acycloguanosine, 523
Adaptation, in host-parasite relationships, 113, 114*f*
Adaptive immune responses, 85
  antibody in
    classes and subclasses, 91, 94*t*
    structure and function of, 91, 91*f*–93*f*
  B cells in
    recirculation of, 92, 95*t*
    subsets of, 92
  innate and, 68*f*, 68
  key facts in, 96*b*
  lymphoid tissues in, 85, 86*f*, 86*t*
  secondary lymphoid organs in, 88, 89*f*–90*f*
  strategies to evade, 161
  subsets of T cells in, 88, 90*f*
  T cells in, 88, 91*f*
    recirculation of, 92, 95*t*
  thymus in, 85, 87*f*–88*f*
Adaptive immune system, 4
Adefovir, 332
Adenosine triphosphate (ATP), 7
Adenovirus infection, 241
Adenylate cyclase toxin, in *Bordetella pertussis* infection, 216
Adjuvants, in vaccines, 543, 544*f*, 545*b*
Adoptive immunotherapy, 559
*Aedes aegypti*
  chikungunya transmitted by, 411
  yellow fever transmitted by, 409
Aflatoxin, in disease, 178*t*
African tick-bite fever, 416
African trypanosomes, gene switching in, 167
AGN. *See* Acute glomerulonephritis
AIDS. *See* Acquired immune deficiency syndrome
Albendazole
  for *Giardia intestinalis* infection, 316
  for lymphatic filariasis, 427

Albert stain, 474
Alcohol disinfectants, 582*t*
Aldehyde disinfectants, 582*t*
Allergic bronchopulmonary aspergillosis (ABPA), *Aspergillus fumigatus* in, 255, 256*f*
Allylamines, 37
Alpha haemolysin, from diffusely adherent *E.coli*, 297
Alpha toxin, *Clostridium perfringens*, 380–381
Alveolar echinococcosis, 441
Alveolar hydatid disease, 441
Alveolar macrophages, destruction by, 119
Amantadine, 528
American trypanosomiasis, 403
Amikacin, 507, 508*t*
Amino acids, 7
Aminoglycoside-modifying resistance, 507, 508*f*
Aminoglycosides, 6–7, 12, 507
  classified by chemical structure, 508*t*
  indications for therapy, 508*b*
  resistance to, 15–16
Amniotic sac, 337
Amoebae, 128
  avoidance strategies for, 41
  CNS and, 156
  *E. histolytica* and, 314
Amoebic dysentery, 3
Amoxicillin for Lyme disease, 418
  for *Pasteurella multocida*, 438
Amphotericin B, 354
  for leishmaniasis, 425
Amplification-based techniques, 480
Amprenavir, 527
Amyotrophic lateral sclerosis, as possible viral etiology, 362
Anaemia iron-deficiency, hookworms and, 319
  severe, malaria and, 419
Anaerobic cellulitis, 380, 380*f*
Anal pruritus, pinworm infection and, 319
Anaphylaxis, 184
*Ancylostoma duodenale*, 317
  entry of, 118*t*
  microbial attachment of, 119*t*
Anergy, 166

*Anopheles*, 130–131, 132*f*
Antagonism, in combined antibacterial agents, 520, 520*f*
Anterior nasal diphtheria, 215
Anthrax, 14, 435, 436*f*
  infection, frequency of, 116*t*
Antibacterial agents, 495
  antibiotic, 495
  assays, 520, 520*b*
  bactericidal, 497
  bacteriostatic, 497
  beta-lactams, 500–501
  cell membrane targets, 497
  cell wall synthesis targets, 497
  chemical structure diversity, 497
  classes of, 499
  classification of, 497
  combinations, 520*b*
  design of, 496*b*
  evolution of resistance, 497*f*
  glycopeptides, 503
  metabolic pathways targets, 497
  nucleic acid synthesis targets, 497
  optimum use of, 500*t*
  in practice, 518
  properties of, 496*b*
  protein synthesis targets, 497
  resistance to, 497
  selective toxicity, 496, 532
  susceptibility tests for, 518
  synergism or antagonism effect of combined, 520, 520*f*
  targets, 497
Antibiotics, 495
  for acute epiglottitis, 211
  assays, 520, 520*b*
  broad-spectrum, *Clostridium difficile* diarrhoea and, 307
  for brucellosis, 440
  for cholera, 303
  for diphtheria toxin, 215
  for enteric fever, 323
  for infective endocarditis, 450
  for leptospirosis, 439
  for Lyme disease, 418

Antibiotics (Continued)
  for plague, 436
  prophylactic, for hospital infection, 574
  for secondary bacterial pneumonia, of measles, 250
  for Shigella diarrhoea, 304
  susceptibility, bacteria and, 472
Antibodies
  adaptor molecule, 98f
  affinity of, 144
  agglutinating and lytic, relapsing fever and, 417
  agglutination of, 145, 145f
  blocking and neutralizing effects of, 144
  for botulism, 365
  classes and subclasses of, 91, 94t, 144
  defect corrections, 564
  dengue haemorrhagic fever/dengue shock syndrome and, 410
  in enhancement of pathology, 188, 188f
  immobilization of, 145
  infection, detection methods for diagnosis of, 481
  monoclonal, 476
  production, 102, 104f
  B cells for, 103, 104f
  T-cell for, 102, 104f
  speed, amount and duration of, 143
  structure and function of, 91, 92f-93f
  type II hypersensitivity reactions and, 185, 185t
  for vaccines, 556
Antibody-dependent cellular cytotoxicity, 145, 146t
Antibody-mediated immunity, 143
Anticytokine antibodies, 563
Antifungals, 532
  applications of, 533t
  for dermatophytes, 386
  resistance to, 533
Antigenic drift, of influenza virus, 167, 242, 550f
Antigenic shift, of influenza virus, 168f, 242
Antigenic variation, 7-8, 167, 167f
  in relapsing fever, 417
  in T. brucei, 423
Antigenicity, inactivation of toxins and, 180
Antigens
  concealment of, 162
  microbial for immune modulation, 166
  noncultural techniques for detection of, 475, 475b
  stage-specific, 168
Antihelminthic drugs, applications of, 536t

Antimetabolites, affecting nucleic acid synthesis, 514
Antimicrobial agents, 495, 539b
  control strategies, 538, 538t
  microorganisms and human host, interactions between, 495f
  for prophylaxis or treatment, 538
  resistance to, 15-16
  selective toxicity, 495, 496b, 532
  susceptibility tests, 518
  targets for, 10, 12
  use and misuse of, 538
Antimicrobial chemicals, sterilization techniques and, 581, 582t
Antimicrobial peptides, in skin, 136
Antimicrobial therapy, for bacterial pneumonia, 226, 227t
Antimonials, for leishmaniasis, 425
Antimyocardial antibody, of group A β-haemolytic streptococcal infection, 186
Antiparasitic agents, 534
  resistance to, 534
Antiprotozoal drugs, applications of, 535t
Antipyretic drugs, 444
Antiretroviral drugs, 525
  for HIV, 267t, 284f, 285
Antiseptics
  definition of, 579
  for urinary tract, 517
Antiserum uses, in passive immunotherapy, 560
Antitoxin
  for diphtheria toxin, 215
  polyvalent, for botulism, 305
Antitrypanosomal antibody, detection of, for human African trypanosomiasis, 423
Anti-TB drugs, 253, 517
Antiviral therapy, 520
Apoptosis, 149
Arbovirus
  haemorrhagic fevers and, 409, 409t
  infections, 408
    arbovirus encephalitis, 412, 412t
    chikungunya virus infection as, 411
    dengue fever as, 410, 412t
    human stage of, 409
    yellow fever as, 409, 412t
    Zika virus as, 411
Arenavirus infections, 429
  diagnosis of, 430, 431b, 431f
  prevention of, 430

Arginine catabolic mobile elements (ACME), 19
Artemisinin combination therapy, 362
Artesunate, for malaria, 422
Arthralgia, 404, 405t
  from Lyme disease, 418
Arthritis, from Lyme disease, 418
Arthropod-borne togaviruses, as cause of meningitis/encephalitis, 360
Arthropods, 47, 129, 132t
  arboviruses and, 409
  blood-feeding, filarial nematodes transmitted by, 426
  conflicts on, 49b
  diseases transmitted by, 48t
  entry of, 118t
  infections, in skin, 390
  infestations, 290
  key facts on, 49b
  Rickettsia and, 414
Arthus reaction, in immune complex deposition, 186f, 187
Ascaris
  immunoglobulin E (IgE) in, 184
  in lower respiratory tract, 257
Ascaris lumbricoides, 317
  intestinal obstruction and, 318
  thick-shelled eggs of, 318, 318f
Asexual reproduction
  in fungi, 35
  in protozoa, 35
Aspergilloma, 255, 256f
Aspergillus fumigatus, 255, 256f
Aspergillus spp., 456, 459t
  in compromised patient, 461, 461f
  in lower respiratory tract, 255
Assays, antibacterial agents, 520, 520b
Astroviruses, diarrhea caused by, 311
Atazanavir, 527
Atmospheric pollution, susceptibility to infectious diseases and, 158t-159t
ATP. See Adenosine triphosphate
Attenuated pathogen, 157, 157t
Atypical lymphocytes, in Epstein-Barr virus, 204, 205f
Autoantibodies to Epstein-Barr virus, 204
  type II hypersensitivity reactions and, 185, 185t
Avian H5 virus infections, 244f

Azidothymidine (AZT), 526
Azithromycin, 267t, 273, 368-369
  for Campylobacter diarrhoea, 300
  for Chlamydia trachomatis, 267t
Azole, 37, 532
Aztreonam, 502-503

B
BCG, 552
Bone marrow transplantation programmes, 559
B subunit, of toxins, 179-180
Bacillary dysentery, 303
Bacille Calmette-Guérin (BCG)
  for leprosy, 383
  for tuberculosis, 552
Bacillus anthracis, 554
  causing anthrax, 435
  entry of, 118t
Bacillus cereus, 292t
  diarrhoeal infection caused by, 296t, 304
  food-associated infection and, 306, 307f
Bacitracin, 499-500
Bacteria, 2, 6, 459t, 462
  antibiotic susceptibility of, 472
  around time of birth infection, 343
  cell membrane, 497
  cell wall of, 7-8
    synthesis, 497
  classification of, 4, 4f
  CNS and, 348
  conflicts on, 26b
  diarrhoeal diseases caused by, 292
    clinical features of, 296t
  DNA in, 6-7
  endospores in, 14, 15f
  flagella in, 7
  gene expression in, 11, 23, 24f
  gene recombination in, 20
  gene regulation in, 12, 13f
  gene transfer in, 20, 22f
  gram-negative bacteria, 3
  gram-positive bacteria, 3, 4f
  growth and division in, 9, 9t, 10f
  growth requirements of, 470
  heterotrophic pathogenic bacteria, 8
  identification of, 470, 471f
  key facts on, 26b
  medically important bacteria, genomics of, 23
  metabolic pathways in, 8, 9f, 497
  mobile genetic elements in, 15
  mutation in, 20, 23, 24f
  nucleic acid synthesis, 497

Bacteria (Continued)
nucleoid in, 6–7
nutrition in, 8
obstetric and perinatal infections, 337
pathogenic bacteria, 8, 14
as pathogens of the gastrointestinal tract, 251t
pili, 7
protein synthesis, 497
repair processes in, 20, 21f
replication in, 10
shapes of, 7, 8f
structure of, 6, 6f
survival under adverse conditions, 14
transcription in, 11
translation in, 11
transposition in, 17
Bacterial colonies, 470f
Bacterial culture, significance of, UTI and, 263
Bacterial endocarditis, 444
Bacterial gyrase, 513f
Bacterial infections persistent, 171t
in skin, 376, 376t
Bacterial meningitis, 349, 349f
clinical features of, 351t
virulence factors in, 350t
Bacterial pneumonia, 223
antimicrobial therapy for, 226, 227t
diagnosis of, 226
in elderly, death in, 225
feeling unwell and fever in, 224
Gram stain and culture in, 225, 226f
prevention of, 226
primary atypical pneumonia, 223, 225f
secondary, in measles, 249, 249f
shadows in lung in, 225
sputum samples in, 225
Streptococcus pneumonia and, 223
Bacterial vaginosis, 276, 277f
Bactericidal antibacterial agents, 497
Bacteriophage (phage) typing, 576
Bacteriophages, 16
life cycle of, 17f
transduction, 21
Bacteriostatic antibacterial agents, 497
Bacteriuria, 262f
Bacteroides fragilis, peritonitis and, 325
Bacteroides spp., 345, 459t
in gut, 58
periodontal disease and, 212
Baghdad boil, 425
Balamuthia mandrillaris, 354
Balanitis, 275

Basic reproduction number (R0), 491, 492t
B-cell lymphomas, Epstein-Barr virus in, 207
Benznidazole, for Chagas disease, 424
Benzylpenicillin, 500
Beta-lactams, 500, 502f
characteristics of, 504t
glycopeptides versus, 503
side effects, 502
Bifidobacterium bifidum, 564
Biliary tract infections, 325
fever of unknown origin and, 444
Biochemical barriers, 69, 69f
Biological response gradient, 116
Biological transmission, 131, 132t
Biting arthropods, 118
Blackheads, 381f
Bladder, 259, 469
defences, 122
Blastocystis hominis, 317
Blastomyces dermatitidis, 388, 389f
skin rashes and, 189t
Blastomycosis, 388
Blocking type I interferons, 160
Blood, 469b
complement system, 482
pneumonia transmission via, 219
spread of infection in, 154, 154f
transmission from, 129
Blood culture, for infective endocarditis, 450
Blood films
for Chagas disease, 424
for malaria, 421
Blood monocytes, 71, 71f
Bloodborne invasion, 347
Blood-brain barrier, 347
structures of, 348f
Blood-CSF barrier, 347
structures of, 348f
Body's mechanical barriers
burns damage, 456
disruption of, 452
Bolivian haemorrhagic fever, 431b, 431f
Bone infections, 404
Bone marrow, 469b
chloramphenicol in, 507
transplant infections, 458
Bone marrow transplantation programmes, 559
Bordetella pertussis, 14, 216. See also whooping cough infection, 216
Borrelia afzelii, 417–418
Borrelia burgdorferi, 356, 417–418
Borrelia garinii, 417–418

Borrelia infections, 416
Lyme disease as, 417
relapsing fever as, 416
Borrelia recurrentis, 268t, 416
Borrelia vincentii, pharyngitis by, 207
Botulinum toxin, in disease, 180
Botulism, 305
Clostridium botulinum and, 305
food-borne, 305
forms of, 306
infant, 305
laboratory diagnosis of, 305–306
mortality rate of, 305
polyvalent antitoxin for, 305
prevention of, 306
wound, 306
Bovine spongiform encephalopathy (BSE), 2
Bradykinin, as inflammatory mediators, 79t
Brain, 347
abscesses, 364, 365t
clinical consequences of mumps in, 210t
congenital rubella in, 339
immune responses and, 159
Brill-Zinsser disease, 416
Bronchiolitis, 218
respiratory syncytial virus in, 218
Bronchitis
acute, 217
chronic, 217
Bronchopneumonia, 219, 220f
Brucella, 501
Brucellosis, 440, 440f
Brugia, 426–427
lymphatic filariasis caused by, 427, 427f
BSE. See Bovine spongiform encephalopathy
Buboes, in plague, 436
Budding, site of, surface/systemic infection and, 153, 153f
Bundle-forming pili, 294
Burkitt's lymphoma Epstein-Barr virus in, 191, 206, 206f
malaria and, 421
Burn wound infections, 456
major pathogens in, 456
BvgS, 14

**C**
C3a, as inflammatory mediators, 76
C5a, as inflammatory mediators, 79t
Calymmatobacterium granulomatis,, 275

Campylobacter
cultural requirements of diarrhoeal infection caused by, 299
azithromycin for, 300
clinical presentation of, 300
cultures for, 300
food-associated infections, 304
and reservoir of, 304
Candida albicans, otitis externa caused by, 211
Candida infection, 275
Candidalysin, 169
Candidiasis, 533t
systemic, 533t
Capsomeres, 27
Carbapenems, 10, 502f
Carbenicillin, 503
Carbon, as bacterial growth requirement
Caries, 212
Case-control studies, 486
'Cassettes' of resistance, resistance to antibacterial agents, 498
Catabolite activator protein (CAP), 12
Catalase, 8–9
Cataract, 340f
Cathelicidin, 70, 136
Catheter-associated infection, of urinary tract, 457
CCHF. See Crimean-Congo haemorrhagic fever
C3 convertase, 76
CD4 glycoprotein, 282
cDNA, 24
C3d receptor (CD21), in Epstein-Barr virus, 204
CDT. See Clostridium difficile transferase
CD8 T cells, 88–89
CD4 T-cell subsets, 90f
Cell differentiation, primary adaptive immunodeficiency from, 453
Cell lysis, viruses and, 32
Cell-mediated immune responses, 187
Cell-mediated immunity (CMI), 146
Cell rupture, in pathologic consequences of infection, 176
Cellular cytotoxicity, antibody-dependent, 145
Cellular prion protein (PrPᶜ), 51–52
Cephalosporins, 10, 211
Cephamycins, 504t
Cercopithecine herpesvirus, 356
Cerebral malaria, as CNS disease, 362
Chagoma, 423–424
Chlamydial infection, 367

Chancroid (soft chancre), 267t, 274
Chemical agents, sterilization techniques and, 581
Chemokine receptor antagonists, 527
Chemokine responses, 282
Chemokines, 93–95
Chiclero ulcer, 425
Chikungunya virus infection (CHIKV), 411
CHIKV. See Chikungunya virus infection
Chlamydia, growth of, 273
Chlamydiaceae
  medically important species of, 273t
Chlamydiae, tetracyclines for, 507
Chlamydial infection, life cycle of, 273
Chlamydia pneumoniae,, 223–224
Chlamydia psittaci,, 134
Chlorinated bisphenol disinfectants, 582t
Chloroquine-resistant antimalarial agents, 534
Cholesterol, 37
Chorioretinitis, CMV causing, 341
Chromosomal mutation, 498
Chronic bronchitis, acute exacerbations of, 217
Chronic mucocutaneous candidiasis, 459
Chronic wasting disease (CWD), 52
Ciclopirox, 533
Cidofovir, 203
Ciprofloxacin, 275
Cirrhosis
  defined, 330
  hepatitis B and, 328
Clavulanate, for Pasteurella multocida,, 438
Clavulanic acid, betalactamases, 502
Clindamycin, 510
Clonal expansion, 102
Cloning and manipulating genes, plasmids for, 16
Clonorchis sinensis,, 44
Clostridium botulinum
  acetylcholine release, 365
  clinical features of, 365
  exotoxins produced by
  food poisoning from, 365
Clostridium difficile transferase (CDT), 307
Clostridium perfringens
  diarrhoeal disease caused by, 380f
  food-associated infection from, 291
Clostridium tetani,, 15f, 345
Clotrimazole, 267t
Coagulase-negative staphylococci, 446t

Coagulase-positive staphylococci, 505
Coccidioides immitis infection, 354
Coccidioidomycosis, 388
Cohort studies, 486
Cold sores, herpes simplex virus infection and, 393
Collagen-vascular disease, fevers and, 444
Collectins, 137
Colorado tick fever, 406t
Combination antiretroviral therapy (cART), 520–521
Combination therapy, for tuberculosis, 253
Combinatorial library, 561
Combined agents, antagonism or synergism effects of, susceptibilities, 520
Commensalism, of symbiotic associations, 59
Community-associated MRSA (CA-MRSA), 568
Complement synthesis, of innate immunity, 452
Complement system, 76
  activation of
    immune complexes in, 186
    in natural immune mechanism, 180
  acute inflammatory response in, 76
Complex intracellular signalling, 101
Confounding bias, concepts, CNS and, 490
Congenital and neonatal listeriosis, 343
Congenital CMV infection, 340
Congenital infections, 338
Congenital rubella, 339
Congenital syphilis, 342
Congenital varicella syndrome, 396
Congo-Crimean haemorrhagic fever, 409t
Conjunctiva, entry by, 118
Conjunctivitis, 367
Contact lenses, eye infection and, 370
Contaminated objects, environmental from, as source of infection, 569
Convalescence, of epidemic typhus, 416
Corneal scarring, 370
Coronavirus 2019 (COVID-19) pandemic, 560
Coronavirus infections, 240
Corticosteroids, 231
  for fever of unknown origin, 444
  for parasitic worm infections, in eyes, 372
Corynebacterium diphtheriae, 214
Co-trimoxazole, trimethoprim and, 515

Councilman bodies, 410
COVID-19 disease, 563
COVID-19 vaccines, 551b, 551
  manufacturers and types, 240t
Coxiella burnetii, causing Q fever, 238
Coxsackie virus infections, 397
C-reactive protein, 137
Creutzfeldt-Jakob disease (CJD), 2
Crimean-Congo haemorrhagic fever (CCHF), 156
CRISPR/Cas9 gene editing, 565f
CRISPR/Cas9 system, 564
Crohn disease, 563
Crude mechanical devices, for attachment, 121
Cryotherapy, 392
Cryptococcosis, 354
Cryptococcus neoformans, 388
Cryptosporidiosis, 535t
Cryptosporidium hominis
Cryptosporidium parvum, 313f
Cutaneous dermatophytes, 384
Cutaneous larval migrans, 389f, 389
Cutaneous mycoses, 388
CWD. See Chronic wasting disease
Cyclic adenosine monophosphate (cAMP)
Cycloserine, 499–500
Cyclospora,, 317
Cyclospora cayetanensis,, 40, 41f, 313
Cysticercosis, of CNS diseases, 363
Cystic fibrosis, as lower respiratory tract infections, 523
Cystic hydatid disease, 324, 363
Cystitis, 260
Cystoisospora,, 317
Cystoisospora belli, AIDS patients infected with, 313
Cytokines, in cell-cell interactions, 103
Cytokine storm, 169
Cytokine synthesis inhibitory factor, 105
Cytomegalovirus infection, 250
Cytoplasm, 73
Cytoplasmic membrane function, inhibitors of, 516
Cytotoxic granules, phagocytic, 140
Cytotoxic T cells, 105
Cytotoxin, in disease, 178t

**D**
Dane particles, 331–332
Dapsone, 514f
  for leprosy, 383
Daptomycin, 516, 517f

Councilman bodies, 410
Dark field microscopy, for laboratory diagnosis of infection, 474, 474f
Darunavir, 527
Deep mycoses, 36, 36f
Deer, chronic wasting disease in, 52, 53f
Defensins, 73–74, 136
Demeclocycline, 509f
Dendritic cells, 98–99
Dendritic ulcer, from keratitis, 332–334, 333f
Dengue fever, 370
  dengue haemorrhagic fever/dengue shock syndrome and, 410, 411f
  transmission of, 410
  vaccine for, 411
Dengue haemorrhagic fever (DHF), 410
Dengue shock syndrome (DSS), 410
Dental caries, 57
Dental plaque, 212f
Deoxynucleotide triphosphate bases (dNTPs), 478–479
Deoxyribonucleic acid (DNA), 6–7
  agents that affect, 516
  CMV, 340
  microarrays, 23, 24f
  molecular typing techniques involve characterizing, 576
  polymerase, prodrugs that target, 523
  repair processes, 20, 21f
  analysis, 577
  in Ebola virus outbreak, 484b
  polymerase chain reaction (PCR) and, 477
  transcription, 11
  transposition, 17
  viral, 30–31, 193–194
Dermacentor variabilis, Rocky Mountain spotted fever transmitted by, 415
Dermatobia, 390
Dermatobia hominis, 47
Dermatophytes, 384–385
  diagnosis of, 385, 386f
  in skin, hair and nails, 385
  skin rashes and, 189t
  treatment of, 386
Dermicidin, 136
Diarrhoea, 292
  antibiotic-associated, 306
  bacterial causes of, 293
    campylobacter as, 299
    clinical features of, 296t
    clostridioides difficile as, 306–307, 307f
    Escherichia coli as, 293
    Salmonella as, 297
    Shigella as, 303
    Vibrio cholerae as, 301

Diarrhoea (Continued)
*Vibrio parahaemolyticus*
as, 304
*Yersinia enterocolitica* as,
304, 304*f*
bacterial toxin-associated,
304
botulism and, 305
*Staphylococcus aureus*
and, 305
in children, mortality in, 292,
294*f*
Cryptosporidia and, 316
deaths from, reductions in,
308, 308*f*
defined, 291*b*
*Entamoeba histolytica*
infection and, 314, 314*f*
*Giardia intestinalis* infections
and, 316
as pathologic consequences
of infection, 180, 181*f*,
181*t*
Trichuris trichiura and,
319*f*
viral causes of, 308
adenoviruses as, 311
astroviruses as, 311
coronaviruses as, 311
noroviruses as, 309
rotaviruses as, 309
sapoviruses as, 311
Dideoxy chain terminator,
sequencing-based
techniques, 478, 479*f*
Dideoxynucleotide (ddNTPs),
478–479
Diethylcarbamazine (DEC), for
filariasis, 427
Diffusely aggregative E. coli
(DAEC), 293
Diffusion susceptibility tests,
518, 518*f*
Diguanide disinfectants, 582*t*
Dihydroxypropoxy-
methylguanine, 525
Dilution susceptibility tests,
518, 519*f*
Dimorphic fungi, 35
Diphtheria, 214, 214*f*
false membrane of, 214–215,
214*f*
immunization for contacts
of, 216
nasopharyngeal, 215
pharyngeal, 214*f*
toxin, 215, 215*b*, 215*f*
antibiotics for, 215
in disease, 178*t*
fatal heart failure by, 215
polyneuritis by, 215
in protein synthesis, 216
vaccine, 546
Diphyllobothrium latum, 320,
320*f*
Dipsticks, for malaria, 421
Direct-acting antivirals, for
hepatitis C, 334

Disinfectants, use in hospitals,
582*t*
Disinfection. *See also*
Sterilization and
disinfection
definition of, 579
Disseminated aspergillosis,
*Aspergillus fumigatus*
in, 255
Disseminated candidiasis, 460,
460*f*
Disseminated intravascular
coagulation, in bacterial
septicaemia, 183
Dolutegravir, 526
Domestic pets, transmission
via, 134, 134*f*
Donovanosis, 275
Double-blinded studies, 490
Doxycycline, 267*t*, 273–274,
507, 509*f*
for Lyme disease, 418
microscopy and treated
with, 275
*Drosophila*, 73
Drugs
congenital infections for, 338
inactivation, mechanism
of resistance to
antibacterial agents, 499
Dry cough, in acute bronchitis,
217
dsDNA, mobile genetic
elements and, 15
dsRNA viruses, 29, 30*f*
Duffy antigen, 419
Duodenal ulcers, *Helicobacter
pylori* and, 312, 312*f*
Dysentery defined, 291*b*
in Entamoeba histolytica
infection, 314, 315*f*, 315*t*
Dysuria, in UTIs, 262

**E**
Ears
CNS and, 347
congenital rubella affecting,
339
Ebola virus disease (EVD), 432,
432*f*, 434*b*
EBV. *See* Epstein-Barr virus
Echinocandins, 532
*Echinococcus*, 441
*Echinococcus granulosus*, 324,
441
in lower respiratory tract,
257
*Echinococcus multilocularis*, 441
'Eclipse phase,' in viruses, 29
Eczema herpeticum, 394, 395*f*
Efavirenz, 527
Effector memory T cells, 106*t*
Effector T cells, 106*t*
El Tor biotype, of *Vibrio
cholerae*, 301
Elephantiasis, 427, 427*f*
ELISA. *See* Enzyme-linked
immunosorbent assay

ELISPOT technique, for cells
secreting antibodies or
cytokines, 483, 483*f*
Elvitegravir, 526
Emetic toxin, 306
Empyema, lung abscess and,
254
Emtricitabine, for hepatitis B,
529
Encephalitis
arbovirus, 409, 412*t*
in genital herpes, 276
HSV, 356
post-infectious, 362
rabies, 358
*Encephalitozoon intestinalis*, 462
Endemic (murine) typhus, 416
Endospores, 14, 15*f*
Endotoxin shock, 182
Endotoxins
in *Bordetella pertussis*
infection, 216
entry of, 122
induced tumour necrosis
factor (TNF), 182, 183*t*
in natural
immunemechanism,
181–182, 182*f*
Enfuvirtide, 527
*Entamoeba coli*, in gut, 57
*Entamoeba histolytica*, 314
four-nucleate cysts of,
instool, 315, 315*f*
infection, 290, 314
complications of, 315
diagnosis of, 315
dysentery in, 315*f*, 315*t*
mild diarrhoea in, 314, 315*f*
treatment for, 315
liver abscess and, 324
in lower respiratory tract,
256–257
metronidazole for, 516
microbial attachment of, 120*t*
transmission of, 314
Entecavir, 299, 530
Enteric fever, 321
antibiotic treatment for, 323
chronic carriers of, 323
complications of, 322, 324*f*
diagnosis of, 323
prevention of, 323
rose spots and, 322, 322*f*
*Salmonella* and, 297
*Salmonella typhi* and
*Salmonella paratyphi* and,
321
transport of, in
macrophages, 321, 322*f*
Enteroaggregative E. coli
(EAEC), 293, 297
*Enterobacteriaceae,,* 459*t*
*Enterobius vermicularis*, 318
anal pruritus and, 319
eggs of, in perianal skin, 319,
320*f*
*Encephalitozoon intestinalis*, 317
Enterocolitis, defined, 291*b*

*Enterocytozoon bieneusi*, 317, 462
Enterohaemorrhagic E. coli
(EHEC), 293, 297*f*
diarrhoeal infection and,
296*t*, 297
Enteroinvasive E. coli (EIEC),
293, 297
Enteropathogenic E. coli
(EPEC), 293, 296*f*
diarrhoeal infection and,
296*t*, 297
Enterotoxigenic E. coli (ETEC),
293, 296*f*
diarrhoeal infection and,
296*t*, 297
Enterotoxins
cholera and, 302, 302*f*
in disease, 178*t*
from enterotoxigenic E.coli,
293
heat-labile (LT-I), 294–296
heat-stable, 294–296
from *Staphylococcus aureus*,
305, 305*t*
Enteroviral infection, 356
Enterovirus 70, 367
Enteroviruses, 200*t*, 347, 397
skin rashes and, 189*t*
Entry, 117, 135*b*
general principle of, in STI,
266
sites of, 117
virus, 360
of viruses, 27–28, 28*f*
Enzyme-linked
immunosorbent assay
(ELISA), 285*f*, 363, 418
Enzymes
in bacteria, 176
mechanisms to counteract,
121
probes and, restriction of,
577, 578*f*
Eosinophilia, tropical
pulmonary, 427
Eosinophils, 140, 141*t*
against large parasites, 80,
80*f*
Epidemic typhus, 416
convalescence of, 416
mortality of, 416
Epidemiology, definition of,
485
*Epidermophyton*, 384, 385*f*
Epstein-Barr virus (EBV)
infections, 29*t*, 32
in cancer, 189*t*, 189, 206
clinical features of, 204, 205*f*
infection
frequency of, 116*t*
lead to tumour
development, 464
persistent, 171*t*
infectious mononucleosisby,
201, 202*f*
latent, 204
in pharyngitis, 204
in saliva, 204

Epstein-Barr virus (EBV)
    infections (Continued)
    skin rashes and, 189t
    treatment of, 206
    viral capsid antigen IgM
        detection for, 206
Eradication, control versus, 538
Ergosterol, 37
Erysipelas, 376, 378, 379f
Erythema migrans, in
        Lymedisease, 418, 418f
Erythema nodosum leprosum,
        383
Erythromycin, 12, 509,
        510f–511f
    for chancroid (soft chancre),
        274
    for streptococcal skin
        infections, 379
    for whooping cough, 216
Escherichia coli, 458
    causing infection, 567, 569b
    as common cause of UTI, 259
    diarrhoeal disease and, 180,
        293
    diffusely aggregative, 293
    in endotoxin shock, 182
    enteroaggregative, 293
    enterohaemorrhagic, 293,
        297f
    enteroinvasive, 293
    enteropathogenic, 293
    enterotoxigenic, 293
    growth and division in, 9
    microbial attachment of, 120t
    nutrition in, 8
    pathotypes of, 293, 295t
    pili in, 7
    shiga-toxin-producing, 293
    tests for, 297
Espundia, 425
Ethambutol, 517
Ethylene oxide gas,sterilization
        techniquesand, 581
Etravirine, 527
Eukaryotes, 2, 2f, 63
EVD. See Ebola virus disease
Exanthem subitum, 398, 398f
Exit, 117, 135b
    general principle of, in STI,
        266
Exotoxins, 178t, 380
    from Clostridium botulinum,
        306
    from Clostridium difficile, 307
    entry of, 122
    mode of action of, 177f
    in serious tissue damage,
        176, 177t
Extracellular
        antimicrobialfactors, 81
Extracellular pathogens, 4
Extrinsic allergic alveolitis, 187
Eye
    congenital rubella affecting,
        339
    infections, 367. See also
        Conjunctivitis

Eye (Continued)
    from bacteria, 370, 371f
    chlamydial infections in,
        367
    from contact lenses, 370
    in deeper layers, 371, 371t
    parasitic worm infections
        in, 372
    toxoplasmosis in, 372, 372f
    transmission of, 370
Eyelid infections, 367

F
FACS. See Fluorescence
        activated cell sorter
'Facultative' oxygen
        requirements, 8
Faecal Helicobacter pylori
        antigen testing, 312
Faecal microbiota
        transplantation, 308
Faecal-oral route
    gastrointestinal infections
        and, 292
    helminths transmission
        through, 43, 43f
    hepatitis A virus transmitted
        by, 326, 327f
    hepatitis E virus spread by,
        327
False membrane, of diphtheria,
        214, 214f
Famciclovir, 370, 395
Fasciola hepatica, 324
Fatal heart disease, Chagas
        disease and, 423, 424f
Fetus, 338
    around time of birth
        infection, 343, 344f
    infections in, 338, 338t
    rubella and, 341b
Fever, 182, 183b, 444
    African tick-bite, 416
    in bacterial pneumonia, 223
    collagen-vascular disease
        and, 444
    dengue, 410, 412t
    fluctuating, malaria and,
        419, 420f
    haemorrhagic, arboviruses
        and, 409, 412t
    as immune defence, 139
    in infective endocarditis, 448
    mechanism of, 445f
    relapsing, 416
    rickettsial infection and, 414
    spotted
        Mediterranean, 415
        Rocky Mountain, 415, 416f
    yellow, 409, 412t
Fever of unknown origin, 444
    causes of, 444, 446t
    definitions of, 444, 445t
    history taking for, 445
    infective causes of, 444
    investigation of, 445, 447b
    non-invasive
        investigationsfor, 446

Fever of unknown origin
        (Continued)
    physical examination for, 445
    screening tests for, 445
    in specific patient group,
        447, 449t
    therapeutic trials for, 447
    treatment of, 447
Fibrin breakdown products,
        as inflammatory
        mediators, 79t
Fibrinopeptides, as inflammatory
        mediators, 79t
Ficolins, 137
Fidaxomicin, 510
Filamentous fungal pathogens,
        35, 37f
Filaria infection, persistent, 171t
Filarial nematodes
    entry of, 118t
    transmission of, by blood-
        feeding arthropod
        vectors, 426
Filariasis, 426
    caused by Brugia and
        Wuchereria, 427, 427f
    lymphatic, 427, 427f
    transmission of, 426
    treatment for, 427
Filtration, sterilization
        techniques and, 580
Fimbrial adhesins, 294
    plasmid-associated, 297
Finger printing, epidemiological,
        molecular techniques
        for, 579
Flagella, 7
Flavivirus infections, 360
Flea, of rats, endemic typhus
        transmitted by, 416
'Flesh-eating bacteria', 380
Flow cytometry, 482f
    for cells secreting antibodies
        or cytokines, 483
    for cytotoxic T cells, 483
Fluconazole, 267t, 275
Flucytosine, 354
    inhibit nucleic acid
        synthesis, 532
Flukes, 44
    schistosomiasis and, 44
    transmission of, 45t
Fluorescence microscopy, for
        laboratory diagnosis of
        infection, 473–474, 475f
Fluorescence-activated cell
        sorter (FACS), 482–483
Fluoroquinolones, 514
    for Campylobacter diarrhoea,
        304
Folic acid, 517f
Folliculitis, 376, 377f
Food poisoning, 304
    botulism and, 305
    in diarrhoea, 180
    versus food-associated
        infection, 291
    Staphylococcus aureus and, 305

Food-associated infection,
        versus food poisoning,
        291
Foreign bodies, susceptibility
        to infectious diseases
        and, 158t–159t
Formalin ethyl acetate, 316
Formalin-ether, 316
Fosamprenavir, 527
Foscarnet, 203, 521f, 525
Francisella tularensis, causing
        tularaemia, 437
Free-living fungi, 36
FTA-ABS test, syphilis and,
        269, 270f
Fungal infections
    in lower respiratory tract,
        254
    on skin, 384
Fungal meningitis, 354
Fungi, 35, 459, 459t
    classification of, 35, 36f
    as common cause of UTI,
        260
    control of infection, 37
    disease-causing, 37t
        major groups of, 35
    growth requirements of, 470
    identifying, 472, 472f
    inhalation of, occupational
        diseases associated
        with, 187
    subcutaneous mycoses, 36
    superficial mycoses, 35–36, 36f
    systemic or deep mycoses,
        35–36, 36f
Fusidic acid, 512
Fusion inhibitors, 527

G
GALT. See Gut-associated
        lymphoid tissue
Gamma irradiation,
        sterilization techniques
        and, 581
Gamonts, 316–317
Ganciclovir, 203, 341, 525
Gangrene, 379
    synergistic bacterial, 380
Gardnerella vaginalis, 276
Gas gangrene, 380–381, 380f
Gastroenteritis, 345
    defined, 291b
    noroviruses and, 309
    Shigella infection and, 303
Gastrointestinal candidiasis, 460
Gastrointestinal tract
    as site of entry, 119,
        120t–121t
    transmission from, 127
Gastrointestinal tract
        infections, 291
    damage resulting from, 292b
    diarrhoeal diseases as, 292
    food-associated, versus food
        poisoning, 291
    gastric ulcer disease as,
        Helicobacter pylori and, 312

Gastrointestinal tract infections (Continued)
grouping of, 293f
host defences against, 291, 292f
parasites in, 313, 313f
protozoan, 313, 313f
worms as, 317
systemic infections and, 321
biliary tract infections as, 325
enteric fevers as, 321
listeriosis as, 323
liver abscesses as, 324
parasitic infections
affecting the liver as, 323
peritonitis and intra-abdominal sepsis as, 325, 325f
viral hepatitis as, 325, 326t
GB virus C. See Hepatitis G virus infections
Gene conjugation, 22, 22f
Gene conversion, 168
Gene expression
altering, 12
in bacteria, 12
DNA microarrays and, 23, 24f
regulation of, 12, 13f
Gene recombination, 20
Gene regulation, in bacteria, 12, 13f
Gene switching, 167
Gene transduction, 21, 22f
Gene transfer, in bacteria, 20, 22f
Gene transformation, 21, 22f
Genes, detection of microbes by, 477
Genital herpes, 266, 267t, 276, 277f
Genital warts, 278
Genome sequencing, 4
Genomes, bacterial, 10
mobile genetic elements and, 19, 19f
Genomics
DNA microarrays and, 23, 24f
of medically important bacteria, 23
'parallel processing' in, 23
Gentamicin, 507, 508t
Germ-free animals, microbiota in, 58
Germinal centre, in antibody production, 102, 103f
Giardia intestinalis, 290, 316
assemblages of, 315
infection, 316
diagnosis of, 316
drugs for, 316
life cycle stages of, 315
metronidazole for, 516
transmission of, 315
trophozoites of, 315, 315f
in stool, 315–316
Giardia intestinalis, microbial attachment of, 120t

Giemsa stain, 276f
Glomerulonephritis, 379
Glutaraldehyde, liquid, sterilization techniques and, 581
Glycopeptides, 10, 503
characteristics of, 505t
resistance, 505
side effects, 505
Gonococcal ophthalmia neonatorum, 345f
Gonococcal-induced inflammatory responses, 270
Gonorrhoea, 266, 270
asymptomatic, 270, 272f
diagnosis of, 271
frequency of infection, 116t
local and systemic spread of, 272f
Gram stain
in bacterial pneumonia, 225, 226f
for laboratory diagnosis of infection, 473, 474f
Gram-negative bacteria, 3
beta-lactamases of, 503f
cell wall of, 7, 7f
nutrition in, 8
resistance issues, 497
Gram-negative opportunist, otitis externa caused by, 211
Gram-negative rod, 259
Gram-positive bacteria, 3, 4f
beta-lactamases of, 503f
cell wall of, 7, 7f
resistance issues, 497
Granuloma formation, 188
Granulysin, 149
Granzymes, 149
Griseofulvin, inhibits nucleic acid synthesis, 532
Group A β-haemolytic streptococcal infection, antimyocardial antibody of, 186
Group B streptococci, 353t
Growth and division, in bacteria, 9, 9t, 10f
Guillain-Barré syndrome, 361
Campylobacter and, 299
Gut bacteria, 58
Gut decontamination regimens, for hospital infection, 574
Gut-associated lymphoid tissue (GALT), 348f

H
H1N1 influenza strain, 243
H5N1 avian influenza, 243
H7N7 influenza, 243
H9N2, influenza A virus, 243
Haemagglutinin, 5
in influenza virus envelope, 241f, 242
Haemagogus, yellow fever and, 410

Haematological malignancy, 458
Haematuria, 262
Haemolysins, 179
in disease, 178t
Haemolytic-uraemic syndrome (HUS), 296
from enterohaemorrhagic E.coli, 296
Haemophilus ducreyi, 267t, 274
Haemophilus influenzae, 458
acute, 352–353
acute epiglottitis caused by, 211
acute otitis media caused by, 211
CNS and, 347
eyelid infections due to, 367
microbial attachment of, 119t
pharyngitis by, 207
strains, inflammation and, 183, 184f
Haemophilus influenzae type b (Hib), vaccination with, 549, 549f
Haemophilus meningitis, 351
Haemopoietic system, infections of, 406, 406t
Haemorrhagic colitis (HC), from enterohaemorrhagic E.coli, 268–270
Haemorrhagic conjunctivitis, 367
Haemorrhagic cystitis, polyomaviruses causing, 165
Haemorrhagic fever
Ebola and Marburg, 432
with renal syndrome, 431–432
Hair, dermatophytes in, 385, 385f
Halogen disinfectants, 582t
Haloprogin, 533
Hand, foot, and mouth disease, 397, 397f
Hand washing, for controlling hospital infection, 573, 573f–574f
Hantavirus pulmonary syndrome (HPS), 219
Healthcare workers (HCWs), hepatitis B virus transmission in, 329
Healthcare-associated infections, 567, 568f
antibiotic susceptibility patterns for, 576
corrective/preventive measures of, 579
in epidemiological terms, 575
investigating, 575
isolation strategies in, 575
outbreak investigations for, 575
phenotypic and genotypic characters for, 576

Haematological malignancy (Continued)
sterilization and disinfection of, 579
surveillance in, 575
tracking, stages in, 575
typing techniques for
bacteriophage, 576
epidemiological, 576
molecular, 576
specialized, 576
Heart
congenital rubella affecting, 339
failure, fatal, by diphtheria toxin, 215
murmur, in infective endocarditis, 449, 450f
Heat, sterilization techniques and, 580
Helicobacter pylori, 299
duodenal ulcers and, 312, 312f
eradication by, 312–313
gastric ulcer disease and, 312
diagnosis of, 312
in gut, 57
neutralization strategy of, 122
persistence of, 312
virulence factors of, 312
Helminth infections, 425, 441
filariasis as, 426
caused by Brugia and Wuchereria, 427, 427f
lymphatic, 427, 427f
transmission of, 427
treatment for, 427
schistosomiasis as, 425
clinical features of, 426
diagnosis of, 426
praziquantel for, 426, 426f
transmission of, 426, 426f
urinary, 426f
Helminths, 43, 463
disease and, 44
identifying, 472
key facts on, 45b
life cycles of, 44
soil-transmitted, 317
transmission of, 318
survival in hosts, 44
transmission of, 43, 43f
Hepadna viruses, 329
Hepatitis
defined, 325
during pregnancy, 337
vaccines against, 553, 553f
viral, 325, 326t
transfusion-associated non-A-non-B, 333
transmission of, 326
Hepatitis A virus infections, 290, 326, 329
in children, 326
clinical and immunological course of, 327f
transmission of, 326, 327f

Hepatitis B immunoglobulin (HBIG), 333
Hepatitis B virus infections, 30–31, 290, 326, 329, 330f, 459t
  antibodies of, 330t
  antigens of, 330t
  antivirals for, 267t, 332, 531
  in cancer, 190t, 192, 193b
  carriers of, 329
  cell infected by, hepatitis D and, 335
  complications of, 331
  diagnosis of, 331, 332t
  immunization for, 333
  pathology of, immune mediated, 329
  prevention of, 333
  transmission of, 329
  treatments, 520–521, 529
Hepatitis C virus infections, 29t, 326, 333, 344, 459t
  antivirals, 531
  in cancer, 190t, 192
  chronic, 331
  direct-acting antivirals for, 334
  genotypes of, 334
  transfusion-associated non-A-non-B hepatitis and, 334
  transmission of, 334
  treatments, 520–521, 530
Hepatitis D virus infections, 326, 335
  hepatitis B virus infected cell and, 335
  spread of, 335
  structure of, 335f
Hepatitis E virus infections, 327
  genotypes of, 328
  incubation period of, 328
  reservoir for, 328
  spread of, 327
Hepatitis G virus infections, 335
Hepatocellular carcinoma, hepatitis B in, 192, 193f, 331
Herd immunity, 451, 542f
Herpes simplex virus infections, 267t, 276, 337
  aciclovir for, 523
  conjunctival infection and, 370, 370f
  infection, persistent, 171t
  on skin, 393, 394f
  in viral pneumonia, 227t
Herpes zoster, 464
Herpesviruses, 30–31, 459t
Heterotrophic pathogenic bacteria, 8
Hib vaccine, 352
Histamine, as inflammatory mediators, 79t
Histoplasma capsulatum infection, 459t
  in immunocompromised patients, 460, 460f

Histoplasmosis, 36
HIV. See Human immunodeficiency virus
HLA. See Human leukocyte antigens
HNIG. See Human normal immunoglobulin
Hodgkin's lymphoma, Epstein-Barr virus (EBV) in, 191
Horizontal transmission, 130, 131f
Hormones, susceptibility to infectious diseases and, 158t–159t
Hospital-acquired infections, 264, 567
  affecting both patient and community, 571
  in air and common vehicle, 570f, 570
  airborne transmission of, control of, 573
  aseptic behaviours, facilitation of, 573
  associated bacteraemias and candidaemias, 574
  associated with indwelling devices, 567, 568f
  boosting specific immunity, 574
  breaking the infection chain, 573
  consequences of, 571
  healthcare setting, seen outside of, 568, 569b
  host factors and, 570
  host resistance to, 574
  important causes of, 567
  invasive devices, care of, 574
  in people and contaminated objects, 569, 570f–571f
  postoperative infection risks of, 572t
  reducing, 574
  prevention of, 572
    strategies for, 572
  prophylactic antibiotics, appropriate use of, 574
  sources and routes of exclusion of, 572
    spread of, 569
  staphylococci, Escherichia coli, 567, 569b
  underlying disease, certain treatments, invasive procedure and, 570, 571t
  UTI, 259
  viral infections, 569
  wound infection factors, 571
Host
  adaptations of, for changes in parasites, 64
  cells of, bacterial parasite in, evolution of, 62, 62f
  controlling parasite development, 61
  evolution of, pressure of infection in, 63, 63t

Host (Continued)
  genetic determinants in, 157
  inflammatory and immune responses of, parasite adaptations in, 63
Host adaptive responses, 110, 113f
Host apoptotic responses, pathogen interference with, 170
Host defence systems
  assessment of, 468, 484b
  against gastrointestinal tract infections, 291
  microbes evolution in, 110, 110t, 113, 114f
  microbial evasion strategies and, 110t, 110, 111t–112t
Host immunodeficiency, correction of, 564
Host specificity, in viruses, 28, 29t
Host-derived molecules, prions as, 51, 53
Host-parasite relationships, 56
  adaptation in, 113, 114b, 114f
  changes in parasites and, 64
  commensalism in, 60
  host adaptive responses, speed with, 110, 113f
  host evolution in, 63, 63t
  microbiota and microbiome in, 56
  mutualism in, 60
  parasitism in, 60
    evolution of, 61
  social and behavioural changes in, 64, 64t
  symbiotic associations in, 59
HPS. See Hantavirus pulmonary syndrome
HPV. See Human papillomavirus
HSV. See Herpes simplex virus infections
Human adenoviruses, in cells, 193
Human African trypanosomiasis, 422
  clinical features of, 422, 423f
  host defence evasion in, 423, 423f
  transmission of, 423
Human antitetanus immunoglobulin, 365
Human bocavirus (hBoV), 241
Human herpesvirus (HHV-6), 391t, 398, 459t, 464
Human herpesvirus-7 (HHV-7), 398, 459t, 464
Human herpesvirus-8 (HHV-8), 32, 398, 459t, 464
Human immunodeficiency virus (HIV), 29t, 260
  antivirals, 495
  clinical features of, 284, 286f
  congenital infection in, 343
  definition of, 279

Human immunodeficiency virus (HIV) (Continued)
  early spread of, 283f
  early stages of, 266
  infection
    frequency of, 116t
    leading to AIDS, 459
    malaria and, 421
    persistent, 171t
    visceral leishmaniasis and, 424
  laboratory tests for, 286
  measures to control spread of, 288, 288f
  personalized medicine for, 481
  Pneumocystis jirovecii in, 484
  during pregnancy
    primary, 284
    replication cycle, 282f
    routes of transmission of, 283, 284f
    skin rashes and, 189t
    structure and genetic map of, 281f
    treatment of, 285, 520–521
    vaccines, 289, 554
Human leukocyte antigens (HLA), 99
Human liver fluke, 323–324
Human memory CD4 T-cell subsets, 106t
Human metapneumovirus infections (hMPV), 241
Human normal immunoglobulin (HNIG), 326–327
Human papillomavirus (HPV) infections, 32–33
  in cancer, 190t, 191
  entry of, 118t
  vaccines, 553
Human parvovirus B19 infections, 29t, 339
Human retroviruses, 280t
Human rhinovirus infections, 29t
Human T-cell lymphotropic virus (HTLV) infections, 344–345
Human T-cell lymphotropic virus type 1 (HTLV-1) infections, 32, 280t
  in cancer, 189, 190t
  infection, 406
Human T-cell lymphotropic virus type 2 (HTLV-2) infections, 407, 280t
HUS. See Haemolytic-uraemic syndrome
Hybridomas, 476
Hydatid cysts, 164f
Hydrogen, as bacterial growth requirement, 9t
5-Hydroxytryptamine (5HT-serotonin), as inflammatory mediators, 79t

Hygiene hypothesis, 184–185
*Hymenolepis nana*, 44, 320, 320*f*
Hyperimmune plasma, for influenza virus infection, 248–249
Hypoglycaemia, malaria and, 421

**I**
'Iceberg' concept, of infectious disease, 116*f*, 116
IL-6 receptor, 563
IL-8 (CXCL8), as inflammatory mediators, 79*t*
Immature T cells, 85
Immediate hypersensitivity, 502–503
Immune complex deposition, in tissues, 183–184
Immune defences, 136
    key facts, 151*b*
Immune modulation, as antigen concealment strategy, 165
Immune responses, 97
    antibody production in, 102
        B cells for, 103
        T cell for, 102
    armies, controlling, 105
    beneficial inflammatory reactions in, 97
    clonal expansion in, 102
    complex intracellular signalling in, 101
    cytokines in, 103
    efficiency in, 97
    immunological memory, 103
    monoclonal antibody in, 103
    opsonization in, 97
    pathologic consequences of, 184
        hypersensitivity, 184
    regulation of, 107*f*
    T cells, activation of, 98
        additional signals for, 100
        with gdTCR, 101
        superantigens in, 101
Immunity, phagocytic activity in, 482
Immunization
    for contacts of diphtheria, 216
    for hepatitis B, 333
    for measles, 250
    passive, as short-term protection, from hospital infection, 574
    for pneumonia, 226
    for tuberculosis (TB), 253
Immunoassay, for antigen concentration, 475
Immunocompromised patients, UTI in, 260

Immunofluorescent preparation, for RSV RNA, 218*f*
Immunoglobulins, 145
    biological properties of, 94*t*
    structure of, 92*f*
    superfamily, 95*t*
Immunoglobulin G messenger RNA (IgG mRNA), 562*f*
Immunological memory, 103
Immunological synapse, 97
Immunomodulators, 169
Immunosuppressed individuals, Epstein-Barr virus (EBV) in, 191
Immunosuppression, 168
Immunotherapy, 559
    active, 564
    adoptive, 559
    key facts of, 566*b*
    passive, 560
    probiotics, 564
    specific, 561
Impetigo, 376
Inactivated vaccines, 542
Incidence (I), definition of, 485
Inclusion conjunctivitis, *Chlamydia trachomatis* causing, 367
Infection control, 467
Infectious diseases, 485
    background to, 110
    biological response gradient in, 116
    causes of, 486
    host-parasite relationships in, 110
    Koch's postulates, 113
    outcome measurements of, 485
    pathogens in, 116
    transmission of, 490
    types of, 486
        case-control studies, 486
        cohort studies, 486
        cross-sectional studies, 486
        intervention studies, 487
Infectiousness, 490*b*, 490
Infective endocarditis, 448
    causative agents of, 449*t*
    oral streptococci and staphylococci and, 448
Inflammasomes, 80
Inflammation, *Haemophilus influenzae* strains and, 183
Inflammatory mediators, 79*t*
Inflammatory response, staphylococcal skin infections, 377
Influenza A (H1N1) virus, 549
Influenza A virus infection, 241
    antigenic variation using, 167
    entry of, 117
    microbial attachment of, 119*t*
    in viral pneumonia, 227*t*
Influenza B virus infection, 242
    in viral pneumonia, 227*t*

Influenza C virus infection, 242
Influenza D virus infection, 242
Influenza vaccines and antigenic drift, 550*f*
Influenza virus
    antigenic variation of, 167
    antivirals targeting, 528
    cell membrane receptors and, 29*t*
    mechanisms of attachment of, 200*t*
Influenza virus infection, 241
    antiviral drugs for, 248
    budding process, 242*f*
    in central nervous system (CNS) complications, 245–246
    diagnosis of, 246
    envelope of, 242
    frequency of, 116*t*
    genetic change of, 242
    outbreaks of, 243
    pandemic, 241
    to respiratory epithelium, 245
    structure of, 245
    transmission of, 245
    types of, 241
    vaccines for, 246
Inhalation, pneumonia by, 219
Innate defences, of body, 68
    adaptive immune defences and, 68
    biochemical and physical barriers in, 69
    complement system, activation of, 76
    against entry, 69
    eosinophils in, 80
    extracellular antimicrobial factors in, 81
    inflammasomes in, 80
    innate lymphoid cells in, 83
    interferons in, 81
    macrophages in, 70
    membrane attack complex in, 76
    natural killer cells in, 71
    phagocytosis in, 70
        killing and, 72
    polymorphs in, 70
    strategies to evade, 70
Innate defences, of body acute phase proteins in, 81
Innate immune system, 4
Innate immunity
    host with deficient, infections of, 456
        burn wound, 456
        due to compromised clearance mechanisms, 458
        of plastic devices in situ, 458
        traumatic injury and surgical wound, 457
    primary defects of, 452
    secondary defects of, 458

Innate lymphoid cells (ILCs), 83*f*, 83
Inosine monophosphate dehydrogenase inhibitor, 528
Insecticides, for prevention of malaria, 422
Insects
    helminths transmission through, 43
    transmission via, 43
Insertion sequences, 17
Integrase inhibitors (INSTIs), 526
Integrins, 95*t*
Integrons, 19, 498–499
Interdigitating dendritic cells (IDC), migration and maturation of, 99*f*
Interferon a (IFNa), 160
Interferon b (IFNb), 160
Interferon gamma (IFNg), 71
    in Epstein-Barr virus infection, 204
Interferon-gamma release assays, for tuberculosis, 250
Interferons (IFNs), 81, 141
    b (IFNb), 160
    gamma (IFNg), 71
        in Epstein-Barr virus infection, 204
    a (IFNa), 81–82
    pegylated
        for hepatitis B, 290
        for hepatitis C, 290
Intermediate host, helminths transmission through, 44
Interstitial pneumonia, 218
Intervention studies, 485
Intestinal infection, transmission of, 127
Intestinal parasites, 4
Intimin, 294
Intra-abdominal sepsis, 325
Intracellular pathogens, 3
Intubation, for acute epiglottitis, 211
'In-use' tests, disinfection and, 582
Invasive devices, care of, to reduce, risk of endogenous infection, 574
Invertebrate vectors
    as intermediate host, 132
    transmission via, 131
Iron-binding molecules, 160
Iron-deficiency anaemia, hookworms and, 319
Irradiation, sterilization techniques and, 580
Isolating patients, for airborne transmission of infection, 573
Isoniazid, 517
Ivermectin
    for lymphatic filariasis, 427
    for onchocerciasis, 427
Ixodes ticks, Lyme disease, 417

**J**

Japanese encephalitis virus infection, 360
Jarisch-Herxheimer reaction, 417
Jaundice, defined, 419
'Jumping genes,' in transposition, 498

**K**

K (capsular) serotypes, 261
Kala-azar, 424
Kaposi's sarcoma, HHV-8 in, 32
Kaposi's sarcoma herpesvirus (KSHV), 32
Kawasaki syndrome, 401
Keratitis, 370
Keratoconjunctivitis, 367
Ketolides, 510
'Kissing contacts,' bacterial meningitis, 351
*Klebsiella granulomatis*, 275
Koch's postulates, in infectious diseases, 115
Koplik's spots, 153f
Kuru, 50

**L**

La Crosse virus infection, 409t
Lactic acidosis, malaria and, 421
*Lactobacillus acidophilus*, 564
Lactoferrin, 74
Lamivudine-resistant HBV, 523
Langerhans cell, 374
Large intestine
  enteroinvasive *E.coli* and, 297
  microorganisms in, 57, 58f
Laryngitis, 214
Lassa fever virus, 430
Latent infections, 173
  reactivation of, 173
Lateral-flow devices, for malaria, 421
LCM. *See* Lymphocytic choriomeningitis
*Legionella pneumophila*, in pneumonia, 225, 226f
*Legionella* spp., 459t, 501
*Leishmania*, 424t
  growth requirements of, 470
  macrophages and, 424, 424f
  transmitted by sandflies, 424
*Leishmania* direct agglutination test, 425
*Leishmania tropica*, skin rashes and, 189t
Leishmaniasis, 389, 424
  cutaneous, 425
  diagnosis of, 425
  immunodeficient patients and, 425
  transmission of, 424
  visceral, 424
  untreated, 424
Lepromatous leprosy, 382, 383f

Leprosy, 381
  BCG for, 383
  dapsone for, 383
  T-cell immunity and, 146, 146t
  treatment of, 383, 518
Leptin, immunity and, 150, 151f
*Leptospira*, entry of, 118t
*Leptospira interrogans*, 106t
  causing leptospirosis, 438, 439f, 439t
Leptospirosis, 438, 439f, 439t
Lesions
  mucocutaneous, 374, 375f
  STIs and, 266
Leukotriene B4 (LTB4), as inflammatory mediators, 79t
Leukotriene D4 (LTD4), as inflammatory mediators, 79t
Levofloxacin, 10
  for UTI, 264t
Lice
  *Borrelia recurrentis* transmitted by, 417
  *epidemic typhus* transmitted by, 416
Light microscopy, for laboratory diagnosis of infection, 473
Lincosamides, 12, 511
Lipid A, in endotoxins, 181–182
*Liponyssoides sanguineus*, rickettsialpox and, 416
Lipopeptides, 516–517
Lipopolysaccharide (LPS)
  in direct activation of complement, 183
  endotoxin, 181–182, 182f
  in gram-negative bacteria, 7
Lipopolysaccharide-rich layer, in gram-negative bacteria, 3
Liquid glutaraldehyde, sterilization techniques and, 581
*Listeria*, 323, 343, 459t
  cell-to-cell spread by, 164, 164f
*Listeria monocytogenes*, 323, 338t, 343
  meningitis, 352
Listeriosis, 323, 338t
Live attenuated measles vaccine, 546
Live attenuated vaccines, 543f
Live vaccines, 541, 543f
Liver
  damage to, yellow fever with, 410
  failure, leptospirosis and, 439
  hydatid disease in, 441f
  parasitic infections affecting, 323
Liver abscesses, 324
  amoebic, 324, 324f
Lobar pneumonia, 219, 220f

Löffler's syndrome, *Ascaris* and, 318
Lopinavir, 527
Lower respiratory tract infections, 214, 215b
  acute bronchitis, 217
  acute exacerbations of chronic bronchitis, 217
  adenovirus infection, 241
  bacterial pneumonia, 223
  bronchiolitis, 218
  cystic fibrosis, 254
  cytomegalovirus infection, 250
  diphtheria, 214, 214f
  fungal infections, 255
  hantavirus pulmonary syndrome (HPS), 219
  human bocavirus, 241
  human metapneumovirus, 241
  influenza virus infection, 241
  laryngitis and tracheitis, 204
  lung abscess, 254
  measles, 249
  parainfluenza virus infection, 240
  pneumonia, 219
  protozoal infections, 256
  respiratory syncytial virus (RSV) infection, 218
  severe acute respiratory syndrome and Middle East respiratory syndrome coronavirus infections, 229
  tuberculosis, 250
  viral pneumonia, 226
  whooping cough, 216f, 217
Lung
  abscess, 219, 220f, 254, 256f
  shadows in, in bacterial pneumonia, 225
Lyme disease, 356, 418
  additional disease from, 418
  antibiotics for, 418
  cause of, 416
  diagnosis of, 418
  erythema migrans in, 418, 418f
  prevention of, 418
  transmission of, *Ixodes* ticks and, 417, 417f
  vaccine for, 418
Lymph nodes
  inguinal lymphadenopathy and, 274
  spread of infection to, 154, 154f
  structure of, 87–88, 89f
  swollen, in tularaemia, 437
Lymphadenopathy, human African trypanosomiasis and, 422, 423f
Lymphatic system, pathogens and, 154
Lymphocytes, 85, 86f, 482

Lymphocytic choriomeningitis (LCM), 431
Lymphogranuloma venereum, 267t, 274, 274f
Lymphoid tissue, 85, 86f, 86t
Lysis, 145
Lysozyme, 7, 73–74, 136, 137f
*Lyssavirus*, 358

**M**

M protein, *Streptococcus pyogenes*, 379
M49, 379
Macrocycle, 510
Macrolides, 12, 510, 510f–511f, 512f
Macroparasites, 3
Macrophages, 141t
  pathogens and, 154
  salmonellae transported in, 321, 322f
  throughout the tissues, 70, 70f, 71f, 72f
Magnetic resonance imaging (MRI), of tuberculomas, 363f
Major histocompatibility complex (MHC) molecules, 99, 100f
Malaria, 418
  avoidance strategies for, 41
  in children, 421
  clinical features of, 419
  drenching sweats in, 419
  fever in, fluctuating, 419
  frequency of, 116t
  HIV and, 421
  immunity to, 421, 422f
  immunosuppressive effect of, 421
  initiation of, by female anopheline mosquito, 418
  parasite of, 419t
    life cycle of, 419, 420f–421f
    species of, patterns of fever in, 419, 420f–421f
  severe anaemia and, 421
  thin and thick blood films for, 421
  vaccines against, 556, 556f
Malarial antigens, 185
*Malassezia furfur*, 383, 384f
*Malassezia* yeast, 384
Malignant transformation, in cells, 190t
Mallon, Mary, 163b
Malnutrition
  causing secondary adaptive immunodeficiency, 455f, 456f
  susceptibility to infectious diseases and, 158t–159t
MALT. *See* Mucosa-associated lymphoid tissue

Mammary glands clinical consequences of mumps in, 210*t*
lactating, 337
Mannose-binding lectin (MBL), 137
Mantoux test, for tuberculosis, 149
Maraviroc, 527
Mass drug administration (MDA) programmes, for schistosomiasis, 426
Mass spectrometry, in identifying microorganisms, 472
Matrix-assisted laser desorption-ionization time-of-flight mass spectrometry (MALDITOF), 4–5, 472
Mature T cells, thymus in, 85, 86*f*–87*f*
MBL. *See* Mannose-binding lectin
Measles virus infection, 249, 249*f*–250*f*, 399, 399*t*
skin rashes and, 189*t*
vaccine, 546
in viral pneumonia, 227*t*
virus, microbial attachment of, 119*t*
Medically important bacteria, genomics of, 23
Mediterranean spotted fever, 415
dog ticks and, 415
Mefloquine-resistant falciparum malaria, 534
Melanocyte, 375*f*
Melarsoprol, for East African trypanosomiasis, 422
Membrane attack complex, 76, 79*f*–81*f*
Meninges, clinical consequences of mumps in, 210*t*
Meningitis, 337, 349
chloramphenicol for, 509
fungal, 354
HIV and encephalitis, 361
listeria monocytogenes, 352
meningococcal, 349
neonatal, 352
neonatal septicaemia progresses to, 343
protozoal, 354
togavirus, 360
tuberculous, 352, 353*f*
Meningococcal meningitis, 349
clinical features of, 351
Meningococcal septicaemia, 351*f*
Meningococcal vaccines, 548
Mepacrine, for *Giardia intestinalis* infection, 316
Meronts, 316
Messenger RNA (mRNA), 2–3
Metabolic pathways in bacteria, 8, 9*f*
targets, antibacterial agents, 497

Methenamine, 517
Methicillin, resistance issues, 499
Methicillin-resistant staphylococci, 501
Methicillin-resistant *Staphylococcus aureus* (MRSA), 19
Methicillin-susceptible *Staphylococcus aureus* (MSSA), 377, 380
Metronidazole, 516
for *Entamoeba histolytica* infection, 315
for *Giardia intestinalis* infection, 316
Metronidazole, for *Trichomonas vaginalis*, 267*t*
MHA-TP test, syphilis and, 269, 270*f*
MHC. *See* Major histocompatibility complex
Microaerophilic streptococci, 380
Microarrays, DNA, 23, 23*f*–24*f*
Microbial disease, in skin, 374, 375*f*
Microbial DNA samples, analysing, 56
Microbial endotoxin, 181
Microbial gene, identification of, 468
Microbial load, in skin, 374, 374*b*
Microbiome
after birth, 56
benefit of various species to host, 58
skin in, 56–57, 57*f*
Microbiota, 56
advantages and disadvantages of, 58
germ-free animals in, 58
identifying and understanding, 56
in pharynx, 57
spread into previously sterile parts of the body, 59
in trachea, 57
Microfilariae, of filarial nematodes, in lower respiratory tract, 256–257
Microimmunofluorescence, for *Rickettsia*, 415
Microorganisms
cultivation of, 470
identification of, 468
infectious in healthy host, 113
obligatory steps for, 110, 110*t*
pathogenicity of, 156
target organs and tissues of, 155, 155*t*
Microparasites, 3

Microscopy
of *C. trachomatis*, 274
diagnosis by, 364
for laboratory diagnosis of infection, 473
of syphilis, 268
of UTI, 263
Microsporidia, 317
*Microsporum*, 384, 386*f*
Middle East respiratory syndrome coronavirus infections, 229, 229*f*–230*f*
Miliary tuberculosis, acute, 352
Milk, transmission in, 128*t*, 129
Miltefosine, for leishmaniasis, 425
Mimicry, as antigen concealment strategy, 164, 165*t*
Minocycline, 507, 509*f*
Mites
larval trombiculid, scrub typhus transmitted by, 417
rickettsialpox and, 416
transmission via, 130, 132*t*
Mitochondria, evolution of, 62, 62*f*
MMR vaccine, 340
Mobile genetic elements, in bacteria, 15
Modified vaccinia virus Ankara (MVA), 542
Molecular cancer biomarkers, personal medicine and, 481
Molecular diagnostic tests, for viruses, in colds, 198
Molecular mediators, stimulate immune system, 563
Molecular typing techniques, 576
*Molluscum contagiosum*, 392, 392*f*
Monobactams, 502, 502*f*
Monoclonal antibodies
in clinical setting, 562
effective therapy provided by, 561
generated by phage display techniques, 561, 562*f*
production of, 103, 105*b*, 105*f*
Monocytes, 349
Mononuclear phagocyte system, 71*f*
*Moraxella catarrhalis*, in pneumonia, 224
Mosquitoes, 47
dengue virus transmitted by, 410
lymphatic filariasis and, 426
malaria transmitted by, 418
West Nile virus transmitted by, 412–413
yellow fever virus transmitted by, 410
Mott cells, 423
Mouth, colonized by bacteria, 57

Moxifloxacin, 513
MRI scans, 356
mRNA, 11, 11*f*
in viruses, 29
MRSA. *See* Methicillin resistant *Staphylococcus aureus*
MSSA. *See* Methicillin susceptible *Staphylococcus aureus*
Mucocutaneous lesions, in skin, 374, 375*f*
Mucosa-associated lymphoid tissue (MALT), 88, 90*f*
Mucus, mechanisms to counteract, 121
Multiple sclerosis, 260, 362
Mumps virus infection, 209, 260
clinical consequences of, 210*t*
enlarged submandibular glands in, 210*f*
pathogenesis of, 209*f*
treatment and prevention of, 209
vaccine, 546
Muscle, infections of, 374
parasitic, 403
viral, 402
Mutation
in bacteria, 20
DNA microarrays and, 23, 23*f*–24*f*
Mutualism, of symbiotic associations, 59*f*–60*f*, 60
MVA *See* Modified vaccinia virus Ankara
Mycelium, 35
Mycetoma (Madura foot), 35, 388
Mycobacteria, acid-fast stains, 473
Mycobacterial diseases, of skin, 383
Mycobacterial infections, prolonged treatment of, 517
Mycobacterial resistance, 518
*Mycobacterium avium intracellulare*, 459*t*
disease, in AIDS, 462
*Mycobacterium leprae*, 338*t*
growth requirements of, 470
skin rashes and, 189*t*
*Mycobacterium marinum*, 383, 384*f*
*Mycobacterium tuberculosis*, 259, 364, 459*t*, 462
infection, persistent, 171*t*
peritonitis and, 325, 325*f*
prolonged treatment of, 517
in tuberculosis, 250
*Mycobacterium ulcerans*, 383
Mycology, 35
*Mycoplasma genitalium*, 275
*Mycoplasma hominis*, 275
Mycoplasma pneumoniae infection, 217, 217*f*
microbial attachment of, 119*t*

Mycoplasmas, tetracyclines for, 507
Mycoses, 35, 384
  subcutaneous, 35
  superficial, 35, 36f
  systemic or deep, 36, 36f
Myiasis, 390
Myocarditis, 402
  Chagas disease and, 424
Myocardium, clinical consequences of mumps in, 210t
Myxomatosis, 114b
Myxomavirus, 114b

**N**

N-acetylneuraminic acid, 528
Naegleria, 354
Nails, dermatophytes in, 385, 385f
Naive T cells, 106t
Nalidixic acid, 513, 513f
Nasopharyngeal carcinoma, Epstein-Barr virus (EBV) in, 207
  and lymphoma, 191
Nasopharyngeal diphtheria, 215
Natural immune mechanism, pathological activation of, 180
  complement, in tissue damaging reactions, 183
  disseminated intravascular coagulation and, 183
  endotoxin shock, 182
  endotoxins and, 181, 182f
  overactivity and, 180
  tumour necrosis factor (TNF) and, 180–181
Natural killer cells, 82, 82f, 138, 139t, 139f
Necator americanus (hookworms), 317
  entry of, 118t
  iron-deficiency anaemia and, 319
  thin-shelled eggs of, 318f, 318
Necrotizing factor 1, from diffusely adherent E.coli, 297
Necrotizing fasciitis, 380, 380f
Necrotizing pneumonia, 219
Needles, spread of infection via, 129
Negri bodies, 360
Neisseria gonorrhoeae, 267t, 270, 271f
  conjunctival infection from, 370
Neisseria meningitidis, 349
  in endotoxin shock, 182
  skin rashes and, 189t

Nematodes, 44, 317
  evolution of, 63
  in lower respiratory tract, 256
  transmission of, 46t
Neomycin, 508t
Nucleic acid inhibitors of, 512b
Nucleic acid synthesis, inhibitors of, 512
Nucleocapsid, 27
Nucleotide-binding and oligomerization leucine-rich repeat receptors (NLRs), 138
Nucleus, 6–7

**O**

O (semantic) serotypes, 261
Obstetric and perinatal infections, 337
  screening programmes of, 339
Occupational diseases, associated with inhalation of fungi, 187
Oesophageal candidiasis, 459–460, 460f
Ofloxacin, for UTI, 513
Onchocerca volvulus infection, causing river blindness, 373, 373f
Onchocerciasis, 389
Oncogenes, viral, 32–33, 33t
Operons, 379
Opisthorchis, 324
Opportunist STIS, 290
Opsonization, 145
Optic neuritis, ethambutol cause, 518
Oral candidiasis, 212
Orf, 392
Organ blockage, in pathologic consequences of infection, 176
OriC, 10
Orientia tsutsugamushi, 416
Oropharyngeal candidiasis, 459–460
Oropharyngeal infections, 128
Oropharynx mechanism, st0150__idx130911_72 transmission from, 123
Oseltamivir, 248
Osler's nodes, in infective endocarditis, 450
Osteomyelitis, 404–405
Otitis externa, 211
Overactivity, host tissue and, 180
Oxazolidinones, 512, 512f
Oxidative killing, 139

**P**

Palivizumab, 218, 523
PAP. See Pyelonephritis associated pili

Papillomavirus infection
  human, 277
  on skin, 391, 391f
Para-aminobenzoic acid, 514f
  sulphonamides versus, 514
Paragonimus westermani, 44
  in lower respiratory tract, 257, 257f
Parainfluenza virus infection, 240
  laryngitis caused by, 214
  mechanisms of attachment of, 200t
  type 1, microbial attachment of, 119t
  in viral pneumonia, 227t
Paralytic poliomyelitis, 358f
Paramyxoviral infections, 358
  persistent, 171t
Paraplegia, UTI, 260
Parasites, 459t
  affecting the liver, 323
  CNS disease caused by, 362
  evasion strategies of, 63, 63t
  gastrointestinal tract and, 313
  living inside or outside cells, 3
  pathogens as, 3
  persistent infections, 160, 171t, 175b
  stages of, 313
  survival strategies, 160, 175b
  transmission of, 313
Parasitic infection
  persistent, 171t
  of skin, 388
Parasitism
  characteristics of, 60
  controlled by the host, 61
  disadvantages of, 61
  evolution of, 61
    changes in, 64, 64t
    host adaptations in, 64
    inside host cells, 62, 62f
    parasite adaptations and, 63
    pressure of infection in, 63, 63t
    through accidental contact, 62
    virus evolution and, 62
  metabolic, nutritional and reproductive advantages of, 61
  in symbiotic associations, 59–60, 60f
  viruses in, 61
Parkinson's disease, as neurologic diseases of possible viral etiology, 362
Paromomycin, for crypto sporidial diarrhoea, 317
Parotitis, 209
Parvovirus B19, 338t, 398
  skin rashes and, 189t
Passive carriage, 131, 132f

Passive immunotherapy, 560
Pasteurella multocida infection, 438
Pasteurization, definition of, 580
Pathogenicity islands, 18f, 19
Pathogens
  genetic determinants in, 157
  with immune response expression in tissues, 170
  immunosuppressive effects of, 169
  ingested, 291
  interference
    with cytotoxic T-cell recognition, 170
    with host apoptotic responses, 170
  as parasites, 2
  persistence of, 162, 173b
  privileged sites against, 163, 163f–164f
  toxin, as immunomodulators, 169, 170f
  varieties of, 2
Pathologic consequences of infection, 176, 177f, 195b
  caused directly by microorganisms, 176, 177t
  blocks protein synthesis, 180
  direct effects of, 176
  enzymes, in bacteria, 176
  exotoxins, 176
  haemolysins, 179
  inactivation of toxins, 180
  loss of water, in intestinal epithelial cells, 180
  in metabolic machinery, 179
  tetanus and botulinum toxins, 180
  toxins as magic bullets, 180
  diarrhoea, 180
  and immune response, 184
  natural immune mechanism, pathological activation of, 180
  skin rashes, 188, 189t
  viruses and cancer, 189, 190t
Pattern recognition receptors, 137
PCR. See Polymerase chain reaction
Pediculosis, 390
Pediculus humanus, 47
  epidemic typhus transmitted by, 416
Penicillin-binding proteins, 498, 500, 503f
Penicillins, 10, 502f
  macrolides versus, 509
  resistance issues, 499
  for streptococcal skin infections, 379
  for syphilis, 269, 267t
Pentamidine, for West African trypanosomiasis, 422

Peptidoglycan, 3, 499–500
  in bacteria, 7
  synthesis of, 501f
Peramivir, 528
Pericarditis, 402
Perinatal transmission, 128
Periodontal disease, 212
Peripheral nerves
  CNS invasions, 347
  spread of infection via, 156
Peritoneal cavity, spread of
    infection via, 156
Peritonitis, 325, 325f
  primary, 325
  secondary, 325
Peritonsillar abscess, as
    complications of
    Streptococcus pyogenes,
    207
Permethrin cream
  for genital scabies, 290
  for Phthirus pubis, 267t
  for Sarcoptes scabiei, 267t
Peroxidase, 8–9, 10f
Pertussis, vaccines against, 546,
    546f
Pertussis toxin
  in Bordetella pertussis
    infection, 216
  in disease, 178t
PFGE. See Pulse-field gel
    electrophoresis
Phagocytes, 70, 139, 139f
  activation of, through PAMP
    recognition, 73, 74f
  chemotaxis in, 75
  intracellular killing by, 139
  non-oxidative killing by,
    139–140, 140t
  sense infection, 72, 73f–74f
  strategies to evade, 160, 161f
Phagocytic activity, immune
    function and, 482
Phagocytic cells, congenital
    defects in, 452
Phagocytic vacuoles,
    antimicrobial
    mechanisms in, 75b
Phagocytosis, 7, 70, 70b, 70f,
    139
  fungi and, 36–37
  internalized pathogen in, 73
  killing and, 72
Pharyngeal diphtheria, 214f
Pharyngitis, 201, 266
  bacterial infections in, 207
  cytomegalovirus infection
    and, 250
    treatment options in, 203
  diagnosis of, 209
  Epstein-Barr virus infection
    in, 204
  microorganisms causing,
    202t
  Streptococcus pyogenes
    infection in, 207
Pharynx, microbiota in, 57
Phenolic disinfectants, 582t

Phosphorus, as bacterial
    growth requirement, 9t
Phthirus pubis, 47
Physical barriers, 69, 71f
Pili, in bacteria, 7
Pinta, 266
Pityriasis versicolor, 384, 384f
PKDL. See Post-kala-azar
    dermal leishmaniasis
Placebo-controlled studies, 490
Plague, 436, 437f
Plant toxin ricin, 180
Plasma cells, 85–86, 86f
Plasma HIV-1 RNA load, 285
Plasmid profiles, 576
Plasmid-encoded dihydrofolate
    reductases, resistance to
    trimethoprim, 516
Plasmid-encoded quinolones,
    513
Plasmids, 2
  cloning and manipulating
    genes in, 16, 16f
  definition of, 15
  resistance to antibacterial
    agents, 498
  virulence genes and, 16
Plasmodia, entry of, 118t
Plasmodium falciparum, 362,
    419t, 419–421
  blood films for, 421
  life cycle of, 419, 420f–421f
Plasmodium knowlesi, 419t
  life cycle of, 419, 420f–421f
Plasmodium malariae, 419t, 419
Plasmodium ovale, 419t, 419
Plasmodium vivax, 419t
  debilitating febrile illness
    from, 419
  infection, persistent, 171t
Plastic devices in situ,
    infections of, 458
Platelet activating factor
    (PAF), as inflammatory
    mediators, 79t
Pleural cavity, spread of
    infection via, 156
Pleural effusion, in pneumonia,
    256
PMNs. See Polymorphonuclear
    leukocytes
Pneumococcal meningitis, 352
Pneumococcal vaccines, 547
Pneumocystis jirovecii, 484,
    36–37, 459t
  causing symptomatic
    disease, 461, 461f
  infection, frequency of, 116t
  in lower respiratory tract,
    251f, 256
Pneumonia, 219
  acquired in hospital, 219
  bacterial, 223
  cause of, 219
  by cytomegalovirus
    infection, 203
  by inhalation, 219
  in plague, 436

Pneumonia (Continued)
  respond to, respiratory tract,
    219, 220f
  types of, 220f
  via blood, 219
  viral, 226
Pneumonitis, hypersensitivity,
    36
Podophyllin, 267t
Point of care (POC) tests,
    480
Polio vaccines, 547, 547t, 548f
Poliomyelitis, frequency of,
    116t
Polioviruses, 29, 347, 348f, 356,
    357f
  infection, 339
  microbial attachment of,
    120t
Polyclonal activation, 169–170
Polyenes, inhibit cell
    membrane function
    targets, 532
Polymerase chain reaction
    (PCR), 4–5, 23, 343, 461f,
    577, 578f
  DNA sequence and,
    477–478
  real-time, 477, 478f
  for Rickettsia, 415
Polymorphonuclear leukocytes
    (PMNs), 70, 136, 141t
Polymyxins, 516
Polyneuritis, by diphtheria
    toxin, 215
Polyomavirus infection, 459t,
    465
  BK virus infection,
    persistent, 171t
  in cells, 193–194
  human, 260
  JC virus infection, persistent,
    171t
Polysaccharide capsules,
    350t
Polyvalent antitoxin, for
    botulism, 305
Pooled serum, antibody in,
    against infection, 561,
    561b
Porins, 7
Postherpetic neuralgia, 397
Post-kala-azar dermal
    leishmaniasis (PKDL),
    424
Postoperative infection risks, of
    hospital infection, 572t
  reducing, 574
Post-transplant
    lymphoproliferative
    disease, Epstein-Barr
    virus (EBV) in, 191
Postviral fatigue syndrome,
    402
Potassium, as bacterial growth
    requirement, 9t
Praziquantel, for
    schistosomiasis, 426

Pregnancy
  chikungunya infection
    during, 411
  HIV-1 infection during, 421
  Listeria and, 323
  on severity of infectious
    disease, 338t
  susceptibility to infectious
    diseases and, 158t–159t
  tetracyclines for, 507
  UTI and, 260
  VZV, 347
Prevalence (P), definition of, 485
Primaquine, for malaria, 422
Primary adaptive
    immunodeficiency, 452,
    454f
Primary atypical pneumonia,
    223
Primary tuberculosis, 252
Prion protein scrapie (PrPSc),
    51
Prions, 2
  animal and, 53b
  conflicts on, 55b
  development of, 52
  diagnosis of, 52
  as host-derived molecules,
    51, 53
  prevention and treatment of
    diseases, 54
  'rogue protein' pathogenesis
    of, 51
  species boundaries and, 53, 54f
  transmission of, 52
Probiotics, 564
Proctitis, 266
Progressive multifocal
    leukoencephalopathy
    polyomaviruses
    causing, 465
Prokaryotes, 2, 2f
Prolonged therapy, for
    tuberculosis, 253
Prostaglandin E2 (PGE2),
    as inflammatory
    mediators, 79t
Prostate, 262, 275
Prostatic hypertrophy, in UTI,
    260
Prostatitis, acute bacterial, 262
Protease inhibitors, 527
Protein synthesis
  inhibitors of, 506, 506f
  targets, antibacterial agents,
    497
  tetracyclines and, 507
Proteins
  absorption of, 122
  viral, 29, 30f
Proteus mirabilis, 259
Protozoa, 41, 260, 463
  avoidance strategies for, 40
  conflicts on, 42b
  evolution of, 63
  identification of, 472, 473f
  occurrence in body, 40, 40f
  transmission of, 41–42, 41t

Protozoal meningitis, CNS and, 354
Protozoan infections, 418
  of gastrointestinal tract, 313, 314f
    Cryptosporidium hominis and Cryptosporidium parvum as, 316, 316f
    Cyclospora, Cystoisospora, and microsporidia in, 317
    Entamoeba histolytica as, 314
    Giardia intestinalis as, 313
    minor, 315
  leishmaniasis as, 424
  in lower respiratory tract, 256
  malaria as, 418
  trypanosomiasis as, 422
  PRP test, syphilis and, 268
Pseudohyphae, 35
Pseudomembranous colitis, clindamycin for, 511
Pseudomonas aeruginosa, 259, 459t
  of burned patients, 456
  cystic fibrosis and, 254, 254f–255f
  quorum sensing and, 14
Pubic louse, 290
Puerperal sepsis, 345
Pulse-field gel electrophoresis (PFGE), 577, 578f
Pyelonephritis, 262, 262f
Pyrazinamide, 518
Pyrimidines, 37
Pyrophosphate analogue, 525
Pyropoptosis, 80–81

Q
QuantiFERON test, 552
Q fever, 435
Quinolones, 303
Quinsy, as complications of Streptococcus pyogenes, 207
Quorum sensing, 14

R
Rabies virus infection, 29t
  clinical features of, 360
  frequency of, 116t
  killed diploid cell-derived virus, 360
  detection of, 360, 360f
  virus
    entry, 118t
    virus replication, 30, 31f
Rabies immunoglobulin (RIG), 360
Radiation, congenital infections, 338
Raltegravir, 526
Randomized controlled studies, 487
Rapid 'hit-and-run' infection, 162

Rashes, skin, 188, 189t
Rat-bite fever, 439
Reactive arthritis, 404, 405t
Reactive oxygen intermediates (ROIs)
  antimicrobial effects of, 140
  cytotoxic lipids and, 140
  oxidative killing with, 139, 140t
Receptor molecules, 117
Reduviid ('kissing') bug, T. cruzi transmitted by, 423
Regulatory T cells (Treg), 105, 166, 166t
Relapsing fever, 106t, 417
  antigenic variation in, 417
  Borrelia recurrentis and, 417
  course of events in, 417f
  diagnosis of, 417, 417f
  epidemics of, 416
  mortality with, 416
  tetracycline for, 417
  tick bites and, 417
  transmission in, 418f
Renal calculi, in UTI, 260
Repair processes, bacterial DNA, 20, 21f
  replication, 152
  in bacteria, 10
  factors affecting, 158, 158t–159t
  genetic determinants of, 156
  key facts, 159b
  in viruses, 29, 30f–31f
Resistance
  to antibacterial agents beta-lactams, 500, 502f
  'cassettes' of resistance, 498, 499f
  chromosomal mutation, 498
  evolution of, 497f
  genetic of, 497
  glycopeptides, 503
  integrons, 498, 499f
  mechanisms of, 499, 500t
  methicillin, 499
  mycobacterial resistance, 518
  by plasmids, 498
  transposons, 497
  to antimicrobials, 15
Respiratory burst, 75f, 139
Respiratory epithelium predisposes, influenza virus infection to, 245
Respiratory infections ciliary activity in, 120t
  transmission of, 125
Respiratory invader, 200t
Respiratory syncytial virus (RSV)
  infection, 218
  bronchiolitis by, 218
  immunopathological basis of, manifestation of, 218
  in infants, 218
  ribavirin in, 218
  RNA, 218, 218f
  in viral pneumonia, 227t

Respiratory syncytial virus (RSV) (Continued)
  mechanisms of attachment of, 200t
  microbial attachment of, 119t
Respiratory tract continuum for infectious agents, 198, 199f
  normal flora of, 199t
  as site of entry, 113, 119t
  transmission from, 125, 126f–127f
  upper, pathogens in, 199t
Respiratory virus infection, 464
Retinal detachment, Toxocara canis causing, 372
Retroviral RNA, 164
Retroviruses, 29, 30f
Reverse transcriptase polymerase chain reaction for Zika virus diagnosis, 411
Revised Jones Criteria, for rheumatic fever, 208t
Rhabdoviridae family, 358
Rheumatic fever, as complications of Streptococcus pyogenes, 208, 208t
Rheumatic heart disease, as complications of Streptococcus pyogenes, 208
Rhinitis, 198, 200t
Rhinovirus infections acute bronchitis by, 217
  mechanisms of attachment f, 200t
  microbial attachment of, 119t
Rhipicephalus sanguineus, Mediterranean spotted fever transmitted by, 415
Ribavirin, 218, 328, 521f, 528
Ribosomes, in bacteria, 6
Rickettsia africae, 416
Rickettsia akari, 415t, 416
Rickettsia conorii, 415t, 416
Rickettsia infections, 414, 415t
  African tick-bite fever as, 416
  clinical symptoms of, 414
  endemic (murine) typhusas, 416
  entry of, 118t
  epidemic typhus as, 416
  events in, 414f
  growth of, 470
  laboratory diagnosis for, 415
  latent, 414
  Mediterranean spotted fever as, 415
  persistent, 414
  rickettsial pox as, 416
  Rocky Mountain spotted fever as, 415, 415f
  scrub typhus as, 416
  serological tests for, 415
  tetracyclines for, 415, 507

Rickettsia prowazekii, 415, 415t
  infection, persistent, 171t
  skin rashes and, 189t
Rickettsia rickettsii, 415t
Rickettsia typhi, 415t
Rickettsial infection, persistent, 171t
Rickettsialpox, 416
Rifampicin, 12, 351, 514
  for leprosy, 518
Rifamycins, 514
Rift Valley fever, 409t
Rilpivirine, 527
Rimantadine, amantadine and, 528
Ritonavir, 527
Rituximab, 206
River blindness, 389
Rocky Mountain spotted fever, 415, 415f
Romaña's sign, 423–424
Rose spots, enteric fever and, 322, 322f
Roseola infantum, 398, 398f
Ross river virus infection, haemorrhagic fevers and, 409t
Rotavirus infection, 292t, 386
  diarrhoea caused by, 180, 308
  fluid and salt replacement for, 311
  microbial attachment of, 120t
  replication and, 309, 309f
  RNA or antigen detection for, 310
  vaccines, 311, 554
Rous sarcoma virus, 32, 33f
rRNA, 23, 23f
RSV. See Respiratory syncytial virus
Rubella virus, 401
  infection, frequency of, 116t
  RNA detection, 339
  skin rashes and, 189t
  vaccine, 546

S
Saliva, 211
  infection transmission via, 128, 129t
Salivary glands, clinical consequences of mumps in, 210t
Salmonella, 290, 292t
  diarrhoeal infection caused by, 180, 296t, 297, 299f
  diagnosis of, 299
  fluid and electrolyte replacement for, 299
  food-associated, 297
  prevention of, 299
  entry of, 298
  excretion of, in faeces, 299
  food-associated infections and, 291
  invasive, 298

*Salmonella (Continued)*
nomenclature of, 297–298
recycling of, 298*f*
transmission of, 299–300
typhoidal, 297–298
*Salmonella enterica*, 297–298
*Salmonella paratyphi*, 298–299
enteric fevers and, 321, 322*f*
*Salmonella typhi*, 259, 299, 553
enteric fevers and, 321, 322*f*
infection, persistent, 171*t*
microbial attachment of, 120*t*
skin rashes and, 189*t*
Sampling sites, in specimen
collection, 469*b*
Sandflies, *Leishmania* parasites
transmitted by, 424
Sandfly fever, 409*t*
Sanger sequencing, 478–479
Sapoviruses, diarrhoea caused
by, 311
Sarcocystis, 404
*Sarcocystis hominis*, 317
*Sarcoptes scabiei*, 47, 48*f*, 290
SARS-CoV-2, 563
SARS-CoV-2 spike protein, 542
SARS coronavirus. *See* Severe
acute respiratory
syndrome coronavirus
infection in lung
immunopathology and
T-cell loss
SBP. *See* Spontaneous bacterial
peritonitis
Scabies mite, 47, 48*f*
Scarlet fever, as complications
of *Streptococcus pyogenes*,
207, 208*f*
Scavenger receptors, 73
*Schistosoma haematobium*, 425, 556
Schistosomal
infection, 389
larvae, in lower respiratory
tract, 256–257
life cycle of, 426, 426*f*
*Schistosoma japonicum*, 320, 425
*Schistosoma mansoni*, 320, 425
infection, persistent, 171*t*
inflammatory responses to,
liver damage and, 323,
324*f*
*Schistosoma* spp., entry of,
118*t*
Schistosomiasis, 44, 425
by cell-mediated immunity,
188
clinical features of, 426
diagnosis of, 426
praziquantel for, 426
transmission of, 426, 426*f*
urinary, 426
Schizophrenia, as neurologic
diseases of possible viral
etiology, 362
Scrapie, 2, 54*f*
Screening programmes, of
obstetric and perinatal
infections, 339

Scrub typhus, 416
Sebaceous follicles, 381
Secondary adaptive
immunodeficiency, 452
causes of, 454–455, 455*f*
infections associated with,
458, 459*t*
Secondary invaders, of
respiratory tract, 198,
200*t*
Secondary lymphoid organs,
88–89, 90*f*
Selectins, 95*t*
Selective bowel
decontamination, for
hospital infection, 574
Selective toxicity, 495, 496*b*, 532
Self-tolerance, mechanisms of,
105, 107*f*
Semen, as source of infection,
128
Sepsis, intra-abdominal, 325
Septic arthritis, 404, 405*t*
Septic shock, 182
Septicaemia, 182
Sequencing by synthesis,
second-generation, 479,
480*f*
Sequencing data, personal
medicine and, 481
Serum sickness, 187, 188*f*
Severe acute respiratory
syndrome coronavirus 2
(SARS-CoV-2), 551
Severe acute respiratory
syndrome coronavirus
infection, 229, 229*f*–230*f*
Severe acute respiratory
syndrome–associated
coronavirus, 563*t*
Sexually transmitted infections
(STIs), 266, 267*t*
adopted by, 267*t*
arthropod infestations, 290
entry/exit/transmission
of, 266
genital herpes of, 276
host factors of, 266
HPV and, 266
inguinal lymphadenopathy
of, 274
opportunist, 290
promiscuous patient of,
271–272
sexual behaviour and, 266
spread of, 266
transmission of, 128
vaccines for, 266
Sheep, scrapie in, 52
Shiga-toxin-producing *E. coli*
(STEC), 296
*Shigella*, 290, 292*t*
culture and serological
typing for, 304
diarrhoeal disease and, 296,
296*t*, 304
antibiotics for, 304
microbial attachment of, 120*t*

*Shigella boydii*, 304
*Shigella dysenteriae*, 304
*Shigella flexneri*, 304
*Shigella sonnei*, 304
Shigellosis, 304, 304*f*
incidence of, 303
Shingles, 395, 396*f*
Single nucleotide
polymorphisms (SNPs),
23
Single-domain variable region
fragments, advantages
of, 562, 563*f*
Single-molecule sequencing,
479
Sinuses, 347
Skin. *See also* Muscle; Soft
tissue as complex
microbiome
helminths transmission
throughc, 43*f*
infections, 374
acne, 381
arthropod infections in,
390, 390*f*
*Candida*, 387, 387*f*
caused by bacteria, 376,
376*t*
cellulitis in, 379, 380*f*
dermatophytes in, 385,
385*f*
fungal, 384
gangrene in, 379
herpes simplex virus, 381,
393, 394*f*–395*f*
measles virus, 399, 399*t*,
400*f*
mycobacterial diseases
in, 381
myonecrosis in, 380
necrotizing fasciitis in,
380
papillomavirus infections
and, 391
parasitic, 389
rashes, 397
rubella in, 401, 401*t*
smallpox, 392, 393*f*
staphylococcal, 377
streptococcal, 378
subcutaneous mycoses,
35–36, 388
varicella-zoster virus, 395
viral infections and, 390,
391*t*
as site of entry, 117, 118*t*
transmission via, 128, 129*t*
Skin rashes, 188, 189*t*
Slapped cheek syndrome, 398
Sleeping sickness, 364
human African
trypanosomiasis and,
422, 423*f*
Small round structured viruses
(SRSV), 309
Smallpox, 392, 393*f*
Snail, schistosomiasis
transmitted by, 425

Sneeze, transmission from, 125,
126*f*
Social changes, in host parasite
relations, 64, 64*t*
Social conditions,
tuberculosis(TB) and,
253
Soft tissue, infections of, 374
Solid organ transplant
infections, 458, 459*t*
Solid-phase immunoassays, for
antibody detection, 481
Spanish influenza pandemic
(H1N1), 242
Species
boundaries, prions and,
52*f*, 53
definition of, 4
Specific immunotherapy, 559
Specimen
collection, 469*b*
processing, handling and
interpretation of results,
469
Spina bifida
CNS and, 347
UTI, 261
Spinal cord, 347
Spiral organisms, of medical
importance, 106*t*
*Spirillum minus*, 439
Spirochetes, dark field
microscopy for, 474,
474*f*
Spleen, structure of, 88, 89*f*
Splenectomy, causing
secondary adaptive
immunodeficiency, 455
Spontaneous bacterial
peritonitis (SBP), 325
*Sporothrix schenckii*, 388, 388*f*
Sporotrichosis, 35–36, 388, 388*f*
Spread, 152
factors affecting, 158,
158*t*–159*t*
genetic determinants of, 156
key facts, 159*b*
mechanism of, 154
Sputum samples, in bacterial
pneumonia, 225
Squamous cell carcinoma,
of skin, human
papillomavirus in, 192
ssRNA viruses, 29, 30*f*–31*f*
Staphylococcal cassette
chromosomes (SCCs), 19
Staphylococcal chromosomal
cassette *mec* (SCC*mec*),
499
Staphylococcal skin infections,
377
scalded skin syndrome, 345*f*,
377, 377*f*
*Staphylococcus aureus*, 259,
377
toxic shock syndrome, 377,
378*f*
Staphylococcal toxins, 169

Staphylococci
  dialysis catheter infections caused by, 458
  entry of, 118t
  infection caused by, 567, 569b
Staphylococcus aureus, 459t
  of burn wounds, 457
  enterotoxigenic strains of, food-borne illness and, 305, 305t
  eyelid infection due to, 367
  food poisoning and, 291, 304
  otitis externa caused by, 211
  surgical wound infection caused by, 457
  virulence in, 14
Staphylococcus epidermidis, 56–57
  dialysis catheter infections caused by, 458
  glycopeptide resistance of, 505
  prosthetic valve and joint infections caused by, 457–458
Staphylococcus haemolyticus, glycopeptide resistance of, 505
Staphylococcus saprophyticus, 259
Stepwise invasion, in systemic infection, 153, 153f
Sterilization and disinfection, 579
  of clean object, 580
  controlling, 582
  definition of, 579
  killing of microorganisms, rate of, 580, 580f
  techniques for, 580
Stevens-Johnson syndrome, sulphonamides cause, 515
Stomach, microorganisms in, 57, 58f
STOP codon, 11, 20
Streptobacillus moniliformis, 439
Streptococcal skin infections, 378f, 379
Streptococci, 459t
  entry of, 118t
Streptococcus mutans
  caries by, 212
  in dental caries, 57
Streptococcus pneumoniae, 547
  acute otitis media by, 211
  in CNS, 352
  eyelid infections due to, 367
  microbial attachment of, 119t
  pneumonia by, 223
Streptococcus pyogenes, 378
  cellulitis and, 379, 379f
  complications of, 207
  gangrene and, 379, 380f
  high transmissibility of, 457
  M proteins in, 379
  penicillin for, 379
  pharyngitis by, 207, 207f
  skin rashes and, 189t

Streptogramins
  chemical structure of, 512f
Streptogramins, 12, 511, 512f
Streptolysin O and S, in disease, 178t
Streptomycin, 508t
  for tularaemia, 438
Stress, susceptibility to infectious diseases and, 158t–159t
String test, for Giardiaintestinalis infection, 316
Strongyloides, 442, 442f
  in lower respiratory tract, 256–257
Strongyloides stercoralis, 3, 43, 43f, 317, 442, 442f, 459t, 463
  eggs of, 318
  in immunosuppressed people, 319
Styes, 367
Subcutaneous mycoses, 35
Sudan black, 474
Sugar metabolism, gene regulation and, 12, 13f
Sulfadiazine, 515f
Sulfanilamide, 515f
Sulphamethoxazole, 515f
  trimethoprim and, 515
Sulphonamides, 514, 515
  resistance to, 15–16
  trimethoprim and, 515f
Sulphur, as bacterial growth requirement, 9t
Superantigens, 169, 170f
  for T cells, 101
Superficial mycoses, 35–36, 36f, 384
Superoxide anion, 73–74
Superoxide dismutase, 8–9, 10f
Suramin, for East African trypanosomiasis, 422
Surface infection, 153, 153f
  features of, 153
  rapid replication in, 154, 154t
Surveillance, of healthcare associated infections, 575
Survival
  of bacteria, 14
  endospores and, 14, 15f
  of helminths, 44
Susceptibility
  immune response and, 157, 157b
  killing curves, 519, 519f
  synergism or antagonism effects of combined agents, 520, 520f
Sustained virological response (SVR), 334
Swine influenza A H1N1 virus, 243–244
Symbiotic associations, 59, 59f–60f

Symbiotic associations (Continued)
  commensalism in, 60
  mutualism in, 60
  parasitism in, 60
Symmers' pipe stem fibrosis, 426
Synergism, in combined antibacterial agents, 520, 520f
Synergistic bacterial gangrene, 380
Synthesis, second-generation, sequencing by, 479, 480f
Synthetic agents gonorrhoea, 270
  syphilis, 266
  diagnosis of, 271
  laboratory diagnosis of, 268
  latent, 269t
  pathogenesis of, 269t
  penicillin for, 342
  penicillins for, 267t, 270
  primary, 268f, 269t
  secondary, 269t
  tertiary, 269t
  treatment of, 270
Syphilis, 266
  diagnosis of, 271
  laboratory diagnosis of, 268
  latent, 269t
  pathogenesis of, 269t
  primary, 268f, 269t
  secondary, 269t
  tertiary, 269t
  treatment of, 270
  for Treponema pallidum, 267t
Systemic infection, 153, 153f
  features of, 153
  initiated in the gastrointestinal tract, 321
  stepwise invasion in, 153, 153f
Systemic mycoses, 35–36
Systems of classification, 4, 4f–5f

T
T cells
  activation of
  additional signals for, 100, 102f
  antigen-presenting cells in, 98
  complex intracellular signalling in, 101
  co-stimulatory signals in, 98, 99f–100f
    for antibody production, 102, 104f
  recirculation of, 88f, 97, 103
  subsets of, 88, 90f
  superantigens and mitogens for, 101
  types of, 90, 91f

Taenia saginata, 320, 320f
Taenia solium (pork tapeworm), 363–364
  infection, 403, 404f
Tapeworms, 44, 45t, 363, 363f
T-cell immunity, leprosy and, 146, 146t
T-cell leukaemia virus infection, persistent, 171t
T-cell loss, SARS-CoV-2 coronavirus in, 188
T-cell receptor (TCR) rearrangement, 86–87, 87f
Teicoplanin, 505
  for gram-positive organisms, 505
  TEM-1, 498
Temperature, surface/systemic infection and, 153
Tenofovir, 526, 530
Termination sites, in transcription, 11
Tetanus, 14, 345f, 364
  clinical features of, 365
  toxin, in disease, 178t
  vaccines, 546
Tetracyclines, 12, 507, 509f
  for relapsing fever, 417
  resistance to, 15
  for Rickettsia, 415
Tetrahydrofolic acid (THFA), 514–515
Th1:Th2 balance, 166
Th17 T cells, 148
Thymus, producing mature T cells, 85, 87f
Thyroid, clinical consequences of mumps in, 210t
Ticks
  arboviruses and, 408
  of dogs Mediterranean spotted fever transmitted by, 415
  Rocky Mountain spotted fever transmitted by, 415
  Lyme disease transmitted by, 417
  relapsing fever transmitted by, 416
  transmission of infection via, 130, 132t
Tigecycline, 509f
Tinea corporis, 386f
Tinea pedis (athlete's foot), 35
Tinea (ringworm), 385, 385f
Tinea versicolor, from Malassezia furfur, 384, 384f
Tipranavir, 527
Tissue fluids, pathogens and, 154
Tissue-resident memory T cells, 106t
Tissues, 469b

Tobramycin, 508t
Toll-like receptors (TLRs), 73, 74f, 138
  signaling pathway, 160
Tolnaftate, 533
Tonsillitis, 201
  diagnosis of, 209
Topoisomerase IV, 513, 513f
Torque Teno virus (TTV) infection, 336
Toxic shock syndrome, 377, 378f
  with staphylococcal infection, 182
Toxic shock syndrome toxin (TSST-1), 178t, 182, 305, 305t
Toxin A, 307
Toxin B, 307
Toxins, 364, 378–379
  inactivation of, 180
  as magic bullets, 180
  noncultural techniques for detection of, 475b
Toxocara canis, 362–363
  infection, retinal detachment from, 372
Toxocara cati, 362–363
Toxocara infection, 362
Toxoids, 180
Toxoplasma gondii, 337, 356, 362, 459t
  infection causing retinochoroiditis, 372, 372f
  persistent, 171t
Toxoplasma tachyzoite, in brain, 356f
Toxoplasmosis
  CNS in, 362
  congenital, 342
  eye infection and, 372
Trachea, microbiota in, 57

Tracheal cytotoxin, in Bordetella pertussis infection, 216
Tracheitis, 214
Trachoma, 367, 369f
Transcription, in bacteria, 11, 11f
Transfusion-transmitted virus, 336
Transient hypogammaglob-ulinaemia, of infancy, 455, 455f
Translation, in bacteria, 11
Translocated intimin receptor (Tir), 294
Transmission, 117, 124t, 135b
  from animals, 130
  between humans, 125, 126f
  stability of, 124, 125t
Transplacental transmission, 130t
Transplant infections bone marrow, 458
  solid organ, 458, 459t
Transposons, 19, 498
Traveller's diarrhea
  enterotoxigenic E.coli and, 294–296
  Giardia intestinalis and, 315
Treponema pallidum, 337
  entry of, 118t
  growth requirements of, 470
  infection, 268
  persistent, 171t
  in syphilis, 266
  transmit, 268
  skin rashes and, 189t
  syphilis and, 267t
Treponema pertenue entry of, 118t
  skin rashes and, 189t
Trichinella, 442, 442f
  infection, 404

Trichinella spiralis, 320
Trichomonas
  growth requirements of, 470
  infection, 275
Trichomonas vaginalis, 41–42, 58, 267t, 275
  metronidazole for, 516

U
Ureaplasma urealyticum, 275
Urethra, 122
Urethritis, 122
Urinary tract, 457

V
Vaccination with a Haemophilus influenzae type b (Hib), 549f
Vaccine-induced immunity, 546–547
Vaccine safety, 544–546
  adjuvants in, 545b
  in current use, 546
  nonspecific beneficial effects, 546
  problems with, 545b
Varicella-zoster virus (VZV) infections, 560, 561t

W
Wart virus, replication in epidermis, 164f
Warts, 31–32, 253, 353–354, 354f
Weil-Felix test, for Rickettsia, 415
West Nile virus infection, 360
West Nile virus (WNV), 347
Western blot analysis, 415

Y
Yeasts, 35, 36f

Yellow fever virus infection, 409, 409t
  clinical diagnosis of, 410
  clinical features of, 410
  with liver damage, 410
  transmission of, 410
Yersinia enterocolitica, 304, 304f
  diarrhoeal infection caused by, 304f, 437
  infection, 437
Yersinia pestis
  entry of, 118t
  plague caused by, 436, 437f

Z
Zanamivir, 528
Zidovudine, 526, 527f
Ziehl-Neelsen stain, 253
  of sputum, in tuberculosis, 226f, 252
Zika virus infection, 411
Zoonoses, 133, 133t
  multisystem, 429, 441
  Yersinia enterocolitica as, 304
Zoster, 395. See also Shingles rash, 396f